The SAGE Handbook of

Healthcare

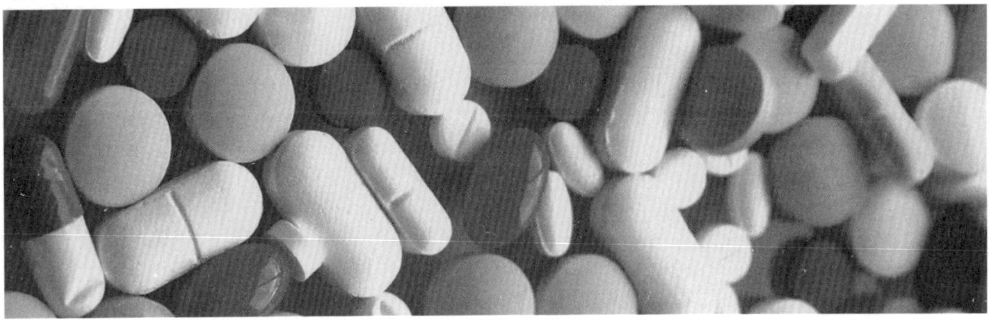

The SAGE Handbook of
Healthcare

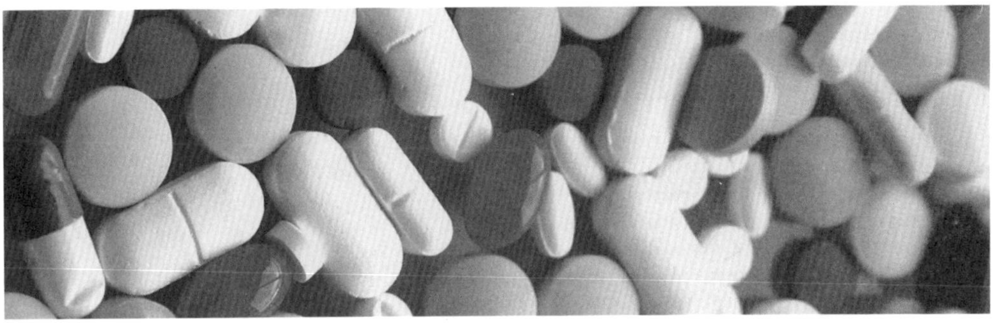

Global Policies • Business Opportunities • Scientific Developments

SAGE

Los Angeles • London • New Delhi • Singapore

First published 2008

SAGE Publications Ltd
1 Oliver's Yard
55 City Road
London EC1Y 1SP

SAGE Publications Inc.
2455 Teller Road
Thousand Oaks, California 91320

SAGE Publications India Pvt Ltd
B 1/I 1 Mohan Cooperative Industrial Area
Mathura Road
New Delhi 110 044

SAGE Publications Asia-Pacific Pte Ltd
33 Pekin Street #02-01
Far East Square
Singapore 048763

Library of Congress Control Number: 2007929747

British Library Cataloguing in Publication data

A catalogue record for this book is available from the British Library

ISBN 978–1–84787–048–3

Typeset by Newgen Imaging Systems (P) Ltd, Chennai, India
Printed in India at Replika Press Pvt Ltd
Printed on paper from sustainable resources

Contents

Preface

Richard G. Frank

Margaret T. Morris Professor of Health Economics, Department of Health Care Policy, Harvard University.

INTRODUCTION

Healthcare spending in the United States was over $2 trillion in 2006 and accounts for roughly 16% of gross domestic product (GDP). In addition, the health sector directly employs nearly 14 million Americans. Many of these people are among the most educated and skilled people in U.S. society. While the United States spends more on healthcare than most other OECD (Organization for Economic Cooperation and Development) nations, other advanced economies spend between 8% and 12% of their GDP on healthcare. Growth in healthcare spending in the United States over the past 50 years has exceeded GDP growth by an average of about 2.5 percentage points. In Europe over the period 1995–2005 increases in healthcare spending have outpaced growth in GDP in nearly every nation. Accompanying these increases in the share of income devoted to healthcare are increases in longevity and declines in age-specific disability. Thus all advanced economies are struggling with the problem of how to control healthcare spending while continuing to enjoy the gains conferred by advances in modern medicine.

As nations try to craft policies that balance a desire to limit the claims that healthcare makes on national income and public budgets, each part of the health sector is scrutinized and determinations are made about the value of the activities taking place in the various subsectors. Making such judgments requires understanding science, the economic dynamics of the sector, and epidemiology and delivery of healthcare. *The Sage Handbook of Healthcare* offers up-to-date focused analysis of a number of key segments of the health sector in the United States and globally. The *Handbook* concentrates on the markets for pharmaceuticals and medical devices and addresses key developments in these areas in considerable depth.

Technology and Healthcare

Advances in medical technology have been blamed for cost growth and hailed for advancing the health and longevity of much of the world's population. Spending on biomedical research in the United States has grown steadily. Total research and development in healthcare grew from $37 billion in 1994 to about

$94 billion in 2003. The products of this research have frequently been dramatic and include vaccines, prescription drugs, diagnostic instruments, and treatment devices that have saved millions of lives. Some have claimed that advances in medicine have improved welfare more than the sum of all other productivity improvements.

The manner in which medical technology is put to work has been pointed to as the most important driver of growth in healthcare spending.[1] For example, US healthcare spending growth has been decomposed into various underlying components. These include economy-wide growth in prices, rises in medical prices, changes in the size and composition of the population, and changes in "intensity." Intensity is widely interpreted as representing changes in technology, know-how, and capability of medical care. For the period 1960–2003, 32% of the growth in healthcare spending was attributed to changes in intensity. Moreover, if one considers the most recent part of that 44-year period, 2000–3, the portion of growth attributable to changes in intensity is 40%.[2]

As noted above drugs and devices are key elements of medical technology. Within those areas there have been important developments in the areas of biopharmaceuticals that now account for about 25% of new drugs, genomic tests, nanotechnologies, and new methods of diagnostic imaging.

The Market and Healthcare Technology

All OECD nations rely on markets to bring new medical products to doctors and patients. Private firms in the pharmaceutical industry, device manufacturers, and biotechnology enterprises make use of basic science (often conducted under government sponsorship), private capital, product development expertise, clinical research, and marketing know-how to bring new treatments to the medical market place. For the most part development of new drugs and devices is a long, costly, and risky process. Thus, the firms in this industry make investments in uncertain projects today that will frequently not begin to pay off until 8–10 years later. These industries, which account for over $260 billion dollars in spending in the United States alone, are important both for the products they create and for the benefits they confer on their communities. These features serve to complicate both the economics and politics of policymaking towards this part of the healthcare sector.

Because healthcare is expensive, complicated, and so important to the lives and well-being of each nation's citizens, all countries regulate markets for healthcare products and their delivery. As the role of drugs and devices has expanded, the policy attention given to this subsector has intensified. While each nation uses a somewhat different array of policy mechanisms to regulate markets for healthcare technology, there are several sets of policy tools most countries have in common. These include law governing intellectual property (e.g., patent law); regulation of market entry based on safety, efficacy, and sometimes cost-effectiveness; pricing (and purchasing arrangements); the regulation of product promotion and distribution channels (wholesaling, retail); and the role of public investments in each area.

The application of these policy levers results in a common set of policy debates. These focus on the tension between what economists refer to as static and dynamic efficiency. In the context of medical technology markets this means that there is a trade-off between getting "good deals" (low prices) today and a flow of new and innovative new treatments tomorrow. Getting low prices today means today's clients benefit from lower claims on their budgets and more money to devote to satisfying wants beyond healthcare. It also means that the returns to investment in innovative technology are reduced, which may mean a reduced flow of innovative medical products in the future. Achieving balance in this policy arena is complicated by the fact that the politics of public budgets tend to make policymakers myopic about long-run gains from maintaining strong incentives to innovate. At the same time assessing the "true" economic costs and hence the economic return to investment in pharmaceutical R&D is very difficult. Hence industry interests, knowing the tendency of policymakers to be myopic, will frequently offset those claims by suggesting that any attempts to rein in prices will drive investment in R&D to levels that are too low.

The *Handbook* covers a tremendous amount of ground aimed at informing these difficult policy debates. It touches on the science; policy toward intellectual property in the United States and Europe; payment policy in the United States, Canada, Europe, and Japan; the R&D process for specific clinical areas and the regulation of market entry in the United States, Europe, and Japan; and finally issues related to the delivery of care. The *Handbook* addresses long-standing debates such as the impact of reference pricing for prescription drugs. It also introduces a relatively new set of policy challenges related to the economics of personalized medicine, and the development of policy towards price competition for "generic" or "follow-on" biologics. These are emerging as hotly debated policy issues that may profoundly shape the cost of care and the flow of new treatments. The authors of the *Handbook* have performed a valuable service by gathering such a comprehensive and informative set of materials in one place. For policymakers and researchers seeking to "get smart" about what is going on in the science, regulations, and economics of the healthcare technology this book represents an ideal starting place.

NOTES

1 Newhouse, J.P. An iconoclastic view of health cost containment. *Health Affairs*, 1993;12:1524–31.
2 www.cms.hhs.gov/statistics/nhe/

Foreword

Gerard J. Wedig

Associate Professor, William E. Simon Graduate School of Business Administration, University of Rochester.

INTRODUCTION

For every person involved in the business of healthcare, one of the most important challenges is the access to information. How does one gain a working knowledge of both the scientific and business sides of the industry? The problem is even more acute in the cases of the pharmaceutical and biotechnology industries, where the science and business models are arguably more complex. Many scientists, who understand the technical possibilities of new therapeutic approaches, still need to understand business models in order to gauge what innovations may be brought to fruition. Conversely, many individuals with business training still need to understand the current trends in medical technology, if only at a basic level.

The present volume lays out both the scientific and technology issues in a manner that enables the reader to gain insights into the industry's future. Each chapter in this book provides either a business or a scientific insight, and in many cases, both. For those with a technical orientation, the book provides a complementary business discussion of issues, including pricing and regulation. For those with primarily a business background, the book provides an effective overview in technical areas that include genomics, oncology, cardiovascular, and other therapeutic areas as well as emerging trends in diagnostics.

PHARMACOECONOMICS

One foundation for understanding what technologies will become commercially feasible is a firm grounding in pharmacoeconomics. Pharmacoeconomics is the study of the cost-benefit ratios of drugs with other therapies or with similar drugs, where costs include both financial and quality-of-life measures. It is a vitally important area of study because in many cases it forms the foundation of what third-party payers will pay for drugs. Third-party payment policy, in turn, is a key "driver" of which drugs will make it to the market and what the future "landscape" of the industry will look like.

The first section of this volume focuses generically on pharmacoeconomics, with a special focus on international pricing and regulatory climates. Pharmaceutical pricing and reimbursement policy show a great deal of variability, worldwide. Most of these differences are driven by government policy. It is well-known, for example, that most governments in Europe use their own novel approaches to control drug costs, by regulating both the price and entry of drugs into the market place. In some cases, drugs that cannot demonstrate adequate efficacy are not covered at all. In cases where the drug is covered, a host of reimbursement mechanisms may be used, including the rate-of-return regulation, reference pricing, strict cost plus reimbursement, plus other approaches. The result is that reimbursement levels vary a great deal.

One result of this is that European drug prices are (on average) only 50% of the price levels achieved in the United States. Furthermore, some analysts estimate that if US pharmaceutical companies were able to receive the same prices abroad as they receive in the United States, they would be able to increase their annual profitability by anywhere from $18 to $27 billion. For this reason alone, it is important to understand the international differences in pricing and reimbursement. It is also well-known that in European countries, much of the profit from a drug must be made upon the drug's introduction. Thereafter, government policy frequently dictates that discounts must be granted. This contrasts with the United States, where, until recently, it has been normal for patented drugs' prices to enjoy year-over-year markups.

There are of course exceptions to these general findings. Drugs in certain areas that qualify as "niche" indications are one example. In the case of niche drugs, European prices are frequently closer to the US levels. For example, Roche indicated that the drug Avastin was introduced in Europe with only a 20% discount relative to US prices.

Of course, differences in international drug prices also have implications for the practice of parallel importation or drug reimportation, which represents the practice of arbitraging drug prices between two countries. The issue has been contentious in the United States, as some individuals have secured drugs from Canada. Moreover, pharmaceutical companies are generally concerned about the same practice originating from Europe, although recent legislative sentiment has been against this.

PHARMACOGENOMICS

Part 2 of this book focuses on pharmacogenomics. Genomics is the study of gene location, structure, regulation, and function. As a business enterprise it provides opportunities in at least two areas: (1) the discovery and marketing of new products and therapies; (2) the development of enabling platforms that consist of new technologies (e.g., equipment), information (e.g., mapping data bases) as well as research capabilities. This section of the volume provides several useful chapters on this topic, which range from discussions of genomics more generally, to specific discussions of pharmacogenomics (e.g., efforts to improve individual responses to drugs), as well as proteomics and nanotechnology.

Genomics lies at the heart of the biotechnology industry. The completion of the human genome project, which provides a complete mapping of the human genome, provides a great opportunity for the development of new targets and clinical therapies. Most analysts, however, expect that the process of developing actual therapies will take a number of years. This is because disease processes and their relation to genes and gene expression is an enormously complex topic. For example, to date only a small percentage of diseases have actually been linked to genes. Still, the opportunities are tremendous. If the more than 1,000 hypothesized "disease genes" can be identified, the potential exists for the development of 5,000–10,000 new disease "targets," representing the proteins expressed by these genes.

Pharmacogenomics uses genomics to study individual responses to drug therapies, based upon individual genetic differences and backgrounds. This increases the potential for the development of personalized medicine, which may increase both drug efficacy and guard against adverse events. Genomics-based "point of care" medicine aims to use genomics to make instant diagnoses of patient-specific immunities and other biological conditions to optimize treatments. One application is in the area of infectious disease. Although this approach has not been made operational, it may be so in the foreseeable future.

Proteomics studies the specific proteins that are expressed by genes. The proteins in turn are implicated in actual diseases and other abnormalities. Ultimately, proteomics allows scientists to understand how individual genes affect basic cellular processes that are at the heart of a disease. Clinical proteomics is the application of proteomics to clinical applications. Thus, it provides a new approach to the diagnosis and treatment of a disease.

The various chapters in this section of the volume offer scientific discussions of developments in these areas, while simultaneously outlining the business opportunities and products that may follow from the scientific developments.

THERAPEUTICS: CASE STUDIES

Oncology

Prior to this century, in the period from 1950–99, virtually all approved cancer drugs could be classified as chemotherapeutic agents. A major drawback of chemotherapy is the associated side effects and toxicity of drugs used. Modern cancer treatments provide the promise of therapies that are more targeted to cancer cells and also less toxic. They do this by being more selective of targets that are located relating to cancer cells. The chapters in this section of the book describe a wide range of clinical and business opportunities in this area, ranging from cancer-vaccine development to antiangiogenesis treatments as typified in the drug Avastin.

There are many cancer treatments in development that target the biological mechanisms underlying the disease. An important class of these is kinase inhibitors. Kinase inhibitors account for the majority of new cancer drugs in development. They work by impeding growth mechanisms in cancer cells, that is by inhibiting kinase, an important protein implicated in cell reproduction.

Another important class of drugs consists of monoclonal antibodies. Monoclonal antibody technology works through the design of antibodies that bind to cancer cells. Once the antibodies bind to cancer cells they effectively kill the cancer cells through a variety of mechanisms. Finally, cancer vaccines hold out the promise of preventing the occurrence or reoccurrence of cancers. They work by stimulating the body's immune system to identify and remove cancers, using cells and antigens.

This section of the book provides many insights into these developments. It also provides updates on reimbursements for cancer treatments as well as updates on novel ways to conduct clinical trials of these developments, through the development and tracking of biomarkers.

Cardiovascular and Other Therapies

This section of the book also includes several chapters that discuss new developments in the therapies for cardiovascular disease, diabetes, hypertension, and inflammatory diseases. Cardiovascular diseases are one of the leading causes of mortality and morbidity. One important treatment for cardiovascular disease is the use of stents and, more recently, drug-eluting stents. Recent years have witnessed significant advances in the technology of this market, with multiple competitors "leapfrogging" one another with their own version of a drug-eluting stent. In addition, there have been great strides in the development of new drugs that address cardiovascular disease, many of which are discussed here.

VLA-4 antagonist drugs are designed to treat inflammatory diseases, such as multiple sclerosis, Crohn's disease, and asthma. A key mechanism in these diseases is the body's inflammatory response. VLA-4 plays an important role in this response and hence presents an intriguing drug target that may be the basis of new therapies. For example, it may be possible to design monoclonal antibodies for this target. Recently, concerns have been raised about the safety of such drugs. These concerns and their likely impact on the treatment of various inflammatory diseases are also discussed in this section of the volume.

Type 2 diabetes is a chronic and progressive disease associated with several morbidities. The incidence of type 2 diabetes has been increasing worldwide as it is associated with the growing incidence of obesity, among other factors. A recent study, referred to as the PROactive study, shows that certain antidiabetic drugs may have favorable effects on the risk of cardiovascular events that are frequently associated with type 2 diabetes. Another recent development in the treatment of diabetes is the development of inhalable insulin. Inhaled insulin eliminates the need for painful injection as a delivery mechanism.

Recent developments in this delivery option are also described in this section.

DIAGNOSTICS

The emergence of genomics offers a new opportunity to combine diagnostics and treatments. Genomic tests may identify individuals who may best benefit from treatments. The same technology that forms the basis of treatment may also form the basis of an effective diagnostic test. Moreover, as it becomes important to personalize treatments, it may eventually be necessary to link diagnostics with treatment. This requires comarketing of diagnostics and therapy. The first two chapters of the final section of this volume describe the challenges of comarketing diagnostics and therapies. For example, the traditional marketing channels for marketing therapies and diagnostics are quite different. It will be important to develop new business models for the challenges associated with comarketing diagnostics and therapies.

The final section of this volume also discusses diagnostic markers for the detection of Alzheimer's disease. To administer effective treatments to Alzheimer's patients in a timely fashion, patients must be diagnosed before severe, cognitive symptoms are evident. Several Alzheimer's markers are in development. The chapters under this section review these potential markers.

PART I

Pharmacoeconomics

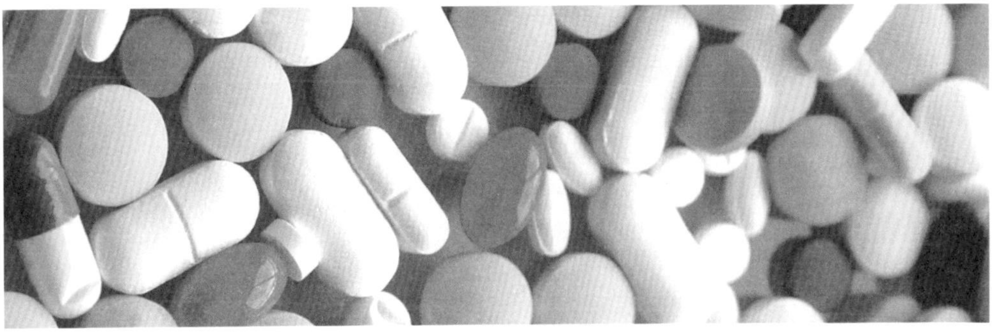

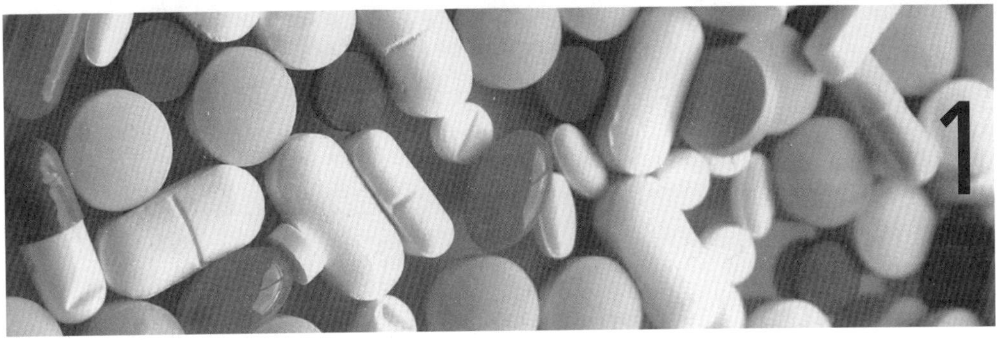

Medicare Part D: An Outlook

OVERVIEW

The Medicare Prescription Drug, Improvement, and Modernization Act of 2003 (more commonly known as the Medicare Modernization Act or MMA) is widely recognized as the most radical reform in the long history of this insurance program. The MMA's most significant achievement is the introduction of Medicare Part D, a wide-ranging new outpatient prescription drug benefit. Yet, the debut of this important new venture was anything but auspicious. The program's launch in January 2006 was beset by problems: a bewildering choice of plans, slow initial enrollment, criticism of the benefit's design (especially the notorious coverage gap), refusal of coverage for some beneficiaries' medicines in the program's first few weeks, and long delays in the reimbursement of pharmacies.

Despite these initial difficulties, the program has steadily gained momentum during the course of the year. Figure 1.1 traces the growth in Medicare Part D enrollment from January to June 2006. According to the Centers for Medicare and Medicaid Services (CMS), overall enrollment increased from 23.8 million in January 2006 to 32.9 million in June 2006, with by far the fastest growth occurring in standalone prescription drug plans (PDPs). Thus, in June 2006, 77% of the 42.5 million Medicare beneficiaries were benefiting from Part D funding in one form or another. In addition, most of the remaining Medicare beneficiaries had drug benefits from an alternative source (e.g., Veterans Administration in active employment with Medicare as the secondary payer, state pharmaceutical assistance programs, Indian Health Service). Figure 1.2 shows the main sources of drug coverage in the Medicare population in June 2006. Disturbingly, 4.4 million beneficiaries (10%) still lacked creditable drug benefits in June 2006. Many of these beneficiaries are younger, healthier seniors who calculated that the costs of membership were likely to exceed the benefits they would derive.

We begin this chapter with a review of key changes to the Medicare Part D plans offered in 2007. We then examine several areas that are likely to be the focus of particular attention from insurers: employer-sponsored health plans, dual-eligible beneficiaries (i.e., beneficiaries who qualify for both Medicare and Medicaid), special needs plans (SNPs), and disease management. We also consider Medicare medical savings accounts – a new provision that, although distinct from Part D, is likely to impact many Medicare beneficiaries. We conclude with a brief assessment of the outlook and implications for biopharmaceutical companies and insurers.

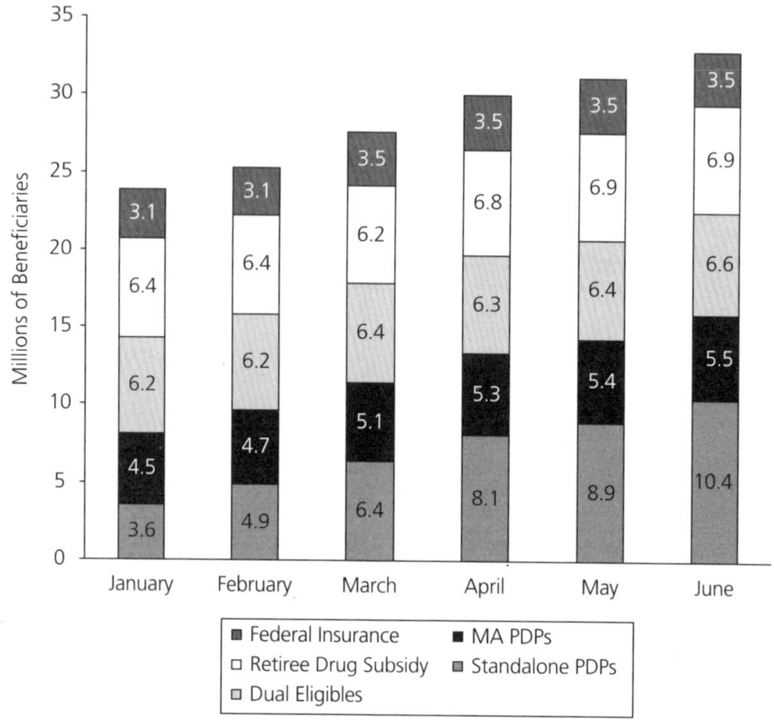

MA = Medicare Advantage
PDP = Prescription drug plan

Figure 1.1 Enrollment in Medicare Part D-Related Plans, January to June 2006

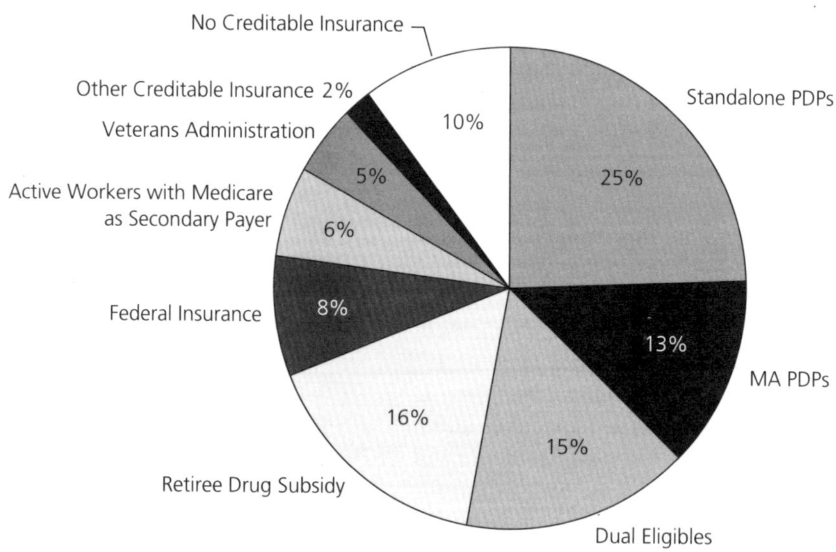

MA = Medicare Advantage
PDP = Prescription drug plan

Figure 1.2 Sources of Prescription Drug Coverage for Medicare Beneficiaries, June 2006

KEY CHANGES IN 2007

The number of companies that offer national PDPs will increase from 9 in 2006 to 17 in 2007 (the original number of national PDPs in 2006 was 10, but UnitedHealthcare and PacifiCare merged). The new national PDP organizations are EnvisionRx Plus, Express Scripts, Health Net, Longs Drug Stores, NewQuest Health Solutions, NMHC Systems, Humana, and Torchmark. The total number of standalone plans will increase from 2,183 (provided by 86 carriers) in 2006 to 2,844 (provided by 97 carriers) in 2007. The number of Medicare Advantage (MA) plans is set to grow even more dramatically – from 36,348 (provided by 316 carriers) in 2006 to 63,391 (provided by 271 carriers) in 2007 (unlike standalone PDPs, MA plans offer a much wider range of services than just the Part D drug benefit, including administration of care under Medicare Part A [inpatient treatment] and Medicare Part B [outpatient treatment]). Because the margins on MA plans are much more generous than on standalone PDPs, insurers that offer both of these plan types would generally like to maximize enrollment in their MA plans.

As required by the MMA, the basic parameters for the standard drug benefit design (e.g., standard deductible, initial coverage limit, threshold for catastrophic coverage) are adjusted annually in line with changes in drug expenses. In 2007, the parameters will be increased by 6.86%. The annual deductible will rise from $250 in 2006 to $265 in 2007. Thereafter, Medicare will cover 75% of the cost of prescription drugs up to an annual total of $2,400. Coverage will then cease until the beneficiary's annual drug costs reach a total of $5,451.25 (and out-of-pocket payments reach a total of $3,850) – a provision known as the "coverage gap" or "doughnut hole." Medicare will then cover 95% of drug costs in excess of the annual threshold of $5,451.25. Table 1.1 summarizes key changes in the standard benefit design from 2006 to 2007.

Table 1.1 Key Features of Standard Medicare Part D Drug Benefit, 2006 and 2007

	Payments ($)	
	2006	*2007*
Annual deductible	250.00	265.00
Initial coverage limit	2,250.00	2,400.00
Out-of-pocket threshold	3,600.00	3,850.00
Drug cost threshold for catastrophic coverage	5,100.00	5,451.25

The open enrollment period for 2007 runs from November 15 to December 31, 2006. Beneficiaries who are already enrolled in a Part D plan and who do not wish to change their plan need take no action. CMS reports that only 5% of beneficiaries who qualify for the low-income subsidy (LIS) will need to change plans to avoid losing this subsidy. Overall, premiums will average $24 per month if beneficiaries remain with their existing plans, but 83% of beneficiaries could reduce their premiums by switching plans. On average, premiums will be 10% lower in 2007 than in 2006. Lower premiums are obviously a competitive advantage, and plans that set their premiums below the benchmark level will benefit from the automatic assignment of dual-eligible beneficiaries.

The 2006 median monthly premium for standalone PDPs is $35.94, but the range is enormous – from a low of $1.87 to a high of $104.89. Seventy-seven percent of plans offer premiums in the range of $20.01–$50.00. In 2007, the median monthly premium will be $33.40, and the range will be $1.90–$135.70. Eighty-three percent of standalone PDPs will offer premiums in the range of $20.01–$50.00. Figure 1.3 compares the distribution of standalone PDPs' monthly premiums in 2006 and 2007.

With the advent of Medicare Part D, most MA plans have added the new drug benefit to their existing range of services. In 2006, most MA plans charged a monthly drug premium of $10.01–$40.00, but 25% of plans waived the drug premium. By comparison, in 2007, 52% of MA plans will waive the drug premium (Figure 1.4). The

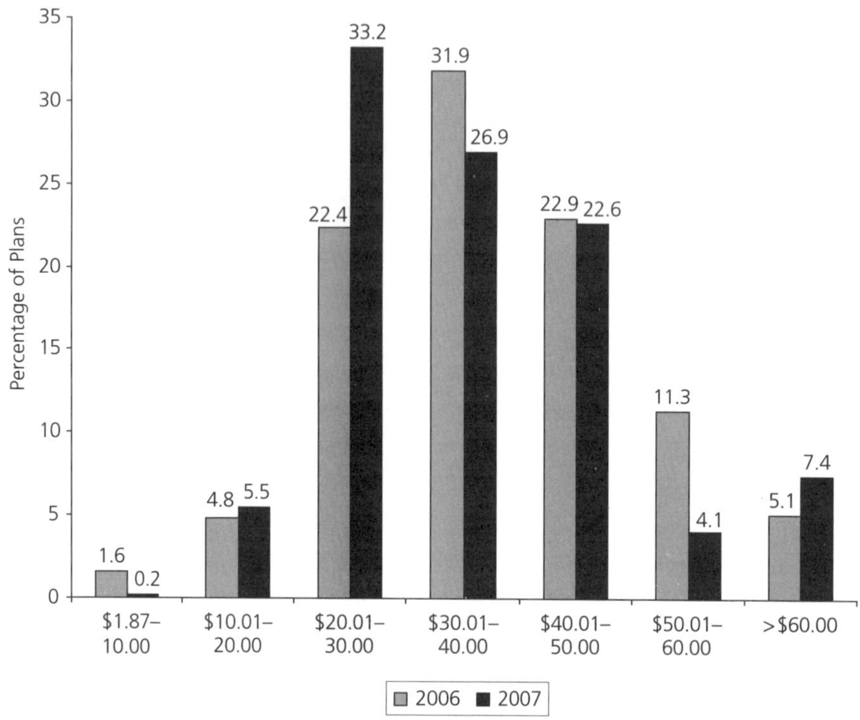

Figure 1.3 Percentage of Standalone Prescription Drug Plans Charging Various Monthly Premiums, 2006 and 2007

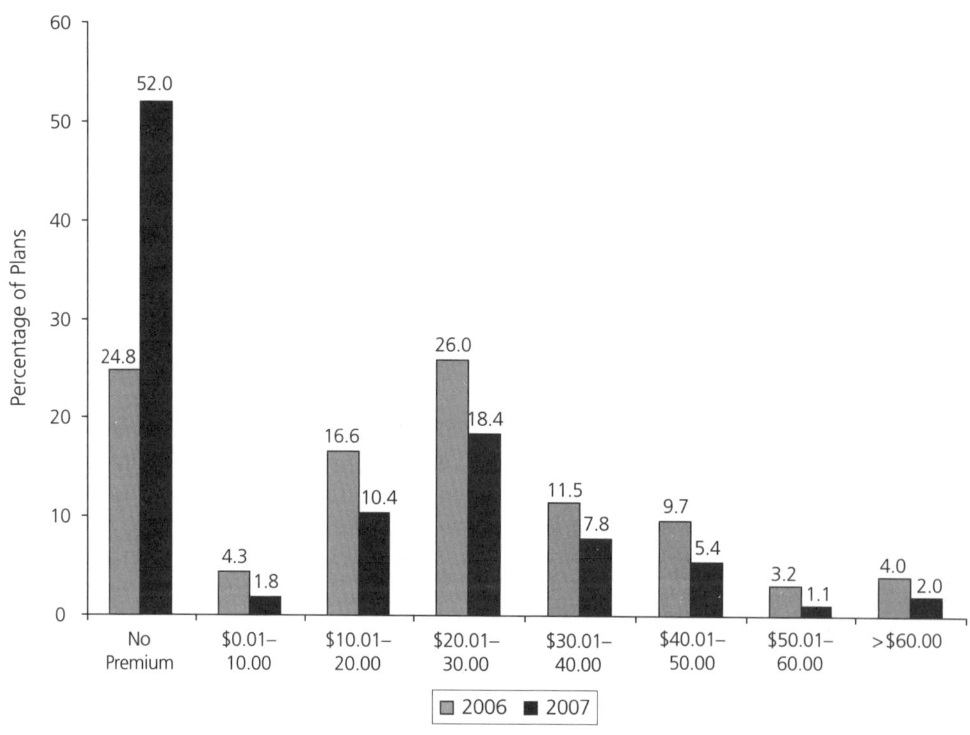

Figure 1.4 Percentage of Medicare Advantage Plans Charging Various Monthly Drug Premiums, 2006 and 2007

median drug premium will decrease from $40.00 in 2006 to $24.40 in 2007.

Most standalone PDPs forgo the annual deductible. Figure 1.5 shows that 58% of plans waived this charge in 2006, a figure that will increase to 60% in 2007. By comparison, only 31% of plans will charge the full deductible in 2007 – down from 34% in 2006. MA plans have been even more decisive in abandoning the annual deductible. Figure 1.6 shows that 91% of MA plans will waive the drug deductible in 2007 – a substantial increase on the 67% of plans that pursued this policy in 2006.

The coverage gap has been one of the most controversial aspects of the Medicare drug benefit – not least because relatively few carriers even offer the option of any form of reimbursement in the gap. At present, 85% of standalone PDPs and 86% of MA plans do not reimburse Part D drugs at all while patients are in the coverage gap, and only 3% of PDPs and 5% of MA plans cover both branded and generic drugs in the gap. However, Figure 1.7 shows signs of a change among PDPs in 2007: only 71% will offer no coverage in the gap, whereas 27% (compared with 13% in 2006) will cover generics. By comparison, MA plan providers are much less inclined to change their coverage gap policies in 2007 (Figure 1.8): 85% will continue to offer no coverage.

EMPLOYER-SPONSORED HEALTH PLANS

Employers that offer their retirees prescription drug benefits that at least match Medicare Part D (e.g., in terms of deductibles, coinsurance, and cost-sharing) can receive a subsidy for Medicare beneficiaries who do not choose to enroll in Part D. In 2006, the tax-free subsidy is equivalent to 28% of retirees' drug costs between $250 and $5,000, with a maximum subsidy per

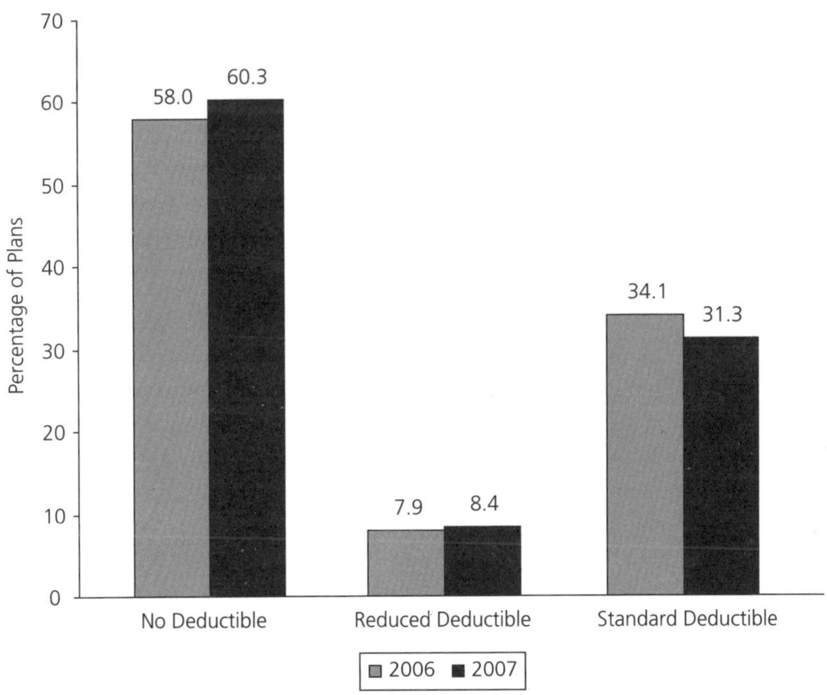

Figure 1.5 Percentage of Standalone Prescription Drug Plans Levying Various Drug Deductibles, 2006 and 2007

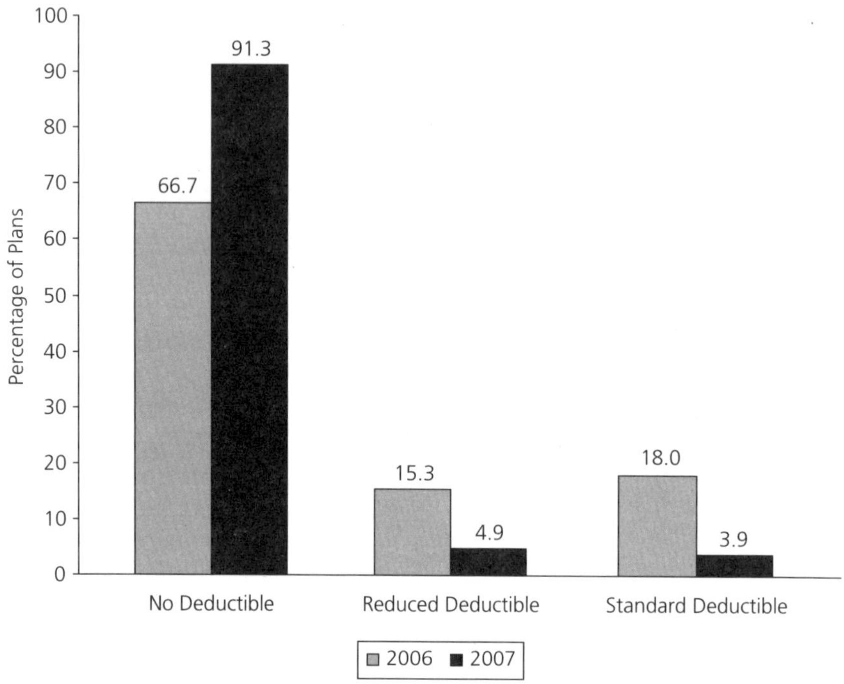

Figure 1.6 Percentage of Medicare Advantage Plans Levying Various Drug Deductibles, 2006 and 2007

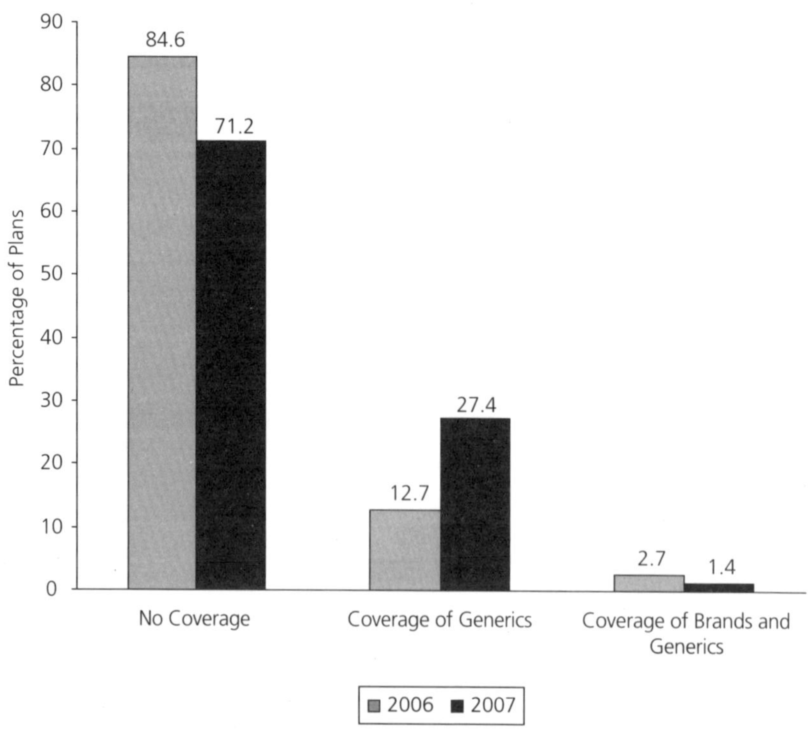

Figure 1.7 Percentage of Standalone Prescription Drug Plans Offering Various Levels of Drug Coverage in the Coverage Gap, 2006 and 2007

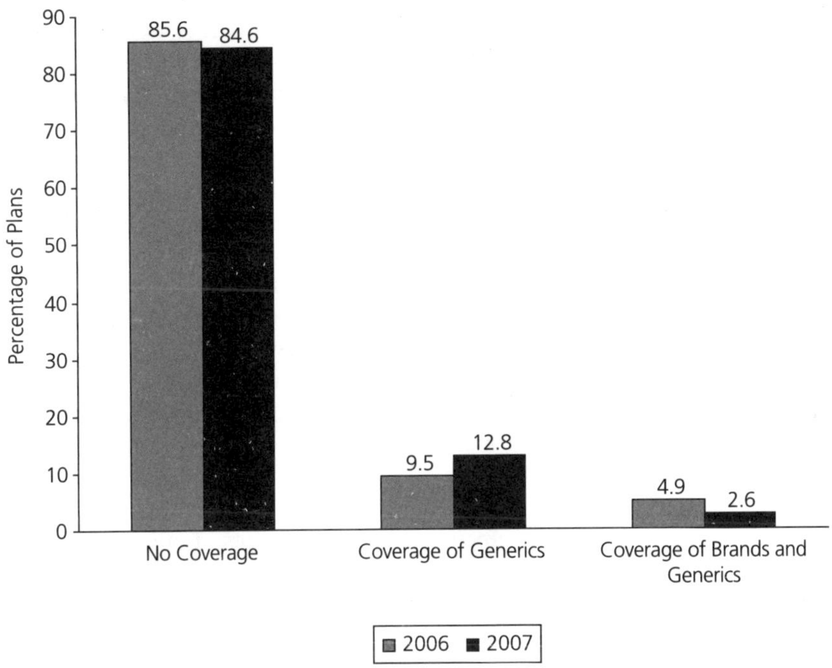

Figure 1.8 Percentage of Medicare Advantage Plans Offering Various Levels of Drug Coverage in the Coverage Gap, 2006 and 2007

beneficiary of $1,330. In 2007, the subsidy will apply to drug costs between $265 and $5,350. To qualify for a subsidy, employers' drug benefits must pass an actuarial equivalence test. Alternatively, companies may decide to pay part or all of the monthly premiums for PDPs or MA plans in which their retirees choose to enroll, contract with CMS to offer an officially approved PDP, or offer their retirees a "wraparound" drug benefit that supplements Medicare Part D.

Between June 21, 2005, and October 7, 2005, the Kaiser Family Foundation and Hewitt Associates conducted a survey of 300 large employers (i.e., companies that each have 1,000 or more employees) that currently offer health benefits to their retired former employees. *Prospects for Retiree Health Benefits as Medicare Prescription Drug Coverage Begins* found that 94% of participating employers believed that their drug benefits were actuarially equivalent or superior to the standard Medicare prescription drug benefit for 2006. Overall, 82% of these employers intended to maintain their prescription drug benefits and take the 28% Medicare subsidy in 2006. Fifteen percent planned to wrap their drug benefits around Medicare Part D, but 11% indicated that they were likely to discontinue drug coverage in 2006.

Beyond 2006, many companies that planned to take the Medicare subsidy for their own drug benefits would consider changing their policies on retiree drug coverage. Fifty percent of these companies considered it very likely and 32% somewhat likely that they would continue to offer their own benefits supported by the Medicare subsidy in 2007, but 3% were very unlikely and 4% somewhat unlikely to follow this course, and 11% did not know what they would do. Not surprisingly, employers' certainty about their intentions diminishes over time. In 2010, only 20% of these companies are very likely and 30% are somewhat likely to continue to offer their own benefits supported by the Medicare subsidy, while 10% are very unlikely and 12% are somewhat unlikely to follow this course, and 28% did not know what they would do.

The Medicare subsidy has been a welcome innovation in the short term, but it is unlikely to have a significant long-term impact on the steady decline in employer-sponsored drug benefits for retirees. Many employers reportedly dislike the complexity and uncertainty associated with applications for the Medicare subsidy. In addition, government accounting standard rules on valuing retiree liabilities will make it more advantageous for employers to contract out their drug benefits.

The Segal Company, a benefits, compensation, and human resources consultancy, found that most of its clients received subsidies of $500–$600 per employee in 2006. However, transferring coverage to a PDP could deliver savings of more than $700 per employee in 2007 and reduce the actuarial and administrative burden and cost of operating a plan. Companies could then give their retirees more generous support (e.g., covering the deductible, paying a proportion of costs in the coverage gap).

In 2007, John Gorman, CEO of the Washington, DC-based Gorman Health Group, expects employers to begin a gradual shift away from the subsidy toward drug plans with private companies. He believes that more generous subsidies would be required to persuade many employers to continue sponsoring their own insurance. Gorman predicts that national and multistate MA plans that have dominant group businesses (e.g., WellPoint, UnitedHealthcare, Humana, Blue Cross/Blue Shield plans) will gain most from the migration from group insurance to PDPs. Public sector employers, labor unions, and tax-exempt and nonprofit organizations are likely to be at the forefront of this movement, a reflection of the relative unimportance of the subsidy to such employers.

Gorman expects many employers to turn to MA plans (e.g., PPOs, private fee-for-service plans, medical savings accounts), which offer retirees more flexible benefits than do HMOs. He believes the Blues plans' large share of the group insurance market among government employers will be a distinct advantage in converting members to PDPs. Midsize employers are expected to follow suit in coming years, followed by the large private-sector employers. Gorman believes that "it's only a matter of time before large employers are out of the retiree health business altogether, as it's becoming a competitive issue."

Pharmacy benefit management (PBM) companies will also benefit from the exodus from employer-sponsored retiree drug benefits. In 2007, four PBMs – EnvisionRx Plus, Express Scripts, Longs Drug Stores, and NMHC Systems – will join Caremark Rx and Medco Health Solutions in offering national standalone PDPs. Dan Mendelson, President of consulting firm Avalere Health, believes the PBMs launched national PDPs specifically to target the employer-sponsored insurance market. This migration is unlikely to be a rapid process. For example, Caremark expects limited change in the retiree market for the year 2007: most of its clients will continue to take the Medicare subsidy. However, two unnamed Caremark clients wrapped their drug benefits around a PDP in 2006.

DUAL-ELIGIBLE BENEFICIARIES

In 2006, an estimated 14.4 million Medicare beneficiaries who had incomes below 150% of the federal poverty level (FPL) qualified to have 85–98% of their prescription drug costs paid by Medicare. The US government laid particular emphasis on encouraging these beneficiaries to sign up for a Medicare PDP or MA plan. Effective January 1, 2006, 6.2 million residents who qualified for both Medicare and Medicaid (the health insurance program for low-income residents) and had an income at or below 100% of the FPL – so-called full-benefit dual-eligible beneficiaries – had their outpatient drug benefits transferred from Medicaid to Medicare Part D. A small minority of these dual-eligible beneficiaries enrolled in a plan of their own choice, however, a majority of 5.9 million dual-eligible beneficiaries were automatically assigned to a plan.

CMS assigned dual-eligible beneficiaries to plans that did not exceed the benchmark for monthly premiums. Carriers that benefited significantly from this process included UnitedHealth (1.1 million automatically assigned beneficiaries), WellPoint (more than 600,000), Humana (595,000), WellCare (570,000), Universal American Financial (328,000), and MemberHealth (260,000). However, dual-eligible beneficiaries were free to switch to a different plan if they wished (e.g., if the automatically assigned plan did not offer generous coverage of their prescribed drugs). WellCare, for instance, expected to lose 20–30% of its automatically assigned beneficiaries to Blue Cross/Blue Shield plans, UnitedHealth, and Humana.

As noted earlier, CMS data indicate that 95% of the low-income beneficiaries will be able to remain with their existing plan and still receive the LIS in 2007. Similarly, Goldman Sachs predicts that more than 90% of dual eligibles will not change their plans in 2007. However, the National Senior Citizens Law Center (NSCLC), in Oakland, California, reports that some plans are leaving the market or no longer meet the benchmark. Jeanne Finberg, the NSCLC's directing attorney, predicts that as many as 30% of the nation's subsidized enrollees could need reassignment. She believes that many of these beneficiaries will stay with the same sponsor but may take on new identification numbers and different formularies.

Plans whose premiums do not exceed the low-income premium subsidy amount by more than $2 in 2007 will keep their LIS-eligible members. At the time of reenrollment, CMS will review plans that have premiums above the benchmark or that are terminating their coverage. CMS will reassign beneficiaries enrolled in such plans to other plans. If a carrier offers other plans in the same region that have premiums below the benchmark level, CMS will switch beneficiaries to such a plan. Otherwise, CMS will reassign beneficiaries randomly among PDP sponsors that offer eligible plans in a given region. Beneficiaries may elect to remain with their existing plan (if still available), but they will then face higher costs.

Following the reassignment process in mid-October 2006, CMS will provide the "losing" PDPs with a preliminary listing of members who will be switched effective January 1, 2007. PDPs gaining new members will also receive a reassignment notification file; by early December, they must send beneficiaries an acknowledgment that their enrollment has been accepted by CMS. According to CMS, 750 plans across the United States will offer a premium waiver to beneficiaries who qualify for the full LIS.

SPECIAL NEEDS PLANS

In preparation for the launch of the Medicare prescription drug benefit, CMS automatically enrolled more than 90% of dual-eligible beneficiaries in standalone PDPs. However, these beneficiaries – and others with special requirements – could benefit from a particular provision of the MMA: SNPs. These plans offer tailored coverage to dual-eligible beneficiaries, residents of long-term care facilities, and beneficiaries who have severe or disabling chronic conditions. Many of these beneficiaries have complex care needs, see multiple physicians, are uneducated, and receive little support from their communities. They could benefit from inclusion in a managed care organization (MCO) instead of being enrolled in plans dedicated solely to Medicare Part D.

Kevin "Kip" Piper, President of Health Results Group and Senior Counselor at Fleishman-Hillard, estimates that there are 3.5 million institutionalized beneficiaries and 7.5 million dual eligibles. CMS data show that 83% of Medicare beneficiaries have at least one chronic condition, but the 23% of beneficiaries who have 5 or more chronic disorders account for 68% of total Medicare spending. According to the recently resigned CMS administrator, Mark McClellan, in the course of a year, these severely ill beneficiaries make an average of 37 physician-office visits, consult 14 different providers, spend 7 days in hospital, and fill 49 prescriptions. By comparison, the average Medicare beneficiary consults just 7 different physicians and fills approximately 20 prescriptions per year. Therefore, Piper believes that SNPs have the potential to exploit "an extraordinarily large, virtually untapped market. We are talking on the order of a quarter-trillion dollars." He added that, "if a plan wants to grow, especially a large plan, they have to get in this business."

In 2005, the first year of the SNP initiative, 125 plans were in operation – mainly managed care plans that had existing MA contracts with CMS. In 2006, the number of SNPs increased to 276. Most of these plans (226) focus on dual eligibles, but 37 care for institutionalized beneficiaries, and 13 address the needs of the chronically ill. Overall, these plans had 550,000 members as of August 1, 2006. According to CMS, the number of SNPs will increase again in 2007, to a total of 471. Piper expects enrollment to grow even faster, reaching 1 million by the end of 2007 and doubling again in 2008. This expected rapid growth is attributable to substantial increases in payments for managing patients with multiple chronic conditions. Plan sponsors have expressed interest in creating specialized SNPs for several chronic conditions, including cardiovascular diseases, osteoarthritis, obesity, mental disorders, end-stage renal disease, and HIV/AIDS.

Before 2005, Medicare beneficiaries with special needs were commonly regarded as an unwelcome liability for health plans. However, the MMA introduced a risk adjustment model that offers greater rewards for managing an increasing number of chronic disorders. The *New York Times* of October 21, 2006, noted that, before the introduction of risk adjustment, a health plan would have received $8,145 per year for the care of a 70-year-old woman. The payment would have varied only according to beneficiaries' age and sex, not their health profile. Under the new system, the basic payment is only $4,075 per year, but this amount increases to $6,197 if the patient is diabetic. If the beneficiary also has circulatory problems, the health plan receives $12,182 per year, and the payment would total $30,126 if the patient additionally had emphysema, congestive heart failure, and depression. These additional payments have made the sickest Medicare beneficiaries a financially attractive target for insurance companies. John Gorman told the *New York Times* that "the people these plans were running from five years ago now become the desirables. It's totally standing the economics of this industry on their head." Notwithstanding these sharp increases in payments for beneficiaries with multiple chronic conditions, some observers see the need for a "frailty adjuster" to cover plans' much higher expenses for the most infirm beneficiaries. CMS is reportedly considering the introduction of such a measure in the future.

SNPs promise to be profitable. Piper forecasts that start-up costs will limit early margins to 4–6%, but improving care and eliminating waste could increase margins to 6–10% in future years. However, government intervention and the need to increase benefits in response to growing competition could trim those margins in the long term.

In the past, differences between Medicare and Medicaid with regard to bidding, contracting, enrollment rate setting, and marketing deterred many plans from entering the special needs market. While Medicare is a federal program, Medicaid is administered at state level, with pronounced policy differences from one state to another. A review of SNPs in Boston (Massachusetts), Miami (Florida), and Phoenix (Arizona) conducted by Mathematica Policy Research found that the most successful plans generally have extensive experience working with both Medicare and Medicaid and can effectively partner with state governments, which have input on the Medicaid business (see Medicare Advantage SNPs site visits, Mathematica Policy Research, June 2006, www.mathematica-mpr.com/publications/pdfs/medadspecial. pdf. Accessed November 15, 2007). The most astute and ambitious plans are creating their own SNPs to service the dual-eligible population. Meanwhile, federal and state governments appear to favor an integrated model for full dual-eligible beneficiaries. Many state governments express a desire for closer collaboration with Medicaid managed care providers in caring for their dual-eligible populations, but Mathematica found that plans were often forced to work primarily with CMS's central office instead of regional offices.

According to Mathematica, approximately a dozen states have passive enrollment in SNPs. In other states, plans must use marketing initiatives to reach out to potential members, but this strategy has had mixed results to date. Data limitations make it difficult for insurers to identify dual-eligible beneficiaries. The Medicare and Medicaid programs have separate enrollment lists, and eligibility for Medicaid changes in line with beneficiaries' income. Insurers do not have contact details for dual eligibles, with the obvious exception of beneficiaries who have been automatically enrolled in their SNPs. Plan sponsors may be able to obtain referrals from network physicians. In addition, MA plans can use claims data to identify members who have specific illnesses that they are targeting.

Aveta has become one of the largest SNP providers in the United States, with almost 100,000 enrollees in total (74,000 chronically ill patients and 23,000 dual-eligible beneficiaries). The Fort Lee, New Jersey-based company has had particular success with its SNPs in Puerto Rico, where it already had a strong presence in MA. In contrast, the company has struggled to raise awareness of its SNPs in Cook County, Illinois, where it has thus far recruited only around 100 members. Consequently, Aveta has requested help from CMS in educating Medicare beneficiaries about the SNP option. Overall, the company expects strong growth, particularly from SNPs for dual-eligible beneficiaries.

HealthSpring, an MCO headquartered in Nashville, Tennessee, was likewise forced to find potential enrollees in the community. However, Craig Schub, the company's senior vice president of marketing, confirms that many dual eligibles cannot be reached through normal marketing channels. Instead, HealthSpring has relied on a strategy of reaching Medicare beneficiaries through trusted organizations in the community, for example, government agencies, community outreach groups, churches and so on (for more information on HealthSpring's future growth strategy, see the sidebar, "HealthSpring: A Regional Player Goes National").

Beginning in the 2008 contract year, CMS will allow SNPs to limit enrollment of dual eligibles to subsets (e.g., the disabled) who are receiving care under Medicaid. This change is intended to provide a more integrated delivery system. CMS will provide further guidance on acceptable subsets and the approval process.

The current legislation governing SNPs runs until December 2008, and Congress will review the impact of this initiative before deciding whether to renew it. However, few observers expect this program to be cancelled.

HealthSpring: A Regional Player Goes National

HealthSpring, an MCO based in Nashville, Tennessee, initially chose to focus its Medicare Part D activities in a handful of regions in southern states – its well-established core market. The company considered it advisable to gain experience in the new program in familiar territory before contemplating nationwide expansion. According to Wendy Richey, the company's vice president of government programs, "the legislative requirements are huge. We're now at a point where we can do national work." Joining the exclusive ranks of national players is a major step for HealthSpring.

At the beginning of 2006, the company received automatic assignments of approximately 90,000 PDP members in the states in which it was active, but many of these beneficiaries subsequently left for competing plans. On May 1, 2006, the company received another 20,000 PDP members, and enrollment in its standalone plan currently stands at 88,000. In 2007, the company hopes a strong focus on customer service will enable it to retain two-thirds to three-quarters of its new automatically assigned members.

Like many other plan sponsors, HealthSpring sees the second year of automatic assignment of dual-eligible beneficiaries as a way to add covered lives and expand into new regions. However, although the company is casting a wide net, it expects to catch far fewer new enrollees than the national companies did last year. Richey predicts that "the migration is not going to be what it was last year because ultimately CMS is going to try to keep duals with who they had this year as long as the premium is within $2 of the national benchmark." The company could benefit from automatic assignment of low-income beneficiaries who become eligible for Medicare in 2007 or whose former plans no longer qualify for the LIS, but this number is expected to be modest. Moreover, HealthSpring will have to contend with more competitive price points from Humana, UnitedHealthcare, and WellCare.

In preparation for the move to nationwide activity, HealthSpring has expanded its resources. The company has moved away from managing each PDP at the state level and will bring that work in-house to the corporate pharmacy. HealthSpring's PBM company has also had an important role to play in broadening the MCO's networks.

DISEASE MANAGEMENT

Historically, Medicare fee-for-service (FFS) enrollees generally lacked access to disease management (DM) programs, unless they had some form of supplementary health insurance. CMS officials have long acknowledged that this situation is a significant problem. In testimony before the House Committee on Ways and Means Subcommittee on Health on May 11, 2004, Mark McClellan offered the following explanation for the dearth of DM activities in the Medicare FFS system:

> The Medicare fee-for-service system is structured and financed to manage acute care episodes, not to manage and support individuals with progressive chronic diseases. Providers of care are organized and paid for services provided in discrete settings (for example, hospitals, physician offices, home health care, long-term care, or preventive services). Patient care can be fragmented and poorly coordinated and patient information difficult to integrate among settings. Providers may lack timely and complete patient clinical information to fully assess their patients' needs and to help prevent complications. Ongoing support to beneficiaries for managing their conditions outside their physicians' offices is rare.

In October 2004, the Congressional Budget Office (CBO) published what has since become a widely publicized review of the clinical effectiveness and cost-effectiveness of commercial DM initiatives. The report, entitled *An Analysis of the Literature on Disease Management Programs*, concluded that "the prevailing evidence appears to be that while disease management programs improve adherence to practice care guidelines and lead to better control of the disease, their net effects on health costs are not clear." The CBO suggested that it might prove difficult to translate the results of successful commercial DM programs to Medicare FFS beneficiaries – a population that is elderly, has multiple illnesses, and consults a wide range of medical providers. The fact that Medicare beneficiaries remain in the program much longer than most employees remain in the same employer-sponsored health plan should enhance the effectiveness of DM in the Medicare population. However, the CBO suggested that the clinical effectiveness of DM programs might actually *increase* Medicare's total costs over a beneficiary's lifetime: "If beneficiaries ended up dying from diseases that are more expensive to treat (such as cancer), the total cost for the program could actually increase."

Section 721 of the MMA mandates by far the largest DM demonstration in history – a voluntary chronic care improvement program, now called Medicare Health Support, to improve the quality of care and life for approximately 180,000 Medicare beneficiaries who have multiple chronic illnesses (e.g., congestive heart failure [CHF], complex diabetes, chronic obstructive pulmonary disorder [COPD]). CMS reports that approximately 14% of Medicare beneficiaries have CHF, but they account for 43% of the program's spending. Similarly, the 18% of Medicare beneficiaries who have diabetes account for 32% of the program's expenditures. The Medicare Health Support Program must reduce health risks, improve participants' quality of life, and achieve savings for Medicare and its beneficiaries. Participating companies are paid monthly fees, but they have to refund some or all of these fees to the federal government if they do not meet agreed standards for quality improvement, save Medicare at least 5% of healthcare costs for enrollees, and improve beneficiary satisfaction.

The MMA made a provision for a wide range of enterprises (e.g., disease management organizations, health insurers, integrated delivery systems, physician group practices, consortia of such entities) to apply to serve as chronic care improvement organizations (CCIOs) in this demonstration project. In December 2004, CMS awarded contracts with a combined value estimated at $100–200 million to 9 CCIOs:

- American Healthways, Washington, DC and Maryland.
- LifeMasters Supported SelfCare, Oklahoma.
- Health Dialog Services, Western Pennsylvania.
- McKesson Health Solutions, Mississippi.
- CIGNA Healthcare, Northwest Georgia.
- Aetna Life Insurance, Chicago, Illinois.
- Humana, Central Florida.
- XLHealth, Tennessee.
- Visiting Nurse Service of New York and United HealthCare Services, Brooklyn/Queens, New York.

If it is apparent before three years have passed that any of the demonstration projects are clearly successful, Medicare will expedite the rollout of these programs to the wider Medicare population. CMS has high expectations for the Medicare Health Support Program. In his aforementioned testimony before the House Committee on Ways and Means Subcommittee on Health in May 2004, McClellan expressed the hope that the Chronic Care Improvement Program (CCIP, now renamed the Medicare Health Support Program) would provide an opportunity to reward disease prevention and health improvement in the Medicare FFS system:

> Currently, Medicare fee-for-service payments do not encourage prevention of diseases, good outcomes and performance. Instead, the payment system provides money for acute events, missing a potential opportunity to prevent these situations which could be beneficial from a cost standpoint, but, more importantly, from a health perspective. In a sense, payment incentives are the opposite of the way they should be. The CCIP seeks to address this problem, as well as others described above, by rewarding efforts to prevent acute episodes and improve health. Under CCIP, awardees will work to increase patient compliance, facilitate communication between patients and providers, and better coordinate care among providers caring for the same individual. In a much more direct way than ever before under fee-for-service Medicare, economic incentives will be directly lined up with prevention and performance. We hope to reward high quality care, rather than high volume and high intensity care.

The DM industry also hopes that the Medicare Health Support Program will give its members the opportunity to penetrate the potentially enormous and lucrative market for Medicare DM. Some analysts suggest that, if the Medicare Health Support Program is judged a success and opens the floodgates to DM, total revenues in this industry could ultimately increase from approximately

$1.2 billion per year at present to $10 billion or even $20 billion per year.

In an interview with the Commonwealth Fund in June 2005, Christobel Selecky, the CEO of LifeMasters Supported SelfCare and President of the Disease Management Association of America, articulated her hopes for this demonstration project:

> Should the Medicare Health Support pilots be successful, and I believe that most of them will be, it will open the door toward a significant expansion of disease management into an as-yet untapped population. Because most of these pilots are built on collaborative models that include disease management organizations, physician organizations, health plans, community organizations, and consumer groups, among others, I hope that their success will serve to more deeply embed disease management into the fabric of our health care system.

Some of the companies involved in the new Medicare Health Support initiative will continue to concentrate on providing DM services in support of health insurers and employers. For example, American Healthways works with more than 50 carriers, including 16 that operate MA plans. On the other hand, some DM organizations have recently shown interest in setting up their own Medicare health plans. For instance, in October 2006, Visiting Nurse Service of New York (VNSNY) launched an MA plan and a standalone PDP under the banner of VNS CHOICE Select. The company plans to target the approximately 250,000 full-benefit dual eligible beneficiaries who live in the five boroughs of New York City. In addition to offering the usual range of MA services, including administration of Medicare Part A and B benefits, VNS CHOICE Select will build on the company's existing program of nurse visits to patients' homes.

In 2006, XLHealth launched a chronic care SNP in its home state of Maryland. In 2007, the company plans to expand this operation to Texas, Arkansas, Missouri, Georgia, and South Carolina. XLHealth chose these states on account of their low overall health scores, lack of MA penetration, and physicians' receptivity to SNPs. The new plans will cover diabetes, COPD, heart failure, and end-stage renal disease. The company estimates the total number of potential enrollees in its target states at 1.2 million, but it would be pleased to sign up 25,000–30,000 members in 2007.

This diversification strategy is not without risks: the launch of the SNP could upset some of the more established plans for which XLHealth has long provided DM services. However, Paul Serini, Executive Vice President at XLHealth, believes "there's plenty of room, plenty of room for others to come in and it would increase awareness of [chronic-care] SNPs in the physician community and in the beneficiary community, and competition is always a good thing." The company has already agreed to form an SNP partnership with an MA plan in New York and is conducting negotiations with three or four major national plans that could lead to alliances in 2008.

MEDICARE MEDICAL SAVINGS ACCOUNTS

The MMA contained a little-known measure to encourage people under age 65 – and their employers – to save toward their current and future healthcare costs: health savings accounts (HSAs). Contributions to an HSA are tax-free if the beneficiary enrolls in a health plan that has a high deductible and a high cap on annual out-of-pocket expenses. Plan enrollees can use funds from their spending account to pay for medical expenses, including prescription and nonprescription medicines. If their spending accounts are exhausted, members must pay all their healthcare expenses out-of-pocket until they reach their plan's deductible. Any money in an HSA that is not spent in a given year may be carried over to the next year and will gain interest tax-free, thereby allowing savers to accumulate substantial funds to cover their healthcare expenses. Approximately 3.2 million US residents have HSAs, and one-fifth of companies (one-third of companies with more than 5,000 employees) offer this type of account to employees.

Under the terms of the MMA, current Medicare beneficiaries cannot sign up for new HSAs, but they can benefit from funds they saved in such accounts before they became eligible for Medicare. However, CMS has been able to sidestep this ban by means of a demonstration project. Beginning in 2007, a provision similar to HSAs – Medicare medical savings accounts (MSAs) – will be offered in a total of 39 states. In addition, more flexible MSAs will be offered in two states. These more flexible accounts will cover preventive services during the deductible period, provide a deductible below the out-of-pocket maximum, impose cost-sharing up to the out-of-pocket maximum, and reduce out-of-pocket payments if enrollees use in-network services.

MSAs cover Medicare Part A and B benefits but exclude Part D: beneficiaries must sign up for a standalone PDP if they wish to receive outpatient drug benefits. Funds in an MSA cannot count as Internal Revenue Service (IRS)-qualified expenses if they are used to pay Part D premiums, but they can be used toward copayments, coinsurance, and deductibles for the Part D drugs. Plans may offer additional benefits for an increased fee, but no plans intend to take advantage of this provision in 2007.

At the beginning of each year, CMS will pay an annual deposit into an interest-bearing account to pay for medical services. After the enrollee has paid the deductible for the year (at least $2,000 in 2007 – far more than the typical Medicare PDP deductible of $265), the insurer will pay for any Medicare-covered services (enrollees whose expenses exceed their annual deductible may be required to share some of the subsequent costs, subject to an out-of-pocket maximum). As with HSAs, unused money in an MSA can be rolled over to the following year, allowing the beneficiary to accumulate money tax-free.

According to CMS, three companies will offer varied MSA plans in 2007:

Blue Cross of California will offer a regular MSA plantargeted at individual and employer group markets in California. Deductibles will range from $2,500 to $4,500, with no cost-sharing after the deductible is met and no coverage of preventive services before the deductible.

Unicare Life and Health Insurance is offering a product similar to that of Blue Cross of California but is focusing on individual and employer group markets in 38 states.

American Progressive, a subsidiary of Universal American Financial, is rolling out a demonstration MSA plan serving the individual market in New York and Pennsylvania, and all 50 states for the employer market. The plans feature a $4,000 deductible, a $4,800 out-of-pocket maximum, 29% cost-sharing after the deducible is met up to the out-of-pocket maximum, and some coverage of preventive services before the deductible.

CMS believes that MSAs will appeal particularly to beneficiaries who are healthier or have experience with HSAs. Federal officials present MSAs as one element in a portfolio of products, ranging from preferred provider organizations (PPOs) to private fee-for-service plans, intended to contain beneficiaries' costs. The National Association of Health Underwriters believes that introducing greater choice and competition into Medicare should foster innovative ideas for controlling costs and improving healthcare delivery.

Before his recent resignation, CMS administrator Mark McClellan predicted that enrollment in Medicare Part D overall and in the MSA demonstration project would grow substantially in 2007 and 2008. Industry observers believe the MSA plans could draw away beneficiaries from the extremely popular Medicare private fee-for-service offerings.

If the high-deductible model takes hold, companies that have long experience in the consumer-directed market (e.g., WellPoint, UnitedHealthcare) could take a substantial share of the market as it matures.

OUTLOOK AND IMPLICATIONS

The massive increase in the number of Medicare Part D plans – especially MA plans – in 2007 demonstrates the health insurance industry's commitment to this new program. Lower premiums, zero deductibles, and an expansion of coverage in the coverage gap are all good news for beneficiaries. However, these changes reflect the intense struggle among insurers to gain an advantage in a highly competitive market.

The large insurers have quickly assumed a dominant position in the Medicare Part D market, leaving other companies to compete for a marginal share of regional markets. In a recent report, Deutsche Bank Securities noted the top-5 PDPs controlled nearly 70% of the Part D market by August 2006. Analysts predict that most of the smaller companies will eventually try to sell their Part D businesses to the large insurers. John Gorman expects smaller companies to reassess their competitive position around the second quarter of 2007, by which time the enrollment figures of all participating insurers will be known. Small companies will then be prime targets for acquisition, and extensive consolidation appears inevitable in the longer term.

With approximately 90% of the Medicare population already enrolled in a Part D plan or equivalent, insurers will need to redouble their efforts to persuade the 4.4 million beneficiaries who still lack drug benefits to sign up in 2007. In addition, successful PDP sponsors will increasingly seek to convert enrollees to MA plans. For example, Humana has stated its ambition to boost its current MA enrollment of close to 1 million by converting many of its 3.5 million PDP members. Almost 70% of Humana's PDP enrollees were not given the option of an MA plan in 2006: they were enrolled through the CMS Web site, Humana's State Farm partnership, or other channels that did not feature MA plans. Humana projects profit margins of 3–5% for its MA business, compared with just 1–3% for its standalone PDPs.

Employer-sponsored insurance for retirees has been in decline in the United States for many years. Research conducted by the Kaiser Family Foundation and the Health Research and Educational Trust found that, among large employers (i.e., companies with 200 or more employees) that offer health insurance to their active employees, the percentage that also offers such a benefit to their retirees has decreased from 66% in 1988 to just 35% in 2006. Medicare's retiree drug subsidy may arrest this decline temporarily, but it is unlikely to stop or reverse the trend in the long term. As noted earlier, many employers would require more generous subsidies to continue to offer these benefits to their former employees in years to come. Medicare Part D will be an invaluable safety net for senior citizens affected by such changes, but the overall quality of retiree drug benefits could be steadily eroded.

The increased emphasis on beneficiaries with special needs – especially chronic illness – will be a positive development. The biopharmaceutical industry could benefit from greater use of its products, particularly in disease prevention. Manufacturers need to look for opportunities to support and sponsor disease management programs linked to this new initiative.

The coverage gap will remain one of the most contentious features of Medicare Part D. The sharp increase in the number of PDPs that offer generics coverage in the gap offers some comfort to beneficiaries who have substantial drug costs, but critics maintain that this provision remains an imperfect solution to a serious problem. Monthly premiums are much higher for plans that offer any form of coverage in the coverage gap. For PDPs, the median monthly premium in 2007 will be $29.00 for plans that offer no gap coverage, $46.90 for plans that cover generics, and $103.20 for plans that cover all formulary drugs (effectively eliminating the gap). Beneficiaries who fell into the doughnut hole in 2006 will likely be interested in plans that fill the gap in future years, but the monthly premiums for plans that cover all formulary drugs may still be unaffordable for some beneficiaries. More significantly, only 38 PDPs will offer coverage of all formulary drugs in the coverage gap in 2007, and some beneficiaries may find that their medications are excluded from these plans' formularies.

The coverage gap presents multiple threats to manufacturers of branded drugs. Nonadherence is one potentially serious problem: faced with a sudden large increase in their out-of-pocket payments, some beneficiaries may discontinue their drug therapy, miss doses, or reduce their dosage to save money. Other beneficiaries may conclude that it is no longer worthwhile to continue paying premiums for Medicare Part D and therefore drop out of the program, losing all drug benefits in the process. Beneficiaries who accept a switch from a branded medicine to a generic one will not necessarily revert to their original medication when they emerge from the coverage gap and are eligible for 95% reimbursement of their drug costs. Physicians may be reluctant to change a patient's medications twice in a year, particularly if the patient has been stabilized on the generic alternative. In that event, the coverage gap could cost manufacturers of branded medicines some of their patients on a permanent basis.

According to CMS, Medicare beneficiaries already rely more heavily on generics than does the US population overall. Prescribing data for the first two quarters of 2006 indicate that generics accounted for 51.9% of prescriptions in the pharmaceutical market as a whole, but 60.1% of prescriptions in the Medicare population. Recent initiatives by retail pharmacies to make inexpensive generics available to all customers – led by Wal-Mart's high-profile promise of generics for $4 per prescription – could reduce the need for generics coverage in the gap. However, the range of drugs included in these programs would need to be expanded substantially to meet the needs of most Medicare beneficiaries.

Most worrisome of all for the biopharmaceutical industry is the renewed focus on drug prices under Medicare Part D. The MMA precludes CMS from using its influence to negotiate price cuts, but many members of Congress remain highly critical of this fundamental aspect of the legislation. Some of the proponents of change cite a study by Dean Baker, an economist at the Center for Economic and Policy Research, which found that direct price negotiation by CMS could deliver total savings more than twice the size of the coverage gap. Following their victories in midterm elections for both the Senate and the House of Representatives, the Democrats have pledged to introduce legislation within the first 100 hours of the new legislative session to empower CMS to bargain for price cuts. The Republicans, led by the Bush administration, remain resolutely opposed to such a change, but it may be difficult for them to withstand the growing pressure for some form of government intervention in Medicare drug pricing.

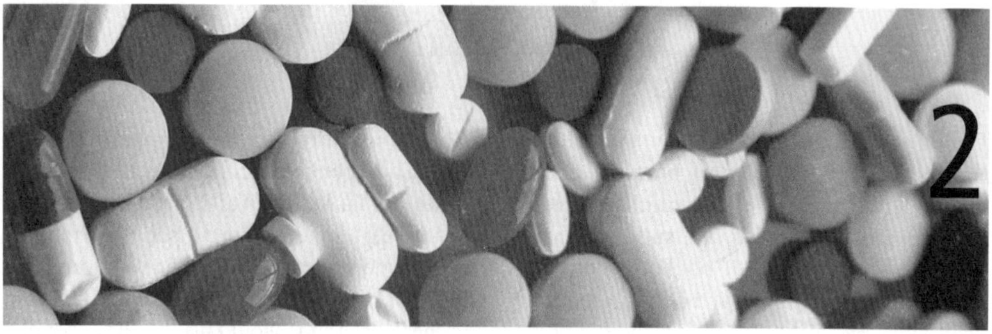

2

Changes in US Oncology Drug Reimbursement: Medicare Sets the Pace

INTRODUCTION

Cancer has a higher profile than almost any other disease. According to the American Cancer Society (ACS), 10.1 million US residents have been diagnosed with cancer at some time in their lives, and approximately 1.4 million US residents were expected to be diagnosed with some form of cancer in 2006. The lifetime risk of developing cancer is 1 in 2 for US men and 1 in 3 for US women. Cancer is also the second most common cause of death in the United States (after coronary heart disease), accounting for one-quarter of all deaths. The ACS forecasted that 564,830 US residents will die from cancer in 2006 (American Cancer Society, 2006).

Providing access to effective cancer therapies is a public health priority, but oncology drugs can cost tens of thousands of dollars per year. Because of the rarity of certain cancers, manufacturers have to recoup their R&D costs from a relatively small patient population. In addition, many of the most efficacious therapies are biologics – agents that have very substantial manufacturing costs. Furthermore, most cancer therapies are intravenous infusions that must be administered by medical professionals – a requirement that adds significantly to the overall treatment costs. Consequently, access to cancer drugs is subject to strict controls.

In most therapeutic areas, patients obtain their own medications from community pharmacies and are reimbursed by their third-party payer (if they have appropriate coverage). Oncology reimbursement in the United States is generally different, however. Approximately 84% of patients receive their cancer therapy in oncologists' offices, and these practices are responsible for collecting patients' out-of-pocket payments and claiming reimbursement for their drug and administrative costs from the relevant payers.

Cancer treatment in the United States is funded by a mixture of public payers (e.g., Medicare, Medicaid, the Department of Veterans Affairs) and commercial payers (e.g., indemnity insurance plans, managed care organizations [MCOs]). The ACS reports that 76% of cancer patients are aged 55 or older, including many Medicare beneficiaries. Data from Verispan's Physician Drug & Diagnosis Audit (PDDA) confirm the important role that Medicare plays in the treatment of cancer in the United States.

Figures 2.1–2.5 show the main sources of insurance coverage for patients who visited a physician for treatment for breast, skin, prostate, lung, and colorectal cancers in the first six months of 2006 (because some patients have more than one form of health insurance, percentages for each indication exceed 100). Medicare was the most common source of funding for all of these cancers except breast cancer, a disease that frequently has an earlier onset than most of the other highly prevalent cancers. Figure 2.6 shows that Medicare and private insurance were the dominant sources of insurance coverage for these five cancers overall. Therefore, our discussion focuses on the reimbursement environment in Medicare and commercial health plans.

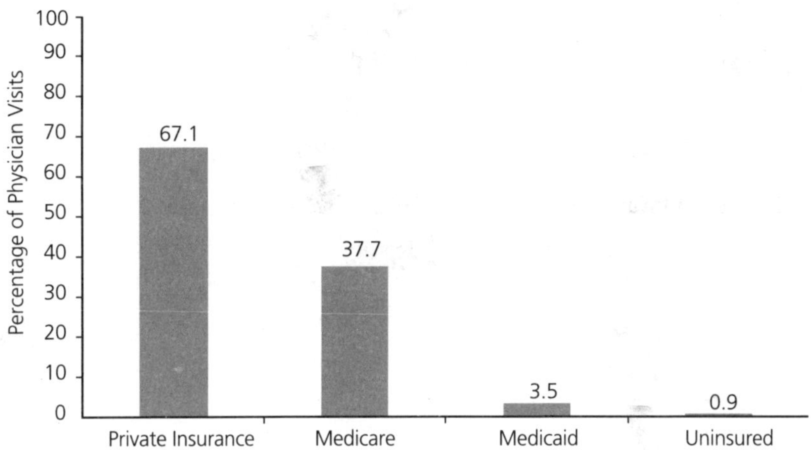

Note: Percentages total more than 100 because some patients have more than one form of insurance

Figure 2.1 Main Sources of Insurance Coverage for Breast Cancer Therapy, 2006

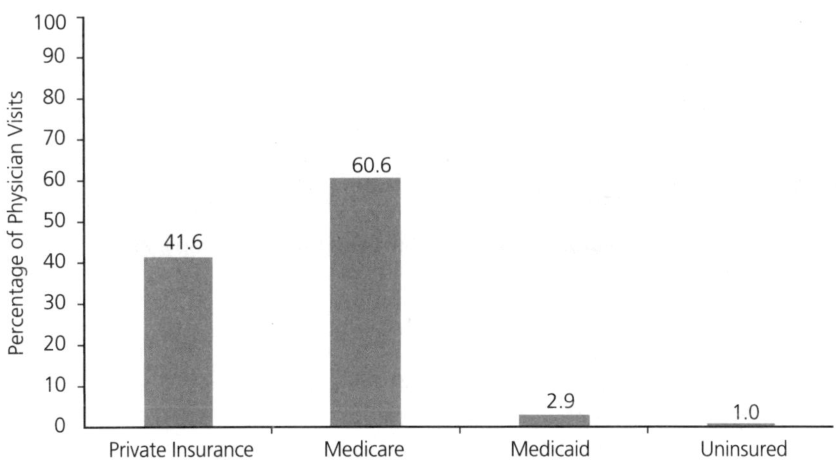

Note: Percentages total more than 100 because some patients have more than one form of insurance

Figure 2.2 Main Sources of Insurance Coverage for Skin Cancer Therapy, 2006

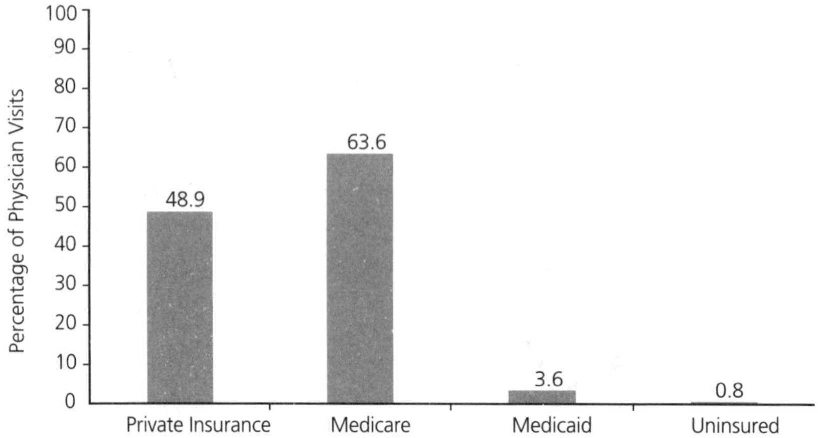

Note: Percentages total more than 100 because some patients have more than one form of insurance

Figure 2.3 Main Sources of Insurance Coverage for Prostate Cancer Therapy, 2006

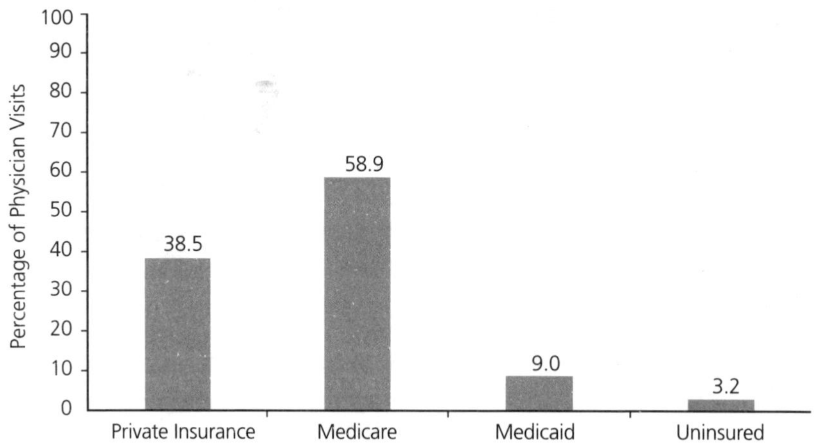

Note: Percentages total more than 100 because some patients have more than one form of insurance

Figure 2.4 Main Sources of Insurance Coverage for Lung Cancer Therapy, 2006

We begin this chapter with a detailed examination of Medicare's reimbursement procedures for office-based treatment, hospital outpatient therapy, hospital inpatient treatment, and self-administered drugs (under the new Medicare Part D prescription drug benefit). We then compare practice in the private sector and review policies on off-label prescribing. We conclude with a brief assessment of the outlook and implications for the pharmaceutical industry.

Medicare

Since its creation in 1965, the Medicare program has become a major source of

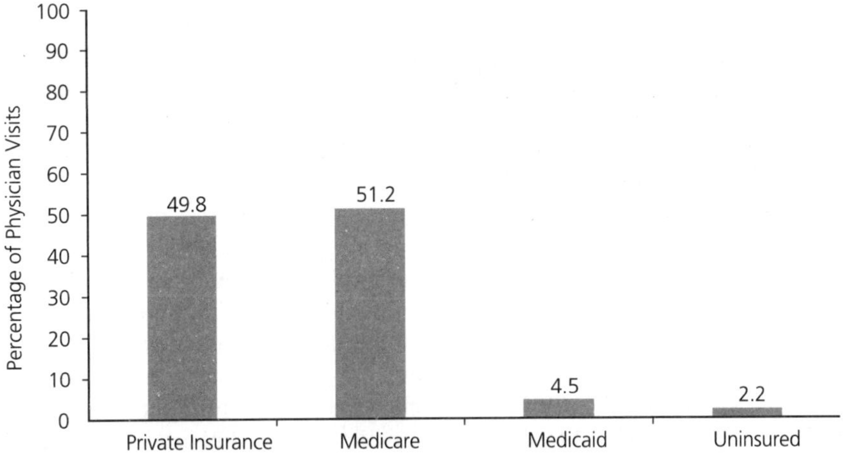

Note: Percentages total more than 100 because some patients have more than one form of insurance

Figure 2.5 Main Sources of Insurance Coverage for Colorectal Cancer Therapy, 2006

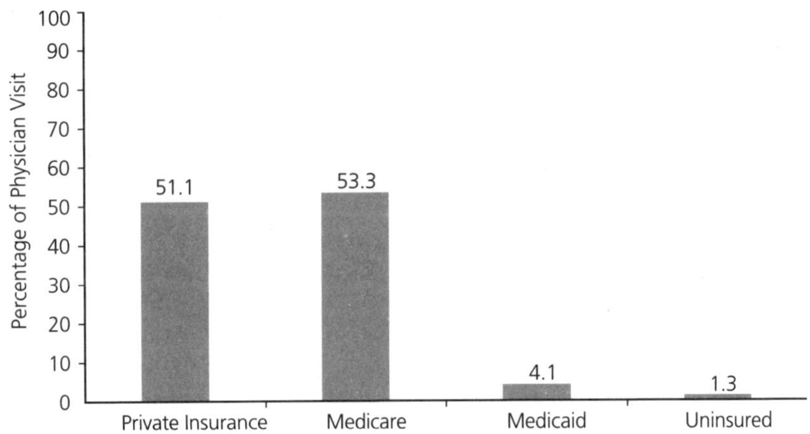

Note: Percentages total more than 100 because some patients have more than one form of insurance

Figure 2.6 Main Sources of Insurance Coverage for Breast, Skin, Prostate, Lung, and Colorectal Cancer Therapy, 2006

healthcare coverage for seniors, the disabled, and patients with end-stage renal disease in the United States. In 2006, approximately 43 million US residents were recipients of at least basic Medicare benefits.

Historically, Medicare offered only limited coverage of prescription medicines: Part A covers inpatient drugs, and Part B (an optional program) covers outpatient drugs that are not usually self-administered (e.g., intravenous infusions, intramuscular injections) but generally excludes oral drugs. In addition, Medicare beneficiaries who can afford the premiums (typically around $140 per month at present) can purchase optional Medigap insurance to increase their level of benefits, including prescription drug coverage. Beginning in 1999, Part C, commonly known as Medicare + Choice (renamed Medicare Advantage in 2004), offered additional services – including prescription drug benefits – through private fee-for-service plans or Medicare MCOs. However, inadequate government funding led to a rapid erosion of benefits and the contraction or closure of many Medicare + Choice plans. To improve beneficiaries' access to outpatient prescription medicines, the Medicare Prescription Drug, Improvement, and Modernization Act of 2003 (commonly known as the Medicare Modernization Act [MMA]) introduced Medicare Part D – a new outpatient drug benefit that began operation on January 1, 2006.

Because most cancer therapies are administered in physician offices in the United States, Part B is currently the most important source of Medicare funding in oncology. However, the shift toward self-administered injections and oral dosage forms will increase the importance of Part D in the future.

In recent years, the US government has broadened Part B prescription drug coverage. The Medicare, Medicaid, State Children's Health Insurance Program (SCHIP), and Benefits Improvement Act of 2000 (BIPA) extended coverage from drugs that are not self-administered to drugs that are not usually self-administered. In May 2002, the Centers for Medicare and Medicaid Services (CMS) clarified this provision: drugs that are delivered by intramuscular injection are covered, but medicines administered by subcutaneous injection are not covered. Oral drugs are excluded from Part B coverage, with the exception of products that also have an injectable dosage form that would be reimbursed if it was administered by a physician. Consequently, innovative oral medicines (e.g., Novartis's Gleevec [imatinib] for chronic myeloid leukemia), which do not also have a dosage form requiring physician administration, are not eligible for reimbursement under Medicare Part B.

Office-Based Treatment

Oncology-related drugs account for the majority of Medicare Part B's pharmaceutical expenditures. Figure 2.7 traces the growth of

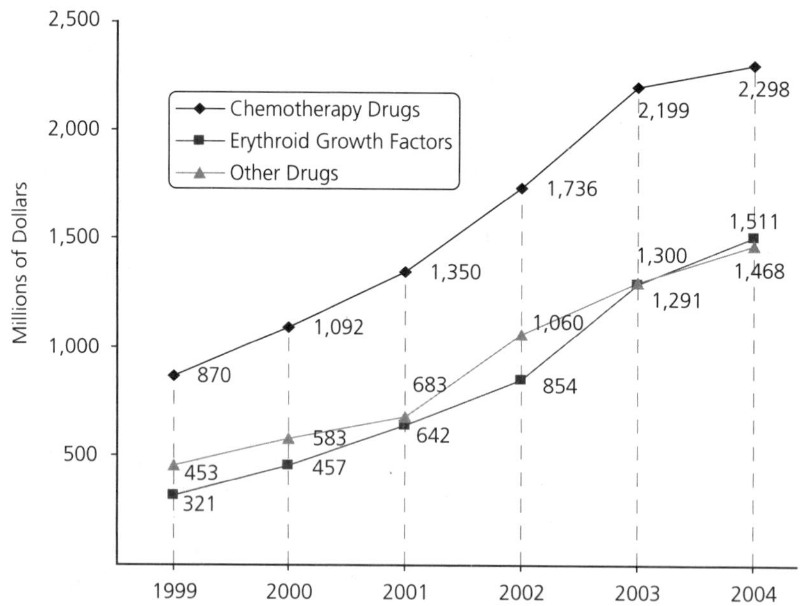

Figure 2.7 Evolution of Medicare Part B Spending on Oncology Drugs, 1999–2004

Medicare spending on oncology-related drugs from 1999 to 2004. Over that period, spending on chemotherapy drugs rose from $870 million to $2.3 billion, a 164% increase (equivalent to 21.4% per year). Spending on erythroid growth factors grew even faster, from $321 million in 1999 to $1.5 billion in 2004, a 371% increase (36.3% per year). Medicare Part B expenditures on other oncology-related drugs rose from $453 million in 1999 to $1.5 billion in 2004, a 224% increase (26.5% per year). Total expenditures on oncology-related drugs grew from $1.6 billion in 1999 to $5.3 billion in 2004, a 221% increase (26.5% per year). Payments for the administration of oncology-related drugs rose relatively slowly, from $180 million in 1999 to $288 million in 2003, but then leapt to $912 million in 2004, following radical changes to the Medicare Part B reimbursement structure (see the next section). Overall, Medicare Part B expenditures on oncology (including evaluation and management services, tests, imaging, and other procedures) grew from $2.5 billion in 1999 to $7.3 billion in 2004, a 191% increase (23.8% per year).

Physician Reimbursement

Historically, Medicare Part B reimbursed physicians for most drugs administered in their offices at 95% of average wholesale price (AWP) – the AWP is the average list price that a manufacturer suggests wholesalers charge pharmacies; in practice, this price is often heavily discounted, particularly for Health Maintenance Organizations (HMOs) and other large purchasers. But actual acquisition costs for most physician-administered drugs were much lower than reimbursement prices. A study conducted by the Government Accountability Office (GAO) found that providers' drug acquisition costs were actually 13–86% below AWP. The GAO and the Office of the Inspector General of the Department of Health and Human Services have independently estimated that the total difference between Medicare Part B drug acquisition costs and reimbursement payments was approximately $1 billion per year (in addition to reimbursing physicians for medications they supply under Medicare Part B, CMS pays these clinicians for providing drug administration services).

Oncologists were the main beneficiaries of the price differential between acquisition costs and reimbursement payments: CMS and the Congressional Budget Office (CBO) estimated that these physicians received $700 million in overpayments for Part B drugs each year. In their defense, physicians argued that overpayments on drug reimbursement offset underpayments by CMS for the cost of administering these drugs. Many oncologists asserted that, without generous reimbursement of drug costs, they could not afford to offer their Medicare patients office-based administration of cancer therapies. Office-based physicians argued that they used the "spread" – the differential between drugs' acquisition prices and their reimbursement prices – to offset the costs of administering these medicines and to subsidize other patient services. CMS estimated that, in 2003, oncologists derived an average of 70% of their Medicare income from the differential between drug acquisition and reimbursement prices.

The MMA mandated radical changes in the method for calculating reimbursement rates for Medicare Part B drugs that are administered in physicians' offices. In 2004, the standard reimbursement rate for office-administered drugs was reduced to 85% of the AWP on April 1, 2003. For certain drugs judged to be subject to particularly aggressive discounting, reimbursement was as low as 80% of AWP. Beginning January 1, 2005, Medicare introduced a new method for reimbursement calculations. Office-administered drugs are generally reimbursed at 106% of the manufacturer's average sales price (ASP). A drug's ASP is the manufacturer's total revenue from the drug divided by the number of units sold. CMS revises its list of ASPs on a quarterly basis. The switch from AWP- to ASP-based reimbursement of drug costs substantially reduced the payments physicians received for providing pharmaceuticals under Medicare Part B.

To mitigate the impact of reduced drug reimbursement, CMS increased its payments for drug administration services (especially chemotherapy) by an average of 110% in 2004. In addition, providers benefited from transitional supplementary payments of 32% of standard drug administration payment rates in 2004 and 3% in 2005. The introduction of new drug administration codes in 2005 also enabled physicians to charge for more services during each session of chemotherapy than had been permitted previously.

CMS calculated that the move to ASP-based reimbursement would reduce oncologists' income from Medicare by an average of 8%. However, in September 2004, the American Society of Clinical Oncology (ASCO) predicted a much more severe impact on its members' incomes. Based on a survey of 93 oncology practices across the United States, ASCO estimated that the average reduction in drug reimbursement rates would be 15% in 2005. With the sharp reduction in the level of the transitional supplementary payment (from 32% to 3%) for drug administration services, ASCO forecast that overall Medicare funding for chemotherapy services would decline by 54%, a cut that would "certainly affect the way oncologists are able to deliver care in the United States."

Three reports published by federal agencies have challenged ASCO's assertions. In December 2004, the GAO published an analysis of Medicare Part B's new drug and administration fees for chemotherapy (Government Accountability Office, 2006). The study reviewed 2003, 2004, and preliminary 2005 acquisition costs and Medicare payments for 16 drugs that together accounted for 75% of Medicare payments to oncologists for physician-administered agents in 2003. Overall, payments for these 16 drugs exceeded acquisition costs by 22.4% in 2004 and 5.5% (projected) in 2005. Extrapolating these figures to the oncology market as a whole, the GAO estimated that Medicare Part B payments for cancer drugs exceeded oncologists' acquisition costs by a total of $790 million in 2004 and by a projected sum of $202 million in 2005.

In September 2005, the Office of Inspector General (OIG) of the Department of Health and Human Services published a report on the adequacy of Medicare Part B's new reimbursement rates, as mandated by the MMA (Office of Inspector General, 2006). The study examined data for 39 reimbursement codes that collectively accounted for more than 94% of Medicare's 2004 payments for hematology, hematology/oncology, and medical oncology. The authors estimated that, overall, Medicare reimbursement rates exceeded acquisition costs for 35 of the 39 codes.

In January 2006, the Medicare Payment Advisory Commission (MedPAC) published a wide-ranging review of the impact of Medicare reimbursement reforms on the practice of oncology in the United States (Medicare Payment Advisory Commission, 2006). The authors' analysis of Medicare Part B claims data showed a 33% increase in the number of chemotherapy drug administration services and a 182% increase in spending on these services in the first half of 2005 compared with the first six months of 2003. The study also reported a 13% increase in the number of chemotherapy sessions in the first half of 2005 compared with the first six months of 2004. However, spending on chemotherapy drugs was 14% lower in the first six months of 2005 than the first half of 2004.

As part of its investigation, mandated by the MMA, MedPAC visited oncology practices in Atlanta, Seattle, Iowa, New Jersey, and New Mexico in 2004, and conducted follow-up interviews in 2005. All physicians contacted in the course of MedPAC's research reported that, following the introduction of the payment reforms, they were devoting more time and resources to sourcing lower-priced drugs. Group purchasing organizations (GPOs) indicated that it had become more difficult to secure substantial discounts from manufacturers – a reflection of the fact that large price cuts would reduce a drug's ASP in subsequent quarters. The new

Table 2.1 Average Price Variations for Select Oncology Drugs Under Medicare Part B, December 2004 and June 2005

	Price Variation (%)	
	December 2004	*June 2005*
Branded drugs	15.6	6.8
Generic drugs	10.4	8.4
Chemotherapy agents	6.9	5.2
Nonchemotherapy agents	25.3	10.3

reimbursement system has significantly reduced the variation in the prices of Part B drugs. Table 2.1 compares price variations for branded and generic oncology drugs, and for chemotherapy and non-chemotherapy agents, in December 2004 and June 2005. The reductions in the price variation of non-chemotherapy agents (from 25.3% to 10.3%) and branded drugs (from 15.6% to 6.8%) are particularly striking.

MedPAC found that oncology practices were generally able to obtain drugs that have lost patent protection relatively recently (e.g., carboplatin, cisplatin) at prices substantially below Medicare's reimbursement rates, but purchasing older generics at prices below 106% of ASP was often more problematic. Price has become a particularly influential factor in the choice of ancillary drugs (e.g., antiemetics, erythroid growth factors), and many practices now tend to stock just one drug in each of these classes. By maintaining smaller drug inventories, practices tie up less capital, can respond quickly to price changes, and can benefit from discounts for prompt payment.

The leading oncology societies and their members are not convinced by the conclusions contained in the GAO, OIG, and MedPAC reports. In July 2006, at a hearing of the Subcommittee on Health of the House Committee on Ways and Means, spokespeople for ASCO and the Community Oncology Alliance (COA), as well as individual oncologists, gave evidence on the damaging effects of Medicare reimbursement reforms. Joseph S. Bailes, ASCO's Executive Vice President, offered the following assessment of the OIG's analysis:

> The OIG's conclusion that reimbursement was "generally adequate" and its analysis based on average drug costs to physicians do not appropriately consider the many situations faced by particular physicians in which the Medicare payment amount does not cover the cost of the drugs. Although the OIG's conclusions did not highlight this problem, the report shows that for 17 of the 39 drugs reviewed, at least 20 percent of physicians incurred an out-of-pocket loss. Only 3 of the 39 drugs could be obtained by all physicians at the Medicare payment amount or less. The OIG's conclusion fails to acknowledge that out-of-pocket losses are incurred by physicians in many circumstances, a situation that threatens access to care for some cancer patients. In some of those circumstances, practices are referring patients to hospital outpatient departments. We have received reports from ASCO members that, in some instances hospitals are not accepting those patients. This is a particular challenge to patients without secondary insurance.

Frederick M. Schnell, the COA's president, expressed a very similar opinion: "Analyzing a clinic's drug acquisition costs in comparison to ASP plus 6% reimbursement and concluding that reimbursement covers cost is a faulty analysis, which is the problem with studies completed by the [OIG] and the [GAO]." In particular, he noted that Medicare's new reimbursement methodology takes no account of patient out-of-pocket payments that are not collected. The COA estimates that such bad debts are, on average, equivalent to 5.3% of Medicare Part B payment rates. In addition, the alliance asserts that Medicare's effective payments are reduced further by a 2% prompt-pay discount that is factored into ASP calculations and by delays in adjusting ASPs to reflect market prices. As a result, the COA calculates that oncologists are effectively reimbursed at ASP minus 3.8%, rather than the headline rate of ASP plus 6%.

> The implications of insufficient reimbursement are that community cancer clinics report sending more patients to the hospital for treatment, closing satellite facilities and practices, reducing staff, and being pressured to factor economic decisions into the cancer treatment plan in order for clinics to continue treating patients. In addition, clinics report considering dropping out of the Medicare program. Already, in 2006, there are reports about access problems from community cancer clinics in over 37 states.

The COA's testimony also included several comments that it had received from some of its members. The clear consensus was that practices could no longer afford to treat Medicare patients who do not have a supplemental insurance. Some of the most disturbing of these quotations are as follows:

- On an average we are sending 25–30 patients to the hospital a month for their chemotherapy treatment and growth factor support due to an overwhelming percentage of 20% coinsurance turning into bad debt. Facilities, however, are providing a very limited number of open chairs for patients which means patients are being delayed a week or two waiting on an open chair.
- We are looking toward closing one of our offices. We can no longer cover the overhead of the practice due to the inadequate payments of ASP plus 6%. The other reimbursement schedules are grossly inadequate. We have already cut staff. Medicare D for oncology patients is a catastrophe. Most cannot afford the co-pays on these very expensive drugs. They are priced out of effective medications such as the [tyrosine kinase] inhibitors, Revlamid, etc. THERE IS A NEW WRINKLE! Medicare is now not denying our claims but "PENDING" all claims for Rituxan, Aranesp, and Herceptin – thus they delay payment for three to four months. This has wiped out all of our money. We cannot purchase any more drugs! We will now be sending all patients to the hospital 10 miles away for chemotherapy. Does Medicare wish to eliminate the private practice of medical oncology?
- We cannot afford to treat patients that cannot pay their 20%. Right now 26 of 64 drugs we commonly give are underwater (i.e., not fully reimbursed) at 100% of Medicare. Also, the hospitals are seeing more and more patients in their outpatient units. We are in a high competition area, and a lot of the oncologists in this area are sending patients to the hospital for treatment.

At the time the MMA was enacted, the CBO forecast that the act's reimbursement reforms would reduce Medicare spending on outpatient cancer therapy by a total of $4.2 billion from 2004 to 2013. However, a more recent study that the COA commissioned from PricewaterhouseCoopers (PwC) forecasts total savings at $13.7 billion over the 10-year period – a reduction in spending that would be a body blow to office-based oncologists.

Patients' Out-of-Pocket Payments

Patients are required to pay 20% of all costs incurred under Medicare Part B, with no limit on the level of out-of-pocket payments. Providers are responsible for collecting these coinsurance payments on CMS's behalf. Medigap covers these payments for beneficiaries who have opted for this form of supplemental insurance.

MedPAC estimates that 9% of Medicare beneficiaries have no form of supplemental insurance. In its investigation of the impact of the MMA on oncologists, the commission found that many oncology practices now employ advisers to check that new patients will be able to meet their out-of-pocket obligations. These advisers may notify patients who do not have supplemental insurance about alternative sources of funding (e.g., Medicaid, manufacturer-sponsored patient assistance programs [PAPs]). However, many physicians have reservations about the value of PAPs in oncology. Because cancer patients frequently require polytherapy, it may be necessary to apply to multiple manufacturers for enrollment in their respective assistance programs. The choice of therapies might then be dictated by the companies that approve the patient for enrollment in their PAPs, a far-from-ideal situation. Furthermore, many physicians dislike the fact that PAPs generally do not cover the cost of medications but replace drugs that have been used. This form of compensation is of little value if a physician has only one patient who requires a particular drug.

Patients who are not eligible for assistance and cannot meet the 20% coinsurance payments are increasingly likely to be referred to hospital outpatient departments or "safety-net facilities" for therapy. From the patients' perspective, treatment in hospital outpatient departments has two major disadvantages compared with therapy in physician offices: it is much more time-consuming (in some cases, 5–6 hours instead of the 1–2 hours required in the office setting) and incurs larger out-of-pocket payments. However, hospital outpatient departments are better placed than office-based practices to accept patients who cannot afford their out-of-pocket payments. Unlike physician offices, hospitals can recover 70% of bad debts on out-of-pocket payments from CMS. Nevertheless, some hospitals have stopped treating Medicare patients without the supplemental insurance, or have even discontinued outpatient chemotherapy altogether.

Competitive Acquisition Program

The MMA called for the creation of a competitive acquisition program (CAP) as an alternative method of supplying providers with Part B drugs. Office-based physicians who did not want to purchase medicines and claim reimbursement from CMS would be able to delegate these responsibilities to Medicare-approved vendors (e.g., pharmaceutical wholesalers, specialty pharmacies). These vendors would buy Part B drugs, deliver required supplies to physician offices, collect patient coinsurance payments, and submit reimbursement claims to CMS.

This initiative was originally scheduled to take effect on January 1, 2006, but implementation was delayed by widespread criticism from both the medical community and potential vendors. The program eventually began operation on July 1, 2006, despite a continued lack of enthusiasm from physicians, wholesalers, and specialty pharmacies. Indeed, only one company – BioScrip – has thus far been registered as a CAP vendor. Other possible applicants have been deterred by the perception that this program offers limited potential for profit. For two main reasons, manufacturers would be reluctant to offer CAP vendors substantial discounts: these discounts would be included in future ASP calculations, and vendors have to supply the drugs prescribed by physicians and cannot promote a switch to an alternative drug.

MedPAC found that physicians had several fundamental reservations about CAP:

- Vendors would be able to discontinue the supply of drugs to patients who did not make their coinsurance payments.
- The administrative burden would increase.
- Practices would have to keep separate drug inventories for each patient treated under the CAP program.
- Practices would not be able to change their vendor mid-year.
- Physicians would be required to appeal all denied claims.
- In rural areas, satellite offices that cannot receive drug deliveries or that mix drugs would be excluded from the program.

Demonstration Projects

In 2005, CMS undertook a one-year demonstration project to assess the side effects of chemotherapy. Oncologists could receive \$130 per patient per day (including a 20% coinsurance payment from each patient) in return for asking three questions on patients' levels of fatigue, nausea, and pain. These payments have been a welcome source of additional income for many practices, but critics question the value of the data gathered in this exercise.

In 2006, CMS launched a new demonstration project. Hematologists and medical oncologists can receive \$23 per patient per day for collecting data on how various cancers are treated at different stages. Participating physicians use new payment codes to indicate the stage of the patient's disease, the purpose of each visit (e.g., disease evaluation, supervision of therapy, disease monitoring, end-of-life care), and the degree of compliance with clinical guidelines (where applicable).

Hospital Outpatient Treatment

When it was established in 1965, Medicare relied entirely on retrospective payment systems for all services – reimbursing providers on the basis of costs incurred. As time passed, the Healthcare Financing

Administration (now CMS) began to realize that this system encouraged inefficiency and undesirable variations in healthcare practice. The Balanced Budget Act of 1997 mandated the introduction of a Medicare outpatient prospective payment system (OPPS), which began operation on August 1, 2000. MedPAC reports that, in 2004, 47% of Medicare beneficiaries received at least one OPPS service, from a total of approximately 4,300 hospitals. The OPPS does not cover beneficiaries who are enrolled in Medicare managed care plans, HMOs, preferred provider organizations (PPOs), or Medicare private fee-for-service plans.

According to CMS, the new payment system is "designed to ensure that Medicare and its beneficiaries pay appropriately for services and to encourage more efficient delivery of care." Under the old cost-based reimbursement system, Medicare payments for outpatient services did not keep pace with prices, with the result that patients' out-of-pocket expenses increased sharply. Prior to the introduction of OPPS, Medicare beneficiaries paid approximately 50% of the total cost of outpatient services. By 2004, this figure had declined to 34%, and it is eventually expected to stabilize at 20%. In addition, Congress has ruled that the patient copayment for a procedure must not exceed the annual inpatient deductible (i.e., $952 in 2006).

The OPPS uses the healthcare common procedure coding system (HCPCS) to assign services to one of approximately 600 ambulatory payment classification (APC) groups. Each group consists of services that are clinically comparable and require similar resources. CMS calculates the national median cost for services and procedures within each group, then adjusts the labor-related proportion of this sum (60% of the national total) to reflect the geographic variations in labor costs. Drugs with median daily costs of less than $50 per day (i.e., the great majority of medicines), along with many other incidental items and services, are bundled into the APC payments. CMS reviews APC payment rates in the fall of each year and makes adjustments, as necessary, to take account of increased costs from new technologies.

New technologies that cannot be readily accommodated within an existing APC group can qualify for reimbursement by one of two other methods: inclusion in a new technology APC group or to be granted transitional pass-through payment status (see further on). A new technology APC is created only for procedures or services that can neither be included in an existing APC group nor meet the conditions for pass-through drugs. Once sufficient time has passed to gather data on hospitals' actual expenditures on these new services and procedures, CMS reassigns these new technologies to standard APC groups as part of its annual review process. Because new technology APC groups are not budget-neutral, they could substantially increase hospitals' treatment costs.

Transitional pass-through payments apply to new drugs, biologics, and medical devices that complement an existing service but are too expensive to be included in existing APC groups. For example, a pass-through payment for a costly new monoclonal antibody may be used to supplement the established base payment that covers the administration of chemotherapy. Table 2.2 lists the technologies that have pass-through status in 2006. To qualify for this status, a new technology must have been on the market for no more than two to three years and must be more expensive than existing therapies. In addition, medical devices (as opposed to drugs) must offer a substantial clinical advantage over established treatments – the same standard that is a condition for add-on payments in the Medicare inpatient prospective payment system (IPPS) that is discussed in the following section. In November 2001, CMS published the following characteristics of a new technology that offers "substantial clinical improvement":

- It offers a treatment option for a patient population unresponsive to, or ineligible for, currently available treatments.
- It offers the ability to diagnose a medical condition in a patient population whose medical condition is currently undetectable or to

Table 2.2 Technologies with Pass-Through Status in the Medicare Outpatient Prospective Payment System, 2006

HCPCS Code	*APC Code*	*Product*
C9220	9220	Sodium hyaluronate
C9221	9221	Graftjacket regular matrix
C9222	9222	Graftjacket soft tissue
C9225	9225	Fluocinolone acetonide
J0128	9216	Abarelix injection
J0878	9124	Daptomycin injection
J2278	1694	Ziconotide injection
J2357	9300	Omalizumab injection
J2503	1697	Pegaptanib sodium injection
J2783	0738	Rasburicase
J2794	9125	Risperidone, long-acting
J7518	9219	Mycophenolic acid
J8501	0868	Oral aprepitant
J9027	1710	Clofarabine injection
J9035	9214	Bevacizumab injection
J9055	9215	Cetuximab injection
J9264	1712	Paclitaxel injection
J9305	9213	Pemetrexed injection
Q4079	9126	Natalizumab injection (1 mg)

HCPCS = Healthcare common procedure coding system (HCPCS)
APC = Ambulatory payment classification

diagnose a medical condition earlier in a patient population than is allowed by currently available methods. There must also be evidence that the use of the technology to make a diagnosis affects the management of the patient.

- Use of the technology significantly improves clinical outcomes for a patient population as compared with currently available treatments. For example, improvements might include the following:

1. Reduced mortality rate.
2. Reduced rate of complications.
3. Reduced rate of subsequent diagnostic or therapeutic interventions (e.g., due to reduced rate of recurrence of the disease process).
4. Decreased number of future hospitalizations or physician visits.
5. More rapid beneficial resolution of the disease process.
6. Less pain, bleeding, or other quantifiable symptom.
7. Reduced recovery time.

Table 2.3 summarizes the similarities and differences of the new technology payment mechanisms in Medicare's prospective payment systems. Critics deplore the inconsistencies of these mechanisms. In a report to Congress published in March 2003, MedPAC made the following assertion:

> The treatment of drugs and devices is inconsistent, in that only newness and cost criteria are applied to pass-through drugs. This difference in the criteria represents unequal treatment between types of technology within the outpatient payment system. It also leads to a discrepancy between the treatment of drugs under the inpatient and outpatient payment systems since the clinical criteria are applied to all technologies, including drugs, on the inpatient side. Furthermore, without considering clinical benefit, the criteria applied to pass-through drugs may overemphasize the goal of paying adequately for new technologies at the expense of prudent purchasing.

Furthermore, MedPAC suggested that "it is appropriate to reserve additional payments for technologies that provide clinical benefit and do not have clinical substitutes. It may even be appropriate to limit payments to technologies that provide additional benefits commensurate with their costs."

Hospital Inpatient Treatment

Medicare Part A provides funding for inpatient hospital treatment. Beneficiaries pay a deductible ($952 in 2006) when first admitted to hospital, but this sum is the only out-of-pocket payment during the first

Table 2.3 Key Features of Medicare Inpatient and Outpatient New Technology Payment Mechanisms

	Inpatient Add-On Payments	*Outpatient Pass-Through Payments*		*Outpatient New Technology APCs*
		Medical Devices	*Drugs and Biologics*	
New technologies eligible for additional payments	New technologies that offer a new procedure or are san input to an existing DRG	New technologies that are an input to an existing DRG	New technologies that are an input to an existing DRG	New technologies that offer a new service
Criteria used by CMS	Clinical benefit, novelty, cost	Clinical benefit, novelty, cost	Novelty, cost	Novelty
Funding method	Budget-neutral	Budget-neutral	Budget-neutral	New expenditures
Unit of payment	Additional costs of treating a case using new technology	Cost of new technology	Cost of new technology	Cost of service
Method of determining payments	Payment = 50% of additional costs (capped at 50% of estimated cost of new technology)	Payment = 100% of reported costs minus device costs already built into base payment rate	Payment = 95% of average wholesale price	Payment = midpoint of payment range for new technology APC group

APC = Ambulatory payment classification

CMS = Centers for Medicare and Medicaid Services

DRG = Diagnosis-related group

60 days of inpatient treatment in a given benefit period. Thereafter, beneficiaries pay an additional $238 per day from day 61 to 90, and $476 per day beyond the 90th day of hospitalization in a benefit period.

In 1983, CMS established the Medicare IPPS, a reimbursement system that pays hospitals according to a patient's diagnosis-related group (DRG) coding at the time of inpatient discharge. DRGs group patients on the basis of factors such as their primary or secondary diagnosis, complications and comorbidities, procedures, age, and sex.

The DRG system that forms the foundation of Medicare's IPPS has been refined repeatedly. The current version is based on the *International Classification of Diseases*, Ninth Revision, Clinical Modification (ICD-9-CM) and comprises a total of 25 major diagnostic categories (MDCs) subdivided into 526 DRGs. Each case is assigned to a particular patient cluster, based on factors such as principal and secondary diagnoses, principal procedures, sex, and discharge status. CMS updates the DRGs, and the related diagnostic and procedural codes, annually, but critics assert that the system is too slow in reflecting changes in medical technology. In April 2006, CMS published proposals for further reform of the IPPS. Among other measures, in fiscal year 2008, the agency plans to introduce a revised version of 3M's All-Patient Refined DRG (APR-DRG) system to take better account of variations in disease severity. CMS intends to consolidate the APR-DRG's 1,258 DRGs into a new system of 861 severity-adjusted DRGs.

The IPPS bundles the costs of most drugs and medical devices into the DRG payment system. New technologies can be added to the standard DRG system through one of three methods:

- A technical advisory panel assigns the new technology an ICD-9-CM code.
- CMS can alter DRG assignments to ensure that a costly new technology is covered by a higher-paying DRG.
- The annual review of DRG case weights is used to adjust payments so that they cover the cost of the new technology.

Particularly expensive new technologies are initially reimbursed by a different method: add-on payments. This procedure applies to drugs and devices that would increase the cost of a case substantially beyond the relevant base DRG payment. In addition, to qualify for add-on payments, technologies must be new (i.e., on the market for less than two to three years) and must offer Medicare beneficiaries a significant clinical advantage over existing therapies. To encourage the prudent use of new technologies, CMS does not reimburse the full cost of these products. Rather, the add-on payment amounts to only 50% of a hospital's costs in excess of the standard DRG payment, to a maximum of 50% of the estimated cost of the new drug or device. Add-on payments are budget-neutral (i.e., they are offset by reductions in base payment rates) and cannot exceed 1% of total operating payments.

Self-Administered Drugs (Medicare Part D)

As of June 11, 2006, 38.2 million out of a total of 42.6 million Medicare beneficiaries enrolled in a Part D program or equivalent, including 6.1 million Medicare-Medicaid dual-eligible beneficiaries who were automatically enrolled in a Medicare prescription drug plan (PDP). At present, Medicare Part D plays a relatively minor role in oncology, but its significance will grow as this program becomes more established and the number of self-administered cancer therapies (e.g., oral dosage forms, subcutaneous injections) increases.

The standard benefit design for Part D requires beneficiaries to pay an average premium of $24 per month and an annual deductible of $250. Thereafter, Medicare covers 75% of the cost of prescription drugs up to an annual total of $2,250. Coverage then ceases until the beneficiary's annual drug costs reach a total of $5,100 (and out-of-pocket payments reach a total of $3,600) – a provision known as the "coverage gap" or, more colloquially, the "doughnut hole." Medicare then covers 95% of drug costs in excess of the annual threshold of $5,100. Variations on the standard benefit design are available, including plans that charge reduced premiums, waive or reduce the annual deductible, or cover drugs (typically generics only) while patients are in the coverage gap. In a recent survey, CMS found that Medicare PDP enrollees who signed up for the lowest-cost plan in their area could save an average of 59%, and a maximum of 72%, on their drug costs (compared with cash prices to patients who have no drug coverage). However, some beneficiaries face the prospect of losing access to PAPs.

PDPs are generally required to cover at least two drugs in each therapeutic category and pharmacological class. CMS expects PDPs to "provide adequate access to medically necessary treatments for Part D enrollees." In particular, plans must cover "all or substantially all" drugs in six classes, including antineoplastic agents. However, relatively few cancer therapies fall within the scope of Part D, a program that focuses primarily on self-administered drugs. CMS notes that "the definition of a covered Part D drug excludes any drug for which, as prescribed and dispensed or administered to an individual, payments would be available under Parts A or B of Medicare for that individual, even though a deductible may apply." Plans cover an average of 75% of Part D oncology drugs. PDPs are not obliged to cover off-label prescribing, and they are permitted to use utilization management controls such as multitier formularies, prior authorization, step therapy protocols, generics substitution, and quantity limits to contain pharmacy costs. However, plans make limited use of these measures in oncology: only 10% of Part D cancer drugs are subject to prior authorization and 4% to quantity limits.

PDPs also exercise restraint in the out-of-pocket payments they impose on cancer patients. The majority of plans levy flat-rate copayments, rather than a percentage coinsurance charge, on most Part D oncology drugs. Moreover, the copayments are generally relatively modest – $30 or less, in most cases. Genentech/OSI Pharmaceuticals' Tarceva (erlotinib) and Gleevec (imatinib) are notable exceptions to this rule: the majority of PDPs require a percentage coinsurance payment for both these drugs.

PRIVATE SECTOR

Physician Reimbursement

Because most oncology drugs are administered by healthcare professionals, private insurers have generally covered these treatments as a medical, rather than a pharmacy, benefit. In their claims for reimbursement, physicians use J codes, a subcategory of HCPCS. These five-digit codes indicate the name and quantity of a prescribed drug, but not the manufacturer, formulation, or strength. CMS updates the HCPCS list annually, but drugs are frequently on the market for 12–18 months before they are assigned a HCPCS code. In the meantime, physicians use a miscellaneous J code in their reimbursement claims. The relatively imprecise nature of HCPCS codes prevents insurers from accurately monitoring the use of these therapies. In addition, covering drugs as a medical benefit makes it difficult to distinguish drug costs and administration fees.

To improve the utilization management and control costs, health plans are increasingly moving oncology drugs from the medical benefit to the pharmacy benefit. In the process, they are replacing HCPCS codes with National Drug Center (NDC) codes. These more detailed 10-digit codes specify a prescribed drug's manufacturer, strength, dosage form, formulation, and pack size. In 2003, Express Scripts, a leading pharmacy benefit management (PBM) company, reported that adoption of NDC coding and stricter biologic formulary control had reduced its medical costs by 10–20%. Covering drugs as a pharmacy benefit enables payers to adjudicate reimbursement claims electronically and to compile long-term data on how these agents are used. In the future, plans will be able to use these data in comparing the cost effectiveness of different therapies. However, the shift to pharmacy benefit coverage of oncology drugs is far from complete: most plans still cover the majority of these agents in their medical benefit.

Private insurers have long followed Medicare's AWP-based model for reimbursing office-based physicians' drug costs – albeit with slightly more generous rates. To determine reimbursement levels in the private sector, MedPAC commissioned a survey of health plans. Between October and December 2002, Dyckman & Associates interviewed representatives of 33 health plans on their use of AWP calculations in setting reimbursement rates for physician-administered drugs. Most health plans paid physicians 90–100% of AWP, and the average reimbursement rate was 98% of AWP. Note, however, that some health plans varied their AWP reimbursement formula by drug class or provider. Respondents were aware that physicians' actual drug acquisition costs were often far below AWP. Some participating health plans were thinking of changing their reimbursement methodology for physician-administered drugs, but many indicated that they would consider increasing fees for drug administration to offset reduced drug reimbursement payments.

MedPAC commissioned a separate study on distribution and payment issues for physician-administered drugs in the private sector from NORC at the University of Chicago. The authors conducted 16 structured interviews with a range of stakeholders, including oncologists, health plans, PBMs, specialty pharmacy companies, consultants, a wholesaler, and a GPO. Representatives of insurers and PBMs believed that the "spread" between acquisition costs and reimbursement payments for physician-administered drugs was a significant source of profit for physicians. Some respondents suggested that cancer therapy reimbursement accounted for 50–60% of oncologists' income. Oncologists, on the other hand, maintained that the spread barely covered their rapidly rising drug administration costs and that they lost money on many chemotherapy procedures. They also insisted that neither a drug's price nor its spread had any influence on their prescribing decisions.

In recognition of the substantial disparities between AWP and drug acquisition prices, many plans have reduced their reimbursement rates as a percentage of AWP. According to the Zitter Group's Managed Care Injectables Index, health plans' average reimbursement rate for specialty pharmaceuticals was 85.8% of AWP in fall 2004 and 84.3% of AWP in fall 2005. Slightly higher rates were available if physicians accepted specialty pharmacy services (Figure 2.8).

Relatively few insurers have yet followed Medicare's move to ASP-based reimbursement. However, the June 2006 issue of *Biotechnology Healthcare* reported that 39.5% of payers that operate Medicare plans intend to adopt ASP-based reimbursement by the end of the year. Some observers believe that oncology drugs will be among the last products to be subjected to ASP-based reimbursement in the private sector. Insurers may be concerned that reduced reimbursement could prompt office-based oncologists to refer more patients to hospital outpatient departments – a more costly situation for the administration of chemotherapy.

Distribution Controls

In most cases, oncologists decide how to obtain the medicines they need. They may buy directly from manufacturers, use general wholesalers or one of several specialist oncology wholesalers, contract with GPOs, or purchase pharmaceuticals from a local retail pharmacy. Recently, however, some

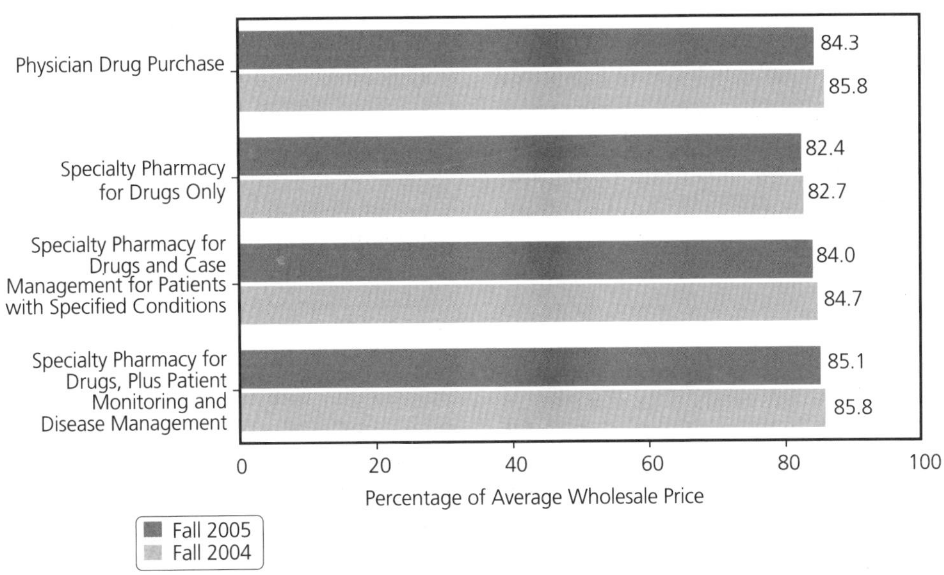

Figure 2.8 Private Health Plans' Average Reimbursement Rates for Onclolgy Drugs, Fall 2004 and 2005

health plans and PBMs have introduced a policy of mandatory vendor imposition, requiring oncologists to use particular distribution channels – typically a specialty pharmacy company.

The origins of specialty pharmacy can be traced back to the mid-1990s, when relatively inexperienced biotechnology companies were looking for assistance in marketing their new products (the term "specialty pharmaceuticals" has various definitions but typically includes drugs that are injected subcutaneously or infused intravenously, as well as oral cancer chemotherapeutics: many of the most widely prescribed specialty pharmaceuticals are biologics). Specialty pharmacy companies acted as intermediaries between biotechnology companies and physicians, patients, insurers, and pharmacies. Over time, many health plans began to contract with specialty pharmacy companies to reduce the health plans' costs for specialty pharmaceuticals. Leading PBMs have also established their own specialty pharmacy services.

Some health plans have adopted a policy known as "brown bagging," requiring patients to take their own medications to their physician's office for administration. Health plans that find an inexpensive wholesaler for specialty pharmaceuticals may insist that patients who are prescribed these drugs have their medications mailed either to their home or to a local retail pharmacy for collection. Patients then carry their medicines to the physician's office in the "brown bag."

Brown bagging may save health plans money, but it has many potential disadvantages for patients and their physicians. Specialty pharmaceuticals (especially biologics) may be temperature sensitive or have other special handling requirements, but some couriers may lack the knowledge or equipment needed to comply with these requirements. Medicines may be damaged in transit or left in unsuitable conditions (e.g., outside the patient's house). Patients may not know how to store their medicines correctly and may, out of embarrassment, mislead their physician about how the drugs have been stored. One or more of these events could render certain drugs useless and thereby compromise patients' treatment. Besides the risks of inappropriate storage, brown bagging is likely to entail some additional inconvenience for seriously ill patients. They may have to make an extra visit to their physician's office for a blood count to ensure that they can tolerate chemotherapy; the physician then orders the drugs for delivery to the patients' home or a nearby pharmacy. If medicines are delivered to the pharmacy, patients have to make an extra journey to collect their drugs prior to administration.

Critics of brown bagging within the medical community argue that this practice is inefficient and imposes a significant burden on their practices. Physicians have to keep separate accounts and other records for each health plan. In some cases, physicians may store brown-bagged drugs in their offices, but these drugs must be kept separate from the practice's regular stock of drugs. Maintaining multiple inventories increases a practice's workload. In addition, high-priced drugs are often wasted: if a patient does not require the full contents of a vial or all the vials in a multivial pack, the remaining medication may not be used to treat another patient.

Cost Sharing

Cancer therapy in the private sector can incur substantial out-of-pocket costs. A recent analysis of 2003 and 2004 pharmacy and medical claims data from 55 employer-sponsored health plans with a combined total of 1.5 million covered lives found that cancer patients had median out-of-pocket expenditures of $1,509 per year, including $336 for medications. In some cases, expenses can be much higher. This survey found that more than 10% of cancer patients had out-of-pocket spending in excess of $18,585, and 5% spent more than $35,660 on their treatment (Goldman, 2006).

For drugs that are covered as medical benefits, insurers generally levy a percentage coinsurance payment – typically 20%. Drugs covered as pharmacy benefits are included in plan formularies. Three-tier formularies are currently the norm, with generic drugs generally assigned to tier 1, preferred brands to tier 2, and nonpreferred brands to tier 3. Plans generally impose flat-rate copayments that increase with each of these tiers. Recently, some health plans have added one or more additional tiers to their formulary designs. Biologics and other high-priced agents, including some cancer therapies, are assigned to a specialty pharmacy tier. Plans frequently levy a percentage coinsurance charge for drugs in the specialty pharmacy tier. Caps on out-of-pocket payments are generally used to protect patients against hardship.

The move from medical to pharmacy benefit coverage of cancer drugs will make it easier for health plans to implement cost-containment strategies. Many plans and/or their PBMs encourage pharmacists to substitute generics for branded versions of off-patent drugs, and some plans and PBMs even promote therapeutic substitution (i.e., switching a patient to a different [and less expensive] compound from the one prescribed). Prior authorization policies exclude certain drugs from reimbursement unless the prescriber justifies the need for these medications and the plan or PBM approves the prescription. Quantity limits restrict the pack size of prescriptions and the frequency of refills. Step therapy protocols reimburse costly drugs only if the patient has first tried, and failed to respond adequately to, less expensive therapies. The Zitter Group's spring 2005 Managed Care Injectables Index found that 64% of payers had increased their use of prior authorization for specialty pharmaceuticals, 42% limited access to these drugs, 33% had increased out-of-pocket payments by more than $20, 30% used differential prior authorization rules to promote the prescription of particular agents, 27% offered higher reimbursement rates for drugs sourced through a particular distribution channel, and 26% had a policy of strict prior authorization with limited cost sharing. It is unclear, however, to what extent such measures are applied specifically to oncology drugs. Given the limited choice of drugs for some cancers and the life-threatening nature of this disease, it is more difficult to impose restrictions on cancer therapies than most other drug classes.

OFF-LABEL PRESCRIBING

In 1991, the GAO published a report titled *Off-Label Drugs: Reimbursement Policies Constraints Physicians in Their Choice of Cancer Therapies*. The authors noted that, "although respondents reported reimbursement problems with many third-party payers, the insurer most frequently cited was Medicare." In an attempt to remedy this situation, the Omnibus Budget Reconciliation Act of 1993 introduced a legal requirement for Medicare to reimburse off-label prescribing that is supported by citations in any of three compendia: *American Hospital Formulary Service Drug Information* (AHFSDI), *United States Pharmacopoeia Drug Information* (USPDI), or the American Medical Association's *Drug Evaluation* (merged into USPDI in 1996). In addition, the act allows Medicare carriers to make local coverage decisions on off-label reimbursement based on supportive clinical evidence published in peer-reviewed medical journals. Data from at least two Phase II clinical trials conducted in different centers are required to support off-label use, but Phase III trial results carry greater weight.

To determine how coverage of off-label usage by both Medicare and private payers affects US oncologists' prescribing behavior, in 2005, the Association of Community Cancer Centers (ACCC), the Biotechnology Industry Organization (BIO), and the Pharmaceutical Research and Manufacturers

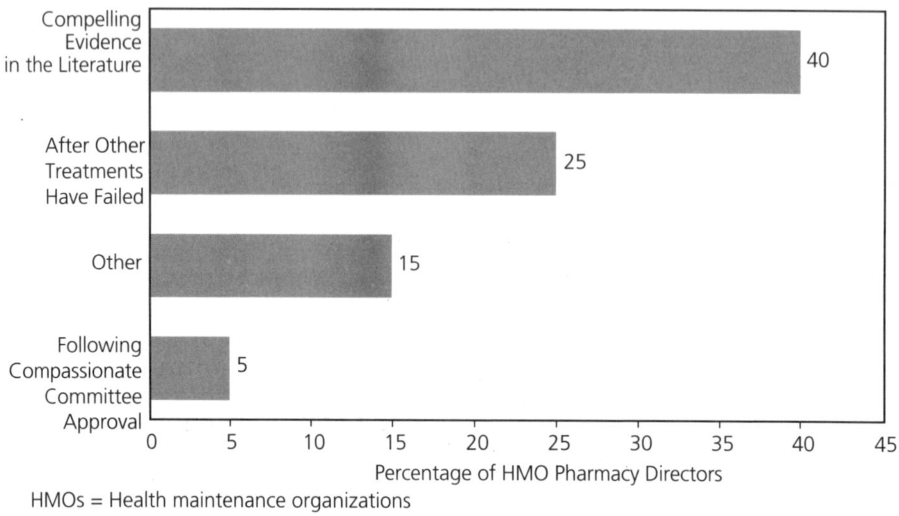

Figure 2.9 Circumstances in Which HMO Pharmacy Directors Would Authorize Off-Label Use of Oral Chemotherapeutic Agents, 2005

of America (PhRMA) jointly commissioned a survey from Covance, a leading drug development service company (Covance Market Access Services, Inc., 2006). Covance interviewed 28 oncologists and 12 oncology practice managers. Respondents identified more than 50 physician-administered therapies that are used off-label. For guidance in off-label prescribing, physicians rely most heavily on peer-reviewed literature (cited by 25 of 28 oncologists), drug compendia (mentioned by 17 oncologists), and manufacturer hot lines and case reports (each cited by seven oncologists). However, reimbursement restrictions deter many oncologists from prescribing cancer therapies off-label, particularly to Medicare patients. Fifteen oncologists (54%) stated that Medicare policies on off-label usage frequently or very frequently interfered with their clinical decision making. By comparison, just eight oncologists (29%) indicated that private payers' policies on off-label usage frequently or very frequently interfered with their clinical decision making.

One participant in Covance's survey commented that "Medicare will deny every off-label indication that is not listed in the two compendia [i.e., AHFSDI, USPDI]. So, at this point, I am only using those products off-label for those indications that are listed in the compendia." The study notes that "listings in recognized compendia are outdated, incomplete, and may not include references to potential off-label uses of new drugs that may be supported by other published clinical evidence." Coverage of off-label prescribing is more restrictive under Part D than Part B. Off-label uses are eligible for reimbursement under Medicare Part D only if they are supported by one or more of three compendia (i.e., AHFSDI, USPDI, and Drugdex); evidence from peer-reviewed literature alone is not adequate for Medicare Part D coverage of off-label prescribing.

Private insurers vary enormously in their policies on reimbursement of off-label prescribing (Figure 2.9), and published research on this subject is extremely limited. Coverage of off-label usage may be subject to one or more of the following conditions:

- The prescribed drug is Food and Drug Administration (FDA) approved and listed on the payer's formulary.
- The patient is diagnosed with a life threatening or otherwise very serious disease.
- The risk-benefit ratio of prescribing the drug for an unlicensed indication justifies this usage.

- Evidence of efficacy is available in designated compendia (e.g., AHFSDI, USPDI) or peer-reviewed journals.
- Therapies approved for the indicated disease are not available, are deemed inappropriate for the patient, or have been tried and found ineffective.
- The payer's medical director approves the off-label usage.

OUTLOOK AND IMPLICATIONS FOR THE PHARMACEUTICAL INDUSTRY

Medicare's recent reimbursement reforms have had a seismic impact on the landscape of oncology in the United States. One immediate effect has been a sharp increase in the number of office-based oncology practices referring Medicare patients who lack supplemental insurance to hospital outpatient departments. Worse still, the reimbursement cuts have reportedly undermined the viability of some office-based oncology practices – especially smaller rural practices. Their problems could be compounded in 2007, if CMS follows through on recently announced proposals to cut physician reimbursement for Part B services by 5.1% and to change the formula for Part B drug reimbursement from ASP plus 6% to ASP plus 5%. If implemented, these changes would be a severe blow to beleaguered oncologists. The CAP was meant to reduce oncologists' financial exposure, but this program appears doomed to failure unless CMS can persuade more companies to become vendors – and more oncologists to use this service.

Other repercussions of the Medicare reforms may take longer to emerge. The MMA explicitly forbids CMS from setting drug prices within Medicare Part D, but CMS has a very powerful influence over prices in Part B – a far more significant factor in the US oncology market. In his testimony to the Subcommittee on Health of the House Committee on Ways and Means, Frederick Schnell of the COA asserted that "Medicare, with its considerable market clout, has set reimbursement rates artificially low for private payers to follow." ASP-based reimbursement has introduced an unprecedented price sensitivity into the US oncology market – a trend that is unlikely to be reversed. Thus far, relatively few private insurers have adopted ASP-based reimbursement, but past experience (and recent surveys) suggests that they will eventually follow CMS's example.

CMS may also set a lead for private insurers in the adoption of health technology assessment and evidence-based medicine. As noted earlier, in its report on the OPPS, MedPAC suggested that "it is appropriate to reserve additional payments for technologies that provide clinical benefit and do not have clinical substitutes. It may even be appropriate to limit payments to technologies that provide additional benefits commensurate with their costs." It will be interesting to see if CMS makes cost effectiveness a condition of reimbursement in the future.

Private payers will continue the recent trend of moving physician-administered drugs from the medical benefit to the pharmacy benefit. The launch of increased numbers of oral or self-injectable drugs will facilitate this migration to the pharmacy benefit. This shift will make it easier to impose cost-containment measures, such as multitier formularies, variable copayments or coinsurance, and prior authorization. However, because of the very specific demands of cancer therapy, oncology drugs will probably be spared from certain forms of cost containment (e.g., generics and/or therapeutic substitution, quantity limits). The adoption of NDC coding will enable health plans to adjudicate claims electronically, perform drug utilization review, and evaluate the long-term impact of drug therapies.

This rapidly changing environment presents manufacturers of oncology drugs with considerable challenges. Companies may need to exercise greater restraint in their pricing policies: when they increase their prices, hard-pressed oncology practices will be penalized by CMS's delay in updating the ASPs that determine reimbursement payments. On the other hand, manufacturers need to be cautious about offering discounts, given that these reductions will be factored into the following quarter's ASP calculations, thereby lowering Medicare reimbursement levels. Companies may find that they experience a significant increase in the number of applications for their PAPs in the future.

The United States has long led the world in terms of the adoption of the most modern cancer therapies. However, unless office-based oncologists receive additional funding by some means as a matter of urgency, innovative medical oncology in the United States could be in jeopardy.

REFERENCES

American Cancer Society. *Cancer Facts & Figures 2006*.www.cancer.org/downloads/STT/CAFF2006PWSecured.pdf. Accessed October 10, 2006.

Covance Market Access Services, Inc. *Off-Label Use of Anticancer Therapies: Physician Prescribing Trends and the Impact of Payer Coverage Policy*. www.bio.org/speeches/pubs/CovanceReport.pdf. Accessed October 10, 2006.

Goldman, D.P., et al. Benefit design and specialty drug use. *Health Affairs*, 2006; 25(5): 1319–1331.

Government Accountability Office. *Medicare Chemotherapy Payments: New Drug and Administration Fees are Closer to Providers' Costs*. December 2004. www.gao.gov/new.items/d05142r.pdf. Accessed October 10, 2006.

Medicare Payment Advisory Commission. *Effects of Medicare Payment Changes on Oncology Services*. January 2006. Accessed at www.medpac.gov/publications/congressional_reports/Jan06_Oncology_mandated_report.pdf. Accessed October 10, 2006.

Office of Inspector General, Department of Health and Human Services. *Adequacy of Medicare Part B Drug Reimbursement to Physician Practices for the Treatment of Cancer Patients*. September 2005. www.oig.hhs.gov/oas/reports/region6/60500024.pdf. Accessed October 10, 2006.

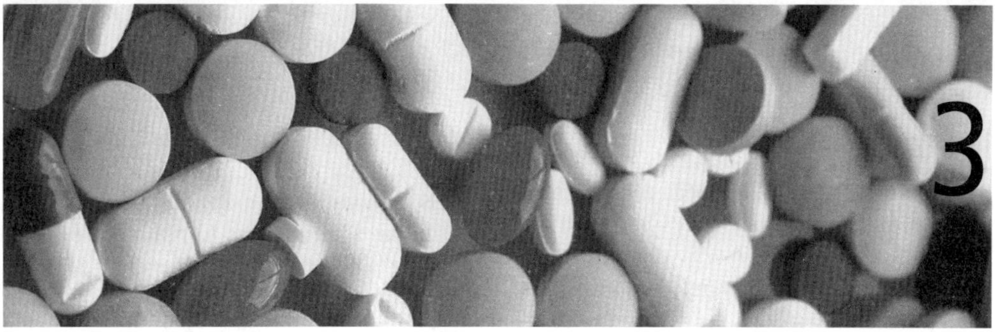

3

Prospective Payment Systems: Opportunities and Threats for the Pharmaceutical Industry

OVERVIEW

In recent years, cost-containment initiatives in the pharmaceutical market have focused primarily on the retail sector. This trend is hardly surprising, given the size and high profile of the retail pharmacy market. In contrast, the hospital sector has received relatively little attention. Indeed, within the constraints of their overall budgets, hospitals have been largely left to their own devices, to define their reimbursement policies and decide how best to control their costs. Today, the climate in the hospital sector is undergoing a marked change. Governments are becoming increasingly concerned about runaway costs and ballooning deficits in their hospitals, a problem that is usually attributed to a combination of inefficiency, waste, inequality, and lack of transparency.

In an attempt to reduce costs and raise the general standard of secondary care, governments in many countries have begun to move from cost-based reimbursement for services rendered to prospective payment systems that pay providers a predetermined amount according to specific definitions. Prospective payment systems are typically based on diagnosis-related groups (DRGs), a system that groups patients on the basis of factors such as their primary or secondary diagnosis, complications and comorbidities, procedures, age, and sex.

Drug manufacturers will need to change in response to this shift from cost-based reimbursement to prospective payment. The high degree of complexity of prospective payment systems precludes an analysis of the intricacies of each system. Rather, this chapter provides an overview of the growth of prospective payment systems in major pharmaceutical markets (the United States, France, Germany, the United Kingdom, and Japan) and assesses the outlook and implications for the pharmaceutical industry.

UNITED STATES

Healthcare in the United States has three main sources of funding: the federal Medicare program for seniors, registered disabled persons, and patients with end-stage renal disease; joint federal/state Medicaid programs for low-income residents; and commercial health plans (sponsored primarily by employers). The use of prospective payment systems varies enormously among these insurance programs.

Medicare

The Medicare program has been the dominant driver of prospective payment systems in the United States. When it was established in 1965, Medicare relied entirely on retrospective payment systems for all services – reimbursing providers on the basis of costs incurred. As time passed, the Healthcare Financing Administration (HCFA; renamed the Centers for Medicare and Medicaid Services [CMS] in 2001) began to realize that this system encouraged inefficiency and undesirable variations in healthcare practice.

Inpatient Prospective Payment System

In an attempt to tackle the deficiencies of cost-based reimbursement, the Omnibus Budget Reconciliation Act (OBRA) of 1980 introduced the ambulatory surgery center benefit. The act stated that "this overhead factor is expected to be calculated on a prospective basis utilizing sample survey and similar techniques to establish reasonable estimated overhead allowances for each of the listed procedures which take account of volume (within reasonable limits)." In 1982, the Tax Equity and Fiscal Responsibility Act introduced measures to calculate Medicare inpatient reimbursement by means of a case-mix system based on DRGs. The following year, Congress revised this act to establish the Medicare inpatient prospective payment system (IPPS). Payments are based on the DRG coding at the time of inpatient discharge.

The DRG system that forms the foundation of Medicare's IPPS has been refined repeatedly. The current version is based on the *International Classification of Diseases*, Ninth Revision, Clinical Modification (ICD-9-CM) and comprises a total of 25 major diagnostic categories (MDCs) subdivided into 1,258 all-patient refined DRGs. Each case is assigned to a particular patient cluster, based on factors such as principal and secondary diagnoses, principal procedures, sex, and discharge status. CMS updates the DRGs, and the related diagnostic and procedural codes, annually, but critics assert that the system is too slow in reflecting changes in medical technology. In April 2006, CMS published proposals for further reform of the IPPS. Among other measures, in fiscal year 2008, the agency plans to replace the 1,258 existing DRGs with 861 severity-adjusted DRGs to take better account of variations in disease severity.

The IPPS bundles the costs of most drugs and medical devices into the DRG payment system. New technologies can be added to the standard DRG system through one of three methods:

- A technical advisory panel assigns the new technology an ICD-9-CM code.
- CMS can alter DRG assignments to ensure that a costly new technology is covered by a higher-paying DRG.
- The annual review of DRG case weights is used to adjust payments so that they cover the cost of the new technology.

Particularly expensive new technologies are initially reimbursed by a different method: add-on payments. This procedure applies to drugs and devices that would increase the cost of a case substantially beyond the relevant base DRG payment. In addition, to qualify for add-on payments, technologies must be new (i.e., on the market for less than two to three years) and must offer Medicare beneficiaries a significant clinical advantage over existing therapies. To encourage the prudent use of new technologies, CMS does not reimburse the full cost of these products. Rather, the add-on payment amounts to only 50% of a hospital's costs in excess of the standard DRG payment, to a maximum of 50% of the estimated cost of the new drug or device. Add-on payments are budget-neutral (i.e., they are offset by reductions in base payment rates) and cannot exceed 1% of total operating payments.

Outpatient Prospective Payment System

Encouraged by the success of the IPPS, in 1988, the HCFA commissioned 3M Health Information Systems to design a prospective payment system for outpatient treatment. The company published the first version of its ambulatory patient group (APG) system in 1990, and a revised version followed in 1995. Medicare and Medicaid carriers in some states adopted one or the other version of the APG system, but the HCFA decided not to use this system.

The Balanced Budget Act of 1997 mandated the introduction of an outpatient prospective payment system (OPPS), which began operation on August 1, 2000. The Medicare Payment Advisory Commission (MedPAC) reports that, in 2004, 47% of Medicare beneficiaries received at least one OPPS service, from a total of approximately 4,300 hospitals. The OPPS does not cover beneficiaries who are enrolled in Medicare managed care plans – HMOs, preferred provider organizations (PPOs), or Medicare private fee-for-service plans.

According to CMS, the new payment system is "designed to ensure that Medicare and its beneficiaries pay appropriately for services and to encourage more efficient delivery of care." Under the old cost-based reimbursement system, Medicare payments for outpatient services did not keep pace with prices, with the result that patients' out-of-pocket expenses increased sharply. Prior to the introduction of OPPS, Medicare beneficiaries paid approximately 50% of the total cost of outpatient services. By 2004, this figure had declined to 34%, and it is eventually expected to stabilize at 20%. In addition, Congress has ruled that the patient copayment for a procedure must not exceed the annual inpatient deductible (i.e., $952 in 2006).

The OPPS uses the healthcare common procedure coding system (HCPCS) to assign services to one of approximately 600 ambulatory payment classification (APC) groups. Each group consists of services that are clinically comparable and require similar resources. CMS calculates the national median cost for services and procedures within each group, then adjusts the labor-related proportion of this sum (60% of the national total) to reflect geographic variations in labor costs. Drugs with median daily costs of less than $50 per day (i.e., the great majority of medicines), along with many other incidental items and services, are bundled into the APC payments. CMS reviews APC payment rates in the fall of each year and makes adjustments, as necessary, to take account of increased costs from new technologies.

New technologies that cannot be readily accommodated within an existing APC group can qualify for reimbursement by one of two other methods: inclusion in a new technology APC group or to be granted transitional pass-through payment status (see further on). A new technology APC is created only for procedures or services that can neither be included in an existing APC group nor meet the conditions for pass-through drugs. Once sufficient time has passed to gather data on hospitals' actual expenditures on these new services and procedures, CMS reassigns these new technologies to standard APC groups as part of its annual review process. Unlike the aforementioned add-on payments under Medicare IPPS, new technology APC groups are not budget-neutral and could therefore substantially increase hospitals' treatment costs.

Transitional pass-through payments apply to new drugs, biologics, and medical devices that complement an existing service but are too expensive to be included in existing APC groups. For example, a pass-through payment for a costly new monoclonal antibody may be used to supplement the established base payment that covers the administration of chemotherapy. Table 3.1 lists the technologies that have pass-through status in 2006. To qualify for this status, a new technology must have been on the market for no more than two to three years and must be more expensive than existing therapies. In addition, medical devices (as opposed to drugs) must offer a substantial clinical advantage over established treatments – the same standard that is a condition for add-on payments in the Medicare IPPS system. In November 2001, CMS published the following characteristics of a new technology that offers "substantial clinical improvement":

- It offers a treatment option for a patient population unresponsive to, or ineligible for, currently available treatments.
- It offers the ability to diagnose a medical condition in a patient population in which their medical condition is currently undetectable or to diagnose a medical condition earlier in a patient

Table 3.1 Technologies with Pass-Through Status in the Medicare Outpatient Prospective Payment System, 2006

HCPCS Code	*APC Code*	*Product*
C9220	9220	Sodium hyaluronate
C9221	9221	Graftjacket Regular Matrix
C9222	9222	Graftjacket Soft Tissue
C9225	9225	Fluocinolone acetonide
J0128	9216	Abarelix injection
J0878	9124	Daptomycin injection
J2278	1694	Ziconotide injection
J2357	9300	Omalizumab injection
J2503	1697	Pegaptanib sodium injection
J2783	0738	Rasburicase
J2794	9125	Risperidone, long acting
J7518	9219	Mycophenolic acid
J8501	0868	Oral aprepitant
J9027	1710	Clofarabine injection
J9035	9214	Bevacizumab injection
J9055	9215	Cetuximab injection
J9264	1712	Paclitaxel injection
J9305	9213	Pemetrexed injection
Q4079	9126	Natalizumab injection (1 mg)

APC = Ambulatory payment classification
HCPCS = Healthcare common procedure coding system

population than allowed by currently available methods. There must also be evidence that the use of the technology to make a diagnosis affects the management of the patient.

- Use of the technology significantly improves clinical outcomes for a patient population as compared with currently available treatments. For example, improvements might include:

1. Reduced mortality rate.
2. Reduced rate of complications.
3. Reduced rate of subsequent diagnostic or therapeutic interventions (e.g., due to reduced rate of recurrence of the disease process).
4. Decreased number of future hospitalizations or physician visits.
5. More rapid beneficial resolution of the disease process.
6. Less pain, bleeding, or other quantifiable symptom.
7. Reduced recovery time.

Table 3.2 summarizes the similarities and differences of the new technology payment mechanisms in Medicare's prospective payment systems. Critics deplore the inconsistencies of these mechanisms. In a report to Congress, which was published in March 2003, MedPAC made the following assertion:

> The treatment of drugs and devices is inconsistent, in that only newness and cost criteria are applied to pass-through drugs. This difference in the criteria represents unequal treatment between types of technology within the outpatient payment system. It also leads to a discrepancy between the treatment of drugs under the inpatient and outpatient payment systems since the clinical criteria are applied to all technologies, including drugs, on the inpatient side. Furthermore, without considering clinical benefit, the criteria applied to pass-through drugs may overemphasize the goal of paying adequately for new technologies at the expense of prudent purchasing.

Furthermore, MedPAC suggested that "it is appropriate to reserve additional payments for technologies that provide clinical benefit and do not have clinical substitutes. It may even be appropriate to limit payments to technologies that provide additional benefits commensurate with their costs."

Medicaid

The Medicare, Medicaid, and SCHIP Benefits Improvement and Protection Act of 2000 (BIPA) opened the way for state Medicaid administrations to establish prospective payment systems for their

Table 3.2 Key Features of Medicare Inpatient and Outpatient New Technology Payment Mechanisms

	Inpatient Add-On Payments	*Outpatient Pass-Through Payments*		*Outpatient New Technology APCs*
		Medical Devices	*Drugs and Biologics*	
New technologies eligible for additional payments	New technologies that offer a new procedure or are an input to an existing DRG	New technologies that are an input to an existing DRG	New technologies that are an input to an existing DRG	New technologies that offer a new service
Criteria used by CMS	Clinical benefit, novelty, cost	Clinical benefit, novelty, cost	Novelty, cost	Novelty
Funding method	Budget-neutral	Budget-neutral	Budget-neutral	New expenditures
Unit of payment	Additional costs of treating a case using new technology	Cost of new technology	Cost of new technology	Cost of service
Method of determining payments	Payment = 50% of additional costs (capped at 50% of estimated cost of new technology)	Payment = 100% of reported costs minus device costs already built into base payment rate	Payment = 95% of average wholesale price	Payment = midpoint of payment range for new technology APC group

APC = Ambulatory payment classification
CMS = Centers for Medicare and Medicaid Services
DRG = Diagnosis-related group

payments to federally qualified health clinics and rural health clinics. Beginning January 1, 2001, states could switch from the established cost-reimbursement system to prospective payment. However, a recent study conducted by the Government Accountability Office (GAO) suggests that many states were slow to embrace prospective payment. On average, states took slightly more than a year to implement Medicaid prospective payment systems, and the GAO found that some states still had not completed this exercise as of June 1, 2004. A survey conducted by the National Association of Community Health Centers (NACHC), assisted by George Washington University, found that 23 of the 42 states that responded excluded pharmacy benefits from their Medicaid prospective payment systems in 2005, compared with just seven states in 2004.

Commercial Health Plans

Commercial insurers observe Medicare's reimbursement practices very closely and often follow CMS's lead (e.g., historically reimbursing office-based clinicians 95% of the average wholesale price of physician-administered drugs). In the matter of prospective payment, however, commercial health plans have generally been reluctant to copy Medicare's example. Adopting a DRG-based IPPS similar to the Medicare model is relatively simple, and some plans have developed such systems in recent years. However, copying Medicare's OPSS would be more challenging. For instance, some APCs are based not on clinical factors but on Medicare reimbursement policies. CMS updates its APC system each quarter, a cycle that would require more frequent changes than many plans would like.

FRANCE

France has traditionally operated a bimodal system of hospital funding. Public and private hospitals working in the public sector receive a *dotation globale* (global budget) that is divided among various areas of expenditure, whereas private hospitals receive *per diem* or activity-based payment. However, as part of its *Plan Hôpital 2007* (Hospital Plan 2007) reform program, the French government wants all hospitals engaged in medicine, surgery, or obstetrics in that country to adopt a system known as *tarification à l'activité* (T2A; activity-based pricing). This new approach to hospital funding in France is based on *groupes homogènes de séjour* (GHSs; uniform hospitalization groups), a system similar to DRGs. The government expects to realize the following key benefits from the T2A system:

- Greater role for clinical factors in funding.
- More responsible behavior by leading players and an incentive for them to change.
- Greater equality of treatment between the (public and private) sectors.
- The development of health economic steering mechanisms (management controls) at the heart of public and private hospitals.

The timetable for the T2A program calls for a steady migration from cost-based reimbursement to activity-based funding. Figure 3.1 shows the government's targets for the percentage of total spending in public and private hospitals working in the public sector that will be derived from activity-based funding in select years from 2004 to 2010, the year when the transition is scheduled for completion.

As a general rule, medicines are included in the GHSs. However, the French government recognizes that certain drugs and other technologies (notably medical devices) are too expensive to fit within the GHSs; therefore, these products will be funded separately. The Ministry of Health and the *Agence Technique de l'Information sur l'Hospitalisation* (ATIH; Technical Agency for Information on Hospitalization) have compiled a list of approximately 80 products that qualify for supplementary reimbursement (Table 3.3). Almost half of these products are oncology-related medicines. The Ministry of Health will update the list annually.

To control spending on drugs that qualify for supplementary reimbursement, ceiling prices will be determined either through negotiations between the manufacturers and the *Comité Economique des Produits de Santé* (CEPS; Economic Committee for Healthcare Products), the organization responsible for setting reimbursement prices

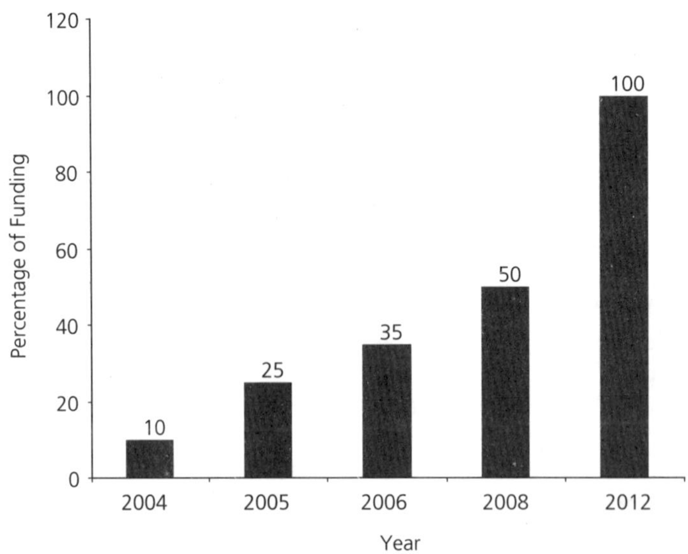

Figure 3.1 Activity-Based Funding in France: Projected Share of Total Budget for Public Hospitals and Private Hospitals Working in the Public Sector in Selected Years, 2004–12

Table 3.3 Drugs Eligible for Supplementary Reimbursement in France, 2005

Drug Class/International Nonproprietary Name	*Brand Name*	*Manufacturer*
Antineoplastic drugs		
Aldesleukin	Proleukin	Chiron
Alemtuzumab	Mabcampath	Schering
Arsenic trioxide	Trisenox	Cell Therapeutics
Bortezomib	Velcade	Janssen-Cilag
Busulfan	Busilvex	Pierre Fabre
Carmustine	Bicnu	Bristol-Myers Squibb
Cladribine	Leustatin	Janssen-Cilag
Daunorubicin	Daunoxome	Gilead Sciences
Docetaxel	Taxot'ere	Sanofi-Aventis
Doxorubicin	Caelyx	Schering-Plough
	Myocet	Elan Pharma
Epirubicin	Farmorubicin	Pharmacia (Pfizer)
Fludarabine	Fludara	Schering
Fotemustine	Muphoran	Servier
Gemcitabine	Gemzar	Lilly France
Ibritumomab-tiuxetan	Zevalin	Schering
Idarubicin	Zavedos	Pfizer
Irinotecan	Campto	Sanofi-Aventis
Oxaliplatin	Eloxatin	Sanofi-Aventis
Paclitaxel	Taxol	Bristol-Myers Squibb
Pemetrexed	Alimta	Lilly France
Pentostatin	Nipent	Wyeth-Lederle
Pirarubicin	Therprubicine	Sanofi-Aventis
Raltitrexed	Tomudex	AstraZeneca
Rituximab	Mabthera	Roche
Tasonermine	Beromun	Boehringer Ingelheim
Topotecan	Hycamtin	GlaxoSmithKline
Trastuzumab	Herceptin	Roche
Vinorelbine	Navelbine	Pierre Fabre
Other oncology-related drugs		
153Sm-samarium-acid	Quadramet	Cis Bio International
89Sr-strontium chloride	Metastron	Amersham Health
Amifostine	Ethyol	Schering-Plough
Darbepoetin alfa	Aranesp	Amgen
Dexrazoxane	Cardioxane	Chiron France
Erythropoietin alfa	Eprex	Janssen-Cilag
Erythropoietin beta	Neorecormon	Roche
Iodine-131 lipiodil	Lipiocis	Cis Bio International
Rasburicase	Fasturtec	Sanofi-Aventis
Porfimer sodium	Photofrin	Isotec
Thyrotrophine	Thyrogen	Genzyme
Yttrium chloride	Ytracis	Cis Bio International
Antifungals		
Amphotericin	Abelcet	Elan Pharma
Amphotericin B	Ambisome	Gilead Sciences
Caspofungin	Cancidas	Merck Sharp & Dohme
Voriconazole	Vfend	Pfizer
Coagulation factors		
Eptacog	Alfa Novoseven	Novo Nordisk
Antihemophilic factor (recombinant)	Advate	Baxter
Factor VII	Factor VII LFB	LFB
Factor VIII	Factane	LFB

(continued)

Table 3.3 Continued

Drug Class/International Nonproprietary Name	*Brand Name*	*Manufacturer*
	Helixate Nexgen	Aventis-Behring
	Hemofilm M	Baxter
	Recombinate	Baxter
	Refacto	Wyeth-Lederle
	Monoclate	Aventis-Behring
	Kogenate Bayer	Bayer Pharma
Factor IX	Betafact	LFB
	Mononine	Aventis-Behring
Factor XI	Hemoleven	LFB
Nonacog	Alfa Benefix	Baxter
von Willebrand factor	Wilfactin	LFB
von Willebrand factor and	Willebrand LFB,	LFB
factor VIII in combination	Innobranduo	LFB
Other blood derivatives		
Activated prothrombic complex	Feiba	Baxter
Antithrombin III	Aclotin	LFB
Factors IX, II, VII, and X in combination	Kaskadil	LFB
Inhibitor C1	Esterasine	Baxter
Protein C	Ceprotin,	Baxter
	Protexel	LFB
Orphan drugs		
Agalsidase alfa	Replagal	TKT Europe 5S
Agalsidase beta	Fabrazyme	Genzyme
Bosentan	Tracleer	Actelion
Carglutamic acid	Carbaglu	Orphan Europe
Epoprostenol	Flolan	GlaxoSmithKline
Iloprost	Ventavis	Schering
Imiglucerase	Cerezyme	Genzyme
Laronidase	Aldurazyme	Genzyme
Miglustat	Zavesca	Actelion
Sodium phenylbutyrate	Ammonaps	Orphan Europe
Treatments for rheumatoid arthritis		
Etanercept	Enbrel	Wyeth-Lederle
Infliximab	Remicade	Schering-Plough
Immunoglobulins		
Antilymphocyte immunoglobulin	Lymphoglobulin	Imtix-Sangstat
Antithymocyte immunoglobulin	Thymoglobulin	Imtix-Sangstat
Immunoglobulin antihepatitis B	Ivhebex	LFB
Polyvalent human	Endobulin	Baxter
immunoglobulins for	Gammagard	Baxter
intravenous administration	Octagam	Octapharma
	Sandoglobulin	OTL Pharma
	Tegelin	LFB
Treatments for severe septicemia		
Drotrecogin	Xigris	Lilly

LFB = Laboratoire Français du Fractionnement et des Biotechnologies

in France, or through a decree from the ministers of health and social security. Manufacturers will also be subject to price/volume constraints, whereby prices will be reduced if sales volume is judged to have grown excessively.

High-priced new drugs can be added to this list as soon as they receive marketing authorization in France. After 12 months on the market, a drug will either be approved to remain on this list, in which case it will become subject to a ceiling price, or it will be removed from the supplementary reimbursement list and covered by the relevant GHS tariff.

Hospitals will be reimbursed for medicines on the supplementary reimbursement list at the level of a drug's ceiling price. To encourage hospital pharmacies to negotiate manufacturer discounts on these medicines, hospitals will be permitted to keep a proportion of any price difference they secure between the ceiling price and their actual purchase price.

Hospitals will also be required to sign a contract for the good use of medicines. Institutions that fail to sign this contract will have their reimbursement rate for drugs on the supplementary reimbursement list reduced to just 70%, leaving them out of pocket. Similarly, if a hospital fails to comply with the terms of its contract for the good use of medicines, the local *agence régionale d'hospitalisation* (ARH; regional hospitalization agency) can call on the health insurance funds to cut the reimbursement rate to 70%.

GERMANY

The German hospital sector has come under intense pressure in recent years. With the exception of Japan, Germany has proportionally more acute hospital beds than any other member of the Organization for Economic Cooperation and Development (OECD): 6.6 per 1,000 population in Germany in 2002, compared with an OECD average of 4.2. Furthermore, hospital stays are longer in Germany than in any other OECD member state except South Korea: an average of 9.2 days in Germany in 2002, compared with an OECD average of 6.7. Not surprisingly, the German healthcare system has struggled to fund this level of hospital care. Healthcare expenditures have risen faster than budgets, with the result that the statutory health insurance system has had deficits in many years since the early 1990s. The implementation of a DRG system is intended to promote greater efficiency in the hospital sector in Germany.

In April 2002, the German Parliament passed the *Gesetz zur Einführung des diagnoseorientierten Fallpauschalensystems* (Act for the Introduction of a Diagnosis-Related Group System). The introduction of this new DRG system began in 2004 and was originally scheduled for completion in 2007, but the government was persuaded to agree that this timetable was too aggressive. The *Zweites Fallpauschalenänderungsgesetz* (second Diagnosis-Related Group Modification Act), enacted in December 2004, extended the deadline for the full implementation of the DRG system to January 1, 2009, with the possibility of a further one-year extension, if necessary (Figure 3.2). As of October 2005, approximately 1,720 acute-care hospitals (94% of the national total) had begun the process of implementing the new DRG system. These hospitals had a total of 494,000 beds, managed 15.3 million cases, and had combined expenditures of €45 billion ($56 billion); for the sake of uniformity of the analysis, the US dollar-to-euro exchange rate used in this chapter is the 2005 average rate, that is, $1 = €0.80453.

Germany's DRG system is an adaptation of the Australian Refined Diagnosis-Related Group (AR-DRG) system. However, the two systems differ significantly in their applications. The Australian system is used essentially as an instrument to manage the supply of healthcare services, but the German system was created as a budgetary control mechanism.

The *Fallpauschalenkatalog* (DRG Catalogue) is updated annually by the *Deutsches Institut für Medizinische Dokumentation und Information* (DIMDI; German Institute for Medical Documentation and Information) and the *Institut für das Entgeltsystem im Krankenhaus* (InEK; Institute for Hospital Reimbursement), in consultation with specialist societies. The total number of DRGs has increased from 664 in 2003 to 954 in 2006 (Figure 3.3). This total is substantially larger than in most other DRG systems and reflects the demand for more nuanced grouping in Germany. Similarly, the number of categories for disease severity was recently increased, from five to eight.

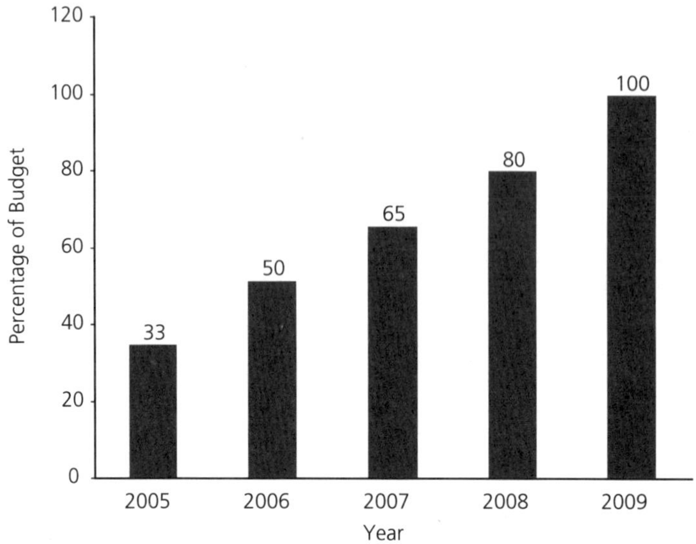

DRG = Diagnosis-related group

Figure 3.2 Percentage of German Hospitals' Budgets to Be Derived from DRG-Based Funding 2005–9

DRG rates vary from state to state. By 2009, payments to all hospitals will be expected to converge on their relevant state rates. High-priced hospitals will lose from this exercise, whereas low-priced hospitals will gain.

A key objective of DRG-based reimbursement is to shorten the length of hospital stays. New cost management systems will measure how effectively a given treatment reduces overall therapy costs while achieving the same clinical outcomes. Product evaluations will need to take account of the following factors:

- Therapy costs that correlate duration of treatment with length of stay.
- Cost of managing side effects.
- Administration and disposal costs.
- Cost of treating therapy failures.

At present, DRGs apply only to inpatient procedures, with the exception of two semi-ambulatory groups related to renal dialysis. However, the government has had plans to introduce DRGs for office-based specialists, a step that is in keeping with the administration's policy of *integrierte Versorgung* (integrated care). Family physicians, specialists, and medical and nonmedical healthcare practitioners in both the primary care and hospital sectors are encouraged to work together to improve the quality of patient care. Hospitals may offer ambulatory care for certain indications and highly specialized services and become involved in disease management programs and the provision of ambulatory care where there is a shortage of office-based specialists. This provision is expected to reduce the need for patients to visit both office- and hospital-based physicians.

In a position statement published in March 2004, the *Verband Forschender Arzneimittelhersteller* (VFA; German Association of Research-Based Pharmaceutical Companies) described the introduction of the new DRG system as "the greatest structural reform in the [German] hospital sector in the last 30 years." The new system presents the pharmaceutical industry with both opportunities and challenges. Drug costs are generally included in the standard DRG rates, but additional funding is available for

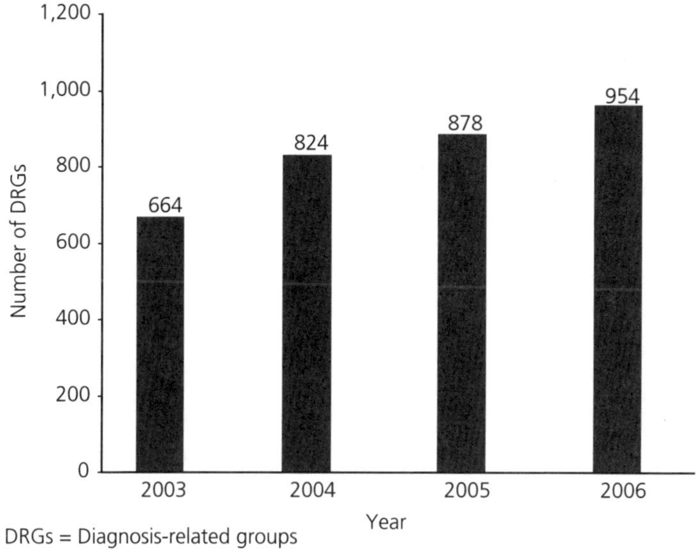

Figure 3.3 Total Number of Diagnosis-Related Groups in Germany, 2003–6

new therapies in specific circumstances. Hospitals can apply for a *Zusatzentgelt* (supplementary payment) for drugs or devices that are not yet covered by DRGs. Supplementary payments are available for technologies that meet any of the following conditions:

- Insufficient data available for inclusion in a DRG.
- Use in multiple DRGs.
- Potentially significant impact on the cost of a given DRG or on the hospital's overall expenditures.

Table 3.4 lists the drugs that are eligible for supplementary payments in 2006. Payments are dose dependent.

Supplementary payments, along with DRGs and days of treatment, are used to set a hospital's revenue budget. The full amount of the supplementary payment is available if hospitals submit their applications to statutory health insurance funds in advance of treatment, but retroactive submissions qualify for only 75% reimbursement. If a hospital exceeds its revenue budget, it must generally repay 65% of the surplus to the statutory health insurance

Table 3.4 Drugs Eligible for Supplementary Payments in Germany, 2006

Code	*Drug*
ZE13	Alemtuzumab
ZE15	Docetaxel
ZE17	Gemcitabine
ZE19	Irinotecan
ZE23	Oxaliplatin
ZE24	Paclitaxel
ZE25	Rituximab
ZE27	Trastuzumab
ZE30	Prothrombin complex
ZE38	Human immunoglobulin for cytomegalovirus
ZE39	Caspofungin
ZE40	Filgrastim
ZE41	Polyvalent human immunoglobulin
ZE42	Lenograstim
ZE43	Liposomal amphotericin B
ZE44	Topotecan
ZE45	Voriconazole (oral)
ZE46	Voriconazole
ZE47	Antithrombin III
ZE48	Aldesleukin
ZE49	Bortezomib
ZE50	Cetuximab
ZE51	Human immunoglobulin for hepatitis B surface antigen
ZE52	Liposomal doxorubicin
ZE53	Pemetrexed

Unless otherwise indicated, coverage relates to parenteral administration funds, but this rate is reduced to 25% for excess revenues derived from supplementary payments for drugs and devices. On the other hand, if a hospital earns less than its revenue budget, it generally receives 40% of the shortfall from the statutory health insurance funds – but nothing for a shortfall in revenues from supplementary payments for drugs and devices. Supplementary payments are a budget-neutral measure – in other words, monies allocated to supplementary payments reduce funding for other areas of the overall budget.

UNITED KINGDOM

The infrastructure of the U.K. National Health Service (NHS) has undergone many changes in recent years. In April 2002, the 95 regional health authorities in England were merged to form 28 new strategic health authorities (SHAs). These SHAs are responsible for strategic development of healthcare services within their areas and for managing the performance of 303 primary care trusts (PCTs) and more than 300 NHS hospital trusts. The SHAs distribute unified budget allocations to the PCTs, the organizations that are now the dominant fund holders in the U.K. healthcare system, managing 75% of the entire NHS budget and 100% of local funds. PCTs have three main roles: (1) to improve the health of the community; (2) to develop primary and community health services; and (3) to commission hospital care for their patients. As the main source of funding for public hospitals, PCTs have enormous influence over the finances and policies of these hospitals. In the spring of 2006, the U.K. government announced plans for further reform of the NHS, reducing the number of SHAs in England to 10 and PCTs to 152.

The government has also made radical changes to hospital funding in England. Until very recently, hospital budgets were set on the basis of historical expenditures. In October 2002, however, the Department of Health published *Reforming NHS Financial Flows*, a blueprint for a new patient-centered funding system known as Payment by Results (PbR). This system gives NHS patients the freedom to choose when and where they receive hospital treatment, a right they had never previously enjoyed. The mechanism has been summarized with the motto "the money follows the patient." Specifically, PbR has the following key objectives:

- Promoting choice and competition.
- Increasing efficiency and value for money.
- Facilitating therapeutic innovation.
- Cutting waiting times and inpatient length of stay.
- Improving equity and transparency in the healthcare system.

The implementation of this new system began on a limited scale in 2004 and was then expanded in 2005 to include all elective inpatients. From 2006 to 2008, the system will be extended to nonelective inpatients, emergency room admissions, and outpatients. Beginning in 2008, PbR will be introduced into the primary care sector.

PbR is based on healthcare resource groups (HRGs), a form of DRG that groups patients who have similar clinical conditions and similar consumption of healthcare resources. The HRG system has been refined repeatedly to make it more discriminating, and a further review is in progress, with the objective of identifying all disease complications and comorbidities. HRGs provide the data that underpin the national tariff for services provided within the PbR system. Efficient hospitals that can provide services for less than national tariff prices will be permitted to keep the surplus. By reinvesting the money saved in their organizations, these hospitals can improve the quality of their services and attract patients away from less-efficient hospitals.

The national tariff does not include procedures that are highly specialized, rarely performed, or subject to price volatility. Furthermore, high-cost drugs (e.g., antiretrovirals, tumor necrosis factor-alpha inhibitors, beta interferons, treatments for hepatitis C, therapies for pulmonary hypertension, some chemotherapy drugs) and devices (e.g., aortic stents, insulin pumps) are excluded from the PbR national tariff. Table 3.5 lists excluded drugs for the 2006–7 financial year. Hospitals that wish to use these drugs have to commission supplementary funding from local PCTs. In addition, new technologies, as well as some existing drugs and devices that have a high price or uneven distribution, may qualify for pass-through status for a maximum of two years. PCTs must notify the Department of Health if they grant pass-through status to drugs used by hospitals in their respective catchment areas.

Since January 1, 2002, PCTs have a statutory obligation to provide funding for therapies endorsed by the National Institute for Health and Clinical Excellence (NICE)

Table 3.5 Drugs Eligible for Supplementary Reimbursement in the United Kingdom, 2006

Drug Class	*Examples*
Cytokine inhibitors	Infliximab (Schering-Plough's Remicade)
Treatments for primary pulmonary hypertension	Bosentan (Actelion's Tracleer), iloprost (Schering's Ventavis), epoprostenol (GlaxoSmithKline's Flolan), phosphodiesterase-5 inhibitors
Antifibrinolytic drugs/hemostatics	Factor VIIa, factor VIII, factor IX, antithrombin III, prothrombin, fibrinogen, factor XI, protein C, von Willebrand factor, factor VIII bypassing products, prothrombin complex, porcine factor VIII, fibrin sealants, thrombin (for topical use only)
Treatments for torsion dystonia and other involuntary movements	Riluzole
Antifungals	Amphotericin (lipid formulations), caspofungin (Merck Sharp & Dohme's Cancidas), voriconazole (Pfizer's Vfend)
AIDS/HIV antiretrovirals	Abacivir with lamivudine and zidovudine (GlaxoSmithKline's Trizivir)
Treatments for viral hepatitis (B and C) and respiratory syncytial virus	Palivizumab (Abbott's Synagis)
Growth hormones and growth hormone receptor antagonists	Somatropin (multisource)
Drugs affecting bone metabolism	Teriparatide (Lilly's Forsteo)
Treatments for multiple sclerosis	Interferon alpha and beta
Somatostatin analogues	Octreotide acetate (Novartis's Sandostatin), lanreotide acetate (Ipsen's Somatuline LA)
Treatments for neutropenia	Filgrastim (Amgen's Neupogen), pegfilgrastim (Amgen's Neulasta)
Drugs used in metabolic disorders	Treatments for carnitine deficiency, Fabry's disease, Gaucher's disease, mucopolysaccharidosis I, nephropathic cystinosis
Treatments for hyperuricemia associated with cytotoxic drugs	Rasburicase (Sanofi-Aventis's Fasturtec)
Dermatological drugs that modify the immune response	Efalizumab (Serono's Raptiva)
Intravenous/subcutaneous human normal immunoglobulins	Baxter BioScience's Subcuvia, ZLB Behring's Vivaglobin

within three months of the institute's publication of its decision. To provide funding for these treatments, the PbR budget was increased by £304 million ($553 million [0.7%]) in financial year 2004–5 and by £328 million ($596 million [0.7%]) in financial year 2005–6 (for the sake of uniformity of the analysis, the U.S. dollar-to-pound sterling exchange rate used in this chapter is the 2005 average rate, that is, $1 = £0.55004). The 0.7% increase was based on national averages and may not have been sufficient to cover increased expenditures in hospitals that had an above-average usage of NICE-endorsed technologies.

A performance assessment known as the annual health check will determine whether hospitals and PCTs are meeting their PbR obligations. These organizations will be required to declare whether they are conforming to NICE's technology appraisals and taking the institute's clinical guidelines into account in the delivery of healthcare. To make such a declaration, hospitals and PCTs must have robust systems to assess, plan for, and monitor the financial impact of implementing NICE's guidance.

JAPAN

In April 2003, the Japanese government introduced a new flat-sum reimbursement system, based on diagnosis-procedure combinations (DPCs), for acute care of inpatients at 82 special-function hospitals and other hospitals that provide advanced medical treatment. The mean fee-per-day determined for each diagnosis group is adjusted according to the mean length of stay at individual hospitals. By fiscal year 2005, 144 Japanese hospitals had adopted the DPC system and 145 other hospitals had introduced it on a trial basis, with more expected to follow in the future. The pharmaceutical industry is concerned that DPC reimbursement might lead to inappropriate prescribing behavior. In an analysis published in June 2004, the Healthcare System Subcommittee of the Federation of Pharmaceutical Manufacturers' Associations of Japan (FPMAJ) suggested that "the expansion of the DPC system is acceptable only to the extent that it does not affect the proper use of drugs." The authors predicted that the DPC system will expand and warned that this trend "will necessarily make medical institutions more strongly concerned about the use of drugs." The DPC system is likely to prompt hospitals to increase their use of generics in order to reduce their drug acquisition costs. To this end, hospitals are introducing electronic prescribing systems that facilitate prescribing by international nonproprietary names.

The Ministry of Health, Labor, and Welfare (MHLW) has ruled that, from July 2005, some expensive therapies (e.g., rituximab for non-Hodgkin's lymphoma) must be excluded from the DPC system and reimbursed on a fee-for-service basis. This decision was prompted by a sizable gap between the treatment costs as calculated in the DPC and fee-for-service systems. Drugs that are more expensive than the DPC cost are funded by medical institutions, a situation that defeats the objective of the DPC system (i.e., cutting the costs of acute inpatient care). The MHLW suggests that such a situation is exceptional and transient, but it has not offered a clear solution to this problem. Therefore, it may be necessary to reserve some expensive therapies for use in the outpatient setting (where the DPC system is not used).

OUTLOOK AND IMPLICATIONS FOR THE PHARMACEUTICAL INDUSTRY

The expansion of prospective payment systems in the world's major pharmaceutical markets appears to offer limited new opportunities for manufacturers of branded medicines. Such systems are meant to improve access to high-quality healthcare and to eliminate geographic inequalities in treatment, but they are also clearly intended to reduce costs – potentially including pharmaceutical expenditures.

Hospitals that can cut their costs below prospective payment system reimbursement levels frequently derive a dual benefit: they can keep part or all of the money they save, and increased resources enable them to improve the quality of their service and attract more patients. This environment increases the pressure on hospitals to use generics wherever possible and to negotiate substantial discounts on branded medicines. On the other hand, hospitals that make above-average use of innovative technologies – in many cases, university hospitals in the vanguard of medical practice – could find themselves penalized for their high costs.

Governments would insist that their measures are not intended to hinder innovation, and all of the prospective payment systems reviewed in this report allow for exceptional coverage of new and/or costly therapies. However, exploiting this provision is not always easy in practice. Hospitals must typically overcome administrative barriers to secure coverage of these therapies. Precise advance planning may be needed to obtain maximum reimbursement – no easy task when new and relatively unfamiliar technologies are involved. Given these obstacles, some hospitals may be deterred from pursuing exceptional coverage of innovative therapies, but such a decision could actually have the effect of delaying the inclusion of these treatments in standard DRGs. Moreover, the fact that funding for new technologies is often diverted from more established products – to ensure a budget-neutral impact – is bad news for both hospitals and pharmaceutical companies.

It will be interesting to observe the growing impact of health economics and health technology assessment on prospective payment systems in the future. NICE is certainly one of the best-known exponents of such research, and many other countries are following suit. Indeed, NICE recently agreed on a triangular collaboration with Germany's *Institut für Qualität und Wirtschaftlichkeit im Gesundheitswesen* (IQWiG; Institute for Quality and Economy in the Healthcare System) and France's *Haute Autorité de la Santé* (HAS; High Authority on Health), in addition to an earlier agreement to exchange information with the Food and Drug Administration (FDA). After largely ignoring health economics and health technology assessment for many years, the United States is slowly beginning to embrace these disciplines. In fact, the Medicare Prescription Drug, Improvement, and Modernization Act of 2003 (MMA) calls on the Agency for Healthcare Research and Quality (AHRQ) to conduct trials to compare the clinical effectiveness and cost-effectiveness of branded medicines that compete within a given drug class. The act directs that cost-effectiveness studies may include "high-cost" healthcare products and services "as well as those which may be underutilized and overutilized and which may significantly improve the prevention, treatment, or cure of diseases and conditions (including chronic conditions) which impose high direct or indirect costs on patients or society." It remains to be seen to what extent the AHRQ's research will influence CMS's decisions on Medicare prospective payment. Furthermore, MedPAC's recommendation that additional payments should be restricted "to technologies that provide additional benefits commensurate with their costs" echoes statements made in some highly cost-conscious European countries.

Continued expansion of prospective payment systems appears very likely. With the steady growth of consumer-directed healthcare, U.S. residents are becoming increasingly aware of opportunities to curb healthcare spending. Commercial health plans may soon decide that the time is right to follow Medicare's lead in establishing prospective payment systems for hospital treatment. European countries look set to overtake the United States in their implementation of prospective payment. Germany plans to extend this system to office-based specialists, and the United Kingdom has an even more radical ambition – to introduce prospective payment in primary care. The trend for closer integration of primary and secondary care may prompt other countries to consider a similar expansion of prospective payment.

If the pharmaceutical industry is to derive some benefit from the growth of prospective payment, it needs to demonstrate clearly and cogently how innovative prescription drugs can add substantial value in such a system. In the past, hospitals had a financial (though not necessarily clinical) incentive to extend a patient's length of stay, but prospective payment essentially inverts this proposition: it is more lucrative to discharge a patient at the earliest appropriate opportunity. If pharmaceutical companies can demonstrate that their products can shorten a patient's length of stay or reduce treatment costs in other ways, their products will surely find a place in even the toughest prospective payment systems.

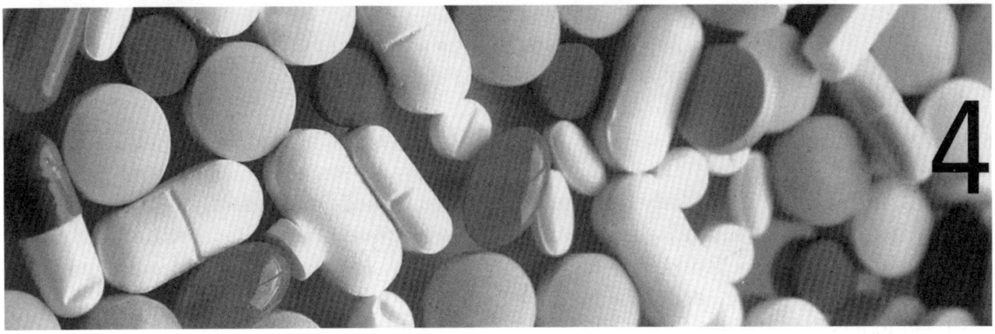

4

Off-label Prescribing: Overcoming the Reimbursement Barrier

OVERVIEW

Off-label prescribing is the practice of using a medicine for a purpose other than that for which it has been officially approved. Off-label usage takes a variety of forms: departing from the dosing range or duration of therapy, using a medicine in an unapproved combination with another agent, prescribing a drug to patients who belong to populations for which the agent is not approved (notably children), and using the product for unlicensed indications.

A drug's initial label is often very narrow, and gaining approval for additional indications can take a long time. Manufacturers are understandably reluctant to conduct expensive clinical trials for new indications on drugs that have lost or will soon lose their patent protection. Furthermore, physicians are often quick to deviate from a new drug's labeling restrictions. Off-label prescribing is frequently prompted by a dearth of effective licensed drugs with which to treat patients. Nevertheless, physicians may expose themselves to an increased risk of litigation if they prescribe medicines off-label. In addition, payers may refuse to reimburse physicians and/or their patients for off-label usage of medicines that does not meet strict conditions.

Anecdotal evidence suggests that off-label prescribing accounts for the majority of uses of certain drugs. Reportedly, this practice is particularly common in oncology, cardiology, neurology, and psychiatry, but few studies have actually measured the frequency of off-label usage. One recent study analyzed prescribing patterns by diagnosis for 160 commonly prescribed drugs in the United States (Radley et al., 2006). The authors found that, of a surveyed total of approximately 725 million prescriptions dispensed in 2001, about 150 million (21%) were for unapproved indications. Off-label prescribing accounted for 46% of prescriptions for cardiac therapies (excluding antihyperlipidemics and antihypertensives) and anticonvulsants, 42% of prescriptions for antiasthmatics, 34% of prescriptions for allergy therapies, 31% of prescriptions for psychiatric therapies (i.e., antidepressants, anxiolytics, antipsychotics), and 30% of prescriptions for peptic ulcer and dyspepsia therapies. Gabapentin was the drug most frequently prescribed off-label: 83% of uses were for unlicensed indications.

Other investigations of off-label prescribing have generally focused on particular drug classes. For example, an analysis of claims data from the Georgia Medicaid program in 1999 and 2000 found that 71% of uses of anticonvulsants were off-label (Chen et al., 2005). An analysis of atypical antipsychotic usage in North Staffordshire, England, from 1994 to 2001 found that 41% of uses of these drugs were for indications that were not approved at the time (Hodgson and Belgamwar, 2006). A 2003 study of atypical antipsychotic usage in seven Italian psychiatric outpatient services found that 52% of prescriptions for these drugs were for off-label indications (Barbui et al., 2002).

Given the time, effort, and cost involved in securing approval for multiple indications, it can be tempting to drug manufacturers to promote off-label prescribing of their products. However, unless carefully controlled, this practice may prove illegal, provoking potentially costly litigation.

This chapter examines the reimbursement barriers to off-label prescribing in the world's six largest pharmaceutical markets: the United States, France, Germany, Italy, the United Kingdom, and Japan. We begin with an analysis of the scale of off-label usage in the United States of four key drug classes: antineoplastic drugs, antidepressants, antipsychotics, and anticonvulsants. We then review the hazards that manufacturers may face when they engage in off-label marketing and explore the reimbursement environment in the United States, focusing on Medicare, Medicaid, and private insurance. Next, we consider the reimbursement challenges in each of the other countries covered in this chapter. We conclude with a brief assessment of the outlook and implications for the pharmaceutical industry.

UNITED STATES

Scale of Off-label Prescribing

To assess the current scale of off-label prescribing in the United States, we analyzed 2005 claims data from Verispan's Physician Drug & Diagnosis Audit (PDDA) database for leading oncology, neurology, and psychiatry drugs. The results of this analysis are presented in the sections that follow. We focused on off-label usage in the form of prescriptions for unlicensed indications and did not examine off-label prescribing by patient age (i.e., the prescription to children of drugs that are not approved for pediatric use). The indications for which drugs were prescribed were based on four-digit codes in the *International Classification of Diseases*, 9th Revision (ICD-9). We deemed prescriptions to be on label in cases where diagnostic codes were more general than, but related to, the approved indication. For example, we considered a diagnosis of "anxiety states" to be compliant with the label for drugs approved for generalized anxiety disorder, social anxiety disorder, or cognate disorders. The PDDA database did not allow us to determine if prescriptions met all of the conditions specified on a given drug's label (e.g., cancer staging, failure to respond to other therapies, use in combination with other agents).

Antineoplastic Drugs

Table 4.1 lists the approved indications in the United States for 14 antineoplastic drugs included in our analysis. Figure 4.1 shows the level of off-label usage for each of these agents. The dearth of effective therapies for some life-threatening cancers is a powerful stimulus to off-label prescribing.

Carboplatin was the antineoplastic drug most frequently prescribed off-label – in 77% of cases. Although this drug is approved for initial and secondary treatment of advanced ovarian cancer, less than 23% of uses were for this indication, compared with 52% for lung cancer, an unlicensed indication. Vinorelbine was also widely prescribed off-label: only 36% of uses were for the approved indication of lung cancer, compared with 47% for breast cancer. The age of these two drugs and the fact that both are off-patent and subject to generics competition may contribute to their very extensive off-label use. At the other end of the spectrum of off-label usage, trastuzumab, oxaliplatin, imatinib, rituximab, and erlotinib were used for unlicensed indications in less than 10% of cases.

Antidepressants

Table 4.2 shows the approved indications in the United States for 10 antidepressants, and

Table 4.1 Approved Indications for Select Antineoplastic Drugs in the United States

INN	*Brand Name*	*Manufacturers*	*Year of First Approval*	*Approved Indications*
Bevacizumab	Avastin	Roche	2004	Metastatic colorectal cancer
Capecitabine	Xeloda	Roche	1998	Colorectal cancer; breast cancer
Carboplatin	Paraplatin; generics	Multisource	1989	Advanced ovarian cancer
Cetuximab	Erbitux	Bristol-Myers Squibb	2004	Metastatic colorectal cancer
Docetaxel	Taxotere	Sanofi-Aventis	1996	Breast cancer; non-small-cell lung cancer; prostate cancer; gastric adenocarcinoma
Erlotinib	Tarceva	Genentech/OSI Pharmaceuticals	2004	Non-small-cell lung cancer; pancreatic cancer
Gemcitabine	Gemzar	Eli Lilly	1996	Breast cancer; non-small-cell lung cancer; pancreatic cancer
Imatinib	Gleevec	Novartis	2001	Chronic myeloid leukemia
Irinotecan	Camptosar	Pfizer	1996	Metastatic colorectal cancer
Oxaliplatin	Eloxatin	Sanofi-Aventis	2002	Colorectal cancer
Paclitaxel	Taxol; generics	Multisource	1992	Advanced ovarian cancer
Rituximab	Rituxan	Genentech/ Biogen Idec	1997	Non-Hodgkin's lymphoma; rheumatoid arthritis
Trastuzumab	Herceptin	Roche	1998	Metastatic HER2-positive breast cancer
Vinorelbine	Navelbine; generics	Multisource	1994	Advanced non-small-cell lung cancer

HER2 = Human epidermal growth factor receptor 2
INN = International nonproprietary name

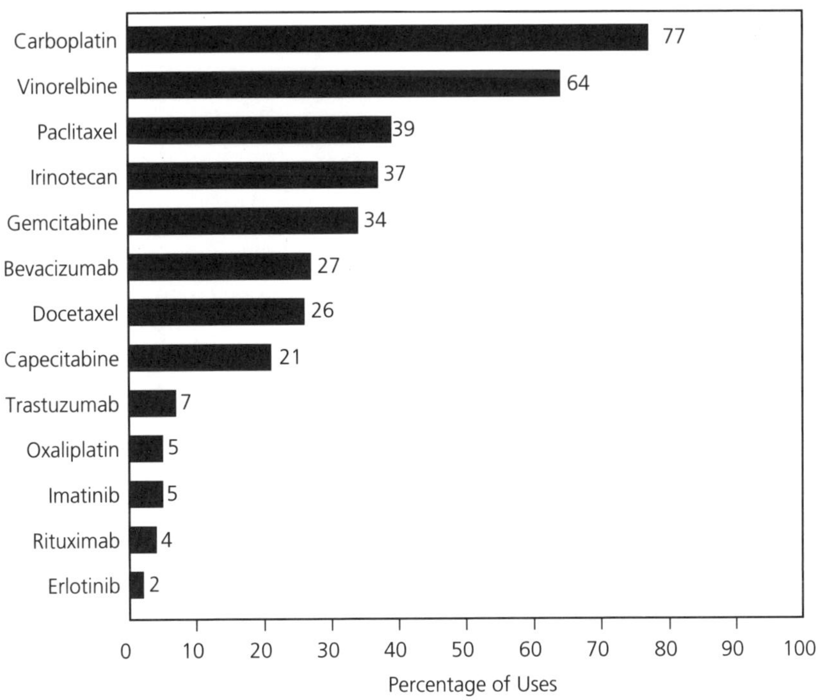

Figure 4.1 Percentage of Off-Label Uses for Select Antineoplastic Drugs in the United States, 2005

Table 4.2 Approved Indications for Select Antidepressants in the United States

INN	*Brand Name*	*Manufacturers*	*Year of First Approval*	*Approved Indications*
Bupropion	Wellbutrin (SL/XR); Zyban; generics	Multisource	1985	Major depressive disorder; smoking cessation
Buspirone	BuSpar; generics	Multisource	1986	Anxiety disorders
Citalopram	Celexa; generics	Multisource	1998	Depression
Duloxetine	Cymbalta	Eli Lilly	2004	Major depressive disorder; diabetic peripheral neuropathic pain
Escitalopram	Lexapro	Forest Laboratories	2002	Major depressive disorder; generalized anxiety disorder
Fluoxetine	Prozac (Weekly); Sarafem; generics	Multisource	1987	Major depressive disorder; obsessive compulsive disorder; bulimia nervosa; panic disorder
Mirtazapine	Remeron; generics	Multisource	1996	Major depressive disorder
Paroxetine	Paxil (CR); generics	Multisource	1992	Major depressive disorder; generalized anxiety disorder; social anxiety disorder; panic disorder; obsessive compulsive disorder; post-traumatic stress disorder; premenstrual dysphoric disorder[a]
Sertraline	Zoloft	Pfizer	1991	Major depressive disorder; social anxiety disorder; panic disorder; obsessive compulsive disorder; post-traumatic stress disorder; premenstrual dysphoric disorder
Venlafaxine	Effexor (XR)	Wyeth	1993	Major depressive disorder; generalized anxiety disorder; social anxiety disorder; panic disorder[b]

[a]Listed indications relate to Paxil CR; other paroxetine products are approved only for major depressive disorder, social anxiety disorder, panic disorder, and premenstrual dysphoric disorder
[b]Listed indications relate to Effexor XR; standard Effexor is approved only for major depressive disorder
INN = International nonproprietary name

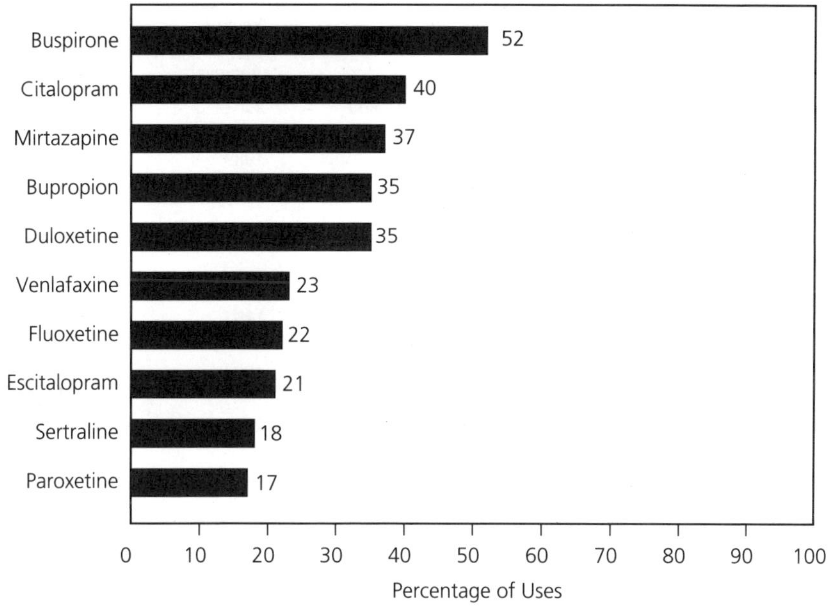

Figure 4.2 Percentage of Off-Label Uses for Select Antidepressants in the United States, 2005

Figure 4.2 summarizes the level of off-label usage for each of these agents. All but one of these drugs (buspirone) are approved for depression or major depressive disorder, and most are additionally approved for other indications – particularly anxiety disorders. Measuring off-label usage of antidepressants and other psychiatric drug classes is complicated by the high degree of diagnostic nuances and the difficulty of selecting a definitive diagnosis. The high prevalence of comorbid psychiatric disorders adds to the difficulties of coding the use of these drugs.

Of the 10 antidepressants included in our analysis, buspirone had the highest level of off-label prescribing (52% of uses) – mainly for depressive disorders, bipolar disorders, and schizoid disorders. Citalopram has a very limited label (i.e., depression), but it was frequently prescribed for anxiety states, bipolar disorder, and schizoid disorders. Similarly, mirtazapine is approved only for major depressive disorder but was widely used to treat other adjustment reactions, schizoid disorders, bipolar disorder, and anxiety states. In contrast, paroxetine and sertraline – both drugs with a wide range of licensed indications – had relatively low levels of off-label usage (17% and 18%, respectively).

The widespread use of antidepressants to treat patients who have bipolar disorder is a cause for concern. Some clinicians believe that these drugs can precipitate the onset of manic episodes in bipolar patients.

Antipsychotics

Table 4.3 lists the approved indications in the United States for six antipsychotics, and Figure 4.3 shows the level of off-label usage for each of these agents. All of these drugs are approved for schizophrenia, and all but one (clozapine) are licensed for aspects of bipolar disorder.

Quetiapine, risperidone, and olanzapine had the highest levels of off-label usage: 48%, 38%, and 37%, respectively. Common off-label uses included depressive disorder, anxiety states, and Alzheimer's disease – all of which may exist as comorbidities of schizophrenia or bipolar disorder. It is

Table 4.3 Approved Indications for Select Antipsychotics in the United States

INN	*Brand Name*	*Manufacturer*	*Year of First Approval*	*Approve Indications*
Aripiprazole	Abilify	Bristol-Myers Squibb	2002	Schizophrenia; bipolar disorder
Clozapine	Clozaril; generics	Multisource	1989	Schizophrenia
Olanzapine	Zyprexa	Eli Lilly	1996	Schizophrenia; bipolar mania; agitation associated with schizophrenia and bipolar mania
Quetiapine	Seroquel	AstraZeneca	1997	Schizophrenia; bipolar mania
Risperidone	Risperdal	Janssen	1993	Schizophrenia; bipolar mania
Ziprasidone	Geodon	Pfizer	2001	Schizophrenia; acute agitation in schizophrenic patients; bipolar mania

INN = International nonproprietary name

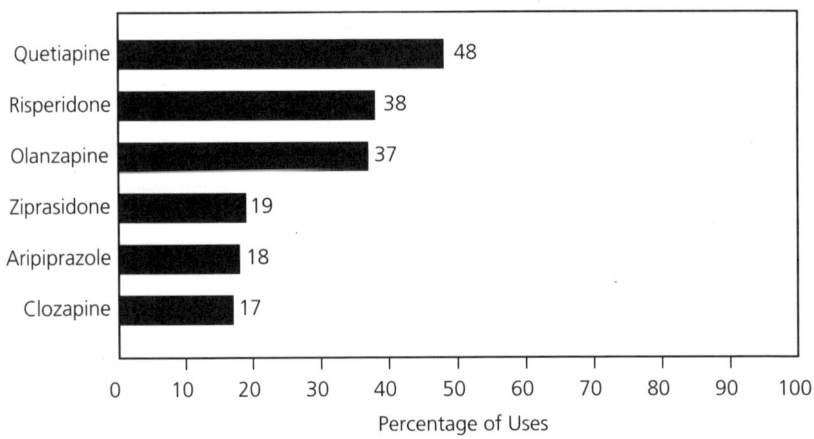

Figure 4.3 Percentage of Off-Label Uses for Select Antipsychotics in the United States, 2005

interesting that clozapine had the lowest level of off-label prescribing of these six antipsychotics (17%). Given that it has the narrowest label – it is approved only for schizophrenia – this agent might be expected to have one of the highest levels of off-label usage in this drug class. However, because of its potentially serious side effects, clozapine is restricted to use in treatment-refractory schizophrenic patients. This restriction likely explains the relatively modest off-label usage of this molecule.

Anticonvulsants

Table 4.4 shows the approved indications in the United States for eight anticonvulsants, and Figure 4.4 summarizes the level of off-label usage for each of these agents. All of these drugs are licensed for epilepsy; in

Table 4.4 Approved Indications for Select Anticonvulsants in the United States

INN	*Brand Name*	*Manufacturers*	*Year of First Approval*	*Approved Indications*
Carbamazepine	Tegretol; generics	Multisource	1968	Epilepsy; trigeminal neuralgia
Divalproex sodium	Depakote (ER); generics	Multisource	1983	Mania; epilepsy; migraine
Gabapentin	Neurontin; generics	Multisource	1993	Epilepsy; postherpetic neuralgia
Lamotrigine	Lamictal	GlaxoSmithKline	1994	Bipolar disorder; epilepsy
Levetiracetam	Keppra	UCB Pharma	1999	Epilepsy
Phenytoin	Dilantin; generics	Multisource	1956	Epilepsy
Pregabalin	Lyrica	Pfizer	2004	Neuropathic pain associated with diabetic peripheral neuropathy; postherpetic neuralgia; epilepsy
Topiramate	Topamax	Ortho-McNeil Neurologics	1996	Epilepsy; migraine

INN = International nonproprietary name

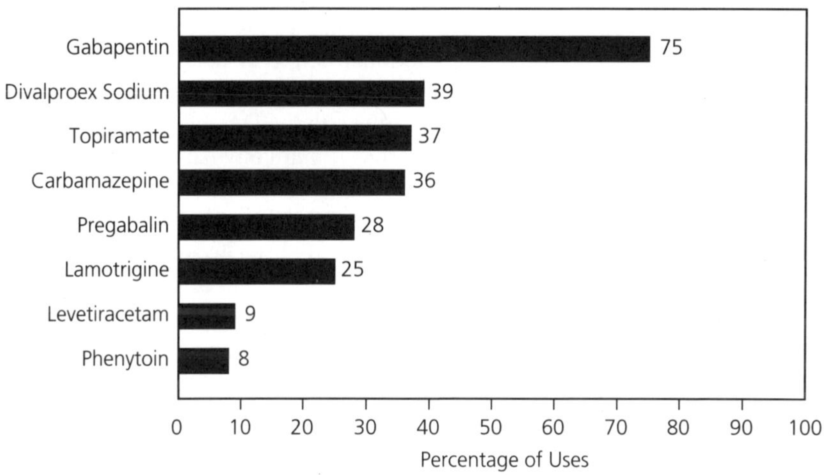

Figure 4.4 Percentage of Off-Label Uses for Select Anticonvulsants in the United States, 2005

addition, three are approved for types of neuralgia, two for migraine, and two for facets of bipolar disorder.

Gabapentin had by far the highest level of off-label prescribing among these anticonvulsants: 75%. The drug is approved for epilepsy and postherpetic neuralgia but was extensively prescribed for the relief of pain resulting from many other causes. In fact, the off-label marketing of gabapentin provoked a high-profile lawsuit that cost Pfizer $430 million in fines and liabilities (see the following section). Divalproex sodium is another drug that is widely used off-label: in 2005, 39% of uses were for unlicensed indications – principally, schizoid disorders.

Perils of Off-Label Marketing

Subject to reimbursement restrictions (discussed further on) and the obligation to accept liability for their decisions, physicians are generally free to prescribe drugs for off-label uses. Pharmaceutical companies, on the other hand, enter a legal minefield when they engage in off-label marketing of their products.

Section 401 of the Food and Drug Modernization Act of 1997 (FDAMA) authorizes strictly limited off-label promotion of medicines. A pharmaceutical company may provide physicians with "enduring materials" – unabridged reprints or copies of studies published in bona fide peer-reviewed scientific or medical journals – as a means of disseminating information on unlicensed uses of drugs, provided that the company has not been involved in the editing or publication of these materials. However, a series of five lawsuits initiated by the Washington Legal Foundation from 1993 to 1998 challenged the legality of restrictions on off-label promotion, arguing that these measures violated the guarantee of free speech under the First Amendment to the U.S. Constitution. Judge Royce C. Lambeth of the United States District Court for the District of Columbia commented: "In asserting that any and all scientific claims about the safety, effectiveness, contraindication, side effects, and the like regarding prescription drugs are presumptively untruthful or misleading until the FDA has had the opportunity to evaluate them, [the] FDA exaggerates its overall place in the universe." The court ruled that the FDA may not restrict pharmaceutical or medical device manufacturers from taking any of the following actions:

- Disseminating or redistributing to physicians or other medical professionals any article concerning prescription drugs or medical devices previously published in a bona fide peer-reviewed professional journal, regardless of whether such article includes a significant or exclusive focus on uses of drugs or medical devices other than those approved by the FDA and regardless of whether such article reports the original study on which FDA approval of the drug or device in question was based.
- Disseminating or redistributing to physicians or other medical professionals any reference textbook (including any medical textbook or compendium) or any portion thereof published by a bona fide independent publisher and otherwise generally available for sale in bookstores or other distribution channels where similar books are normally available, regardless of whether such reference textbook or portion thereof includes a significant or exclusive focus on uses of drugs or medical devices other than those approved by the FDA.
- Suggesting content or speakers to an independent program provider in connection with a continuing medical education seminar program or other symposium, regardless of whether uses of drugs and medical devices other than those approved by the FDA are to be discussed.

Freedom to disseminate peer-reviewed information on unlicensed uses of their drugs does not mean that manufacturers may engage in unrestrained off-label marketing, however. Some pharmaceutical companies have been criticized for aggressive off-label marketing, and Pfizer paid a high price for an off-label promotional strategy pursued by Warner-Lambert, a subsidiary acquired in 2000.

In 1993, the FDA approved Warner-Lambert's anticonvulsant Neurontin (gabapentin) as an adjunctive therapy for partial seizures in adults and children. The drug has subsequently been awarded an additional license for the treatment of postherpetic neuralgia. However, Warner-Lambert actively marketed Neurontin for a wide range of unlicensed indications – including monotherapy for seizures, bipolar disorder, migraine, restless legs syndrome, attention deficit hyperactivity disorder, amyotrophic lateral sclerosis, alcohol withdrawal seizures, and various pain disorders – that were not supported by clinical data. The company used medical liaison experts, preceptorships, consultant and advisory board meetings, dinner meetings and teleconferences, continuing medical education initiatives, ghostwritten articles, and payments to approximately 3,000 physicians to promote off-label prescribing. All of this activity helped to boost the off-label usage in the United States from 40% of Neurontin's prescriptions in 1995 to 94% in 2002. U.S. sales of Neurontin peaked at $2.2 billion in 2003 (the drug is now off-patent and subject to generics competition).

Warner-Lambert's off-label marketing strategy was eventually stopped by a whistleblower lawsuit initiated by David Franklin, who had briefly worked as a medical liaison expert for Neurontin. In Franklin versus Pfizer, the manufacturer was charged with violating the False Claims Act, a law that prohibits any person from making a false or fraudulent claim for payment from the U.S. government. The lawsuit accused Pfizer of causing substantial losses to federal and state governments as a result of Medicaid payments for off-label usage of Neurontin based on fraudulent claims. In May 2004, Pfizer pleaded guilty to the civil and criminal charges and agreed to pay penalties totaling $430 million: a federal criminal fine of $240 million, federal civil liabilities of $152 million, and state civil liabilities of $38 million.

In a statement on the outcome of this lawsuit, the Department of Justice expressed its commitment:

> to rooting out and prosecuting healthcare fraud. It is of paramount importance that the Department use every legal tool at its disposal to assure the health and safety of the consumers of America's healthcare system, and to pursue companies and individuals that steal from the taxpayers and inflict suffering on patients and families. The Department's commitment to effective healthcare fraud enforcement is driven by a mandate that wrongdoers be brought to justice, to deter conduct which threatens the safety and welfare of all Americans, and the need to protect the resources of the Medicare Trust Fund, state Medicaid programs, and other government health programs.

The introduction of the Medicare prescription drug benefit beginning January 2006 will expand the impact of the False Claims Act on fraudulent off-label marketing.

Pharmaceutical companies also face the threat of litigation instigated by private insurers. In March 2006, a group of union and employer insurance funds simultaneously filed lawsuits against Pfizer in the U.S. District Court for the District of New Jersey and in federal courts in Illinois, Ohio, Indiana, New York, and Florida for improper off-label marketing of Lipitor (atorvastatin). The complaint seeks to secure class-action certification on behalf of health and welfare funds and third-party payers, including Medicaid plans. Managed care organizations also stand to benefit from this class action, but none had joined at the time the lawsuits were filed. The lawsuits allege that, from January 2002 onward, Pfizer promoted the use of Lipitor beyond the terms of the drug's label. The plaintiffs assert that Pfizer's "Get to Goal", campaign encouraged physicians to prescribe Lipitor to low-risk patients who, according to the Adult Treatment Panel III (ATP III) guidelines of the National Cholesterol Education Panel quoted on the drug's label, did not require such therapy. The lawyers representing the plaintiffs suggest that 14.6 million dyslipidemic patients fall into this low-risk category and estimate that the cost of unnecessary Lipitor prescriptions may exceed $800 million per year. In addition, the lawyers plan to include the costs of regular liver function tests (a requirement for patients on statin therapy) in their claims for restitution. The lawsuits contend that Pfizer was able to conduct this allegedly illegal promotional campaign because managed care organizations rarely checked the usage of Lipitor, a drug that had preferred brand status on most formularies. If successful, this litigation would set a precedent that could severely restrict manufacturers' marketing freedom.

Reimbursement

Patients in the United States receive prescription drug benefits from three main sources: Medicare, Medicaid, and private insurers. Policies on coverage of off-label prescribing vary enormously from one payer to another.

Medicare

Medicare, established in 1965, is a federal program that provides basic healthcare coverage to the U.S. population aged 65 or older, some disabled people, and patients with end-stage renal disease. In 2004, 85% of the total population of 42 million Medicare beneficiaries were aged 65 or older.

Medicare now comprises four distinct programs, three of which (Parts B, C, and D) are generally optional and require the payment of premiums. Beneficiaries are automatically enrolled in Medicare Part A, a program that covers inpatient expenses, including medicines. Part B covers outpatient drugs that are not usually self-administered (e.g., intravenous infusions, intramuscular injections). Oral drugs are excluded from Part B coverage, with the exception of products that also have a parenteral dosage form that would be reimbursed if administered by a physician. Part C, more commonly known as Medicare Advantage (previously Medicare + Choice), offers beneficiaries a wider range of healthcare options, including HMOs and other managed care plans, private fee-for-service plans, and medical savings accounts. The majority of Medicare Part C enrollees receive some level of prescription drug benefits. Beginning January 1, 2006, many Medicare beneficiaries are receiving outpatient prescription drug benefits through Medicare Part D. As of April 3, 2006, approximately 27 million beneficiaries were receiving Medicare Part D benefits, either through automatic enrollment (e.g., as Medicaid beneficiaries or members of an employer-sponsored health plan subsidized by Medicare) or by voluntarily signing up for the drug benefit.

In 1991, the U.S. General Accounting Office (GAO; now renamed the Government Accountability Office) published a report titled *Off-Label Drugs: Reimbursement Policies Constrain Physicians in Their Choice of Cancer Therapies*. The authors noted that, "although respondents reported reimbursement problems with many third-party payers, the insurer most frequently cited was Medicare." In an attempt to remedy this situation, the Omnibus Budget Reconciliation Act of 1993 introduced a legal requirement for Medicare to reimburse off-label prescribing that is supported by citations in any of three compendia: *American Hospital Formulary Service Drug Information* (AHFSDI), *United States Pharmacopoeia Drug Information* (USPDI), or the American Medical Association's *Drug Evaluation* (merged into USPDI in 1996). In addition, the act allows Medicare carriers to make local coverage decisions on off-label reimbursement based on supportive clinical evidence published in peer-reviewed medical journals. Data from at least two Phase II clinical trials conducted in different centers are required to support off-label use, but Phase III trial results carry greater weight.

To determine how the coverage of off-label usage by both Medicare and private payers affects U.S. oncologists' prescribing behavior, in 2005, the Association of Community Cancer Centers (ACCC), the Biotechnology Industry Organization (BIO), and the Pharmaceutical Research and Manufacturers of America (PhRMA) jointly commissioned a survey from Covance, a leading drug development service company (see *Off-Label Use of Anticancer Therapies*, 2006). Covance interviewed 28 oncologists and 12 oncology practice managers. Respondents identified more than 50 physician-administered therapies that are used off-label. For guidance in off-label prescribing, physicians rely most heavily on peer-reviewed literature (cited by 25 of 28 oncologists), drug compendia (mentioned by 17 oncologists), and manufacturer hotlines and case reports (each cited by seven oncologists). However, reimbursement restrictions deter many oncologists from prescribing cancer therapies off label, particularly to Medicare patients. Fifteen oncologists (54%) stated that Medicare policies on off-label usage frequently or very frequently interfered with their clinical decision making. By comparison, just eight oncologists (29%) indicated that private payers' policies on off-label usage frequently or very frequently interfered with their clinical decision making.

One participant in Covance's survey commented that "Medicare will deny every off-label indication that is not listed in the two compendia [i.e., AHFSDI, USPDI]. So, at this point, I am only using those products off-label for those indications that are listed in the compendia." The study notes that "listings in recognized compendia are outdated, incomplete, and may not include references to potential off-label uses of new drugs that may be supported by other published clinical evidence."

Most cancer therapies remain covered by Medicare Part B, but orally administered antineoplastic drugs that are not also available in a parenteral dosage form are now covered by Part D. Medicare prescription drug plans (PDPs) must cover "all or substantially all" antineoplastics (except for agents covered by Medicare Part B), antidepressants, antipsychotics, anticonvulsants, immunosuppressants, and HIV/AIDS therapies. However, coverage of off-label prescribing is more restrictive under Part D than Part B. Off-label uses are eligible for reimbursement under Medicare Part D only if they are supported by one or more of three compendia (i.e., AHFSDI, USPDI, and Drugdex); evidence from peer-reviewed literature alone is not adequate for Medicare Part D coverage of off-label prescribing. PDPs may use cost-containment measures (e.g., increased copayments, prior authorization, step therapy protocols) to control off-label prescribing.

Medicaid

Medicaid is a joint federal/state program that provides healthcare coverage to low-income residents of the United States. The Medicaid population increased from 33.2 million as of June 30, 1996, to 44.4 million as of June 30, 2004 (the most recent year for which data are available). The percentage of Medicaid beneficiaries enrolled in managed care health plans grew from 40.1% in 1996 to 60.7% in 2004.

States are not legally bound to offer Medicaid prescription drug benefits, but all states do offer coverage of outpatient medicines to at least some of their Medicaid beneficiaries. The Congressional Research Service reports that, in 2004, Medicaid payments for outpatient prescription drugs totaled $30.4 billion (net of the federal rebates that manufacturers are required to pay to the Medicaid program). State Medicaid administrations develop their own formularies for fee-for-service beneficiaries, but they are required to cover nonformulary drugs subject to a prior authorization process and to cover all drugs manufactured by companies that have signed federal rebate agreements with the secretary of health and human services. Managed care organizations that offer Medicaid health plans are generally required to cover all drugs included in state Medicaid formularies.

States may use prior authorization procedures to control the prescription of some or all medicines to Medicaid beneficiaries. Congress granted states this power to enable them to control the use of drugs that have narrow labeling or significant potential for abuse. According to a survey conducted by the National Pharmaceutical Council (NPC) in 2004, every state except Arizona operates some form of prior authorization within its Medicaid program. Thirty-nine states provided the NPC with data on the percentage of prior authorization requests that they granted, ranging from 27% in Nebraska to 100% in New York and South Dakota, with a national mean of 81% and a median value of 82%. Off-label usage is likely to be subject to prior authorization in most cases. Decisions on prior authorization requests are generally based on medical necessity.

In addition, all state Medicaid administrations are required to establish a drug utilization review (DUR) program to improve the quality of patient care and to contain costs. Both prospective and retrospective DUR procedures are used to combat inappropriate prescribing practices.

Private Insurers

Private insurers vary enormously in their policies on reimbursement of off-label prescribing, and published research on this subject is extremely limited. Coverage of off-label usage may be subject to one or more of the following conditions:

- The prescribed drug is FDA-approved and listed on the payer's formulary.
- The patient is diagnosed with a life-threatening or otherwise very serious disease.
- The risk-benefit ratio of prescribing the drug for an unlicensed indication justifies this usage.
- Evidence of efficacy is available in designated compendia (e.g., AHFSDI, USPDI) or peer-reviewed journals.
- Therapies approved for the indicated disease are not available, are deemed inappropriate for the patient, or have been tried and found ineffective.
- The payer's medical director approves the off-label usage.

FRANCE

Physicians are permitted to prescribe off label in France but must overcome some substantial hurdles. Clinicians must assume responsibility for the medical consequences of prescribing a drug for an unlicensed indication and could face criminal charges in the event that such a decision is judged to have harmed a patient. Prescribers must also inform the patient of the risks of using the proposed drug. Outpatient prescriptions for off-label indications are generally not reimbursed by the French social security system – a significant deterrent to this practice. Consequently, physicians must also notify their patients that they (the patients) would have to pay the full cost of medications prescribed off label. The letters "NR," for *non remboursable* (not reimbursable), must be written on all off-label prescriptions.

In addition, the French healthcare system imposes strict limits on the prescribing of certain drugs. Since 1993, physicians in France have been subject to *références médicales opposables* (RMOs; medical guidelines) on the appropriate use of a wide range of common medical procedures and treatments. Separate lists exist for general practitioners and specialists. Prescribers are expected to mark both patient records and prescription forms with either "R" for *référence* to show that they are complying with the guidelines or "HR" for *hors référence* (outside the guidelines) for therapies that are not subject to RMOs. Social security medical advisers conduct spot checks on physician compliance with RMOs, and prescribers who persistently flout the guidelines may face fines or even exclusion from working within the national healthcare system.

In some cases, the government limits reimbursement to specific indications or populations. For example, influenza vaccine is reimbursed only for patients older than age 65, and acetylcholinesterase inhibitors are covered only for Alzheimer's disease sufferers who satisfy strict eligibility criteria.

In 1994, the French government introduced a measure that is unique in Europe: the *autorisation temporaire d'utilisation* (ATU; temporary authorization for use) for medicines that treat serious or rare diseases for which no appropriate registered therapy is available. AFSSAPS grants an ATU for one year. Drugs qualify for an *ATU de cohorte* (group temporary authorization for use) if they have strong evidence to support their efficacy and safety. Alternatively, an *ATU nominative* (individual temporary authorization for use) can be issued if a physician assumes responsibility for prescribing a given drug to a designated patient. In 2000, approximately 60,000 patients were treated with a range of 35 group temporary authorizations for use, and about 27,000 patients were treated with a total of 213 individual temporary authorizations for use. In 2004, approximately 24,000 patients were treated with more than 180 individual temporary authorizations for use (details on the number of group temporary authorizations for use granted in 2004 are not available).

GERMANY

Off-label prescribing has been the subject of considerable controversy in Germany in recent years. Several landmark court cases, together with decisions by official bodies that formulate national healthcare policy, have progressively defined the circumstances in which it is acceptable for physicians to prescribe off label.

A judgment by the *Bundessozialgericht* (Federal Social Court) on March 19, 2002, first focused attention on the issue of off-label prescribing. The case concerned the use of intravenous immunoglobulin to treat visual impairment suffered by a female patient as a side effect of cortisone therapy for multiple sclerosis. The woman's health insurance fund had refused to reimburse the immunoglobulin therapy, arguing that the efficacy of this treatment was unproven. The court ruled that the health insurance fund was not obliged to cover off-label prescribing in this case but defined three circumstances in which statutory health insurance funds should be required to reimburse off-label therapy:

- The disease to be treated is a condition that is life threatening or causes chronic impairment of quality of life.
- No other therapy is available.
- There is reasonable evidence that the treatment in question could achieve therapeutic success (remedial or palliative). Such evidence could take one of two forms:
  1. The manufacturer has already applied for an extension of the drug's label for the intended indication and the results of a controlled Phase III clinical trial (using standard therapy or placebo as the comparator) have been published and have demonstrated clinically relevant efficacy and acceptable risks.
  2. Published data, gathered outside the scope of a licensing application, provide reliable, scientifically verifiable evidence of the quality and efficacy of the drug in its new indication, thereby creating a consensus in the relevant community of experts on the proposed new usage.

If all three of these conditions are satisfied, health insurance funds are obliged to reimburse off-label prescribing.

In December 2005, the *Bundesverfassungsgericht* (Federal Constitutional Court) strengthened the grounds for off-label prescribing. The court ruled that it is unlawful to refuse reimbursement of an alternative therapy to patients who have a life-threatening disease for which no approved treatments are available, as long as the alternative offers at least some prospect of a cure or an appreciable effect on the course of the disease. Given that the overwhelming majority of residents in Germany are legally obliged to enroll in – and contribute to – the statutory health insurance system, the court reasoned that they should not be forced to fund their own treatment if they develop a serious disease. This ruling is likely to have an impact not only on physicians' freedom to prescribe off label but also on the future development of treatment guidelines and on the composition of reference pricing groups. Disease severity and the range of available therapies will exercise an increased influence on decision making in the future.

The German government has sought to rationalize off-label prescribing. In September 2002, the Ministry of Health established the *Expertengruppe Off-Label* (Off-Label Expert Group) within the *Bundesinstitut für Arzneimittel und Medizinprodukte* (BfArM; Federal Institute for Medicines and Medical Devices), with a brief to focus on oncology. In August 2005, the ministry created additional expert groups to evaluate off-label prescribing in neurology/psychiatry and infectious disease (with an emphasis on HIV/AIDS). The original group has been criticized for being too slow in its deliberations, but it has recently published decisions on the off-label use of three cancer therapies. The group endorsed reimbursement for the use of 5-fluorouracil as adjuvant therapy in breast cancer but opposed reimbursement of irinotecan for small-cell lung cancer and inhaled interleukin-2 for metastatic renal cell carcinoma.

Since 2004, the *Gemeinsamer Bundesausschuß der Ärzte, Zahnärzte, Krankenhäuser und Krankenkassen* (GBA; Joint Federal Committee of Physicians, Dentists, Hospitals, and Health Insurance Funds) has been responsible for deciding whether a given therapy should be reimbursed by the *Gesetzliche Krankenversicherung* (GKV; statutory health insurance) system. The GBA's reimbursement decisions are binding on all physicians contracted to the GKV and on all statutory health insurance funds. In April 2006, the GBA identified three prerequisites for off-label prescribing:

- An off-label indication should be positively assessed by one of the aforementioned expert groups. Their evaluations form the basis of the GBA's subsequent appraisal of drugs.
- The manufacturer should confirm the appropriateness of off-label usage of a drug.
- Drugs that meet the two preceding requirements will be added to a new appendix (9A) to the official pharmaceutical guidelines. Medicines that are not judged suitable for off-label usage – on clinical or economic grounds – will be added to appendix 9B of the official pharmaceutical guidelines.

Physicians can face substantial fines for improper off-label prescribing. For example, in July 2005, the *Sozialgericht Berlin*

(Berlin Social Court) ordered a cardiothoracic surgeon to refund a sum of €53,000 ($65,877) to a statutory health insurance fund as a penalty for improper off-label prescribing (the U.S. dollar-to-euro exchange rate used in this chapter is the 2005 average rate [i.e., $1 = €0.80453]). In 1999, the surgeon had prescribed a total of 11 courses of iloprost (Schering AG's Ilomedin) to a patient diagnosed with advanced chronic obstructive pulmonary disease and secondary pulmonary hypertension. At that time, the drug was approved in Germany only for the treatment by intravenous administration of advanced thromboangiitis obliterans (Buerger's disease). Inhaled iloprost (Schering AG's Ventavis) was approved for advanced pulmonary hypertension in Germany only in September 2003, but the surgeon considered inhaled iloprost to be the best therapy available to his patient in 1999. This decision was based on evidence from numerous articles in medical literature. However, the patient's health insurance fund objected to this off-label prescription on the grounds that, in the absence of any Phase III clinical trial data, the efficacy of this treatment for pulmonary hypertension was unproven and the GKV was under no obligation to reimburse the treatment. The court ruled against the surgeon, arguing that physicians working under contract to the GKV automatically oblige health insurance funds to reimburse treatments they prescribe. In the event that physicians prescribe therapies that should not be covered, they may be required to refund part of the cost of such treatment to health insurance funds. This threat is likely to be a powerful deterrent to unrestrained off-label prescribing in Germany.

ITALY

The *Agenzia Italiana del Farmaco* (AIFA; Italian Medicines Agency), established in 2004, oversees all aspects of Italy's national pharmaceutical policy, including spending on prescription drugs. Among the measures it employs to control pharmaceutical expenditures are *note limitative* (restrictive notes), which impose strict conditions on the use of certain drugs. Drugs subject to such restrictive notes are typically limited to specific indications, patient subpopulations, or care settings. Physicians are required to write the reference number of any applicable restrictive note next to the product name. Physicians who do not comply with this system may, in theory, have to repay the cost of any drugs that they have prescribed inappropriately; however, this sanction is seldom imposed.

Off-label prescribing is also strictly controlled in Italy, and the following conditions must be satisfied:

- The physician assumes direct responsibility for prescribing the drug for an unlicensed use.
- The drug is prescribed to an individual patient and only in the absence of therapeutic alternatives.
- Usage is outside clinical trials or for a patient who is not eligible for a trial.
- Off-label usage is supported by evidence published in accredited international scientific journals.
- The patient is provided with detailed information on the off-label usage and gives informed consent to the treatment.
- The method of prescription allows for the prescribing physician to be identified.

The *Servizio Sanitario Nazionale* (SSN; National Health Service) generally reimburses off-label prescriptions only if they are provided by means of a clinical trial.

UNITED KINGDOM

Prescribing medicines off label is, in theory, relatively straightforward in the United Kingdom. The *British National Formulary* (BNF) states that "unlicensed use of medicines becomes necessary if the clinical need cannot be met by licensed medicines; such use should be supported by appropriate evidence and experience." The BNF warns physicians that "prescribing medicines outside the recommendations of their marketing authorisation alters (and probably increases) the doctor's professional responsibility."

In practice, however, off-label prescribing can be extremely difficult and inconsistent in the U.K. National Health Service (NHS). Primary care trusts (PCTs), the organizations that control 75% of the NHS budget, have a high degree of autonomy in determining both hospital and primary care prescribing policies in their respective catchment areas (however, PCTs in England and Wales are required to fund all therapies that have been approved by the National Institute for Health and Clinical Excellence [NICE]). Many PCTs refuse to fund off-label treatment, especially for new or risky therapeutic approaches. The typical rationale for such decisions is that it would be unethical to endorse unlicensed drug usage, but critics suggest that PCT decision makers are motivated more by financial than ethical considerations: providing wider access to new therapies – especially high-priced biologic treatments for cancer and other severe or life-threatening diseases – would substantially increase their pharmaceutical expenditures. PCTs' varying policies on off-label prescribing have contributed to the so-called postcode lottery – geographic inequalities in access to care. It is theoretically possible for one person to receive coverage for a treatment while a neighbor living in a different PCT catchment area is denied reimbursement for the same therapy.

Some patients have protested this situation by taking legal action against their local PCTs. For instance, in recent months, the media has given extensive coverage to several lawsuits initiated by breast cancer patients who have been denied access to trastuzumab (Roche's Herceptin) for the treatment of early-stage human epidermal growth factor receptor 2 (HER2)-positive breast cancer. Notwithstanding the fact that trastuzumab was not yet approved for early-stage HER2-positive breast cancer, in November 2005, the Department of Health indicated that PCTs should fund the drug for this indication on a case-by-case basis. Jane Kennedy, a junior health minister, went even further, suggesting that patients denied access to new cancer therapies should consider legal action against their PCTs if the patients believe that the refusal of treatment is "inappropriate." If widely heeded, this advice could stimulate a substantial increase in litigation against the NHS and in off-label prescribing in the United Kingdom.

JAPAN

The Japanese public health insurance system reimburses medicines only if they are prescribed for approved indications. Indeed, patients who receive off-label therapy or treatment with drugs that are not yet approved in Japan may forfeit their right to reimbursement for all treatments for the prescribed indication, not just for the off-label or unregistered therapy. This penalty can impose a heavy financial burden on patients. Consequently, Japanese physicians tend to avoid off-label prescribing.

These prescribing restrictions present a particularly severe challenge in oncology. Many treatment options that are accepted as standard practice in the United States and Europe are not yet available in Japan. Manufacturers might be expected to pursue approval for additional indications for their drugs, but many companies appear content with the status quo. Although the public health insurance system forbids off-label reimbursement, individual institutions or payers may cover off-label prescribing to cancer patients on an ad hoc basis. Consequently, manufacturers have not been strongly motivated to spend time, energy, and money on pursuing additional indications for their oncology drugs.

To promote the approval of oncology drugs for broader indications, the Ministry of Health, Labor, and Welfare (MHLW) established the *Koganzai Heiyo Ryohoni Kansuru Kentokai* (Committee for Combination Therapy with Anticancer Drugs) in December 2003. Considering suggestions from academic societies and/or patients' groups, a working group identifies drugs that could be used in additional indications and gathers evidence on the efficacy and safety of these drugs from the literature and other sources. The group then discusses the data with the relevant company. The *Yakuji Shokuhin Eisei Shingikai* (Council on Drugs and Food Sanitation [CDFS]) also evaluates the data that have been gathered; if it decides in favor of additional indications, the MHLW asks the manufacturer to submit an application for the new indications.

These applications receive priority review, which takes approximately four months. Approval, if granted, is conditional on post-marketing safety measures. Drugs approved by this procedure are eligible for reimbursement under the aforementioned specified medical care coverage provision that covers all medical costs except the cost of the drug itself. This coverage is available from the time a candidate drug receives its preliminary evaluation from the CDFS.

Of 61 therapies that have been reviewed for use in additional indications, 7 proposed therapies had already reached an advanced stage in the regular approval process and therefore completed that process, and 20 therapies in great demand have undergone the new procedure for approval of additional indications. Table 4.5 shows that, by September 2005, all 20 of these therapies had been approved for additional indication(s). The remaining therapies were not judged to be in great demand and therefore were not approved through this framework. After completing its evaluation of the 20 therapies in great demand, the committee was dissolved in February 2005.

The committee is generally considered to have fulfilled its role to improve the status of off-label use of anticancer drugs. Some officers of the MHLW have suggested that the framework for off-label use drugs could continue after the dissolution of the committee, but no official announcement on future policy for off-label use of oncology agents has been made. Based on the perceived success of the Committee for Combination Therapy with Anticancer Drugs, we believe that the MHLW could set up a similar ad hoc committee in the future to handle off-label issues as they arise.

Table 4.5 Oncology Drugs Approved for Additional Indications in Japan

Drug	*Additional Indication*	*Date of Approval*
Pamidronate	Breast cancer	November 2004
Doxorubicin	Breast cancer	February 2005
Ifosfamide	Soft tissue and bone sarcomas	February 2005
Doxorubicin	Soft tissue and bone sarcomas	February 2005
Ifosfamide/doxorubicin	Soft tissue and bone sarcomas	February 2005
Doxorubicin	Solid tumors of childhood	February 2005
Etoposide	Solid tumors of childhood	February 2005
Cisplatin	Osteosarcoma	February 2005
Doxorubicin/cisplatin (AP)	Endometrial cancer	February 2005
Vincristine, doxorubicin, dexamethazone (VAD)	Multiple myeloma	February 2005
5-fluorouracil (5-FU) infusion	Head and neck cancer	February 2005
Procarbazine	Malignant astrocytoma/ oligodendroglioma	February 2005
Vincristine	Malignant astrocytoma/ oligodendroglioma	February 2005
Infusional 5-FU/leucovorin (l-LV)	Colorectal cancer	February 2005
Cyclophosphamide	Breast cancer	September 2005
Cisplatin	Malignant lymphoma	September 2005
Cisplatin	Solid tumors of childhood	September 2005
Carboplatin	Solid tumors of childhood	September 2005
Actinomycin-D	Solid tumors of childhood	September 2005
Epirubicin/cyclophosphamide (EC, CEF)	Breast cancer	September 2005
Dexamethasone	Chemotherapy-induced nausea and vomiting	September 2005

OUTLOOK AND IMPLICATIONS FOR THE PHARMACEUTICAL INDUSTRY

Off-label prescribing has enormous untapped clinical potential, but the regulatory and reimbursement environment for this practice does not appear promising. The definition of new diseases and the segmentation of established disorders have contributed to the growth of off-label prescribing in recent years. Furthermore, the launch of numerous biologics has enlarged the scope for off-label therapy, given that these agents frequently have a very wide range of possible uses. However, the potentially enormous cost of extensive off-label prescribing motivates payers to take action to curb this practice; these measures are predominantly targeted at manufacturers and prescribers.

Off-label marketing by pharmaceutical companies is likely to become increasingly hazardous, especially in the United States. Public and private payers have demonstrated their determination to limit this activity, particularly if it relates to completely unfounded uses for medicines, and further litigation can be expected. The potentially enormous rewards that the False Claims Act offers whistleblowers could incentivize more employees of pharmaceutical companies to report illegal marketing activities. For example, David Franklin received a payment of $26.6 million for alerting the authorities to Warner-Lambert's illicit promotion of Neurontin. In the future, manufacturers will engage in questionable off-label marketing practices at their peril. Nevertheless, the financial rewards of off-label promotion are undeniably enticing. Neurontin's peak-year off-label sales dwarfed the $430 million in fines imposed on Pfizer. Companies might conclude that the monetary benefits amply outweigh the possible costs of off-label marketing. On the other hand, the damage done to an individual company's reputation from a lost lawsuit, and to the image of the pharmaceutical industry if such events become commonplace, is much more difficult to calculate.

In many countries, pharmaceutical pricing and reimbursement terms are increasingly influenced by health economic calculations, including detailed projections of the potential drug-treated populations for approved indications. If extensive off-label usage stimulates sales far in excess of original forecasts, manufacturers may be forced to cut their prices. Regulatory authorities would undoubtedly like manufacturers to conduct clinical trials for major new indications for medicines, but the cost of such research will remain a substantial obstacle.

Payers will also try to exercise stricter control over physicians' behavior, for example, by restricting the type of evidence that can be used to justify off-label prescribing. As discussed earlier, physicians generally regard peer-reviewed journals as the most useful source of guidance on off-label therapy, but the Medicare Part D rules preclude off-label prescribing that is based solely on this type of evidence. Many prescribers are concerned that relying entirely on several compendia for information on off-label therapy could severely hamper their clinical options. Compendia may not be comprehensive, and they can rapidly become dated. The German solution – commissioning expert groups to assess off-label prescribing in key therapeutic areas – may produce more robust results but is likely to be time consuming and highly bureaucratic.

Cost-containment measures will be employed to limit off-label therapy. Prior authorization is likely to remain the most important method of control, complemented by DUR or prescribing audits. The growth of computerized prescribing will help payers in their efforts to enforce limits on off-label prescribing and to monitor and manage physicians who disregard these restrictions.

Physicians are concerned about the liability risks of off-label prescribing, but they must also pay increasing attention to the financial costs of this practice. Their patients may face the prospect of paying the full cost of drugs prescribed off label – a burden that many patients would struggle to bear, particularly if prescribed costly biologics. Physicians in some countries might also have to pay a high price for inappropriate off-label prescribing, namely substantial refunds. These sanctions already exist in Germany and Italy, and physician accountability can be expected to grow in other countries too.

As a consequence of all these pressures, the use of medicines for unapproved indications will become more difficult. Ultimately, off-label prescribing may be limited to severe diseases and/or conditions that lack effective licensed therapies.

REFERENCES

Barbui C, et al. Prescribing second-generation antipsychotics and the evolving standard of care in Italy. *Pharmacopsychiatry*, 2002;35(6): 239–243.

Chen H, et al. An epidemiological investigation of off-label anticonvulsant drug use in the Georgia Medicaid population. *Pharmacoepidemiology* and Drug Safety, 2005;14(9):629–638.

Hodgson R, Belgamwar R. Off-label prescribing by psychiatrists. *Psychiatric Bulletin*, 2006;30:55–57.

Off-Label Use of Anticancer Therapies: Physician Prescribing Trends and the Impact of Payer Coverage Policy. www.bio.org/speeches/pubs/ CovanceReport.pdf. Accessed April 20, 2006.

Radley DC, et al. Off-label prescribing among office-based physicians. Archives of *Internal Medicine*, 2006;166:1021–1026.

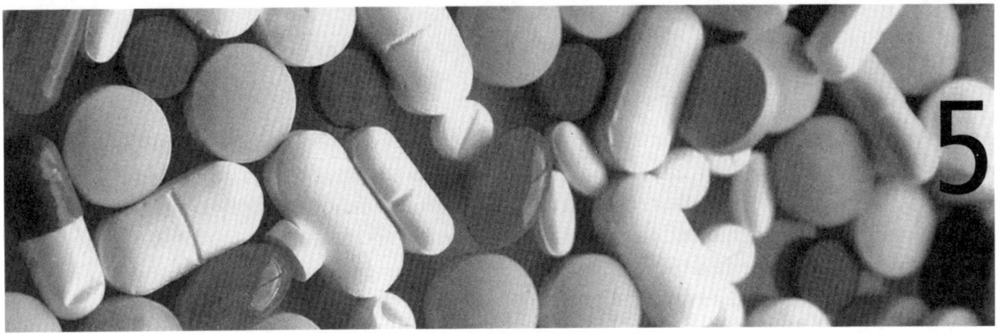

Pricing and Reimbursement Issues in Neurology

INTRODUCTION

Neurological disorders are common and highly disabling conditions that will impose a growing burden on aging societies in industrialized nations. We estimate that, in the United States, France, Germany, Italy, Spain, the United Kingdom, and Japan alone, the number of people afflicted with Alzheimer's disease, epilepsy, multiple sclerosis, and Parkinson's disease will increase from approximately 15 million in 2005 to 17 million in 2015. Spending on drug therapies for these four disorders will grow even faster, increasing from $11 billion in 2005 to $18 billion in 2015.

The size of this market is attributable in part to high drug prices, especially in the United States. The rising cost of routine polytherapy and long-term use of these drugs has prompted payers to impose increasingly stringent cost-containment measures (e.g., price controls, prescribing budgets, formulary restrictions, increased cost-sharing). To secure favorable pricing and reimbursement terms in the future, manufacturers will need to demonstrate that their drugs offer significant advantages over existing therapies.

This chapter addresses key pricing and reimbursement issues in four major neurological drug classes – dementia therapies, Parkinson's disease therapies, multiple sclerosis therapies, and antiepileptics – in seven major pharmaceutical markets: the United States, France, Germany, Italy, Spain, the United Kingdom, and Japan. We begin with an analysis of the prices of select branded and generic agents within the aforementioned drug classes. We then examine the reimbursement environment, in general terms and with specific reference to the four drug classes, in each of the markets under review. We conclude with an assessment of the outlook and implications for the manufacturers of neurology drugs.

INTERNATIONAL PRICE COMPARISONS FOR NEUROLOGY DRUGS

Overview

The United States has the highest prices overall of any of the major pharmaceutical markets under study. An analysis of the 2005 ex-manufacturer prices of 150 of the world's best-selling branded drugs found that US prices were, on average, 138% higher than prices in the six other markets under review. In the United States, manufacturers are free to set drug prices in negotiation with third-party payers (the US government does, however, require discounts for certain government-sponsored health insurance programs [e.g., Veterans Affairs, Medicaid]). By comparison, Japan and most European countries exercise strict control over pharmaceutical prices, in many cases comparing a manufacturer's proposed price for a new drug with the prices of existing therapies in their markets and the new agent's price in other countries. Increasingly, price premiums are available only to drugs that are deemed to be innovative. For example, in 2001, edaravone (Mitsubishi Pharma's Radicut), a free-radical scavenger neuroprotectant used in the treatment of acute ischemic stroke, qualified for a 20% "innovativeness" price premium in Japan – only the second drug ever to receive such an accolade in that country, and one of the very few agents ever approved as a neuroprotectant. The price premium for innovativeness stimulated rapid uptake of this drug – a survey of 285 medical institutions found that 66% had adopted it by 2002 – but safety concerns and new contraindications have since eroded sales.

Prices for neurology drugs vary widely across the major markets. Table 5.1 lists the international nonproprietary names, brand names, and manufacturers of key drugs in the four classes covered in our analysis. Table 5.2 shows the ex-manufacturer prices of these drugs in Europe and Japan as a percentage of the equivalent US prices. European prices for the neurology drugs in our survey averaged 59% of US prices for branded products and 169% of US prices for the lowest-priced generics. The very high average price of generic neurology drugs in Europe as a percentage of US prices reflects the speed of generic price erosion in the United States. Japanese prices averaged 93% of US prices for branded products and 141% of US prices for generics, but it is important to bear in

Table 5.1 Brand Names and Marketing Companies of Select Neurology Drugs

	Brand Name(s)	*Marketing Companies*
Dementia therapies		
Donepezil	Aricept	Eisai, Pfizer
Rivastigmine	Exelon, Prometax	Novartis, Sigma Tau
Galantamine	Reminyl, Razadyne	Shire Pharmaceuticals, Janssen-Cilag
Memantine	Axura, Ebixa, Namenda	Merz, Lundbeck, Forest Laboratories
Parkinson's disease therapies		
Carbidopa/levodopa	Sinemet, generics	Bristol-Myers Squibb, multisource
Cabergoline	Dostinex, generics	Pfizer, multisource
Pramipexole	Mirapex	Boehringer Ingelheim
Ropinirole	Requip	GlaxoSmithKline
Pergolide	Permax, generics	Eli Lilly, multisource
Entacapone	Comtan	Novartis
Carbidopa/levodopa/ entacapone	Stalevo	Novartis
Selegiline	Eldepryl, generics	Somerset Pharmaceuticals, multisource
Multiple sclerosis therapies		
Interferon-beta-1b	Betaseron, Betaferon	Schering AG
Interferon-beta-1a	Avonex	Biogen Idec
Interferon-beta-1a	Rebif	Serono
Glatiramer acetate	Copaxone	Teva
Antiepileptic Agents		
Phenytoin	Dilantin, generics	Pfizer, multisource
Valproic acid	Depakene, generics	Abbott Laboratories, multisource
Gabapentin	Neurontin, generics	Pfizer, multisource
Lamotrigine	Lamictal, generics	GlaxoSmithKline, multisource
Carbamazepine	Tegretol, Carbatrol, generics	Novartis, Shire, multisource
Levetiracetam	Keppra	UCB Pharma
Pregabalin	Lyrica	Pfizer
Topiramate	Topamax	Ortho-McNeil Pharmaceutical

Note: This list does not cover every brand name in all markets

Table 5.2 Exmanufacturer Prices of Select Neurology Drugs in Europe and Japan as a Percentage of the US Price, 2005

	Dosage	*France*	*Germany*	*Italy*	*Spain*	*United Kingdom*	*European Average*	*Japan*
Dementia therapies								
Donepezil	5 mg	86	82	64	69	92	79	91
Rivastigmine	3 mg	78	73	61	62	86	72	N.A.
Galantamine	8 mg	74	97	65	71	97	81	N.A.
Memantine	10 mg	98	92	93	96	107	97	N.A.
Parkinson's disease therapies								
Carbidopa/levodopa (brand)	25–100 mg[a]	13	23	11	15	25	17	48
Carbidopa/levodopa (generic)	25–100 mg[a]	38	113	81	81[b]	106	84	69
Cabergoline (brand)	0.5 mg	17	27	18	15	21	20	N.A.
Pramipexole	0.18 mg[c]	35	75	39	35	89	55	137
Ropinirole	1 mg	38	85	29	37	67	51	N.A.
Pergolide (brand)	0.25 mg	31	44	28	18	46	33	134
Pergolide (generic)	0.25 mg	N.A.	64	N.A	21	37	41	159
Entacapone	200 mg	59	74	55	55	60	61	N.A.
Carbidopa/levodopa/ entacapone	25–100–200 mg	54	80	N.A	57	64	51	N.A.
Selegiline (brand)	5 mg[d]	26	20	12	16	12	17	125
Selegiline (generic)	5 mg	364	382	230	245	173	279	N.A.
Multiple sclerosis therapies								
Interferon-beta-1b	0.3 mg[e]	108	125	99	111	91	107	123
Interferon-beta-1a (Avonex)	30 μg	101	116	91	102	102	103	N.A.
Interferon-beta-1a (Rebif)	44 μg	85	121	101	117	109	107	N.A.
Glatiramer acetate	20 mg	131	141	114	129	113	127	N.A.
Antiepileptic agents								
Phenytoin (brand)	100 mg	16	16	34	13	23	20	N.A.
Phenytoin (generic)	100 mg	N.A.	31	N.A	23	162	72	N.A.
Valproic acid (brand)	250 mg[f]	6	10	5	7	6	7	10
Valproic acid (generic)	250 mg	54	100	62	N.A.	77	73	38
Gabapentin (brand)	300 mg	54	50	33	43	76	51	N.A.
Gabapentin (generic)	300 mg	318	436	291	309	745	420	N.A.
Lamotrigine (brand)	25 mg	15	22	14	14	21	17	N.A.
Lamotrigine (generic)	25 mg	N.A.	5	N.A	13	23	13	N.A.
Carbamazepine (brand)	200 mg	45	39	29	19	39	34	35
Carbamazepine (generic)	200 mg	333	300	200	167	300	260	267
Levetiracetam	500 mg	66	84	63	69	72	71	N.A.
Pregabalin	75 mg	61	81	51	53	116	72	N.A.
Topiramate	50 mg	21	47	29	29	33	32	N.A.
Average for all branded drugs		57	71	51	53	67	59	93
Average for all generic drugs		226	189	178	113	212	169	141

[a]10–100 mg in France, 100 mg in Spain and Japan
[b]Controlled-release formulation
[c]0.25 mg in the United States, 0.5 mg in Japan
[d]2.5 mg in Japan
[e]0.25 mg in Germany and Japan
[f]300 mg in Germany, Italy, and Japan
N.A. = Product not available

Notes: Prices relate to standard formulations. Newer reformulations (e.g., liquids, orally disintegrating tablets, extended-release formulations) were not included
Generic prices relate to the lowest-priced product in each market

mind that only 9 of the 24 compounds included in our survey were available in Japan in 2005. The impact of exchange rate movements must also be considered when assessing international prices as a percentage of US prices. From 2001 to 2005, the US dollar depreciated by 28% against the euro, 21% against the pound sterling, and 9% against the Japanese yen (Table 5.3).

Dementia Therapies

Sales of treatments for Alzheimer's disease in the seven major markets totaled almost $2.3 billion in 2005. This market was dominated by three acetylcholinesterase inhibitors (AChEIs) – donepezil (Eisai/Pfizer's Aricept), galantamine (Shire Pharmaceuticals' Reminyl, Janssen Pharmaceutica's Razadyne), and rivastigmine (Novartis's Exelon, Sigma Tau's Prometax) – and the N-methyl-D-aspartate (NMDA) receptor antagonist memantine (Merz's Axura, Lundbeck's Ebixa, Forest Laboratories Namenda). With sales of $2 billion, these four drugs accounted for 90% of the Alzheimer's disease therapy market in 2005.

Figure 5.1 shows the average prices of the three AChEIs and memantine in each market as a percentage of US prices in 2005. European prices averaged 82% and Japanese prices 91% of US prices, although donepezil is the only one of these drugs available in Japan. Italy had the lowest average prices for dementia therapies among the major markets (71% of US average prices), and the United Kingdom had the highest prices outside the United States (96% of US average prices). With sales of $1.2 billion in the major markets, donepezil had a 71% share of the AChEI market in 2005. The drug owed its dominance to several factors: its earlier

Table 5.3 Average Annual Exchange Rates Against the US Dollar, 2001–5

	Euro	*Pound Sterling*	*Yen*
2001	1.11691	0.69434	121.55551
2002	1.06106	0.66641	125.21937
2003	0.88540	0.61229	115.97995
2004	0.80510	0.54604	108.17451
2005	0.80453	0.55004	110.12445

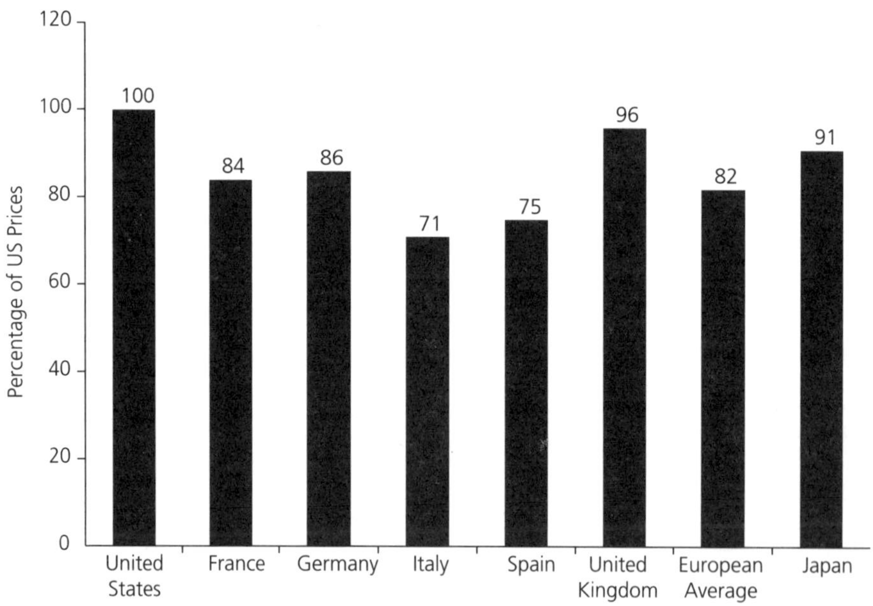

Note: The drugs included are donepezil, galantamine, rivastigmine, and memantine

Figure 5.1 Average Exmanufacturer Prices of Dementia Therapies as a Percentage of US Prices, 2005

launch and greater familiarity, its tolerability, the convenience of once-daily dosing, and its proven safety and efficacy in combination with memantine. In addition, donepezil had a lower daily cost of therapy than the two other AChEIs. The average European price of the three AChEIs was 77% of the average US price, whereas the average European price of memantine was 97% of the US price, and the UK price was 7% higher than the US price (see the sidebar "Memantine: New Life – and a New Price – for an Old Drug").

Memantine: New Life – and a New Price – for an Old Drug

The N-methyl-D-aspartate (NMDA) receptor antagonist memantine was originally launched in Germany in 1982 as a treatment for cognitive disorders. Under the brand name Akatinol, this relatively inexpensive drug gained a loyal following among German physicians and became the most widely prescribed chemical dementia therapy in Germany. (Ginkgo biloba products were, until very recently, by far the most frequently prescribed treatments overall for dementia in Germany.)

In the 1990s, Merz began investigating the potential of memantine in the treatment of moderate-to-severe Alzheimer's disease. The agent was approved for this indication in 2002, and Merz relaunched it under the brand name Axura in Europe. Memantine is also marketed in Europe by Lundbeck (as Ebixa) and in the United States by Forest Laboratories (as Namenda). Merz took advantage of the new indication and the relaunch under a new brand name to set the German price of Axura at roughly twice the level of Akatinol (now withdrawn from the market). However, memantine is priced below donepezil in all countries except Italy, where it is currently not reimbursed (and is therefore subject to free pricing). This pricing policy is intended to avoid economic barriers to the widespread use of this agent.

The experience of memantine offers valuable lessons for other companies that hope to launch an established drug for a new indication. For instance, Grupo Ferrer is developing the membrane-stabilizing agent citicoline (Somazina), a drug first launched as Nicholin by Takeda in Japan in the 1960s. Largely on the strength of unsubstantiated data, many Spanish neurologists have long prescribed this inexpensive drug as a neuroprotectant for acute ischemic stroke. Phase III trials of an oral version of the drug in acute stroke failed in the United States in 2001, but positive outcomes of a meta-analysis of several clinical trials have inspired repeat Phase III testing for stroke in Spain and Portugal. If the new indication is approved, citicoline would join a very limited list of approved neuroprotectants and stroke therapies, possibly allowing Ferrer to negotiate a substantial price increase. However, the company's pricing strategy would need to take account of the fact that citicoline would likely be used in combination with very expensive thrombolytic agents.

Parkinson's Disease Therapies

Sales of Parkinson's disease therapies in the seven major markets totaled approximately $800 million in 2005. Table 5.1 lists the drugs that are most commonly used in the management of this disease, several of which are available in generic form. Figure 5.2 shows average prices of branded versions of these drugs in each market as a percentage of US prices in 2005. European prices averaged 40% of US prices, but ranged from 27% of US prices in Italy to 53% in Germany. It is interesting that Germany has the highest European prices overall for Parkinson's disease therapies despite the reference pricing of several agents: carbidopa/levodopa, pergolide, and selegiline. The price of branded selegiline in Italy and the United Kingdom was just 12% of the US price. By comparison, the UK price of pramipexole (Boehringer Ingelheim's Mirapex) was 89% of the US price. Japanese prices for branded Parkinson's disease therapies averaged 111% of US prices in 2005, although four of the eight drugs in our survey were not available in Japan.

In 2005, three of the Parkinson's disease therapies in our sample were available in generic form in at least some of the major markets: carbidopa/levodopa, pergolide, and selegiline. Figure 5.3 shows average prices of the lowest-priced generic versions of these three agents in each market as a percentage

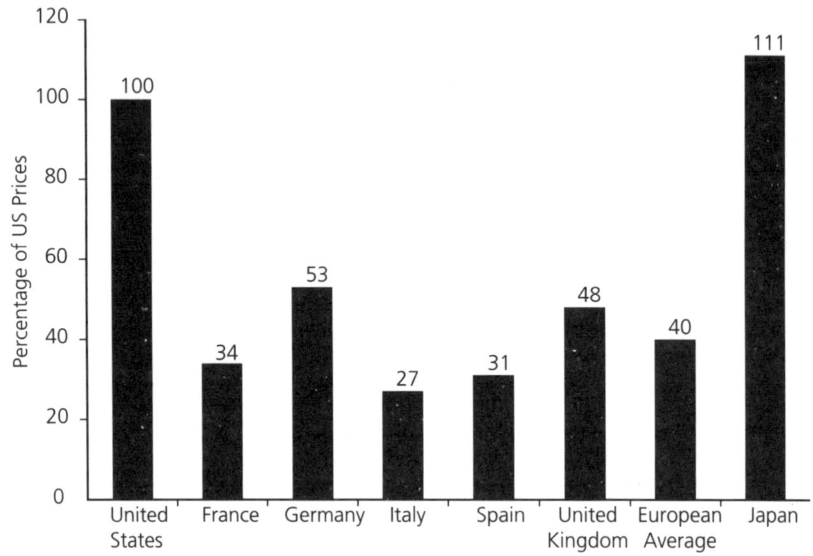

Note: The drugs included are branded versions of cabergoline, carbidopa/levodopa, carbidopa/levodopa/entacapone, entacapone, pergolide, pramipexole, ropinirole, and selegiline

Figure 5.2 Average Exmanufacturer Prices of Select Branded Parkinson's Disease Therapies as a Percentage of US Prices, 2005

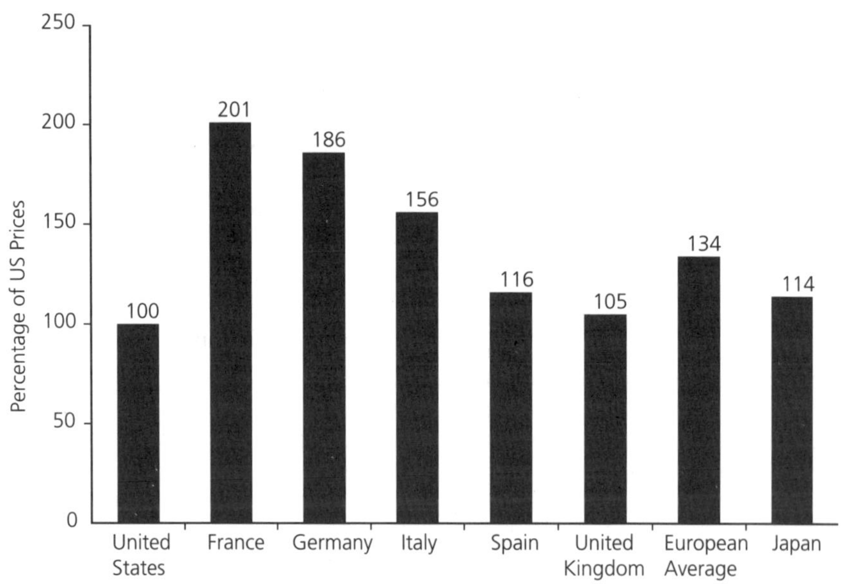

Note: The drugs included are the lowest-priced generic versions of carbidopa/levodopa, pergolide, and selegiline

Figure 5.3 Average Exmanufacturer Prices of Lowest-Priced Generic Versions of Select Parkinson's Disease Therapies as a Percentage of US Prices, 2005

of US prices in 2005. Whereas the European average price of branded Parkinson's disease therapies was just 40% of the US average price, the European average price of the lowest-priced generic drugs in this class was 34% higher than the US average price. Prices of generic Parkinson's disease therapies in France were, on average, double US prices; only the United Kingdom had prices close to US generics prices (a 5% differential). The substantial price differentials between generic prices in most European markets and the United States reflect the much more aggressive price erosion that characterizes the US generics market.

Polytherapy is routine in the management of Parkinson's disease, with some advanced patients receiving 10 or more tablets a day. The high cost of treatment can be a significant deterrent to the use of expensive brands when numerous generic alternatives are available. For instance, US sales of branded carbidopa/levodopa (Bristol-Myers Squibb's Sinemet), the cornerstone of Parkinson's disease treatment since its launch in 1975, declined by 83% from 2000 to 2005, whereas sales of generic versions of this molecule increased by 59% over the same period. However, neurologists and payers are willing to accept increased costs in return for improved safety. Unlike pergolide, the non-ergot-derived dopamine agonists pramipexole and ropinirole do not carry the risk of fibrosis, but they are significantly more expensive than pergolide. Nevertheless, uptake of these newer dopamine agonists has been swift. From 2000 to 2005, US sales of pramipexole doubled (to $250 million) and sales of ropinirole tripled (to $160 million), whereas sales of pergolide declined by 60%.

Multiple Sclerosis Therapies

The market for multiple sclerosis therapies is dominated by four drugs: two interferon beta-1a products (Biogen Idec's Avonex, Serono/Pfizer's Rebif), interferon beta-1b (Schering-Plough's Betaseron/Betaferon), and glatiramer acetate (Teva's Copaxone). Sales of these four drugs in the seven major markets totaled $4 billion in 2005, an increase of 12% over 2004.

Figure 5.4 shows average prices of these drugs in each market as a percentage of US

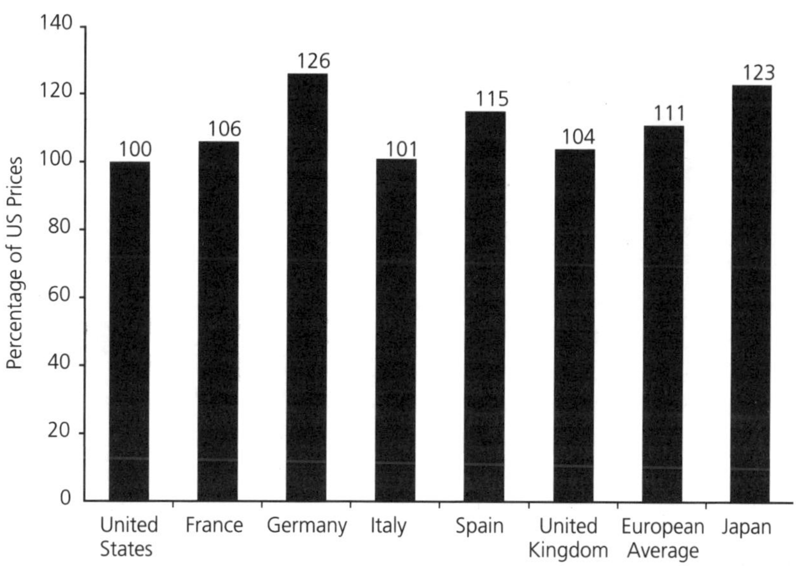

Note: The drugs included are interferon-beta-1a (Avonex and Rebif), interferon-beta-1b, and glatiramer acetate

Figure 5.4 Average Exmanufacturer Prices of Disease-Modifying Multiple Sclerosis Therapies as a Percentage of US Prices, 2005

prices in 2005. It is striking that European prices for multiple sclerosis therapies were, on average, 11% higher than US prices. The percentage price differential was even greater for glatiramer acetate – European prices were, on average, 27% higher than US prices, and the drug was 41% more expensive in Germany than in the United States. The price differential for interferon-beta products was much smaller: European prices were, on average, just 6% higher than US prices. In only four instances were multiple sclerosis therapies less expensive in European markets than in the United States: Rebif in France, Avonex in Italy, and Betaferon in Italy and the United Kingdom. Only one of the four leading multiple sclerosis therapies is currently available in Japan – Betaferon. In 2005, this drug cost 23% more in Japan than in the United States.

Antiepileptic Agents

Table 5.1 lists the most commonly prescribed antiepileptics, several of which are available in generic form. Sales of these drugs in the seven major markets totaled approximately $7 billion in 2005, a decline of 6% over 2004. This decrease is attributable primarily to growing generics competition in the US market for gabapentin products. Several other drugs in this class – carbamazepine, lamotrigine, phenytoin, valproic acid – are also available in generic form in most of the major markets.

Figure 5.5 shows average prices of branded antiepileptics in each market as a percentage of US prices in 2005. On average, European prices for branded antiepileptics were just 38% of US prices, and the two antiepileptics available in Japan (carbamazepine and valproic acid) had an average price that was just 23% of US prices. The price of branded valproic acid in Italy was only 5% of the US price. The only instance of a branded antiepileptic that was more expensive in Europe than the United States was pregabalin in the United Kingdom – 16% higher than the US price and more than twice the Italian and Spanish prices.

Five leading antiepileptics – carbamazepine, gabapentin, lamotrigine, phenytoin, valproic

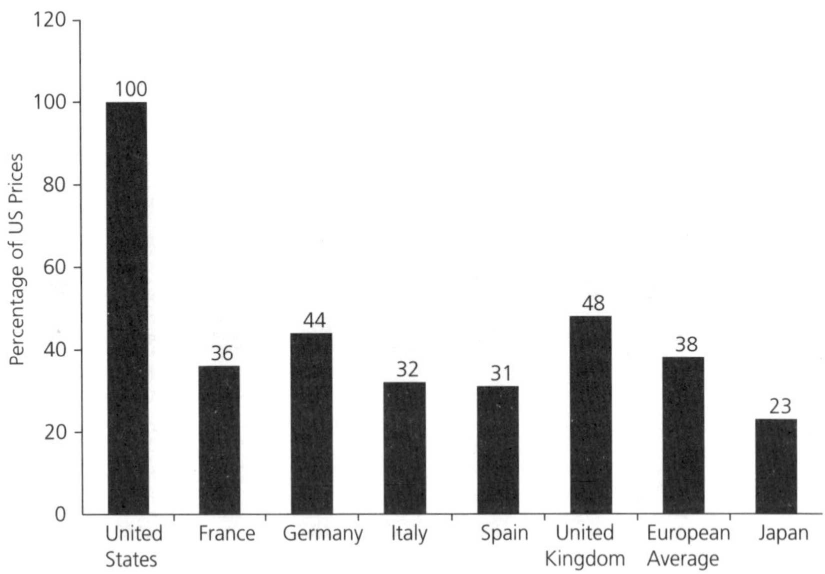

Note: The drugs included are branded versions of carbamazepine, gabapentin, lamotrigine, levetiracetam, phenytoin, pregabalin, topiramate, and valproic acid

Figure 5.5 Average Exmanufacturer Prices of Select Branded Antiepileptic Agents as a Percentage of US Prices, 2005

acid – are available in generic forms in at least some of the major markets. Figure 5.6 shows average prices of the lowest-priced generic versions of these agents in each market as a percentage of US prices in 2005. Generics were substantially more expensive in Japan and all European markets than in the United States. The average European price of the lowest-priced generics was 68% higher than the average US price of the least expensive generics. Unusually, the United Kingdom had the highest prices for generic antiepileptics – 261% of the lowest US prices overall, but the lowest-priced gabapentin product in the United Kingdom was 745% of the US price. However, price is seldom the main factor in prescribing decisions for antiepileptics. For instance, despite being one of the most expensive antiepileptics on the market, topiramate achieved sales of $1.5 billion in the seven major markets in 2005. Neurologists are willing to accept the higher cost of newer antiepileptic drugs in return for their improved tolerability and reduced drug interactions compared with first-generation antiepileptics. Moreover, concerns about poor bioequivalence have limited the use of generic antiepileptics.

Reformulations and "Me-too" Drugs

Reimbursement authorities in Europe have generally been less willing than third-party payers in the United States to accept price premiums on line extensions or reformulations (e.g., liquids, rapid disintegration tablets, once-daily forms). For example, new formulations of the four main dementia therapies have been launched or are pending: orally disintegrating donepezil tablets, a once-daily dosage and a liquid formulation of galantamine, liquid and transdermal patch formulations for rivastigmine, and an oral solution of memantine. Table 5.4 shows the prices of these reformulations (where available) as a percentage of the price in each market of the drug's original formulation. Manufacturers generally charge relatively substantial price premiums for reformulations in the United States, with the notable exception of galantamine oral solution, which is priced at just 71% of the price of the

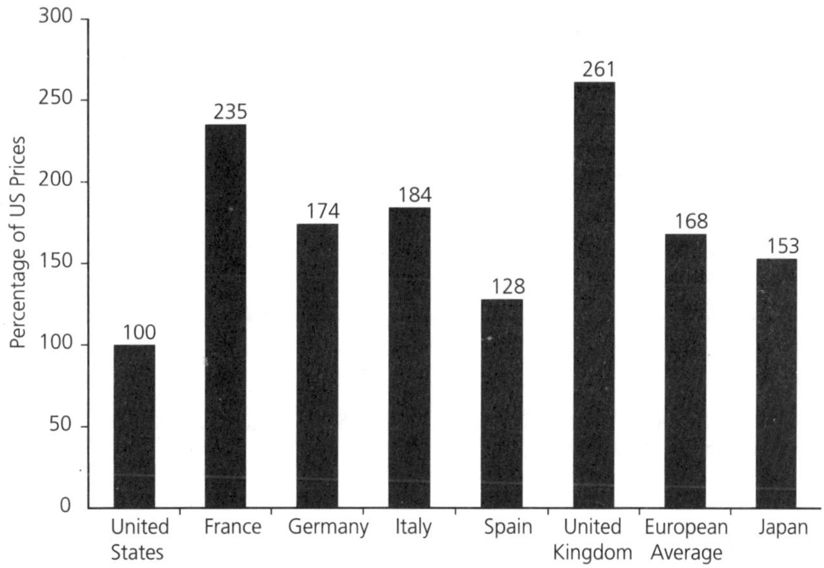

Note: The drugs included are the lowest-priced generic versions of carbamazepine, gabapentin, lamotrigine, phenytoin, and valproic acid

Figure 5.6 Average Exmanufacturer Prices of the Lowest-Priced Generic Version of Select Antiepileptic Agents as a Percentage of US Prices, 2005

original tablet formulation. The picture in Europe is much more varied. With just one exception (the once-daily tablet formulation of galantamine in Germany), reformulations of dementia therapies are less expensive than their respective original formulations in France and Germany. The oral solution of galantamine was also much less expensive than the original formulation in Spain, but other reformulations of dementia therapies were more costly than their respective original formulations in that country. Modest prime premiums for reformulations were permitted in Italy, and manufacturers used their price-setting freedom to charge substantial premiums for most reformulations in the United Kingdom.

European reimbursement authorities tend to be less inclined than US payers to countenance price premiums for "me-too" drugs. Table 5.5 expresses the prices of the maximum approved daily dosages of dementia therapies as a percentage of the price of donepezil, the dominant brand in this market. In the United States, the maximum approved daily dosages of rivastigmine and galantamine are, respectively, 16% and 10% more expensive than the maximum daily dosage of donepezil, but Forest Laboratories set the price of memantine 5% below the price of donepezil. By comparison, later entrants to the European market for dementia therapies are generally priced below the level of donepezil, with the exception of memantine in Italy and galantamine in France, Germany, and Italy. In the United Kingdom – a market in which the price of dementia therapies has provoked considerable controversy – rivastigmine and memantine are almost a quarter less expensive than donepezil.

REIMBURSEMENT ENVIRONMENT

United States

General Environment

The majority of US residents have private health insurance, but government-sponsored programs (e.g., Medicare, Medicaid, military programs) also play an important role in healthcare funding. According to the US Census Bureau, in 2004, 245.3 million US residents (84.3% of the population) had some form of health insurance, and 45.8 million (15.7%) were uninsured throughout that year. Table 5.6 shows the main sources of

Table 5.4 Prices of Reformulations of Dementia Therapies in the United States and Europe as a Percentage of the Price of the Original Formulations in Each Market, 2005

Drug	*Dosage Form*	*United States*	*France*	*Germany*	*Italy*	*Spain*	*United Kingdom*
Donepezil	Orally disintegrating tablets	108	—	—	—	—	—
Rivastigmine	Oral solution	143	82	94	113	106	120
Galantamine	Once-daily tablet	206	—	162	—	—	155
Galantamine	Oral solution	71	62	47	—	57	122
Memantine	Oral solution	169	—	—	—	—	—
Memantine	Oral drops	—	97	99	102	102	100

Table 5.5 Prices of Dementia Therapies in the United States and Europe as a Percentage of the Price of Donepezil in Each Market, 2005

Drug	*Dosage (mg)*	*Year of First Launch*	*United States*	*France*	*Germany*	*Italy*	*Spain*	*United Kingdom*
Donepezil	10[a]	1996	100	100	100	100	100	100
Rivastigmine	6[b]	1997	116	96	84	87	76	76
Galantamine	12[b]	2000	110	103	104	100	86	94
Memantine	10[b]	2002	95	99	87	109	89	77

[a]Once daily
[b]Twice daily

Table 5.6 Health Insurance Coverage of the US Population, 2002–4

	2002		*2003*		*2004*	
	Millions of Residents	*Percentage of Population*	*Millions of Residents*	*Percentage of Population*	*Millions of Residents*	*Percentage of Population*
Private insurance						
Any private plan	200.4	69.6	199.5	68.6	198.3	68.1
Employment-based insurance	176.5	61.3	175.6	60.4	174.2	59.8
Direct-purchase insurance	26.8	9.3	26.8	9.2	27.0	9.3
Government insurance						
Any government plan	74.0	25.7	77.4	26.6	79.1	27.2
Medicare	38.6	13.4	39.8	13.7	39.7	13.7
Medicaid	33.4	11.6	36.1	12.4	37.5	12.9
Military healthcare	10.1	3.5	10.2	3.5	10.7	3.7
No Insurance	43.8	15.2	45.4	15.6	45.8	15.7

Note: Some residents have more than one type of insurance coverage

health insurance from 2002 to 2004. Employer-sponsored insurance for current employees and many retirees remains the dominant source of healthcare funding, but the number of US residents who have such insurance is declining steadily. Conversely, enrollment in Medicare (the federal health insurance program for seniors, the registered disabled, and patients with end-stage renal disease) and Medicaid (the federal/state program for low-income residents) is growing steadily, as are the ranks of the uninsured. Private health plans generally offer extensive prescription drug coverage, albeit with substantial out-of-pocket payments in some cases, and Medicare now covers outpatient prescription drugs. Thanks to these relatively generous drug benefits, neurologists in the United States tend to adopt new therapies more quickly than their counterparts in other countries. On the other hand, the use of generic drugs is also more widespread in the United States than most other markets.

Private Insurance

Pharmacy benefits offered by private insurers tend to be considerably more generous than the coverage provided by Medicare and Medicaid, but cost-containment measures are proliferating. Formularies have grown ever more complex: three-tier designs are now the norm, but formularies with additional tiers for "lifestyle drugs" and specialty pharmaceuticals (principally biologics and some other injectable/infused therapies) are increasing. Copayments continue to rise steadily, and plans are increasingly applying coinsurance (a percentage of the cost of medications) to the highest formulary tiers. The positioning of generics in the lowest tier of formularies is intended to maximize use of these products, but many plans and/or their PBMs encourage pharmacists to substitute generics for branded versions of off-patent drugs, and some plans and PBMs even promote therapeutic substitution (i.e., switching a patient to a different [and less expensive] compound from the one prescribed). Prior authorization policies exclude certain drugs from reimbursement unless the prescriber justifies the need for these medications and the plan or PBM approves the prescription. Quantity limits restrict the pack size of prescriptions and the frequency of refills. Step therapy protocols reimburse costly drugs only if the patient has first tried, and failed to respond adequately to, less expensive therapies.

Table 5.7 summarizes the coverage of widely prescribed neurology drugs in the standard three-tier formularies of five of the largest insurers in the United States: Aetna, Cigna, Humana, UnitedHealth, and WellPoint. Aetna, Cigna, and Humana cover all of the drugs in our sample, albeit with prescribing restrictions on some agents. WellPoint excludes several Parkinson's disease therapies (mainly branded products) and Lyrica from its formulary. UnitedHealth has the most limited coverage of neurology drugs among these five insurers: only one dementia therapy (Aricept) is included

Table 5.7 Formulary Positioning of Select Neurology Drugs in Five Leading Managed Care Organizations

	Tier				
	Aetna	*Cigna*	*Humana*	*UnitedHealth Group*	*WellPoint*
Dementia therapies					
Donepezil (Aricept)	3	2	2	2[a]	N.S.
Rivastigmine (Exelon)	2	3	2	—	N.S.
Galantamine (Razadyne)	3	3	2	—	N.S.
Galantamine (Razadyne ER)	3	3	2	—	N.S.
Memantine (Namenda)	2	3	2	—	N.S.
Parkinson's disease therapies					
Carbidopa/levodopa (Sinemet)	3	3	3	—	—
Carbidopa/levodopa (generic)	1	1	1	1	N.S.
Pergolide (Permax)	3	3	3	—	—
Pergolide (generic)	1	1	1	—	N.S.
Cabergoline (Dostinex)	3	3[a]	2	3	—
Cabergoline (generic)	1	1[a]	1	2	—
Pramipexole (Mirapex)	2	2	2	3	N.S.
Ropinirole (Requip)	2	—	2	2	N.S.
Entacapone (Comtan)	2	3	2	—	N.S.
Carbidopa/levodopa/ entacapone (Stalevo)	3	3	2	—	—
Selegiline (Eldepryl)	3	2	2	—	—
Selegiline (generic)	1	1	1	—	N.S.
Multiple sclerosis therapies					
Interferon-beta-1b (Betaseron)	3		3[a,b]	3[a]	N.S.
Interferon-beta-1a (Avonex)	2	3[b]	3[a,b]	2[a]	N.S.
Interferon-beta-1a (Rebif)	3	3[b]	3[a,b]	3[a]	N.S.
Glatiramer acetate (Copaxone)	2	2[b]	3[a,b]	2[a]	N.S.
Antiepileptic agents					
Valproic acid (Depakene)	3	3	3	—	N.S.
Valproic acid (generic)	1	1	1	—	N.S.
Phenytoin (Dilantin)	3	2	2	2	N.S.
Phenytoin (generic)	1	1	1	1	N.S.
Gabapentin (Neurontin/Gabarone)	3[a,c]	3	3[a]	3	—
Gabapentin (generic)	1[a]	1	1[a]	1	N.S.
Lamotrigine (Lamictal)	2	2	3	2/3	N.S.
Lamotrigine (generic)	1	1	1	—	N.S.
Carbamazepine (Carbatrol)	3	3	2	3	N.S.
Carbamazepine (generic)	1	1	1	1	N.S.
Levetiracetam (Keppra)	2	2	3	2	N.S.
Pregabalin (Lyrica)	3[a]	3	3[a]	—	—
Topiramate (Topamax)	3	2	3	2	N.S.

[a]Quantity limits
[b]Prior authorization
[c]Step therapy
N.S. = Tier not specified

in its formulary, and several Parkinson's disease therapies and anti-epileptics are excluded.

Medicare

The US Census Bureau calculates that, in 2004, Medicare provided healthcare benefits to 95% of seniors and 2.5% of the nonelderly population in the United States. The Centers for Medicare and Medicaid Services (CMS) reports somewhat higher enrollment in the Medicare program than the US Census Bureau – 41.7 million versus 39.7 million, respectively, in 2004.

Historically, Medicare offered only limited coverage of prescription medicines. Part A covers inpatient drugs; Part B (an optional program) covers outpatient drugs that are not usually self-administered (e.g., intravenous infusions, intramuscular injections) and oral drugs that also have a parenteral dosage form that would be reimbursed if it were administered by a physician. Beginning in 1999, Part C, more commonly known as Medicare + Choice (renamed Medicare Advantage in 2004), offered additional services – including prescription drug benefits – through private fee-for-service plans or Medicare managed care organizations. The most recent expansion of the Medicare program, Part D, offers outpatient drug coverage to all Medicare beneficiaries who choose to enroll. As of June 11, 2006, 38.2 million out of a total of 42.6 million Medicare beneficiaries were enrolled in a Part D program or equivalent, including 6.1 million Medicare-Medicaid dual-eligible beneficiaries who were automatically enrolled in a Medicare prescription drug plan (PDP). Given that neurodegenerative disorders (e.g., Alzheimer's disease and other forms of dementia, Parkinson's disease) are most prevalent among the elderly, the introduction of the Medicare drug benefit is a very significant development in the US market for neurology drugs.

The standard benefit design for Part D requires beneficiaries to pay an average premium of $24 per month and an annual deductible of $250. Thereafter, Medicare covers 75% of the cost of prescription drugs up to an annual total of $2,250. Coverage then ceases until the beneficiary's annual drug costs reach a total of $5,100 (and out-of-pocket payments reach a total of $3,600) – a provision known as the "coverage gap" or, more colloquially, the "doughnut hole." Medicare then covers 95% of drug costs in excess of the annual threshold of $5,100. Variations on the standard benefit design are available, including plans that charge reduced premiums, waive or reduce the annual deductible, or cover drugs (typically generics only) while patients are in the coverage gap. In a recent survey, CMS found that Medicare PDP enrollees who signed up for the lowest-cost plan in their area could save an average of 59%, and a maximum of 72%, on their drug costs (compared with cash prices to patients who have no drug coverage). However, some beneficiaries face the prospect of losing access to patient assistance programs (PAPs) that provide free medications to low-income patients who lack adequate insurance coverage (see the sidebar "Patient Assistance Programs – An Important Source of Drug Funding").

Patient Assistance Programs – An Important Source of Drug Funding

Manufacturer-sponsored patient assistance programs (PAPs) play a significant role in the supply of medicines to needy patients (including many Medicare beneficiaries) in the United States. According to the Pharmaceutical Research and Manufacturers of America (PhRMA), the number of prescriptions filled through PAPs increased from 22 million in 2004 to 35 million in 2005, and the total cost of these programs increased from $4 billion in 2004 to $5.1 billion in 2005. PhRMA estimates that senior citizens account for approximately one-quarter of the beneficiaries of PAPs.

PAPs are available for all the leading dementia therapies (i.e. Aricept, Exelon, Namenda, Razadyne) and all the leading multiple sclerosis therapies (i.e. Avonex, Betaseron, Copaxone, Rebif). Other neurology drugs covered by PAPs include Comtan, Stalevo, Mirapex, Requip, Lamictal, and Keppra.

In 2006, some manufacturers decided to exclude Medicare Part D enrollees from their PAPs to avoid any risk of violating the federal antikickback statute and incurring substantial fines. However, a recent advisory opinion from the Office of Inspector General (OIG) of the Department of Health and Human Services concluded that PAPs present "minimal risk of fraud and abuse" provided that they do not seek payment from Medicare and they base eligibility purely on financial need. The Centers for Medicare and Medicaid Services has indicated that it would like manufacturers to continue to include eligible Medicare beneficiaries in their programs.

PDPs are generally required to cover at least two drugs in each therapeutic category and pharmacological class. CMS expects PDPs to "provide adequate access to medically necessary treatments for Part D enrollees." In particular, plans must cover "all or substantially all" drugs in six classes, including antiepileptic agents. However, PDPs are not obliged to cover off-label prescribing, and they are permitted to use mechanisms such as multitier formularies, prior authorization, step therapy protocols, generics substitution, and quantity limits to control pharmacy costs.

Medicare plans have taken advantage of these provisions. An analysis of CMS data shows that 98% of PDPs place a prior authorization or step therapy restriction on at least one of the 100 drugs most frequently prescribed to Medicare beneficiaries. On average, Medicare PDPs include 93.5 of the top 100 drugs in their formularies and subject 9.5 of these medicines to prior authorization or step therapy restrictions. Some plans require physicians to submit detailed laboratory test results, comprehensive office notes, and other data to demonstrate the clinical need for certain medicines. In addition, PDPs may have 25–30 different forms for prior authorization of various drugs.

Additionally, Medicare PDPs appear to be much more inclined than private health plans to assign medicines to the specialty tier of their formularies, a positioning that incurs the heaviest copayments or coinsurance rates. Avalere Health calculates that Medicare plans have an average of 88 drugs in the fourth tier of their formularies, compared with an average of 15–20 drugs for private health plans.

To assess Medicare Part D coverage of neurology drugs specifically, we analyzed the formularies of the 10 national stand-alone PDP organizations. Table 5.8 shows the number of these plans that assign select neurology drugs to particular formulary tiers and impose prior authorization or quantity limit restrictions. Generics, where available, are usually assigned to tier 1 (i.e., the tier that incurs the lowest copayment), though several plans exclude generic cabergoline and lamotrigine from their formularies. Branded Parkinson's disease therapies and antiepileptics that have generic equivalents are commonly excluded from the national PDPs' formularies. With the notable exception of injectable multiple sclerosis therapies, relatively few neurology drugs are assigned to a specialty formulary tier. Prior authorization and quantity limits are applied primarily to multiple sclerosis therapies and, to a lesser extent, dementia therapies and some antiepileptics.

Medicaid

The Medicaid program was established in 1965 to provide medical coverage to the neediest US residents. Federal and state governments jointly finance the standard program, but state governments must provide full funding for any supplementary state programs. According to data from CMS, the Office of the Actuary, and the National Health Statistics Group, Medicaid spent approximately $33.7 billion in 2003 on prescription drugs.

Every state's Medicaid program offers coverage for prescription drugs, but most have instituted cost-saving mechanisms, such as preferred drug lists, prior authorization, quantity limits on brand-name drugs, and mandatory use of generics. Table 5.9 traces the growing use of cost-cutting measures in state Medicaid programs, based on data from the most recent edition of a survey commissioned by the Kaiser Commission on Medicaid and the Uninsured (KCMU) (see Crowley J.S., et al. *State Medicaid Outpatient Prescription Drug Policies: Findings from a National Survey, 2005 Update*. Kaiser Commission on Medicaid and the Uninsured, October 2005). All of the 37 states that replied to the 2005 survey indicated that they practiced some form of prior authorization in their Medicaid programs, 95% used dispensing limits by quantity per prescription, and 92% operated a policy of mandatory generics substitution.

State Medicaid programs have a legal obligation to cover all drugs manufactured by companies that have signed federal rebate agreements, but they are permitted to promote the use of particular drugs by means of preferred drug lists (PDLs). Table 5.10 shows

Table 5.8 Formulary Coverage of Select Neurology Drugs in National Medicare Prescription Drug Plans

	Formulary Status					*Prescribing Restrictions*	
	Tier 1	*Tier 2*	*Tier 3*	*Specialty Tier*	*Nonformulary Status*	*Prior Authorization*	*Quantity Limits*
Dementia therapies							
Donepezil (Aricept)	—	10	—	—	—	3	3
Donepezil (Aricept ODT)	—	4	—	—	—	—	1
Rivastigmine	—	5	5	—	—	3	2
Rivastigmine (solution)	—	—	—	1	—	—	—
Galantamine (Razadyne)	—	6	3	—	1	2	3
Galantamine (Razadyne ER)	—	4	2	—	—	2	3
Memantine	—	9	1	—	—	3	3
Memantine (solution)	—	2	—	—	—	2	—
Parkinson's disease therapies							
Carbidopa/levodopa (Sinemet)	—	—	3	—	7	—	—
Carbidopa/levodopa (generic)	10	—	—	—	—	—	—
Pergolide (Permax)	—	—	3	—	7	—	—
Pergolide (generic)	9	—	—	—	1	—	—
Cabergoline (Dostinex)	—	4	3	—	3	1	1
Cabergoline (generic)	3	—	—	—	7	—	—
Pramipexole	—	8	2	—	—	—	—
Ropinirole	—	8	2	—	—	—	—
Entacapone (Comtan)	—	8	2	—	—	—	—
Carbidopa/levodopa/entacopone (Stalevo)	—	7	2	—	1	—	—
Selegiline (Eldepryl)	—	—	3	—	7	—	—
Selegiline (generic)	10	—	—	—	—	—	—
Multiple sclerosis therapies							
Interferon-beta-1b (Betaseron)	—	1	3	6	—	7	2
Interferon-beta-1a (Avonex)	—	3	1	6	—	7	2
Interferon-beta-1a (Rebif)	—	1	4	3	2	5	2
Glatiramer acetate (Copaxone)	—	5	—	5	—	6	2
Antiepileptic agents							
Valproic acid (brand)	—	2	2	—	6	1	—
Valproic acid (generic)	10	—	—	—	—	—	—
Phenytoin (brand)	—	8	—	—	2	—	—
Phenytoin (generic)	10	—	—	—	—	—	—
Gabapentin (brand)	—	6	3	—	1	—	2
Gabapentin (generic)	10	—	—	—	—	—	2
Lamotrigine (brand)	—	7	3	—	—	2	—
Lamotrigine (generic)	5	—	—	—	5	—	—
Carbamazepine (brand)	—	6	3	—	1	—	—
Carbamazepine (generic)	10	—	—	—	—	—	—
Levetiracetam	3	7	—	—	—	—	1
Pregabalin	—	4	2	—	3	1	—
Topiramate	—	7	3	—	—	3	—

Note: Figures refer to the number of the 10 national prescription drug plan organizations that apply a particular formulary status or prescribing restriction to each drug

that 42 states currently operate such lists. Increasingly, states require manufacturers to pay them supplemental rebates in return for inclusion of their drugs in state PDLs. Drugs that are not included in PDLs are frequently subject to prior authorization restrictions. Table 5.11 shows the PDL status of neurology drugs in the five states that have the largest Medicaid populations. Most of the leading therapies are included in these PDLs, though generics are typically favored when drugs are off patent.

Table 5.9 Percentage of State Medicaid Programs Using Various Pharmaceutical Cost-Containment Measures, 2000, 2003, and 2005

	2000 (n = 44)	*2003 (n = 43)*	*2005 (n = 37)*
Dispensing limits by quantity per prescription	91	98	95
State preferred drug list	N.A.	42	68
Any form of prior authorization	82	95	100
Mandatory generics substitution	36	70	92
Patient copayments	66	81	81
Supplemental rebates on drug purchases	N.A.	21	43

N.A. = Not available

Table 5.10 State Medicaid Programs' Use of Preferred Drug Lists, August 2006

State	*PDL Status*	*State*	*PDL Status*
Alabama	PDL in operation	Montana	PDL in operation
Alaska	PDL in operation	Nebraska	No known plans
Arizona	No known plans	Nevada	PDL in operation
Arkansas	PDL in operation	New Hampshire	PDL in operation
California	PDL in operation	New Jersey	No known plans
Colorado	Legislation pending	New Mexico	PDL in operation
Connecticut	PDL in operation	New York	PDL in operation
Delaware	PDL in operation	North Carolina	PDL in operation
Florida	PDL in operation	North Dakota	Legislation defeated in 2005
Georgia	PDL in operation	Ohio	PDL in operation
Hawaii	PDL in operation	Oklahoma	PDL in operation
Idaho	PDL in operation	Oregon	PDL in operation
Illinois	PDL in operation	Pennsylvania	PDL in operation
Indiana	PDL in operation	Rhode Island	Legislation enacted, July 2006
Iowa	PDL in operation	South Carolina	PDL in operation
Kansas	PDL in operation	South Dakota	No known plans
Kentucky	PDL in operation	Tennessee	PDL in operation
Louisiana	PDL in operation	Texas	PDL in operation
Maine	PDL in operation	Utah	Legislation defeated in 2005
Maryland	PDL in operation	Vermont	PDL in operation
Massachusetts	PDL in operation	Virginia	PDL in operation
Michigan	PDL in operation	Washington	PDL in operation
Minnesota	PDL in operation	West Virginia	PDL in operation
Mississippi	PDL in operation	Wisconsin	PDL in operation
Missouri	PDL in operation	Wyoming	PDL in operation

PDL = Preferred drug list

The introduction of the new Medicare prescription drug benefit will have a major impact on Medicaid pharmacy provision: dual eligible beneficiaries now receive their prescription drug coverage through Medicare rather than Medicaid. The resulting substantial cut in the states' pharmaceutical spending will reduce their bargaining power with drug manufacturers. Seventy-two percent of states that responded to the KCMU survey expected reduced manufacturer rebates as a result of the introduction of the Medicare prescription drug benefit. To compensate for reduced rebates, states might form multistate purchasing pools to increase their negotiating strength with pharmaceutical companies. Alternatively, individual states might pool their Medicaid members with other state-funded groups (e.g., state workers, prisoners) to gain critical mass. The effectiveness of such tactics in reducing costs remains to be seen.

Table 5.11 Status of Select Neurology Drugs in Five States' Preferred Drug Lists

	California	*Texas*	*Florida*	*Michigan*	*Pennsylvania*
Dementia therapies					
Donepezil	Included[a]	Included	Included	Included	Included
Rivastigmine	Included[b]	Included	Included	Included	Included
Galantamine	Included[c]	Included	Included	Included	N.A.
Memantine	N.A.	Included	Included	Included	Included
Parkinson's disease therapies					
Carbidopa/levodopa	Included[d]	Included	Included	Included	Included
Pergolide	Included	Included	N.A.	Included	Included
Cabergoline	N.A.	N.A.	Included	Included	N.A.
Pramipexole	Included	Included	Included	Included	Included
Ropinirole	Included	Included	N.A.	N.A.	Included
Entacapone	Included	Included	Included	Included	Included
Carbidopa/levodopa/entacopone	Included[d]	Included	Included	Included	Included
Selegiline	Included	Included	Included	Included	Included
Multiple sclerosis therapies					
Interferon-beta-1b	N.A.	Included	Included	Included	Included
Interferon-beta-1a (Avonex)	N.A.	Included	Included	Included	Included
Interferon-beta-1a (Rebif)	N.A.	Included	Included	Included	Included
Glatiramer acetate	N.A.	Included	Included	Included	Included
Antiepileptic agents					
Valproic acid	Included	N.A.	Included	Included	Included
Phenytoin	Included	N.A.	Included	Included	Included
Gabapentin	Included	N.A.	Included	Included	Included
Lamotrigine	Included	N.A.	Included	Included	Included
Carbamazepine	Included	N.A.	Included	Included	Included
Levetiracetam	Included	N.A.	Included	Included	Included
Pregabalin	N.A.	N.A.	N.A.	Included	Included
Topiramate	Included	N.A.	N.A.	Included	N.A.

[a]Prior authorization
[b]Restricted to mild-to-moderate Alzheimer's disease
[c]Solution restricted to mild-to-moderate Alzheimer's disease
[d]Quantity limits
N.A. = Not preferred

Dementia Therapies

To determine the principal sources of funding for the main classes of neurology drugs in the United States in 2005, we analyzed data from Verispan's Prescription Drug and Diagnosis Audit (PDDA). Figure 5.7 shows the percentage of patients younger than 65 diagnosed with Alzheimer's disease or other dementias, Parkinson's disease, epilepsy, and multiple sclerosis who had private insurance, Medicare or Medicaid coverage, or no insurance. Figure 5.8 presents the same data for patients aged 65 or older, and Figure 5.9 shows summary data for all ages. Note that, because some patients have more than one type of insurance (e.g., private insurance and Medicaid, Medicare and Medicaid), percentages may total more than 100.

We calculate that 93% of patients diagnosed with Alzheimer's disease or other dementias were aged 65 or older. According to PDDA data, 84% of patients in this age group had health coverage from Medicare (though not necessarily Part D drug benefits), 30% from private insurance, and 16% from Medicaid. No Alzheimer's disease or dementia patients aged 65 or older were uninsured. Data from the 2002 Medicare Current Beneficiary indicate that 3% of Medicare beneficiaries had Alzheimer's disease and 26% had some form of cognitive impairment.

Formulary guidelines for Medicare Part D require all PDPs to cover at least two AChEIs and memantine. Table 5.8 shows that all 10 plans grant the standard formulation of donepezil preferred brand status (i.e., tier 2), and 9 plans do the same for memantine,

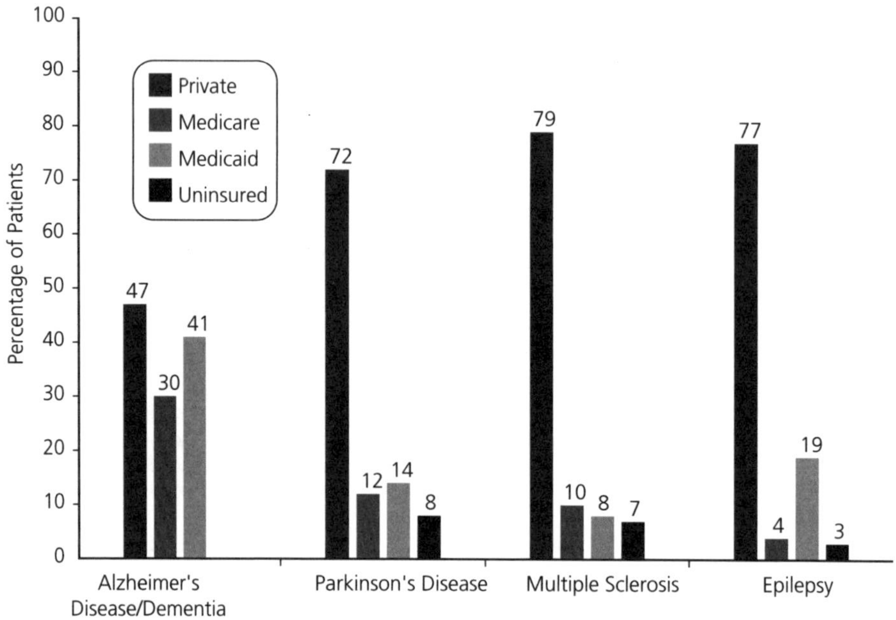

Figure 5.7 Sources of Healthcare Funding for US Residents Younger Than Age 65 by Neurological Disease, 2005

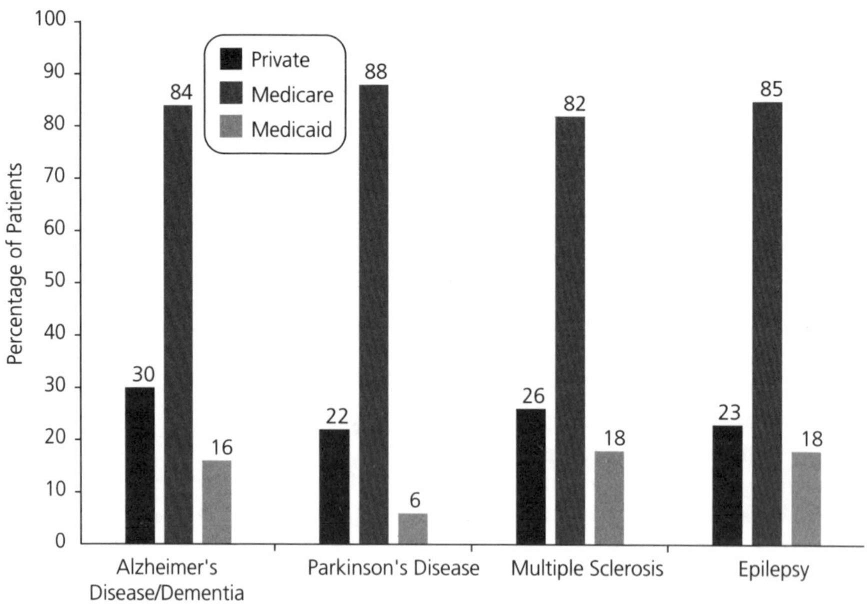

Figure 5.8 Sources of Healthcare Funding for US Residents Aged 65 or Older by Neurological Disease, 2005

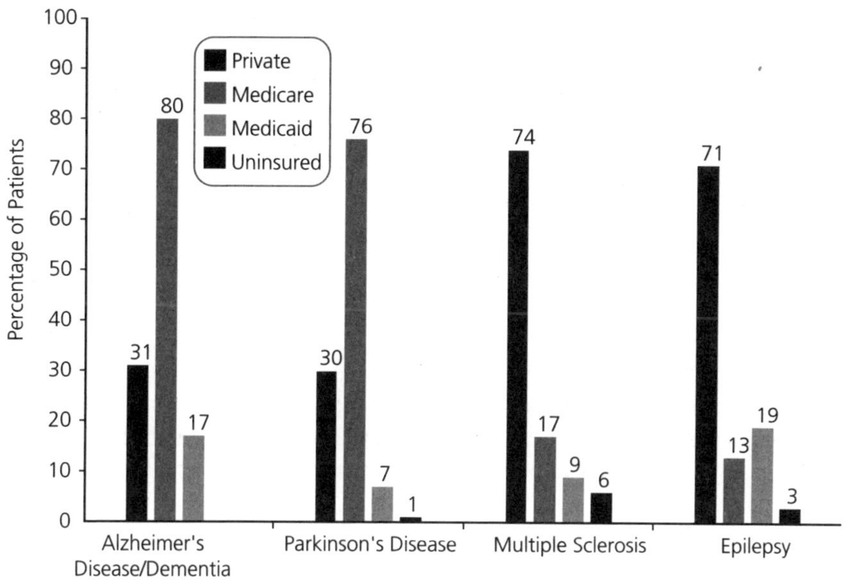

Figure 5.9 Sources of Healthcare Funding for US Residents by Neurological Disease, 2005

whereas several plans accord galantamine and rivastigmine nonpreferred status (i.e., tier 3). Several plans use prior authorization or quantity limits to restrict the use of dementia therapies. The United States Pharmacopeial Convention also recommends the inclusion of generic ergoloid mesylates in Medicare Part D formularies, but the side-effect profiles of these drugs deter most plans from covering them and most physicians from prescribing them.

Table 5.7 shows the formulary status of the AChEIs and memantine in the standard three-tier formularies of five leading private insurers. Donepezil is the only one of these agents covered by all five insurers, and it has preferred brand status (tier 2) in all formularies except Aetna's. UnitedHealth covers none of the other leading dementia therapies.

Parkinson's Disease Therapies

Parkinson's disease, like Alzheimer's disease, is overwhelmingly a disease of the elderly. We calculate that 84% of patients diagnosed with Parkinson's disease in the United States in 2005 were aged 65 or older. Figure 5.6 shows that, according to PDDA data, 88% of senior patients with Parkinson's disease had Medicare coverage, 22% had private insurance, and 6% were covered by Medicaid.

In 2006, Medicare Part D formulary guidelines require coverage of at least two drugs in each of the following: catechol-O-methyltransferase (COMT) inhibitors, dopamine agonists, and other anti-Parkinson agents. Table 5.8 shows that the 10 national PDPs almost invariably assigned generic carbidopa/levodopa, selegiline, and pergolide to the first tier of their formularies, but only three of these plans covered generic cabergoline. Most of the national PDPs assigned pramipexole, ropinirole, entacapone, and carbidopa/levodopa/entacapone preferred drug status. The majority of national PDPs excluded branded pergolide, cabergoline, and selegiline from their formularies. Beginning in 2007, Parkinson's disease therapies will be reclassified into five formulary key drug types (FKDTs): anticholinergics, COMT inhibitors, direct dopamine agonists, dopamine precursors, and other anti-Parkinson agents. Plans will be expected to cover at least one drug in each FKDT, a change that could lead to more limited coverage of Parkinson's disease therapies.

Polypharmacy is the norm in Parkinson's disease, and patients in the advanced stages of the disease may consume as many as 8–10 tablets a day to manage their Parkinson's symptoms alone. In addition, many elderly Parkinson's disease patients require complicated multi-drug regimens to treat a host of other chronic comorbidities. The cumulative cost of all these medications can be very substantial. Medicare Part D enrollees who are switched to less expensive generic drugs when they enter the coverage gap may respond poorly to their new medications. The possibility that patients who enter the coverage gap will limit, or even discontinue, drug therapy to cut costs is a disturbing prospect.

Table 5.7 shows the status of Parkinson's disease therapies in the formularies of leading private insurers. With a few exceptions, coverage follows the standard pattern for three-tier formularies: generics in tier 1, patent-protected branded drugs in tier 2, and off-patent branded drugs subject to generics competition in tier 3.

Multiple Sclerosis Therapies

We calculate that 90% of multiple sclerosis patients in the United States in 2005 were younger than 65. Figure 5.5 shows that 79% of patients younger than 65 had private insurance, 10% qualified for Medicare (primarily on the grounds of disability), 8% received Medicaid assistance, and 7% were uninsured. In the overall population of multiple sclerosis patients, 74% had private insurance, 17% were enrolled in the Medicare program, 9% qualified for Medicaid, and 6% were uninsured (Figure 5.7).

Private health plans that use three-tier formularies (the current norm in the United States) generally assign the leading multiple sclerosis therapies to either the second or third tiers of their formularies (Table 5.7). However, plans frequently impose quantity limits, prior authorization restrictions, or both these cost-containment measures. In addition, plans are increasingly using specialty pharmacy services (often provided by their PBMs) to regulate the use of multiple sclerosis therapies and other very costly parenteral drugs.

The introduction of Medicare Part D has expanded the Medicare program's coverage of multiple sclerosis therapies. Prior to January 1, 2006, Medicare Part B covered Avonex (a drug usually administered by intramuscular injection in the physician's office) but not the subcutaneously injectable agents Rebif, Betaseron, and Copaxone. Part D covers all four of these drugs, though Avonex is still funded by Part B if it is administered in the physician's office. For 2006, Medicare Part D formulary guidelines classify multiple sclerosis therapies simply as "immunomodulators" – a very broad pharmacologic class that includes, without distinction, interferon-alfa, interferon-beta, and interferon-gamma products, as well as other agents (e.g., leflunomide, lenalidomide, omalizumab, thalidomide). PDPs are required to cover only two agents in this class, but most offer more generous coverage. Beginning in 2007, the guidelines will recognize four distinct FKDTs within this pharmacologic class: interferon-alfa, interferon-beta, and interferon-gamma products, and other immunomodulators. Plans will be required to cover at least one agent in each FKDT.

The change in the Medicare formulary guidelines is unlikely to have a major impact on the coverage of multiple sclerosis therapies. Table 5.8 shows that, in 2006, all of the 10 national PDPs cover Avonex, Betaseron, and Copaxone, and 8 cover Rebif. With the exception of Copaxone, however, these drugs are usually assigned to the specialty pharmaceutical or third tiers of formularies, thereby incurring substantial copayments. Moreover, the majority of the national PDPs subject all multiple sclerosis therapies to prior authorization restrictions, and two impose quantity limits on these drugs. However, even if their medications are covered by a Medicare PDP, multiple sclerosis patients who depend on Medicare Part D for subsidy of their treatment face the challenge of the coverage gap. Because of the relatively high price of all multiple sclerosis therapies, patients reach the coverage gap earlier in the year than for most other disorders. Indeed, the National Multiple Sclerosis Society reported that some patients reached the coverage gap as early as February 2006. Loss of access to patient assistance programs has compounded problems for some Medicare beneficiaries.

Antiepileptic Agents

We calculate that 89% of epileptic patients in the United States in 2005 were younger than 65. Figure 5.5 shows that 77% of patients younger than 65 had private insurance, 19% received Medicaid assistance, 4% qualified for Medicare (primarily on the grounds of disability), and 3% were uninsured. In the overall population of multiple sclerosis patients, 71% had private insurance, 19% qualified for Medicaid, 13% were enrolled in the Medicare program, and 6% were uninsured (Figure 5.7).

Because antiepileptic agents generally have very specific indications (e.g., monotherapy, adjunctive therapy, a particular epileptic syndrome), securing reimbursement can be problematic sometimes. Neurologists use broad diagnostic coding to circumvent these obstacles. For instance, PDDA data indicate that approximately 50% of epilepsy prescriptions are coded for "epilepsy not otherwise specified."

The leading private health plans cover most antiepileptic agents. Table 5.7 shows that Aetna, Cigna, Humana, and WellPoint cover all the antiepileptic drugs in our sample, but UnitedHealth offers more limited coverage. In keeping with standard industry practice, the leading plans assign generic antiepileptics to the first tier of their formularies and branded drugs to the second or third tiers. Aetna and Humana apply quantity limits to gabapentin and pregabalin.

The Medicare Part D formulary guidelines classify anticonvulsants as a therapeutic category subdivided into five pharmacologic classes – calcium-channel modifying agents, gamma-aminobutyric acid (GABA) augmenting agents, glutamate-reducing agents, sodium-channel inhibitors, and other anticonvulsants. However, instead of the usual requirement for PDPs to cover at least two agents in each pharmacologic class, CMS directs plans to cover "all or substantially all" antiepileptics. This rule recognizes the fact that antiepileptic agents are not as easily interchangeable as drugs in most other classes. Table 5.8 summarizes the 10 national PDPs' coverage of antiepileptics. All of these plans assign generic valproic acid, phenytoin, gabapentin, and carbamazepine to the first tier of their formularies, but only five of these plans cover generic lamotrigine. Six plans exclude branded valproic acid from their formularies. Most of the other antiepileptics in our survey are generally assigned to the second tier of national PDPs' formularies. Prior authorization restrictions and quantity limits are relatively uncommon for antiepileptic agents.

France

General Environment

France operates a positive list of reimbursable drugs for both outpatient and hospital medicines. Drugs dispensed in public hospitals are fully reimbursed. Outpatient drugs that qualify for social security coverage are reimbursed at one of three rates, determined by disease severity and drug efficacy:

- 100% reimbursement for indispensable drugs for life-threatening or disabling conditions.
- 65% reimbursement for drugs for severe diseases.
- 35% reimbursement for symptomatic treatments for diseases that are not generally serious.

With very few exceptions, neurology drugs qualify for 65% reimbursement. However, patients diagnosed with any of 30 *affections de longue durée* (ALD; chronic disorders) receive full reimbursement of the cost of drugs used specifically to treat the ALD itself (since April 2006, patients diagnosed with an ALD are meant to pay standard copayments for all their other medications). The ALD list includes Alzheimer's disease, Parkinson's disease, multiple sclerosis, and severe epilepsy.

In some cases, the government limits reimbursement to specific indications or populations. For example, acetylcholinesterase inhibitors are covered only for Alzheimer's disease sufferers who satisfy strict eligibility criteria. Costly new drugs (especially therapies that were once restricted to hospital use) are subject to strict prescribing controls. For patients to receive reimbursement for these *médicaments d'exception* (drugs for exceptional use), the prescription must be issued on a special form.

The Commission de la Transparence (CT; Transparency Commission) evaluates new drugs on the basis of three main measures: (1) the *service médical rendu* (SMR; medical benefit); (2) the *amélioration du service médical rendu* (ASMR; improvement in medical benefit); and (3) the target population. The CT uses the following criteria to determine an SMR:

- The nature and severity of the disease for which the product is intended.
- The drug's efficacy/side-effect profile.
- The drug's importance in the treatment strategy (e.g., first- or second-line therapy).
- Whether the drug is preventive, curative, or symptomatic.
- The existence (and number) of therapeutic alternatives.

Based on its degree of clinical utility, a drug is given an SMR rating: major, important, moderate, weak, or insufficient. The SMR rating determines a drug's reimbursement rate. In the case of new drugs awarded a "major" or "important" SMR rating, the reimbursement rate also depends on the seriousness of the indicated disorder. The ASMR rating compares a drug's medical benefit with that of competing therapies. A new drug's degree of improvement is measured on a six-point scale, from I (major improvement) to VI (unfavorable opinion). The ASMR is an important influence on a new drug's price. A rating of I or II offers the potential of price premiums and concessions on sales volume restrictions. Conversely, a rating of V necessitates lower prices and a rating of VI precludes reimbursement. The CT also considers a new drug's target population. The agency evaluates both quantitative and qualitative data on the patients likely to benefit from treatment with the agent under review. Table 5.12 shows the SMR and ASMR ratings and target populations of select neurology drugs. With the exception of selegiline, all the drugs in our sample received an SMR rating of important, but the assessment of their degree of improvement over existing therapies was much more variable: only the multiple sclerosis therapies received the highest rating for innovation.

Dementia Therapies

Donepezil, galantamine, and rivastigmine are reimbursed in France only for mild-to-moderate Alzheimer's disease (i.e., Mini-Mental State Examination [MMSE] score of greater than 10 and/or a score of 1 or 2 on the Clinical Dementia Rating [CDR] scale). Memantine is reimbursed only for moderate-to-severe Alzheimer's disease. All four drugs are *médicaments à prescription restreinte* (drugs subject to prescribing restrictions). In a patient's first year of treatment, only specialists (e.g., neurologists, psychiatrists, gerontologists) are permitted to prescribe these agents.

Parkinson's Disease Therapies

As noted earlier, Parkinson's disease is classified as an ALD, allowing patients full reimbursement of their medications for this disorder. However, the Haut Comité Médical de la Sécurité Sociale (National Social Security Medical Committee) notes that the initial phase of Parkinson's disease is frequently prolonged and that many patients experience minimal disability at this stage. Therefore, the committee recommends that exemption from prescription copayments should be deferred until the patient's condition can no longer be controlled with a low-dose combination product.

Multiple Sclerosis Therapies

Interferon-beta products and glatiramer acetate are reimbursed for patients diagnosed with

Table 5.12 Assessment of Select Neurology Drugs by France's Medicines Evaluation Commission

	SMR	*ASMR*	*Target Population*
Dementia therapies			
Donepezil	Important	II	260,000–400,000
Rivastigmine	Important	II	260,000–400,000
Galantamine	Important	V	260,000–400,000
Memantine	Important	II/V[a]	270,000–435,000
Parkinson's disease therapies			
Carbidopa/levodopa	Important	III	
Pramipexole	Important	V	84,000–105,000
Ropinirole	Important	IV/V[b]	84,000–105,000
Pergolide	Weak[c]	V	84,000–105,000
Entacapone	Important	III	—
Carbidopa/levodopa/entacapone	Important	V	45,000–65,000
Selegiline	Moderate	—	—
Multiple sclerosis therapies			
Interferon-beta 1b	Important	I	12,000–15,000
Interferon-beta 1a (Avonex)	Important	I	11,500–13,500
Interferon-beta 1a (Rebif)	Important	I	12,000–15,000
Glatiramer acetate	Important	I	8,000–10,000
Antiepileptic agents			
Valproic acid	Important	IV	—
Lamotrigine	Important	II	—
Levetiracetam	Important	IV	47,840–84,300[d]
Pregabalin	Important	V	42,000–72,000[e]
Topiramate	Important	III	115,000–160,000

[a]ASMR rating of II for severe dementia, V for moderately severe dementia
[b]ASMR rating of IV for monotherapy, V for use as an adjunct to levodopa
[c]SMR rating was originally "important," but was amended to "weak" in 2005, following a change in the terminology of the indication
[d]Target population of 42,000–72,000 adults and 5,840–12,300 children
[e]Figures relate only to epilepsy; an additional 250,000–420,000 patients are targets for the treatment of peripheral neuropathic pain
ASMR = Amélioration du service médical rendu (improvement in medical benefit)
SMR = Service médical rendu (medical benefit)

progressive relapsing multiple sclerosis who have had at least two attacks in the previous two years (three years for Avonex) and are able to walk. Betaferon is additionally reimbursed for secondary progressive multiple sclerosis if the patient's Expanded Disability Status Scale (EDSS) score is 6 or lower. As *médicaments d'exception*, multiple sclerosis therapies are subject to prescribing restrictions: they may be prescribed only by neurologists and their use must be monitored throughout treatment.

Antiepileptic Agents

Given the number of antiepileptic agents that are off patent, it is not surprising that the French government is encouraging greater use of generic agents. In particular, it has identified gabapentin as one of 20 targets for a rapid increase in generics dispensing rates. In December 2005, generics accounted for only 11% of the total prescriptions dispensed for gabapentin, but this figure increased to 20% in April 2006. The government is targeting a generics dispensing rate of 40% in December 2006.

Germany

General Environment

The *Gesetzliche Krankenversicherung* (GKV; statutory health insurance) system covers approximately 90% of the German population. Manufacturers are free to set their own prices for new drugs, and medicines generally qualify for automatic reimbursement unless they treat relatively trivial disorders or are deemed inefficient.

Since the 1980s, successive German governments have introduced major reforms to curb pharmaceutical spending within the statutory health insurance system. The current cost-containment strategy includes measures such as a negative list of drugs excluded from reimbursement, a general price freeze, price cuts on off-patent drugs, industry rebates, reference pricing, indicative prescribing amounts, prescribing guidelines, generics substitution, the promotion of parallel imports, patient copayments, and dereimbursement of most nonprescription medicines.

Reference pricing, introduced in 1989, has been the most enduring cost-containment measure in Germany. If a drug's retail price exceeds its reference price, the patient must pay the difference – a powerful incentive for the manufacturer to reduce the price. From 1996 to 2004, patent-protected drugs approved in Germany after December 31, 1995, were excluded from reference pricing. In 2005, however, the German government began the gradual reintroduction of reference prices for some drug classes that include patent-protected agents – most notably statins and proton-pump inhibitors.

No patent-protected neurology drugs are subject to reference pricing at present, but carbamazepine, gabapentin, carbidopa/levodopa, pergolide, phenytoin, selegiline, and valproic acid are all reference-priced. Table 5.13 compares the retail and reference prices of select dosages and pack sizes of reference-priced neurology drugs. None of these drugs exceed their reference prices, and many products have retail prices more than 20% lower than their reference prices. Figure 5.10 shows mean reference prices for these compounds as a percentage of their reference prices. Phenytoin is unusual in having a mean reference price exactly in line with its reference price, but competition is limited in this market, with only three companies marketing products. By comparison, much more intense competition in the gabapentin market has reduced the mean retail price to just 72.5% of the reference price, and the lowest-priced product costs just 68.5% of its reference price.

Since July 1, 2006, drugs in 79 reference pricing groups that are priced at least 30% below their respective reference prices are exempt from any patient copayments. Table 5.14 shows the new out-of-pocket payment structure for reference-priced drugs in Germany. The 79 affected reference pricing groups contain approximately 7,200 distinct product presentations. According to the Bundesverband der Betriebskrankenkassen (BKK; Federal Association of Occupational Health Insurance Funds), as of August 15, 2006, 2,638 reference-priced product presentations were exempted from copayments, including 755 neurology product presentations (148 carbamazepine product presentations, 219 gabapentin product presentations, 87 carbidopa/levodopa product presentations, 76 selegiline product presentations,

Table 5.13 Reference and Retail Prices of Select Doses and Pack Sizes of Neurology Drugs Subject to Reference Pricing in Germany, August 2006

Drug	*Dosage (mg)*	*Pack Size (tablets/ caplets)*	*Reference Price (€)*	*Mean Retail Price (€)*	*Median Retail Price(€)*	*Retail Price Range(€)*
Carbamazepine	200	200	29.79	27.80	27.41	23.65–29.79
Gabapentin	300	200	129.83	94.17	93.70	88.98–129.83
Carbidopa/levodopa	25–100	100	28.28	23.96	22.62	22.60–28.28
Pergolide	0.25	100	81.42	71.14	70.26	69.98–74.23
Phenytoin	100	200	17.45	17.45	17.45	17.45–17.45
Selegiline	5	100	54.44	41.88	40.92	40.91–54.44
Valproic acid	300	200	46.03	35.85	35.02	34.75–46.03

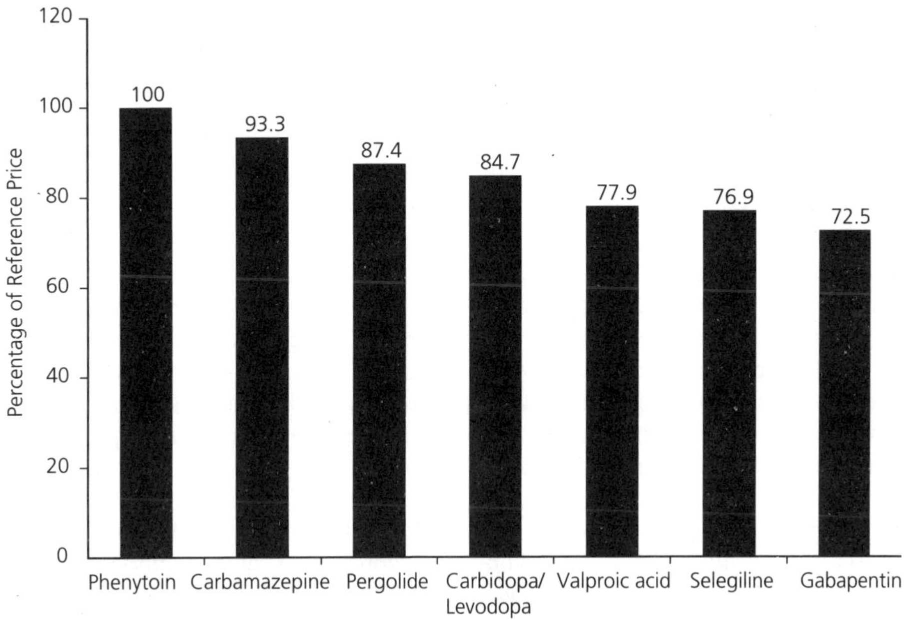

Figure 5.10 Mean Retail Prices for Select Neurology Drugs as a Percentage of Reference Prices in Germany, 2006

Table 5.14 Out-of-Pocket Payments for Reference-Priced Drugs in Germany

Retail Price Level	*Out-of-Pocket Payment*
At least 30% below reference price	0
Reference price	10% of retail price (within the range €5–10)
Above reference price	10% of retail price (within the range €5–10) plus the difference between the reference price and the retail price

and 225 valproic acid product presentations). Such numerous exemptions are somewhat surprising, given that relatively few neurology drugs are priced at least 30% below their respective reference prices. This reform is likely to have a major impact on branded versions of molecules that are subject to reference pricing. Drugs that are not subject to reference pricing but have therapeutic alternatives that are within the reference-pricing system could also lose sales.

Since the early 1990s, the German government has tried to curb pharmaceutical spending by a succession of budgetary limits on physicians. At present, physicians are subject to *Richtgrößen* – indicative prescribing amounts that determine the maximum expenditure on medicines per patient per quarter. Physicians who exceed these amounts by more than 25% face the prospect of heavy fines. Indicative prescribing amounts are set at state level and vary substantially by physician specialty. The allowances are much higher for senior citizens than for nonelderly patients. For example, in Berlin, GPs' indicative prescribing amounts in 2006 are €39.46 ($49.05) per quarter for each nonelderly patient and €112.83 ($140.24) for senior citizens. (The US dollar-to-euro exchange rate used in this chapter is the 2005 average rate, i.e., $1 = €0.80453.) By comparison, neurologists' indicative prescribing amounts are €96.62 ($115.12) per quarter for each nonelderly patient and €128.82 ($160.12) for senior citizens. These amounts are averages for all patients who visit physicians within a quarter. Concessions are granted to practices that have a disproportionately large number of patients who require costly treatments, and some expensive therapies are excluded from indicative prescribing amounts.

Beginning January 1, 2007, a new measure known as the *Bonus-Malus* (bonus/fine) rule will allow health insurance funds to set daily cost of therapy limits (by indication) for drugs that have substantial sales and a range of clinically comparable therapies. Physicians whose average prescribing costs exceed the daily cost of therapy limits in a quarter could face fines equivalent to as much as 50% of the excess cost. On the other hand, physicians whose prescribing averages less than the daily cost of therapy limit could qualify for a bonus. Physicians can draw some comfort from the fact that drugs that are subject to the *Bonus-Malus* rule are automatically exempt from indicative prescribing amounts. Alternative methods of controlling expenditures on best-selling drugs may be negotiated at state level, but physicians would still have to recompense the health insurance funds if their spending exceeded daily cost of therapy limits. The list of drugs to be included in this system has not yet been finalized, but high-priced neurology drugs (e.g., dementia therapies, multiple sclerosis therapies) could be targeted.

Dementia Therapies

The treatment of Alzheimer's disease and other forms of dementia in Germany has changed enormously over the past decade. Plant-derived therapies and nootropics have been progressively superseded by more costly AChEIs and memantine. In 1995, the statutory health insurance system reimbursed 260 million defined daily doses (DDDs) of ginkgo biloba extracts, 89 million DDDs of ergot alkaloid products, and 61 million DDDs of piracetam. In 2004, the number of DDDs of ginkgo biloba extracts declined to just 32 million, and ergot alkaloid and piracetam prescriptions amounted to 18 million and 14 million DDDs, respectively. Conversely, the volume of prescriptions for AChEIs and memantine has increased from a total of 25 million DDDs in 2001 to 37 million in 2004.

These statistics indicate that the number of patients receiving any form of drug therapy for dementia has declined sharply. According to GKV data, in 1992, a total of 516 million DDDs of dementia therapies were dispensed – sufficient to treat 1.4 million patients. In 2004, a total of 104 million DDDs of dementia therapies were enough to treat only 285,000 patients. Some comfort can be drawn from the fact that the dramatic reduction in the overall number of drug-treated dementia patients has been partially offset by an increase in the number of patients treated with the most modern drugs (i.e., AChEIs and memantine). However, the majority of dementia patients remain untreated. According to data compiled by Insight Health, only 290,000 of the 600,000 Alzheimer's disease patients in Germany receive drug therapy. The company reports that a total of 43.6 million DDDs of medication were dispensed in 2005 – enough to treat 120,000 patients according to guidelines. The undertreatment of Alzheimer's disease appears to be due in large measure to physicians' lack of conviction of the value of drug therapies for this disorder. GPs, in particular, are often wary of diagnosing Alzheimer's disease and do not always persevere with drug treatment. In addition, Insight Health found that 34.5% of drug-treated patients discontinued therapy within the first quarter of treatment, and 49.9% dropped out within two years.

Several factors explain Germany's historic reliance on traditional medicines in the management of dementia. Traditional remedies, especially plant-based products, are highly regarded by both the public and many physicians. These therapies have comparable status to modern synthetic drugs: they are licensed medicines, can be prescribed by physicians, and are reimbursed by the statutory health insurance system. Furthermore, traditional remedies are generally less than one-fifth the price of AChEIs and memantine. Cost is a very significant consideration in Germany not merely because of patients' out-of-pocket payments, but also because indicative prescribing amounts strongly influence physicians' prescribing behavior. The retail price of AChEIs and memantine – close to €4 ($4.97) per DDD – substantially exceeds GPs' and neurologists' indicative prescribing amounts for both nonelderly patients and senior citizens. Traditional medicines are much more affordable, even if their efficacy is now widely disputed. However, some states include dementia therapies in the list of *Praxisbesonderheiten* (practice special cases) that are exempt from indicative prescribing amounts.

In February 2005, the Institut für Qualität und Wirtschaftlichkeit im Gesundheitswesen (IQWiG; Institute for Quality and Economy in the Healthcare System), Germany's new health technology assessment (HTA) authority, began an assessment of the long-term use of AChEIs in Alzheimer's disease. The institute's preliminary report, published on September 8, 2006, concluded that in patients who have mild-to-moderate Alzheimer's disease, these drugs delay slightly the loss of cognitive faculties and the ability to perform activities of daily living. However, the authors found no proof of benefit in terms of disease-related quality of life and prevention of institutionalization. In a press release on the preliminary report, IQWiG mentioned the prevailing uncertainty in the international HTA community about the value of AChEIs. The press release specifically mentioned the repeated changes in the recommendations of the United Kingdom's National Institute for Health and Clinical Excellence (NICE) on the treatment of Alzheimer's disease (see further on), but also noted a key difference between these two HTA organizations – IQWiG does not take health economic considerations into account in its deliberations. Following a four-week public review period, IQWiG will prepare a final report for the Gemeinsamer Bundesausschuß der Ärzte, Zahnärzte, Krankenhäuser und Krankenkassen (GBA; Joint Federal Committee of Physicians, Dentists, Hospitals, and Health Insurance Funds), the authority that will ultimately decide whether the reimbursement terms for AChEIs in Germany should be altered. The GBA has also commissioned IQWiG to review other dementia therapies: memantine, ginkgo biloba, and nonpharmacological treatments.

Parkinson's Disease Therapies

The treatment of Parkinson's disease in Germany has changed radically since the mid-1990s. In 1995, anticholinergic drugs were the most widely prescribed agents, with 34 million DDDs reimbursed by the statutory health insurance system. That same year, 26 million DDDs of levodopa products (including combinations) and 4 million DDDs of dopamine agonists were dispensed. In 2004, levodopa products dominated the market, with 43 million DDDs, compared with 22 million DDDs of dopamine agonists and just 17 million DDDs of anticholinergics.

As with other neurological disorders, cost is a significant influence on prescribing decisions in Parkinson's disease. Anticholinergics typically cost less than €1 ($1.24) per DDD and levodopa products less than €3 ($3.73), compared with a daily cost of more than €7 ($8.70) for most dopamine agonists. Physicians – especially GPs – who are anxious about exceeding their indicative prescribing amounts may be reluctant to prescribe newer drugs. However, some states exempt Parkinson's disease therapies from indicative prescribing amounts.

Multiple Sclerosis Therapies

National guidelines on the treatment of multiple sclerosis direct physicians to prescribe interferon-beta products or glatiramer acetate to patients who have had at least two attacks in the previous two years, or after one attack if clinical evidence demonstrates disease progression. A neurologist should supervise treatment with these drugs and review each case within two years of the start of therapy.

States generally exempt multiple sclerosis therapies from indicative prescribing amounts. Therefore, the cost of disease-modifying drugs should not deter physicians from prescribing these drugs to patients who meet the basic requirements. However, in November 2002, the Deutsche Multiple Sklerose Gesellschaft (German Multiple Sclerosis Society) estimated that only 25% of patients were treated with these agents, a situation that the society attributed directly to cost-containment pressures.

Antiepileptic Agents

First-generation agents dominate the German antiepileptic market. According to GKV prescribing data, in 2004, 64.7 million DDDs of carbamazepine and 42.5 million DDDs of valproic acid were dispensed. A total of 54.3 million DDDs of second-generation agents were prescribed in 2004, including 18.5 million DDDs of gabapentin. Generics accounted for the majority of prescriptions for off-patent drugs: 74.7% for carbamazepine, 61.7% for valproic acid, 60.7% for phenytoin, and 53.2% for gabapentin.

Not surprisingly, cost is the main factor in the dominance of older antiepileptics. As with other neurology drug classes, German physicians are concerned that prescribing relatively expensive antiepileptics could cause them to exceed their indicative prescribing amounts. However, antiepileptics are exempt from such limits in some states.

Italy

General Environment

Italy's Servizio Sanitario Nazionale (SSN; National Health Service) uses a variety of supply- and demand-side restrictions to curb pharmaceutical expenditures: price controls, budgets, prescribing restrictions, reference pricing, promotion of generics dispensing, dereimbursement, and regional copayments. In 2001, the government streamlined the reimbursement structure by abolishing class B – the 50% reimbursement rate. Since that time, drugs that are included in the Prontuario Nazionale Farmaceutico (National Formulary) are assigned to class A and fully reimbursed. All other drugs are assigned to class C, which is not reimbursed at all. The vast majority of neurology drugs are in class A.

Reference pricing is an important element in the government's strategy to stimulate the immature Italian generics market. Bromocriptine, carbamazepine, gabapentin, carbidopa/levodopa, and valproic acid are the neurology drugs currently subject to reference pricing.

Dementia Therapies

The Italian healthcare system spent €73 million ($91 million) on AChEIs in 2005, a 6.5% increase over 2004. Donepezil, galantamine, and rivastigmine are fully reimbursed in Italy, but they are subject to prescribing restrictions. The Agenzia Italiana del Farmaco (AIFA; Italian Pharmaceutical Agency) operates a system of *note limitative* (restrictive notes) to control the prescription of certain drugs. *Nota limitativa* 85 governs the use of the AChEIs. The drugs may be prescribed only by neurologists working in approximately 500 *unità di valutazione Alzheimer* (Alzheimer's evaluation units) to patients who have mild-to-moderate Alzheimer's disease and an MMSE score higher than 10. Patient response is reviewed after three months of treatment and then every six months. Continued reimbursement is contingent on proof of benefit (cognitive stabilization as demonstrated by MMSE), patient compliance, and tolerability. If the patient's MMSE score falls to 10 or lower, treatment must be discontinued.

At present, memantine is not reimbursed in Italy. Launched in October 2004, the drug reached the Italian market too late to be included in Progetto CRONOS (Project CRONOS), a nationwide postmarketing surveillance study to evaluate the efficacy and safety of the AChEIs in the treatment of mild-to-moderate Alzheimer's disease. Consequently, few Italian physicians prescribe memantine, despite the fact that it is the only drug approved for moderate-to-severe Alzheimer's disease. However, health authorities in some regions (e.g.,

Lombardy) are reportedly seeking to introduce reimbursement for this agent. Manufacturers of other innovative medicines have launched drugs in Italy with class C status as a stepping stone to inclusion in the National Formulary.

Parkinson's Disease Therapies

In 2005, SSN spending on Parkinson's disease therapies totaled €146 million ($181 million), a 10.3% increase over 2004. Most drugs for this indication are fully reimbursed, but selegiline products and the 60-tablet pack size of entacapone are in class C (curiously, the 100-tablet pack size of entacapone is in class A).

Neurologists treat the majority of Parkinson's disease patients in Italy. Many patients are referred to one of 30 certified Parkinson's disease centers for treatment.

Multiple Sclerosis Therapies

All four disease-modifying therapies for multiple sclerosis are fully reimbursed by the SSN, but they are subject to stringent prescribing restrictions. *Nota limitativa* 65 specifies that these drugs may be prescribed only in specialist, university, or health authority centers. Any of the disease-modifying drugs may be prescribed to patients who have relapsing–remitting multiple sclerosis and an EDSS score of 1–5.5. Betaseron alone may be prescribed to patients who have been diagnosed with secondary-progressive multiple sclerosis, have an EDSS score of 3–6.5, and have had at least two relapses or an increase of at least one point in their EDSS score in the preceding two years. Regional health authorities may monitor the prescription and dispensation of the drugs at their discretion.

Antiepileptic Agents

The SSN spent €243 million ($302 million) on antiepileptics in 2005, an increase of 1.5% over 2004. Pregabalin is the only notable drug in this class that is not reimbursed in Italy. Although several first-generation antiepileptics are now off patent, generics typically account for a relatively modest share of this market. However, unbranded generics accounted for 89% of SSN spending on gabapentin in 2005.

Spain

General Environment

The Sistema Nacional de Salud (SNS; National Health System) provides healthcare coverage to 99% of the Spanish population; fewer than 10% of residents have supplementary private health insurance. Although drug prices in Spain are among the lowest in Europe, escalating pharmaceutical expenditure has prompted the government to introduce a variety of cost-cutting measures in recent years, including negative and positive lists, reference pricing, price cuts and freezes, a sales tax, prescribing restrictions and budgets, patient copayments, prior authorization, and the promotion of generics. Legislation enacted in June 2006 will expand the reference-pricing system, reduce the prices of older drugs by 20%, expedite the launch of generics, introduce health economic evaluation into reimbursement decision making, and limit reimbursement to drugs that meet strict criteria.

The standard out-of-pocket payment for outpatient prescription drugs is 40% of the retail price. The copayment is reduced to 10% of the retail price, with a maximum charge of €2.64 ($3.28) per pack, for certain drug classes or patient groups (e.g., statins prescribed to patients with heterozygous familial hypercholesterolemia). Senior citizens, pensioners, and some other groups are exempt from copayments. As a result of these concessions, patients' share of pharmaceutical spending in Spain has declined from roughly 18% in 1982 to less than 7% at present.

Dementia Therapies

The AChEIs and memantine are classified as *diagnóstico hospitalario* (DH; hospital diagnosis) products in Spain: the initial diagnosis and prescription must be made by a hospital-based neurologist or psychiatrist. In addition, the AChEIs are subject to *visados de inspección* (inspection visas), a form of prior authorization. Approval by the Servicio de Inspección (Inspection Service) generally requires a long-term clinical protocol prepared by an SNS neurologist. The visa must be renewed at least annually. Therapy is discontinued in patients who do not demonstrate an adequate response to treatment.

When dispensed in the hospital setting, AChEIs and memantine are fully reimbursed, but prescriptions dispensed in the community are subject to the *aportación normal* (normal copayment) of 40%. However, the majority of dementia patients are senior citizens, all of whom automatically qualify for full reimbursement of outpatient prescription drugs. Therefore, relatively few Spanish patients are required to make substantial copayments for dementia therapies.

Parkinson's Disease Therapies

Parkinson's disease patients in Spain are generally diagnosed and treated by neurologists. Therapies for this disorder (i.e., drugs that have the anatomical therapeutic chemical [ATC] codes N04A and N04B) are generally subject to the *aportación reducida* (reduced copayment) of 10%. However, differential reimbursement rates apply to cabergoline products: Kenfarma's Dostinex is subject to the normal copayment but Pfizer's Sogilen to the reduced payment.

Multiple Sclerosis Therapies

Spanish patients who present to their GPs with symptoms of multiple sclerosis are generally referred to a neurologist for diagnosis. Most patients are subsequently managed in specialized care settings.

Disease-modifying therapies for multiple sclerosis are restricted to *uso hospitalario* (hospital use, designated as category H products). In common with other drugs dispensed in the hospital setting, these agents are fully reimbursed. Early treatment with these drugs has become more common in Spain following the revision of national regulations to allow therapy after one demyelinating event.

Antiepileptic Agents

Spanish neurologists typically use first-generation antiepileptics (e.g., valproic acid, phenytoin, carbamazepine) as first-line therapies for epilepsy. Second-generation agents are widely prescribed to patients who fail to respond adequately to initial treatment.

The cost of antiepileptics is not a significant factor in prescribing decisions in Spain. Products with ATC code N03 are reimbursed at the 90% rate in Spain. The Spanish generics market as a whole is immature by international standards, and neurologists are particularly reluctant to prescribe generic antiepileptics.

United Kingdom

General Environment

A pricing system that allows manufacturers freedom to set their own prices for branded prescription drugs but limits their overall profits has contributed to the United Kingdom's position among the highest-priced pharmaceutical markets in Europe. Drugs can be launched as soon as they are licensed, and most are immediately reimbursable by the National Health Service (NHS). However, reimbursability does not guarantee use. Primary care trusts (PCTs), the organizations that now control 80% of the NHS budget, are frequently reluctant to add new drugs to their formularies before these products have been evaluated by the National Institute for Health and Clinical Excellence (NICE), one of the world's foremost HTA organizations.

The influence of NICE on the healthcare system in England and Wales can scarcely be overstated. (Scotland has its own HTA and reimbursement authorities – the Scottish Intercollegiate Guidelines Network [SIGN] and the Scottish Medicines Consortium [SMC].) The delayed adoption of drugs undergoing or awaiting evaluation by NICE – a problem commonly known as "NICE blight" – is a major factor in the exceptionally slow penetration of new therapies in the UK pharmaceutical market. The creation of NICE was expected to combat the "postcode lottery" of variations in PCTs' coverage of innovative therapies, but inequalities persist. Notwithstanding their legal obligation to cover NICE-approved treatments within three months of the institute's decision, some PCTs reportedly continue to restrict access to certain therapies.

The UK government has explicitly focused its healthcare policy (and resources) on several clinical priority areas, namely cancer, coronary heart disease, mental illness, diabetes, and geriatric medicine. NICE's program of technology appraisals and clinical guidelines has concentrated on these disease areas. In addition, the government has published national service frameworks that provide GPs with broad guidance on how best to manage disorders in these therapeutic areas. Since 2004, a general medical services (GMS) contract rewards GPs who meet defined performance targets in the prevention and/or treatment of several key disorders, including epilepsy and transient ischemic attacks.

Despite allowing relatively high prices for branded drugs, the United Kingdom is a highly price-sensitive market. The government's cost-containment strategy includes price controls on generic drugs, profit controls on branded drugs, price cuts, primary care prescribing budgets, prescribing audits, patient copayments, promotion of parallel imports, and a strong culture of generic prescribing and dispensing. In 2004, generics accounted for 58% of all prescriptions dispensed in England.

Patient copayments are not a major factor in prescribing decisions in the United Kingdom. In England and Scotland, patients pay a flat sum of £6.65 ($12.09) per prescription item; in Wales, the charge is £3.00 ($5.45) per item. (The US dollar-to-pound sterling exchange rate used in this chapter is the 2005 average rate, i.e., $1 = £0.55004.) However, approximately half of all UK residents – including senior citizens and patients with low incomes and/or particular medical conditions – are exempt from copayments. These patients account for approximately 86% of all prescriptions dispensed within the NHS.

Dementia Therapies

The AChEIs and memantine are reimbursable by the NHS, but their use has been curtailed by restrictions contained in NICE guidance. In January 2001, NICE published an appraisal that recommended the use of AChEIs for the adjunctive treatment of mild and moderate Alzheimer's disease in patients who have an MMSE score above 12 points, subject to the following conditions:

- A specialist clinic must make the diagnosis of Alzheimer's disease and should assess the patient's cognitive, global, and behavioral functioning, activities of daily living, and likelihood of compliance with treatment.
- Treatment should be initiated by specialists but may be continued by general practitioners under a shared-care protocol.
- Caregivers should be consulted before and during drug treatment for their view of the patient's condition.
- Two to four months after a maintenance dose is established, the patient's condition should be reassessed and drug treatment should continue only if the MMSE score has improved or has not deteriorated and if behavioral or functional assessment shows evidence of improvement.
- The patient should be reassessed every six months, and drug treatment should normally continue only if the MMSE score remains above 12 points and if treatment is judged to have a worthwhile effect on the patient's global, functional, and behavioral condition.

NICE estimated that approximately 50,000 new cases of Alzheimer's disease would be diagnosed each year, of which roughly 30,000 might be expected to receive a prescription for an AChEI for six months, at a total cost to the NHS of £12 million ($21.8 million). If half of this group (i.e., 15,000 patients per year) continued drug therapy for an average of three years (until they progressed to severe Alzheimer's disease or succumbed to another disease), total costs to the NHS would increase to approximately £42 million ($76.4 million) per year. However, NICE acknowledged that this figure, which assumed that no patients would discontinue treatment, may have been an overestimate. In addition to estimating the direct costs of prescribing AChEIs, NICE noted that increased use of these drugs could deliver indirect savings in the cost of caring for Alzheimer's disease patients. For example, delaying a patient's admission to a nursing home by 12 weeks could save social services approximately £4,500 ($8,181).

In February 2005, NICE published a preliminary decision on its review of the AChEIs for mild-to-moderate Alzheimer's disease, with the addition of an assessment of memantine for moderately-severe-to-severe Alzheimer's disease. To the surprise of most observers, the institute reversed its earlier decision in favor of prescribing the AChEIs for the mild-to-moderate stages of the disease and advised against the use of memantine other than in new clinical trials. However, NICE did not oppose the continued use of any of these dementia therapies by patients who were already taking them in a clinical trial or as part of their established therapeutic regimen. NICE's objections to these drugs were based mainly on doubts about some outcomes (notably, functional outcomes, quality of life, and behavioral symptoms) and disagreements with the manufacturers' health economic data.

In June 2006, NICE published its final appraisal document on the AChEIs and memantine. The report recommended that the NHS should reimburse AChEIs only for patients with moderate Alzheimer's disease, despite the fact that these drugs are also approved for the mild stages of this disorder – the time of maximum clinical impact, in the opinion of many physicians. The institute also reaffirmed its view that memantine should be reimbursed only for participants in approved clinical trials.

Eisai, Shire Pharmaceuticals, and Lundbeck all registered appeals, as did several patient organizations and medical societies. Novartis, on the other hand, did not appeal NICE's judgment. Lundbeck argues that memantine is needed because AChEIs are unsuitable for up to half of Alzheimer's disease patients: the company calculates that NICE's decision would deny 309,000 patients in England and Wales the possibility of effective therapy. In a press statement, Paul Hooper, the managing director of Eisai Limited, notes that, "in every other disease, doctors are encouraged, even instructed, to find and treat patients early. However, with Alzheimer's disease, NICE is saying wait until patients deteriorate before you treat them. It makes no sense medically, it makes no sense economically, and it makes no sense in improving the lives of patients and their carers." The manufacturers involved are also critical of NICE for refusing to disclose the model that it used in its appraisal, thereby denying them the opportunity to run their own simulations.

A final decision on the status of AChEIs and memantine will be made after the appeals process is completed. This final ruling, along with key elements of NSFs on long-term care and older people, will be incorporated into new guidelines on the cost-effective treatment of dementia that are being developed by the National Collaborating Centre for Mental Health.

Parkinson's Disease Therapies

All Parkinson's disease therapies are reimbursed in the United Kingdom, but newer agents are prescribed relatively rarely. NHS prescribing data indicate that levodopa products (mainly carbidopa/levodopa and levodopa/benserazide) accounted for almost 70% of all Parkinson's disease therapies in England in 2005. Because of concerns over bioequivalence, generics were used much less frequently than for most other off-patent medicines: generics accounted for 76% of all prescriptions for carbidopa/levodopa.

In June 2006, NICE published clinical guidelines on the management of Parkinson's disease. The report contained no comments about the cost of drug therapy for this disorder and concluded that there is no single drug of choice in the treatment of either early or more advanced Parkinson's disease. NICE recommended that patients who present to their GPs with symptoms of Parkinson's disease should be referred untreated to a neurologist for diagnosis and therapy. However, a recent survey of 203 GPs conducted by the Parkinson's Disease Society suggests that many physicians in primary care disregard such recommendations and seek to manage patients with Parkinson's disease themselves. The survey found that, although more than 90% of GPs conceded that they lacked specialist knowledge of Parkinson's disease, approximately 20% chose not to refer patients with symptoms of this disorder to a specialist, and around one-quarter changed patients' medications without consulting a specialist.

Multiple Sclerosis Therapies

Access to disease-modifying multiple sclerosis therapies in the United Kingdom has been severely hampered by NICE's assessment of these agents. In July 2000, the institute concluded that interferon beta products were too expensive and therefore should not be prescribed at NHS expense. The committee deferred assessment of glatiramer acetate pending its marketing authorization.

Eight consultees, representing companies and interest groups, appealed against various aspects of the final appraisal determination (FAD); in November 2000, the appeals committee upheld some objections but rejected others. The main area of contention was NICE's assessment of cost-effectiveness. In December 2000, NICE commissioned new economic models for interferon beta products and glatiramer acetate, which had by then been granted marketing authorization. In October 2001, a second FAD, based on the revised economic models, questioned the cost-effectiveness of these therapies. In January 2002, NICE announced that a second appeal hearing, in November 2001, had upheld the appraisal committee's recommendations. In February 2002, NICE issued its final guidance, reiterating its original advice that these multiple sclerosis therapies should not be prescribed to NHS patients.

In a draft decision in August 2001, NICE had also recommended that the manufacturers of interferon beta products and glatiramer acetate negotiate price cuts with the DH to make their drugs more cost-effective for the NHS. Not surprisingly, the companies reacted angrily: they criticized the NICE appraisal process and the DH's prolonged lack of communication. To break the stalemate between NICE and the pharmaceutical companies and ensure patient access to the new multiple sclerosis therapies, the Department of Health negotiated a new risk-sharing program with manufacturers. Since May 2002, designated neurologists can enroll all patients who satisfy the multiple sclerosis criteria of the Association of British Neurologists in this new program. The NHS is paying agreed prices for these drugs but will be entitled to cut the prices if they exceed a cost-effectiveness threshold of £36,000 ($65,450) per quality-adjusted life year (QALY). The drugs' performance will be measured by their progressive impact on patients' disability scores, measured against baseline and monitored annually for 10 years or more.

By November 2003, the program aimed to offer interferon beta therapy to 7,500–9,000 additional patients, including 5,500–7,000 patients in a formal monitoring cohort. However, enrollment has been slow. In May 2002, before the program began, 2,977 patients were taking disease-modifying agents for multiple sclerosis. To date, approximately 6,500 patients have been treated in the risk-sharing program.

In a June 14, 2004, debate in the House of Lords, Earl Howe, the opposition health spokesman who tabled the debate, noted that only approximately 8% of multiple sclerosis patients in the United Kingdom receive disease-modifying therapies, compared with an EU average of roughly 35% and 50% in the United States. In the course of this debate,

Lord Clement-Jones, another opposition spokesman on health, commented: "Many PCTs are treating MS as low priority, although . . . there is a mandatory requirement to fund medicines under the risk-sharing scheme. Funding levels also vary between regions, pointing continually to the problems with addressing specialist care at PCT level. It is clear that PCTs are not treating specialist conditions as a priority."

Howe suggested that a shortage of qualified specialists in the NHS is a major factor in the slow enrollment in the risk-sharing scheme. For example, he noted that the United Kingdom has one neurologist for every 177,000 inhabitants, compared with one for every 38,000 inhabitants in France. Given the lack of neurologists, it is hardly surprising that a survey commissioned by the Multiple Sclerosis Society in 2003 found that almost 20% of respondents and potentially eligible patients were still awaiting an appointment for assessment of their condition. Moreover, 55% of respondents reported difficulties in obtaining an initial assessment. These findings indicate that inadequate capacity in the NHS may be a major factor in the slow uptake of NICE-approved therapies.

Experts report that NICE's generally negative assessment of disease-modifying therapies has damaged these agents' reputation and credibility in the United Kingdom. One physician suggested that the utility of disease-modifying drugs

> is still considered very modest, but what's changed is the context in which they've been introduced. I don't think many people really believe the risk-sharing scheme is going to change our view of the efficacy of these agents. It is a political fudge by which both or all three parties get something that they want: the government gets cost control, the patient gets access to the medication, and the drug companies get access to a market.

In November 2006, NICE plans to review its guidance on the use of disease-modifying therapies in the light of data from the risk-sharing program. However, even if the institute recommends a relaxation of the restrictions on the use of these agents, the conservative climate that has been created will likely limit the future growth of this market in the United Kingdom.

Antiepileptic Agents

Unlike most of the other major pharmaceutical markets, the United Kingdom manages the majority of epileptic patients at the primary care level. This practice reflects the aforementioned shortage of neurologists within the NHS. Specialists express reservations about GPs' ability to diagnose the type of epileptic syndrome accurately.

All antiepileptic drugs are reimbursable within the NHS, but prescribing budgets prompt many GPs to use less expensive older drugs in preference to second-generation agents. NICE also exerts an important influence on the management of epilepsy in England and Wales. The institute had published technology appraisals of the use of newer antiepileptic drugs for adults and children in March and April 2004, respectively. Furthermore, in October of that year, NICE had also published a broader clinical guideline entitled "The Epilepsies: The Diagnosis and Management of the Epilepsies in Adults and Children in Primary and Secondary Care." The technology appraisal on the use of newer antiepileptics for adults directs that second-generation antidepressants can be tried if older drugs (e.g., valproic acid, carbamazepine) provoke serious side effects, fail to prevent seizures, or are unsuitable for a patient (e.g., because of contraindications or drug interactions). NICE recommends the use of adjunctive therapy only if various forms of monotherapy have first proved unsuccessful.

As noted earlier, the GMS contract rewards GPs for meeting specified targets on the management of epilepsy. Practices are measured on four indicators:

- Maintaining a register of patients aged 18 and older who receive drug therapy for epilepsy.
- The percentage of drug-treated adult epileptics who have a record of seizure frequency over the preceding 15 months.
- The percentage of drug-treated adult epileptics who have a record of medication review with the

patient and/or a caregiver over the preceding 15 months.

- The percentage of drug-treated adult epileptics who have been free of seizures for the last 12 months recorded in the preceding 15 months.

The inclusion of epilepsy in the GMS contract demonstrates the importance that the UK government attaches to the effective management of this disorder. However, the general price sensitivity of the NHS, reinforced by NICE's recommendation of older drugs as first-line therapy, suggests that the untapped market potential for second-generation antiepileptics in the United Kingdom is limited.

Japan

General Environment

Japan is the world's largest price-controlled market for prescription drugs. Drugs that are to be prescribed by physicians in office- or hospital-based practice under any social health insurance program must be listed with a *yakka* (reimbursement price) in the National Health Insurance (NHI) tariff. The most distinguishing feature of the Japanese market is the biennial NHI price-revision process, an exercise intended to narrow the gap between reimbursement prices and actual market prices. In addition, the Ministry of Health, Labor, and Welfare (MHLW) sometimes cuts the prices of individual brands or entire classes in response to, or even in anticipation of, increased sales.

Because the Japanese government exercises such strict control over prices, it has not needed to employ the wide range of cost-containment measures that have been imposed in most other markets. However, patients are required to pay part of the cost of their healthcare: salaried workers and their dependents generally pay 30% of their outpatient treatment costs, while seniors benefit from reduced coinsurance rates – currently 10–20%. Forty-five "intractable diseases," including multiple sclerosis and Parkinson's disease, are subject to reduced copayments: depending on their income, patients pay ¥0–11,550 ($0–104.88) for outpatient treatment. (The US dollar-to-yen exchange rate used in this chapter is the 2005 average rate, i.e., $1 = ¥110.12445.)

As in most other therapeutic areas, the range of neurology drugs available in Japan is much more limited than in the other major pharmaceutical markets. Many drugs that have been available in the United States and Europe for several years have yet to reach the Japanese market, and some agents are unlikely ever to be launched in Japan.

Dementia Therapies

Donepezil, a drug developed by a Japanese company (Eisai), is the only AChEI currently available in Japan. The drug is subject to standard reimbursement terms within the NHI. The MHLW has removed nootropic agents (e.g., aniracetam [Toyamakagaku's Sarpul, Nippon Roche's Draganon]) from the NHI reimbursement list.

Parkinson's Disease Therapies

The NHI reimburses most drug treatments for Parkinson's disease on the market in Japan. Because this disorder is classified as an intractable disease, patients can benefit from full reimbursement of the cost of their medications, provided that they have a Hoehn-Yahr score of at least 3. Patients who do not qualify for full reimbursement may face substantial out-of-pocket costs for the more expensive Parkinson's disease therapies (e.g., dopamine agonists).

Multiple Sclerosis Therapies

Only one disease-modifying multiple sclerosis therapy – interferon beta-1b – is currently available in Japan. Sales are modest by international standards – just $36 million in 2005. Because of Japan's small population of multiple sclerosis patients, this agent has orphan-drug status in Japan. Patients who meet the intractable disease conditions for multiple sclerosis receive full reimbursement of the cost of their medications for this disorder.

Antiepileptic Agents

Only one second-generation antiepileptic drug – zonisamide (Dainippon's Excegran, Elan's Zonegran) – is currently available in Japan. Therefore, neurologists in Japan tend to rely more heavily than their counterparts in the other major pharmaceutical markets on first-generation agents (especially valproic acid, carbamazepine, and phenytoin). A special reimbursement plan covers 95–100% of epileptic patients' treatment costs (except hospitalization). Generic usage is generally limited in Japan, and demand for generic antiepileptic drugs has been particularly hampered by physicians' doubts about the bioequivalence of these products.

OUTLOOK AND IMPLICATIONS FOR THE PHARMACEUTICAL INDUSTRY

Our analysis of neurology drug prices confirms the conventional wisdom that branded-drug prices are generally substantially higher in the United States than in Europe or Japan, whereas US prices for generics tend to be much lower than prices in other major markets. However, our data highlight some interesting variations in the pricing of branded neurology drugs. While the average European prices for branded Parkinson's disease therapies and antiepileptics were, respectively, 40% and 38% of US average prices, the average European price for branded Alzheimer's disease therapies was 82% of the US average price. Moreover, the average European price for multiple sclerosis therapies was 11% higher than the US average price. In assessing these price differentials, it is important to bear in mind that the Parkinson's disease therapy and antiepileptic drug classes both contain several older drugs that are off patent and subject to generics competition, a development that generally prompts a reduction in the originator brands' prices. Nevertheless, it is noteworthy that European reimbursement authorities have been prepared to accept prices in some drug classes that approach, or even exceed, US prices. In particular, manufacturers of biologics have been able to secure relatively high prices in most therapeutic areas in Europe.

Of course, high prices do not guarantee commercial success. Negotiating generous reimbursement terms and persuading physicians to prescribe the new therapy can be difficult, particularly in an increasingly price-sensitive environment. Funding for neurology drugs will come under increasing pressure in most markets, especially at the upper end of the pricing spectrum (notably biologics).

The US market will be boosted by massive investment in Medicare Part D, but the benefits to the pharmaceutical industry may be largely offset by larger discounts and rebates and a continued decline in employer-sponsored insurance. Medicare prescription drug plans have thus far demonstrated a much greater propensity than private insurers to use cost-containment measures such as prior authorization, quantity limits, step therapy protocols, and assigning drugs to the specialty pharmacy tier of their formularies. The pharmaceutical industry could face serious difficulties if insurers use the experience they gain from Medicare Part D to introduce similarly aggressive cost-containment strategies in their commercial health plans. In addition, generics substitution and therapeutic interchange (i.e., switching a patient from a prescribed drug to a completely different compound) will become more common, often at the instigation of PBMs.

European healthcare systems have generally regulated the use of neurology drugs by limiting the prescription of these agents, at least initially, to specialists – often in the hospital setting. Safety considerations are a major factor in the imposition of prescribing restrictions on neurology drugs, but payers are not averse to the savings that come from more restrictive use. The common requirement to review the clinical impact of therapy at frequent intervals and to discontinue treatment if outcomes targets are not achieved confirms that cost is a very important influence on prescribing policies for neurology drugs. Physicians in Europe can expect increasingly close scrutiny of their prescribing activity with a view to providing feedback, rewarding economical prescribing, or even penalizing what is perceived to be extravagant prescribing. Budgetary pressures will prompt many physicians to prescribe lower-priced drugs, particularly as further drugs lose patent protection and face generics competition. Because of wide-ranging exemptions, patient copayments have had limited impact as a cost-containment measure in Europe, but governments are likely to control exemptions more strictly in the future.

In Japan, the greatest challenge for the future evolution of the neurology drug market is the need to expand the range of available drugs. Because of lower prevalence, diagnosis, and drug treatment rates than in most of the other major pharmaceutical markets, the Japanese market for neurology drugs is not especially attractive to foreign companies.

Increasing generics competition is likely to impact all markets in the next decade. Although numerous generic anti-epileptic drugs and Parkinson's disease therapies are available, concerns about their bioequivalence have limited their use. The dementia and multiple sclerosis therapy markets offer potentially greater rewards to generics companies, and some manufacturers are trying to accelerate the launch of generics in these drugs classes. (See the sidebar "Generic Neurology Drugs – An Increasingly Competitive Market.") However, Table 5.15 shows that most patent-protected neurology drugs are unlikely to face the threat of generics competition before 2010.

Generic Neurology Drugs – An Increasingly Competitive Market

While generics have long been an important feature of the US market for Parkinson's disease therapies and antiepileptics, branded dementia and multiple sclerosis therapies have yet to face generics competition. However, this situation could change in the near future – at least if generics companies have their way. The market for dementia therapies is a particularly attractive target for generics manufacturers. In 2005, the FDA tentatively approved Ranbaxy's generic donepezil (5 and 10 mg), but Eisai reached an agreement with the generics company to delay the launch until the expiry of the product patent in 2010. In August 2006, however, Mutual Pharmaceutical and United Research Laboratories filed abbreviated new drug applications (ANDAs) against Aricept ODT, only a year after its US launch. Similarly, generics manufacturers Dr Reddy's Laboratories, Sun Pharmaceuticals and Watson Pharmaceuticals have filed Paragraph IV challenges against the product patent on rivastigmine tablets and solution. This patent was originally scheduled to expire in 2007, but the FDA has reportedly granted an extension until 2012.

Barr Laboratories filed an ANDA against Janssen's method of use patent for galantamine on February 28, 2005, precisely one year before the expiration of the drugís marketing exclusivity. Janssen and Synaptech jointly sued in June 2005, thereby delaying the launch of generics by at least 30 months (unless litigation is resolved before this period ends). Between April and May of that year, six other generics manufacturers (Teva, Mylan, Dr. Reddy's Laboratories, Purepac Pharmaceutical, Roxane Laboratories and Mutual Pharmaceutical) filed ANDAs for the drug. Then, in March 2006, generics manufacturers again filed ANDAs against Razadyne ER, the extended-release formulation of galantamine launched in May 2005. Janssen's prospects of successfully defending its patent on galantamine may be undermined by the number of generics companies challenging a relatively weak primary patent (i.e. a method of use patent).

The launch of generic disease-modifying multiple sclerosis therapies will be more challenging for generics manufacturers. Developing generic versions of biologic agents is a very new and unfamiliar exercise that will be costly, time-consuming and fraught with regulatory difficulties. Europe leads the United States in this particular field. The European Union has established a regulatory framework for the licensing of "similar biologic medicinal products." Sandoz's Omnitrope (somatropin) made biogeneric history when it became the first official biogeneric – or biosimilar, as it is known in Europe – to receive EMEA approval, on April 19, 2006. The following month, the FDA also approved biogeneric Omnitrope, albeit following a long regulatory delay and litigation. However, the agency maintains that it does not have the legal authority to approve biogenerics that reference biologic agents marketed under biologic license applications (BLAs). The FDA believes that new legislation is required for biogeneric versions of products approved under the Public Health Service Act (PHS Act). The only sure resolution to the possibility of biogenerics marketed under BLAs would need to come from the US Congress, which would have to amend the PHS Act to allow an abbreviated pathway.

Undeterred by the regulatory hurdles and the potential cost of conducting clinical trials to satisfy the FDA, several generics manufacturers – GeneMedix, Bioceuticals Arzneimittel, and Prolong Pharma – are developing interferon beta products. The first product is expected to be launched in Europe in 2008, but a potential launch date in the United States remains uncertain. In addition, the temporary withdrawal from the market of Elan/Biogen Idec's Tysabri (natalizumab) following the death of several patients has made the FDA more cautious about the regulation of biologics. As a condition of the relaunch of Tysabri, Elan and Biogen Idec must conduct post-marketing surveillance studies. This development will likely heighten physicians' reservations about the safety and efficacy of biogenerics. To offset the costs of the additional studies, Elan and Biogen Idec increased Tysabri's average wholesale price by 21% when they relaunched the drug in the United States.

In the future, the pricing and reimbursement terms for new drugs will depend heavily on their degree of innovation. France, Italy, and Japan have used this methodology for price-setting for several years, and Germany and Spain plan to adopt innovation as a key criterion in reimbursement decision making. "Me-too" drugs and reformulations will be at a disadvantage in this climate. For instance, payers may be reluctant to pay a premium for GlaxoSmithKline/SkyePharma's controlled-release formulation of ropinirole or Novartis's Exelon TDS (transdermal system patch). On the other hand, drugs that offer a major clinical advance could benefit from higher prices, more favorable reimbursement terms, and wider prescribing. For example, Neurochem's NC-758 and Myriad Genetics' R-flurbiprofen are expected to be the first disease-modifying dementia therapies to reach the market – a potentially significant breakthrough that could be rewarded with generous price premiums. Similarly, oral multiple sclerosis therapies could offer a considerable improvement in convenience and garner higher prices, provided that advanced clinical trials dispel current concerns about the safety of these agents.

Increasingly, new and established therapies will be subjected to HTA and health economic evaluation. The United Kingdom has been a pioneer in this field, but other countries are following suit. Germany's IQWiG and France's Haute Autorité de Santé (National Health Authority) have recently agreed on a collaboration with NICE, and Italy's AIFA publicizes NICE judgments. In the United States, the Medicare Prescription Drug, Improvement, and Modernization Act of 2003 (MMA) calls on the Agency for Healthcare Research & Quality (AHRQ) to conduct trials to compare the clinical effectiveness and cost-effectiveness of branded medicines that compete within a given drug class. The act directs that cost-effectiveness studies may include "high-cost" healthcare products and services "as well as those which may be underutilized and overutilized and which may significantly improve the prevention, treatment, or cure of diseases and conditions (including chronic conditions) which impose high direct or indirect costs on patients or society." The Department of Health and Human Services has identified dementia including Alzheimer's disease as one of the ten priority conditions for AHRQ research on effective healthcare.

As noted in the introduction to this chapter, the burden on society from neurological disorders – especially diseases associated with aging – will grow in coming years. The costs of treating these conditions are likely to increase steadily, an unwelcome

Table 5.15 Patent Expiration Calendar for Select Neurology Drugs

	United States	*France*	*Germany*	*Italy*	*Spain*	*United Kingdom*	*Japan*
Dementia therapies							
Donepezil	11/2010[a,b]	2/2012[a]	6/2012[a]	2/2012[a]	2/2012[a]	2/2012[a]	9/2011[a]
Rivastigmine	8/2012[a,c]	7/2012[a]	2/2008[a]	3/2013[a]	3/2013[a]	7/2012[a]	3/2008[a]
Galantamine	12/2008[a,d]	1/2012[a]	1/2012[a]	1/2012[a]	1/2012[a]	1/2012[a]	1/2007[a]
Memantine	4/2010[a,e]	8/2012[e]	8/2012[e]	8/2012[e]	8/2012[e]	8/2012[e]	Post-2015[e]
Parkinson's disease therapies							
Cabergoline	N.A.	Expired	Expired	Expired	Expired	Expired	12/2006
Entacapone	10/2013	11/2012[f]	11/2012[f]	11/2012[f]	11/2007[g]	11/2012[f]	11/2010
Carbidopa/levodopa/entacapone	10/2013	11/2010[g]	11/2010[g]	11/2015[f]	1/2010	11/2010[h]	2012[i]
Pramipexole	12/2011	12/2010	12/2010	12/2010	12/2010	12/2010	11/2010
Ropinirole	12/2008[j]	Expired	11/2011[f]	11/2008[f]	11/2005	11/2008[f]	12/2003
Multiple sclerosis therapies							
Interferon-beta-1b	2007[a]	2008[a]	2008[a]	2008[a]	2008[a]	2008[a]	2008[a]
Interferon-beta-1a (Avonex)	2013[a]	2005[a]	2005[a]	2005[a]	2005[a]	2005[a]	2005[a]
Interferon-beta-1a (Rebif)	2013[a]	2013[a]	2013[a]	2013[a]	2013[a]	2013[a]	2013[a]
Glatiramer acetate	2014[a]	2015[a]	2015[a]	2015[a]	2015[a]	2015[a]	2015[a]
Antiepileptic agents							
Gabapentin	Expired	4/2009	Expired	Expired	Expired	Expired	5/2009
Levetiracetam	8/2009[a,k]	5/2010[a]	5/2010[a]	5/2010[a]	2/2012[a]	5/2010[a]	5/2005
Pregabalin	Post-2014	5/2013[g]	5/2013	5/2013[g]	5/2013	Post-2014[a]	5/2013
Topiramate	9/2008[a,k]	9/2009[a]	9/2009[a]	9/2009[a]	7/2005	9/2009[a]	Expired

[a]Expiry of key patent (includes any relevant extensions, e.g., Hatch-Waxman, SPC, or Japanese patent extension)
[b]Ranbaxy Laboratories filed a Paragraph IV certification for the 5 mg and 10 mg formulations of donepezil in October 2003. The 30-month stay following the ANDA filing is estimated to expire in 2006. In February 2005, the FDA tentatively approved Ranbaxy's abbreviated new drug application (ANDA), but we believe this to be a judgment on the safety of the drug, not an approval to begin its manufacture. In December 2005, Eisai filed a patent infringement lawsuit against Teva regarding the latter's ANDA submission to the FDA for a generic version of Aricept. In February 2006, Par Pharmaceutical Companies received tentative approval for its 5 and 10 mg generic donepezil tablets. In August 2006, Mutual Pharmaceutical and United Research Laboratories filed ANDAs against Aricept ODT; Eisai has countersued
[c]Paragraph IV certifications were filed in April 2004 and November 2004 for the capsule and oral solution formulations of rivastigmine, respectively. The compound patent for rivastigmine has qualified for a patent term extension in the United States until 2012. Dr. Reddy's, Sun Pharmaceuticals, and Watson Pharmaceuticals have filed applications to market generic Exelon in the United States. In December 2005, the FDA's Office of Generic Drugs granted tentative approval for generic Exelon; patent infringement litigation is pending
[d]In January 2004, the key patent expiry was extended 1,064 days from the original expiration date of January 2006, yielding a new expiry date of December 2008
[e]We anticipate generics companies will file a Paragraph IV challenge against memantine's method-of-use patents in 2007, one year before the new chemical entity (NCE) exclusivity ends in October 2008. We believe that a generic form of memantine is an attractive option, so the Paragraph IV is likely. Paragraph IVs were systematically filed for donepezil, galantamine, and rivastigmine one year before these drugs' exclusivity was up, suggesting that memantine would follow suit. The Paragraph IV challenge starts an automatic 30-month stay to resolve the litigation, during which time no generic can be approved unless the litigation is resolved beforehand. We anticipate generics will be approved, leading to a possible entry in 2010 in the United States. New drugs in Europe have 10 years of data exclusivity from a drug's first approval date. Although memantine was originally launched in Germany in 1982, the drug was officially launched for AD in the *European Union* in 2002, yielding a date of 2012 for generic entry. In Japan, new drugs get six years of exclusivity from launch; because we anticipate a launch in 2010, the patent expiration date falls outside of our forecast time frame
[f]Supplementary protection certificate (SPC) granted. This certificate will provide a maximum of 15 years of protection from the date of the first marketing approval in a EU member state. The SPC will come into effect when the cited patent expires and will extend protection for a maximum of five years
[g]SPC filed
[h]SPC filed and withdrawn, November 2005
[i]Predicted data exclusivity (five year)
[j]FDA new indication exclusivity (three year)
[k]Paragraph IV certification filed; we do not assume early generic entry
N.A. = Not available

prospect for third-party payers, but the costs of failing to manage these diseases adequately could be even greater, in both human and economic terms. Effective treatment can help reduce or postpone disability and unemployment, delay hospitalization or nursing home care, and improve the quality of life of patients and their caregivers. The fundamental challenge facing the pharmaceutical industry is to present this message clearly and cogently to third-party payers in all markets.

REFERENCE

Crowley J.S. et al. *State Medicaid Outpatient Prescription Drug Policies: Findings from a National Survey*, 2005.

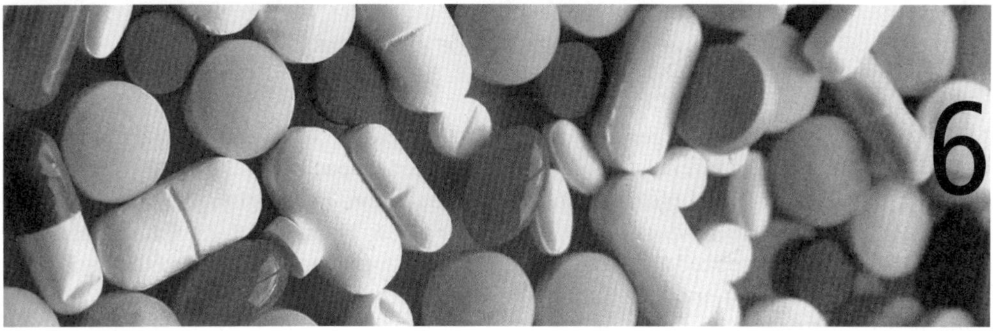

6

Authorized Generics: Look Before You Leap

PARAGRAPH IV CHALLENGES: AN OVERVIEW

In an effort to help retain revenue and lessen the impact of generic erosion, research-based pharmaceutical companies have used a variety of tactics to extend the life of a patented drug with varying degrees of success. One such tactic that has garnered a lot of attention – and spurred a lot of debate – is the use of authorized generics. The term *authorized generic* refers to a brand-name drug that the originating company repackages and markets as a generic, to ward off pending generic competition.

The 1984 Hatch-Waxman amendments to the Food, Drug, and Cosmetic Act encourage early generic entry by providing an incentive for generics companies to challenge brand-name drug patents. During a 180-day exclusivity period, the successful challenger alone is allowed to market its generic product – in essence, an *exclusive generic* – and compete with the brand-name product and the authorized generic, if there is one. This exclusivity period can bring a huge payday for the generics company, especially when the brand-name drug is a blockbuster (i.e., with billions of dollars in sales). By bringing its product to market, which is priced at a minor discount to the brand product, the marketer of the exclusive generic can generate substantial market share and revenue.

How successful have generics companies been with these so-called paragraph IV challenges? In a word, very. According to the Federal Trade Commission's (FTC's) July 2002 Generic Drug Study, generics companies prevailed 73% of the time in patent litigation initiated between 1992 and 2000. According to attorney Gregory Glass, editor of the *Paragraph Four Report*, this percentage has declined since 2003, and generics companies are prevailing 50–55% of the time – still a healthy success rate. Of course, the outcome of paragraph IV litigation will vary on a case-by-case basis, but the general success enjoyed by generics companies certainly creates an even greater incentive for them to challenge brand-name drug patents.

On the other side of the equation, the loss of a paragraph IV lawsuit can have a huge negative impact on the pharmaceutical company that originally developed the brand-name drug. If the drug is a key product for the company, the result is usually a major loss in revenue as a result of competition entering the market sooner than expected. Some brand-name products may weather the storm of generic entry if they have enough complex attributes – for example, if the drug has a narrow therapeutic index (e.g., Bristol-Myers Squibb's Coumadin [warfarin]), if the drug has a fairly complex formulation (e.g., asthma inhalers), or if physicians and patients remain loyal to the brand version.

For many drugs, however, generic entry equates to a major loss in revenue and market share for the research-based pharmaceutical company. When generic products enter the market, they are usually priced at a significant discount to the branded product. Coupled with payers' tendency to adopt generics immediately, this factor erodes the market share of the brand product.

In this chapter, we examine the current climate for authorized generics, a topic that remains the subject of hot debate. To date, much has been written and said about this issue from the opposing viewpoints of brand and generics companies as well as regarding the impact of paragraph IV challenges on consumers. This chapter seeks to provide insight, regardless of the proposed legislation and ongoing studies, about how and to what extent the authorized generics help or hinder the product life-cycle strategies of brand companies.

Specifically, we address the following questions:

- What are the generic-erosion dynamics during the first 180 days of generic entry when there is one exclusive generic versus when there is an exclusive generic and an authorized generic?
- Which scenarios offer the best outcomes for brand companies that choose to follow an authorized generic strategy? Which are not beneficial from a revenue standpoint?

In addition, we examine recent experiences with authorized generics to highlight the dynamics of the first 180 days, when a limited number of companies can market a particular drug. Finally, we discuss which circumstances are essential for success and suggest when authorized generics might not be a good option for brand companies.

THE CURRENT LANDSCAPE FOR AUTHORIZED GENERICS

In the wake of a paragraph IV challenge, authorized generics represent a way for research-based pharmaceutical companies to retain market share and revenue, albeit in a reduced capacity, and create "three-party competition." Currently, the law does not prevent a brand company from creating a generic version of its own product and marketing the product at any point, including during the 180-day marketing exclusivity period awarded to a successful generic challenger. In his July 20, 2006 statement before the Special Committee on Aging of the US Senate, Gary Beuhler, director of the Office of Generic Drugs, stated:

> The term *authorized generic* is generally used to describe an instance when an innovator company, in the face of pending generic competition, repackages its own product and markets it as a generic. Prior FDA approval is not needed for the innovator company to do this, as review and approval occur under the auspices of the innovator's approved NDA. Generic drug companies, through citizen petitions and lawsuits, have sought the FDA's intervention to halt the marketing of authorized generics. The FDA determined, and the courts upheld, that the FD&C Act does not give the FDA authority to intervene in the matter.

Thus the current landscape provides a way for pharmaceutical companies to launch generic versions of their own brand-name products in the face of generic competition. For those brand companies that go the route of authorized generics, the mantra is "If you can't beat 'em with the brand, bring a close friend to help."

The story does not end there, however. Generics companies' success with paragraph IV challenges and brand companies' countermoves with authorized generics, settlements, and other legal mechanisms have spawned strong opinions about whether authorized generics are anticompetitive and have led to calls to update the Hatch-Waxman legislation. In his own statement before the Special Committee on Aging of the US Senate, FTC commissioner Jon Leibowitz both lauded the short-term benefits of authorized generics to consumers and warned about the negative long-term effects on consumers as a result of reduced competition. According to Leibowitz, the FTC is studying the anticompetitive effects of authorized generics using data from the FDA, brand manufacturers, generics manufacturers, authorized generics manufacturers, and other sources. Although the results of the FTC study have yet to be determined, some people are already convinced that authorized generics should be prohibited. For example, Senators Jay Rockefeller (D-W.V.), Charles Schumer (D-N.Y.), and Patrick Leahy (D-Vt.) introduced a bill in July 2006 that would update the FDC Act to prohibit authorized generics. The proposed legislation (S.3965) states:

> SECTION 1. PROHIBITION OF AUTHORIZED GENERICS
>
> Section 505 of the Federal Food, Drug, and Cosmetic Act (21 U.S.C. 355) is amended by adding at the end the following:
>
> (o) Prohibition of Authorized Generic Drugs—
>
> (1) IN GENERAL: Notwithstanding any other provision of this Act, no holder of a new drug application approved under subsection (c) shall manufacture, market, sell, or distribute an authorized generic drug, directly or indirectly, or authorize any other person to manufacture, market, sell, or distribute an authorized generic drug.
>
> (2) AUTHORIZED GENERIC DRUG: For purposes of this subsection, the term "authorized generic drug"
>
> (A) means any version of a listed drug (as such term is used in subsection (j)) that the holder of the new drug application approved under subsection (c) for that listed drug seeks to commence marketing, selling, or distributing, directly or indirectly, after receipt of a notice sent pursuant to subsection (j)(2)(B) with respect to that listed drug; and
>
> (B) does not include any drug to be marketed, sold, or distributed
>
> (i) by an entity eligible for exclusivity with respect to such drug under subsection (j)(5)(B)(iv); or
>
> (ii) after expiration or forfeiture of any exclusivity with respect to such drug under such subsection (j)(5)(B)(iv).

The Generic Pharmaceutical Association (GPhA) would certainly like to see such legislation enacted, and it has gone on record on its Web site as not being in favor of authorized generics. The GPhA's main argument is that the long-term outcome of greater reliance on authorized generics could be fewer paragraph IV challenges, ultimately leading to less competition. Nevertheless, not all generic manufacturers advocate the ban of authorized generics. In particular, those companies that have benefited from authorized generics deals do not support this view. Clearly, the GPhA position is not a consensus position among all of the group's members.

STRATEGIES FOR DEALING WITH EXCLUSIVE GENERICS

Consolidation and Integration of Brand and Generic Activities

Although the continued introduction of authorized generics might ultimately lead to less competition (the GPhA position), there is an opposing view that leverage might be realized by some brand and generics companies which work together in a different way. Under the current system, a generics firm has a clear incentive to be the first successful paragraph IV challenger. As an alternative to going through court proceedings, however, a generics company might work more closely with the brand company by partnering with it, thereby avoiding a long and expensive lawsuit. Although the current environment is sometimes portrayed as "us against them," several brand and generics companies are already looking at ways to work together rather than against one another. Indeed, a number of generics companies have already benefited from such arrangements. For example, in 2003, Par Pharmaceutical entered into an authorized generic arrangement for Paxil (paroxetine) with GlaxoSmithKline. According to Par's 2003 annual report, the authorized generic, which was launched in September 2003, generated sales of $192 million over the rest of the year – certainly a solid influx of revenue over a short period of time.

Another key dynamic at play in this arena is the consolidation that has occurred in both the generics industry and the research-based pharmaceutical industry. The line between a brand firm and a generics company has become increasingly blurred – some large brand companies participate in the generic arena by establishing subsidiaries and affiliates (Table 6.1 lists examples). This trend is important because whether a company falls into the brand bucket, the generic bucket, or both buckets could potentially affect the firm's willingness to pursue paragraph IV challenges.

These factors become important when one considers whether authorized generics should be prohibited. For example, might the proposed legislation inspire brand companies with generic subsidiaries to file paragraph IV challenges on behalf of those subsidiaries against their brand-company rivals? If such challenges prove successful, they could essentially extend the product life cycle further. Although this extension would amount to only six months, it is nevertheless a change that opponents of authorized generics would most assuredly not welcome.

Discounting and Price Negotiations

If authorized generics are prohibited, brand companies have other options. Merck, for example, offered Zocor (simvastatin) at favorable prices to major managed care organizations (MCOs) once the agent's patent was close to expiration. By contracting and maintaining a favorable formulary position for Zocor, Merck was able to prevent a significant loss of revenue to generics. In several plans that accepted Merck's offer, the generic versions were "disadvantaged" with higher copays relative to the price paid for the brand-name drug. Zocor competed in a dynamic market, jockeying with other statins for formulary positioning. As such, several contracts were probably already in place for Zocor that brought the net cost to these plans down to a level that was well below the prices that the generics would charge. This fact, in all likelihood, prompted some plans to take steps to favor Zocor.

How long can Merck continue to pursue this discount strategy and stave off generic competition for Zocor? In December 2006 and January 2007, several more generic versions of simvastatin are expected to enter the market. Most observers expect the prices of these generics to plummet to less than $1 per day. At that point, MCOs will begin to establish a maximum allowable cost (MAC) – the reimbursement rate set by payers, which is traditionally 150% of the lowest generally available price for generics. At that price point, many payers are likely to forgo the Merck discounts in anticipation of the long-run savings offered by the lower-cost generics. Certainly, Zocor is a high-volume

Table 6.1 Select Brand Companies and Their Generic Subsidiaries

Brand Company	*Generic Subsidiaries*
Pfizer	Greenstone
Schering-Plough	Warrick
Novartis	Sandoz[a]
Forest	Inwood
Boehringer Ingelheim	Roxane
Johnson & Johnson	Patriot
Schwarz Pharma	Kremers Urban

[a]Sandoz has acquired or integrated a number of generics companies into its activities, including Geneva, Hexal, and Eon Labs. A full history of Sandoz acquisitions can be found on the U.S. Sandoz Web site (www.us.sandoz.com/site/en/company/profile/history/content.shtml)

product – according to EvaluatePharma, a US company, it's reported sales for Zocor exceeded $3 billion in 2005 and topped $1.5 billion in the first two quarters of 2006 – so a lot of money is at stake for the MCOs. The "Merck strategy" made good financial sense for both Merck and the payers during the 180-day period of exclusivity. However, once the rapid price erosion begins, managing the Zocor/simvastatin category as an exception will be less attractive and more costly to most MCOs.

Similar price cuts and aggressive negotiations with payers could become even more attractive to brand companies if authorized generics are prohibited. In his recent presentation to the Intellectual Property, Healthcare, and Federal Civil Enforcement Committees of the American Bar Association's Antitrust Section, Jerome Swindell, senior counsel for Johnson & Johnson, alluded to another potential outcome of banning authorized generics: At the end of his presentation, he asked whether generics companies and legislators will pursue legislation to prevent innovator companies from lowering their prices in response to competition (presentation at orangebookblog.com, accessed October 10, 2006). In looking at the big picture, the actions of brand and generics companies are very much interrelated, so any actions must be considered in terms of their impact and the resulting behavior at multiple points in the system.

GENERIC EROSION

Historic Patterns: Multiple Generics Enter the Market upon Patent Expiry

Before examining various exclusive and authorized generic scenarios, it is important to understand historical generic erosion in the context of generics entering the market upon a brand-name drug's patent expiry.

In cases where more than one generic enters the market, the rate of erosion is quick. For example, no generics received exclusivity for Forest's Celexa (citalopram) and Bristol-Myers Squibb's Glucophage (metformin), so several generic competitors were available in the first month after their patent expiration. In these cases, prices fell dramatically in a short period of time. Pfizer's Zithromax (azithromycin), which recently began to face multiple generic competition, has lost share at an even faster rate than brand-name drugs from only two or three years ago. Sanofi-Aventis and Bristol-Myers Squibb's Plavix (clopidogrel bisulfate) has reportedly lost share at a rate roughly the same as that experienced by Zithromax (though no data are available at this time). We believe this faster rate of loss is now the norm.

For these drugs, brands lost sales to generics at a relatively consistent rate. Although this pattern still holds true for markets in which multiple generics are present during the first month of exclusivity loss, a different pattern emerges when a generics firm has exclusive access to the market for a period of time.

Generic Erosion with 180-Day Exclusivity: One Brand, One Generic

As mentioned earlier, the first successful paragraph IV challenger has 180 days of marketing exclusivity – in other words, the firm does not have to compete with other generics companies. As a result, it can price its generic product close to the price of the brand-name drug. This pricing is the key incentive for a generics firm to be the first successful challenger. During its 180-day exclusivity period, a generics firm can realize a substantial short-term gain, though its advantage diminishes when the 180 days pass and other generics enter the market and begin to compete on price. In theory, one would expect a generics firm with an exclusive generic to rapidly become the dominant player if it prices its product at even a slight discount of 10–20%. In reality, other factors come into play, such that the brand erosion may not occur as quickly as expected during this 180-day period.

The erosion curve for a brand product might differ depending on whether it faces multiple generic products during the first 180 days or a single generic product during the first 180 days. At this time, we cannot point with complete confidence to the reason for such differences.

The Payer Perspective: Can a Generic That Is Priced Lower Result in Less Savings?

When an exclusive generic is priced lower than the brand by only a small amount, few potential savings are available to MCOs and pharmacy benefit managers (PBMs). When factoring in the loss of rebates provided by the brand and the lower copay, exclusive generics can actually hike payers' expenditures. Not all payers respond in the same way to generic entry, however. In this section, we discuss key payer segments and describe how some payers have begun to consider more than price when making reimbursement decisions.

Table 6.2 lists some of the key payer segments. These groups employ generic "strategies" in very different ways. The MCOs that perform a thorough analysis are likely to withhold reimbursement of new generics until these drugs' prices have dropped to levels that result in real savings to their plans. These plans implement National Drug Code (NDC) blocks or place these generics on a higher tier (i.e., they charge a higher copay). Those payers that adopt generics as a point of principle simply allow generic substitution to occur and wait until the savings begin. Medicaid plans are likely to do the same, as most feel bound by the rules of the Omnibus Reconciliation Act (OBRA) of 1990, which mandate generic substitution without regard to financial questions.

Maintaining brand sales through the mail-order segment is simply a matter of contracting. Because mail-order pharmacies have absolute control over what they buy and dispense, a branded manufacturer can always maintain sales in that channel through price negotiations and contracts with these pharmacies as well as with closed-system HMOs.

Table 6.2 Key Payer Segments

MCOs that adopt generics after a thorough cost analysis of the 180-day exclusivity period (including Medicare PDPs)
MCOs that adopt generics as a point of principle and wait for the cost savings to occur (including Medicare PDPs)
Mail-order pharmacies and other closed-payer systems (e.g., Kaiser's staff model HMO)
Medicaid

HMO = Health maintenance organization; MCOs = Managed care organizations; PDPs = Prescription drug plans

Generalizable Rates of Erosion for Brands

As the preceding discussion suggests, the rate of generic erosion for a brand depends on the dynamics of the generic market. In the first scenario, there is a single generic available for a period of time; in the second, multiple generics enter the market simultaneously. Table 6.3 estimates the brand-name drug's share of the market under these two scenarios. It is not only based on an analysis of

Table 6.3 Brand-Name Drug's Share of the Market Under Two Scenarios

Month	*Single High-Priced Generic Enters the Market (Scenario A) (%)*	*Multiple Generics Enter the Market Simultaneously (Scenario B) (%)*
1	70	55
2	60	20
3	50	10
4	40	5
5	35	5
6	30	5

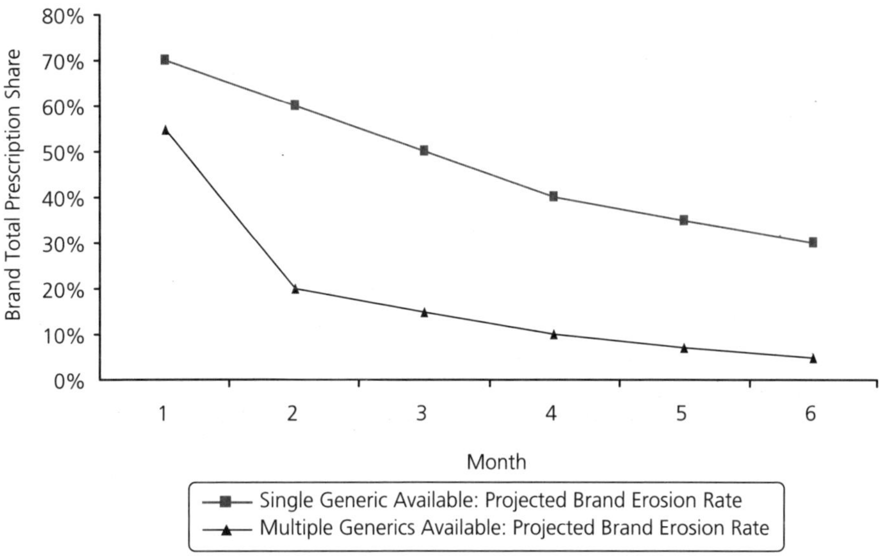

Figure 6.1 General Projected Brand Erosion to Generics during the First 180 Days of Generic Entry

historical data but also takes into account the fact that the rate of generic erosion has accelerated in recent years. Naturally, any particular drug might have a different experience given that generic erosion rates vary on a drug-by-drug basis.

Figure 6.1 presents these generic erosion rates in graphical form, showing the rate of share loss to generics during each of the first six months under the two scenarios. Under scenario A (an exclusive generic), the brand's share loss occurs gradually. When additional generics enter the market, the rate of share loss picks up and soon matches the loss seen in month 1 of scenario B (when multiple generics enter the market simultaneously).

IMPLICATIONS FOR AUTHORIZED GENERICS

Generic Erosion and the Authorized Generic Strategy

We now turn our attention to three basic scenarios that help illustrate potential outcomes of implementing an authorized generic strategy:

- *Scenario 1*: A paragraph IV challenger is successful and enters the market with an exclusive generic. The brand product represents the only competition.
- *Scenario 2*: A paragraph IV challenger is successful and enters the market with an exclusive generic. The competition consists of not only the brand but also an authorized generic that has been licensed by the brand company to another generics company; the brand company and the licensee company split the revenue stream from the authorized generic in an equal manner.
- *Scenario 3*: A paragraph IV challenger is successful and enters the market with an exclusive generic. The competition consists of not only the brand product but also an authorized generic that is marketed by a generic subsidiary of the brand company (e.g., Pfizer can market authorized generics through its Greenstone division).

All three scenarios include the following assumptions: The total volume is 10 million prescriptions, the price of the brand product is $100 per prescription and does not fluctuate, and the scenario covers only the first 180 days after generic entry. These assumptions can, of course, be altered depending on the specific nuances of the competitive climate. Readers are encouraged to input different numbers based on their own assumptions.

The Three Competitive Scenarios: Example 1

In Table 6.4, scenario 1 assumes that the generic is priced at a minor discount of 15%, which is in line with historical discounts. The scenario also uses an average generic erosion rate, such that the brand maintains a 35% share of the market during the 180-day generic-exclusivity period. In this scenario, the brand company realizes $350 million in revenue.

Scenario 2 assumes that there will be more price competition – namely, the authorized and exclusive generic products will compete on price. In this situation, the discount amounts to 35% of the brand drug's price. Both the authorized generic and the exclusive generic pick up larger shares of the market owing to their lower prices; the brand product is left with only a 15% share. The brand company receives revenue from the authorized generic, which helps offset the brand drug's share loss, but the gain is not enough that the brand company has the same revenue stream it achieved under scenario 1. Also, under scenario 2, the brand company has to share its revenue from the authorized generic with its licensee.

Table 6.4 Generic Erosion: Three Competitive Scenarios

	Price	*Total Volume*	*Share (%)*	*Revenue*
Scenario 1: One Brand, One Exclusive Generic				
Brand product	$100.00	10,000,000	35	$350,000,000
Exclusive generic	$85.00	10,000,000	65	$552,500,000
			100	$902,500,000
Assumption: Exclusive generic is priced at 15% of the brand-name drug's price during the first 180 days.		Revenue for Parent Company		$350,000,000
Scenario 2: One Brand, One Authorized Generic (Licensed to Another Company), One Exclusive Generic				
Brand product	$100.00	10,000,000	15	$150,000,000
Authorized generic product (revenue stream for licensor)	$65.00	10,000,000	21	$138,125,000
Authorized generic product (revenue stream for licensee)	$65.00	10,000,000	21	$138,125,000
Exclusive generic	$65.00	10,000,000	43	$276,250,000
			100	$702,500,000
Assumptions: Two generic products – an authorized and an exclusive – compete on price. In this example, both are priced at 65% of the brand-name drug's price during the first 180 days.		Revenue for Parent Company		$288,125,000
Scenario 3: One Brand, One Authorized Generic (from Subsidiary), One Exclusive Generic				
Brand product	$100.00	10,000,000	15	$150,000,000
Authorized generic product (revenue stream for licensor)	$65.00	10,000,000	43	$276,250,000
Exclusive generic	$65.00	10,000,000	43	$276,250,000
			100	$702,500,000
Assumptions: Two generic products – an authorized and an exclusive – compete on price. In this example, both are priced at 65% of the brand-name drug's price during the first 180 days.		Revenue for Parent Company		$426,250,000

Scenario 3 makes the same price assumptions as in scenario 2, but now the brand company receives all of the authorized generic revenue because this product is marketed by one of its subsidiaries. In this case, the brand company has higher revenues than it received under either scenario 1 or scenario 2.

These scenarios suggest that a brand company should not automatically be inclined toward launching an authorized generic in the face of generic competition during the first 180 days; under scenario 2, it is at a decided disadvantage. Changing the dynamics of the market and altering the assumptions slightly cause a different picture to emerge. For example, if the brand company averages a 25% share during the first 180 days in scenario 1, then scenario 2 becomes more attractive. In that case, launching an authorized generic through a licensing agreement would be worthwhile, assuming a 50–50 revenue-sharing deal (which might not be realistic). Alternatively, if the authorized generic and the exclusive generic in scenario 3 were priced at a lesser discount and the brand drug's share fell to only 25%, then either launching an authorized generic through a subsidiary or not launching an authorized generic at all is a more attractive proposition.

Of course, the decision whether to launch an authorized generic may also be influenced by other company objectives. For example, authorized generics might be part of a broader plan for a brand company to expand into the generic arena, a step that several companies have already taken.

The Three Competitive Scenarios: Example 2

Table 6.5 uses total prescription shares to illustrate the outcomes under the three competitive scenarios. That is, it indicates the average total prescription share over the first six months following the introduction of the generic drugs. In general, when examining the performance of generics when they first enter a market, it is important to evaluate them using a measure of total prescriptions, and not new prescriptions, because the way in which the new prescriptions are recorded distorts the actual product use. It is very uncommon for the use of a molecular entity to increase after generics enter a market, but the new prescription data disguise that fact. Instead, the generic will always show an extremely large new prescription share relative to other agents in the market because every prescription for the generic in the first month (indeed, for most of the first three months) will be new – for the generic. Many of those prescriptions, however, represent switches from the brand-name drug rather than new therapy. Using total prescription data avoids the confusion caused by this short-term distortion in prescription volumes.

In scenario 2, the brand company had to split the revenue from the authorized generic. In this example, the agreement between the licensor and the licensee calls for them to distribute the revenues from the generic drug's sale in a 50–50 manner. If the authorized generic deal favored the licensee – for example, if the licensee received 60–65% of the revenue – then the brand company would have to average approximately 35% of the total prescription share to make scenario 2 as attractive as scenario 1.

Scenario 3 is by far the most attractive scenario, assuming the brand company could launch an authorized generic through a subsidiary company. In this example, the brand maintained an average of about 27% of the total prescription share during the first six months, the authorized generic picked up a 43% share, and the generic claimed 30% of the market. According to Table 6.5, the brand company would have had to believe that it could maintain, on average, a 41% share without launching an authorized generic during the 180-day exclusivity period to make scenario 1 be at least as attractive as what occurred in scenario 3.

Table 6.5 Generic Erosion: Three Competitive Scenarios: Another Example

	Price	*Total Volume*	*Share (%)*	*Revenue*
Scenario 1: One Brand, One Exclusive Generic				
Brand product	$100.00	10,000,000	41	$410,000,000
Exclusive generic	$85.00	10,000,000	59	$501,500,000
			100	$911,500,000
Assumption: Exclusive generic is priced at 15% of the brand-name drug's price during the first 180 days.		Revenue for Parent Company		$410,000,000
Scenario 2: One Brand, One Authorized Generic (Licensed to Another Company), One Exclusive Generic				
Brand product	$100.00	10,000,000	27	$270,000,000
Authorized generic product (revenue stream for licensor)	$65.00	10,000,000	22	$139,750,000
Authorized generic product (revenue stream for licensee)	$65.00	10,000,000	22	$139,750,000
Exclusive generic	$65.00	10,000,000	30	$195,000,000
			100	$744,500,000
Assumptions: Two generic products – an authorized and an exclusive – compete on price. In this example, both are priced at 65% of the brand-name drug's price during the first 180 days.		Revenue for Parent Company		$409,750,000
Scenario 3: One Brand, One Authorized Generic (from Subsidiary), One Exclusive Generic				
Brand product	$100.00	10,000,000	27	$270,000,000
Authorized generic product (revenue stream for licensor)	$65.00	10,000,000	43	$279,500,000
Exclusive generic	$65.00	10,000,000	30	$195,000,000
			100	$744,500,000
Assumptions: Two generic products – an authorized and an exclusive – compete on price. In this example, both are priced at 65% of the brand-name drug's price during the first 180 days.		Revenue for Parent Company		$549,500,000

A Recent Example of an Authorized Generic Strategy

A real-world example of a company that is pursuing an authorized generic strategy can be found in Pfizer's launch of an authorized generic version of Zoloft (sertraline). This move came in response to generic competition from Teva. It appears that Pfizer and its generic subsidiary, Greenstone, combined for an average of 72% of the total prescription data. It may be a bit early to tell how the strategy will pay off for Pfizer. The story is promising, however, in that the authorized generic is being marketed by Pfizer's generic subsidiary, so the entire revenue stream from the authorized generic will ultimately accrue to Pfizer.

Authorized Generics: Not the Only Option

Regardless of the proposed legislation that threatens to ban authorized generics, employing an authorized generic strategy should not always be the first reaction of a brand company when competition from an exclusive generic is imminent. A key consideration should be how quickly erosion will occur during the first 180 days given the parameters of the situation. If its share is not expected to slip quickly during that time period, the pharmaceutical company might be better off not pursuing an authorized generic strategy; instead, it should work more closely with third-party payers with the goal to help those plans realize savings during this period. When an exclusive generic becomes available, the third-party payers must assess whether a discounted brand-name drug or a relatively high-priced exclusive generic is a better deal and make formulary decisions accordingly. Therefore, no matter what the outcome of the debate over authorized generics, brand companies would still have a number of competitive options available to them during the 180-day exclusivity period.

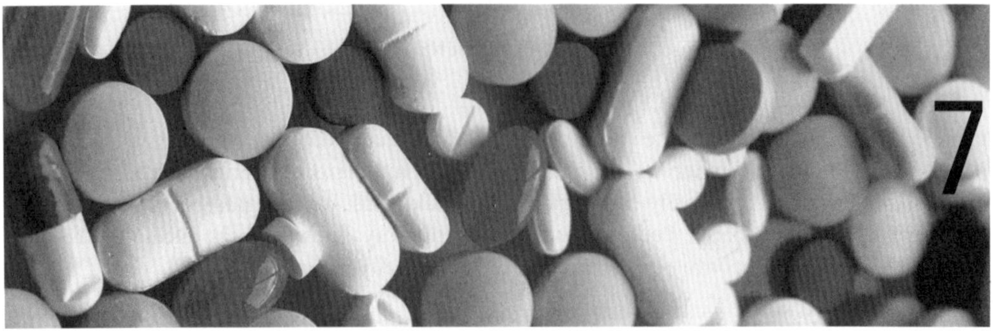

Pharmaceutical Pricing and Reimbursement in Canada

OVERVIEW

Canada is the world's eighth largest pharmaceutical market (after the United States, Japan, Germany, France, the United Kingdom, Italy, and Spain). In 2004, according to IMS Health, pharmaceutical sales in Canada totaled US $10 billion (at ex-manufacturer prices), equivalent to 2.9% of total sales in major world markets. Canada's market share has been rising steadily, reflecting sales growth that has outpaced that of other markets. In 2004, Canada's pharmaceutical sales grew 9% (in local currency terms), while sales grew 8% in the United States, 7% in the United Kingdom and Spain, 5% in France, 3% in Italy, and 1% in Germany. The Canadian Institute for Health Information (CIHI) estimates that the total expenditure for prescription and nonprescription drugs in 2004 was C$21.8 billion (US $16.7 billion), up from C$18.4 billion (US $14.1 billion) in 2002. (The US-to-Canadian dollar exchange rate used in this report is the 2004 average rate [i.e., US $1 = C$1.30151].) The Organization for Economic Cooperation and Development (OECD) reports that in 2003, Canada had the third highest total drug expenditure per capita (after the United States and France).

Drugs dispensed in hospitals are fully covered by Medicare, Canada's universal public health insurance system, but outpatient prescription drug coverage varies. Each province has its own drug-plan budget and controls its own formulary. In 2004, the public sector funded 47.3% of spending on prescribed drugs, up from 45% in 2002. The Common Drug Review (CDR) process established in 2003 by federal, provincial, and territorial governments is helping to standardize the lists of new drugs reimbursed by public plans across the country.

Canadian ex-manufacturer prices for brand-name drugs are close to median European prices but lower than US prices. After many years of static prices, manufacturers have begun to raise patented drug prices in Canada, but the US/Canadian price differential is still substantial. This price gap has stimulated a flourishing cross-border trade, notwithstanding the fact that this practice is technically illegal in the United States. For several years, US consumers seeking lower-priced prescription drugs have been purchasing pharmaceuticals by mail order from "Internet pharmacies" based in Canada. However, action by some manufacturers to limit the number of drugs they supply to cross-border pharmacy outlets has hampered this trade. In addition, the Canadian government is proposing to restrict bulk exports and to monitor the Canadian drug supply to prevent shortages.

We begin this chapter with an overview of the Canadian healthcare system and pharmaceutical market. We then focus on drug pricing and reimbursement procedures and provide an update on the cross-border trade situation. We conclude with a brief assessment of the prospects for change in the Canadian pricing and reimbursement environment.

ORGANIZATION AND FUNDING OF THE CANADIAN HEALTHCARE SYSTEM

In 2003, according to the OECD, Canada spent 9.9% of its gross domestic product (GDP) on healthcare. Among the major industrialized countries, only the United States, Switzerland, Germany, and France invested a higher proportion of GDP in healthcare. CIHI forecast that spending on healthcare would rise to C$130.3 billion (US $100 billion) in 2004, with the public sector financing 70% of expenditures.

The Canadian healthcare system has a complex structure: the federal government, the ten provinces, and the three territories are all involved in different aspects of the system.

The federal government's responsibilities are as follows:

- Setting and administering national principles or standards for the healthcare system through the Canada Health Act.
- Assisting in the financing of provincial healthcare services through fiscal transfers.
- Delivering health services to specific groups, including veterans, native Canadians, people living on reserves, military personnel, inmates of federal penitentiaries, and the Royal Canadian Mounted Police.
- Fulfilling other health-related functions such as health protection, disease prevention, and health promotion.

The provincial and territorial governments' responsibilities include the following:

- Managing and delivering health services.
- Planning, financing, and evaluating the provision of hospital care and physician services.
- Managing some aspects of prescription drug care and public health.

Under the Canada Health Act, all Canadians have access to medically necessary hospital care and physician services that are fully funded by the government. All services are billed directly to the provincial government; the patient does not have to make any payments.

Pharmaceuticals dispensed in hospitals are covered under the Canada Health Act and publicly funded with no copayment. However, Canada has no national insurance program for outpatient prescription medicines. Instead, outpatient prescription drugs are funded from many different sources, including provincial, territorial, and federal governments (largely financed through taxes); employer-sponsored private insurance plans; and individual consumers.

The federal government administers the Patent Act, which provides intellectual property protection for drugs. Under this act, prices of patented drugs are regulated by the Patented Medicine Prices Review Board (PMPRB). Canada is the only country where the patent status of a medicine determines whether the product is subject to government price controls.

The federal government reviews the safety and efficacy of drugs and approves them for sale through Therapeutic Products Directorate of Health Canada (the country's national health department). It also monitors the safety of drugs on the market.

After receiving its Notice of Compliance (marketing approval) from Health Canada, a new branded drug must be reviewed for clinical-effectiveness and cost-effectiveness by the CDR before provincial and federal drug plans will reimburse it. Prior to the establishment of the CDR in September 2003, each plan conducted its own reviews of new chemical entities and new combination drugs and had its own committee of experts to provide listing recommendations. The CDR reduces duplication and streamlines the system for reviewing new drugs. Each of the drug plans that participates in CDR makes its own formulary listing and benefit- coverage decision, based on the CDR's recommendation and the drug plan's mandate, priorities, and resources. Only

Quebec maintains an independent review process for new chemical entities.

The 2002 Commission on the Future of Healthcare in Canada recommended creation of a national drug agency to perform many functions, including drug reviews, postmarketing surveillance, pharmacoeconomic evaluations, and price monitoring – functions that are currently divided among Health Canada, provincial governments, the PMPRB, and the Canadian Coordinating Office for Health Technology Assessment (CCOHTA). However, this recommendation has not been implemented.

THE CANADIAN PHARMACEUTICAL MARKET

CIHI estimates that total spending on prescription and nonprescription drugs increased from C$18.4 billion (US $14.1 billion) in 2002 to C$21.8 billion (US $16.7 billion) in 2004. Pharmaceuticals' share of total health expenditures grew from 9.5% in 1985 to 17% in 2004 (Canadian Institute for Health Information [CIHI], *Drug Expenditure in Canada, 1985 to 2004.* Ottawa. April 2005. www.cihi.ca).

The PMPRB reports that in 2004, ex-manufacturer sales of all drugs totaled C$15.9 billion (US $12.2 billion), an increase of 5.3% from the previous year. The rate of growth in sales was markedly less than the 15.2% recorded in 2003 and was the lowest growth rate seen since 1996. Ex-manufacturer sales of patented drugs increased by 7.9% to C$10.9 billion (US $8.4 billion). Over the last decade, the patented drug sector has grown significantly: its share of total sales increased from 45% in 1996 to more than 68% in 2004. Nonpatented brand-name products made up 18.9% of sales, and generics accounted for 12.6%.

Spending on prescription drugs continues to increase and now accounts for 82.5% of total pharmaceutical expenditure. Spending has been rising rapidly because of increased utilization and a shift in prescribing to newer, more expensive treatments. CIHI projected private sector spending on prescribed drugs in 2004 at C$9.5 billion (US $7.3 billion). The private sector share of spending on prescription drugs has been declining slowly in the recent years and now accounts for 52.7% of spending, down from 57.5% in 1998.

Generics are widely used in Canada. Pharmacists are required to substitute generic equivalents for branded drugs that are off patent unless the physician specifies that no substitution is allowed. For multisource products, most provincial drug plans and many private plans will reimburse only up to the cost of the lowest-cost alternative treatment, usually a generic.

The Canadian Generic Pharmaceutical Association reported that for the 12 months ending June 2005, sales of generics accounted for 16.8% of the total prescription drug market – that is, nearly C$2.7 billion (US $2.1 billion) of retail and hospital sales. The generics share of retail prescriptions filled was 42.7% (almost 161 million generic prescriptions). Growth in the volume of generic prescriptions was 13.3%, compared with the previous 12-month period (Canadian Generic Pharmaceutical Association, *Market Trends*, www.cdma acfpp.org/en/resource/market_trends.shtml).

Canada's generic drug industry has also built a successful international business. Approximately 20% of the industry's sales volume comes from exports to 120 countries.

PRICING OF PRESCRIPTION MEDICINES

As mentioned previously, Canadian prices for brand-name prescription medicines tend to be much lower than US list prices and are generally closer to European prices. (It should be noted that discounts and rebates in the US market often result in large US purchasers paying prices much lower than published list prices.)

Ex-manufacturer prices of patented drugs in Italy and France are well below Canadian prices, but average prices in the United Kingdom and Switzerland are substantially higher. The price gap between

Canada and the United States continues to widen. In 2002, US prices were on average 56% higher than Canadian prices; they are now 79% higher.

The PMPRB maintains the Patented Medicine Price Index (PMPI), which measures the annual change in ex-manufacturer prices of patented pharmaceuticals in Canada. As measured by the PMPI, patented drug prices fell by 0.2% in 2004. Canadian prices were, on average, 91% of the median international price. As in previous years, US prices were substantially higher than prices in both Europe and Canada.

The Patented Medicine Prices Review Board

In 1987, the Canadian Parliament established the PMPRB with a mandate to ensure that the prices of patented medicines sold in Canada are not excessive. The PMPRB fulfills this assignment by regulating the maximum price at which patented drugs can be sold. The PMPRB's jurisdiction includes both prescription and nonprescription medicines that are subject to patents. The PMPRB has no authority to regulate the prices of nonpatented drugs (including generic drugs sold under compulsory licenses), and it does not have jurisdiction over prices charged by wholesalers or retailers or over pharmacists' professional fees.

The Patent Act defines the PMPRB's mandate, authority, and jurisdiction, and determines the factors it must consider in deciding whether a price is excessive:

- The drug's price in the relevant market.
- Prices of other drugs from the same therapeutic class in the relevant market.
- Prices of the review drug and other drugs from the same therapeutic class in other countries.
- Changes in the Consumer Price Index (CPI).
- Other factors specified in Section 85(1) of the Patent Act.

The Patent Act also defines the penalties for excessive pricing. The PMPRB can order price reductions prospectively and can also order price cuts retrospectively through recovery of excess revenues from past periods. Double damages can be imposed if the PMPRB concludes that a manufacturer had a policy of excessive pricing; these penalties can be applied only after a formal public hearing into the price of the medicine. The PMPRB has established a system of voluntary compliance whereby a company can forgo this formal process by agreeing to reduce the price of a medicine to a nonexcessive level and to repay any excess revenues deemed to have accrued. This mechanism is termed a "voluntary compliance undertaking" (VCU).

Excessive Price Guidelines for Existing and New Medicines

The PMPRB has developed Excessive Price Guidelines that take account of the factors defined in the Patent Act. These pricing rules are used in reviewing prices of all patented medicines, both newly launched drugs and established products. Under the guidelines, the PMPRB limits price increases on existing patented medicines to changes in the CPI. In addition, the price of a patented medicine may never exceed the medicine's highest international price. The reference countries are France, Germany, Italy, Sweden, Switzerland, the United Kingdom, and the United States.

Launch prices for new patented medicines are subjected to one of a series of price tests, determined by the new drug's category. Table 7.1 shows the relevant tests and price limits for the three categories of new medicines:

- Line extensions (category 1).
- Products that offer a breakthrough or substantial improvement (category 2).
- Products that offer moderate or no improvement (category 3).

The concept behind the Reasonable Relationship Test is that the price of a new strength or comparable formulation of an existing medicine should bear a reasonable relationship (i.e., the association between the

Table 7.1 Price Tests Used by the Patented Medicine Prices Review Board

Medicine Type	*Primary Test*	*Secondary Test*[a]
New medicine category		
1. Line extension	Reasonable Relationship Test	Therapeutic Class Comparison
2. Breakthrough/substantial improvement	Higher of Therapeutic Class and International Median	—
3. Moderate/no improvement	Therapeutic Class Comparison	International Median
Existing medicines	CPI Test: Three-year cumulative change in CPI One-year "cap" (1.5 × CPI)	

[a]If primary test is not possible or not appropriate
CPI = Consumer Price Index

Note: International Price Comparison Test is used to determine the international maximum price

strength of the medicine and its price) to the prices of the existing presentations of the medicine.

Under the Therapeutic Class Comparison Test, the price of the new medicine on a cost-per-day or course-of-therapy basis should not exceed the prices of other medicines in the same therapeutic class. PMPRB reviews the actual average selling price (transaction price) of each product. The average selling price is the list price net of rebates, discounts, and free goods.

The International Price Comparison Test is used to establish the overall price ceiling for all patented medicines sold in Canada. Manufacturers' prices for patented medicines in Canada cannot be higher than the corresponding highest international price in the seven comparator countries listed in the Patented Medicines Regulations. The net effect is that, on average, the prices of all patented medicines in Canada are below the international median.

According to the PMPRB, reviews of 90 new patented drug products introduced in 2004 had been completed as of March 31, 2005. Sixty-eight products were within the guidelines, and twenty-two products were subject to ongoing investigations.

Recent Price Increases in Patented Medicines

Although the PMPRB Guidelines allow manufacturers to increase prices of patented drugs up to the level of the CPI to take into account inflation, governments in Ontario and Quebec (the most populous provinces) have had price-freezes in place since 1994 for drugs reimbursed under their provincial drug plans. These provincial policies have effectively prevented manufacturers from taking increases allowed by the PMPRB. Consequently, many brands have not had any price increases since they were launched. However, in 2003, several manufacturers began to raise their prices after many years with no increases. Manufacturers are reacting to these constraints:

- Long-standing (more than 10 years) price-freeze policies in Ontario and Quebec.
- The US/Canadian price gap and potential for cross-border trade.
- Need to generate revenue following the expiration of patents on several best-selling brands.

A review of prices of the best-selling brands revealed that slightly more than half have had at least one increase since 2001 (with most increases occurring in 2003 and 2004). The PMPRB reports that, in 2004, 48% of patented drug prices rose by 0–1% and 52% increased between 1% and 3.3% (i.e., 1.5 times CPI) – the maximum price increase allowed by the PMPRB in 2004 (PMPRB Annual Report 2004).

Increases largely remain within the PMPRB's guidelines but may trigger an investigation into excessive pricing. The PMPRB reacted to the increases by proposing amendments to the Patented Medicines

Regulations and launching a review of the guidelines with respect to price increases.

Proposed Changes to the Patented Medicines Regulations

The Patented Medicines Regulations set out patentees' filing requirements with respect to the PMPRB and have not had any substantial amendments since 1994. The regulations require that patentees file extensive details on pricing information semiannually for existing drugs and for the first 30 days of sales for new products. The PMPRB issued a Notice and Comment in January 2005 advising stakeholders of proposed amendments to the Patented Medicines Regulations. (PMPRB Notice and Comment: Proposed Amendments to the Patented Medicines Regulations January 2005, www.pmprb-cepmb.gc.ca/MFiles/jan05notice-e15OAH-272005–2828.pdf) The PMPRB says that the proposed changes will improve the timeliness of price reviews. However, industry stakeholders doubt that the speed of price reviews will actually increase because existing provisions already require companies to submit pricing information early in the review process, and it is unlikely that adding to the filing requirements will increase efficiency.

The following proposed amendments are related to pricing:

- Notification of the intended price of a new medicine 60 days prior to its launch date.
- Notification of a proposed price increase to an existing medicine for any class of customer in any market in Canada at least 120 days in advance of implementing the increase.
- Provision of details of any amounts used in the calculation of net quantities, net revenues, and average selling price, in relation to all price and sales data filed under the regulations.

If the proposed amendments are implemented, they will increase the regulatory burden on companies. The increased detail and frequency of reporting the pricing data will also add to the workload of the PMPRB and will likely lengthen price-review period. Industry is arguing that the PMPRB does not have authority to issue regulations for "proposed" prices because the Patent Act refers only to those prices of medicines that are being sold or have been sold. Parliament has authorized the PMPRB to obtain the proposed pricing for new medicines only on an exceptional basis.

The proposed amendment that would require a manufacturer to notify the PMPRB 120 days in advance of a proposed price increase is another area of concern for industry. As it stands now, patentees are required to file their sales and price information within 30 days of the end of each six-month reporting period, but no provision in the regulations requires patentees to notify the board of price increases between reporting periods. This proposal appears to go beyond the current provisions of the Patent Act.

The PMPRB applies the Excessive Price Guidelines to the average selling prices, but not to the list prices. A manufacturer may not only increase the list prices but may also intend to manage average transaction prices so that they remain within the guidelines. It appears that the PMPRB may now be moving toward regulating list prices, although the board does not have the statutory authority to do so.

Currently, the regulations require patentees to report only net sales and net revenues. Detailed information on the processes leading to the determination of these figures is not required, but the PMPRB can request further details on a case-by-case basis when needed. The PMPRB says that more detailed information is necessary to better understand how the patentee arrived at its calculation of the average price per package.

The PMPRB requested written comments from stakeholders on the proposed changes, and the responses have been published on the PMPRB web site (www.pmprb-cepmb.gc.ca/english/View.asp?x = 400&mp-68). The PMPRB says that there was a divergence of opinion between industry and nonindustry stakeholders when it came to the proposals requiring patentees to file a proposed price in advance of a first sale and an advance notice of a price increase. The board notes, "While a number of stakeholders were in favor of such changes, patentees saw the change as problematic given the mechanisms of a competitive market." It went on to say that "for those proposed amendments related to the type of information required of patentees, many stakeholders saw the changes as an effective tool for the PMPRB to gain a more complete insight into the pharmaceutical market and pricing. Patentees, on the other hand, were concerned about the potential impact of the increased regulatory burden. There was also confusion over the mechanism of reporting" (*PMPRB NEWSletter*, 2005).

As yet, the PMPRB has not announced whether the proposed regulatory amendments will be modified to reflect feedback received from stakeholders. If the PMPRB approves the proposed amendments, there will be a further opportunity for comment during the Canada Gazette process. (The gazette is a publication by the government of Canada that is used to publish official announcements of acts, regulations or proposed regulations, orders in council, proclamations, and other government notices.)

Review of the Guidelines with Respect to Price Increases

The PMPRB has expressed concerns over the recent price increases, saying that they raise the question of whether Canada is on the verge of experiencing a change in the pricing of the patented medicines that would bring an end to the past decade of price stability. The industry believes that the board is laying the groundwork for tighter price controls, even though the recent increases have generally been within the guidelines (less than CPI) and that the PMPRB reports that Canadian prices are still below the international median. It may be that the PMPRB is coming under pressure from provincial governments, which are facing rising drug-plan costs, to move toward a more restrictive pricing environment.

The PMPRB announced in late 2004 that it is reviewing its guidelines on price increases. Under the Patent Act, the PMPRB's pricing guidelines cannot be changed without the stakeholder consultation. To facilitate this dialogue, the PMPRB issued a discussion paper in March 2005 that outlines price trends, how the guidelines for price increases have evolved over time, and the factors that suggest it may be time for a change. The PMPRB asked stakeholders to submit comments and to choose one of three regulatory frameworks:

- The current system, where patentees are allowed to take an automatic price increase in a given period up to a predetermined maximum (CPI), with price reviews taking place after the fact.
- Patentees would be required to apply to the PMPRB in advance of any price increase, allowing a review of the proposed price increase before it is implemented to ensure that the new price is within the guidelines.
- Patentees would be required to apply in advance for a price increase and would also be required to provide justification for the proposed increase and the extent of the increase. The PMPRB would make a determination on both the appropriateness of the increase and on the extent of the increase up to a nonexcessive maximum.

The PMPRB has published the responses received to the discussion paper from the industry and other stakeholders on its web site. The PMPRB says that "respondents chose to focus primarily on two issues in their submissions: the establishment of a system of prior approval for price increases and changes to the factors used to gauge the appropriateness of price increases. Some submissions favored a system of prior approval for price increases. Others questioned the need for such a major change given the lack of clear evidence of a problem. Some stakeholders recommended a more thorough use of all the existing factors outlined in the Patent Act. Still others advocated the review of price increases based on new factors such as R&D expenditures or promotional spending by patentees" (*PMPRB NEWSletter*, 2005). The board discussed strategic options as to how it will proceed on the matter of reviewing price increases at its September meeting, but as yet, no announcements have been made.

These consultations represent the first major review of the PMPRB's guidelines and of the Patented Medicines Regulations since the implementation of the international price guideline in 1994 and the cap imposed on CPI-related price increases instituted in 1996. The issues for discussion have the potential to seriously impact the allowable pricing of patented medicines in Canada and to increase the filing burden as mandated by the regulations. Amendment to the Patent Act may be necessary if the PMPRB wishes to limit price increases to something less than the change in the CPI, a pricing factor outlined in Section 85(1) of the act.

REIMBURSEMENT

Canada has a mix of private and public coverage for prescription drugs. Provincial and territorial plans subsidize the cost of prescription drugs for their residents, particularly social assistance recipients and seniors. The federal government provides drug coverage for registered First Nations and eligible Inuit through the Non-Insured Health Benefits Program (NIHB) for drug needs that are not covered by provincial and territorial plans. Many Canadians are covered under private, employer-sponsored group insurance plans.

Canada provides a lower proportion of public funding for outpatient prescription drugs than most European countries, and private insurers play a significant role in the Canadian market. CIHI estimates that public plans funded 47.3% of prescribed drugs expenditure in 2004, private insurance plans covered 33.5% of costs, and patients paid 19.2% of prescription costs out of pocket. (See *Drug Expenditure in Canada, 1985 to 2004*. Canadian Institute for Health Information. Ottawa. April 2005.) The Atlantic provinces offer much less generous insurance coverage for prescription drugs than the rest of the country. Provinces with a large industrialized base, such as Ontario and Quebec, tend to have more generous employer-sponsored drug insurance programs, while smaller, less-industrialized provinces are less likely to have private insurance that covers expenses not reimbursed by the public plan.

National Pharmaceuticals Strategy and Catastrophic Drug Coverage

There have been repeated calls for the creation of a national "Pharmacare" program that will give all Canadians equal access to publicly funded prescription drugs. However, the cost of implementing such a program and the impact on the private insurance sector have so far prevented the federal government from adding outpatient prescription medicines to the essential healthcare benefits included under the Canada Health Act. Instead, the federal, provincial, and territorial governments are attempting to fill the gaps in the existing system by developing a program intended to cover high drug costs for any Canadians who lack insurance coverage.

At the first ministers' conference in September 2004, the prime minister and the provincial and territorial leaders agreed on a Health Accord that will involve increased federal funding to the provinces and territories for the delivery of healthcare. A ministerial task force was established to develop and implement a national pharmaceuticals strategy as one component of the Health Accord. The task force is cochaired by the federal health minister and the British Columbia minister of health services and includes representatives from all provinces and territories except Quebec. The task force has been working on the following nine objectives of the national pharmaceuticals strategy:

- To develop, assess, and cost options for catastrophic pharmaceutical coverage.
- To establish a common national drug formulary for participating jurisdictions based on safety and cost-effectiveness.
- To accelerate access to breakthrough drugs for unmet health needs through improvements to the drug approval process.

- To strengthen the evaluation of real-world drug safety and effectiveness.
- To pursue purchasing strategies to obtain best prices for Canadians for drugs and vaccines.
- To enhance action to influence the prescribing behavior of healthcare professionals so that drugs are used only when needed and the right drug is used for the right problem.
- To broaden the practice of electronic prescribing through accelerated development and deployment of the electronic health record.
- To accelerate access to nonpatented drugs and achieve international parity on prices of nonpatented drugs.
- To enhance analysis of cost drivers and cost-effectiveness, including best practices in drug-plan policies.

The task force is expected to report on its progress in June 2006.

Provincial and Federal Government Reimbursement

Canada has a fragmented public reimbursement system: eligibility, coverage levels, and lists of reimbursable drugs vary by plan. Most provincial plans cover people aged 65 or older, social assistance recipients, and people with high drug costs. Some provinces have special programs for people with specific diseases that require expensive treatments, such as cancer and HIV/AIDS.

Because of its large population, Ontario has the largest drug-benefit program in Canada. The plan reimburses prescription costs for all Ontario residents aged 65 or over, with small deductibles and copayments. It also provides benefits to people receiving social assistance and to other people with high drug costs relative to income. Although most Ontario residents do not qualify for the provincial plan, drug-plan costs continue to rise; people covered by the provincial plan tend to use more medicines and have higher per-capita costs.

Quebec is the only province that requires all residents to have prescription drug coverage. Private employers with group plans must provide prescription drug coverage for all active employees and must cover all drugs listed on the formulary of the *Régie de l'assurance maladie du Québec* (RAMQ; Quebec Health Insurance Authority). Quebec residents who are not eligible for an employer plan are required to join the provincial plan and must pay the applicable premiums.

Some of the provinces are moving increasingly toward providing income-based benefits in an effort to concentrate resources on people with the greatest financial needs. This type of program has the effect of excluding most people whose drug costs are low to moderate, unless they are social assistance recipients or have extremely low family incomes.

Each province has developed its own formulary that lists drug products (primarily prescription medicines) that are reimbursable by the public plan. Formularies not only list the medicines that the province will reimburse, but they also set reimbursement levels, limits for drug-ingredient costs, and limits for markups and professional fees. Formularies are becoming more and more restrictive as provinces try to control rising costs for new technologies. Provinces frequently establish criteria to restrict reimbursement. In some cases for which the only treatment available is a nonlisted product, a request for special authorization/coverage may be made; for example, Ontario's Section 8 mechanism allows for reimbursement of nonformulary drugs on a case-by-case basis at the physician's request. For multisource products, most plans will reimburse only up to the level of the lowest-cost alternative treatment, usually a generic.

Decisions on which drugs will be reimbursed are based on therapeutic value and cost-effectiveness. Usually, generic products are quickly added to formularies in order to reduce plan costs.

Until recently, each province conducted an independent review of new brand-name drugs, and manufacturers were obliged to complete separate submissions for each provincial and federal drug plan. However, the establishment of the CDR in September 2003 has helped to streamline the review process, reduce duplication, and harmonize reimbursement procedures across the country.

Drug plans are reacting to rising drug expenditures by tightening reimbursement of new drugs (more limited listings, increasingly stringent criteria for reimbursement, and more case-by-case assessments at physician request), increasing premiums and copayments, speeding up the reimbursement of lower-priced generics, and in some instances, expanding the maximum allowable cost policies to include not only the multisource drugs with generics, but also some single-source brands.

Common Drug Review

The CDR is a federal/provincial/territorial initiative intended to reduce duplication and streamline the system for reviewing new drugs for public reimbursement. It is managed and overseen by the CCOHTA, located in Ottawa. Before September 2003, each publicly funded drug plan conducted its own reviews of new chemical entities and new combination drugs and had its own committee of experts to provide listing recommendations.

Currently, only new chemical entities and new combinations are being submitted to the CDR for review. All other submissions – that is, new dosage forms and strengths of existing drugs and new generics – will be directed to the drug plans. The CDR's recommendations with respect to clinical-effectiveness and cost-effectiveness will impact the reimbursement decisions made by public payers outside of Quebec. Table 7.2 shows the time frames for the CDR. Key steps in the process include the following:

Table 7.2 Time Frames for Common Drug Review Procedures

Task	*Time Frame (in business days)*	*Weeks*
Review process		
1. Checking submission for completeness	5	1
2. Assignment of submission coordinator, contracting reviewers	10	2
3. Internal staff review of search strategy and research	10	2
4. Review time for reviewers	20	4
5. Quality assessment of reviewers' reports by submission coordinator	5	1
6. Manufacturer's review of reviewers' reports	7	1.5
7. Reviewers' replies to comments	7	1.5
8. Preparation of CEDAC brief	5	1
9. Placement on CEDAC agenda	10–40	2–8
10. Sending out CEDAC recommendation and reasons for recommendation	5	1
11. Embargo period	10	2
12. Sending out final recommendation (no request for reconsideration or clarification)	5	1
Total review time	99–129 days	20–26 weeks
Reconsideration process (manufacturers)		
1. Examination of reconsideration request	5	1
2. Preparation of reconsideration brief	5	1
3. Placement on CEDAC agenda	Next CEDAC agenda	Next CEDAC agenda
4. Sending out CEDAC final recommendation	5	1
Clarification request (drug plans)		
1. Providing clarification and sending out CEDAC final recommendation	5	1

CEDAC = Canadian Expert Drug Advisory Committee

Note: Time frames assume that the most expedient method of delivering data is used. Schedule of CEDAC meetings will be posted on the CEDAC Web site

- A drug manufacturer, a drug plan, or the Advisory Committee on Pharmaceuticals files a submission for a new drug to the CDR.
- A systematic clinical review of the drug is prepared by pharmacists or physicians; a review of the pharmacoeconomic data is prepared by health economists.
- The reviewers consider the drug submission plus information retrieved through an independent literature search conducted by an information specialist.
- Guidelines and templates are used in preparing the reviews to ensure a consistent and rigorous, high-quality approach.
- CDR staff edit and assess the reviews for quality.
- Reviews are sent to the manufacturer for comments and to drug plans for information.
- Reviewers prepare a reply to the manufacturer's comments on the reviews.
- A brief is prepared for the Canadian Expert Drug Advisory Committee (CEDAC).
- CEDAC members meet to consider the submission. Their deliberations are based on the CEDAC brief; they may also request the input of other experts or the CDR reviewers.
- The initial CEDAC formulary-listing recommendation is sent to the manufacturer and the drug plans in confidence. The manufacturer may request reconsideration, and the drug plans may request clarification of the recommendation.

CEDAC, which meets monthly, is an independent advisory body of health and other professionals with expertise in drug therapy and drug evaluation. The committee may recommend that a drug be listed, a drug be listed with criteria or conditions, a drug not be listed, or that a recommendation be deferred pending clarification of information (Table 7.3). Criteria and factors that CEDAC considers in making its recommendations include the following:

- Clinical studies that demonstrate the safety and efficacy of the drug in appropriate patient populations.
- Therapeutic advantages and disadvantages of the drug relative to accepted therapy.
- Cost effectiveness of the drug relative to accepted therapy.

Each of the drug plans that participates in CDR will make its own formulary listing and benefit-coverage decision based on the CEDAC recommendation and the plan's mandate, priorities, and resources.

Impact of Price Increases on Provincial Drug Plans

Provinces differ considerably in their policies on drug price increases. While some provincial drug plans reimburse actual acquisition costs and are impacted by price changes as soon as pharmacies submit claims at a higher price, other plans reimburse the drug-benefit prices listed on their formularies and do not allow increases until the formulary price is updated.

Quebec and Ontario have had long-standing policies of refusing to accept price increases for drugs listed on their provincial formularies, or to allow increases only if they are offset by reductions on other products.

Price increases are a major concern for governments because an increase in the price of a best-selling drug can have a large impact on public drug-plan budgets. For example, the Ontario Drug Programs Branch says that if it had allowed a 4% increase in the reimbursement price of Pfizer's Lipitor (atorvastatin) in 2004, it would have cost the province C$7.8 million (US $6 million) in one year.

Table 7.3 Common Drug Review Final Recommendations

Year	*Number of Reviews Completed*	*CDR Final Recommendation*		
		Drug Should Be Listed	*Drug Should Be Listed with Criteria or Conditions*	*Drug Should Not Be Listed*
2004	15	0	6	9
2005	16	2	4	10
Total	31 (100%)	2 (7%)	10 (32%)	19 (61%)

When new drug submissions are reviewed, provinces look at cost-effectiveness and the projected budget impact of listing the new drug. If a price increase is proposed for a drug already listed on the formulary, Ontario has suggested that evidence of the medicine's increased value and cost effectiveness may be required. Ontario also supports changing the PMPRB Guidelines to require prior approval and justification for price increases of patented drugs.

Prices are still frozen on the Ontario formulary. For the most part, pharmacists are absorbing the increases or are submitting "cost-to-operator" claims to the Ontario government if a drug's new price is greater than the formulary price plus the allowed 10% markup. These cost-to-operator claims are now having a significant budget impact in Ontario.

In Quebec, manufacturers' contracts stipulate that they will not increase the guaranteed selling price of their products above the price listed in the current *Liste de Médicaments* (the Quebec drug list). In an effort to maintain prices at 2003 levels, the Quebec minister of health did not issue a new edition of the drug list from October 2003 to February 2005. In the summer of 2005, the minister announced that the "no increases" policy will remain in effect throughout 2006. It is expected that the province's new pharmaceutical policy (intended to establish rules for price increases and other pharmaceutical matters) will be completed by that time.

Most manufacturers have not implemented price increases in Quebec, and as a result, Canada now has differential pricing: for many products, prices are lower in Quebec than in other provinces.

Quebec's Pharmaceutical Policy

Quebec has traditionally provided a supportive environment for the innovative pharmaceutical industry, and many companies, including several biotech firms, have located their Canadian headquarters in Quebec. The province is in the process of developing a new pharmaceutical policy through a consensus approach with government, industry, and other stakeholders. The government released a draft policy paper in December 2004, and manufacturers and other stakeholders – including the pharmacists' association, medical association, and patient advocacy groups – have appeared before the *Commission des Affaires Sociales* (Social Affairs Commission) to provide their views on the policy. (Schedule of hearings and stakeholders appearing before the commission: www.assnat.qc.ca/fra/37legislature1/commissions/cas/ho-cas-2005-04-19-Politique%20médicament.pdf) The commission hearings were completed in September 2005; the final version of the pharmaceutical policy is now being prepared. Proposals in the draft policy include the following:

- End the nonincreasing drug price policy (the price-freeze that has been in force for many years) and set up a mechanism to manage drug price increases. Some of the measures proposed to manage increases include limiting the average price increase of all products in a manufacturer's line to the CPI increase rate minus a 0.5% correction factor, limiting the rate of price increase for each product to no more than 1.5% of a defined maximum rate, and restricting price indexation to products that have been on the formulary for five years or more.
- Allow agreements for setting up compensation measures to minimize or prevent the impact of price increases on the public system and give more latitude to manufacturers in the case of drugs that represent a significant innovation.
- Tighten the rules governing wholesalers so as to ensure equity between them. The province is proposing to unfreeze wholesalers' markups and establish a maximum markup of 6.0%. Place a ceiling of C$24 (US $18) on products costing more than C$400 (US $307).
- Promote the innovative pharmaceutical industry by keeping the "15-year rule" in its current form, instead of setting up a reference-based pricing system. This proposal seeks to guarantee innovative companies that the purchase price of their products will be fully reimbursed for 15 years after listing on the drug formulary, even if the patent has expired or a less- expensive generic equivalent is available.

Private Drug Plan Reimbursement

Just over half of Canadians are covered through employer-sponsored drug plans or individual drug insurance plans. CIHI reports that 33.5% of prescription drug expenditures were funded through private insurance plans in 2004.

Private plans range from very liberal plans that reimburse all prescription drugs, and even over-the-counter products if prescribed by a physician, to more restrictive plans with closed formularies. Most private plans cover all prescription drugs as soon as they are approved by Health Canada, with a few exceptions. It is fairly common for plans to exclude or limit reimbursement for "quality-of-life" products, such as oral contraceptives, weight-loss treatments, erectile-dysfunction treatments, smoking-cessation products, and fertility treatments. Most plans require employee contributions through payroll deduction. Deductibles and copayments are generally low – for example, C$100 (US $77) annual deductible and 20% coinsurance per prescription.

Most private plans do not use managed formularies. However, rising plan costs in recent years have forced many plans to consider formularies and other approaches to cost-containment. Many insurers are connected to third-party administrators that process drug claims (often electronically through a pay-direct network linked to pharmacies) and manage costs. Generics substitution plans are common, with the plan reimbursing only up to the cost of the lowest-priced generic available. Some plans have formularies that mirror provincial drug plans, but they usually reimburse nonformulary drugs at a higher copayment. Some plans are beginning to adopt the types of multitier plans that are already common in the United States. Under these arrangements, a high copayment is applied to nonformulary brand-name drugs, a smaller copayment to formulary brands, and no copayment to generics. Some plans use dispensing-fee caps to control costs. Third-party administrators and insurers also provide plan sponsors with regular reports on plan costs and utilization. Savings from cost-containment initiatives are generally passed along to the plan sponsor or insurer. The third-party administrator will receive an administration fee based on the number of transactions processed and the complexity of the plan design. The US system of managed care rebates does not exist in Canada.

When private plans use formularies, manufacturers must prepare reimbursement submissions for new drugs that include details of clinical benefits and projected budget impact. Insurance companies and the third-party administrators sometimes receive presentations from drug manufacturers who are trying to have new products reimbursed. This type of presentation is often provided by manufacturers of products that are expected to have many claimants and to incur high plan costs or products that may be considered quality-of-life drugs.

Private insurance plans tend to cover brand-name drugs as soon as they reach the market, unlike public plans, which decline to list new medicines or provide limited reimbursement after a lengthy review process. Because they typically reference provincial drug- plan prices when determining the drug cost payable, private plans are affected by the price increases that have occurred in all provinces except Quebec. In addition, private plans generally charge smaller deductibles and copayments than public plans.

Hospital Formularies

Medicare provides full funding for drugs administered in hospitals. Individual provinces and territories plan, finance, and evaluate the provision of hospital care. Hospitals are funded largely through prospective global budgets negotiated with or imposed by provincial governments. Hospitals have control over the day-to-day allocation of resources, provided they stay within the operating budgets established by the regional or provincial health authorities.

Manufacturers negotiate contracts with hospitals to have their products listed on hospital formularies, which vary from hospital to hospital. Generics are widely used, and bulk purchase discounts are expected. In reports to the PMPRB, manufacturers are required to report average selling prices of products sold to hospitals and their retail sales in separate categories.

Although hospitals account for the largest share of healthcare spending in Canada, the share is declining as a result of both cost-shifting and cost-containment measures enacted in response to the constrained global budgets (e.g., the closure of emergency rooms or entire hospitals, the merging of services, reductions in bed numbers). The availability of effective new medicines has also progressively reduced the importance of hospitalization in the healthcare system. The shift from hospital-based care to community care has added to the strain on provincial drug plans because more patients are being treated on an outpatient basis and their drug costs are not covered by hospital budgets.

CROSS-BORDER TRADE OF PRESCRIPTION DRUGS TO THE UNITED STATES

For several years, residents of the United States have been taking advantage of the much lower branded-drug prices in Canada to purchase medicines from Canadian pharmacies either through the Internet or by mail order. Since 2001, more than 100 Internet pharmacies have been established in Canada with the purpose of filling prescriptions for US customers; most of these are located in Manitoba, Alberta, and British Columbia. Although the US federal law prohibits prescription drug imports for personal or commercial use without the permission of the manufacturer, the US authorities have generally allowed cross-border sales for individuals.

Several Internet pharmacies have grown into thriving businesses that employ hundreds of people, including pharmacists, pharmacy technicians, customer call-center staff, mail-room staff, and other employees. At the height of the boom in early 2004, the industry employed as many as 4,000 people. However, the cross-border trade has been declining for the past year. IMS Health reports that cross-border sales of prescription drugs peaked in the first quarter of 2004 and have since declined. According to IMS Health, sales in the fourth quarter of 2004 were estimated at C$128.5 million (US $98.7 million), down almost 20% from C$159.9 million (US $122.9 million) in the first quarter of 2004.

Supply restrictions imposed by some manufacturers and wholesalers are making it more difficult for Canadian pharmacies to supply US customers. Some cross-border pharmacies are managing to remain in business by obtaining small supplies from other pharmacies, but this is a costly arrangement and reduces their profit margin. Health Canada has notified pharmacies that it is illegal to supply drugs to other retailers without a wholesaler establishment license. Some pharmacies are directing US customers to pharmacies in other countries, including the United Kingdom and New Zealand, if they do not have sufficient supply of a drug.

The continuing strength of the Canadian dollar compared with the US dollar also means that pharmacies are raising prices for US customers, thereby reducing the savings available. However, despite the rise in prices, many brand-name drugs are still available at much lower prices from Canada than from US pharmacies.

The US federal government and the FDA remain opposed to parallel imports of prescription drugs from Canada and elsewhere. The Medicare Prescription Drug, Improvement, and Modernization Act of 2003 will provide drug benefits for US seniors beginning January 1, 2006, and it is anticipated that this benefit will reduce the demand for lower-priced drugs from Canada. However, the US federal regulators face growing resistance from state governments that have set up programs to make it easier for government employees – and in some cases, other residents – to purchase drugs from Canada and Europe. Minnesota and New Hampshire were at the forefront of this movement. In 2004, Illinois, Kansas, Missouri, and Wisconsin set up a program called I-SaveRx that connects patients with 45 pharmacies and wholesalers in Canada, Ireland, and the United Kingdom. In 2005, Vermont also joined this program, which offers enrollees 100 of the most commonly prescribed branded drugs for chronic conditions. Several other states – Maine, Nevada, Texas, Virginia, and Washington – enacted legislation in 2005 that is designed to facilitate drug importation. The governors of Minnesota, Wisconsin, Utah, Kansas, Maine, and North Dakota sent a letter to the Canadian prime minister in early 2005 stating that the health of their citizens would suffer if Canada restricted the cross-border trade in prescription drugs. Some municipalities (e.g., the Massachusetts cities of Boston, Springfield, and Worcester) have also implemented drug importation programs.

Canadian authorities have expressed concerns that continued cross-border trade could lead to supply shortages and higher prices in Canada. Health Canada has come under pressure from various sources including patient groups, provincial regulatory authorities that oversee pharmacists and physicians, and the pharmaceutical industry to outlaw exports to the United States. However, cross-border trade is supported by the pharmacies involved (which employ several thousand Canadians) and by the Manitoba government, which views the trade as a growth industry because many cross-border businesses are based in Manitoba. Health Minister Ujjal Dosanjh has started public consultations on three proposed measures intended to protect Canadians' access to safe and affordable prescription drugs:

- Establish a drug supply network to provide Health Canada with more comprehensive data on Canada's drug supply.
- Draft legislative and regulatory amendments to the Food and Drugs Act and its regulations to provide new authority for the minister to restrict the export of drugs deemed to be in actual or potential shortage.
- Strengthen existing federal regulations to require that prescription drugs be sold pursuant to a prescription issued within an established patient-practitioner relationship.

The consultation process is expected to continue through fall 2005. It is likely that bulk exports of prescription drugs for commercial use will be prohibited, but it is unclear how the Internet pharmacies will be impacted. The health minister is not expected to introduce legislation preventing Canadian pharmacies from filling prescriptions for individual patients who reside in the United States. However, doctors who cosign prescriptions for patients they have not seen and pharmacists who fill the prescriptions may be subject to stricter regulation by provincial authorities.

OUTLOOK FOR THE CANADIAN PHARMACEUTICAL MARKET

Although Canadian prices for patent-protected medicines are, on average, only 91% of median international prices and have been very stable, the cost of prescription drugs in Canada has provoked intense debate. National, provincial, and territorial governments, the PMPRB, and private insurers are all concerned about the recent upward trend in prices, even though increases have generally been within the PMPRB's guidelines and below the general rate of inflation. It will be interesting to see if these stakeholders will intensify their efforts to curb price increases and pharmaceutical expenditures.

The PMPRB has been particularly critical of rising drug prices and has called for the introduction of tighter price controls and stricter reporting requirements. The proposed amendments to the Patented Medicines Regulations, if implemented, will likely extend price-review times and increase the administrative burden on pharmaceutical companies. The PMPRB's proposals for future procedures for increasing prices could also be bad news for drug manufacturers, particularly if the model that requires advance application and justification of the proposed increase is adopted. The pharmaceutical industry has cause to be concerned about the PMPRB's growing influence in the Canadian pharmaceutical pricing and reimbursement environment.

Differences in provincial and territorial drug benefits and formulary coverage have led to considerable geographic disparities in access to prescription medicines. The proposed national, publicly funded Pharmacare program would tackle these inequalities by providing universal drug coverage across the country, but the cost of such a program may prove to be a major stumbling block.

Private insurers have generally been much more generous than the public sector in the provision of prescription drug benefits. However, growing cost pressures are forcing private health insurance plans to intensify their cost-containment strategies. Measures such as multitier formularies, generics substitution, and drug utilization reviews will probably become more common in the future.

The export of prescription drugs to US consumers has been a highly controversial practice, not least because of its actual or potential impact on the pharmaceutical supply system in Canada. The government has expressed its willingness to introduce tougher regulations if it believes that exports are harming public health in Canada.

The pharmaceutical pricing and reimbursement climate in Canada is likely to remain challenging for research-based pharmaceutical companies for the foreseeable future. However, staying out of the world's eighth-largest pharmaceutical market, and one of the fastest-growing markets, is not an option for multinational companies.

REFERENCE

PMPRB Newsletter, July 2005; 9(3).

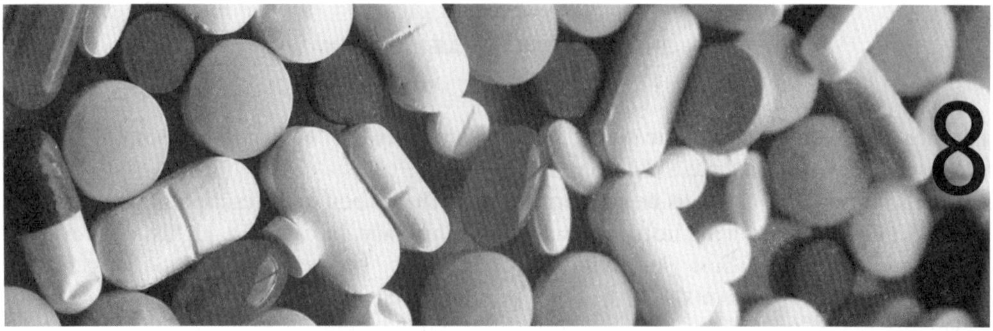

Contrasting European and US Patent Laws: Issues for the Pharmaceutical Industry

OVERVIEW

Patents have become the lifeblood of the biopharmaceutical industry, which depends heavily on intellectual property (IP) protection (especially patents and trade secrets) to justify and support its investment in R&D. Without IP protection, generic drug companies could develop products that match the physical and chemical specifications of innovator products and behave in a comparable manner and enter the market within only a few years of the introduction of a new drug product. Such a short period of exclusivity would not give developers of new molecular entities enough time to recoup their investments in R&D.

In addition to supporting laws protecting patents, most industrialized nations also recognize the importance of protecting data generated from preclinical and clinical studies. Both Europe and the United States provide periods of data or marketing exclusivity for such data.

An effective IP system must provide an incentive to seek a patent. No inventor is *required* to patent an invention; as a way of benefiting from the invention, an inventor could simply keep it secret. Indeed, this option is widely used in all industries. Trade secrets do not expire, but special measures are required to ensure continued secrecy; should such measures be violated, there is little legal protection for the owner. In the drug industry, however, many aspects of the business are subject to regulatory and public scrutiny, making secrecy a difficult option.

In the European and US patent systems, in exchange for complete disclosure of the invention, patent law creates and enables the enforcement of a right to exclude others from practicing the invention, often referred to as a *limited monopoly*. This right to exclude allows an inventor time to recoup R&D investments and encourages further investment of time and resources.

Few patents truly give an inventor a monopoly in an area; indeed, patent systems encourage competitors to design around or improve on patented inventions. However, in recent decades, legislatures, courts, and patent offices in Europe and the United States have generally increased patent protection for inventors, and there has been pressure on all government entities to attract and support R&D-intensive industries in increasingly knowledge-based economies.

Although the fundamentals of IP law in the United States and Europe are similar, there are key differences with regard to issues of special concern to the pharmaceutical and biotechnology industries. Decisions of the European Patent Office Board of Appeals in the area of biotechnology have been largely consistent with those of the US Patent and Trademark Office (PTO), though the bodies of law have developed at different paces and differences exist that may have consequences in the future. In this chapter, we discuss the fundamentals of IP law on both sides of the Atlantic, highlighting those trans-Atlantic differences that affect pharmaceutical companies operating in both regions.

US PATENT LAW

The framers of the US Constitution considered inventions and technological progress sufficiently important to include a clause for IP protection, and Congress has enacted laws to confer a time-limited right to exclude others from making, selling, using, or importing a patented invention. The US Patent Act of 1790 granted patents to the "first and true inventor"; as a result, the United States has a first-to-invent system of awarding patents. In the United States (as in Europe), patent protection is limited to inventions in the fields of *applied* technology. It is not possible to patent basic scientific research, discovery of a law of nature, discovery of physical phenomena, abstract ideas, or the discovery of something found in nature (in that natural state).

US law allows the patenting of design and utility inventions; design patents protect ornamental features of an article of manufacture and utility patents protect a composition, process, assembly, or arrangement of steps. Utility patents are of two types: process and product. Process patents protect a process but not the end result or product made by it (others may achieve the same result by a different process), while product patents provide broader protection by preventing others from making or using the final product, regardless of how it is made. According to US law, the following key requirements must be satisfied to obtain a patent on an invention:

- Novelty
- Nonobviousness
- Utility
- Enablement
- The best mode of practicing the invention

The novelty and nonobviousness requirements mandate a comparison between the invention and the prior art (everything that is known, published, and publicly available *before* the invention). It is fundamental that to be patentable, an invention must be novel or not already exist.

A proposed patent claim is obvious "if the differences between the subject matter sought to be patented and the prior art are such that the subject matter as a whole would have been obvious at the time the invention was made to a person having ordinary skill in the art."

The utility requirement means simply that the invention has some known use. The threshold for this requirement is low; almost any use will do, so long as it is functional and not solely aesthetic.

To be enabling, a patent specification must teach one skilled in the art how to make or use the invention, without undue experimentation. A key question in determining whether a specification is enabling is the predictability of the art. Because biotechnology is an unpredictable art, an inventor is likely to be held to the higher enablement standard and required to provide data showing that an invention works as claimed, in contrast to inventions in more predictable areas, such as some fields of engineering, where hypothetical examples often suffice. The written description requirement is related, but distinct, from enablement. It requires sufficient disclosure in the claims and specification to demonstrate to a person of skill in the art that the applicant was in possession of the invention when the application was filed.

Under US law, an applicant must disclose the best mode of practicing the invention; the inventor cannot seek a patent and still keep some important aspect secret (there must be *full* disclosure). Despite the absence of this requirement in Europe, leaving it out of a European patent application that is subsequently filed in the United States can preclude patentability in the United States. An inventor may not be able to obtain a US patent on the same invention if there is an intermediate disclosure by another that renders the invention obvious (i.e., the European filing will be incomplete as a priority document for the US filing).

EUROPEAN PATENT LAW

In Europe, whoever files a patent application first is deemed to be the inventor (first-to-file rule). Aside from this difference between US and European patent law, the fundamentals of both systems are similar. Table 8.1 lists key European Union (EU) directives and regulations affecting the pharmaceutical/biotech sector.

Table 8.1 Key EU Directives and Regulations Affecting the Pharmaceutical/Biotech Sector

Directive/Regulation	*Year*	*Outcome*
Directive 65/65/EEC	1965	Required member states to establish systems for premarket approval of drugs and to detail what information would be required for marketing authorization
Directive 75/318/EEC	1975	Established detailed requirements for the scientific information to be submitted in marketing authorization applications
Directive 75/319/EEC	1975	Established a multinational approval procedure and set up the Committee for Proprietary Medicinal Products (CPMP) to implement it
Directive 87/21/EEC	1986	Amended Directive 65/65, permitting abridged applications subject to data protection periods. The basic data protection period was six years, but states could provide a 10-year period or no data protection after patent expiry
Directive 93/39/EEC	1993	Established a mutual recognition procedure to replace the old multistate system of Directive 75/319. It came into effect on January 1, 1995
Regulation (EEC) No. 2309/93	1993	Created a centralized approval system for biotechnology products and provided a 10-year protection period for such products. This procedure came into effect on January 1, 1995, and is administered by the European Medicines Agency (EMEA). Marketing authorizations are granted by the European Commission on the advice of the CPMP, now part of the EMEA
Directive 98/44/EC	1998	The "Biotech Directive" required member states to harmonize their laws, providing broad protection for biotechnology inventions involving biological materials, biotechnological processes, and products concerning genetic information. The directive also provided a legal right to patents on plants and animals
Regulation 141/2000	1999	The Orphan Drug Regulation, providing 10 years of marketing exclusivity for such products, was adopted in 1999 and went into effect in January 2000
Directive 2004/27/EC	2004	Amends Directive 2001/83/EC and creates a Bolar-like provision, exempting generics companies preparing abridged applications from patent infringement. Member nations have until October 2005 to implement this provision

EC = European Community
EEC = European Economic Community

A Brief History

The three landmarks in European patent legislation are the Paris Convention (1883), the Strasbourg Convention (1963), and the European Patent Convention (EPC or the Munich Convention; 1977), as shown in Table 8.2. Implementing the EPC resulted in the first-to-file patent system and the requirement that the pending application be published, and it established a centralized system by which an applicant can obtain national patents. It did not create a single-patent system for Europe, only a single-granting system. Patents granted under the EPC do not become Europe-wide; instead, they become a bundle of national patents in the countries chosen by the applicant, and these patents can then be enforced in the national courts of those countries. Following the EPC, signatory nations revised their patent laws. As a result, at least with regard to the patent application and the examination procedure, Europe has unified patent rules.

European Patent Explained

An inventor seeking to patent an invention in one or more European nations can either file an application with a national patent office and subsequently file the application in other countries, claiming priority from the first filing, or file the patent with the European Patent Office (EPO) to receive a European patent, which is then converted to national patents in designated EPC states. The effect of both routes is the same, and the patent(s) obtained expire at the same time.

Article 52 of the EPC provides that "European patents shall be granted for any inventions which are susceptible of industrial application, which are new, and which involve an inventive step." These requirements – novelty, inventive step, and industrial application – parallel the novelty, nonobviousness, and utility requirements of US law. Novelty is defined as "not forming a part of the state of the art" (Article 54). Article 56 relates to the inventive step, which is essentially the same as the US nonobviousness requirement and states, "An invention shall be considered as involving an inventive step if having regard to the state of the art, it is not obvious to a person skilled in the art." Article 57 of the EPC, relating to industrial applicability, states that the invention will be considered if it "can be made or used in any kind of industry, including agriculture."

An invention must also be of "technical nature" to be patentable. Article 52(2) of the EPC considers the following inventions to be nontechnical and, therefore, unpatentable:

- Discoveries, scientific theories, and mathematical methods.
- Aesthetic creations.
- Schemes, rules, and methods for performing mental acts, playing games or doing business, and programs for computers.
- Presentations of information.

Table 8.2 Landmarks in European Intellectual Property Law Legislation

Legislation	*Year*	*Description*
Paris Convention for the Protection of Industrial Property	1883	Required parties to treat foreign and domestic patent holders in the same way and to respect international priority dates
Strasbourg Convention on the Unification of Certain Points of Substantive Law on Patents for Invention	1963	Part of the effort toward the establishment of a common market in Europe, it harmonized aspects of substantive patent law, including the concepts of novelty and inventive step
European Patent Convention (EPC)	1973 (signed) 1977 (enforced)	Created the European Patent Office (EPO) in Munich, Germany, and established procedural rules for the examination of patent applications

The EPC does not address many issues of substantive patent law. For example, the EPC is silent regarding employed inventors, co-ownership of inventions, and remedies (such as injunctions and damages and how they are calculated). These and many other matters are left to the laws of the individual European states.

This situation creates several important problems; most obviously, the views of national courts are not always uniform. Each nation's courts interpret the EPC in accordance with its own body of law; each EPC signatory country uses the powers of its highest court to unify interpretation of the EPC. Only a common European patent court, at least one of last resort, could coordinate such differing interpretations.

Conflicting results, where courts in different countries in parallel cases have come to differing interpretations of the EPC and/or the "same" patent, have occurred because there is no supranational harmonizing mechanism. The best-known examples of these varying interpretations, often cited when criticisms are leveled at Europe's current patent system, are the "Epilady" cases. The patents in question concerned a hair-removal product for women. The patent owner filed infringement suits against the same party in courts in various European states where an allegedly infringing device was being sold. Different national courts reached differing, sometimes opposite, decisions in the various cases. Such varying and even conflicting decisions make it difficult to conduct business across Europe. A uniform interpretation of the EPC and European patent law in general would represent a major advance in the current patent system.

Community Patent Stalls

The EPC was intended only as a first step in the harmonization of European patent law; the next step was the proposed Community Patent, which was to provide a set of rules to integrate laws promulgated under the EPC, completing the harmonization process begun by the EPC. The Community Patent legislation would reduce the powers of national courts and the role of national patent offices and would hand these powers over to a new, pan-European patent court. Although a Community Patent Convention (the Luxembourg Convention) was held in 1975, the Community Patent has yet to become effective. Intense political debate and discussion ever since the 1975 convention, including renegotiations of the convention in 1985 and 1989, have failed to resolve even basic features of the Community Patent, such as in which language(s) it will be written. In 2000, a diplomatic conference was held to discuss modernizing the European patent system so as to make procedures before the EPO quicker, clearer, and more efficient and to discuss advancing toward a Community Patent.

In 2003, the Council of the European Union reached an agreement on the structure of courts to try patent infringement and validity cases. The agreement was intended to create a new jurisdictional system for the Community Patent, including a new court – the Community Patent Court within the European Court of Justice – which was scheduled to be in place by 2010. The Community Patent Court will have exclusive jurisdiction over many patent issues, including validity, infringement, and prior rights. However, many details of the court remain unresolved, not least the issues of language(s), sovereignty, and the transfer of powers from the national courts, details of patent-office fees, the appointment of judges to the Community Patent Court, and translation of applications and issued patents.

Most recently, in March 2004, the European Union (EU) Competitiveness Council failed to reach agreement on the details of the Community Patent Regulation, which will govern the proposed Community Patent, will apply to all EU member states, and is intended to build on the EPC for substantive patent law. Applicants will apply for patents through the EPO but will be able to designate the EU as a single territory. The EPO will examine the application in one of its existing three languages (English, French, and German). After the patent is granted, the patent holder will translate the patent claims into every language used in the EU.

The Community Patent is not intended to replace national patent systems or even the existing European patent. Instead, applicants will choose between national patents, national patents granted via the existing European patent system, and the new Community Patent.

Although recent momentum toward implementing a Community Patent and Community Patent Court has been encouraging, there is some doubt whether the necessary agreements will ever be reached. The matter is complicated by the EU's continuing expansion and the need to reach unanimity or consensus among a growing group of nations with an ever-increasing number of languages for translation.

US AND EUROPEAN PATENT LAW: IMPORTANT DIFFERENCES

Ordre Public and Morality

US law has historically considered moral issues, but the current view is that morality has nothing to do with patents or patenting. In 1817, regarding the patentability of a water pump in *Lowell v. Lewis*, the US Supreme Court stated that for an invention to be useful, it must not conflict with the "sound morals of society," referred to as the "moral utility doctrine." Although US courts have relied on *Lowell*, in recent years it is usually in relation to inventions of specious utility rather than questions of moral utility.

In contrast, the concepts of *ordre public* and morality are unique to European patent law. Article 53 of the EPC states that patents will not be granted for "inventions the publication or exploitation of which would be contrary to *ordre public* or morality, provided that the exploitation shall not be deemed so contrary merely because it is prohibited by law or regulation in some or all of the Contracting States." The EPC does not define *ordre public* or morality, nor does it state what is contrary to public morality.

The EPO has interpreted *ordre public* to cover "the protection of public security and the physical integrity of individuals as part of society." Thus, inventions will be unpatentable if their exploitation is "likely to breach public peace or social order (e.g., through acts of terrorism) or to seriously prejudice the environment." Issues of *ordre public* and morality were not an issue of great concern in European patent law until the concept was used to challenge several important biotechnology patents, including the attempt made to patent the "Harvard mouse," discussed further on, and genetically modified cells and organisms generally.

Candor

US patent law imposes a duty of candor on inventors in prosecuting US patent application. This duty applies to the inventors, their patent attorneys or agents, and anyone else associated with the inventors or the assignee who is substantively involved with the application. The duty requires that information material to patentability be disclosed to the examiner during prosecution.

European law has no such duty of candor for applicants, inventors, or their representatives, and the burden is on the EPO examiner to find relevant prior art. However, European inventors seeking US patents, especially based on a European priority filing, should keep the duty of candor in mind and not leave prior art skeletons in the closet. A breach of the duty may result in a finding of inequitable conduct, rendering any US patent resulting from the application unenforceable in US courts. A US examiner might not find them, but a competitor in a lawsuit will be much more motivated and likely to do so.

Disclosure

In the United States, because of the first-to-invent system, there is a one-year grace period during which an application must be filed following the publication or the first commercial use of an invention. This grace period is strictly enforced, and disclosure of the invention can lead to forfeiture of patent protection even if the following occurs:

- Delivery occurred subsequent to the disclosure (within the one-year grace period).
- The sale of the product containing the invention was not public.
- The sale of the product containing the invention was not consummated.
- The prospective purchaser did not know that the article for sale embodied an invention.

If publication or commercial use of an item embodying the invention is made by someone other than the applicant during the year, the applicant may "swear behind" the publication or use, demonstrating an earlier invention date but only if the activities forming the basis of this swearing behind occurred in the United States.

By contrast, there is no grace period in Europe, and an invention is deemed unpatentable if it is made available to the public anywhere in the world before the filing or the priority date of the application. "Available to the public" is generally taken to mean any dissemination of information concerning the invention to the public in an uncontrolled manner.

Oppositions and Reexamination

Apart from the 1999 American Inventors Protection Act introduction of *inter partes* reexamination into the US patent system, the US patenting process is essentially *ex parte*, that is, solely between the Patent and Trademark Office (PTO) and the inventor. Some experts do not believe that this system imposes a sufficiently rigorous review of patent and nonpatent prior art, leading to patents of excessive breadth and poor quality. Currently, in the United States, a party can challenge the validity of a patent in a district court if the party has been sued for infringement or in the PTO through patent reexamination procedures. Patent reexamination was established in 1980 to address concerns over the quality of patents; Congress sought to provide a less-expensive and quicker way to resolve patent-validity disputes than via district courts and to use the expertise of the PTO.

To begin a reexamination, "any person at any time may cite to the [Patent] Office in writing prior art consisting of patents or printed publications which that person believes to have a bearing on the patentability of any claim of a particular patent." Within three months of the filing of such a request, the PTO determines whether the request raises a substantial new question of patentability. It may also, on its own initiative, determine whether a substantial new question of patentability is raised by patents and publications discovered by the PTO or cited by any person.

Although a reexamination is conducted according to the same standards of patentability as the initial examination, the issues that can be considered are more limited than during the initial examination. Patentability issues examined during reexamination are typically novelty and/or obviousness. If the PTO allows the request for reexamination and the requesting party is not the owner of the challenged patent, the PTO provides a copy of the request to the patent holder. The patent holder can submit statements, including amendments or new claims, for consideration during reexamination. If the owner does submit such statements, the challenger has an opportunity to respond but cannot participate further. The major difference between *ex parte* and *inter partes* reexamination is that the latter allows the challenger to participate and to respond to everything the patent owner says.

If, in an *inter partes* reexamination, any claim of the challenged patent is found valid after exhaustion of appeal, the third-party challenger cannot at a later time call into question the validity of such claim in a civil trial based on any ground the challenger raised or could have raised during the reexamination proceedings. This estoppel is an important consideration for third-party challengers.

In both types of reexamination, when the time for appeal has expired or any appeal has ended, the PTO issues a certificate indicating the status of the reexamined patent. Any claim, including claims added or amended during reexamination, can be found patentable, unpatentable, or patentable after amendment.

The patent owner in either an *ex parte* or an *inter partes* reexamination can appeal an adverse decision to the Board of Patent Appeals and Interferences and, if not satisfied, to the Court of Appeals for the Federal Circuit (the Federal Circuit). Congress created this court in 1982 to promote uniformity across the country. It has nationwide jurisdiction over all appeals from district court patent cases and from the PTO. There has been much recent discussion about strengthening the US reexamination system into a full, postgrant open-review system, similar to the EPO opposition system (discussed in the following paragraphs).

Although the national courts of European countries can invalidate patents, most challenges take place at the EPO through the opposition procedure, the most convenient and inexpensive method for challenging patent validity. The pan-European scope of a successful opposition's effect and the participation of the opponent as an adversary make the opposition system attractive to patent challengers. Anybody can oppose a pending or granted European patent; the legal framework for the opposition process is contained in the EPC. Oppositions are handled by the Opposition Division, which assists the EPO in discovering prior art of which competitors are most likely to be aware. A third party may file an opposition within nine months of the granting of a patent by the EPO. Admissible reasons for an opposition are as follows:

- The subject matter is not patentable because the three key criteria (novelty, inventive step, commercial applicability) have not been met.
- Disclosure of the invention is insufficient to enable somebody skilled in the art to practice the invention.
- The scope of the patent as granted exceeds the scope of the original application.

An opposition proceeding has three potential outcomes: the patent may be revoked; the opposition may be rejected; or the patent may be narrowed, in which case the EPO will publish a modified patent. Any party to the opposition who is adversely affected by the decision of the opposition may appeal. The other parties to the opposition have the right to be parties in any appeal. The Board of Appeals examines the appeal and can either make a decision or remand the case to the Opposition Division for further examination. The entire opposition procedure, including appeals, can take up to five years or more.

Right to Exclude and Compulsory Licenses

In the United States, the patentee's right to prevent anyone from using the invention (right to exclude) is almost absolute – its exercise is limited only by antitrust laws. A patent holder can simply sit on a patented invention without exploiting it and prevent others from doing so.

In contrast, many countries in Europe have provisions for compulsory licensing of nonexploited inventions. The EPC does not address the issue, and national laws apply. France, Germany, and the United Kingdom for example, have compulsory license statutes.

US patent law recognizes compulsory licensing only when the patent resulted from federal government-funded research. In principle, these provisions apply to many fundamental inventions, particularly those arising from university-based research funded by federal grants to academic scientists and physicians. The National Institutes of Health, for example, could make such inventions available if a patent holder fails to do so. The funding agency has the right to grant a compulsory license, if that is necessary, for reasons including the following:

- Because the patent holder has not taken, or will not achieve, practical application of the invention.
- To alleviate health or safety needs not reasonably satisfied by the patent holder.
- To meet requirements for public use of the invention.

Arguably, these provisions are of intellectual and not practical concern, and, in fact, they have *never* been exercised, despite several high-profile attempts to persuade the government to invoke them (most famously, the 1997 Johns Hopkins University/CellPro case regarding stem-cell separation technology).

BIOPHARMACEUTICAL INDUSTRY PATENT ISSUES

Specific differences between US and European patent law exist that may have consequences for the operations of the biopharmaceutical industry in the future. First, the issues of *ordre public* and morality in European patent law mean that the EPO must determine whether an invention is contrary to morality before a patent can be granted. Second, the EPO cannot grant patents for new plant or animal "varieties." Third, the EPO cannot grant a patent for an essentially biological process for the production of plants or animals. We explore in this section patent issues unique to the pharmaceutical and biotechnology industries.

Patenting Life Itself

Because biotechnology enables scientists to genetically engineer cells, plants, and animals, opponents of patents on living organisms argue that living organisms are not patentable inventions but products of nature, objections that have failed in both the United States and Europe. The issue of patents on living organisms is not new; in 1873, Louis Pasteur obtained a US patent for a yeast (US Patent No. 141,072). Although the statutory definition of an invention has not changed since that time, in the 1970s, the PTO rejected claims for genetically engineered organisms because living organisms and cells were considered unpatentable products of nature.

Diamond v. Chakrabarty: *A Landmark Case*

In 1980, the issue of whether genetically engineered organisms were patentable reached the US Supreme Court, which decided the landmark case of *Diamond v. Chakrabarty*. The court held that a living organism – a genetically modified bacterium – *was* patentable under US law. In the *Chakrabarty* case, the microbiologist challenged the PTO's denial of a patent for a bacterium into which plasmids had been introduced, enabling it to break down components of crude oil. The PTO had rejected the patent application on the grounds that microorganisms were nonpatentable products of nature and living organisms were not patentable under the Patent Act (35 U.S.C. §101).

On appeal, the Board of Patent Appeals decided that the new bacterium was not a product of nature because bacteria containing such plasmids did not occur naturally but affirmed the rejection based on the argument that Congress had not intended living organisms to be patentable. However, the Supreme Court held that a genetically altered living organism *could* be patented. Chakrabarty had created "a new bacterium with markedly different characteristics from any found in nature." It was "not nature's handiwork, but his own; accordingly, it is patentable subject matter." Indeed, according to a congressional report quoted by the Supreme Court, Congress intended patentable subject matter to "include anything under the sun that is made by man."

Oyster Patent Broadens Scope

Few areas of IP law have generated more attention than the realization that it is now possible to use utility patents to protect rights in genetically modified higher animals, as long as they otherwise meet the criteria for patentability. On the back of the *Chakrabarty* decision, the patentability of multicellular animals was also resolved (settled law) in the United States in the 1980s. In *Ex Parte Allen* (1987), the issue was the patentability of genetically engineered polyploid Pacific-coast oysters containing an extra set of chromosomes. The applicant sought to patent the oysters and a method of inducing polyploidy.

Following *Chakrabarty*, the PTO held that such genetically modified oysters could be patented and issued a notice saying that altered multicellular animals were patentable subject matter within the scope of the Patent Act.

Far more controversial than the *Allen* decision was the granting of a US patent (US Patent No. 4,736,866, issued in April 1988) to Harvard University. The patent covered the so-called Harvard mouse or oncomouse – a genetically engineered cancer model. Two notable features of claim 1 of the patent are that it covers all mammals, not just mice, and it covers the progeny of the animals that first received the oncogene. The PTO applied *Chakrabarty* broadly, granting a patent for the oncomouse less than four years after the application was filed.

Europe Follows US Lead, Eventually

The Harvard mouse patent was at the center of controversy surrounding patenting life in Europe. Harvard University also sought a European patent for the invention. Interpreting Article 53(b) of the EPC as excluding animals *per se* from patentability, the EPO Examining Division rejected the application for failure to constitute patentable subject matter. Although the Examining Division had not rejected the patent under Article 53(a) as being immoral, the Board of Appeals reversed the decision, broadly interpreting the scope of patentable subject matter under the EPC, but it remanded the case for examination of whether the patent violated *ordre public* or morality; on remand, the Examining Division decided that the invention did not. The grant of the patent was hardly the end of the issue; *17 parties* filed oppositions with the EPO. Ultimately, in 2001, the Opposition Division ruled that the patent should bc amended, limiting it "to transgenic rodents containing an additional cancer gene" and the patent was issued.

Two other decisions by the EPO have contributed to the developing law on the patentability of inventions involving genetic engineering and address the issue of the EPO's prohibition on inventions that are contrary to morality or *ordre public*. In the first case, *Plant Genetic Systems v. Greenpeace*, relating to the patentability of genetically engineered plants, the appeals board remained unconvinced that granting the patents would be immoral or contrary to *ordre public* and could see no moral distinction between modifying plant characteristics by genetic engineering and modifying them by traditional selective breeding. We discuss the second case – the Relaxin/Howard Florey Research Institute case – later.

DNA Sequences Are Patentable

Genetic material such as genes, gene fragments, and single nucleotide polymorphisms (SNPs) can be patented under US law, and thousands of patent applications have been filed with the PTO for human genetic material. Patents have been issued on whole genes whose function is known, so long as the gene is isolated and purified from its natural state. Such patents on gene sequences cover the isolated and purified gene but not the gene as it occurs naturally.

Three seminal cases addressed the patentability of DNA sequences under the US law: *Amgen v. Chugai Pharmaceutical* (1991), *Fiers v. Revel* (1993), and *The Regents of the University of California v. Eli Lilly* (1997).

Amgen v. Chugai Pharmaceutical

This case concerned Amgen's patent claims covering complementary DNAs (cDNAs) encoding erythropoietin; the claims were broad and included all erythropoietin cDNAs, including those from other animals. The only limitation on the claim was that the encoded erythropoietin must be able to stimulate red blood cell production. That is, the gene was defined with regard to function and not its structure (sequence). The Federal Circuit held that the genus claim, to cDNAs encoding all erythropoietins that stimulate red blood cell production, was permissible only if the specification disclosed a sufficient number of DNA sequences to demonstrate that the inventors were in possession of the genus of erythropoietin DNAs the claim sought to cover. In fact, the patent's specification disclosed only a few examples, and the court held that Amgen was not entitled to a claim covering the genus. The court required that a gene be described by its structure (sequence), not by its function, and ruled that the scope of enablement was not as broad as the scope of the claims sought.

Fiers v. Revel

In this case, which arose out of an interference to determine who was first to invent and therefore who should get the patent, it was held that for complete conception of an invention of a DNA sequence encoding a particular protein, a written description of the complete DNA sequence is required. The Federal Circuit affirmed the PTO's holding that Fiers did not conceive of the invention because his original priority application described a method for isolating a DNA encoding interferon-beta but not a DNA sequence encoding interferon-beta. The court reaffirmed that a gene must be described by its sequence and not by its function and that "Conception of a substance claimed *per se* without reference to a process requires conception of its structure, name, formula, or definitive chemical or physical properties."

The Regents of the University of California v. Eli Lilly

In this case, the university's patent contained claims for recombinantly produced human insulin. However, at issue in *Lilly* was the validity of a patent broadly directed to recombinant insulin DNA, where the specification disclosed only a DNA sequence for rat insulin. The university argued that the provided rat sequence, along with the level of skill in molecular biology for obtaining cDNAs, enabled one of skill to clone the human insulin cDNA by routine experimentation. The Federal Circuit disagreed, affirming that DNA be described by its sequence and not by its function and holding that one of ordinary skill in the art would not recognize that the patent holder was "in possession" of the broader invention at the time of filing the application.

More recently, inventors have sought patents on DNA fragments, a move that has sparked controversy among scientists, many of whom have urged the PTO not to grant patents to applicants who have neither characterized the genes nor determined their function or uses. In 1999, the PTO developed guidelines on how to deal with these fragments; it stated that more usefulness – specifically how the product functions in nature – must now be shown before gene fragments are considered patentable. The patenting of such DNA fragments presents the issue of whether an inventor trying to patent a larger fragment or the entire gene that contains the already partial-patented sequence will need to obtain a license from the first or whether the inventor can obtain the patent without the first patent holder's permission.

The Federal Circuit's 2005 *In re Fisher* ruling may not be the last word on the subject, but it rejected the patenting of gene fragments (ESTs, expressed sequence tags) when the gene from which the fragment came and the encoded protein were unknown. The court held that the ESTs had no specific and substantial utility and thus failed to satisfy 35 U.S.C. §101.

European Stance

In contrast to the US court ruling, English courts allowed Amgen to claim all the variant sequences that could encode an erythropoietin molecule. Although there are millions of such variant sequences, the court held that given the level of skill in molecular biology at the time, it was possible to perform the invention with *routine* methods (thus, the patent disclosures were adequate because one skilled in the art can practice the invention with only *routine* experimentation). The decision was affirmed on appeal.

In the 1995 Relaxin/Howard Florey Research Institute case, the EPO's Opposition

Division approved the grant of a patent for a DNA sequence encoding a protein produced by pregnant women (European Patent No. 0112149 B1). The European Parliament's Green Party opposed the issuing of the patent for relaxin on the grounds that the DNA sequence claimed was a discovery, not an invention, and that the issuing of a patent for a human gene offended *ordre public*. The Opposition Division held that "if a substance found in nature has first to be isolated from its surroundings and a process for obtaining it is developed, that process is patentable" and that the substance itself may be patentable if it "can be properly characterized by its structure and it is new in the absolute sense of having no previously recognized existence." Thus, the Opposition Division dismissed the argument that the invention claimed was a mere discovery on the grounds that such an argument is incompatible with long-standing EPO practice in respect to the patentability of other natural substances as set out in the guidelines. On the question of morality, the Opposition Division rejected all arguments submitted and noted that exceptions to the grant of patents for inventions because they were "immoral" should occur only "in those very limited cases in which there appears to be an overwhelming consensus that the exploitation or publication of an invention would be immoral."

Contrasting Laws for Generic Drugs

Hatch-Waxman Act

Before the Drug Price Competition and Patent Term Restoration Act of 1984 in the United States (also known as the Hatch-Waxman Act after its congressional sponsors), the FDA regarded safety and efficacy data generated by the innovator company as trade secrets that could neither be disclosed nor used by any other company to obtain approval of a generic product. Generics companies were required to file new drug applications (NDAs) with the Food and Drug Administration (FDA), but because of the huge expense and the limited profits available to a generic drug company, very few did. In conceiving the act, Congress intended to make available more low-cost generic drugs through a simplified abbreviated NDA (ANDA) procedure and to provide incentives to pharmaceutical companies for increased R&D by granting patent-term extensions and guaranteeing periods of marketing exclusivity for new products.

Following the implementation of the act, generics companies received a new, expeditious route to approval for their products. Under the act's ANDA provisions, after the appropriate data-exclusivity period, generic drug makers can rely on the safety and efficacy studies performed by the innovator of the drug and do not have to repeat them; they are required to provide only bioequivalence data.

The Hatch-Waxman Act limited the term of exclusivity for data submitted in support of the approval of a new chemical entity to five years and three years for other data, after which a generics company can use the safety and efficacy data to seek approval for its product. In most cases, these five- and three-year data-exclusivity periods have proven to be of relatively little value when compared with patents because they run concurrently with the patents and typically expire long before the patent does.

If the innovator company has relevant patents, the generic applicant must either wait for those patents to expire or provide notice to the patent holder. The patent holder can then sue the generics company, forcing it to prove invalidity or noninfringement of its patents or to keep its product off the market until the patents expire.

The Hatch-Waxman Act also provides a mechanism for challenging patents, initiated by filing an ANDA containing a certification of noninfringement or patent invalidity. NDA filings now include patent information, which the FDA publishes in the so-called *Orange Book*. The filer is required to submit a list of those patents that cover the drug product (formulation, composition, or method of use of the drug). Each ANDA must contain a certification relating to any patents that are listed in the *Orange Book* for the pioneer drug. Once an ANDA is filed containing such a challenge (a paragraph IV certification) and it is accepted by the FDA, the applicant must notify the patent holder and NDA holder, providing "the factual and legal basis" for its claim of invalidity or non-infringement. The patent owner/NDA holder then has 45 days to initiate infringement litigation or the ANDA may be approved as soon as FDA review is satisfactorily completed. If the innovator sues, forcing the generics company to prove noninfringement or patent invalidity, the ANDA may not be approved until the suit is resolved or 30 months has elapsed, whichever is shorter. The 30-month stay provides time for the patent infringement litigation, ideally without delaying the approval of the ANDA, review of which continues during the litigation.

Bolar Amendment

The 1984 case of *Roche v. Bolar* was overruled by a provision in the Hatch-Waxman legislation, commonly referred to as the "Bolar amendment" (35 U.S.C. §271[e]). Roche had sued Bolar for infringement of its flurazepam hydrochloride patent after Bolar had used a small amount of the drug for studies necessary for a "paper" NDA to the FDA before the relevant patent expired.

Under the Federal Circuit's *Bolar* ruling, the generics company could not obtain FDA approval immediately upon the expiration of the innovator's patent(s) because the company could not begin the required bioequivalency testing of the generic product until the patent expired. Consequently, the company had to wait typically three to five years after patent expiry for FDA approval before it could sell its generic drug. Thus, the innovator gained an informal, competition-free extension of its expired patent for this period.

The so-called Bolar amendment overruled the court decision, enabling generics companies to do work toward their regulatory submission on a drug before the expiry of the innovator company's patent(s). In return, the 1984 act gave innovator pharmaceutical companies patent- term extensions to compensate for the time "lost" during the FDA's regulatory review, which reduces their effective patent life. The scope of the Bolar amendment and its implications for drug company R&D efforts have been the focus of much recent discussion.

The Federal Circuit held in *Integra Lifesciences v. Merck* that the Bolar amendment requirement "solely for uses reasonably related to the development and submission" of information to the FDA for approval of a new drug "does not globally embrace all experimental activity that at some point, however attenuated, may lead to an FDA approval process." The court held that Merck KgaA was not protected by the Bolar amendment when it used Integra's patented peptides as part of its search for new pharmaceutical compounds.

The US Supreme Court disagreed with this assessment. In 2005, it ruled unanimously that the Bolar amendment allows biomedical research using patented inventions "as long as there is a reasonable basis for believing" the studies would yield information that could be used to gain regulatory approval. The Supreme Court stated that the Bolar amendment "provides a wide berth for the use of patented drugs in activities related to the federal regulatory process . . . . Properly construed, [the statute] leaves adequate space for experimentation and failure on the road to regulatory approval."

Thus, it is now clear that the Bolar amendment does not apply *only* to generic drug companies conducting bioequivalency studies for an ANDA filing, as drug companies, generic and innovator alike, are exempt from US patent-infringement charges, to the extent that their work is related to the FDA regulatory process.

European Laws

Abridged marketing-authorization applications (MAAs) are the European equivalent of US ANDAs, but the generic situation differs in many important ways in Europe. Article 4.8 of the Council of the European Economic Community Directive 65/65 requires a drug's MAA to contain results of pharmacological, toxicological, and clinical studies, but Article 4.8.a.(iii) provides for an exception when an applicant can demonstrate that the product is "essentially similar to a product which has been authorized within the Community, in accordance with Community provisions in force, for not less than six years, and is marketed in the Member State for which the application is made." Unlike its US equivalent, the Hatch-Waxman Act, where approvals depend on patents – either the generics company has to wait for them to expire or has to prove noninfringement/invalidity – Article 4.8.a.(iii) is not connected to the patent status of the innovator product. In Europe, once a data-protection period has expired, regulatory agencies can approve abridged applications for products with valid, unexpired patents. It is then up to the patent holder to bring an action for infringement against the generics company. Table 8.3 provides details on the data-protection periods in the European Union.

Until recently, Europe had no Bolar-like provision allowing generics manufacturers to conduct tests necessary for regulatory approval before patent expiry, although several nations had adopted such measures, encouraging generics companies to do bioequivalency testing there to generate data for regulatory submissions. However, in 2004, Directive 2001/83/EC of the European Parliament and the Council of the European Union was amended, enabling generics companies throughout the European Union to use patented drugs for development and regulatory testing before the patent(s) expires.

Europe also has no official listing of products eligible for abridged applications and their associated patents that is equivalent to the United States' *Orange Book*. Indeed, generic applicants sometimes have difficulty identifying a reference product and may have to consult unofficial documents, such as European versions of the *Physicians' Desk Reference*.

European Biotechnology Directive

The following sources of European IP law are of particular relevance to biotechnology:

- The EPC, discussed previously.
- Directive 98/44/EC of the European Parliament and the Council of the European Union on the Legal Protection of Biotechnological Inventions.
- The national laws of the individual states (EU member states and/or EPC signatories).

Table 8.3 EU Data Protection Periods

Length of Data Protection Period	*Applicable Member States/Products Protected*
Ten years	Applies in all member states for products approved under the "centralized procedure," the approval process of Council Regulation (EEC) No. 2309/93 (see Table 8.1)
Ten years	Applies in all member states for products approved under the earlier "concentration procedure," the approval process of EEC Directive 87/22
Ten years	Applies for all other products in Belgium, France, Germany, Italy, the Netherlands, Sweden, and the United Kingdom
Six years	Applies for all other products in Austria, Denmark, Finland, Ireland, and Luxembourg
Six years	Applies for all other products in Greece, Spain, and Portugal, but this protection period will not be applied beyond the expiry of a patent protecting the original product

EEC = European Economic Community

Note: More than one data protection period may apply under Article 4.8.a(iii) of EEC Directive 65/65

Biotechnology IP in Europe has been continually undermined by the lack of harmony between these sources, the need for morality and *ordre public* assessments by the EPO, and the ability of European citizens to challenge a patent.

In an attempt to correct this situation, the European biotech directive of 1998 required EU member states to harmonize their laws, providing broad protection for biotechnology inventions involving biological materials, biotechnological processes, and products concerning genetic information. The directive also provided a legal right to patents on plants and animals, despite the EPO's prior interpretation of EPC Article 53 regarding plant and animal varieties, which stated that patents should not be granted in respect to "plant or animal varieties or essentially biological processes for the production of plants or animals." (This provision did not apply to microbiological processes or resulting products.)

The directive reaffirmed the long-standing view of the EPO (and the US PTO) that naturally occurring substances (e.g., proteins, DNA) can be patented *provided* they are isolated or purified. Because of the EPC's prohibition on patenting inventions whose exploitation is contrary to *ordre public* or morality, inventions in the following categories are not patentable:

- Processes for cloning human beings.
- Processes for modifying the germ line genetic identity of human beings.
- Uses of human embryos for industrial or commercial purposes.
- Some types of stem cells.
- Processes for modifying the genetic identity of animals that are likely to cause them suffering, without any substantial medical benefit to man or animal, and animals resulting from such processes.

The EPO incorporated the provisions of the directive into its Implementing Regulations in 1999.

Medical-Use Patents

Historically, the medical profession and the courts have been hostile to medical-process patents on the grounds that nobody should patent medical procedures that might prevent them from being used on a patient. Indeed, European law expressly prohibits the patenting of medical processes. Specifically, Article 52(4) of the EPC states that "methods for the treatment of the human or animal body by surgery or therapy and diagnostic methods practiced on the human or animal body shall not be regarded as inventions which are susceptible of industrial application." Europe is not alone in this view: approximately 80 countries do not allow medical method patents. Under the General Agreement on Tariffs and Trade and the North American Free Trade Agreement, member countries may exclude "diagnostic, therapeutic, and surgical methods for the treatment of humans or animals" from patentability.

In the United States, there had also been a general notion that medical and surgical procedures were not patentable as processes, but in 1954, in *Ex parte Scherer*, the US Patent Office Board of Appeals reversed its long-standing position. Focusing on the utility of a new method for injecting a medication with a pressure jet (Scherer's US Patent No. 2,704,543), the board held that "[t]here is nothing in the patent statute which categorically excludes [methods of treating the human body]." The ruling opened the door for medical-procedure patents. Nevertheless, US patents on medical and diagnostic procedures have rarely been enforced. Patents obtained by researchers and physicians on medical procedures are primarily used to claim credit and recognition. Although infringement of patents for devices or drugs can be readily detected by the presence of the infringing product, enforcement of patents for medical procedures is much more difficult; it requires locating and suing each infringer (i.e., the physician or surgeon) individually. The availability of medical insurance company and other databases of information regarding patients and the treatment they received may enable enforcement of such patents on a larger scale.

OUTLOOK

The pharmaceutical industry faces many – at least potential – legislative and regulatory challenges. Although fundamental aspects of biotech IP have been resolved, new issues lie ahead.

The recent introduction of a Bolar-like provision in Europe establishes a new regime, and nobody yet knows how that system will work. EU member states had 18 months beginning on April 30, 2004, to implement the change into their national law, bringing us to the present. The provision provides that conducting studies required for regulatory approval is not infringing activity. A near-term problem will likely arise from the arguably general or, less generously, vague wording of the clause. Is it as broad as the US Supreme Court recently ruled that the US provision is? Or does it apply *only* to generic drug companies conducting bioequivalency testing? Its scope will likely have to be defined in the courts.

The Community Patent and Community Patent Court may yet come to pass; of course, a follow-up issue is whether anyone will care. Clearly, for the Community Patent and Community Patent Court to be successful, inventors will have to choose to file Community Patents and to litigate in the Community Patent Court. Whether inventors and patent owners will make this choice or continue to file European patents will probably be determined by their view of validation costs, renewal fees, and the effectiveness of patent enforcement via the Community Patent Court. Validation costs involve the costs of translating the claims of a Community Patent into the official languages of *all* EU member states. Will it be worth translating a Community Patent in every state versus filing a European patent and paying only for translations in designated states of interest? Renewal costs or maintenance fees for an issued Community Patent are another issue. Again, will it be worth paying the Community Patent fees versus obtaining a European patent, converting it to national patents in countries of interest, and then being able to *selectively* allow them to lapse, by not paying fees, in nations where it no longer makes economic sense?

It is obviously difficult to assess in advance the effectiveness of enforcement under a new regime in a new court. The present system of litigating country by country is hardly ideal, as the Epilady cases well illustrate. The proposed system gives exclusive jurisdiction over the determination of infringement and validity of Community Patents and the relief to be granted to the European Court of Justice (ECJ).

The Community Patent Court is to be established within the ECJ to hear trials. The new court will apply substantive law relating to infringement and validity as set out in the commission's proposed regulation on the Community Patent. So far, the judges have not been chosen and the rules of procedure have not been written. Obviously, it will take time for inventors and applicants to see how the Community Patent Court operates.

Another issue of industry and political concern is that of biogenerics or follow-on proteins. Patents on many of the biologics developed by the early biotechnology industry during the 1980s (e.g., growth hormone, insulin, erythropoietin) have already expired or will expire soon. These expiries potentially open a huge new market to generic competition and reduced prices for these products. On both sides of the Atlantic, regulatory agencies are scrambling to cope with this eventuality.

Recombinant biologics barely existed in 1984 when the Hatch-Waxman Act was written, and they were not included in its provisions. Under the current US law, there cannot be a generic biologic. A full clinical program is necessary for approval, and such a product would not be substitutable for the existing product, absent further clinical studies establishing bioequivalence.

Europe is somewhat further along and has established a legal framework for "biosimilar" drug applications and guidelines. There is a genuine technical issue here, not just protectionism by the brand industry. In contrast to chemically synthesized drugs, it *is* difficult to develop quality standards for biologics. Consequently, determining bioequivalence is problematic. Seemingly minor changes in a biologic production process can significantly affect a product's safety and efficacy.

Various proposals are under review in the current (2005) session of Congress to move away from the first-to-invent system of awarding patents and to add an EPO-like post-grant opposition procedure to US patent law. The changes are supposed to make the process of obtaining a US patent less expensive and less prone to litigation. It remains to be seen which, if any, of the various proposals will make it into legislation and whether the proposal will be enacted. Discussions are also continuing about patent quality, patent pendency, and funding for the PTO, which has a backlog of unexamined applications and an inadequate number of examiners.

In short, the biotechnology and pharmaceutical industries as well as their lawyers in both Europe and the United States will be busy arguing for and against patentability for many years to come.

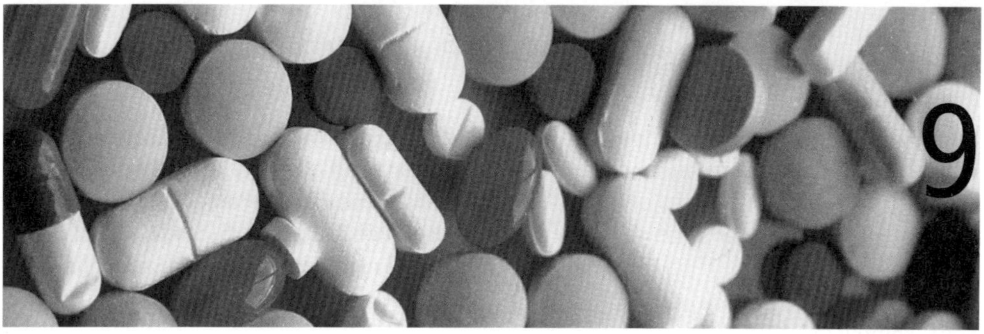

9

The Changing Face of European Drug Registration

INTRODUCTION

Until the mid-1990s, drug registration in Europe was the prerogative of regulatory authorities in each country. On January 1, 1995, however, the countries of the European Economic Area (EEA) (the member states of the European Union [EU] plus Iceland, Liechtenstein, and Norway) inaugurated the European Agency for the Evaluation of Medicinal Products (commonly known as the European Medicines Evaluation Agency [EMEA]). The European Commission states that the EMEA is charged with "pooling the scientific expertise of member states in order to ensure a high degree of protection for public health, ensuring free movement of pharmaceuticals, and making certain that Europeans have access to new generations of medicinal products." The creation of the EMEA was arguably the first significant milestone on the long road to a single European market for pharmaceuticals.

After almost a decade of activity, the EMEA has transformed the drug registration process in Europe, and this evolution will continue in the coming years. On March 31, 2004, the European Parliament enacted the EU Pharmaceutical Review, a package of radical reforms of the legal framework for the supply of medicines in the EU. Beginning November 2005, this legislation will introduce extensive changes to the drug registration system in Europe.

We begin this chapter with a brief overview of drug-licensing procedures in the EEA and a discussion of key findings from the EMEA audit survey of 2000. We then consider the EMEA's recent performance and changes resulting from the EU Pharmaceutical Review. We conclude with an assessment of the outlook and implications for the pharmaceutical industry.

OVERVIEW

National Procedures

In the EEA, national regulatory agencies are important because an applicant must approach at least one such agency for authorization to market a drug anywhere in the EEA, unless the centralized procedure (CP) is used. Until 1998, companies could apply for multiple national approvals. Currently, a product approved in one member state may be sold only in that country, unless that country is to be used as the reference member state (RMS) in the mutual recognition procedure (MRP). All marketing authorization applications that are subject to any regulatory procedure in the EEA are harmonized so that the same format is used, as described in the "Notice to Applicants" (the official guidelines for marketing authorization applications). The approved marketing authorization application is valid for five years and then must be renewed. Companies use the national procedure extensively for generic and OTC products that will be marketed in only one member state.

Centralized Procedure

The CP came into operation in 1995 and is now compulsory for medicinal products derived from a biotechnological process (known as "Part A products"). For other innovative products and products with a new active substance (known as "Part B products"), a company can currently choose to register the product using either the CP or the mutual recognition procedure. Since July 1, 2003, all new CP marketing authorization applications must use the common technical document (CTD) developed by the International Conference on Harmonisation of Technical Requirements for Registration of Pharmaceuticals for Human Use (ICH).

Table 9.1 Illustrative Timetable for the Centralized Procedure

Timeline	*Steps*
Day −180 to day −120	*Notification of intention to submit an application* Applicant notifies EMEA of its intention to apply to register a drug through the centralized procedure
Day −120 to day −90	*Selection of rapporteur, corapporteur, and European experts* CHMP selects a rapporteur and corapporteur for the application
Day −90 to day −1	Rapporteur and corapporteur select European experts to provide scientific advice and then notify the applicant of their choices
Day −15	*Submission of application: 15 days* Applicant submits dossier to EMEA
Day −10	EMEA validates the submission
Day 1	*Preliminary review of dossier: 120 days* Rapporteur and corapporteur begin to review the dossier
Day 70	Rapporteur and corapporteur submit assessment report to CHMP and EMEA
Day 120	CHMP sends a list of questions to the applicant
	Stopclock: 6 months Applicant responds to CHMP's questions
Day 121	*European step: 90 days* Rapporteur and corapporteur review applicant's responses to its questions
Day 150	Rapporteur and corapporteur publish joint response assessment report
Day 170	Deadline for comments from CHMP members
Day 180	CHMP decides whether an oral explanation from the applicant is necessary. If so, the clock stops, usually for up to 30 days, but exceptionally for 60–90 days
Day 181 to day 210	Applicant submits final draft of English SmPC, labeling, and package leaflet
Day 210	CHMP adopts opinion and assessment report
Day 270	*Translation: 60 days* Translation of product information from English into all official EU languages, Norwegian, and Icelandic
Day 300	*European Commission decision: 30 days* European Commission decides whether to approve the application
Day 330	*Issuance of national marketing authorizations: 30 days* Each national regulatory authority issues its own marketing authorization

CHMP = Committee for Medicinal Products for Human Use; EMEA = European Medicines Agency; SmPC = Summary of product characteristics

Table 9.1 presents an illustrative timetable for the CP. Applicants can nominate the member states they would ideally like to serve as their rapporteur and corapporteur (i.e., the states that will review the application on behalf of all member states), but they cannot be certain that their choices will be granted. The rapporteur generally uses the expertise available within its own national regulatory agency in preparing the assessment report, a document that is subsequently distributed to all members of the EMEA's Committee for Medicinal Products for Human Use (CHMP, formerly the Committee for Proprietary Medicinal Products [CPMP]). The CHMP has a maximum of 210 days to review the dossier, reach a final decision, and draft its assessment report. This timetable may be interrupted and the review time clock stopped to give the company the opportunity to answer questions prior to drafting the assessment report. Companies are sometimes allowed to provide an oral explanation of the submitted data at a hearing, in which case the review time clock stops again.

The entire CP review process – including translations, finalization of the assessment report, European Commission opinion, and finalization of the European public assessment report (a version of the assessment report that has all commercially confidential information removed) – should be completed within 300 days. The final opinion of the CHMP is sent to the European Commission, the member states, and the applicant. If the opinion is positive, these three groups also receive the finalized summary of product characteristics (SmPC), labeling, and patient package leaflet in all EEA official languages.

The European Commission has 30 days to draft a decision but usually accepts the opinion of the CHMP in its entirety. The decision is circulated to member states, which are given 30 days in which to submit objections. If any such objections are new scientific issues, the Commission refers the application back to the CHMP for reconsideration within 60 days. The Standing Committee on Medicinal Products for Human Use (with representatives from each member state) assists the Commission in the decision-making process. Nonscientific issues are also referred to this committee. If no objections are raised, the Commission either approves or rejects the MA. Details of new marketing authorizations issued are published in the EU's *Official Journal*.

Mutual Recognition Procedure

The mutual recognition procedure (MRP; often also called the decentralized procedure [DP]) consists of several steps designed to acquire identical nationally based marketing authorization approvals in the applicant-selected member states. The first member state the applicant designates to carry out the investigative work is called the RMS.

Since July 1, 2003, all new dossiers submitted to RMSs under the mutual recognition procedure must use the ICH's common technical document. From January 1, 2005, the CTD will also become mandatory for dossiers submitted to concerned member states (CMSs).

The mutual recognition procedure's evaluation parameters are similar to those of the CP (i.e., evaluation and approval based on efficacy, quality, and safety). Table 9.2 presents an illustrative timetable for the mutual recognition procedure. The RMS is the first EEA country to approve the medicinal product and submit its assessment report to other member states that the applicant selects for identical approval. These countries, known as CMSs, are given 90 days to approve or reject the RMS's decision. A CMS may oppose the authorization only on the grounds of a risk to public health.

The applicant needs to select an RMS with which it can work harmoniously and which will submit a robust assessment report and negotiate effectively with CMS rapporteurs. When using this approval procedure, the RMS rapporteur is the applicant's expert for the medicinal product.

If the countries cannot agree, the EMEA and the CHMP are responsible for deciding the matter by arbitration. The RMS rapporteur

Table 9.2 Illustrative Timetable for the Mutual Recognition Procedure

Timeline	*Steps*
	Submission of application to RMS Applicant submits dossier to RMS
	Review of dossier: 210 days RMS sends its assessment report to applicant
	Issuance of marketing authorization in RMS: 30 days RMS issues a marketing authorization
	Update of final assessment report: 90 days RMS updates its final assessment report and produces an SmPC in English
	Submission of application to CMSs Applicant requests mutual recognition of marketing authorization issued by RMS Applicant submits application to CMSs and guarantees that dossier is identical to the one approved by the RMS CHMP is notified of this submission RMS distributes its assessment report to all CMSs
Day −15	*Validation of the application: 10 days* Regulatory agencies in CMSs validate the application
Day −5	*Confirmation of validity of application* Regulatory agencies in CMSs confirm that the application is valid
Day 1	*Mutual recognition procedure: 90 days* CMSs begin to review RMS's assessment report
Day 50	RMS forwards CMSs' comments to applicant
Day 60	Applicant sends its responses to RMS and all CMSs
Day 75	If necessary, MRFG holds a breakout session to discuss CMSs' concerns and questions. Applicant may be invited to attend this meeting
Day 76 to day 85	If necessary, MRFG coordinates further discussions among CMSs. Applicant suggests SmPC amendments to RMS and CMSs
Day 85	RMS notifies applicant of CMSs' final position Applicant submits revised SmPC to RMS and CMSs
Day 90	MRP is completed
Day 91 to day 120	*Issuance of national marketing authorizations: 30 days* CMSs issue national marketing authorizations

CHMP = Committee for Medicinal Products for Human Use; CMS = Concerned member state; MRFG = Mutual Recognition Facilitation Group; MRP = Mutual recognition procedure; RMS = Reference member state; SmPC = Summary of product characteristics

and corapporteurs from the CMSs prepare a consolidated statement of issues. Then they forward this statement, along with all assessment reports, summaries of product characteristics, and labeling, to the EMEA with a full copy of the dossier the applicant submitted. The CHMP nominates experts to consider the objections and make a decision within 90 days. The CHMP decision is binding on all member states concerned, including the RMS.

EMEA AUDIT SURVEY

Regulation EEC 2309/93 – the act that paved the way for the establishment of the EMEA – mandated a review of that agency's activity within six years of its inception. Cameron McKenna and Andersen Consulting were commissioned to audit the EMEA's procedures and operations. The report of this survey – *Evaluation of Community Procedures for the Authorisation of Medicinal Products* – was published in October 2000. It was based on interviews with and/or questionnaire responses from trade associations, national drug registration authorities, professional and patient associations, national ministries with an interest in drug approval, and pharmaceutical companies. The audit report contained the following summary of survey responses:

> The centralised and decentralised procedures are both perceived to have contributed . . . to the creation of a harmonised Community market in medicinal products. There is criticism of particular aspects of both systems and in the case of the decentralised system, a level of real concern about the willingness of regulatory authorities to operate the central principle of mutual recognition. However, in general, the rationale underlying both the centralised and decentralised procedures is viewed as sound and such that, provided there is the necessary political will, the two systems provide a strong foundation for future progress to a harmonised and efficient regulatory environment. Because of their different attributes, there is a strong desire on the part of both applicants for marketing authorisations and the competent regulatory authorities to maintain the parallel systems.

The survey examined many aspects of both the centralized and mutual recognition procedures. The auditors did not limit their research to the EMEA's activities, but they also investigated member states' responses to EMEA decisions. In this review, we focus on the perceived performance of the European drug registration system.

Centralized Procedure

The audit survey examined the level of satisfaction with the CP. Of the 32 companies that had obtained marketing authorizations by this route, 28 (88%) were satisfied with the system and 1 (3%) was very satisfied. Member states' regulatory authorities were even more enthusiastic about the CP: 11 (73%) were satisfied and 3 (20%) were very satisfied with its operation.

Companies had many reasons for using the CP to register new drugs. Respondents were asked to rate the importance of several factors on a scale of 1–9, where 1 denoted the greatest importance and 9 the least. Table 9.3 shows the mean scores for each of these factors plus other (unspecified) factors. These scores do not take account of the fact that some respondents did not express an opinion on certain factors. With the exception of "other factors" (cited by seven respondents), the most important reason for using the centralized therapies was that the therapies in question were Part A products (with a mean score of 1.85). Access and speed of access to the entire EU market were also judged very important. On the other hand, the cost of the CP relative to the mutual recognition procedure was unimportant.

Despite the generally high degree of satisfaction with the CP, many companies considered the number of application withdrawals and rejections that occur to be a problem. The audit survey found that 46% of companies regarded the number of withdrawals as a significant problem and 29% a minor problem. Manufacturers expressed particular concern

Table 9.3 Manufacturers' Most Important Reasons for Using the Centralized Procedure

	Number of Respondents[a]	*Mean Score*[b]
Other factors	7	1.43
Part A product	13	1.85
Speed of access to entire EU market	21	2.33
Access to entire EU market	21	2.62
Single procedure	23	3.00
Quality of scientific assessment	16	4.25
Ten years' protection against abridged applications	20	4.25
Only one authorization to maintain	20	4.65
Gaining experience of centralized procedure	12	6.25
Cost relative to mutual recognition procedure	10	7.90

[a]Number of respondents that expressed an opinion on each factor
[b]Ranking scale runs from 1 (greatest importance) to 9 (least importance). Scores do not take account of respondents who did not express an opinion on a given factor

about withdrawals of drugs that had already been approved in the United States on the basis of the same data. Thirty-two percent of the participating companies had withdrawn at least one application from the CP, including 16% that had withdrawn their last application. Companies indicated that they withdrew applications because data were deemed incomplete, proof of efficacy was judged inadequate, or trial design was criticized. Among companies that had withdrawn a CP application, 82% did not resubmit it. However, the small size of this sample suggests that caution is advisable in drawing conclusions from this last result. Furthermore, although only one participating company had ever had a CP application rejected, 25% considered the general level of rejections to be a significant problem, and 39% considered it a minor problem.

Interestingly, regulatory authorities did not generally share manufacturers' concerns about withdrawals and rejections from the CP. Only 7% regarded the level of withdrawals as a significant problem, and 40% considered it a minor problem. They identified concerns about safety and efficacy as the two main reasons for withdrawals. None of the regulatory authorities considered the level of rejections a significant problem, and only 11% viewed it as a minor problem. These figures suggest that regulatory authorities are either unaware of or unsympathetic toward manufacturers' concerns about CP application withdrawals and rejections.

Mutual Recognition Procedure

Pharmaceutical companies cited three main reasons for using the mutual recognition procedure. By far the most common was the fact that the product in question was not eligible for the CP: 51% gave this factor as the most important reason. Speed of launch and flexible access to the EU market (i.e., the freedom to launch the product only in selected member states) were both cited by 9% of companies as the main reason for choosing the mutual recognition procedure and by 13% as the second most important reason for following this route.

Interestingly, among the 51% of respondents who indicated that their ineligibility for the CP was the main reason for using the mutual recognition procedure, opinion was evenly divided on whether they would have chosen the mutual recognition procedure even if the CP had been accessible to them. Respondents who would have chosen the CP if available gave the following reasons for their preference: the advantages of dealing with a single agency and receiving a single marketing authorization, superior scientific assessment, better data protection, greater speed and efficiency of the process, access to the entire EU market, and the fact that national regulatory authorities could not obstruct authorizations for political motives. Companies that would still have used the mutual recognition procedure said that they would have done so because of its greater flexibility (particularly for commercial arrangements), the freedom to choose the RMSs and to establish an early dialog with regulators, and the fact that not all EU markets were of interest to them.

The United Kingdom was the overwhelming favorite choice for RMS – selected by 40% of participating companies. Sweden, Denmark, and the Netherlands were also popular – chosen by 12%, 10%, and 10% of companies, respectively. The choice of RMS was influenced by the following factors: reputation for efficiency (29%), location (27%), reputation for scientific expertise (26%), and previous favorable experience with the regulatory authority (23%).

Pharmaceutical manufacturers were generally much less satisfied with the mutual recognition procedure than the CP. The audit survey found that 2% were very satisfied and 42% were satisfied, but 48% were dissatisfied and 8% were very dissatisfied. In contrast, regulatory authorities had a much higher opinion of this system: 80% were satisfied and only 20% were dissatisfied.

One reason for pharmaceutical companies' dissatisfaction with the mutual recognition procedure is the number of changes to the SmPC that the process requires them to make. The audit survey found that 94% of the applicants had been forced to alter their SmPCs. Some companies reported that they had to make extensive changes to almost every section of their SmPCs. One respondent suggested that the result was a document that represented "the lowest common denominator." Common changes included deleting indications, adding contraindications and warnings, and altering dosage regimens.

These changes are necessary because CMSs are often reluctant to compromise. The audit report contained the following criticisms of the limitations of the mutual recognition procedure:

> The core impediment to the efficient performance of the decentralised system appears to be that there is no real pressure nationally to converge and many member states pay scant regard to the basic principle of recognition. Rather than encourage harmonisation and efficient use of regulatory resources, one regulator stated that the system "entrenched disharmony" and wasted resources. Consistent with this, over a third of authorities reported that they frequently or always analyse the whole dossier, rather than rely upon the reference member state's assessment and judgment. Over 50% of the authorities reported carrying out a full assessment of significant parts of the dossier.

Pharmaceutical companies also complained that CMSs frequently abused the safeguard of concerns over risk to public health (the only basis for opposing the RMS's recommendation of approval). Manufacturers suggested that national authorities sometimes invoked public health concerns for reasons of national interest – for example, to force an applicant to "vertically harmonize" its product with existing local products or with a view to negotiating pricing terms more favorable to payers. In the audit survey, several regulatory authorities acknowledged that their objections often related less to serious public health issues than to national preferences. Indeed, one authority admitted that it liked the vagueness of the definition of "risk to public health" precisely because the imprecision enabled the authority to raise a variety of objections.

However, manufacturers – and even some regulatory authorities – would welcome a clearer definition of "risk to public health." The audit survey found that 24% of the MRP authorization holders agreed and 71% strongly agreed with the need for a better definition of this concept. Similarly, 32% of the CP authorization holders agreed and 68% strongly agreed that it should be more clearly defined. Manufacturers generally believed that CMSs should be required to provide a detailed and substantiated explanation of their objections to an application.

Pharmaceutical companies also expressed the view that, pending the outcome of arbitration initiated by a CMS, manufacturers should be permitted to market the drug in question in the RMS and in states that have no objection to the marketing authorization. Among the 50 MRP authorization holders that responded, 30% agreed and 66% strongly agreed with this idea. Likewise, among the 22 CP authorization holders that answered this question, 50% agreed and 46% strongly agreed with this suggestion. Not surprisingly, regulatory authorities were less enthusiastic about this idea: two (14%) strongly agreed with it and seven (50%) agreed, but four (29%) disagreed and one (7%) strongly disagreed.

Participating companies that had faced the prospect of MRP arbitration had invariably decided instead to withdraw their application in the CMS that opposed the authorization. The most common reason for this decision, as cited by 44% of respondents, was that the arbitration procedure would delay product launch in other member states. A further 13% indicated that the CMSs that objected were not major markets for them, and 11% intended to resubmit their application with additional data. Concern that the arbitration procedure might have a negative effect on a company's existing marketing authorizations was another reason for withdrawing an application in an opposing CMS.

Data Protection and Generics Competition

Pharmaceutical companies were generally pleased with the standard of data protection in the CP: 84% of the CP marketing authorization holders and 79% of the MRP marketing authorization holders considered the level of protection to be either satisfactory or very satisfactory. However, manufacturers were much less content with the mutual recognition procedure's data protection: no MRP authorization holders regarded this system's level of protection as very satisfactory, and only 37% judged it to be satisfactory, compared with 34% who considered it unsatisfactory and 10% very unsatisfactory. The CP authorization holders were even more critical of the mutual recognition procedure's data protection: none viewed it as very satisfactory, only 10% considered it satisfactory, while 40% dismissed it as unsatisfactory and 47% as very unsatisfactory.

The survey asked respondents if drug originators should be granted an additional period of marketing exclusivity as a reward for enhancing their products. Overall, 69% of manufacturers agreed and 23% disagreed. However, originator companies and generics manufacturers had contrasting views on this question: 50% of generics companies disagreed with extended marketing exclusivity, whereas originator companies unanimously supported this idea. Regulatory authorities were much less supportive of this idea, and only 41% expressed agreement. Among companies that favored extended marketing exclusivity, 92% believed that such a provision should cover new indications, 73% new methods of delivery, 60% new dosage forms, and 40% new dose or dosage schedules.

The principle of a uniform data protection period throughout the EU commanded wide support: all originator companies, 93% of regulatory authorities, and 86% of generics manufacturers agreed with this idea. However, opinions on the appropriate length of this period ranged from 1 year to 15 years. Overall, 79% of respondents (though only 56% of generics manufacturers) believed that the data protection period should be harmonized at 10 years.

Originator companies and generics manufacturers were sharply divided on the question of whether the EU should follow the example of countries such as the United States and Canada by introducing a Bolar provision to allow the development in the EU of generic versions of a drug before its patent expires. While 83% of generics manufacturers agreed with this idea, only 20% of originators were in favor of such a reform. Generics companies noted that they can already submit applications before a patent expires, but a Bolar provision would allow them to begin development, testing, and experimental work on their drugs in the EU while patent protection is still in force. Regulatory authorities had mixed views on this subject: some believed that a Bolar provision would stimulate increased competition, reduce the price of generics, and encourage testing in the EU, but others cautioned that the law must afford drug originators adequate data protection.

RECENT PERFORMANCE OF THE EMEA

In April 2004, the EMEA published a review of its performance. The report examined several broad areas, including review times, failure rates for applications, major objections to applications, and the influence of EMEA scientific advice on an application's prospects for success.

Review Times

Overall, the average time taken to review a marketing authorization application through the CP has remained relatively stable since the agency's inception. However, the average review time for Part B products has fluctuated significantly, rising from 229 days in 1995 to a peak of 391 days in 1999, but then declining to 302 days in 2002. Table 9.4 shows average review times overall and for Part A and Part B products. In its first eight years, the EMEA registered a total of 79 Part A products and 110 Part B products through the CP, a mean of 9.9 Part A products and 13.8 products per year. Over the eight-year period, total review times averaged 332 days

Table 9.4 Average Review Times for Drugs Licensed Through the EMEA's Centralized Procedure, 1995–2002

	Number of Marketing Authorizations Issued		*Average Total Review Time (Days)*			*Division of Average Total Review Time (Days)*	
	Part A Products	*Part B Products*	*Part A Products*	*Part B Products*	*All Products*	*Active Time*	*Stop Clock*
1995	8	6	373	229	311	181	131
1996	6	14	363	255	288	165	122
1997	13	19	372	282	319	185	134
1998	7	19	352	382	374	188	186
1999	16	12	338	391	361	178	183
2000	10	16	335	327	330	183	147
2001	16	15	373	321	348	182	166
2002	3	9	395	302	325	177	148
Annual mean	10	14	363	311	332	180	152

Notes: All data relate to the years in which marketing authorization applications (MAAs) were submitted. Reviews of some MAAs were not completed in the calendar year in which they were started

MAAs submitted before January 1, 2003, but not completed until after October 31, 2003 (the cutoff date for the EMEA study), may subsequently alter some results, particularly for 2002

Table 9.5 Outcomes of Centralized Procedure Applications, January 1995–October 2003

	Applications	*Percentage*
Positive by consensus	181	63.7
Positive by majority	25	8.8
Positive after appeal	3	1.1
Withdrawn prior to opinion	69	24.3
Withdrawn after appeal	2	0.7
Negative after appeal	3	1.1
Negative by majority	1	0.4
Total	284	100.0

Source: Based on data from the European Medicines Agency

(363 days for Part A products and 311 for Part B products). The mean active time spent on reviewing marketing authorization applications was 180 days, compared with a mean stopclock of 152 days.

The recent sharp increase in average review times for Part A products is a disturbing trend. The EMEA attributes this development to "the increased 'innovativeness' and hence complexity of [Part A] products." However, the EMEA also notes that review times for certain drugs in clinical priority areas (e.g., oncology, HIV/AIDS) are much shorter than average. For instance, imatinib (Novartis's Glivec) required no stopclock time and was approved after 119 days. New medicines that clearly satisfy unmet clinical needs are less likely to face objections and delaying tactics than drugs that are similar to existing products (i.e., "me-too" drugs) or that have questionable quality, safety, or efficacy.

Unsuccessful Applications

Since 1995, the percentage of unsuccessful CP applications (i.e., applications that were withdrawn or ultimately received negative opinions) has generally remained in the range of 25–30% per year. Table 9.5 shows that, from January 1995 to October 2003, 69 out of a total of 284 applications (24.3%) were withdrawn before an opinion was issued. The CHMP expressed a negative opinion in only nine cases (3.2%). According to the EMEA, issues related to the clinical development process often led to the rejection of an application. In particular, a lack of adequate randomized controlled clinical trials (RCTs) reduced the probability of a successful outcome by more than 50%.

On the other hand, 181 applications (63.7%) received a unanimously positive opinion, 25 applications (8.8%) were given a positive opinion by a majority of CHMP members, and 3 (1.1%) received a positive opinion on appeal. Forty applications (14.1%) were given an approval under exceptional circumstances. Therapies for metabolic

Table 9.6 Percentage of Centralized Procedure Applications That Encountered Major Objections, January 1998–October 2003

	1998 (n = 49)	*1999 (n = 32)*	*2000 (n = 45)*	*2001 (n = 36)*	*2002 (n = 36)*	*2003[a] (n = 25)*	*Mean*
Inadequate clinical efficacy	41	31	49	31	36	40	38
Dose regimen justification	39	53	40	22	28	32	36
Lack of adequate RCTs	35	53	31	39	17	32	35
Analysis/robustness of clinical data	45	34	33	36	28	20	33
Choice of end points	37	31	29	19	22	36	29
Pharmacokinetics/pharmacodynamics	16	16	24	17	8	16	16
Insufficient patient enrollment	18	6	7	17	8	0	9

[a]Data cover January–October 2003
RCTs = Randomized clinical trials

disorders, oncology drugs, immunomodulators, and anti-infectives were among the drug classes most likely to benefit from an approval under exceptional circumstances.

Major Objections

The EMEA reports that most CP applications are nonapprovable by the CHMP after the initial review. Table 9.6 shows that inadequate clinical efficacy, poor dose-regimen justification, and a lack of RCTs are the most common major objections. Problems with the analysis or robustness of clinical data and poor choice of end points were also frequently cited as major objections. The EMEA hopes that better communication between applicants and the CHMP will reduce the frequency of major objections related to study design issues (especially a lack of adequate RCTs).

CHANGES RESULTING FROM THE EU PHARMACEUTICAL REVIEW

The EU Pharmaceutical Review was first proposed in 2001 but underwent numerous revisions at the hands of the European Commission, the European Parliament, and the European Council of Ministers. The finalized legislative package, passed by the European Parliament on March 31, 2004, consists of one regulation (on the authorization of medicines) and two directives (one each on human and veterinary pharmaceuticals) that have different timetables for implementation. Title IV of the regulation, which governs the composition of the management board and committees of the European Medicines Agency (a new name for the European Agency for the Evaluation of Medicinal Products, but the acronym EMEA will be retained), took effect on May 20, 2004. In addition, the directives must be incorporated into the national law of each member state. The new legislation will impact many aspects of pharmaceutical registration, but we will focus primarily on changes to the drug registration process and data protection.

Terms and Conditions of Marketing Authorizations

In the past, marketing authorizations had to be renewed every five years. Under the new legislation, marketing authorizations will be renewed after a drug has been on the market for five years; the review will be based on an updated assessment of the product's risk–benefit balance. Thereafter, the marketing authorization should normally be of unlimited validity.

Manufacturers will be incentivized to market drugs for which they hold marketing authorizations. Products that are not marketed for three consecutive years will usually forfeit their marketing authorizations (a provision commonly known as the "sunset clause").

Centralized Procedure

The CP will remain mandatory for products developed by the following methods:

- Recombinant DNA technology.
- Controlled expression of genes coding for biologically active proteins in prokaryotes and eukaryotes including transformed mammalian cells.
- Hybridoma and monoclonal antibody methods.

The CP will also become mandatory for orphan drugs and all new medicines for AIDS, cancer, neurodegenerative disorders, and diabetes. Beginning May 20, 2008, the CP will also become mandatory for all new medicines for viral diseases, autoimmune diseases, and other immune dysfunctions. The CP will be extended, as an option, to nonprescription medicines that are judged to be of "community interest." Manufacturers of innovative nonprescription drugs will have to make a case for using the CP for the approval of their products.

The CP will also be an option for generic drugs if the respective originator drugs were registered using this procedure. If an originator drug was registered using the mutual recognition procedure or a national registration procedure, generics manufacturers will not be able to use the CP to register generic versions of the drug. "Biosimilar" products (i.e., generic versions of biologics) will be required to undergo approval by means of the CP.

Manufacturers will be able request a new accelerated assessment procedure for drugs that are of "major interest from the point of view of public health and in particular from the viewpoint of therapeutic innovation." Under this arrangement, the time-limit for the completion of CHMP's review would be reduced from the standard 210 days to 150 days.

Mutual Recognition Procedure and Decentralized Procedure

Although the term *decentralized procedure* (DP) is widely used as an unofficial synonym for the mutual recognition procedure, the new legislation introduces a formal distinction between these two procedures. If a manufacturer already has a license for a particular drug in one member state and wants to market it in other member states, the mutual recognition procedure is mandatory. However, if the drug is not yet on the market anywhere in the EU, the new DP may be an alternative: if the CP is not mandatory or the manufacturer decides not to use either the CP or the mutual recognition procedure, the DP can be used to license a new medicine in multiple member states. The new procedure should allow more time for discussion of the dossier, reduce the risk of arbitration, and expedite marketing authorization in many cases.

An applicant will choose an RMS and submit its dossier to that country and the CMSs simultaneously. The RMS will have 120 days in which to review the submission, circulate a preliminary assessment report, collate initial feedback from the CMSs, and send a consolidated list of questions to the applicant. A stopclock period will then begin, during which time the applicant will respond to the RMS's questions and the RMS will prepare and distribute a draft assessment report, SmPC, package leaflet, and label. Ninety days will then be allowed for the CMSs to review the application and submit questions that will be forwarded in a consolidated list to the applicant. By day 210 (counting from the start of the review process), the RMS and CMSs will either agree to approve the product or, if they cannot reach a consensus, refer the product to the newly established Coordination Group. If the product is approved, national regulatory authorities will have 30 days in which to issue a marketing authorization for their territories. In the event that the RMS and CMSs cannot reach agreement, the Coordination Group will have 60 days in which to try to resolve the impasse. If this exercise also fails to break the stalemate, details of the disputed matters will be forwarded to the EMEA for arbitration. Member states that accept the assessment report and SmPC may immediately authorize the product for sale in their territories.

The only legitimate grounds for a CMS to reject a favorable assessment of an application by the RMS will be the evidence that the product under review presents a "serious risk to public health." The European Commission, in collaboration with the Mutual Recognition Facilitation Group and the Veterinary Mutual Recognition Facilitation Group, has to define what constitutes a "serious risk to public health." This task is a matter of considerable importance. The use of the adjective "serious" suggests that the European Commission wants to discourage frivolous objections. As noted earlier, the EMEA audit survey found evidence to confirm manufacturers' suspicions that the national regulatory authorities sometimes misused the mutual recognition procedure's "risk to public health" provision to block marketing authorization applications that did not suit their national interests. The pharmaceutical industry is hoping that the DP will be less susceptible to such abuses.

Data Protection

Directive 2004/27/EC includes new rules on the data protection of medicinal products. The data protection period for all new products will be standardized at eight years, but manufacturers will enjoy a further two years of marketing exclusivity before they face generics competition. Generics manufacturers will be allowed to begin developing generic versions of a drug and to submit marketing authorization applications after the originator brand has had eight years of data protection. An additional year of marketing exclusivity will be available to companies that gain approval for a significant new indication for a drug within eight years of the issuance of the marketing authorization. This measure is commonly known as the "8 + 2 + 1" formula. The harmonized data protection period will not be applied retroactively to products that were approved in any of the existing or candidate member states before this legislation was implemented. The 10 accession countries that joined the EU on May 1, 2004 – Cyprus, the Czech Republic, Estonia, Hungary, Latvia, Lithuania, Malta, Poland, the Slovak Republic, Slovenia – will be able to seek a derogation from the "8 + 2 + 1" formula but will have to justify their request to the European Commission.

A "global marketing authorization," issued at the time of a new drug's first marketing authorization, will become the starting point for data protection. Product variations (e.g., new dosage forms, line extensions) will be subject to the original marketing authorization, thereby preventing manufacturers from using superficial changes to extend their data protection period.

Products that are switched from prescription to nonprescription status on the basis of significant preclinical and clinical studies will benefit from a year of data exclusivity (a reduction from the original proposal of two years).

Generics

Directive 2004/27/EC suggests that "since generics account for a major part of the market in medicinal products, their access in the Community should be facilitated in the light of experience acquired." To that end, the directive broadens the definition of generic drugs:

> "Generic medicinal product" shall mean a medicinal product which has the same qualitative and quantitative composition in active substances and the same pharmaceutical form as the reference medicinal product, and whose bioequivalence with the reference medicinal product has been demonstrated by appropriate bioavailability studies. The different salts, esters, ethers, isomers, mixtures of isomers, complexes or derivatives of an active substance shall be considered to be the same active substance, unless they differ significantly in properties with regard to safety and/or efficacy. In such cases, additional information providing proof of the safety and/or efficacy of the various salts, esters or derivatives of an authorised active

substance must be supplied by the applicant. The various immediate-release oral pharmaceutical forms shall be considered to be one and the same pharmaceutical form. Bioavailability studies need not be required of the applicant if he can demonstrate that the generic medicinal product meets the relevant criteria as defined in the appropriate detailed guidelines.

The introduction of "European reference products" will allow generics manufacturers to launch a generic version of a drug in a particular member state even if the originator brand is not currently registered in that country. The applicant will have to indicate where the reference product is or has been authorized, and the regulatory authorities in that member state will then have a month to confirm the marketing authorization and disclose the reference product's full composition.

The new data protection rules will likely expedite the launch of generics. Unless the manufacturer of the originator brand obtains approval for a new indication, generics companies should be able to launch competing products 10 years after the original drug receives its marketing authorization.

OUTLOOK AND IMPLICATIONS FOR THE PHARMACEUTICAL INDUSTRY

The research-based pharmaceutical industry can draw encouragement from the fact that the EU Pharmaceutical Review fulfilled several of the wishes expressed by drug manufacturers in the EMEA audit survey. For example, pharmaceutical companies that participated in the EMEA audit survey were generally in favor of a uniform period of data protection throughout the EEA and the granting of an additional period of marketing exclusivity to manufacturers that enhance their products. The new "8 + 2 + 1" formula standardizes the data protection period and offers an extra year of marketing exclusivity to companies that gain approval for a significant new indication for a drug. Manufacturers also indicated that, in situations where a CMS rejects a marketing authorization application, they would like to be able to launch the drug in question in the RMS and in CMSs that have no objection to the marketing authorization. The DP will give companies this freedom. In the EMEA audit survey, drug manufacturers expressed their frustration at the uncertain definition of "risk to public health" and the tendency of some regulatory agencies to misuse this provision to obstruct certain MRP applications. The adoption of "serious risk to public health" as the only ground for CMSs to reject a favorable assessment in the DP, and the commitment to provide a clear definition of this term, suggest that the European Commission recognizes the need to promote greater transparency and to combat abuses of the system by some national agencies.

The Pharmaceutical Review contains other measures that will expedite drug registration. The introduction of an accelerated assessment procedure will benefit manufacturers of drugs that are highly innovative or particularly important for public health. This innovation will give the pharmaceutical industry in Europe a procedure similar to the United States' fast-tracking system. The early involvement of CMSs in the DP should also help cut the number of objections raised and reduce the frequency of arbitration.

On the other hand, the Pharmaceutical Review contains some reforms that research-based manufacturers will not necessarily welcome. The Bolar-type provision will permit earlier development of generic versions of drugs. Originator companies will also find it harder than in the past to impede the launch of generics. The advent of European reference products will nullify the strategy of withdrawing a drug from a particular market as a way of forestalling generics competition. Global marketing authorizations for a compound will also make it more difficult to use new dosage forms and line extensions to extend a branded drug's marketing exclusivity, and a broader definition of generics (to include all salts, esters, ethers, isomers, mixtures of isomers, complexes, or derivatives of an active substance) will frustrate attempts to use product variations as a defense strategy.

The extension of mandatory use of the CP to include all new medicines for AIDS, cancer, neurodegenerative disorders, and diabetes, and, from May 2008, all new drugs for viral diseases, autoimmune diseases, and other immune dysfunctions will not be good news for manufacturers of these products. In many cases, companies would choose to register these drugs through the CP, but most would value the option of using the mutual recognition procedure or the DP.

Manufacturers may decide that they do not want to launch certain drugs in particular member states, but the requirement to use the CP could oblige companies to register these products throughout the EEA. Given the use of increasingly draconian price controls (e.g., the imposition of reference prices on patent-protected drugs), companies might be forced to accept a very low price in some European countries, a situation that could fuel parallel trade. On the other hand, manufacturers may face the risk that concerns about the potential cost of an expensive new therapy, which will prompt some member states to oppose the registration of such a drug.

The recent enlargement of the EU will also have significant implications for drug registration in Europe. On the positive side, approval of a drug through the CP will guarantee the manufacturer access to 28 countries. However, this benefit will depend on the regulatory agencies in every member state accepting the EMEA's recommendation to approve the drug. An objection from one or more member states could impede the registration process throughout the EEA, even though the manufacturer may not plan to market the drug in the countries that raise the objection. In addition, manufacturers using the CP may be assigned a rapporteur or corapporteur from an accession country that has limited experience of the EMEA's working practices. Furthermore, the need to translate documentation from English into nine new official EU languages (in addition to the languages of the 15 established EU member states, Norway, and Iceland) will increase manufacturers' costs and administrative burden.

Table 9.7 Preferred Reference Member States for Mutual Recognition Procedure

Member State	*Number of Times Chosen as RMS*
Denmark	1,097
United Kingdom	987
Netherlands	761
Sweden	699
Germany	531
Finland	424
France	250
Ireland	191
Austria	73
Spain	45
Italy	23
Norway	21
Belgium	13
Portugal	6

RMS = Reference member state

EU enlargement may also complicate and prolong the mutual recognition procedure. Manufacturers will have a wider choice of potential RMSs, but experience suggests that most will choose the regulatory authorities that have earned a reputation for speed and efficiency. Table 9.7 shows that Denmark, the United Kingdom, the Netherlands, Sweden, and Germany are the preferred RMSs. In contrast, southern European countries (e.g., Greece, Portugal, Italy, Spain) are rarely chosen as RMSs. Accession countries may also be overlooked as potential RMSs, at least until they demonstrate their ability to compete with the current favorites.

Further changes to Europe's drug registration system can be expected in the years ahead. Whatever reforms are introduced, it is very likely that factors beyond a drug's quality, safety, and efficacy will play an increasingly influential role in decision making in the future.

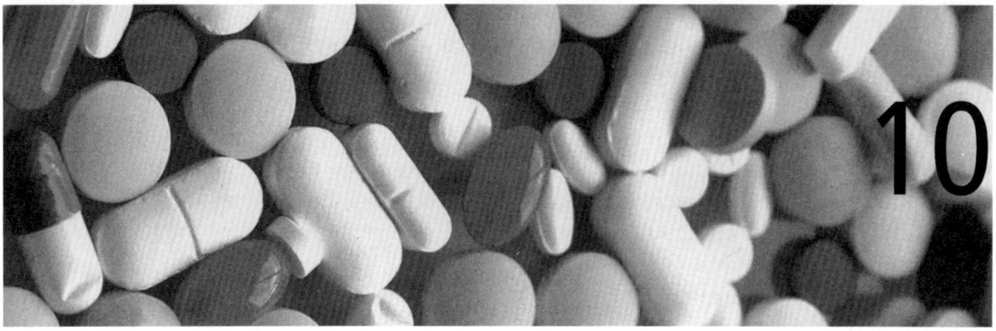

10

The Impact of Reference Pricing in Europe

OVERVIEW

European governments have tried many different methods to control spending on pharmaceuticals, with varying results. One of the oldest of these cost-containment measures is reference pricing – the practice of setting a maximum reimbursement price, in most cases only for off-patent medicines, and then requiring patients to pay any excess if the manufacturer sets the retail price above the reference price. This measure directly penalizes patients who use medicines that exceed their reference prices, but it also indirectly penalizes pharmaceutical companies in one of the two ways, that is, either lower prices or a reduction in the volume of prescriptions (if patients are switched to an alternative drug). Reference pricing may appear to target consumers, but its objective is to force manufacturers to reduce their prices.

Evidence of the success of reference pricing in curbing costs has prompted an increasing number of European countries to adopt this practice in recent years. Furthermore, some governments have expanded their reference pricing systems or made them more aggressive. However, the expected savings from reference pricing can easily overshadow the potential costs of this approach to pharmaceutical cost containment.

In this chapter, we review the use of reference pricing in four major European markets: Germany, Spain, Italy, and France. We conclude with an assessment of the outlook and implications for the pharmaceutical industry.

GERMANY

Germany pioneered the concept of reference pricing in 1989, when it implemented the Gesundheitsreformgesetz (Health Reform Act). A *Festbetrag* (reference price) is the maximum sum that the *Gesetzliche Krankenversicherung* (GKV; statutory health insurance) system will reimburse for a drug that is subject to reference pricing. (Privately insured patients, who account for approximately 10% of the German population, are not subject to reference prices on their prescription drugs.) If a drug is more expensive than its reference price, the patient must pay the excess. This charge is in addition to the standard 10% coinsurance payment (with a minimum payment of €5.00 [$6.21] and a maximum of €10.00 [$12.42]). (For the sake of uniformity of the analysis, the dollar-to-euro exchange rate used in this report is the 2004 average rate [i.e., $1 = €0.80510].) Furthermore, there are no concessions on excess payments and no cap on these payments.

The objective of this cost-containment measure is to induce manufacturers to cut their prices to reference price or lower levels. As of July 1, 2005, of a total of 27,908 reference-priced product presentations (i.e., individual dosages, dosage forms, and pack sizes of a product) in Germany, only 1,973 product presentations (7.1%) exceeded their reference price. The government's strategy has succeeded in curbing costs. From January 1, 1989, to December 31, 2003, the price index for reference-priced drugs declined by 33% (2.6% per year). Conversely, over the same period, the price index for drugs that were not subject to reference pricing increased by 27% (1.6% per year). Since its introduction, the reference-pricing system is estimated to have reduced pharmaceutical expenditures in Germany by an average of €1.2 billion ($1.5 billion) per year. Savings for 2004 are estimated at €2.5 billion ($3.1 billion). Table 10.1 shows the growth of savings from reference pricing.

There are three different reference-pricing groups in Germany:

1 Level 1 Drugs that have the same active ingredient and bioavailability (if therapeutically relevant).
2 Level 2 Drugs that have pharmacologically and therapeutically comparable active ingredients (particularly chemically related agents).
3 Level 3 Drugs that have therapeutically comparable effects (particularly combination agents).

Table 10.1 Evolution of Savings from Reference Pricing in Germany, 1989–2004

Year	*Savings (€ Billion)*	*Index (1989 = 100)*
1989	0.2	100
1990	0.4	200
1991	0.5	250
1992	0.7	350
1993	0.8	400
1994	0.9	450
1995	1.0	500
1996	1.2	600
1997	1.5	750
1998	1.6	800
1999	1.6	800
2000	1.6	800
2001	1.7	850
2002	2.0	1,000
2003	2.1	1,050
2004	2.5[a]	1,250[a]

[a]Projected

Level 1 groups are defined (and reference prices set) when an originator product's patent has expired and several generic versions of the compound are on the market. Level 2 and 3 groups and reference prices for older drugs can be defined at any time. In 1996, the German government suspended level 2 and 3 reference pricing for all patent-protected drugs approved in Germany after December 31, 1995, and effectively restricted this cost-containment measure to off-patent medicines.

The *Spitzenverbände der Krankenkassen* (leading associations of the health insurance funds) are responsible for setting reference prices, which are generally reviewed annually. Not surprisingly, however, drug manufacturers have misgivings about the fact that health insurance funds, as principal payers for healthcare, are also responsible for setting reference prices for the products they reimburse. In the mid-1990s, the pharmaceutical industry initiated a protracted legal action to challenge the legitimacy of the health insurance funds' role in setting reference prices. In July 2001, pending the outcome of this lawsuit, the government temporarily transferred authority for determining reference prices to the Ministry of Health. On March 16, 2004, the European Court of Justice (ECJ) ruled that the involvement of the health insurance funds in setting reference prices does not violate EU competition law. The ECJ judged that health insurance funds are not enterprises; rather, they "fulfill an exclusively social function" that is "founded on the principle of national solidarity and is entirely nonprofit making." In essence, they act as administrative agents for the national government. The task of setting reference prices has reverted to the *Spitzenverbände der Krankenkassen*.

Notwithstanding the use of reference pricing and other cost-containment measures for many years, spending on healthcare, including prescription drugs, has increased steadily – to the growing alarm of the German government. In an effort to curb expenditures, in October 2003, the government enacted the *Gesetz zur Modernisierung der Gesetzlichen Krankenversicherung* (GMG; Statutory Health Insurance Modernization Act), a major overhaul of healthcare funding in Germany. One of the GMG's most controversial measures is the gradual reintroduction of reference pricing for many patent-protected drugs. The only products that will be safe from the threat of reference pricing will be those that have demonstrable therapeutic superiority over existing therapies. Speaking at a press conference in September 2003, health minister Ulla Schmidt justified this change as follows: "The healthcare system can no longer permit the reimbursement of high-priced sham innovations that have little benefit. Therefore, in future, patent-protected medicines that provide no significant therapeutic improvement will be included in the reference pricing regulation."

The *Gemeinsamer Bundesausschuß der Ärzte, Zahnärzte, Krankenhäuser und Krankenkassen* (GBA; Joint Federal Committee of Physicians, Dentists, Hospitals, and Health Insurance Funds) is now responsible for defining reference-pricing groups but receives advice from the *Institut für Qualität und Wirtschaftlichkeit im Gesundheitswesen* (IQWiG; Institute for Quality and Economy in the Healthcare System). Both organizations are the product of the GMG. In addition, another body, the *Arzneimittelkommission der Deutschen Ärzteschaft* (Pharmaceutical Commission of the German Medical Profession), has been given the task of identifying patent-protected medicines launched from 1996 onward that could be assigned to existing reference-pricing groups.

On January 1, 2005, new reference pricing groups for proton pump inhibitors, sartans, triptans, and statins took effect in Germany. The imposition in these four drug classes of reference prices that are, on average, 16.2% below 2004 retail prices is expected to save the statutory health insurance funds a total of €340 million ($422 million) in 2005.

Initial evidence suggests that the new reference-pricing groups have had a significant impact on prescribing patterns in Germany, though not necessarily in line with the expectations of the GBA and the German government. For example, Insight Health (formerly NDC Health) reports that, in the first half of 2005, the volume of prescriptions for proton-pump inhibitors increased by 20.9% (relative to the first six months of 2004). This growth was partially offset by a 10.4% decrease in the volume of prescriptions for H_2 antagonists. Overall, the combined volume of prescriptions for these two drug classes increased by 14.6% in the first six months of 2005. The reasons for this strong growth in the use of antiulcerants are unclear, but the consequence is that the savings from reference pricing have been largely negated.

The pharmaceutical industry is particularly critical of what it considers to be an unduly narrow definition of "therapeutic improvement" and the GBA's policy of combining patent-protected and off-patent medicines in "jumbo" reference-pricing groups. The *Verband Forschender Arzneimittelhersteller* (VFA; German Association of Research-Based Pharmaceutical Companies), the association that represents Germany's largest drug manufacturers, argues that the GBA should accept any of the following enhancements as the evidence of therapeutic improvement:

- Superior efficacy with demonstrable effects.
- Less-severe side effects.
- Improved tolerability.
- Less-severe interactions with other drugs.
- A significant additional indication.
- More rapid effects.
- A new mechanism of action.
- A new dosage form.

Several companies affected by the imposition of reference pricing on patent-protected drugs decided to challenge the legality of this reform in court by filing lawsuits against the health insurance funds in Berlin's Sozialgericht (Social Court). The cases concerned Altana's Pantozol (pantoprazole),

AstraZeneca's Nexium (esomeprazole), Boehringer Ingelheim's Micardis (telmisartan), Merck & Co.'s Maxalt (rizatriptan), and Pfizer's Sortis (atorvastatin). Because each company manufactures separate products, a joint case was not possible. However, all but one of these companies – Pfizer – have since abandoned their legal action and aligned their prices for these drugs with the respective reference prices. The first hearing in Pfizer's lawsuit is expected to take place in fall 2005.

Pfizer has been the most vociferous critic of the new reference-pricing groups. The company objects to the inclusion of atorvastatin (Sortis) in the same reference-pricing group as all other statins (including off-patent lovastatin, pravastatin, and simvastatin). In addition to its lawsuit challenging the reference pricing of atorvastatin, Pfizer refused to cut the drug's price and undertook a controversial advertising campaign that has provoked a fierce backlash from the government and a range of organizations involved in the healthcare system.

The extension of reference pricing to patent-protected medicines may also deter manufacturers from launching certain new drugs in Germany. For example, in November 2004, AstraZeneca revealed that it had suspended its plans to launch Crestor (rosuvastatin) in Germany in 2005. The company is concerned that rosuvastatin, if not judged to be innovative, would immediately be subject to reference pricing. The drug's price in countries in which it is already marketed is, on average, 40% higher than German reference prices. AstraZeneca warned that launching the drug in Germany at the same price as generic statins would deny it an adequate return on its investment and might open the door to massive parallel trade. Withholding a major new drug from the market to avoid the threat of reference pricing is without precedent in Germany and sends an ominous message to manufacturers regarding the future access to innovative medicines in that country.

Undeterred by such findings, the GBA and the German government are intent on further expansion of the reference-pricing system. In July 2005, the GBA introduced six new reference-pricing groups: antianemic agents, fluoroquinolones, heparins, macrolides, serotonin (5-HT_3) receptor antagonists, and triazole antimycotics. These drug classes have combined annual sales of approximately €800 million ($994 million); the government hopes that reference pricing could reduce this total by approximately €50 million ($62 million). The GBA is expected to introduce further waves of new reference-pricing groups in January and July 2006 and January 2007. Ultimately, the government hopes that the new reference-pricing groups will save the German healthcare system approximately €1 billion ($1.2 billion) per year.

Table 10.2 summarizes reference-priced drugs' role in the German pharmaceutical market. As of July 1, 2005, a total of 436 active substances and combinations were subject to reference pricing. These drugs were available in 27,908 different product presentations. Level 1 products (i.e., drugs that have the same active substance and bioavailability) accounted for the majority of product presentations (15,429) subject to reference pricing and the greatest number of prescriptions (221.6 million). However, the number of level 2 products (i.e., drugs that have pharmacologically and therapeutically comparable active substances) subject to reference pricing increased substantially, and these products had the greatest sales as of July 1, 2005: €5.1 billion ($6.3 billion), equivalent to 24.1% of total pharmaceutical sales within the statutory health insurance system. This growth has been driven primarily by the new reference-pricing groups implemented on January 1, 2005.

SPAIN

Reference pricing was introduced in Spain on December 1, 2000, and soon became the mainstay of the government's cost-containment strategy. Drugs within the system were assigned to "homogeneous groups" – medicines that were therapeutically equivalent

Table 10.2 Reference-Priced Drugs' Place in the German Pharmaceutical Market

	Level 1[a]	*Level 2*[b]	*Level 3*[c]	*Total*
Status as of July 1, 2004				
Active substances/combinations subject to reference pricing	189	174	28	391
Product groups subject to reference pricing	306	55	55	416
Packages subject to reference pricing	14,117	5,447	4,117	23,681
Sales (€ billion)	4.5	2.5	1.2	8.2
Share of total GKV drug sales (%)	19.7	10.9	5.2	35.8
Prescriptions (millions)	284.2	88.7	72	444.9
Share of total GKV prescriptions (%)	38.4	12.0	9.7	60.2
Status as of July 1, 2005				
Active substances/combinations subject to reference pricing	200	208	28	436
Product groups subject to reference pricing	326	65	59	450
Packages subject to reference pricing	15,429	8,304	4,175	27,908
Sales (€ billion)	4.1	5.1	1.0	10.2
Share of total GKV drug sales (%)	19.4	24.1	4.7	48.2
Prescriptions (millions)	221.6	120.1	46.2	387.9
Share of total GKV prescriptions (%)	39.4	21.3	8.2	68.9

[a]Drugs that have the same active substance and bioavailability (if therapeutically relevant)
[b]Drugs that have pharmacologically and therapeutically comparable active substances (particularly chemically related agents)
[c]Drugs that have therapeutically comparable effects (particularly combination agents)
GKV = Gesetzliche Krankenversicherung (statutory health insurance)

and had the same qualitative and quantitative composition, pharmaceutical form, dosage form, and route of administration. All homogeneous groups had to contain at least one generic drug. The *Sistema Nacional de Salud* (SNS; National Health System) reimbursed reference-priced drugs only to the level of the reference price for the respective homogeneous group.

The first wave of reference pricing assigned 590 products to 114 homogeneous groups. These products accounted for approximately 10% of public spending on medicines. Manufacturers were obliged to reduce the prices of 193 copy products that lacked proof of bioequivalence to reference-price levels. In April 2002, the government assigned a further 113 products to 28 homogeneous groups and obliged pharmaceutical companies to cut the prices of 25 copy products to reference-price levels.

Originally, the reference price was the average of the prices of the least expensive drugs that collectively accounted for 20% of the sales within each homogeneous group. In May 2003, however, the Ley de Cohesión y Calidad del Sistema Nacional de Salud (Law on the Coherence and Quality of the National Healthcare System) changed the method for calculating reference prices: reference prices were thereafter based on the average price of the three products in a homogeneous group that have the lowest daily-treatment costs. Each of the three products used in setting a reference price had to be marketed by a different manufacturer. Products that had an ex-manufacturer price of less than €2.00 ($2.48) were excluded from these calculations. Prices for generics were not allowed to exceed the group's reference price.

If pharmacists received a prescription for a product that was in a generics group but exceeded its reference price, they were required to substitute a product that did not exceed the reference price. In the event that a product less expensive than the reference price was not available, the pharmacist dispensed the prescribed product but charged the patient the reference price. The manufacturer was then required to reimburse the pharmacist the difference between the reference price and the retail price of its drug.

In October 2003, the government published the new Orden de Precios de Referencia de Medicamentos (Pharmaceutical Reference Pricing Order). On January 1, 2004, the reference prices of 2,070 different presentations of 62 frequently prescribed compounds were reduced by an average of

28%, but some products were subjected to cuts of as much as 80%. In 2002, SNS spending on the targeted drugs totaled €1.64 billion ($2.04 billion), a sum that the government hoped to reduce by €463 million ($575 million) per year.

In March 2004, the *Federación Empresarial de Farmaceúticos Españoles* (FEFE; Business Federation of Spanish Pharmacists) suggested that reference pricing was not achieving the level of savings that the government had expected. FEFE attributed this situation to the fact that many physicians were prescribing more-expensive innovative therapies in place of drugs that are subject to reference pricing. A study conducted by IMS Health on behalf of the Ministry of Health supported the belief that Spanish physicians often avoided prescribing reference-priced drugs. For example, sales of simvastatin, a drug that was subject to reference pricing, grew by 4.6% in 2003 as a whole but declined by 14.3% in December 2003, shortly after reference price cuts were announced. Conversely, sales of atorvastatin, a drug that was excluded from reference pricing, increased by 13.1% in December 2003 and by 23% in the year as a whole. Similarly, sales of the proton-pump inhibitor pantoprazole, which was not subject to reference pricing, grew much faster than sales of omeprazole, a drug that was reference priced.

On May 19, 2004, nine additional molecules became subject to reference pricing in Spain: bisoprolol, cefaclor, fluvoxamine, loratadine, lormetazepam, spironolactone, terazosin, tramadol, and zolpidem. Manufacturers of these products were given two months to reduce their prices to reference-price levels. Approximately 45 companies were affected by this extension of reference pricing. The Ministry of Health forecasted that this action would reduce pharmaceutical expenditures by a total of €12.94 million ($16.07 million), producing savings of €12.04 million ($14.95 million) for the healthcare system and €0.9 million ($1.1 million) for patients. The reference price cuts were expected to cost the pharmaceutical industry a total of €8.1 million ($10.1 million).

On August 1, 2004, the Ministry of Health cut the reference prices of 281 products containing 15 different active ingredients. The list of affected drug classes included antibiotics, antidepressants, antihistamines, antineoplastics, antiulcerants, beta blockers, diuretics, hypnotics and anxiolytics, and opioid analgesics.

In September 2004, the Ministry of Health announced plans to subject four additional molecules – amlodipine, cefazolin, ofloxacin, and pravastatin – to reference pricing beginning March 1, 2005. A total of 82 product presentations would be affected, 32 of which were priced above the proposed reference-price levels.

In early October 2004, however, the Ministry of Health surprised observers by announcing plans for radical changes to the reference-pricing system. Since coming to power in March 2004, the new Socialist government has been disappointed by the savings achieved by the reference-pricing system – €210 million ($261 million) instead of the €430 million ($534 million) forecasted in 2003. Furthermore, the government is concerned that the reference-pricing system causes what it describes as "collateral damage." Some domestic manufacturers and generics companies have lost as much as 25% of their sales as a result of reference pricing, whereas the impact on multinationals has been much smaller (0.5–3%). The government stated that it wanted to save money "without suffocating pharmaceutical companies." Pending reforms, the government suspended the reference-pricing system, on the grounds that this system was unpredictable and arbitrary – penalizing some companies but largely excluding the manufacturers of certain drugs that were judged to be innovative.

In June 2005, the Spanish government gave regional authorities the opportunity to comment on the draft of its proposed Ley de Garantías y Uso Racional de los Medicamentos y Productos Sanitarios (Law on the Security and Rational Use of Medicines and Medical Devices). A Ministry of Health press release explained that "the objective is to ensure quality, security, transparency, and universality in pharmaceutical services, driving the rational use of medicines and the financial sustainability of the system." The proposed medicines law would establish a new reference-pricing system. The Ministry of Health states that this new reference-pricing system will "generate greater savings for the National Health System, will be predictable, objective, and stable, will have a gradual impact on the pharmaceutical industry, will make it possible to keep generics as the most economical option, and will affect all drugs that are in a mature stage of market development." The reference-pricing system would have the following key features:

- Reference prices would be the average of the three lowest-priced versions of compounds.
- In the event that a reference price is more than 30% below a drug's retail price, the manufacturer may either reduce the price in one step or in stages of at least 30% per year until the reference price is reached. If the manufacturer opts for staged price cuts, the drug will not be formally added to the reference-pricing system until its price falls to the reference-price level.
- In exceptional cases, new reference-price groups and reference prices will be set immediately (in agreement with the Comisión Interministerial de Precios de los Medicamentos [CIPM; Interdepartmental Commission on Drug Pricing]) when three generic versions of a compound are approved. This provision will expedite the reference pricing process.
- Reference-priced drugs will be dispensed in the following circumstances:

    1. When a physician prescribes a drug that belongs to a reference-pricing group and that has a price equal to or less than its reference price, the pharmacist will dispense the prescribed drug.
    2. When a physician prescribes a drug that belongs to a reference-pricing group and that has a price higher than its reference price, the pharmacist must substitute the lowest-priced generic of identical composition.
    3. When a physician prescribes, by its international nonproprietary name, an active substance that is subject to reference pricing, the pharmacist will dispense the lowest-priced generic.

In late September 2005, the government responded to widespread criticism of this bill by announcing plans to soften some of the proposed reforms. Among other changes, the government may postpone the introduction of the new reference-pricing system until March 2007, a year later than the original schedule. Products that offer useful "incremental innovations" (e.g., a beneficial new formulation) may qualify for a temporary premium 25% above the relevant reference price. This premium would then be reduced to 15% after one year, 10% after two years, and 5% after three years. Thereafter, the prices of these products would be aligned with their reference prices.

ITALY

Italy's 1994 Finance Act made provision for reference pricing, but the system was not actually established until September 2001. The program initially covered approximately 1,000 patent-expired products containing 38 multisource substances categorized by anatomic therapeutic chemical (ATC) classifications. The price ceiling was set as the weighted average of all products in the group that are at least 20% less expensive than the originator product. The SSN reimbursed the full cost of drugs that did not exceed the reference price, but patients had to pay the excess for drugs that were priced above the reference price.

Just weeks after the program was inaugurated, the government adopted a decree law that radically changed the system. Since November 1, 2001, reference prices are set at the level of the least-expensive available generic rather than based on a weighted average. In addition, if a prescribed drug appears on the reference list, pharmacists are authorized to substitute the least- expensive generic equivalent unless the prescribing physician explicitly forbids substitution. Furthermore, physicians who prescribe products that exceed reference prices must inform their patients about the excess they would have to pay and advise them if less-expensive options are available. As of May 2005, 138 compounds are included in the Italian reference-pricing list. Regional governments have some discretion in deciding reimbursement terms in their territories for reference-priced medicines.

In addition to reference pricing for off-patent medicines, Italy imposes strict reimbursement ceilings on patent-protected drugs. The *Prontuario Farmaceutico Nazionale* (PFN; national formulary) determines reimbursement status on the basis of a drug's cost effectiveness. Drugs dispensed by retail pharmacies are assigned to *categorie terapeutiche omogenee* (homogeneous therapeutic categories) based on ATC fourth-level classification. A homogeneous therapeutic category is defined as "a group of drugs that, in relation to the main therapeutic indication, share the same mechanism of action and are characterized by similar clinical efficacy and profile of undesired side effects. Individual drugs, however, may differ in terms of additional therapeutic indications." For example, in the antiulcerants drug class, H_2 antagonists and proton-pump inhibitors are assigned to different homogeneous therapeutic categories as a result of their different mechanisms of action.

Products that do not exceed their price ceilings in the PFN are included in reimbursement class A (100% reimbursement), but products that are priced above this level are assigned to class C (no reimbursement at all). The threat of dereimbursement is a powerful incentive for manufacturers to cut their prices. In January 2003, when the government introduced its reform of the PFN, only 21 product presentations (out of a total of 4,039 that were eligible for class A status) were assigned to class C because their manufacturers refused to reduce their prices to the level of the reimbursement ceiling.

FRANCE

On October 1, 2003, *tarifs forfaitaires de responsabilité* (reference prices) were introduced in France. The government had hoped to implement this new cost-containment measure on July 1, 2003, but postponed the start date to give manufacturers ample time to reduce their prices to reference price-levels if they wished to do so. Any product that is subject to reference pricing but does not show its reference price on its label is not reimbursed by the social security system.

The first wave of products to undergo reference pricing comprised all substances that were available as generics but that had a generics substitution rate in April 2003 of 10–45%. Products containing a total of 29 substances, divided into 72 generics groups, fell within the government's target range in that month and therefore became subject to reference pricing from October 1, 2003. Before that deadline, many manufacturers reduced their prices to reference-price levels to ensure that patients would not have to pay the excess or accept an alternative product. *Les Entreprises du Médicament* (Leem; Pharmaceutical Companies), the association that represents the French pharmaceutical industry, warned that reference-pricing could cost its members €100 million ($124 million) per year in lost sales.

On June 1, 2005, the *Comité Economique des Produits de Santé* (CEPS; Economic Committee for Healthcare Products) implemented France's second wave of reference prices, which comprised 11 compounds and 17 product presentations. These drugs have combined annual sales of €158 million ($196 million); branded drugs account for 73% of the sales total and generics for 27%. Subjecting these drugs to reference pricing is expected to save the French health insurance system €42–€45 million ($52.2–$55.9 million) per year. Seven compounds that were at risk of reference pricing were unexpectedly spared this fate: aciclovir cream, clomipramine, lactulose, nitrendipine, norfloxacin, rilmenidine, and roxithromycin. The generics dispensing rates for some of these compounds (e.g., clomipramine, nitrendipine) were reportedly as low as 25%, a fact that makes the decision not to impose reference prices surprising. Gilles Bonnefond, the secretary general of the *Union des*

Syndicats de Pharmaciens d'Officine (USPO; Amalgamated Union of Retail Pharmacists), suggested that the CEPS showed favoritism to certain manufacturers.

In July 2004, the French Parliament passed the Projet de Loi Relatif à l'Assurance Maladie (the Health Insurance Bill), a bill that introduced radical reforms in the funding of healthcare in France. Among its many measures, this bill made the reference-pricing system much more aggressive: The Comité de Suivi des Génériques (Generics Monitoring Committee) will meet monthly to review the generics-dispensing rates of drugs that have been off patent for a year or longer. Reference prices will be imposed if a drug's generics-dispensing rate does not reach 50% (60% in the case of drugs with substantial sales) within one year of patent expiration and 70% (80% in the case of drugs with substantial sales) within two years of patent expiration. These conditions may be relaxed if generics dispensing is growing strongly but has not reached the targeted rates, or if the range of generics on the market is limited. However, in early October 2005, the government published the *Projet de Loi de Financement de la Sécurité Sociale* (PLFSS) 2006 (Social Security Finance Bill 2006). In an effort to reduce the deficit in the healthcare budget from an estimated €8.3 billion ($10.3 billion) in 2005 to €6.1 billion ($7.6 billion) in 2006, the government plans to impose a wide range of stringent cost-cutting measures, including the automatic imposition of reference pricing two years after the patent on a compound expires.

In October 2004, the CEPS reported that sales of generics in France grew from €609 million ($756 million) in 2002 to €871 million ($1.1 billion) in 2003, a 43% increase. The greater use of generics saved the French healthcare system an estimated €130 million ($161 million) in 2003. However, the government has much more aggressive ambitions for savings from generics in the future: in the three-year period 2005–7, the government hopes that generics will reduce pharmaceutical spending by approximately €1 billion ($1.2 billion).

The growth of the French generics market continued in 2004. In November 2004, Leem reported that, in the 12 months to September 2004, total sales of off-patent products (both branded and generic) included in the official *répertoire des produits génériques* (generics list) totaled €2.3 billion ($2.9 billion) in 2003, a 10.3% increase in one year. Generic and branded products included in the generics list had contrasting fortunes in the 12 months to September 2004; sales of generic versions of these drugs increased by 32% to €1.1 billion ($1.4 billion), whereas sales of branded versions of these medicines declined by 2.9% to €1.3 billion ($1.6 billion). By comparison, total sales of reimbursed medicines in France amounted to €16.7 billion ($20.7 billion) in the 12 months to September 2004, an increase of 7.3% over the 12 months to September 2003.

The introduction of reference pricing in France has helped to moderate the prices of off-patent medicines. The CEPS reports that, in 70% of cases, manufacturers of branded medicines that were subjected to reference pricing reduced their prices to the level of the reference prices. Overall, very few drugs have not had their prices aligned with their respective reference prices. Of 541 reference-priced products, only 34 (6.3%) exceeded their reference prices. Table 10.3 lists the products that are priced above their reference prices. The mean price difference between the reference prices and retail prices of these drugs was 41.5%, a surprisingly large margin. Manufacturers of these products presumably concluded that the potential loss of sales from refusing to cut their prices was greater than the reduction in revenues that would result from lower prices. These companies may have hoped that established patients would remain loyal to familiar brands, even if they had to pay a premium to continue taking them. Note that all but three of the products that exceed their reference prices are originator brands. The only exceptions are Dexo's Spironone, a generic spironolactone product, and two generic timolol products from Alcon.

Table 10.3 Drugs That Exceeded Their Reference Prices in France as of June 1, 2005

Compound	*Product Name*	*Dosage*	*Pack Size*	*Manufacturer*	*Reference Price (€)*	*Retail Price (€)*	*Price Difference (€)*	*Price Difference (%)*
Bisoprolol	Soprol	10 mg	28 tablets	Wyeth Lederle	7.07	10.67	3.60	50.9
Cimetidine	Tagamet	200 mg	30 tablets	Axcan Pharma	6.89	9.97	3.08	44.7
Cimetidine	Tagamet	200 mg	60 effervescent tablets	Axcan Pharma	13.87	19.59	5.72	41.2
Cimetidine	Tagamet	400 mg	30 tablets	Axcan Pharma	14.69	20.8	6.11	41.6
Cimetidine	Tagamet	800 mg	15 tablets	Axcan Pharma	14.69	20.75	6.06	41.3
Disodium cromoglycate	Nalcron	100 mg/5 mL	30 ×5 mL solution	Sanofi-Aventis	10.82	15.23	4.41	40.8
Fluvoxamine	Floxyfral	50 mg	30 tablets	Solvay	6.5	10.47	3.97	61.1
Fluvoxamine	Floxyfral	100 mg	15 tablets	Solvay	5.9	9.47	3.57	60.5
Imidazole	Pevaryl	1% cream	30 g	McNeil	2.84	4.79	1.95	68.7
Imidazole	Pevaryl	1% emulsion	30 mL	McNeil	3.12	4.98	1.86	59.6
Imidazole	Pevaryl	1% solution	30 g vial	McNeil	3.63	5.58	1.95	53.7
Imidazole	Pevaryl	1% powder	30 g bottle	McNeil	4.66	6.68	2.02	43.3
Indapamide	Fludex	2.5 mg	30 tablets	Servier	8.98	12.6	3.62	40.3
Ketoprofen	Profenid	50 mg	24 capsules	Sanofi-Aventis	2.48	3.3	0.82	33.1
Ketoprofen	Profenid	100 mg	30 tablets	Sanofi-Aventis	5.12	7.1	1.98	38.7
Ketoprofen	Profenid LP	200 mg	14 tablets	Sanofi-Aventis	6.08	8.26	2.18	35.9
Ketoprofen	Profenid LP	200 mg	14 tablets	Sanofi-Aventis	6.08	8.67	2.59	42.6
Metoprolol	Lopressor	100 mg	30 tablets	Sankyo Pharma France	3.37	4.58	1.21	35.9
Metoprolol	Seloken	100 mg	28 tablets	AstraZeneca	3.19	4.12	0.93	29.2
Molsidomine	Corvasal	2 mg	30 tablets	Sanofi-Aventis	3.52	4.82	1.30	36.9
Molsidomine	Corvasal	2 mg	90 tablets	Sanofi-Aventis	8.83	12.38	3.55	40.2
Molsidomine	Corvasal	4 mg	30 tablets	Sanofi-Aventis	5.53	7.66	2.13	38.5
Propranolol	Avlocardyl	40 mg	50 tablets	AstraZeneca	2.6	3.48	0.88	33.8
Spironolactone	Aldactone	50 mg	30 tablets	Pfizer	5.97	8.9	2.93	49.1
Spironolactone	Aldactone	75 mg	30 tablets	Pfizer	8.06	12.84	4.78	59.3
Spironolactone	Spironone	75 mg	30 coated tablets	Dexo	8.06	9.32	1.26	15.6
Terazosin	Dysalfa	5 mg	28 tablets	Fournier	19.33	27.38	8.05	41.6
Terazosin	Hytrine	5 mg	28 tablets	Abbott	19.33	27.38	8.05	41.6
Ticlopidine	Ticlid	250 mg	30 tablets	Sanofi-Aventis	18.94	26.81	7.87	41.6
Timolol	Timolol Alcon	0.25%	5 mL liquid	Alcon	4.75	5.16	0.41	8.6
Timolol	Timolol Alcon	0.5%	5 mL liquid	Alcon	5.03	5.53	0.50	9.9
Timolol	Timoptol	0.1%	3 mL liquid	Merck Sharp & Dohme Chibret	2.89	3.91	1.02	35.3
Timolol	Timoptol	0.25%	3 mL liquid	Merck Sharp & Dohme Chibret	3.06	4.52	1.46	47.7
Timolol	Timoptol	0.5%	3 mL liquid	Merck Sharp & Dohme Chibret	3.23	4.82	1.59	49.2

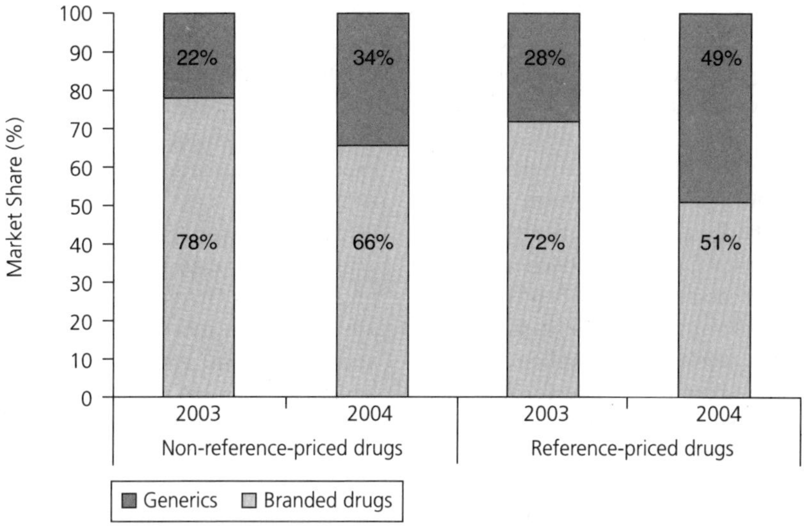

Figure 10.1 Generic and Branded Medicines share prescription, for off-patent Drugs in France, 2003–2004

In November 2004, Leem estimated that the first wave of reference pricing in France had saved the social security system approximately €115 million ($143 million) to date. Most of this savings (€95 million [$118 million]) came from manufacturers' price cuts, while increased use of generics saved €20 million ($25 million). Figure 10.1 shows that, from 2003 to 2004, generics' share of the market for off-patent drugs increased among both reference-priced and non-reference-priced drugs, but the growth rate was much faster among reference-priced drugs. In 2004, generics accounted for 49% of prescriptions for reference-priced drugs, compared with only 34% of prescriptions for off-patent drugs that were not subject to reference pricing.

OUTLOOK AND IMPLICATIONS FOR THE PHARMACEUTICAL INDUSTRY

The spread of reference pricing across Europe in recent years is a disturbing trend for the pharmaceutical industry, and not just for manufacturers of branded medicines; generics companies are also disadvantaged by this cost-containment measure. By pressuring manufacturers of branded medicines to cut their prices to the level of generics, reference pricing erodes generics' key selling point – their price advantage. Given a choice between a familiar brand and an unfamiliar generic, both of which are similarly priced, many physicians and patients would favor the branded product. Reference pricing can trigger a downward spiral in prices – a prospect that is bad news for manufacturers (both branded and generic) but good news for payers. Governments are often impervious to generics manufacturers' complaints that reference pricing hurts them. As a rule, governments are not concerned whether savings on pharmaceutical spending come from increased use of generics or price cuts on branded medicines.

The German reference-pricing system, being the oldest in the world, is observed closely by other European governments. Therefore, it is worrying for the pharmaceutical industry that Germany has taken the lead in extending reference pricing to some drug classes that include patent-protected medicines. The prospect that new drugs launched in these classes could be immediately subject to reference pricing is especially alarming. AstraZeneca's decision to suspend plans for the launch of Crestor in Germany may set an ominous precedent for the German pharmaceutical market. Patients in Germany could find that they are increasingly denied access to novel drugs that are available in other European countries.

Two events are likely to have a major bearing on the future of reference pricing in Germany. Following the inconclusive outcome of the general election on September 18, 2005, a coalition government has been formed after weeks of wrangling. Angela Merkel, the chancellor designate, has expressed reservations about the GMG. She has indicated that she regards reform of the new reference-pricing system as a priority. Her party's working group on health has also expressed the opinion that the GBA sometimes takes too narrow a view of innovation, ignoring benefits such as additional indications or improved side-effect profiles. However, the likely fragility of her coalition government may frustrate her desire for change. The outcome of Pfizer's legal challenge against the reference pricing of atorvastatin will also have lasting repercussions for the pharmaceutical industry as a whole in Germany – and beyond, if other European countries decide to follow the German lead in extending reference pricing to patent-protected medicines.

As noted previously, Italy's PFN already excludes from reimbursement patent-protected drugs that exceed the reimbursement ceiling for their homogeneous therapeutic category. The Italian government is pursuing an aggressive cost-cutting strategy, but it has not focused on reference pricing in the past year or two and has given no indication that it plans to escalate this cost-containment measure in the foreseeable future. In Spain, the government has proposed major changes to the reference-pricing system, including disturbing plans to require pharmacists to substitute the lowest-priced generic version of a drug if a physician prescribes a drug that exceeds its reference price. If the reforms contained in the new medicines law do not achieve the savings that the government wants, it might consider more radical reforms, possibly along German lines. The French government is the most recent convert to reference pricing and remains cautious about the benefits of this cost-cutting strategy. Reference pricing has been regarded in France as a last resort, to be invoked only if physicians and pharmacists collectively fail to meet the government's requirements for generics dispensing. However, the pharmaceutical industry has condemned the proposal in the PLFSS 2006 for automatic reference pricing of drugs two years after patent expiration.

Both the European Union and national governments have expressed their determination to bolster Europe's pharmaceutical industry, especially by reversing the sharp decline in Europe's importance in research and development. However, reference pricing could undermine investment in R&D. The pharmaceutical industry in Germany attributes the decline in R&D activity in that country primarily to the government's aggressive cost-containment strategies. Some governments would like to dichotomize the pharmaceutical market – allowing relatively free pricing and price premiums for drugs that are deemed to be innovative, but subjecting other drugs to reference pricing. However, governments might ultimately find that aggressive reference pricing comes at a high price: a decline in the number of innovative drugs reaching the market.

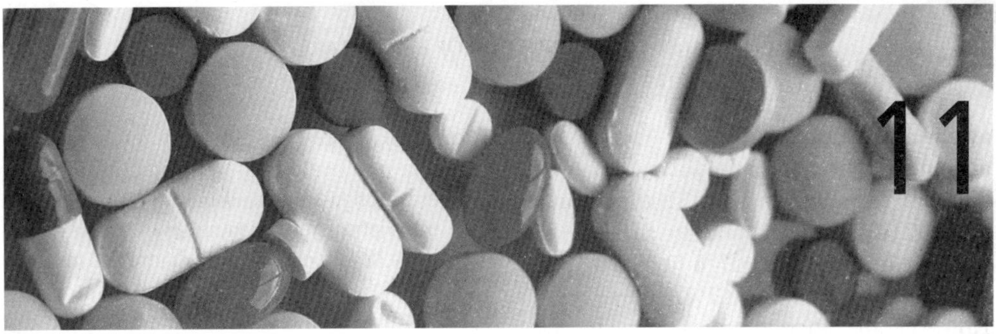

Pharmaceutical Pricing, Reimbursement, and Prescribing in the United Kingdom

INTRODUCTION

In 1948, the United Kingdom established a pioneering universal healthcare system: the National Health Service (NHS). In the visionary words of its founders, the NHS was intended to offer all UK citizens comprehensive medical care "from the cradle to the grave." The original concept was based on the principle that all healthcare provision – prescription medicines, primary care, dental and ophthalmic treatment, and hospitalization – should be free at the point of delivery. However, inexorably rising costs necessitated the progressive imposition of a range of patient copayments. In the 1960s, for example, the government introduced prescription charges in a bid to restrain the growth in NHS pharmaceutical expenditures.

The United Kingdom is the world's fifth-largest market for prescription drugs and, thanks to a relatively liberal regulatory environment, one of the most accessible of all European markets in terms of product registration, price setting, and reimbursement. Pharmaceutical prices are higher in the UK market than in most other European countries. However, tough supply- and demand-side restrictions, together with a flourishing generics market, severely limit the uptake of innovative new drugs. The United Kingdom therefore remains one of the most conservative pharmaceutical markets in Europe.

ORGANIZATION AND FUNDING OF THE UK HEALTHCARE SYSTEM

In 1948, the NHS had a budget of £437 million ($714 million) – equivalent to approximately £9 billion ($14.7 billion) in current terms. (For the sake of uniformity of the analysis, the dollar-to-pound-sterling exchange rate used in this report is the 2003 average rate: $1 = £0.61229.) By the 2001–2 financial year, NHS spending had increased to £59.6 billion ($97.3 billion). According to the Organization for Economic Cooperation and Development, in 2002 (the most recent year for which data are available), the United Kingdom spent 7.7% of its gross domestic product (GDP) on healthcare – less than the European Union (EU) mean of 8.5% and substantially less than Germany's 10.9% and France's 9.7%. However, the Labor government elected in May 1997 has pledged to increase investment to at least the EU average (as a share of GDP). In April 2002, it announced plans to increase investment in the NHS from £65 billion ($106 billion) in the 2002–3 financial year to £105 billion ($171 billion) in the 2007–8 financial year – an increase of almost 62% in five years. However, the pharmaceutical industry will receive only a modest share of this increased spending.

The NHS is the dominant source of healthcare financing and provision in the United Kingdom. Direct taxation generates 86% of NHS finances, employee contributions through a payroll-levied national insurance scheme provide 12% of the budget, and patient copayments account for just 2% of funding.

The private sector accounts for a relatively small share of total healthcare provision. Private healthcare focuses primarily on areas where waiting times for NHS interventions are long (e.g., elective surgery for conditions that are not life-threatening) and areas where NHS-funded services are severely restricted (e.g., optical and dental care). For most indications, pharmaceutical sales to the private sector are small compared with sales to the NHS.

The infrastructure of the NHS has undergone many changes in recent years. In July 2000, the government published the NHS Plan, which outlines its program for future investment and reform. A key reform is the decentralization of power within the NHS. On April 1, 2002, the 95 regional health authorities in England were merged to form 28 new strategic health authorities (SHAs). These SHAs are responsible for the strategic development of healthcare services within their areas and for managing the performance of 304 primary care trusts (PCTs) and more than 300 NHS hospital trusts. PCTs have three main roles: (1) improve the health of the community; (2) develop primary and community health services; and (3) commission hospital care for their patients.

PHARMACEUTICAL CLASSIFICATION

All registered medicines marketed in the United Kingdom are assigned to one of the following three classes:

- Prescription-only medicines (POM) require a prescription from a physician or a dentist and must be dispensed by a pharmacist (retail or hospital).
- Pharmacy-only medicines (P) are available without a prescription but are restricted to pharmacy distribution.
- General Sales List (GSL) products are available without a prescription and may be sold in any retail outlet.

P and GSL products may be prescribed and reimbursed. However, most prescriptions are for POM products.

PHARMACEUTICAL PRICES IN THE UNITED KINGDOM

On average, pharmaceutical prices in the United Kingdom are higher than in most other European countries but much lower than in the United States. High prices in comparison with most of the rest of Europe have encouraged parallel importing (discussed further on).

The Department of Health (DH) monitors the prices of the most frequently prescribed drugs in the United Kingdom, several other European markets, and the United States. Table 11.1 uses the United Kingdom as a benchmark and expresses average pharmaceutical prices in several leading markets as a percentage of average UK prices in a given year. Besides the impact of price reductions or increases in individual markets, exchange rate fluctuations are a significant factor in relative pricing trends in these markets. In the late 1990s, sterling appreciated strongly against most European currencies (thereby inflating UK prices in comparison with prices in those countries) but lost value against the US dollar (thereby reducing UK prices in comparison with prices in the United States). In 2002 and 2003, however, these trends reversed: sterling appreciated against the dollar and lost value against the euro. *Pharmaceutical Price Regulation Scheme: Seventh Report to Parliament,*

Table 11.1 Multilateral Comparison of Average Exmanufacturer Prices of Branded Medicines in Select Markets as a Percentage of UK Average Exmanufacturer Prices, 1992–2002

Year	*France (%)*	*Germany (%)*	*Italy (%)*	*Spain (%)*	*United States (%)*	*United Kingdom (%)*
1992	93	158	108	95	172	100
1993	96	158	100	89	202	100
1994	100	143	90	88	192	100
1995	107	130	83	89	179	100
1996	105	125	93	89	191	100
1997	85	101	86	74	184	100
1998	85	109	88	77	188	100
1999	86	103	82	72	213	100
2000	83	94	82	70	241	100
2001	81	90	85	72	205	100
2002	83	94	86	77	194	100
Average percentage, 1998–2002[a]	83	94	86	77	197	100

[a]Based on 2002 price data but converted to pounds sterling using average exchange rates for the period 1998–2002

a study published in December 2003, expressed concern that because of the steady appreciation of the pound sterling, the United Kingdom moved from the middle of the European price range for prescription medicines in the mid-1990s to the very top of the European price range in 2002. However, US prices are, on average, twice as high as UK prices, and the price differential between the United States and continental Europe is even larger.

REIMBURSEMENT OF OUTPATIENT MEDICINES

General Features

In the United Kingdom, all marketed drugs are automatically eligible for full reimbursement unless they are included in Schedules 10 or 11 of the Drug Tariff, the official list of drugs, devices, dressings, and appliances that general practitioners (GPs) in England and Wales may prescribe at NHS expense. Reimbursement applies only to products dispensed by a licensed pharmacy under contract to the NHS. Products purchased at other outlets or without a prescription are not reimbursed. Most drugs prescribed in the primary care setting are dispensed by private pharmacies and reimbursed as part of the General Pharmaceutical Services of the NHS. A small proportion of drugs is prescribed and dispensed by "prescribing physicians" – mainly in rural areas where patients do not have easy access to a pharmacy. A recent regulatory change allows NHS physicians to issue private prescriptions for drugs that are not reimbursed – a practice that was previously illegal. However, this practice remains very uncommon.

Prices listed in the Drug Tariff are discounted by a small percentage (known as *clawback*) to reflect possible discounts to the pharmacy from wholesalers, and they are further adjusted for patient copayments collected in the pharmacy. As an incentive to seek low-cost sources of supply, such as parallel imports, retail pharmacists are allowed to retain the difference between their drug acquisition price and the reimbursed price based on the Drug Tariff.

Admission to Reimbursement

Application

Admission of a product to reimbursement in the United Kingdom is generally straightforward. Manufacturers advise the DH of their intention to launch a product and request that it be added to the Drug Tariff. The drug is added automatically unless the DH objects.

Listing

Products listed in the Drug Tariff are reimbursed if prescribed by a GP and dispensed by a licensed pharmacy or other approved supplier. More restricted lists apply to NHS dentists and prescribing nurses. The Drug Tariff states the price of the product, which may be subject to periodic variations.

Entry to the Drug Tariff is granted to all drugs approved for marketing unless they are included in Schedule 10 of the NHS (General Medical Services) Regulations 1992, commonly referred to as the *black list*. Introduced in 1985, this negative list now encompasses products in 17 drug classes, including contraceptives, benzodiazepines, and categories that have acceptable OTC alternatives (e.g., mild to moderate analgesics, laxatives, indigestion remedies). Blacklisted products are excluded from reimbursement on the grounds that expert opinion indicates they have no clinical or therapeutic advantage over other, less-expensive drugs.

Government ministers ultimately decide which drugs are included in the black list. They receive advice from the Advisory Committee on NHS Drugs (ACD), an independent body of physicians, dentists, and pharmacists. Schedule 10 is published in the NHS Drug Tariff (Parts XVIIIA and B).

In practice, voluntary price cuts by manufacturers generally avert blacklisting. The last compulsory new addition to the black list occurred in 1997. Moreover, since the establishment of NICE in April 1999, the ACD has met less frequently. In April 2002, however, Merck Sharpe & Dohme took the unusual step of *voluntarily* having a drug – finasteride (Propecia), a treatment for male pattern baldness – added to Schedule 10. The company's decision may have been influenced by the fact that minoxidil (Pfizer's Rogaine), an over-the-counter treatment for male pattern baldness, was already blacklisted.

The existence of Schedule 10 gives the DH some influence over drug prices – especially in categories already covered by the black list. Companies planning to launch drugs that are similar to existing products or that have generics competition may have to justify their requested price or even negotiate a price that is more acceptable to the DH. If manufacturers charge a price that the DH deems excessive, they face the implicit threat of blacklisting. Anecdotal evidence suggests that in recent years, the DH has become more inclined to challenge companies that propose prices it considers excessive.

The Drug Tariff also contains Schedule 11, a *grey list* of products for which reimbursement is restricted to particular patient groups and/or specific indications. The grey list is rarely used in practice and contains only 12 drugs. The best-known drug on Schedule 11 is probably sildenafil (Pfizer's Viagra), a treatment for erectile dysfunction that attracted enormous media attention when it was launched in 1998. Alarmed by predictions that this drug might cost the NHS as much as £100 million ($163 million) a year, the government decided to restrict prescribing. The Schedule 11 criteria for the prescribing of sildenafil limit use of the drug to approximately 17% of the total population of impotent men.

Another list in the Drug Tariff contains a large number of nutritional supplements and "borderline substances." Although not normally regarded as drugs, these products may be prescribed to individual patients who have specified disorders.

Northern Ireland and Scotland have separate Drug Tariff Sections, but they follow the lead of the London-based Drug Tariff Section. Products are added to Scotland and Northern Ireland's Drug Tariffs approximately one month after a decision is made in London.

Financial Data Requirements

Companies that have not previously sold branded pharmaceuticals to the NHS are expected to submit annual financial returns (AFRs) to the DH (see the section Profit Control).

Supply-Side Restrictions

The UK government seeks to limit NHS pharmaceutical expenditures by several measures designed to influence drug prices.

Price Control

Launch prices of new branded prescription drugs are not subject to formal control in the United Kingdom. However, the existence of the aforementioned black list allows the DH to influence entry prices. Changes to the prices of branded prescription drugs are governed by the Pharmaceutical Price Regulation Scheme (PPRS) (described further on in the section Profit Control).

In August 2000, the government introduced a maximum price scheme for certain generic drugs in response to a supply crisis that inflated the NHS drug bill by approximately £200 million ($327 million) in 1999. This scheme applies only to unbranded products with sales in excess of £750,000 ($1.2 million) or sales of more than £100,000 ($163,321) if the price has increased materially since January 1999. This initiative was expected to save the NHS £240 million ($392 million) in 2000–1, but savings have actually amounted to £330 million ($539 million) per year. Encouraged by the program's success, the government extended the initiative in October 2001 and again in December 2002.

In September 2003, the DH published draft proposals for a new system of "free-market" pricing for generics. The draft includes the following recommendations:

- Generics companies would be free to set their own prices but would need to justify any price increases that exceed approximately 10% in a six-month period.
- In markets characterized by limited supply (i.e., three or fewer manufacturers), companies would need the DH's permission to increase their prices. Manufacturers would need to give the DH at least eight weeks' notice of the proposed change and would need to provide evidence of their manufacturing costs.
- Manufacturers of new generics would be able to set their own prices as long as those prices were less than the Drug Tariff prices for the relevant originator brand.
- Manufacturers and wholesalers would have to provide the DH with quarterly data on their income revenues, cost of purchases, and transaction volumes.

The DH has presented the proposed changes as the restoration of pricing freedom in the UK generics market, but manufacturers remain unconvinced. Generics companies particularly dislike the prospect of having to obtain permission for the price increases that may be substantial in percentage terms but are relatively modest in absolute terms. Manufacturers are also concerned that, because of the volatility of the generics market, they will be unable to meet the DH's exacting requirements for pricing forecasts.

Profit Control

Since its introduction in 1957, the PPRS has been used to control the level of profit companies may make on sales of branded prescription drugs to the NHS. The PPRS now covers approximately 80% of the branded drugs dispensed in the United Kingdom. For many years, the program was voluntary, but it recently became compulsory. The DH and the Association of the British Pharmaceutical Industry (ABPI) periodically renegotiate the terms of the program.

The PPRS is intended to balance the NHS's need for an affordable and dependable supply of medicines with drug manufacturers' need for a reasonable profit margin. It allows companies to make a maximum level of profit either as a percentage of capital used (the return on capital [ROC] method) or as a percentage of sales (the return on sales [ROS] method). Companies are free to choose their method of assessment. The ROS method is generally preferable for manufacturers that have only limited investment in the United Kingdom because it allows them to retain a higher level of profit.

Profit targets relate to a company's total NHS business, not to individual products. The target ROC is either 17% (when considering possible price increases) or 21% of capital invested (when considering whether annual profitability is excessive). The target ROS is 6–6.5%.

To ensure that accountants do not try to manipulate their companies' profit levels, the PPRS contains detailed regulations that restrict the following:

- The level of R&D expenditure that may be offset against NHS profits. This figure is generally 20% of NHS sales, but the allowance may be increased or reduced by up to 3%, depending on the number of products a company markets and whether it is seeking a price increase.
- Promotional spending that may be offset against NHS profits. The standard allowance for sales promotion is 6% of NHS sales. This figure is reduced when companies propose a price increase. However, the scheme includes tiered cash allowances related to a company's total number of products. Smaller companies additionally benefit from a fixed element in the sales promotion allowance.
- How the costs of fixed assets may be allocated between NHS sales and other sales. UK fixed costs are divided between home and export sales. A figure of 7.5% is allocated to home NHS sales, and the balance is then divided according to the proportion of a company's home and export sales.
- Transfer prices for products imported into the United Kingdom.

Under PPRS regulations, manufacturers are free to set the prices of new entities and line extensions launched within five years of the original therapy. However, they must give the DH advance warning if profit is likely to exceed 140% of the target ROC/ROS. If profit exceeds this upper limit (i.e., a company makes profits of more than 29% of capital or more than 9% of sales), the company is expected to reduce prices, delay price increases, or directly repay the excess to the DH.

Profits are calculated using AFRs. AFRs are accounts, prepared in an agreed format, that identify a company's NHS sales, costs, and trading profit. They must be submitted within set periods at the end of each financial year. AFRs are not complex documents, but they must contain sufficient financial information for the DH to assess whether the company is exceeding its permitted profit level. Companies that have NHS sales of less than £25 million ($41 million) may submit audited accounts in place of AFRs, and companies that have NHS sales of less than £1 million ($1.6 million) are not required to provide financial information.

The PPRS also requires foreign companies with UK subsidiaries to submit their accounts. Allowances against NHS sales (as opposed to other business, such as exports) are calculated on the basis of capital employed.

The government takes the submission of financial data under the PPRS very seriously. Companies that fail to provide the necessary information may suffer financial penalties.

Price increases are subject to DH approval. The DH generally allows price increases only if a company's profit is less than 50% of the target ROS/ROC. Price increases are therefore permitted only if a company's profit is less than 8.5% of capital employed, or less than 3% of sales. Manufacturers are generally free to reduce the prices of reimbursed medicines at any time.

The 1999 PPRS settlement imposed a 4.5% price cut on all marketed products and a price-freeze that was in effect until 2001. The *Fifth Report to Parliament on the Pharmaceutical Price Regulation Scheme*, published in December 2001, reported that this price-cut saved the NHS approximately £200 million ($327 million) between October 1999 and December 2000. Since 2001, price increases have been permitted (subject to DH approval), but they may not exceed the August 1999 levels by more than 20%.

The PPRS is a complex system that is open to abuse. For example, a company could manipulate its UK capital base to increase the basis for its profit calculations. Because of the complexity of the system, negotiations between manufacturers and the DH can sometimes be protracted, particularly if a company is close to the upper limit of permitted profit. Overseas companies have sometimes complained that the PPRS lacks transparency and, because of its complexity, allows the DH to manipulate the system in favor of UK companies.

In the fall of 2003, well before the current five-year agreement ends, the government invited submissions to an eight-week consultation exercise on the future of the

PPRS. The government's discussion paper for this consultation identified several significant advantages to the PPRS as a method of price regulation:

- [It] is relatively flexible and has been adopted over the years to take account of changes in the NHS and elsewhere.
- [It] has provided a stable regulatory environment for the industry and stable prices for the NHS.
- [It] allows doctors and patients a wide choice of medicines.
- [It] is a relatively light touch form of regulation compared to that in some other countries and is relatively cheap to operate.
- [It] is a voluntary scheme and has avoided the legal challenges that have occurred under the statutory schemes in some other countries.

The discussion paper also identified several drawbacks to the PPRS:

- Until five years ago, UK medicine prices were in the mid-range of comparable European countries and significantly lower than those in the United States. Now, largely as a result of the appreciation of the pound sterling, UK prices are at the top end of comparator countries though still significantly lower than US prices.
- The increased globalization of the pharmaceutical industry is making it more difficult to identify capital and costs relating to the supply of medicines to the NHS, thereby making administration of the scheme more complex.
- As reported in the Fifth and Sixth Reports to Parliament on the PPRS, some member companies continue to be reticent in providing information provided for under the scheme to DH[the Department of Health].

The discussion paper acknowledged that the current PPRS agreement, negotiated in 1999, "has largely achieved the objectives Government set for the new scheme." Nevertheless, to prepare for future needs, the government invited comments on four main options: (1) continuing the 1999 PPRS agreement without change; (2) amending key aspects of the current PPRS agreement; (3) potential deregulation of drug pricing; and (4) alternative proposals suggested by respondents.

On the subject of possible deregulation of prescription-drug pricing, the discussion paper cites key findings from *PPRS: The Study into the Extent of Competition in the Supply of Branded Medicines to the NHS*, a study conducted jointly by the DH and the ABPI. This study, which was published in December 2002, found that the UK pharmaceutical market is not highly concentrated, but later entrants to a drug class often struggle to challenge more established brands. Physicians are not very aware of pharmaceutical prices and are influenced more by efficacy than by price when making prescribing decisions. The discussion paper notes that "the operation of this market has been affected by the PPRS. However, where price changes have occurred, the study was unable to find consistent volume responses to such changes. Over half of price changes triggered no response from competitors. In the majority of cases, the launch of new products provoked no price response from competitor products." This evidence of the price stability of the UK market may help explain the government's willingness to consider deregulation of branded prescription drug pricing.

Demand-Side Restrictions

The UK government also uses several demand-side restrictions to control overall expenditure on drugs.

Primary Care Budgets and Cost Consciousness

In the United Kingdom, GPs have always been the gatekeepers to the NHS, controlling access to specialist and inpatient care, and the government is increasing its emphasis on the primary care sector. In England, PCTs now control 75% of the overall NHS budget and 100% of local funds. PCTs spend an average of £18 million ($29 million) per year on medicines (i.e., 16% of their total expenditures).

PCTs are required to forward details of their prescribing budgets to the Prescription Pricing Authority (PPA), which monitors prescribing patterns and disseminates prescribing analysis and cost (PACT) reports to

SHAs, PCTs, and primary care practices. These reports enable GPs to compare their own prescribing costs with the prescribing costs of their practice as a whole, with SHA averages, and with national averages. The National Tracker Survey of Primary Care Groups and Trusts 2000–1 (known as the Tracker Survey), conducted in December 2000 by the National Primary Care Research and Development Centre and the King's Fund, found that 96% of primary care groups and trusts used PACT prescribing indicators to monitor prescribing patterns and that 93% used them to identify poorly performing practices.

An Audit Commission report published in March 2003 found that PCTs had increased their drug budgets for the 2002–3 financial year by an average of 10%, compared with the preceding financial year, an increase that was unlikely to be sufficient to cover the growth in pharmaceutical spending. In January 2003, the DH issued guidelines to PCTs on setting prescribing budgets for the next three financial years (April 6, 2003 to April 5, 2006). The DH recommended that the starting point in budgeting should be the current growth rate for prescription drugs (11–13% per year), thereby indicating that the government expects recent growth rates to continue. The DH guidelines also explicitly emphasize the need for PCTs to take into account several other factors that could substantially increase their prescribing costs; the following relevant passages are quoted from the guidelines:

- *The National Institute for Clinical Excellence* (NICE): PCTs are reminded that they are under a statutory obligation to provide funding for clinical decisions within recommendations from NICE contained in Technology Appraisal Guidance. It is important that mechanisms are in place to assess the impact of NICE guidance on both primary and secondary care . . . Additionally, PCTs are reminded about the statutory requirements to fund the provision of disease-modifying therapies for multiple sclerosis in accordance with HSC 2002–4.
- *National Service Frameworks* (NSFs): NSFs are clearly leading to additional expenditure as more patients are treated. (National service frameworks (NSFs) are clinical guidelines designed to improve the quality of patient care in clinical priority areas [e.g., mental health, coronary heart disease, oncology, geriatric medicine].) For instance, national expenditure on statins continues to increase by approximately 30% year on year. The financial implications of NSFs have been factored into unified allocations and PCTs should ensure adequate provision [for them] in primary care budgets. (Health authorities and PCTs now have overall budgets from which they have to fund hospital and community health services, primary care infrastructure, and prescribing.) Additionally, PCTs should consider the feasibility of arrangements to monitor patients' compliance with and benefit from the treatment prescribed for them.
- *Newly Licensed Drugs*: Most significant new drugs will be referred to NICE for appraisal, but plans should recognize the scope for prescribing during the interim period between the reference and NICE providing their guidance (see para. 5 of HSC 1999/176). Underlying trends of new drugs are picked up in the drugs-bill forecast but any large spending may need to be factored in. To help with these assessments, the National Prescribing Centre (NPC) has distributed the document "On the Horizon" to all PCTs. This document provides information about potentially significant new developments to aid the capacity planning round.
- *Primary Care/Secondary Care Collaboration*: It is important to ensure a common understanding between primary and secondary care about a consistent approach to clinical responsibilities and funding. For example, it is probable that patients (and their GPs) will benefit if Hospital Pharmacy Services supply greater quantities [of drugs] on discharge. Such arrangements can only be facilitated by a realignment of funding between primary and secondary care.

The DH's reminders underscore the government's commitment to increasing the use of effective new drug therapies. PCTs are expected to set aside adequate funds to meet their NHS prescribing obligations. However, anecdotal evidence indicates that many PCTs have considerable room for improvement in these areas.

In 2002, the Prescribing Research Group (PRG) at the University of Liverpool interviewed 60 key NHS stakeholders about the influence of various cost factors on clinical practice and prescribing behavior. (Interviews were conducted with eight GPs, eight hospital physicians, six health authority pharmaceutical advisers, four PCT prescribing advisers, four practice nurses/advanced nurse practitioners, and an undisclosed number of pharmacists and PCT managers.) Prescribing advisers expressed concern about convincing physicians to comply with budgets and reconciling cost-containment with effective prescribing. Physicians were more interested in making clinically effective decisions than in minimizing costs. Indeed, because of the absence of sanctions, prescribers were generally unconcerned about exceeding their prescribing budgets. Some interviewees from the primary care sector believed that the NHS would not risk harming patient care by penalizing practices that exceed their budgets. The PRG researchers found that many primary care practices deliberately overspend their budgets in order to secure increased funding in subsequent years. Some practices reported that in the past, their efforts to contain costs had been rewarded with budget reductions, while more profligate practices had received increased funding. Similarly, GPs who try to prescribe economically and to remain within their budgets often lose out on financial rewards because colleagues within the same practice exceed their budgets.

The PRG study also found that GPs were not always familiar with the relative costs of various medications. GPs were asked either to rank drugs by price within each of several classes – statins, angiotensin-converting enzyme (ACE) inhibitors, selective serotonin reuptake inhibitors, and proton-pump inhibitors – or to estimate the cost of a 28-day course of therapy with each medicine. All the GPs chose to rank the drugs rather than estimate their price. Their rankings were reasonably accurate for statins and proton-pump inhibitors but poor for other drug classes. When they occasionally do want drug price information, GPs tend to consult their PCT, health authority, or pharmaceutical company representatives. Prescribers regarded measures such as cost-effectiveness and cost-benefit as too complex for use in clinical practice but expressed interest in national guidance based on health economic evaluation.

Influence of the National Institute for Clinical Excellence

In April 1999, the UK government established NICE to guide the NHS in England and Wales in the optimal use of medical technologies. (Northern Ireland and Scotland have their own advisory bodies.) NICE appraises the clinical-effectiveness and cost-effectiveness of health technologies, including pharmaceuticals, medical devices, and medical procedures. Its stated goals include promoting the faster uptake of new interventions and eliminating inequalities in patient access to healthcare.

Since January 1, 2002, PCTs have a statutory obligation to provide funding for NICE-approved therapies within three months of NICE's publication of its decision. However, the PPA has consistently reported that "NICE guidance is not a major driver of growth in volume." Table 11.2 shows the sales evolution from 2001 to 2003 of a selection of drugs that have been appraised by NICE. Pioglitazone, sibutramine, the acetylcholinesterase inhibitors (donepezil, rivastigmine, and galantamine), and rosiglitazone had the largest increases in percentage terms but because of their relatively modest sales in 2001, they made only a minor contribution to overall sales growth in 2003. Combined sales of the drugs listed in Table 11.2 grew by £228 million ($372 million) in 2002, a trend that the PPA attributes largely to NICE's endorsement of most of these therapies.

Conversely, an unfavorable appraisal by NICE can limit a drug's sales potential in the United Kingdom, as illustrated by the experience of influenza therapies. In October 1999, NICE judged that zanamivir (GlaxoSmithKline's Relenza) was not cost effective and therefore should not be prescribed at NHS expense. Based on additional clinical trial data, NICE revised its

Table 11.2 Sales Evolution of Select Drugs Appraised by the United Kingdom's National Institute for Clinical Excellence, 2001–3

Drugs/Drug Class	*Indications*	*Publication Date*[b]	*Sales (£ Million)*[a]			*Prescriptions (Thousands)*		
			2001	*2003*	*Change (%)*	*2001*	*2003*	*Change (%)*
Proton-pump inhibitors	Dyspepsia	July 2000	364.4	419.6	15.2	13,211	17,374	31.5
Rosiglitazone	Type 2 diabetes	August 2000[c]	10.0	26.9	168.8	237	571	141.4
Donepezil, rivastigmine, galantamine	Alzheimer's disease	January 2001	11.0	30.7	179.1	122	351	187.1
Pioglitazone	Type 2 diabetes	March 2001[c]	1.7	8.3	379.8	42	193	356.4
Orlistat	Obesity	March 2001	17.6	21.1	19.7	416	486	16.7
Selective COX-2 inhibitors	Osteoarthritis, rheumatoid arthritis	July 2001	47.8	103.7	116.9	1,944	4,113	111.6
Sibutramine	Obesity	October 2001	2.0	8.5	316.1	53	204	282.3
Atypical antipsychotics	Psychotic disorders	June 2002	114.3	178.1	55.8	1,842	3,089	67.7

[a]Sales at net ingredient cost (i.e., pharmacy acquisition prices)
[b]Publication date of relevant guidance from NICE
[c]Superseded guidance published in October 1999 and November 2000

opinion in November 2000 and recommended use of the drug in "at-risk patients." However, the initial adverse judgment caused lasting damage to this drug class, and the PPA reports that NHS sales of zanamivir and oseltamivir (Roche's Tamiflu) totaled only £25,400 ($41,500) in 2003.

The PRG study found that the NHS stakeholders they interviewed had a high level of awareness of NICE guidance but had some misgivings about its impact on clinical practice. Interviewees were concerned about a lack of funding to support the implementation of NICE recommendations. Respondents also disagreed with some of NICE's decisions. Similarly, a 2001 survey published in *BMA News*, the newsletter of the British Medical Association, found that 74% of UK physicians disagreed with at least one NICE decision and 85% were prepared to ignore NICE guidance if they considered it wrong.

One of the UK government's key objectives in establishing NICE was to eliminate the "postcode lottery" – the problem of geographic inequalities in access to innovative medicines. However, notwithstanding the PCTs' statutory obligation to provide funding for NICE-approved therapies, access to novel therapies remains highly variable.

Another problem is the phenomenon known as "NICE blight," a twofold restraint on prescribing. Health authorities and PCTs may impose prescribing restrictions on a therapy either because they are awaiting the outcome of a NICE appraisal currently in progress or because they expect NICE to appraise the therapy in the future. Data compiled by the DH indicate that a favorable NICE appraisal can stimulate a sudden surge in demand for a therapy, a tendency that appears to confirm the existence of NICE blight. For instance, hospital prescriptions for paclitaxel, vinorelbine, docetaxel, and gemcitabine increased exponentially following NICE's favorable appraisal of the use of these drugs in ovarian cancer and advanced breast cancer.

Focus on Clinical Priority Areas

In April 1998, as part of its NHS modernization agenda, the UK government initiated a continuous program of NSFs. These guidelines are designed to improve the quality of care and reduce variations in service in the following ways:

- Setting national standards and defining service models for a defined service or care group.
- Putting in place strategies to support implementation.
- Establishing performance milestones against which progress will be measured.

Thus far, the government has published NSFs for mental health (September 1999); coronary heart disease (CHD, March 2000); cancer (September 2000); the treatment of older patients (March 2001); diabetes (December 2001 and January 2003); the first part of the guidelines on children's services (April 2003); and renal services (January 2004). An NSF on long-term conditions (with emphasis on neurological disorders) is in preparation. The DH estimates that NSFs were largely responsible for increasing the growth rate in pharmaceutical expenditures from an average of 8% in the preceding five years to 10% in the 2001–2 financial year.

Because PCTs are audited on their compliance with NSFs, these guidelines have a significant bearing on primary care prescribing practice. The Tracker Survey found that 71% of primary care organization prescribing leads (key decision makers in local primary care prescribing policy) considered NSFs to be a strong influence on their practices' prescribing targets and priorities, particularly the CHD framework. An NHS Alliance survey in 2001 reported that 46% of primary care personnel (including GPs) believed that clinical decisions are or may be compromised by the need to observe NSFs. Furthermore, 36% believed that NSFs placed them under "undue or inappropriate pressure." The PRG study also found that NHS stakeholders believed that NSFs can increase the workload in primary care practices and, by raising costs, intensify the pressure on GPs.

Use of Generics

The UK generics market is the second largest in Europe. The DH reports that in 2002 net ingredient costs for generics dispensed in England totaled £1.3 billion ($2.1 billion), equivalent in monetary terms to 19.9% of the total pharmaceutical market. Generics penetration rates are also among the highest in Europe. In 1991, 41% of prescriptions in England were written generically, and 35% were dispensed generically. By 2002, the generics prescribing rate in England had risen to 76%, and the generics dispensing rate had risen to 53%. Figure 11.1 shows the evolution of generics prescribing and dispensing rates in England.

The NHS encourages rather than compels physicians and pharmacists to use generics whenever possible. Trainee physicians are taught to prescribe drugs using their international, nonproprietary name, even if products are still patent-protected. Computerized prescribing systems notify physicians of generic alternatives to drugs they propose to prescribe. In addition, pharmacists have financial incentives to source the lowest-priced generics available.

Price differentials between originator drugs and generics tend to be much greater in the United Kingdom than in other European countries. The extremely low prices in the United Kingdom are attributable in part to the dominance of unbranded generics in this market. Ex-manufacturer prices in the United Kingdom often drop by 70–80% within four years of a drug's patent expiration, compared with an average decline of just 30% in Germany and even less in other major markets in Europe. Price reductions in the United Kingdom can be extremely dramatic. For instance, the day after captopril's UK patent expired, competition from 13 generics reduced prices by 50–60%. Within a week of patent expiration, generic captopril was available at just 20% of the original branded price. Similarly, the price of fluoxetine declined by 77% within nine months of that molecule's patent expiration.

Parallel Imports

The United Kingdom is Europe's largest parallel import market, and this trade has

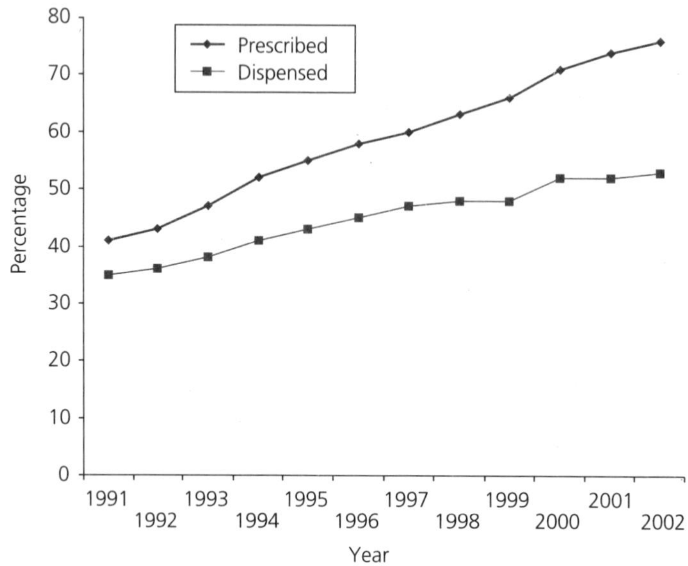

Figure 11.1 Percentage of Prescriptions Prescribed and Dispensed Generically in England, 1991–2002

flourished in recent years. A study by authors at the York Health Economics Consortium (West and Mahon, 2003) reported that parallel imports jumped from £462 million ($755 million) in 1998 to £1.35 billion ($2.2 billion) in 2002, an increase of 191% in just four years. Parallel imports' share of the total pharmaceutical market grew from 9.5% in 1998 to 19.8% in 2002. Recently, however, the growth of parallel imports has slowed. According to IMS Health, parallel imports into the United Kingdom in 2003 increased by just 1%. The parallel import market focuses on a limited number of drugs but is becoming less concentrated: in 2002, just 12 products accounted for 50% of total sales of parallel imports, but in 2003, 15 products accounted for 50% of this market.

The NHS actively promotes parallel importing. As we explained earlier in the report, prices listed in the official Drug Tariff are discounted by a small percentage (the clawback) to reflect possible discounts to the pharmacy from wholesalers and further adjusted for patient copayments collected in the pharmacy. As an incentive to seek low-cost sources of supply, such as parallel imports and the least expensive generics, retail pharmacists are allowed to retain the difference between their drug acquisition price and the reimbursed price based on the Drug Tariff. Clawback recoups for the NHS some of the savings that come from the use of parallel imports. The DH surveys the average level of discounts and sets a high clawback rate for all pharmacies, regardless of how many (if any) parallel imports they have dispensed. This clawback payment is then automatically deducted from pharmacists' reimbursement payments for the following year. Pharmacists who do not dispense any parallel imports are in effect required to pay back a discount they never received. This plan provides pharmacists with a powerful incentive to dispense parallel imports whenever possible, a situation that accounts for parallel imports' substantial market share in the United Kingdom.

The benefits of parallel trade are hotly disputed throughout Europe. Pharmaceutical manufacturers argue that parallel traders are the main beneficiaries of this trade, but parallel traders insist they save healthcare payers substantial sums on their pharmaceutical expenditures. Recent studies have merely served to fuel the debate. For instance, the authors of the York Health Economics Consortium study calculated that parallel imports saved the NHS €342 million ($386 million) in 2002. (For the sake of uniformity of the analysis, the euro-to-dollar exchange rate used herein is the 2003 average rate [i.e., $1 = €0.8854].) However, a study by the London School of Economics (LSE) estimated that, if the effect of the clawback is included, parallel imports saved the NHS €55.9 million ($63.1 million). Moreover, if the effect of the clawback is excluded, the savings to the NHS amounted to only €6.9 million ($7.8 million). By comparison, the LSE study reported that parallel trade's net benefits to parallel traders totaled €518 million ($585 million) if the effect of clawback is included and €469.5 ($530.3 million) if the effect of clawback is excluded.

Patient Copayments

Drugs and devices prescribed by GPs are subject to a patient copayment for each item on the prescription. This flat fee is independent of the cost of the product. The fee has risen from 20 pence (33 cents) in 1979 to £6.40 ($10.45) in April 2004. Approximately 60% of prescriptions cost less than the current prescription charge. However, most prescriptions are exempt from copayments. For example, patients aged 60 or older, children younger than age 16, students aged 16–18 in full-time education, pregnant women and mothers of children less than a year old, the unemployed, and patients suffering from certain chronic diseases (e.g., diabetes) are all exempt. About half of the UK population belongs to one of these categories, but because these patients include the most frequent consumers of pharmaceuticals, they accounted for more than 85.7% of all prescriptions in 2002. Consequently, patient copayments in the United Kingdom are probably more important as a revenue source for the NHS than as a cost-containment measure. We estimate that prescription charges contributed £550 million ($898 million) to NHS funds in 2002.

General Medical Services Contracts

Since April 1, 2004, GPs are subject to a new contract for general medical services (GMS). This agreement is intended to increase the level of support for the primary care sector and thereby improve the quality of patient care. One element of this contract is "a quality and outcomes framework which [provides] resources and rewards GPs on the basis of how well they care for patients rather than simply the number of patients they treat, leading to good chronic disease management in the community and relieving pressures on hospitals." The quality and outcomes framework will cover the following disorders:

- Secondary prevention in coronary heart disease
- Stroke or transient ischemic attacks
- Hypertension
- Diabetes
- Chronic obstructive pulmonary disorder
- Epilepsy
- Hypothyroidism
- Cancer
- Mental health
- Asthma

Most of these indications coincide with the NSFs, confirming the government's policy of prioritizing diseases that cause the greatest burden to society. To qualify for maximum rewards, GPs will likely need to make extensive use of drug therapy, and the government accepts that prescription volume and cost may therefore increase.

REIMBURSEMENT OF HOSPITAL MEDICINES

General Features

Based on data from IMS Health and the DH, we estimate that ex-manufacturer sales of pharmaceuticals in hospitals in the United Kingdom totaled £1.9 billion ($3.1 billion) in 2002. This sum was equivalent to 21% of the total UK pharmaceutical market in that year.

As we mentioned previously, the DH and the ABPI published a joint study in

December 2002 entitled *PPRS: The Study into the Extent of Competition in the Supply of Branded Medicines to the NHS*. This wide-ranging report included an analysis of the hospital sector. The authors found that the hospital market was less concentrated than the retail pharmaceutical market: in the 12 months up to and including April 2002, the top-10 manufacturers of branded medicines had a collective market share of 45.2% in the hospital sector, compared with a combined market share of 58.8% for the top-10 companies in the retail sector.

Products used exclusively in hospitals are not subject to drug tariff listing. These products therefore have automatic admission to reimbursement.

Supply-side Restrictions

The PPRS regulates the profitability of branded medicines sold to hospitals in exactly the same manner as drugs sold in retail pharmacies.

Demand-side Restrictions

NHS hospitals receive most of their funding from their local PCTs, and hospital budgets are divided among the various clinical directorates. In the case of the drug budget, the hospital pharmacy seeks to monitor and control spending by each clinical directorate, but most hospitals exceed their overall pharmaceutical budgets. A survey conducted by the Audit Commission in 2001 found that one-third of NHS trusts exceeded their pharmaceutical budgets by more than 10% in the 2000–1 financial year and 6% of trusts were more than 25% over budget. (See A Spoonful of Sugar: Medicines Management in NHS Hospitals. Audit Commission/ Her Majesty's Stationery Office, 2001.) Figure 11.2 shows the level of overspending in NHS trusts. If a budget is exceeded, hospital managers must decide whether they can balance the budget internally or need to approach the local SHA or PCT with a request for additional funding.

Because their budgets are fixed, NHS hospitals have an incentive to seek low-cost sources of supply. Most hospitals operate formularies that restrict prescribing, and hospital pharmacies demand significant discounts on Drug Tariff prices as a condition of admission to their formularies. The drug and therapeutics committee (DTC) in each hospital is usually responsible for deciding the composition of the formulary. A subcommittee, the new drugs committee, may assess novel therapies in some institutions. In some

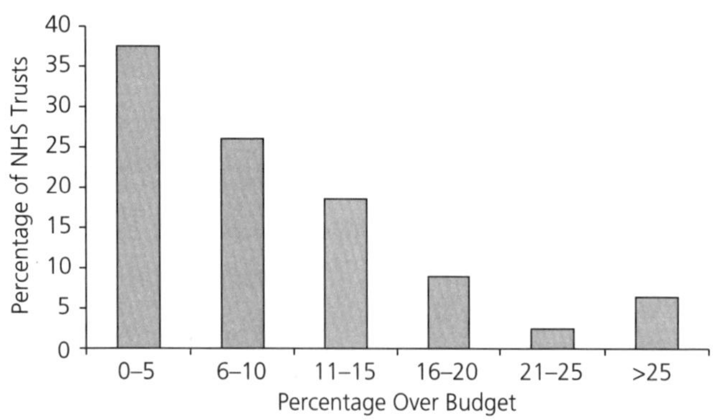

NHS = National Health Service
Note: Based on a sample of 157 NHS trusts

Figure 11.2 Percentage of NHS Trusts That Overspent Their Pharmaceutical Budgets by Various Margins, 2000–1

hospitals, a committee of senior managers makes formulary decisions based on the DTC's evidence-based recommendations.

Pharmaceutical companies are motivated to offer discounts by the prospect of securing greater sales in the much larger primary care market, given that GPs usually keep patients on the medication originally prescribed in hospital. A study conducted by the Audit Commission in 1994 found that approximately 18% of GP prescribing was initiated in the hospital and about 40% was strongly influenced by hospital prescribing. (See A Prescription for Improvement – Toward More Rational Prescribing in General Practice. Audit Commission/Her Majesty's Stationery Office, 1994.) However, respondents to the DH/ABPI survey generally expressed the view that, thanks to improvements in the quality of prescribing guidance available in the primary care sector, "GPs were much less likely [than in the past] to slavishly follow hospital prescribing." As a result, some companies had begun to question the benefits of heavy discounting and consequently to moderate the level of their discounts. The DH/ABPI study reported that the unweighted mean discount offered to hospitals in March 2000 was 28%. The level of discounting depended on the general value of a given market, the availability of generics, and a hospital's negotiating power. If no generic was available, the mean discount was 16.2% in low-value markets and 22.7% in high-value markets. However, if generics were available, the mean discount rose to 28.3% in low-value markets and 44.3% in high-value markets.

In 1994, the DH began a process to encourage greater cooperation between the primary and secondary care sectors in prescribing practice. A key feature of this initiative was the creation of area-prescribing committees (APCs) – bodies that brought together hospital clinicians and pharmacists, GPs, and representatives of local healthcare management to provide guidance on good prescribing practice. Most APCs originally reported to the 95 health authorities that existed at the time. A survey of 77 APCs conducted by the NPC in 2000 found that 50% of these committees formally reported to their local health authority board and another 16% reported to the health authority's executive or management team. In the future, however, PCTs – as the dominant fund holders in the NHS – are likely to become the key stakeholders in APCs. The NPC survey found that 53% of APCs met bimonthly, 32% quarterly, and 7% monthly.

Hospitals and PCTs are increasingly developing joint formularies. A survey conducted by Pharmacy Management in May and June 2003 found that of the 223 participating PCTs, 47% shared a formulary with a local hospital.

In January 2003, the DH issued guidelines to PCTs on setting prescribing budgets for the next several years. The document stated, "It is important to ensure a common understanding between primary and secondary care about a consistent approach to clinical responsibilities and funding. For example, it is probable that patients (and their GPs) will benefit if Hospital Pharmacy Services supply greater quantities of drugs on discharge. Such arrangements can only be facilitated by a realignment of funding between primary and secondary care." Consequently, the boundary between primary and secondary care is likely to become increasingly blurred in the coming years.

SALES AND PRESCRIBING TRENDS

Market Overview

According to IMS Health, 2003 ex-manufacturer pharmaceutical sales in UK retail pharmacies totaled $12.9 billion, a 19% increase if the depreciation of the US dollar against the pound sterling is taken into account. Using constant exchange rates, the market grew by 9% – a faster rate than all other major European markets except Spain.

Using data from the DH and the Office of Health Economics, we estimate that the net ingredient costs (i.e., pharmacy acquisition costs) of medicines dispensed by retail

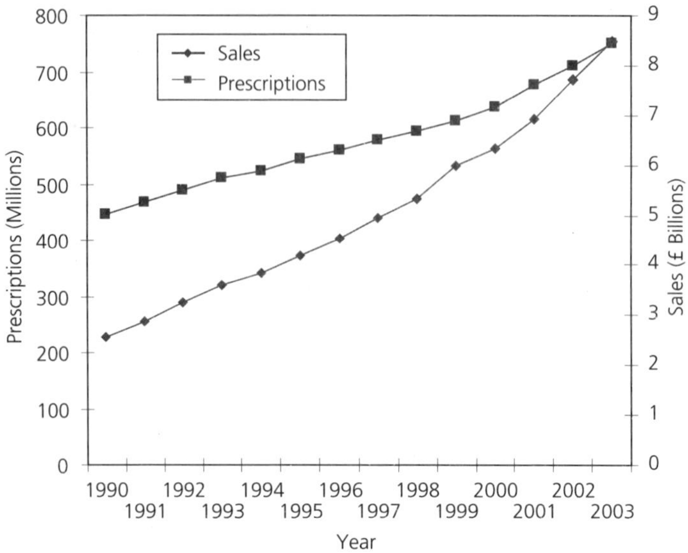

Note: Figures for 2003 are estimates. Sales are expressed at the level of net ingredient costs

Figure 11.3 Evolution of Sales and Prescriptions in UK Retail Pharmacies, 1990–2003

pharmacies in the United Kingdom in 2003 totaled £8.5 billion ($13.8 billion), a 10% increase over the preceding year. If the standard 12.5% wholesaler margin is deducted from this figure, sales amounted to $12.3 billion at ex-manufacturer prices, a sum comparable with IMS Health's calculation. Figure 11.3 shows the evolution of sales (at net ingredient costs) and prescriptions in UK retail pharmacies from 1990 to 2003. We estimate that the total number of prescriptions grew from 447 million in 1990 to 750 million in 2003, an increase of 68% in 13 years, equivalent to a compound growth rate of 4.1% per year. However, sales grew more than twice as fast as prescriptions, rising from £2.6 billion ($4.2 billion) in 1990 to £8.5 billion ($13.8 billion) in 2003, an increase of 231%, or 9.6% per year. The PPA has attributed recent growth in the volume of prescriptions largely to the stimulus of NSFs.

We estimate that the average net ingredient cost of prescriptions dispensed by retail pharmacies in the United Kingdom increased from £5.74 ($9.37) in 1990 to £11.30 ($18.46) in 2003, an increase of 97% in 13 years, or 5.4% per year. Figure 11.4 traces the evolution of average net ingredient costs for prescriptions over this period.

Despite the steady growth in prescribing, NHS per capita spending on pharmaceuticals amounted to only £137 ($224) per year in 2002, a much lower figure than in the United States, Japan, and most other EU countries. On its web site, the ABPI notes that per capita annual pharmaceutical expenditure was significantly higher in most other major pharmaceutical markets (e.g., £437 [$714] in the United States, £292 [$477] in Japan, £203 [$332] in France). The United Kingdom also lags behind other leading pharmaceutical markets in the adoption of new medicines. Figure 11.5 shows the 2002 market share in several major pharmaceutical markets of drugs that were launched in the preceding five years. New drugs' market share was much lower in the United Kingdom (15.5%) than in almost all other

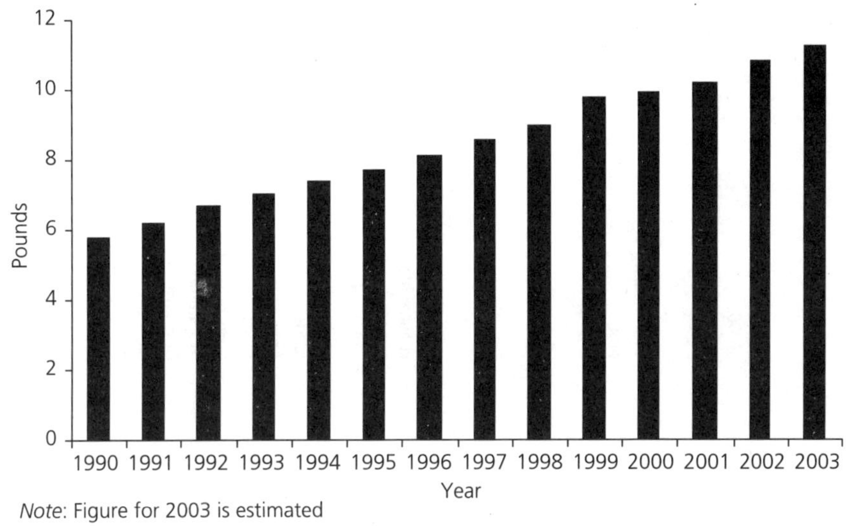

Figure 11.4 Average Net Ingredient Cost of Prescriptions Dispensed by Retail Pharmacies in the United Kingdom, 1990–2003

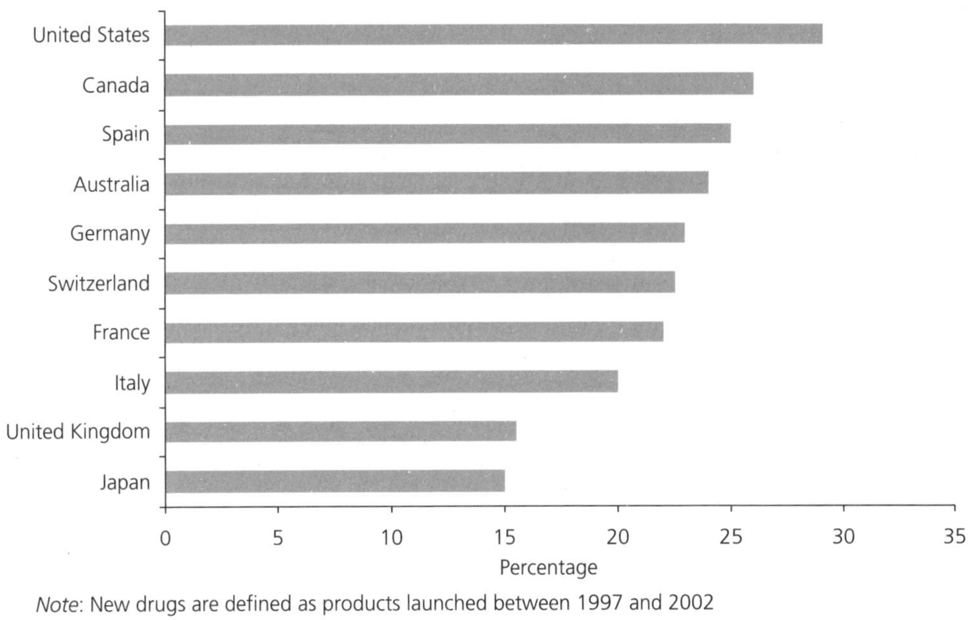

Figure 11.5 New Drugs' Market Share in Select Countries, 2002

major pharmaceutical markets and was barely half the penetration rate in the United States (29%). The systematic bias in favor of low-priced, unbranded generics and the enormous price advantage of these drugs help explain the United Kingdom's generally conservative prescribing culture and its slow adoption of new therapies.

Although the pharmaceutical industry, physicians, and patients frequently express frustration at this conservatism, some influential observers of the NHS believe that it

Table 11.3 Top 20 Drug Classes in England, Ranked by Annual Sales, 1998–2003

Rank	*1998*		*1999*		*2000*	
	Drug Class	Sales (*£ MM)*	*Drug Class*	Sales (*£ MM)*	*Drug Class*	*Sales (£ MM)*
1	Ulcer-healing drugs	432.2	Ulcer-healing drugs	448.9	Ulcer-healing drugs	412.9
2	Nitrates, calcium-channel blockers, potassium-channel activators	309.0	Nitrates, calcium-channel blockers, potassium-channel activators	338.5	Antihypertensives	362.6
3	Antihypertensives	280.1	Antihypertensives	336.1	Nitrates, calcium-channel blockers, potassium-channel activators	348.2
4	Antidepressant drugs	279.0	Antidepressant drugs	315.3	Lipid-regulating drugs	326.1
5	Corticosteroids (respiratory)	266.9	Corticosteroids (respiratory)	274.5	Antidepressant drugs	310.4
6	Bronchodilators	220.0	Lipid-regulating drugs	256.4	Corticosteroids (respiratory)	283.2
7	Lipid-regulating drugs	190.0	Bronchodilators	230.9	Drugs used in diabetes	230.3
8	Analgesics	186.8	Analgesics	213.7	Bronchodilators	230.3
9	Drugs used in rheumatic diseases and gout	168.0	Drugs used in diabetes	201.0	Analgesics	224.6
10	Drugs used in diabetes	167.0	Drugs used in rheumatic diseases and	188.0	Drugs used in rheumatic diseases and gout	195.0

			gout			
11	Antibacterial drugs	163.0	Antibacterial drugs	177.1	Antibacterial drugs	172.2
12	Sex hormones	146.8	Sex hormones	154.4	Sex hormones	157.0
13	Vaccines and antisera	94.4	Sex hormones and antagonists in malignant disease	106.1	Sex hormones and antagonists in malignant disease	122.4
14	Sex hormones and antagonists in malignant disease	88.2	Vaccines and antisera	96.0	Vaccines and antisera	107.8
15	Beta-adrenoceptor-blocking drugs	76.5	Beta-adrenoceptor-blocking drugs	90.2	Drugs used in psychoses and related disorders	100.2
16	Antiepileptics	74.9	Antiepileptics	86.5	Antiepileptics	99.1
17	Drugs used in psychoses and related disorders	60.5	Drugs used in psychoses and related disorders	81.3	Beta-adrenoceptor-blocking drugs	91.6
18	Drugs affecting the immune response	53.8	Diuretics	77.2	Diuretics	84.5
19	Hypothalamic and pituitary hormones and antiestrogens	49.1	Drugs for genitourinary disorders	64.1	Drugs for genitourinary disorders	81.3
20	Laxatives	47.0	Drugs affecting the immune response	61.2	Drugs affecting the immune response	64.3

(continued)

Rank	2001		2002		2003	
	Drug Class	*Sales (£ MM)*	*Drug Class*	*Sales (£ MM)*	*Drug Class*	*Sales (£ MM)*
1	Lipid-regulating drugs	438.8	Lipid-regulating drugs	571.0	Lipid-regulating drugs	715.0
2	Antihypertensives	420.6	Antihypertensives	506.5	Antihypertensives	575.8
3	Ulcer-healing drugs	418.9	Ulcer-healing drugs	455.4	Ulcer-healing drugs	466.5
4	Nitrates, calcium-channel blockers, potassium-channel activators	366.7	Nitrates, calcium-channel blockers, potassium-channel activators	383.1	Nitrates, calcium-channel blockers, potassium-channel activators	403.9
5	Antidepressant drugs	341.7	Antidepressant drugs	380.9	Antidepressant drugs	395.2
6	Corticosteroids (respiratory)	308.7	Corticosteroids (respiratory)	338.1	Drugs used in diabetes	391.1
7	Drugs used in diabetes	278.6	Drugs used in diabetes	335.9	Corticosteroids (respiratory)	363.2
8	Bronchodilators	238.5	Analgesics	253.3	Analgesics	273.9
9	Analgesics	234.4	Bronchodilators	239.6	Drugs used in rheumatic diseases and gout	247.1
10	Drugs used in rheumatic diseases and gout	196.1	Drugs used in rheumatic diseases and gout	220.2	Bronchodilators	245.6

11	Sex hormones	164.9	Drugs used in psychoses and related disorders	165.3	Drugs used in psychoses and related disorders	197.3
12	Antibacterial drugs	162.8	Antibacterial drugs	164.4	Sex hormones and antagonists in malignant disease	181.1
13	Sex hormones and antagonists in malignant disease	140.0	Sex hormones and antagonists in malignant disease	161.7	Antibacterial drugs	168.8
14	Drugs used in psychoses and related disorders	132.8	Sex hormones	161.1	Antiepileptics	165.8
15	Antiepileptics	120.4	Antiepileptics	142.2	Drugs for genitourinary disorders	137.9
16	Vaccines and antisera	107.0	Drugs for genitourinary disorders	121.1	Sex hormones	137.7
17	Drugs for genitourinary disorders	100.7	Vaccines and antisera	106.9	Vaccines and antisera	111.9
18	Beta-adrenoceptor-blocking drugs	81.6	Beta-adrenoceptor-blocking drugs	88.8	Antiplatelet drugs	110.8
19	Drugs affecting the immune response	69.4	Antiplatelet drugs	81.1	Drugs affecting bone metabolism	97.8
20	Treatment of glaucoma	65.6	Drugs affecting the immune response	73.6	Beta-adrenoceptor-blocking drugs	94.5

Notes: Drug classes are classified according to paragraph definitions in the *British National Formulary* (*BNF*). Sales figures are net ingredient costs in millions of pounds has certain merits. In April 2002, Derek Wanless, the author of *Securing Our Future Health: Taking a Long-Term View*, a government commissioned, independent review of NHS resource requirements, suggested that "it is, of course, possible that some other countries adopt new technologies too quickly. Being quick is not necessarily a good thing if the technology is found not to be effective. The appropriate response to new technologies is for rapid and consistent diffusion across the health service once robust evidence of their cost-effectiveness is available." If the NHS heeds this advice, NICE's influence on prescribing patterns is likely to grow substantially in the coming years.

Leading Drug Classes

The UK pharmaceutical market is dominated by a limited number of drug classes. Indeed, the 20 best-selling drug classes (as defined by the *British National Formulary*) consistently account for more than 70% of total sales, and their share is growing steadily. According to PPA data, the top-20 drug classes' combined share of pharmaceutical sales in England increased from 71.3% in 1998 to 73% in 2003. Their combined share of the total volume of prescriptions in England increased from 56.8% in 1998 to 60.9% in 2003.

Table 11.3 lists the 20 best-selling drug classes in England in each year from 1998 to 2003. Most of the 20 best-selling drug classes in 1998 remained among the top-20 in 2003. Only drugs affecting the immune response, hypothalamic and pituitary hormones and antiestrogens, and laxatives – ranked 18 to 20, respectively, in 1998 – were displaced in 2003, by drugs for genitourinary disorders, antiplatelet drugs, and drugs affecting bone metabolism. However, some rankings *within* the 20 best-selling drug classes changed substantially. In particular, lipid-regulating drugs and antihypertensives overtook ulcer-healing drugs and nitrates, calcium-channel blockers, and potassium-channel activators as the best-selling drug classes in England in 2003.

Table 11.4 traces the sales evolution from 1998 to 2003 of the 20 best-selling drug classes (in monetary terms) in 2003. Sales of all but one of these drug classes (i.e., sex hormones) grew over the period under review, but some classes grew vigorously while others managed only very small increases. Figure 11.6 illustrates the differing fortunes of the five best-selling drug classes in 2003.

Not surprisingly, drug classes that fall within the clinical priority areas targeted by the NSFs – notably coronary heart disease, mental health, cancer, and diabetes – have experienced the greatest growth in recent years. Among the top-20 drug classes in England, sales of drug classes that are promoted in NSFs increased from £1.5 billion ($2.4 billion) in 1998 to £3.2 billion ($5.2 billion) in 2003: lipid-regulating drugs, antihypertensives, nitrates, calcium-channel blockers and potassium-channel activators, antidepressants, drugs used in diabetes, drugs used in psychoses and related diseases, sex hormones and antagonists in malignant disease, antiepileptics, antiplatelet drugs, and beta-adrenoceptor-blocking drugs. If drugs outside the 20 best-selling BNF drug classes and drugs related to other NSFs were included, NSF-promoted medicines would make an even larger contribution to the overall growth of the market.

Lipid-regulating drugs achieved by far the largest growth in absolute terms: a sales increase of £525 million ($857 million) in five years. As noted earlier, the DH's guidelines to PCTs on setting prescribing budgets draw attention to the fact that "national expenditure on statins continues to increase by around 30% year on year." The government appears sanguine about increased spending on drug classes that are promoted by NSFs. The prescribing budget guidelines state that "the financial implications of NSFs have been factored into unified allocations and PCTs should ensure adequate provision [for them] in primary care budgets."

Ulcer-healing drugs, the top-ranked drug class in 1998, fared less well than

Table 11.4 Sales Trends, 1998–2003, of the 20 Best-Selling Drug Classes in England in 2003

Drug Class[a]	*Total Net Ingredient Costs (£ millions)*							
	1998	*1999*	*2000*	*2001*	*2002*	*2003*	*Change*[b] *(%)*	*CGR (%)*
Lipid-regulating drugs	190.0	256.4	326.1	438.8	571.0	715.0	276.4	30.4
Antihypertensives	280.1	336.1	362.6	420.6	506.5	575.8	105.6	15.5
Ulcer-healing drugs	432.2	448.9	412.9	418.9	455.4	466.5	7.9	1.5
Nitrates, calcium-channel blockers, potassium-channel activators	309.0	338.5	362.6	366.7	383.1	403.9	30.7	5.5
Antidepressant drugs	279.0	315.3	310.4	341.7	380.9	395.2	41.6	7.2
Drugs used in diabetes	167.0	188.0	230.3	278.6	335.9	391.1	134.1	18.5
Corticosteroids (respiratory)	266.9	274.5	283.2	308.7	338.1	363.2	36.1	6.4
Analgesics	186.8	213.7	224.6	234.4	253.3	273.9	46.6	8.0
Drugs used in rheumatic diseases and gout	168.0	201.0	195.0	196.1	220.2	247.1	47.1	8.0
Bronchodilators	220.0	256.4	230.3	238.5	239.6	245.6	11.6	2.2
Drugs used in psychoses and related disorders	60.5	81.3	100.2	132.8	165.3	197.3	226.4	26.7
Sex hormones and antagonists in malignant disease	88.2	106.1	122.4	140.0	161.7	181.1	105.2	15.5
Antibacterial drugs	163.0	177.1	172.2	162.8	164.4	168.8	3.6	0.7
Antiepileptics	74.9	86.5	99.1	120.4	142.2	165.8	121.5	17.2
Drugs for genitourinary disorders	45.3	64.1	81.3	100.7	121.1	137.9	204.1	24.9
Sex hormones	146.8	154.4	157.0	164.9	161.1	137.7	(6.2)	(1.3)
Vaccines and antisera	94.4	96.0	107.8	107.0	106.9	111.9	18.5	3.4
Antiplatelet drugs	10.4	20.9	35.1	51.0	81.1	110.8	967.7	60.6
Drugs affecting bone metabolism	32.0	38.3	43.3	55.0	73.5	97.8	206.1	25.1
Beta-adrenoceptor-blocking drugs	76.5	90.2	91.6	81.6	88.8	96.8	26.6	4.8

[a]Drug classes are classified according to paragraph definitions in the *British National Formulary (BNF)*
[b]Percentage change from 1998 to 2003
CGR = Cumulative growth rate

NSF-promoted drug classes. Sales of ulcerzhealing drugs grew from £432.2 million ($705.9 million) in 1998 to £466.5 million ($761.9 million) in 2003, a 7.9% increase, equivalent to 1.5% per year. In July 2000, NICE published a technology appraisal that recommended more conservative use of proton-pump inhibitors in the management of dyspepsia. But this guidance has done little to slow the prescription of ulcer-healing drugs. Indeed, the total number of prescriptions for ulcer-healing drugs in England increased from 15.1 million in 1998 to 22.4 million in 2003, a 48.2% increase. However, this drug class's modest growth in monetary terms was attributable to a decline in the average net ingredient cost of a prescription from £28.60 ($46.71) in 1998 to £20.83 ($34.02) in 2003, a decline of 27.2%. The expiration in May 2002 of the patent on the leading proton-pump inhibitor, AstraZeneca's Losec (omeprazole), contributed to the downward trend in prices of ulcer-healing drugs.

Table 11.5 shows prescribing trends from 1998 to 2003 for the 20 drug classes that achieved the highest sales in England in 2003. Drugs affecting bone metabolism had the fastest growth rate: 293.8% in five years, equivalent to 31.5% per year. Antihypertensives had a slower growth rate (16.9% per year) but had the strongest growth in absolute terms, increasing from 15.4 million prescriptions in 1998 to

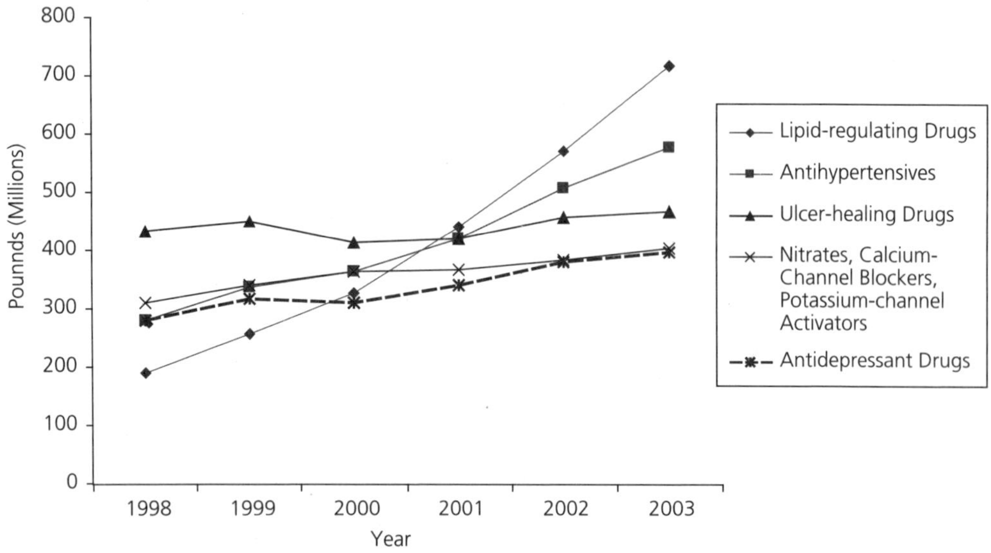

Note: Sales are expressed at the level of net ingredient costs

Figure 11.6 Sales of the Five Best-Selling Drug Classes in England, 1998–2003

Table 11.5 Table 11.5 Prescribing Trends, 1998–2003, of the 20 Best-Selling Drug Classes in England in 2003

	Millions of Prescriptions							
Drug Class[a]	*1998*	*1999*	*2000*	*2001*	*2002*	*2003*	*Change*[b] *(%)*	*CGR (%)*
Lipid-regulating drugs	6.0	7.9	10.3	13.5	17.6	22.7	278.7	30.5
Antihypertensives	15.4	17.9	21.1	25.0	29.6	33.8	118.7	16.9
Ulcer-healing drugs	15.1	16.1	17.2	19.0	20.6	22.4	48.2	8.2
Nitrates, calcium-channel blockers, potassium-channel activators	23.4	24.3	21.1	26.8	28.0	29.2	24.7	4.5
Antidepressant drugs	18.4	20.1	22.0	24.3	26.3	27.7	50.1	8.5
Drugs used in diabetes	12.7	21.3	15.9	18.1	20.3	22.3	75.7	11.9
Corticosteroids (respiratory)	11.9	11.9	12.0	12.4	12.8	12.9	8.9	1.7
Analgesics	41.5	42.7	42.8	44.0	44.7	45.8	10.2	2.0
Drugs used in rheumatic diseases and gout	21.0	14.2	21.7	22.5	23.2	23.9	14.1	2.7
Bronchodilators	24.2	7.9	24.3	24.9	25.0	24.6	1.9	0.4
Drugs used in psychoses and related disorders	5.4	5.6	5.9	5.7	6.0	6.4	18.1	3.4
Sex hormones and antagonists in malignant disease	1.7	1.7	1.8	1.9	1.9	2.0	17.6	3.3
Antibacterial drugs	42.6	38.6	36.9	37.9	37.0	37.6	(11.8)	(2.5)
Antiepileptics	6.1	6.4	6.7	7.2	7.6	8.1	32.0	5.7
Drugs for genitourinary disorders	2.3	2.9	3.6	4.2	4.8	5.3	137.2	18.9
Sex hormones	7.2	7.3	7.5	7.6	7.4	6.5	(10.2)	(2.1)
Vaccines and antisera	10.8	11.3	13.0	12.9	12.6	13.1	21.1	3.9
Antiplatelet drugs	12.2	14.6	16.6	18.9	21.6	24.4	100.7	14.9
Drugs affecting bone metabolism	0.7	0.9	1.0	1.4	2.1	2.9	293.8	31.5
Beta-adrenoceptor-blocking drugs	15.3	16.6	18.3	20.4	22.4	24.3	58.9	9.7

[a]Drug classes are classified according to paragraph definitions in the *British National Formulary (BNF)*
[b]Percentage change from 1998 to 2003
CGR = Cumulative growth rate
Note: Drugs are listed in the order of their sales rankings, not their volume of prescriptions

33.8 million prescriptions in 2003. A comparison of Tables 11.3 and 11.4 reveals that, in addition to the aforementioned ulcer-healing drugs, many other drug classes had significant disparities between their growth rates for sales and prescriptions. Drugs used in diabetes, respiratory corticosteroids, analgesics, drugs used in rheumatic diseases and gout, bronchodilators, drugs used in psychoses and related disorders, sex hormones and antagonists used in malignant disease, antiepileptics, drugs for genitourinary disorders, and antiplatelet drugs all experienced much stronger growth in sales than in prescriptions, indicating that the average cost of prescriptions in these drug classes increased over the review period. On the other hand, ulcer-healing drugs, antidepressants, antibacterial drugs, drugs affecting bone metabolism, and beta-adrenoceptor-blocking drugs all had higher growth rates for prescriptions than sales, indicating that the average cost of prescriptions in these classes declined from 1998 to 2003.

Leading Molecules

The 20 best-selling molecules in England together account for approximately one-third of total sales of prescription drugs in England. In 2003, their market share amounted to 32.9%. Total net ingredient costs of the 20 best-selling molecules increased from £1.6 billion ($2.6 billion) in 1998 to £2.5 billion ($4.1 billion) in 2003, a 56% increase.

The list of the top-20 molecules is much more volatile than the list of the top-20 drug classes. Table 11.6 shows that only 11 of the drugs that ranked among the 20 best-selling molecules in 1998 were still among the top-20 five years later: omeprazole, beclomethasone, simvastatin, amlodipine, lansoprazole, salbutamol, paroxetine, salmeterol, lisinopril, fluticasone, and goserelin. Ranitidine, fluoxetine, diclofenac, enalapril, nifedipine, budesonide, isosorbide mononitrate, sertraline, and biphasic isophane insulin all dropped out of the list of the 20 best-selling molecules by 2003. They

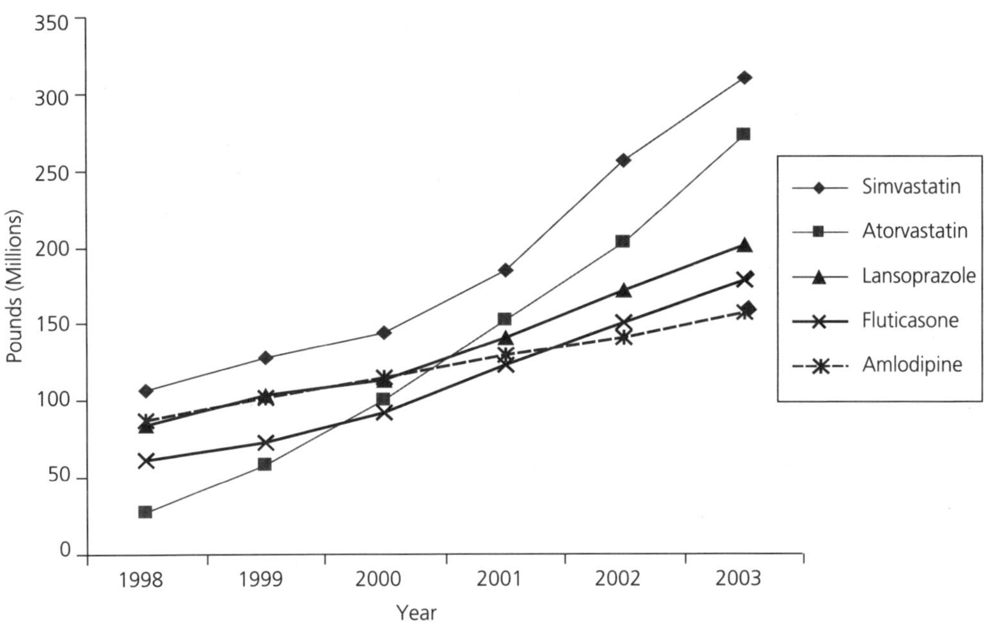

Note: Sales are expressed at the level of net ingredient costs

Figure 11.7 Sales Evolution, 1998–2003, of the Five Best-Selling Molecules in England in 2003

Table 11.6 Top 20 Molecules in England, Ranked by Annual Sales, 1998–2003

Rank	*1998*		*1999*		*2000*	
	Molecule	*Sales (£MM)*	*Molecule*	*Sales (£ MM)*	*Molecule*	*Sales (£ MM)*
1	Omeprazole	196.7	Omeprazole	201.4	Omeprazole	183.5
2	Beclomethasone	144.3	Beclomethasone	143.9	Simvastatin	144.1
3	Simvastatin	106.3	Simvastatin	128.4	Beclomethasone	138.9
4	Ranitidine	104.5	Lansoprazole	104.1	Amlodipine	115.5
5	Amlodipine	87.6	Amlodipine	102.0	Lansoprazole	113.4
6	Fluoxetine	86.1	Fluoxetine	91.4	Atorvastatin	99.7
7	Lansoprazole	85.0	Ranitidine	84.8	Fluticasone	92.4
8	Salbutamol	81.8	Paroxetine	82.7	Paroxetine	83.3
9	Diclofenac	81.7	Salbutamol	82.6	Salmeterol	79.8
10	Enalapril	72.9	Diclofenac	82.4	Salbutamol	79.2
11	Paroxetine	72.0	Lisinopril	76.6	Diclofenac	74.3
12	Nifedipine	71.7	Salmeterol	76.2	Lisinopril	73.3
13	Salmeterol	68.9	Fluticasone	73.7	Doxazosin	65.0
14	Lisinopril	68.3	Enalapril	71.8	Nifedipine	62.1
15	Fluticasone	62.2	Nifedipine	67.5	Fluoxetine	61.1
16	Budesonide	60.4	Isosorbide mononitrate	59.2	Goserelin	60.4
17	Isosorbide mononitrate	49.2	Atorvastatin	59.1	Isosorbide mononitrate	58.5
18	Goserelin	46.1	Budesonide	56.9	Ranitidine	53.0
19	Sertraline	39.2	Goserelin	53.1	Budesonide	51.8
20	Biphasic isophane insulin	38.5	Doxazosin	47.3	Enalapril	49.6

Rank	*2001*		*2002*		*2003*	
	Molecule	*Sales (£MM)*	*Molecule*	*Sales (£ MM)*	*Molecule*	*Sales (£ MM)*
1	Simvastatin	184.8	Simvastatin	255.7	Simvastatin	309.1
2	Omeprazole	174.7	Atorvastatin	201.9	Atorvastatin	272.5
3	Atorvastatin	152.5	Lansoprazole	171.6	Lansoprazole	201.6
4	Lansoprazole	140.3	Omeprazole	162.9	Fluticasone	178.5
5	Beclomethasone	135.1	Fluticasone	150.6	Amlodipine	156.7
6	Amlodipine	129.0	Amlodipine	140.2	Omeprazole	131.2
7	Fluticasone	123.1	Beclomethasone	131.8	Beclomethasone	122.1
8	Paroxetine	93.3	Doxazosin	93.0	Ramipril	113.8
9	Salmeterol	84.7	Lisinopril	88.2	Doxazosin	98.7
10	Doxazosin	82.6	Paroxetine	86.8	Olanzapine	98.4
11	Lisinopril	82.4	Salmeterol	85.5	Venlafaxine	92.2
12	Salbutamol	78.8	Ramipril	83.7	Pravastatin	91.6
13	Goserelin	67.6	Olanzapine	81.2	Salmeterol	84.1
14	Diclofenac	67.1	Pravastatin	80.7	Lisinopril	80.4
15	Olanzapine	62.6	Salbutamol	77.9	Citalopram	80.0
16	Nifedipine	60.4	Goserelin	73.4	Clopidogrel	79.6
17	Pravastatin	58.9	Venlafaxine	73.1	Goserelin	78.6
18	Isosorbide mononitrate	58.2	Citalopram	69.8	Salbutamol	76.0
19	Biphasic isophane insulin	57.2	Diclofenac	63.7	Losartan	64.9
20	Ramipril	54.1	Biphasic isophane insulin	62.6	Paroxetine	64.3

Note: Sales figures are net ingredient costs in millions of pounds were replaced by atorvastatin, ramipril, doxazosin, olanzapine, venlafaxine, pravastatin, citalopram, clopidogrel, and losartan. Figure 11.7 illustrates the differing fortunes of the five best-selling molecules in 2003. Sales trends for the leading molecules help explain the aforementioned growth of lipid-regulating drugs (e.g., simvastatin, atorvastatin, pravastatin); antihypertensives (e.g., amlodipine, ramipril, doxazosin, lisinopril, losartan); respiratory corticosteroids (e.g., fluticasone); antiplatelet drugs (e.g., clopidogrel); bronchodilators (e.g., salmeterol, salbutamol); antidepressants (e.g., venlafaxine, citalopram); and drugs for psychoses and related disorders (e.g., olanzapine).

Table 11.7 traces the sales evolution from 1998 to 2003 of the 20 best-selling molecules (in monetary terms) in 2003. Only 4 of the top-20 molecules in 2003 – omeprazole, beclomethasone, salbutamol, and paroxetine – lost sales over our review period. Conversely, 12 drugs – simvastatin, atorvastatin, lansoprazole, fluticasone, ramipril, doxazosin, olanzapine, venlafaxine, pravastatin, citalopram, and losartan – experienced sales growth of more than 100%. Clopidogrel, which was launched in the United Kingdom in July 1998, had by far the highest growth rate: 44,827% in five years. However, atorvastatin had the largest growth in absolute terms: sales increased from £28.2 million ($46.1 million) in 1998 to £272.5 million ($445 million) in 2003.

Table 11.8 shows prescribing trends from 1998 to 2003 for the 20 molecules that achieved the highest sales in England in 2003. A comparison of Tables 11.7 and 11.8 reveals that 10 of the 20 best-selling molecules in 2003 – simvastatin, atorvastatin, lansoprazole, doxazosin, olanzapine, pravastatin, lisinopril, citalopram, clopidogrel, and losartan – had stronger volume growth than sales growth, indicating that the average net ingredient cost of prescriptions for these molecules declined over the review period. Olanzapine suffered a particularly sharp reduction in the average net ingredient cost of a prescription, from £109.37 ($178.62) in 1998 to £79.51 ($129.86) in

Table 11.7 Sales Trends, 1998–2003, of the 20 Best-Selling Molecules in England in 2003

Molecule	*Total Net Ingredient Costs (£ million)*							
	1998	*1999*	*2000*	*2001*	*2002*	*2003*	*Change*[a] *(%)*	*CGR (%)*
Simvastatin	106.3	128.4	144.1	184.8	255.7	309.1	190.7	23.8
Atorvastatin	28.2	59.1	99.7	152.5	201.9	272.5	866.5	57.4
Lansoprazole	85.0	104.1	113.4	140.3	171.6	201.6	137.2	18.9
Fluticasone	62.2	73.7	92.4	123.1	150.6	178.5	186.9	23.5
Amlodipine	87.6	102.0	115.5	129.0	140.2	156.7	78.9	12.3
Omeprazole	196.7	201.4	183.5	174.7	162.9	131.2	(33.3)	(7.8)
Beclomethasone	144.3	143.9	138.9	135.1	131.8	122.1	(15.4)	(3.3)
Ramipril	16.4	22.3	34.2	54.1	83.7	113.8	592.7	47.3
Doxazosin	32.7	47.3	65.0	82.6	93.0	98.7	201.7	24.7
Olanzapine	20.0	33.3	44.2	62.6	81.2	98.4	391.1	37.5
Venlafaxine	19.6	28.1	38.1	52.9	73.1	92.2	369.5	36.2
Pravastatin	24.8	33.9	41.4	58.9	80.7	91.6	269.4	29.9
Salmeterol	68.9	76.2	79.8	84.7	85.5	84.1	22.0	4.1
Lisinopril	68.3	76.6	73.3	82.4	88.2	80.4	17.7	3.3
Citalopram	12.8	23.5	38.2	53.9	69.8	80.0	525.9	44.3
Clopidogrel	0.2	3.7	10.8	26.0	52.4	79.6	44,827.1	>1,000
Goserelin	46.1	53.1	60.4	67.6	73.4	78.6	70.3	11.2
Salbutamol	81.8	82.6	79.2	78.8	77.9	76.0	(7.0)	(1.5)
Losartan	20.5	28.5	35.0	41.8	53.0	64.9	216.7	25.9
Paroxetine	72.0	82.7	83.3	93.3	86.8	64.3	(10.7)	(2.2)

[a]Percentage change from 1998 to 2003

CGR = Cumulative growth rate

Table 11.8 Prescribing Trends, 1998–2003, of the 20 Best-Selling Molecules in England in 2003

Molecule	*Millions of Prescriptions*							
	1998	*1999*	*2000*	*2001*	*2002*	*2003*	*Change*[a] *(%)*	*CGR (%)*
Simvastatin	3.0	3.6	4.2	5.3	7.1	9.4	215.3	25.8
Atorvastatin	0.8	1.7	2.9	4.4	6.5	8.6	953.1	60.1
Lansoprazole	2.8	3.6	4.7	6.2	7.7	9.1	227.0	26.7
Fluticasone	1.5	1.8	2.2	2.7	3.1	3.6	130.5	18.2
Amlodipine	4.2	4.9	5.6	6.3	6.8	7.4	78.0	12.2
Omeprazole	5.1	5.3	5.1	4.8	4.6	4.6	(10.4)	(2.2)
Beclomethasone	8.4	8.4	8.2	8.2	8.1	7.6	(9.7)	(2.0)
Ramipril	1.1	1.5	2.5	3.9	5.7	7.5	563.7	46.0
Doxazosin	1.1	1.7	2.3	2.9	3.5	4.0	255.1	28.8
Olanzapine	0.2	0.3	0.5	0.7	1.0	1.2	575.6	46.5
Venlafaxine	0.6	0.8	1.1	1.5	2.1	2.6	339.5	34.5
Pravastatin	0.7	0.9	1.2	1.7	2.3	2.6	277.4	30.4
Salmeterol	1.8	2.0	2.1	2.2	2.3	2.2	20.1	3.7
Lisinopril	3.9	4.6	5.2	5.9	6.3	6.5	65.3	10.6
Citalopram	0.5	1.2	2.0	2.8	3.6	4.2	710.1	52.0
Clopidogrel	0.0	0.1	0.3	0.6	1.2	1.9	N.M.	N.M.
Goserelin	0.2	0.2	0.2	0.3	0.3	0.3	38.3	6.7
Salbutamol	15.8	15.8	15.8	16.2	16.3	15.9	0.6	0.1
Losartan	0.7	1.0	1.2	1.4	1.8	2.3	221.2	26.3
Paroxetine	2.7	3.1	3.5	3.8	3.7	2.9	5.5	1.1

[a]Percentage change from 1998 to 2003
CGR = Cumulative growth rate
N.M. = Not meaningful
Note: Drugs are listed in the order of their sales rankings, not their prescription volumes

2003. The average net ingredient cost of a prescription for citalopram also fell sharply, from £24.59 ($40.16) in 1998 to £19.00 ($31.03) in 2003.

OUTLOOK FOR THE UK PHARMACEUTICAL MARKET

Improving the UK healthcare system is a high priority for the current government – hence the decision to increase annual investment in the NHS by 62% from financial year 2002–3 to 2007–8. Drug manufacturers stand to benefit significantly from this increased investment. The government believes that the pharmaceutical industry can make an important contribution to both healthcare and the economy in the United Kingdom. As a demonstration of its commitment to a strong UK pharmaceutical industry, the government established the Pharmaceutical Industry Competitiveness Task Force in 2000.

The relatively free pricing environment (by European standards, at least) created by the PPRS has probably been a major factor in the competitiveness of the UK pharmaceutical market. At this writing, however, the future direction of pharmaceutical pricing in the United Kingdom is unclear. The government may decide to renew the PPRS when it expires in October 2004, perhaps using the opportunity to impose a price- cut similar to the 4.5% reduction that it implemented in 1999. An alternative option would be deregulation of pharmaceutical pricing – a reform that would move the UK pharmaceutical market away from its European neighbors and closer to the United States. However, the UK government's deliberations could be superseded if the EU adopts a proposal to introduce uniform ex-manufacturer pricing for prescription medicines. In that event, the pharmaceutical industry would have to negotiate national rebates or discounts with the governments of the United Kingdom and other EU member states.

Drug manufacturers are likely to face significant challenges as well as attractive opportunities in the future UK pharmaceutical market. In particular, pharmaceutical companies will have to cope with some paradoxical trends. For example, the government is determined to end the postcode lottery and achieve more uniform standards of medical care and access to innovative therapies across the country. Initiatives such as the NSF program, mandatory funding of NICE-approved therapies, and the introduction of GMS contracts are intended to harmonize and improve standards. On the other hand, the government has devolved enormous powers to PCTs, which now control 75% of the entire NHS budget. Conflicts between national and local policy are likely to occur in the future, and it is unclear how these differences will be resolved.

The government is also seeking to balance a policy of increasing NHS expenditures on pharmaceuticals, especially innovative medicines, with its instinct for cost containment. To maximize the funds that are available for novel drugs, the NHS will continue to promote generics prescribing and dispensing whenever possible. The expiration of patents on many blockbuster drugs in the next few years will increase the scope for using generics. The UK pharmaceutical market could become increasingly polarized, with innovative medicines and generics flourishing while "me-too drugs" lose out.

NHS pharmaceutical policy is likely to focus increasingly on the clinical priority areas that the government has targeted in its NSF program to date, namely mental health, CHD, cancer, geriatric medicine, and diabetes. GPs will have strong incentives to comply with NSF requirements, and the new GMS contracts will reinforce the emphasis on these chronic diseases. NICE's future activity will prioritize the same disease areas. In the past, NICE has concentrated mainly on technology appraisals, but its future program will be biased more heavily toward broader clinical guidelines. The list of proposed guidelines focuses on cardiovascular disease (e.g., atrial fibrillation, familial hypercholesterolemia, hyperlipidemia and cardiovascular risk, hypertension, postmyocardial infarction, venous thromboembolism); cancer (e.g., brain tumors, breast cancer, child and adolescent cancer, colorectal cancer, familial breast cancer, head and neck cancers, lung cancer, prostate cancer, sarcoma, and skin tumors, including melanoma); and mental health (e.g., bipolar disorder, dementia, depression, depression in children, generalized anxiety disorder, obsessive compulsive disorder, post-traumatic stress disorder). The disadvantage of the overriding emphasis on clinical priority areas is the risk that other important diseases will be neglected.

As traditional gatekeepers to the NHS – controlling access to both primary and secondary healthcare services – GPs are arguably the most powerful decision makers in the UK healthcare system. However, the government is increasing the powers of other healthcare professionals (e.g., nurses, pharmacists). For example, nurses now have the freedom to run primary care centers – potentially employing salaried GPs to perform certain services. The government has also approved supplementary prescribing by eligible pharmacists, nurses, and midwives. (The government defines supplementary prescribing as "a voluntary prescribing partnership between an independent prescriber and a supplementary prescriber, to implement a patient-specific clinical management plan with the patient's agreement." The independent prescriber must be a physician or dentist. Supplementary prescribers will be permitted to prescribe most pharmaceuticals marketed in the United Kingdom but not controlled drugs.)

By 2008, the PPA, physicians, and pharmacists will exchange prescribing data in a bid to improve patient compliance and reduce waste. Pharmacists will become increasingly conscious of cost-effectiveness and the need to contain local pharmaceutical expenditures. Some expert observers predict that pharmacists will ultimately replace GPs as the most important pharmacy decision makers in the NHS – especially in the management of chronic conditions. This trend will challenge the traditional divide between physicians as prescribers and pharmacists as dispensers. Pharmaceutical companies will therefore need to adapt their marketing strategies for the primary care pharmacy market. In particular, manufacturers will need to invest more time, effort, and resources in communicating with pharmacists.

Pharmaceutical companies will also need to be prepared for increasing collaboration between the primary and secondary care sectors. APCs and joint formularies are likely to become more influential in the future.

With few formal hurdles to negotiate and high prices, the general pricing and reimbursement climate in the United Kingdom is relatively benign. While other European countries that have traditionally been generous in their funding of prescription drugs adopt increasingly aggressive cost-containment measures, the UK government appears relatively relaxed about the steady growth in its pharmaceutical expenditures. Thus, the outlook for the pharmaceutical industry is highly promising in the United Kingdom.

REFERENCE

West, P. and Mahon, J. *Benefits to Payers and Patients from Parallel Trade*. York Health Economics Consortium. May 2003.

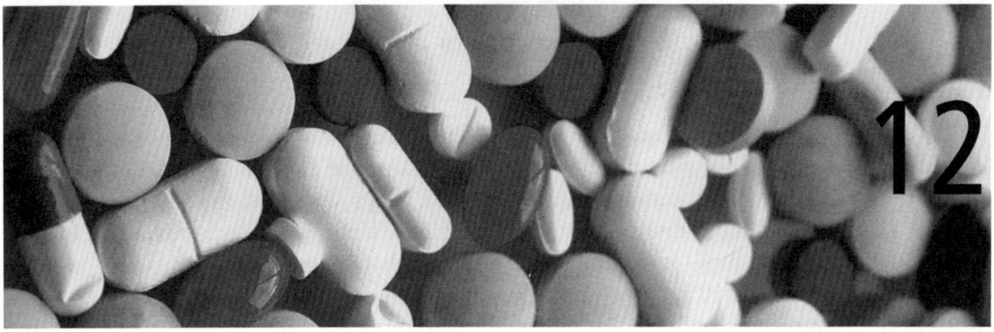

Pharmaceutical Pricing, Reimbursement, and Prescribing in Italy

INTRODUCTION

The Italian pharmaceutical market is the fourth largest in Europe and the sixth largest in the world. Steady growth in the second half of the 1990s lifted the Italian market to third place in Europe and fifth place in the world. As recently as 2001, pharmaceutical sales grew by 32%.

These trends may suggest that the pharmaceutical market in Italy is a favorable environment for drug companies. However, pharmaceutical manufacturers face many challenges in doing business in Italy. The government exercises strict control over drug prices, uses a wide range of cost-containment measures to curb spending, and is now taking greater account of pharmacoeconomic data than in the past. Public expenditures on prescription drugs declined in 2003. The government has also recently decentralized responsibility for the healthcare system, a development that has begun to fragment the Italian pharmaceutical market.

In this chapter we present a brief overview of the Italian healthcare system, discuss the pricing and reimbursement of both outpatient and hospital medicines, review recent sales and prescribing trends in Italy, and assess the outlook for the Italian pharmaceutical market.

ORGANIZATION AND FUNDING OF THE ITALIAN HEALTHCARE SYSTEM

According to the Organization for Economic Cooperation and Development, Italy spent 8.5% of its gross domestic product (GDP) on healthcare in 2002 – in line with the European Union (EU) mean of 8.5%. The share of GDP invested in healthcare in Italy fluctuated only slightly over the course of the 1990s, declining from 8.0% in 1990 to 7.7% in 1995 but then increasing again to 8.1% in 2000.

The national healthcare system is a relatively recent innovation in Italy. Until the 1970s, healthcare was coordinated by approximately 100 health insurance funds and was highly fragmented. In 1978, however, Law 833/1978 created the *Servizio Sanitario Nazionale* (SSN; National Health Service). The fundamental objective of the SSN is to provide a healthcare service based on the principles of equal dignity, health need, equity, protection of citizens' health, solidarity with the most vulnerable members of society, effective and appropriate treatments, and cost effectiveness. The system is intended to be subject to "popular democratic control" at national, regional, and local levels.

Funding for the SSN originally came from general taxation and payroll taxes collected by the national government. Each year, the government determined the size of the *fondo sanitario nazionale* (FSN; national health budget), which was then divided among Italy's 21 regions. In turn, regional health departments allocated global budgets (to cover all areas of healthcare expenditure, including pharmaceuticals) to each of the country's *aziende sanitarie locali* (ASLs; local health authorities). However, legislation in 1992 (Law 502/92) and 1993 (Law 517/93) transformed the organization of the SSN by devolving extensive powers from national government to the regions. Funding remained a national responsibility, but the regions became responsible for any deficits that might occur. The new legislation also required regional health departments to restructure their healthcare services. For example, many ASLs were amalgamated into larger bodies, and some large and/or highly specialized hospitals became self-governing public entities known as *aziende ospedaliere* (AOs; hospital authorities). Regional health departments also had to define new funding criteria and introduce competition and modern management methods.

The government made further radical changes to the SSN in 2001, when it introduced a federalist structure for the healthcare system. The national government still defines standards for the SSN, but regional authorities are now responsible for collecting the taxes that fund the service. A solidarity fund helps to offset inequalities between regions. Until 2003, each region had to meet nationally defined "essential and uniform levels of care." Beginning in 2004, however, regions are free to determine how much they spend on healthcare (provided that they have an adequate monitoring system).

PHARMACEUTICAL PRICES IN ITALY

In January 2002, the Ministry of Health declared that drug prices in Italy were too high – 5% above the European average. However, Farmindustria, the Italian pharmaceutical industry association, disputed this figure, arguing that Italian prices were at least 6% below the European average. Other studies have also found that pharmaceutical prices in Italy are generally lower than in most other European markets. For example, Table 12.1 shows the results of an international price comparison conducted by the UK Department of Health, which monitors prices of the most frequently prescribed drugs in the United Kingdom, several other European markets, and the United States. (The analysis uses the United Kingdom as a benchmark for a multilateral comparison of average prices of branded prescription medicines in these

Table 12.1 Multilateral Comparison of Average Exmanufacturer Prices of Branded Medicines in Select Markets as a Percentage of UK Average Exmanufacturer Prices, 1992–2002

Year	*France (%)*	*Germany (%)*	*Italy (%)*	*Spain (%)*	*United States (%)*	*United Kingdom (%)*
1992	93	158	108	95	172	100
1993	96	158	100	89	202	100
1994	100	143	90	88	192	100
1995	107	130	83	89	179	100
1996	105	125	93	89	191	100
1997	85	101	86	74	184	100
1998	85	109	88	77	188	100
1999	86	103	82	72	213	100
2000	83	94	82	70	241	100
2001	81	90	85	72	205	100
2002	83	94	86	77	194	100
Average percentage, 1998–2002[a]	83	94	86	77	197	100

[a]Based on 2002 price data but converted to pounds sterling using average exchange rates for the period 1998–2002

markets. Fluctuations from year to year are attributable primarily to exchange rate movements. In the late 1990s, the pound sterling appreciated strongly against most European currencies [thereby inflating UK prices in comparison with prices in those countries] but lost value against the US dollar [thereby reducing UK prices in comparison with prices in the United States]. Conversely, the pound sterling has appreciated against the US dollar but lost value against the euro.) This study found that from 1998 to 2002, Italy had the third-lowest average prices of the major European markets (Spain and France had lower average prices).

A more recent analysis conducted by Farmindustria found that in 2003, average pharmaceutical prices in Italy were 25.2% below the average for the eight largest European markets. Prices in France were 27.1% below the eight-country average, and prices in Spain were 41.2% below the eight-country average.

Until recently, the pricing procedure for a new drug to be launched in Italy depended on whether the agent was registered through the national procedure or by the European Medicines Agency (EMEA; formerly the European Agency for the Evaluation of Medicinal Products). Drugs registered through the national procedure were subject to a requirement that their ex-manufacturer prices in Italy should not exceed the average European price (AEP) for the compound in question. However, the government has now abolished this requirement.

In May 1997, the Italian government introduced a contractual model for the pricing of innovative drugs registered through the EMEA's centralized procedure. In 1998, the government extended this model to products registered through the EMEA's mutual recognition procedure (MRP). From January 1, 2004, this model applies to all branded medicines marketed in Italy.

Until recently, the *Commissione Unica del Farmaco* (CUF; National Pharmaceutical Committee), an agency of the Ministry of Health, worked with a group of government-appointed experts in evaluating all new drugs and determining acceptable prices for inclusion in the SSN reimbursement list. In June 2004, however, a powerful new national medicines agency, the *Agenzia Italiana del Farmaco* (AIFA; Italian Medicines Agency), took over the CUF's responsibilities. (See the sidebar, "Creation of a New Medicines Agency.") At this writing, it is not known whether the government will change the procedures for setting pharmaceutical prices.

Creation of a New Medicines Agency

In November 2003, the Italian parliament approved a package of major pharmaceutical reforms contained within an annex to the *Legge Finanziaria 2004* (Finance Act, 2004). The centerpiece of the reform program was the creation of the *Agenzia Italiana del Farmaco* (AIFA; Italian Medicines Agency), which will take over the functions previously performed by the Ministry of Health's *Direzione Generale dei Farmaci e dei Dispositivi Medici* (Directorate General for Medicines and Medical Devices) and the *Commissione Unica del Farmaco* (CUF; National Pharmaceutical Committee). The AIFA will oversee all aspects of national pharmaceutical policy, including drug approvals, pharmacovigilance, pricing and reimbursement, promotional spending, and pharmaceutical expenditures.

The AIFA will have the following responsibilities:

- Preparing prescribing guidelines for new therapies.
- Monitoring the prescribing volume and cost (public and private) of drugs dispensed in the community and in hospitals.
- Reviewing whether drugs meet the cost-effectiveness conditions for inclusion in the list of reimbursable medicines. This review will generally be an annual exercise but will be conducted on a quarterly basis in the case of drugs that exceed spending limits.
- Assessing whether new drugs qualify for a price premium on the grounds of therapeutic superiority.
- In the case of new drugs that are not therapeutically superior to established therapies, authorizing reimbursement only

if prices are less than or equal to the lowest price of drugs in the relevant homogeneous therapeutic category.

- Ensuring that pharmaceutical expenditures do not exceed their designated maximum share of the total SSN health care budget (i.e., 13%). If spending does exceed this limit, the AIFA will require the excess to be refunded by the pharmaceutical industry (60%) and regional authorities (40%).

The first step in the price negotiation process requires the marketing company to submit an application to the Italian Ministry of Health. The dossier of required data includes the drug's therapeutic class, information on whether it is similar to or equivalent to any existing drugs, pharmacoeconomic data (if available), and the proposed price. Representatives of the CUF and several government ministries review this documentation, taking into account the drug's likely impact on SSN pharmaceutical spending (except in the case of orphan drugs). Innovative compounds are frequently compared with existing therapies for the same indication (many of which may be much less expensive than the proposed price of the new agent). The following factors are generally the key considerations in price setting.

- Degree of innovation and therapeutic value.
- Comparative efficacy and price of any competing or similar drugs.
- Price and reimbursement status of the same or similar products in other EU countries.
- Sales forecasts (including market share in Italy after two years and sales through any licensees).
- Projected number of prescriptions and patient population using the drug.
- Company investment in the Italian economy in developing or manufacturing the drug.

Since spring 2001, companies are expected to demonstrate the cost-effectiveness profile of a new drug in any of the following circumstances: (1) the drug is indicated for a disease that has no available therapy; (2) existing treatments are inadequate; and (3) the new drug is claimed to have a cost-benefit profile that is better than that of established therapies. Companies may also have to offer commitments on sales volume, discounts to hospitals and other healthcare facilities, and possible concessions on the sales volume and price of other drugs in their product ranges. Companies that do not honor their commitments could face price-cuts, delisting, or other penalties.

Pharmacoeconomic data are required only for orphan drugs or highly innovative pharmaceuticals. However, manufacturers have the option of including cost-effectiveness, cost-utility, or cost-benefit data in their applications for other kinds of drugs. A guide published by the *Comitato Interministeriale per la Programmazione Economica* (CIPE; Interdepartmental Committee for Economic Planning) defines the requirements for pharmacoeconomic studies (e.g., the use of comparators, efficacy indicators, methods for calculating comparative cost data, and general statistical methodology).

The pricing review should last no longer than 90 days. The law permits reviewers to stop the process once if they require additional data and/or clarification of data, but additional interruptions may sometimes occur in practice. The applicant company may withdraw its application at any time during the assessment.

Assuming that the regulatory authorities and the company reach agreement, an ex-factory price is set for two years and the drug becomes eligible for SSN reimbursement. This "contract" is automatically renewed unless either party submits any changes to the terms of the agreement at least 90 days before its expiration. For example, if a drug's sales are expected to grow as a result of approval for increased dosing or a new indication, the manufacturer may need to start renegotiating its price before the pricing contract expires.

If a manufacturer does not agree with the CUF's proposed price for a given drug, it can ask for the drug to be assigned to class C – drugs that are excluded from reimbursement and therefore eligible for generally free pricing (discussed further on). However, given that exclusion from reimbursement reduces a drug's sales, companies are understandably reluctant to take such action. Furthermore, the CUF may exceptionally decide to refuse a request for class C status, in which case the pricing negotiation process must continue until an agreement is reached. The agreed price is then approved by the CUF and the *Conferenza Stato-Regioni* (State and Regional Conference) and certified by the *Comitato Interministeriale Prezzi* (CIP; Interdepartmental Committee on Prices). It is then published in the *Gazzetta Ufficiale della Repubblica Italiana* (Official Bulletin of the Italian Republic).

In addition, the CUF has the authority to reassess (and potentially reduce) prices two years after a product's launch or if the drug is approved for new indications that might increase its total sales. This rule presents pharmaceutical companies with a formidable additional hurdle in the market.

The *Legge Finanziaria 2003* (2003 Finance Act) holds out the prospect of premium prices as a reward for "innovation." However, the government's definition of "innovation" is rather unusual and appears to be determined with an eye toward supporting the Italian economy and pharmaceutical industry. Eligibility for premium prices is based on the following criteria:

- Manufacturing investment in the current year compared with average investment in the three preceding years.
- Increases in exports compared with the preceding year.
- The number of employees working in research compared with the preceding three years.
- Increases in research investment in Italy compared with sales in preceding years.

Even if many companies should satisfy these criteria, the impact of this measure would be extremely limited. The 2003 Finance Act indicates that premium pricing must not increase total pharmaceutical spending by more than 0.1%.

A relatively recent innovation that may help to boost sales of innovative drugs is the provision for companies to negotiate higher prices for new products in return for price cuts on older therapies. This mechanism is reminiscent of the United Kingdom's Pharmaceutical Price Regulation Scheme.

REIMBURSEMENT OF OUTPATIENT MEDICINES

Prontuario Farmaceutico Nazionale *(National Formulary)*

In 1978, the Italian government introduced a positive list of pharmaceuticals that qualified for reimbursement by the newly created SSN. In 1994, however, the authorities replaced the positive list with the *Prontuario Farmaceutico Nazionale* (PFN; national formulary). The PFN assigned all registered medicines in Italy to one of four reimbursement categories: classes A, B, and C covered products available from community pharmacies and class H consisted of hospital-only products. The SSN reimbursed the full cost of class A products and of class H drugs dispensed to inpatients. (However, patients had to pay the full cost of class H medicines they received after their discharge from hospital.) Class B drugs were reimbursed at a rate of 50%. The SSN provided no reimbursement for class C drugs. Table 12.2 summarizes the reimbursement categories.

On January 1, 2001, however, the government altered the reimbursement structure by abolishing class B – the category that offered patients 50% reimbursement. All drugs that were previously in this category were reassigned to either class A or class C. Drugs that were deemed of minor therapeutic value were generally moved to class C (i.e., dereimbursed).

On January 16, 2003, the Italian government introduced a radical new PFN that determined reimbursement status on the basis of a drug's cost effectiveness. The CUF assigned drugs dispensed by retail pharmacies to *categorie terapeutiche omogenee* (homogeneous therapeutic categories) based on anatomic therapeutic chemical (ATC) fourth-level classification. (These categories

Table 12.2 Pharmaceutical Reimbursement Categories in Italy

Category	*Characteristics*	*Reimbursement Rate*
Class A	Drugs with documented efficacy for the treatment of severe and chronic disorders	100%
Class B[a]	Other drugs with documented efficacy (drugs "of therapeutic relevance") Drugs excluded from Class A on account of a high cost-benefit ratio	50%
Class C	Drugs without proven efficacy Drugs with documented efficacy for minor disorders	0%
Class H	Hospital-only drugs requiring specialist supervision	100%[b]

[a]Abolished in 2001; drugs formerly in this category were assigned to either class A or class C
[b]Patients pay the full cost of these drugs after they are discharged from hospital

had been defined in 1999.) A homogeneous therapeutic category is defined as "a group of drugs that, in relation to the main therapeutic indication, share the same mechanism of action and are characterized by similar clinical efficacy and profile of undesired side effects. Individual drugs however may differ in terms of additional therapeutic indications." For example, in the antiulcerants drug class, H_2 antagonists and proton-pump inhibitors are assigned to different homogeneous therapeutic categories as a result of their different mechanisms of action. The CUF then set a *cut-off*, or price ceiling, for each homogeneous therapeutic category based on 50% of SSN spending and 60% of prescribing volume in the respective category in 2001. This method of calculating the price ceiling for each class required relatively few substantial price cuts to meet the price ceiling. In any event, the maximum price cut would have been 20%, and companies had the option of transferring part of any price reduction (i.e., up to 7%) to other SSN-reimbursed branded medicines that they marketed.

Products that do not exceed their price ceilings in the new PFN are included in reimbursement class A (100% reimbursement), but products that are priced above this level are assigned to class C (no reimbursement at all). The threat of dereimbursement proved to be a powerful incentive for manufacturers to cut their prices. The new PFN contains 4,017 product presentations in class A; only 21 product presentations that might have been eligible for class A status were assigned to class C because their manufacturers refused to reduce their prices to the level of the reimbursement ceiling. The Italian government forecasted that this restructuring of the PFN would save the SSN €285 million ($322 million) in 2003. The government plans to update the PFN every September.

Supply-side Restrictions

As discussed earlier, the Italian government exercises strict control over the prices of new medicines that will be reimbursed by the SSN. In addition, the government periodically imposes restrictions on drugs that are already on the market.

Price Control

The Italian government has repeatedly used mandatory price freezes or cuts to reduce pharmaceutical spending. For example, in January 1999, the authorities imposed a 15% price reduction on the reference AEP of many drugs. In 2000, prices of reimbursable branded drugs not covered by patents were reduced by 5%.

In January 2002, the government imposed a 5% price cut on all pharmaceuticals (except products costing less than €3 [$3.39], blood derivatives, and products derived from recombinant DNA techniques). (For the sake of the uniformity of the analysis, the US dollar-to-euro exchange rate used in this report is the 2003 average rate [i.e., $1 = €0.8854].) In January 2003, the government increased the level of the price cut to 7%.

Because class C drugs are excluded from SSN reimbursement, the government allows manufacturers a high degree of freedom in setting the prices of these drugs. However, the authorities will intervene to reduce prices that they consider to be excessive. In April 2004, the Ministry of Health expressed concern about rising prices for class C drugs. In 2003, sales of class C drugs totaled €3.1 billion ($3.5 billion), a 13% increase in one year. According to Farmindustria, prices increased by an average of 3.3% and consumption grew by 9%. However, Farmindustria notes that average prices of class A drugs (i.e., fully reimbursed prescription medicines) declined by 5%, more than offsetting the price increases for class C products.

Demand-side Restrictions

The Italian government also uses a variety of demand-side restrictions to control public spending on pharmaceuticals.

Budgets

In 1994, the government introduced a national pharmaceutical budget enforced by the threat of dereimbursement if the spending cap was exceeded. However, although the annual budget was consistently exceeded, the government carried out its threat of dereimbursement only once, in 1996.

In 1998, the government replaced the threat of dereimbursement with the prospect that the pharmaceutical industry, wholesalers, and pharmacists would have to pay back 60% of any future deficit in the annual prescribing budget. Other penalties, such as price cuts, have also been proposed, but little has been done to enforce the budget. Indeed, in recent years, SSN pharmaceutical expenditures – and the prescribing budget deficit – have grown rapidly.

Regional authorities have been given greater autonomy in healthcare policy, but they also have increased responsibility for enforcing the pharmaceutical budget. Consequently, regional governments are making increasing use of their powers to impose pharmaceutical cost-containment measures within their area of authority.

In fall 2003, the Italian government passed legislation to penalize the pharmaceutical industry and regional governments if SSN spending on medicines exceeds the national target of 13% of the SSN budget. In that event, the pharmaceutical industry would have to pay a penalty equivalent to 60% of the excess, and the regional governments would have to repay 40% of the excess. Pharmaceutical companies would pay their penalties by reducing their ex-manufacturer prices. In June 2004, the Italian government announced that pharmaceutical expenditures were projected to be €1.3 billion ($1.5 billion) over budget in 2004, an overspend that would require the industry to pay back €745 million ($841 million). However, after protests from drug manufacturers, the government reduced the industry's projected penalty to €495 million ($559 million), a decision that provoked fierce criticism from Federfarma, the association of Italian pharmacists.

Prescribing Restrictions

Even if a drug is approved for SSN reimbursement, it may be subject to one of a number of prescribing restrictions.

One of the most common prescribing constraints is the CUF's note limitative (restrictive notes), which impose strict conditions on the use of certain drugs. Drugs subject to such restrictive notes are typically limited to specific indications, patient subpopulations, or care settings. Physicians are required to write the reference number of any applicable restrictive note next to the product name. Physicians who do not comply with this system may, in theory, have to repay the cost of any drugs that they have prescribed inappropriately; however, this sanction is seldom imposed.

In February 2001, however, the government abolished many of these restrictive notes and relaxed others. This action stimulated a dramatic increase in the use of these agents. For example, CUF note 80 formerly restricted SSN reimbursement of new-generation antidepressants to patients who could not tolerate tricyclic antidepressants. The ending of this restriction contributed substantially to a 130% increase in SSN expenditures on new-generation antidepressants in 2001. Similarly, the abolition of CUF note 81 helped to increase SSN spending on low-molecular-weight heparin by 182% in 2001.

The Ministry of Health controls the use of certain drugs by a procedure known as *File F*, a mechanism for financing certain hospital medicines from ASL funds rather than from hospital budgets. For example, under File F, ASLs cover the cost of intravenous drug infusions administered in hospital outpatient clinics. File F also provides ASL funding for expensive inpatient therapies that would not be covered by hospital budgets.

In January 2003, the government imposed new restrictions on the indications for which certain products may be prescribed and reimbursed. These restrictions are expected to save the SSN approximately €150 million ($169 million) per year.

Reference Pricing

Italy's 1994 Finance Act made provision for reference pricing, but the system was not actually established until September 2001. The program initially covered approximately 1,000 patent-expired products containing 38 multisource substances categorized by ATC classifications. The price ceiling was set as the weighted average of all products in the group that are at least 20% less expensive than the originator product. The SSN reimbursed the full cost of drugs that did not exceed the reference price, but patients had to pay the excess for drugs that were priced above the reference price.

Just weeks after the program was inaugurated, the government adopted a decree law that radically changed the system. Beginning November 1, 2001, reference prices were set at the level of the least-expensive available generic rather than based on a weighted average. In addition, if a prescribed drug appeared on the reference list, pharmacists were authorized to substitute the least-expensive generic equivalent unless the prescribing physician explicitly forbade substitution. Furthermore, the decree law required physicians who prescribed products that exceeded reference prices to inform their patients about the excess they would have to pay and to advise them if less-expensive options were available. Regional governments have some discretion in deciding reimbursement terms in their territories for reference-priced medicines.

Promoting Greater Use of Generics

The Italian generics market is extremely small by international standards. This weakness is attributable in large measure to historically poor patent protection and the existence of numerous copy products that were usually priced at the same level as originator brands. Price competition in the Italian pharmaceutical market was therefore almost unknown.

In August 1996, the Italian government took action to boost the generics market. Law 425/96 created a framework for greater use of generics:

- *Denomination*: the international nonproprietary name (INN) followed by the name of the marketing authorization holder.
- *Price*: must be at least 20% below the price of the originator/reference product.
- *Substitution*: permissible unless the prescriber specifies a manufacturer.

On its own, this legislation had little impact on demand for generics. For example, in 1999, only approximately one million packs of unbranded generics were dispensed in Italy, with a total value of less than $5 million. In 2001, however, the market grew rapidly. Total sales in that year were estimated at $120 million – still very modest by international standards, but a huge increase on Italian sales in 1999. The market share of unbranded generics in 2001 was 1.3% in monetary terms and 2.1% in volume terms.

In January 2002, the government introduced additional measures to promote greater use of generics. It reduced the duration of supplementary protection certificates (a mechanism for extending the benefits of patent protection) from 18 to 15 years. The government also introduced a Bolar-type provision that allows generics manufacturers to begin drug development one year before patent expiration, thereby expediting the launch of generics. Furthermore, the government decreed that, from January 2003, all pharmaceutical packs must bear the product's generic name and ATC classification code in addition to the brand name, which must be printed at least 20% smaller than the lettering of the generic name.

Yet despite these measures, the Italian generics market remains underdeveloped by international standards. The *Osservatorio Nazionale sull'Impiego dei Medicinali* (OsMed; National Observatory on the Use of Medicines) reports that in 2002 *genericabili* (molecules that are available as generics, that is, both branded and unbranded drugs that are off patent) accounted for 14% of the SSN pharmaceutical market in volume terms and 7% in monetary terms. In 2003, *genericabili* increased their share of the SSN pharmaceutical market to 20.8% in volume terms and to 9.8% in monetary terms. The availability of a wider range of off-patent drugs contributed to this growth.

The Italian market for unbranded generics is much smaller than the total market for off-patent medicines. OsMed reports that, in 2003, branded off-patent drugs accounted for 8.1% of total sales in the SSN pharmaceutical market, compared with a 1.7% share for unbranded generics. These figures indicate that government initiatives have not yet stimulated major growth in the Italian market for low-priced, unbranded generics.

Regional Patient Copayments

In January 2001, the Italian government abolished patient copayments and the fixed prescription charge for all reimbursed drugs. This move was made in preparation for the introduction of the new reference-pricing system. It had a dramatic effect on pharmaceutical expenditures, which were 36.5% higher in the first six months of the year than in the corresponding period in 2000.

However, regional governments now have the authority to impose a range of cost-containment measures, including prescription charges and restrictions. Ten of Italy's 21 regions – Bolzano, Calabria, Lazio, Liguria, Lombardy, Molise, Piedmont, Puglia, Sicily, and Veneto – currently impose their own cost-containment measures. (Sardinia revoked its regional cost-containment measures in April 2004.) Copayments vary from region to region, but most charge a standard fee of €1–€2 ($1.13–$2.26) per prescribed product, usually with a maximum charge per prescription (typically €3–€4 ($3.39–$4.52). Copayments are generally lower for certain drug classes, treatments for particular disorders, or patient groups; disabled patients, pensioners, and low-income patients are often exempt from regional copayments altogether. In 2003, regional copayments contributed a total of approximately €480 million ($542 million) to SSN coffers.

Dereimbursement

In January 2003, the government dereimbursed 78 "nonessential" active substances, including certain antibiotics, allergy treatments, and anti-inflammatory drugs. This action was expected to save the SSN approximately €282 million ($319 million) per year.

REIMBURSEMENT OF HOSPITAL MEDICINES

Information regarding the size of the Italian hospital pharmacy market is scarce. Based on data published by IMS Health, we estimate that ex-manufacturer sales of pharmaceuticals in Italian hospitals totaled $2.8 billion in 2002. This sum was equivalent to 20% of the total pharmaceutical market in Italy.

In many European countries, manufacturers are allowed much greater freedom in setting drug prices in the hospital sector than in retail pharmacies. Italy is an exception to this rule. In the Italian hospital pharmacy market, manufacturers are legally obliged to offer substantial discounts relative to the retail prices of drugs in classes A and H. In the case of drugs registered through Italy's national registration procedure, manufacturers must reduce their prices to hospitals by at least 50% of the retail prices (net of value-added tax). In the case of hospital-only drugs approved by the EMEA, manufacturers must reduce their prices to hospitals by at least 40% of the retail prices (net of value-added tax). The *Comitato Interministeriale per la Programazzione Economica* (CIPE; Interdepartmental Committee for Economic Planning) publishes hospital acquisition prices for hospital-only drugs on its web site (www.cipecomitato.it/Documentazione/farmaci/Elenco_farmaci_ospedalieri_contrattati.pdf).

Hospitals favor the prescribing of drugs listed in their own *prontuario terapeutico ospedaliero* (PTO; hospital formulary). A typical hospital formulary includes approximately 1,000 drugs, contrast media, and diagnostics. The addition of new drugs to a formulary often takes 12–18 months, but innovative therapies with exceptional clinical value tend to achieve much faster formulary inclusion. In addition, hospitals may sometimes allow the use of new drugs before they are listed in their formularies – especially if these drugs appear to be superior to more established therapies.

Hospital physicians usually initiate the evaluation of new drugs by requesting their addition to the formulary. Their submission is often supported by a recommendation from their head of department and a clinical summary document or compilation of references to demonstrate a new drug's advantages over products already listed in the hospital formulary. In response, one of the hospital's pharmacists generally conducts research to identify any opposing evidence. Decisions on formulary inclusion are usually made by the *commissione terapeutico ospedaliero* (CTO; hospital therapeutic commission). In 2003, a survey commissioned by the *Società Italiana di Farmacia Ospedaliera e dei Servizi Territoriali* (Italian Society for Hospital Pharmacy and Territorial Services) found that more than 80% of Italian hospitals had a CTO.

In addition to local hospital formularies, many of Italy's regions have introduced a *prontuario terapeutico ospedaliero regionale* (regional hospital formulary) for all public hospitals within their territories. Cost-containment is an important objective of such regional formularies. For example, the *Bolletino Ufficiale della Regione Campania* (Official Bulletin of the Region of Campania) states that "over the years, publishing a formulary has become not just a choice of medical specialties and diagnostics but also a task of great political and social responsibility because the scarcity of financial resources dedicated to healthcare demands that [these resources] are used in the most rational way possible."

SALES AND PRESCRIBING TRENDS

Market Overview

IMS Health reports that pharmaceutical sales in Italian retail pharmacies grew from $10.4 billion at ex-manufacturer prices in 2002 to $12.8 billion in 2003, a 23% increase. However, this growth in dollar terms is almost entirely attributable to the depreciation of the US dollar against the euro. Using constant exchange rates, sales in Italy increased by only 2%, the slowest growth rate of the world's leading pharmaceutical markets. The sluggishness of the Italian market is attributable largely to the effects of the government's tough cost-containment measures. Figure 12.1 shows how the Italian pharmaceutical market has evolved since 2000, based on average exchange rates for each year.

According to OsMed, overall spending on prescription and nonprescription pharmaceuticals totaled €18.2 billion ($20.6 billion) at retail prices in 2003, a 2% increase over the preceding year. Gross public expenditures declined by 2.3%, from €12.6 billion ($14.2 billion) in 2002

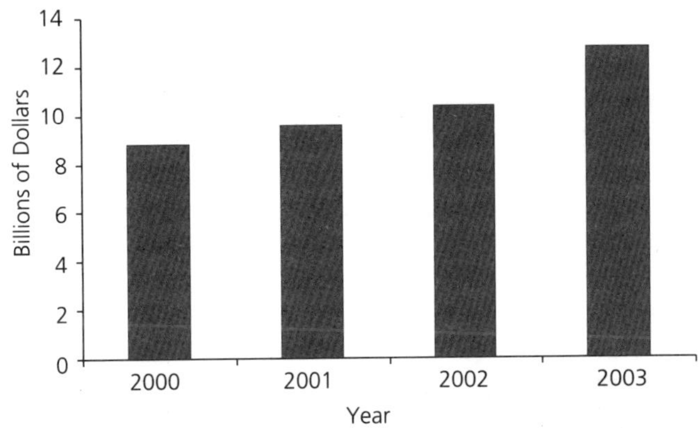

Figure 12.1 Evolution of the Italian Pharmaceutical Market at Exmanufacturer Prices, 2000–3

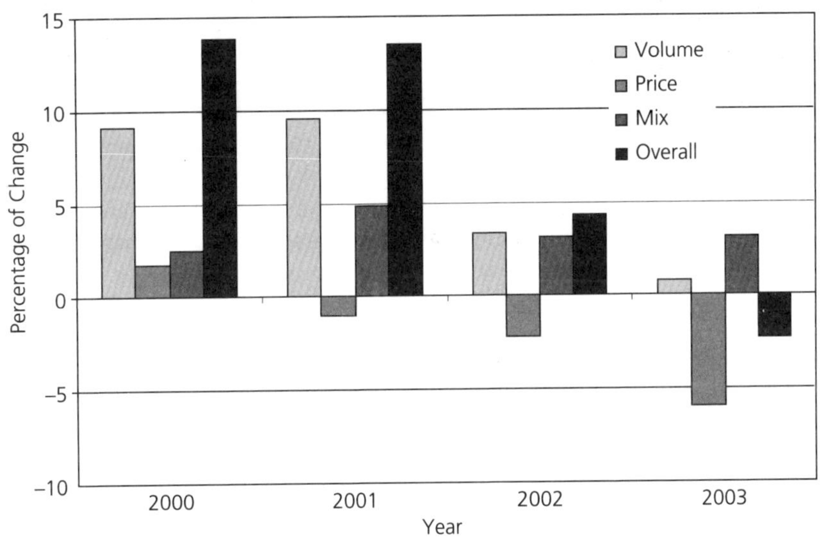

Figure 12.2 Effect of Changes in Prescription Volume, Drug Prices, and Product Mix on Gross Pharmaceutical Expenditures in Italy, 2000–3

to €12.4 billion ($14 billion) in 2003. Several factors contributed to this trend:

- A general reduction in pharmaceutical prices.
- Price adjustments for single active substances as a result of the introduction of new reference prices.
- The transfer of certain drugs from class B to class C.
- The imposition of a restrictive note on the prescribing of topical nonsteroidal anti-inflammatory drugs.

Figure 12.2 shows how changes in the volume of medicines prescribed, drug prices, and product mix contributed to gross pharmaceutical expenditures in Italy from 2000 to 2003. In 2000 and 2001, increased prescription volume was by far the most important stimulus to the growth of pharmaceutical sales. In 2002, however, volume growth slowed sharply, and in 2003, changes in the mix of products prescribed (i.e., a shift toward more expensive medicines) was the most important driver of sales growth. Despite widespread criticism of the harm caused by runaway pharmaceutical prices, OsMed's analysis shows that average drug prices increased only very modestly in 2000 and declined in the three following years.

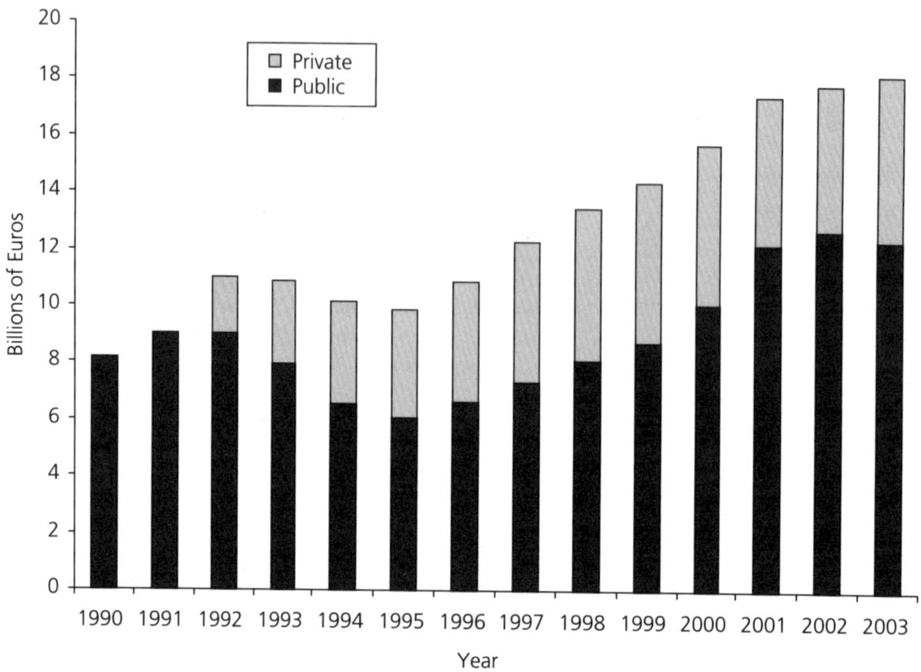

Figure 12.3 Private and Gross Public Expenditure on Prescription and Nonprescription Pharmaceuticals in Italy, 1990–2003

In contrast to the recent decline in gross public expenditures on medicines, private spending on prescription and nonprescription drugs grew from €5.2 billion ($5.9 billion) in 2002 to €5.9 billion ($6.7 billion) in 2003, a 12.4% increase. Figure 12.3 traces the evolution of public and private spending on pharmaceuticals in Italy from 1990 to 2003.

Federfarma, the association that represents Italian pharmacists, reports that approximately 439 million prescriptions were dispensed in Italy in 2003, a 2.7% decline compared with the preceding year. The average price of drugs dispensed per prescription also declined by 2.7% to €25.26 ($28.53). Pharmaceuticals' share of overall government spending on healthcare declined from 16.3% in 2001 to 15.5% in 2002 and to 13.8% in 2003 – close to the government's target of a 13% maximum share.

Rebates paid by the pharmaceutical industry to the SSN totaled €617 million ($697 million) in 2003. The government asserts that savings have been used to improve coverage of innovative medicines. However, drug manufacturers are predictably unhappy at the erosion of their profitability.

Leading Drug Categories, Classes, and Compounds

According to data published by OsMed, the top-10 drug classes, as defined by level 1 of the ATC classification system, account for more than 97% of SSN gross expenditures on pharmaceuticals. Table 12.3 shows public expenditures on these drug classes from 2000 to 2003. (OsMed does not publish detailed data on patients' spending on medicines.)

Cardiovascular drugs dominate the Italian pharmaceutical market. In 2003, this ATC level 1 drug category accounted for 33.2% of total SSN expenditures on medicines and an even higher percentage (48%) of SSN prescriptions. Public spending on this drug category increased by 28.4% in three years, equivalent to annual growth of 8.7%. However, CNS drugs experienced the most

Table 12.3 Evolution of Public Expenditures, 2000–3, on the 10 Best-Selling Drug Categories in Italy in 2003

Drug Categories[a]	*Sales (millions of euros)*				*Percentage Growth*	*CGR*
	2000	*2001*	*2002*	*2003*	*(2000-3)*	*(%)*
Cardiovascular drugs	3,267	3,771	4,079	4,195	28.4	8.7
Systemic antimicrobials	1,684	1,768	1,678	1,599	(5.1)	(1.7)
Gastrointestinal and metabolic agents	1,289	1,542	1,639	1,583	22.8	7.1
CNS therapies	554	928	1,131	1,148	107.3	27.5
Respiratory medicines	672	953	949	759	13.0	4.1
Antineoplastics and immunomodulators	672	716	753	736	9.5	3.1
Blood and hemopoietics	549	722	702	692	26.1	8.0
Genitourinary products and sex hormones	487	553	566	579	19.0	6.0
Musculoskeletal agents	404	599	565	561	38.7	11.5
Systemic hormone preparations[b]	220	244	248	236	7.1	2.3
Total	9,799	11,795	12,310	12,088	23.4	7.2

[a]Drug categories accord with definitions used in level 1 of the ATC classification system
[b]Excludes sex hormones
CGR = Cumulative growth rate
CNS = Central nervous system

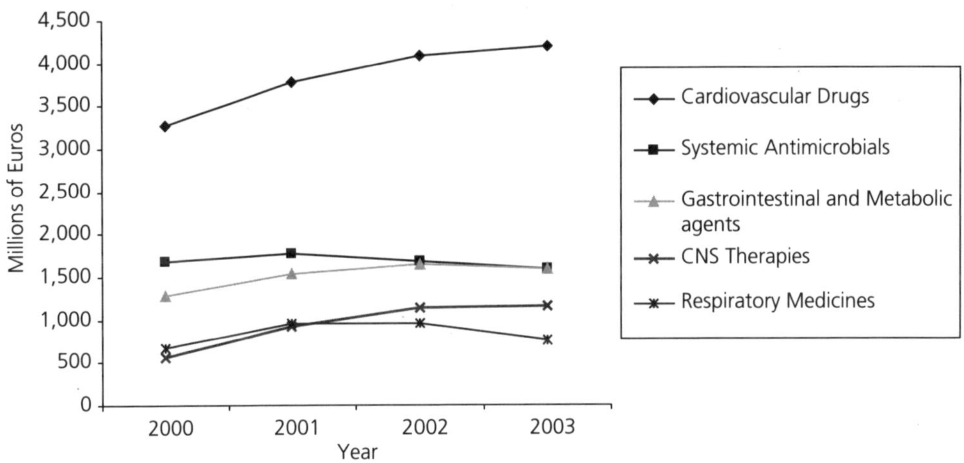

CNS = Central nervous system
Note: Drug categories accord with definitions used in level 1 of the ATC classification system

Figure 12.4 Evolution of Public Expenditures on the Five Best-Selling Drug Categories in Italy in 2000–3

vigorous growth in the period under review: public expenditures on this drug category more than doubled between 2000 and 2003, a cumulative growth rate of 27.5%. Increased sales of selective serotonin reuptake inhibitors (SSRIs) and antiepileptics were the main stimulus to this drug category. Public spending on musculoskeletal agents also grew rapidly – by 38.7% in three years, or 11.5% per year – a trend that is attributable largely to the success of the selective cyclooxygenase-2 (COX-2) inhibitors. Systemic antimicrobials were the only drug category that suffered a decrease in sales from 2000 to 2003: public expenditures declined by 5.1%. This trend is consistent with guidelines that recommend more conservative use of antibiotics. Figure 12.4 illustrates the trend in public expenditures on the five best-selling ATC level 1 drug categories in Italy.

An analysis of OsMed data on ATC level 4 drug classes shows that the 20 best-selling drug classes accounted for 60% of total SSN pharmaceutical expenditures in 2003. Table 12.4 shows public spending from 2000 to 2003 on the 20 drug classes that achieved the highest sales in 2003. In 2000, angiotensin-converting enzyme (ACE) inhibitors, calcium antagonists, and cephalosporins were the three largest drug classes in terms of SSN spending. Three years later, proton pump inhibitors and statins had become the best-selling drug classes in Italy, thanks to cumulative growth rates of more than 28%. However, several smaller drug classes had even faster annual growth rates: antiepileptics (32.3%); angiotensin II antagonists plus diuretics (39.2%); SSRIs (42.4%); low-molecular-weight heparins (62.6%); and beta blockers (91.8%). Figure 12.5 illustrates the trend in public expenditures on the five best-selling ATC level 4 drug classes in Italy.

The leading drugs grew much faster than the Italian pharmaceutical market as a whole. Table 12.5 shows that public spending on the 30 best-selling compounds in 2003 increased by 66.9% in three years, equivalent to 18.6% per year. Omeprazole (AstraZeneca's Losec) was the clear leader in 2000 and maintained this position throughout our review period. Indeed, its sales increased sharply in 2001 and 2002. In 2003, however, omeprazole's sales slumped as physicians increasingly switched patients to esomeprazole (AstraZeneca's Nexium), the single isomer of omeprazole. Statins – notably simvastatin (Merck's Zocor), atorvastatin (Pfizer's Lipitor), and pravastatin (Bristol-Myers Squibb's Pravachol) – all made strong gains. However, Girolamo Sirchia, the Italian minister of health, has recently criticized what he considers to be the widespread overuse of statins in Italy. Following their launch in the third quarter of 2000, the selective COX-2 inhibitors rofecoxib (Merck's Vioxx) and celecoxib (Pfizer's

Table 12.4 Evolution of Public Expenditures, 2000–3, on the 20 Best-Selling Drug Classes in Italy in 2003

Drug Classes[a]	*Sales (millions of euros)*				*Percentage Growth (2000–3)*	*CGR (%)*
	2000	*2001*	*2002*	*2003*		
Proton pump inhibitors	390	617	799	835	114.0	28.9
Statins	366	552	654	774	111.6	28.4
ACE inhibitors	593	635	668	626	5.6	1.8
Calcium antagonists	592	626	622	547	(7.6)	(2.6)
ACE inhibitors plus diuretics	449	456	458	451	0.4	0.1
Cephalosporins	570	419	470	431	(24.4)	(8.9)
Angiotensin II antagonists	237	301	344	377	59.1	16.7
Selective serotonin reuptake inhibitors	125	297	372	362	188.7	42.4
Angiotensin II antagonists plus diuretics	119	196	271	322	169.9	39.2
Macrolides and lincosamides	326	359	354	316	(3.0)	(1.0)
Combination respiratory agents	N.A.	199	270	289	N.M.	N.M.
Penicillins	239	270	274	266	11.4	3.7
Inhaled corticosteroids	N.A.	307	296	256	N.M.	N.M.
Selective Cox 2 inhibitors	N.A.	234	241	245	N.M.	N.M.
Quinolones	215	253	253	242	12.8	4.1
Alpha blockers	147	179	196	227	54.3	15.6
Beta blockers	32	201	212	223	605.6	91.8
Antiepileptics	96	136	193	221	131.3	32.3
Nitrates	238	248	237	213	(10.5)	(3.6)
Low-molecular-weight heparins	46	131	182	199	329.9	62.6
Total	4,778	6,616	7,366	7,422	55.3	15.8

[a]Drug classes accord with definitions used in level 4 of the ATC classification system

ACE = Angiotensin-converting enzyme; CGR = Cumulative growth rate; N.A. = Not available; N.M. = Not meaningful

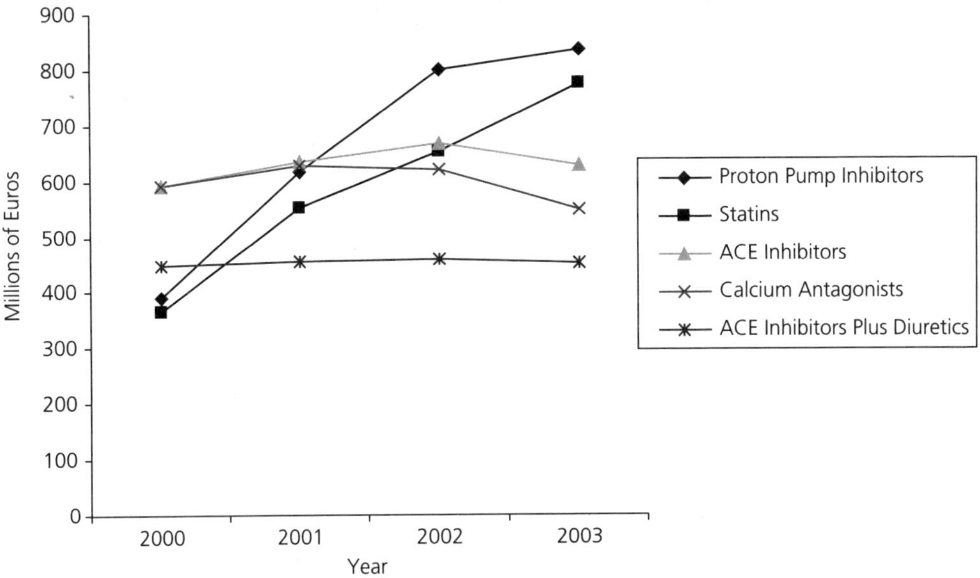

ACE = Angiotensin-converting enzyme
Note: Drug classes accord with definitions used in level 4 of the ATC classification system

Figure 12.5 Evolution of Public Expenditures on the Five Best-Selling Drug Classes in Italy, 2000–3

Celebrex) made a dramatic impact on the Italian market for anti-inflammatory drugs. SSRIs – notably citalopram (Lundbeck's Celexa) and paroxetine (GlaxoSmithKline's Seroxat) – also grew strongly. Figure 12.6 shows public expenditures on the five best-selling compounds in Italy.

OUTLOOK FOR THE ITALIAN PHARMACEUTICAL MARKET

In recent years, the Italian pharmaceutical market has suffered from the government's fluctuating policies on cost containment. From 1991 to 1994, public spending on pharmaceuticals declined by an average of 9.3% per year. However, in the next four years, public expenditures grew by an average of 9.5% per year. The growth rate in public pharmaceutical spending accelerated to 14.6% in 2000 and peaked at 21% in 2001. The growth rate then slowed to 4% in 2002, and public expenditures on medicines declined by 2.3% in 2003. Renewed growth in the pharmaceutical market in the first few months of 2004 could prompt the government to impose further draconian cost-cutting measures in the near future. In the first four months of 2004, public spending on pharmaceuticals increased by 10.1% compared with the corresponding period in 2003. In April 2004, public pharmaceutical expenditures were 16.5% higher than in April 2003. However, the growth rate declined to just 2.9% in May 2004. Consequently, from January to May 2004, public spending on pharmaceuticals was 7% higher than in the first five months of 2003. As noted earlier, the government has predicted that SSN pharmaceutical spending will be €1.3 billion ($1.5 billion) over budget in 2004, an overspend that will incur a €495 million ($559 million) penalty for the pharmaceutical industry.

Measures such as the aggressive reference-pricing system for off-patent drugs and the new PFN's price ceilings for homogeneous therapeutic categories have been severe blows to the pharmaceutical industry.

Table 12.5 Evolution of Public Expenditures, 2000–3, on the 30 Best-Selling Compounds in Italy in 2003

Compounds	*Sales (millions of euros)*				*Percentage Growth (2000–3)*	*CGR (%)*
	2000	*2001*	*2002*	*2003*		
Omeprazole	260	405	443	349	34.1	10.3
Simvastatin	149	221	268	291	95.0	24.9
Atorvastatin	110	173	223	274	149.1	35.6
Amlodipine	244	266	285	255	4.4	1.4
Amoxicillin/clavulanate	136	160	182	200	47.2	13.8
Salmeterol plus fluticasone[a]	—	149	183	199	N.M.	N.M.
Enalapril	209	211	207	191	(8.7)	(3.0)
Esomeprazole[b]	—	—	81	186	N.M.	N.M.
Nitroglycerine	178	187	184	171	(4.0)	(1.4)
Clarithromycin	160	181	179	165	3.4	1.1
Doxazosin	135	153	167	163	20.9	6.5
Pravastatin	58	105	133	160	174.5	40.0
Ceftriaxone	122	132	131	144	18.1	5.7
Omega 3[c]	—	—	—	140	N.M.	N.M.
Bicalutamide	50	71	117	138	175.4	40.2
Ramipril	63	82	113	137	116.1	29.3
Tamsulosin	81	108	116	127	56.1	16.0
Citalopram	28	73	105	124	349.0	65.0
Rofecoxib[d]	41	99	110	124	203.4	44.8
Celecoxib[d]	31	134	131	121	289.1	57.3
Paroxetine	51	118	144	120	134.2	32.8
Lansoprazole	56	88	107	115	107.1	27.5
Pantoprazole	53	73	98	110	107.5	27.5
Hydrochlorothiazide plus enalapril	128	124	120	109	(14.9)	(5.2)
Levofloxacin	69	83	95	105	52.9	15.2
Losartan plus hydrochlorothiazide	53	61	87	104	95.5	25.0
Finasteride	92	103	100	101	9.3	3.0
Somatropin	107	111	107	100	(6.5)	(2.2)
Azithromycin	85	96	99	95	11.3	3.6
Beclomethasone	73	104	98	94	28.3	8.7
Total	2,824	3,872	4,413	4,712	66.9	18.6

[a]Launched in the fourth quarter of 2000
[b]Launched in the second quarter of 2002
[c]Launched in the first quarter of 2001
[d]Launched in the third quarter of 2000
CGR = Cumulative growth rate

In June 2003, IMS Health reported that average pack prices for off-patent drugs in Italy had declined by 40% since the introduction of reference pricing in September 2001. Together with the 7% price cut, the government's imposition of tough controls on reimbursement prices could precipitate a downward spiral in drug prices that will make pharmaceutical companies think twice about launching new drugs in Italy and investing in R&D in that country. Italy's recent reimbursement restrictions have set an alarming precedent for other countries that operate similar systems. Germany is currently extending its reference-pricing system, and France may do the same with its new reference-pricing system. The best defense against restrictions on reimbursement prices is evidence that a drug is therapeutically superior to established therapies. However, it remains to be seen if the Italian government will really reward innovation with generous price premiums. The government has certainly indicated that it does not expect price premiums to have a substantial impact on overall SSN pharmaceutical expenditures.

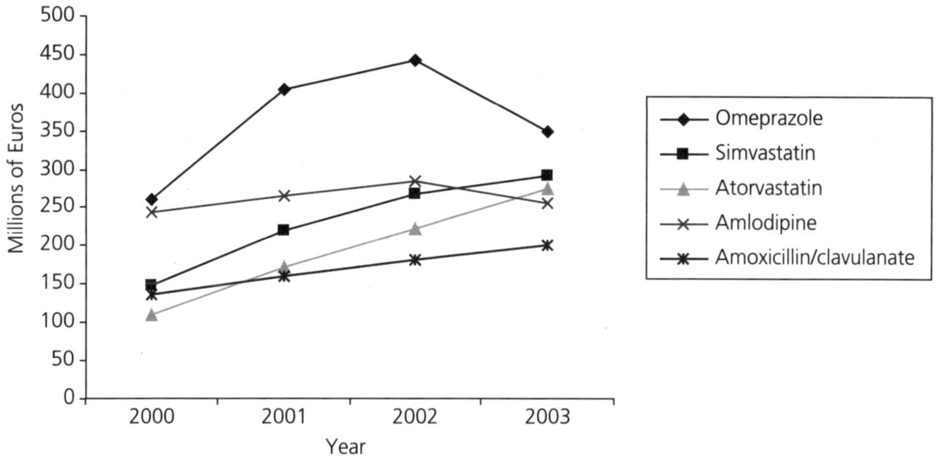

Figure 12.6 Evolution of Public Expenditures on the Five Best-Selling Drug Compounds in Italy in 2000–3

The research-based pharmaceutical industry can derive some comfort from the fact that generics continue to pose little threat to branded medicines. Despite the government's repeated efforts to stimulate greater use of generics, unbranded medicines still account for less than 2% of sales. However, the sluggish response of the generics market could induce the government to take a more aggressive stance on promoting the use of generics.

In the coming months, the pharmaceutical industry will have to learn to work with the new *Agenzia Italiana del Farmaco (AIFA)*. It remains to be seen what approach this organization will take to regulating the pharmaceutical market. Given the thrust of government policy, it appears almost certain that the AIFA will place considerable emphasis on price and cost-effectiveness.

Italy has also shown increasing interest in health technology assessment and evidence-based medicine. On June 18, 2004, the minister of health and Dr. Nello Martini, the director general of the AIFA, were among the eminent participants at a seminar and round-table discussion in Milan entitled "The NICE Impact on Drug Evaluation and Use in the U.K." This event suggests that the Italian government may be giving serious consideration to establishing an Italian organization similar to the United Kingdom's National Institute for Clinical Excellence (NICE).

The decentralization of responsibility for healthcare could prove to be one of the most important influences on the future evolution of the Italian pharmaceutical market. Several regional governments have already introduced prescription charges, while another has dereimbursed many "nonessential" drugs and imposed quantity limits per prescription. Growing pressure on regional authorities to comply with spending targets will likely result in further differences in healthcare policy between the regions. The pharmaceutical industry could therefore face the challenge of an increasingly fragmented market in Italy.

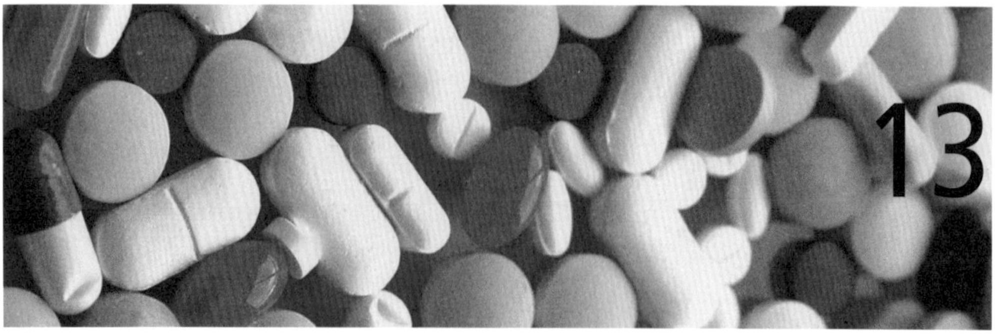

13

Pharmaceutical Pricing, Reimbursement, and Prescribing in Spain

OVERVIEW

The Spanish healthcare system has traditionally offered its beneficiaries very generous reimbursement terms for prescription drugs, the result being that Spain has a high level of pharmaceutical consumption. Nevertheless, the Spanish market has always been challenging for pharmaceutical companies: prices are among the lowest in Europe, and manufacturers face tough negotiations to set pricing and reimbursement terms for drugs that are covered by the national healthcare system. Despite these low prices, the Spanish government has imposed a wide range of cost-containment measures on the pharmaceutical industry. The Socialist government, elected in April 2004, has shown signs that its pharmaceutical cost-containment strategy may focus increasingly on multinational pharmaceutical companies.

ORGANIZATION AND FUNDING OF THE SPANISH HEALTHCARE SYSTEM

According to the Organization for Economic Cooperation and Development, Spain spent 7.6% of its gross domestic product (GDP) on healthcare in 2002 – significantly less than the European Union (EU) average of 8.5%. In 2000, the *sistema de seguridad social* (social security system) spent a total of €27.4 billion ($30.9 billion) on healthcare. (For the sake of uniformity of the analysis, the dollar-to-euro exchange rate used in this report is the 2003 average rate: $1 = $0.8854.)

The *Sistema Nacional de Salud* (SNS; National Health System) is based on the constitutional principle of universal and equal access to healthcare. The SNS covers 99.5% of the Spanish population, and all employees (except for civil servants and certain other exempt groups) are required to contribute to the SNS. (Civil servants are covered by a program known as the Mutualidad General de Funcionarios Civiles del Estado [MUFACE; General Mutual Benefit Society for State Civil Servants]. General taxes account for 97.4% of SNS funding.

Approximately 10% of Spanish citizens either supplement their SNS coverage with private insurance or rely exclusively on private insurance. Private healthcare accounts for approximately 20% of total healthcare spending in Spain – a share that is expected to remain constant for the foreseeable future.

On January 15, 2002, Spain reformed its healthcare system by devolving authority for many policy areas to the country's

17 autonomous regions. Before that date, seven regions (Andalucia, the Basque Country, Catalonia, the Canary Islands, Galicia, Navarre, and Valencia), covering 65% of the national population, had independent healthcare administrations. Healthcare provision in the other 10 regions was coordinated by the *Instituto Nacional de la Salud* (INSALUD; National Health Institute), an agency of the Ministry of Health and Consumer Affairs. In August 2002, the government replaced INSALUD with the *Instituto Nacional de Gestión Sanitaria* (National Institute for Healthcare Management), a much smaller organization with limited powers.

Governments in the 17 autonomous regions are now responsible for determining and implementing healthcare policy within their regions. Most of their funding comes from central SNS finances, but regional governments have the freedom to allocate additional funds to the healthcare system within their territories. Increasing regional fragmentation of the Spanish healthcare system can be expected in the years ahead.

However, the national government retains ultimate authority over healthcare regulation and policy. The Ministry of Health now concentrates on strategic issues, such as cost containment, product approvals, drug safety, implementing EU directives, and drug pricing and reimbursement.

PHARMACEUTICAL PRICES IN SPAIN

Pharmaceutical prices in Spain are among the lowest in the European Union. Table 13.1 shows the results of an international price comparison conducted by the UK Department of Health, which monitors prices of the most frequently prescribed drugs in the United Kingdom, several other European markets, and the United States. (The analysis uses the United Kingdom as a benchmark for a multilateral comparison of average prices of branded prescription medicines in these markets. Fluctuations from year to year are attributable largely to exchange rate movements.) This study found that, from 1998 to 2002, among the major European markets, Spain had by far the lowest prices.

The *Ley del Medicamento 25/90* (Pharmaceutical Law 25/90) of December 20, 1990, is the main law governing drug pricing and reimbursement. It defines the criteria for including or excluding medicines from the SNS-reimbursable list. Since 1998, pharmaceutical companies have been free to set the prices of drugs that the SNS does not cover. However, given that a lack of reimbursement can severely restrict a new drug's sales potential, few manufacturers are willing to launch a new product without SNS coverage. Pharmaceutical companies therefore have to negotiate an acceptable price for reimbursement.

Table 13.1 Multilateral Comparison of Average Exmanufacturer Prices of Branded Medicines in Select Markets as a Percentage of UK Average Exmanufacturer Prices, 1992–2002

	France	*Germany*	*Italy*	*Spain*	*United States*	*United Kingdom*
1992	93	158	108	95	172	100
1993	96	158	100	89	202	100
1994	100	143	90	88	192	100
1995	107	130	83	89	179	100
1996	105	125	93	89	191	100
1997	85	101	86	74	184	100
1998	85	109	88	77	188	100
1999	86	103	82	72	213	100
2000	83	94	82	70	241	100
2001	81	90	85	72	205	100
2002	83	94	86	77	194	100
Average, 1998–2002[a]	83	94	86	77	197	100

[a]Based on 2002 price data but converted to pounds sterling using average exchange rates for the period 1998–2002

The *Dirección General de Farmacia y Productos Sanitarios* (DGFPS; General Directorate of Pharmacy and Health Products) and its agencies are responsible for setting the prices of SNS-reimbursable drugs. Pharmaceutical companies must include the following information in their pricing application to the DGFPS:

- Scientific and clinical data.
- Degree of innovation relative to similar drugs on the Spanish market.
- Copy of marketing authorization.
- Proposed ex-manufacturer and retail prices.
- Detailed production and R&D costs.
- Transfer costs (if applicable).
- Company financial statements.
- Estimated product sales in Spain.
- Prices in the country of origin and in other EU countries.

The DGFPS's *Subdirección General de Economía del Medicamento y Productos Sanitarios* (SGEMPS; General Subdirectorate of Pharmaceutical and Health Product Economics) reviews the application and produces a summary dossier. This dossier forms the basis for pricing negotiations between the manufacturer and the *Comisión Interministerial de Precios de los Medicamentos* (CIPM; Interdepartmental Committee on Pharmaceutical Prices), the body that ultimately determines the prices of SNS-reimbursable drugs.

The pricing of new pharmaceuticals in Spain is based on a cost-plus formula. Under this system, the maximum price for an SNS-reimbursable drug covers a manufacturer's production costs (including raw materials), promotional costs (to a maximum of 16%), and administrative and general costs (including R&D) and allows a margin for profit (calculated on the basis of projected sales volume). The agreed price should provide a profit in the range of 12–18% on invested capital. If a product later exceeds its projected sales volume, its price may be reduced to restore profits to the acceptable range.

Several other factors can have a particularly important bearing on a new drug's price in Spain:

- Prices in other EU countries (especially France, Italy, Germany, and the United Kingdom).
- Prices of comparable existing therapies.
- Prices of comparable existing therapies in foreign markets.
- R&D activity and manufacturing investment in Spain.
- Degree of therapeutic innovation.
- Existence of licensing agreements with local research-based companies.

REIMBURSEMENT OF OUTPATIENT MEDICINES

Drugs covered by the SNS are reimbursed (In Spain, "reimbursement" does not refer to the repayment of expenses that patients incur out of their own pockets at the time of purchase. Rather, the SNS either covers the full cost of medication or requires a nonrefundable patient copayment for part of the cost.) at one of three rates:

- 100% for hospital-only medicines.
- 90% for therapies for chronic disorders. (Patients pay a maximum of €2.64 [$2.98] per prescription item.)
- 60% for all other reimbursable drugs.

The *Comisión Nacional para el Uso Racional del Medicamento* (CNURM; National Committee for the Rational Use of Medicines), an agency of the DGFPS, is the body responsible for deciding reimbursement terms for pharmaceuticals in Spain. The CNURM consists of the following: representatives from the *Administración General del Estado* (State General Administration), the 17 autonomous regions, the pharmaceutical industry, the medical profession, consumer organizations, and trade unions, together with external experts nominated by the Ministry of Health. The *Ley del Medicamento 25/90* defines the following criteria for reimbursement decisions:

- Price agreed on by the DGFPS.
- Severity, duration, and effects of the indicated disease.

- Needs of particular patient populations.
- Clinical and social value of the therapy.
- Cost and efficacy relative to similar products.
- Total cost to the SNS and pharmaceutical budget limits.
- Potential role in therapeutic strategy.
- Existence of similar therapies with lower prices or treatment costs.

The law does not yet require pharmacoeconomic data, but they may be included in the submission if they are available.

Supply-side Restrictions

The Spanish government has implemented several supply-side restrictions, as discussed in the following sections.

Negative List

Like other EU countries, Spain excludes from public reimbursement drugs that have minimal or questionable efficacy, as well as drugs that are not deemed cost effective or could prove too expensive for the healthcare system. A Socialist government created the negative list in 1993. Five years later, the *Partido Popular* (Popular Party) added a further 834 products in 39 therapeutic groups to the list. Critics asserted that dereimbursement decisions in 1998 were motivated primarily by cost-containment considerations, whereas pharmacological criteria had been more influential in 1993. Further products have been added to the negative list in subsequent years.

The negative list has shifted prescribing away from older (and in many cases less-expensive) drugs of questionable efficacy toward newer (and frequently more-expensive) therapies that are still covered by the SNS. Many of the drugs on the negative list are now available over the counter, a development that has stimulated the practice of self-medication in Spain. However, a substantial minority of products on the negative list have been withdrawn from the market. At the beginning of 2002, approximately 40% of drugs excluded from reimbursement in 1993 and 25% of medicines added to the negative list in 1998 had been withdrawn from the market.

Positive List

Spain also operates a positive list – a catalogue of products that are approved for SNS reimbursement. This list is updated monthly. The Real Decreto 83/1993 (Royal Decree 83/1993) defines the criteria by which a drug is assessed for possible inclusion in the positive list:

- Disease characteristics.
- Characteristics of patient population.
- Clinical utility.
- Public spending limits.
- Existence of alternative therapies.

Products that offer only symptomatic relief or that treat relatively minor conditions do not qualify for inclusion in the positive list. Drugs that are not economically justifiable or that are deemed unnecessary are also excluded.

Reference Pricing

Reference pricing was introduced in Spain on December 1, 2000, and soon became the mainstay of the government's cost-containment strategy. Drugs within the system are assigned to "homogeneous groups" – medicines that are therapeutically equivalent and have the same qualitative and quantitative composition, pharmaceutical form, dosage form, and route of administration. All homogeneous groups must contain at least one generic drug. The SNS reimburses reference-priced drugs only to the level of the reference price for the respective homogeneous group.

The first wave of reference pricing assigned 590 products to 114 homogeneous groups. These products accounted for approximately 10% of public spending on medicines. Manufacturers were obliged to reduce the prices of 193 copy products that lacked proof of bioequivalence to reference price levels. In April 2002, the government assigned a further 113 products to 28 homogeneous groups and obliged pharmaceutical companies to cut the prices of 25 copy products to reference-price levels.

Originally, the reference price was the average of the prices of the least-expensive drugs that collectively accounted for 20% of sales within each homogeneous group. In May 2003, however, the *Ley de Cohesión y Calidad del Sistema Nacional de Salud* (Law on the Coherence and Quality of the National Healthcare System) changed the method for calculating reference prices: reference prices are now based on the average price of the three products in a homogeneous group that have the lowest daily treatment costs. Each of the three products used in setting a reference price must be marketed by a different manufacturer. Products that have an ex-manufacturer price of less than €2.00 ($2.26) are excluded from these calculations. Prices for generics may not exceed the group's reference price.

If pharmacists receive a prescription for a product that is in a generics group but exceeds its reference price, they are required to substitute a product that does not exceed the reference price. In the event that a product less expensive than the reference price is not available, the pharmacist dispenses the prescribed product but charges the patient the reference price. The manufacturer must then reimburse the pharmacist the difference between the reference price and the retail price of its drug.

This law could trigger a relentless downward spiral in prices as manufacturers seek to ensure that their prices are among the bottom three in each group. The *Asociación Española de Fabricantes de Sustancias y Especialidades Farmacéuticas Genéricas* (AESEG; Spanish Association of Manufacturers of Generic Pharmaceutical Substances and Specialties) predicted that generics prices could fall by an average of 30%. Manufacturers of products that exceed reference prices will not welcome the extra bureaucracy and expense involved in reimbursing pharmacists the differential between the reference price and their products' retail price.

In October 2003, the government published the new *Orden de Precios de Referencia de Medicamentos* (Pharmaceutical Reference Pricing Order). On January 1, 2004, the reference prices of 2,070 different presentations of 62 frequently prescribed compounds were reduced by an average of 28%, but some products were subjected to cuts of as much as 80%. In 2002, SNS spending on the targeted drugs totaled €1.64 billion ($1.85 billion), a sum that the government hoped to reduce by €463 million per year. Such a drop in sales would reduce the annual growth rate for SNS pharmaceutical spending from 11% to 8%.

Not surprisingly, the pharmaceutical industry was fiercely critical of the new reference prices. Farmaindustria, the Spanish pharmaceutical industry association, predicted that the reform could reduce employment levels in the Spanish pharmaceutical sector by 2.6% and slash R&D investment in Spain by as much as 35%. The association recently reported that some companies have been forced to reduce the prices of more than 60% of their products and is also concerned that multinationals will be deterred from investing in Spain in future. Farmaindustria threatened to take legal action to challenge the new reference prices.

In March 2004, the *Federación Empresarial de Farmaceúticos Españoles* (FEFE; Business Federation of Spanish Pharmacists) suggested that reference pricing was not achieving the level of savings that the government had expected. FEFE attributed this situation to the fact that many physicians were prescribing more-expensive innovative therapies in place of drugs that are subject to reference pricing. A study conducted by IMS Health on behalf of the Ministry of Health supports the belief that Spanish physicians often avoid prescribing reference-priced drugs. For example, sales of simvastatin, a drug that is subject to reference pricing, grew by 4.6% in 2003 as a whole but declined by 14.3% in December 2003, shortly after the latest reference price cuts were announced. Conversely, sales of atorvastatin, a drug that is currently excluded from reference pricing, increased by 13.1% in December 2003 and by 23% in the year as a whole. Similarly, sales of the proton-pump inhibitor pantoprazole, which is not subject to reference pricing, grew much faster than sales of omeprazole, a drug that is reference priced.

However, government data indicate that the reference price cuts imposed on January 1,

2004, had an immediate effect on pharmaceutical expenditures. Spending on medicines in the first month of 2004 increased by just 1.89% compared with January 2003, the smallest increase recorded since 1995.

On May 19, 2004, nine additional molecules became subject to reference pricing in Spain: bisoprolol, cefaclor, fluvoxamine, loratadine, lormetazepam, spironolactone, terazosin, tramadol, and zolpidem. Manufacturers of these products were given two months to reduce their prices to reference price levels. Approximately 45 companies were impacted by this extension of reference pricing. The Ministry of Health forecasted that this action would reduce pharmaceutical expenditures by a total of €12.94 million ($14.6 million), producing savings of €12.04 million ($13.6 million) for the healthcare system and €0.9 million ($1 million) for patients. The reference price cuts were expected to cost the pharmaceutical industry a total of €8.1 million ($9.1 million).

On August 1, 2004, the Ministry of Health cut the reference prices of 281 products containing 15 different active ingredients. The list of affected drug classes included antibiotics, antidepressants, antihistamines, antineoplastics, antiulcerants, beta blockers, diuretics, hypnotics and anxiolytics, and opioid analgesics.

In September 2004, the Ministry of Health announced plans to subject four additional molecules – amlodipine, cefazolin, ofloxacin, and pravastatin – to reference pricing from March 1, 2005. A total of 82 product presentations (i.e., individual dosages, dosage forms, and pack sizes of a product) would be affected, 32 of which are currently priced above the proposed reference-price levels. Several pravastatin products would require price cuts of more than 50% to meet reference prices. For example, Bristol-Myers Squibb's Lipemol and Esteve's Liplat both currently cost €23.89 ($26.98) for twenty-eight 10 mg tablets, but their prospective reference price is just €11.48 ($12.97).

In early October, the Ministry of Health surprised observers by announcing plans for radical changes to the reference-pricing system. The new Socialist government has been disappointed by the savings achieved by the reference-pricing system – €210 million ($237 million) instead of the €430 million ($486 million) forecasted in 2003. Furthermore, the government is concerned that the reference-pricing system causes what it describes as "collateral damage." Some domestic manufacturers and generics companies have lost as much as 25% of their sales as a result of reference pricing, whereas the impact on multinationals has been much smaller (0.5–3%). At this writing, the government has not revealed how it plans to overhaul the reference-pricing system, but it has said that it wants to save money "without suffocating pharmaceutical companies."

Price Cuts and Freezes

Several times in recent years, the Spanish government has imposed either price freezes or price cuts on established drugs. In 1999, for instance, the government imposed a 6% reduction in the price of all drugs that cost more than PTA 350 ($2.38). In 2001, the government reduced the prices of five successful drugs – atenolol (Alter's Atenolol Alter), ciprofloxacin (multisource), enalapril (multisource), famotidine (multisource), and omeprazole (multisource) – by 15%. Such measures have driven Spain's already low drug prices even lower. The industry therefore has to rely on increased prescription volumes and a shift toward innovative drugs for sales growth.

Sales Tax

In September 2004, the government announced that a new tax on sales of prescription drugs to the SNS would take effect from January 1, 2005. The tax will be calculated on the basis of a company's sales to the SNS every four months. The level of the tax will increase in line with each company's sales to the SNS. Table 13.2 shows the tax thresholds. The government hopes that this measure will raise revenues of more than €200 million ($226 million) per year. Half of the revenues will be used to fund research projects conducted by the Instituto Carlos III and the rest will be used, in as yet unspecified ways, to

Table 13.2 Thresholds for Company Tax on Sales to the SNS

SNS Sales (€Million)	*Tax (%)*
0–3	1.5
3–6	2.0
6–15	2.5
15–20	3.0
30–60	3.5
60–120	4.0
120–300	4.5
>300	5.0

SNS = Sistema Nacional de Salud (National Healthcare System)

Note: Sales totals relate to each four-month period in the year

promote rational prescribing and continuing education of physicians. The opposition *Partido Popular* intends to challenge the new sales tax as unconstitutional.

Demand-side Restrictions

In an effort to curb pharmaceutical consumption, the Spanish government has also introduced several demand-side restrictions.

Prescribing Restrictions and Budgets

To curb excessive prescribing, the government has introduced restrictions on the number of drugs that general practitioners may prescribe on a single prescription. A national prescription monitoring system – the *Terminal Autónomo de Identificación de Recetas* (TAIR; Independent Prescription Identification Terminal) – is being introduced to identify and warn physicians who are judged to be overprescribing.

Several autonomous regions have implemented their own cost-containment measures. For example, some authorities encourage primary care centers to implement prescribing budgets by allowing them to retain 20% of the savings they achieve (subject to maintaining acceptable clinical standards). Another approach is paying general practitioners, or in some cases all medical personnel, bonuses at year end if their practices remain within their prescribing budget and meet certain other targets. Some regions have experimented with rewarding physicians for increased prescribing of generics. However, they abandoned these initiatives when they discovered that, instead of using generics in place of branded medicines (as intended), some physicians were prescribing generic versions of drugs in addition to the branded originals to receive the incentive payment for generic prescribing.

Patient Copayments

As noted earlier, the SNS requires patients to make a copayment for certain drugs. In theory, patients pay 10% of the cost (to a maximum of €2.64 [$2.98]) for drugs that treat chronic disorders and 40% of the cost of most other reimbursed medicines. In practice, however, only a minority of patients are required to make these copayments. Seniors and certain other groups are exempt from all pharmaceutical copayments. As a consequence, patient contributions account for only a very modest share of the total cost of prescription medicines. Indeed, patients' share of pharmaceutical spending has declined steadily, from roughly 18% in 1982 to less than 7% at present. These figures illustrate the limited effectiveness of patient copayments as a pharmaceutical cost-containment measure.

Prior Authorization

To control the prescription of certain drugs, the government sometimes imposes a *visado de inspección* (inspection visa). For such drugs to be dispensed at the expense of the SNS, the prescribing general practitioner must justify the prescription and the inspection service must authorize its use. The system aims to promote more rational use of drugs that are subject to *Especial Control Médico* (Special Medical Control), to limit the prescription of costly therapies, and to prevent off-label prescribing. Selective cyclooxygenase-2 (COX-2) inhibitors, acetylcholinesterase inhibitors, interferons, and many antimicrobials and vaccines are among the list of more than 600 drugs that are subject to inspection visas. In September 2004, the

Ministry of Health added atypical antipsychotics to this list. Almost 90% of medicines subject to an inspection visa require an initial hospital diagnosis (see further on). The impact of an inspection visa on sales can be dramatic. The pharmaceutical industry is highly critical of the lack of clarity about the criteria for imposing inspection visas on medicines. Manufacturers also argue that this control increases bureaucracy and frequently denies patients access to innovative new medicines.

Promoting Greater Use of Generics

For several reasons, multiple versions of most drugs have long been common in the Spanish pharmaceutical market. (See the sidebar, "The Spanish Market for Multisource Pharmaceuticals: A Complex Picture.") However, the market for true generic drugs has remained underdeveloped compared with such markets in the United States, Germany, and the United Kingdom.

The Spanish Market for Multisource Pharmaceuticals: A Complex Picture

One of the defining features of the Spanish pharmaceutical market is the prevalence of multisource pharmaceutical products. However, true generic drugs account for only a very modest share of total sales. This paradox is attributable primarily to the countryís historically weak intellectual property protection laws.

Spain joined the European Patent Convention in 1986, when it became a member of the European Communities (now the European Union [EU]). However, pharmaceutical patent protection in Spain remained relatively weak until a transition period expired on October 8, 1992. Until that date, pharmaceuticals in Spain were covered by process patents, rather than product patents. Provided they used different manufacturing processes, companies were free to reproduce molecules originally developed by other companies. Manufacturers of such copy products did not need to demonstrate bioequivalence with the original drug. Copy products could be marketed under either a brand name or the international nonproprietary name (INN) for the molecule in question followed by the manufacturer's name. If a manufacturer decided to use the INN plus company name, the product would be termed a *falso genérico* (false generic), because it lacked proof of bioequivalence.

In 1997, the Spanish government created a classification known as *especialidades farmacéuticas genéricas* (EFGs; generic pharmaceutical specialties) for products that have identical composition, dosage form, and indications to those of original drugs that have been on the market in Spain for at least ten years and/or that have generic equivalents in other EU countries. EFGs also require proof of bioequivalence and therapeutic equivalence to the reference drug. They are marketed under the INN plus manufacturer's name, and the packaging bears the abbreviation "EFG." Prices tend to be significantly lower than those of branded versions of the same molecule.

The Spanish market is further complicated by the widespread practice of one or more companies signing comarketing agreements with the developer of a new drug while the molecule is still subject to patent protection. Thus, it is common for several branded versions of a patent-protected drug to compete with one another in the Spanish market. Price differences among these competing brands are typically very small.

Because of these different drug categories, some older molecules may be available in four different classifications in Spain:

- The originator product.
- Licensed products (i.e., products that are identical to the originator product but marketed under different brand names through an agreement with the original developer).
- Copy products (i.e., products developed by a different process from that of the originator product and marketed under a different brand name or the INN).
- EFGs (i.e., products that are identical to the originator product, have proof of therapeutic equivalence and bioequivalence, and are marketed under the INN).

In an effort to stimulate greater use of generics, the Spanish government has implemented a series of reforms in recent years. In 1997, it created a new classification for generics: *especialidades farmacéuticas genéricas*

(EFGs; generic pharmaceutical specialties). The number of EFGs on the market has increased from 307 in 1999 to 1,870 in September 2004. Since 1999, the government has promoted a policy of generics substitution. Pharmacists are required to substitute an alternative therapy if the prescribed drug is not readily available, exceeds a reference price (where applicable), is prescribed using its international nonproprietary name [INN], or is a specifically named EFG. (If a physician prescribes a particular EFG by name, a pharmacist may substitute only another EFG, not a branded medicine.) Physicians cannot forbid generics substitution.

In 2001, the government of the time set a target for generics to account for 15% of all prescriptions in Spain by 2005. At this writing, it appears highly unlikely that this goal will be met. According to the AESEG, in 2003, EFGs had a market share of 5.1% in volume terms and 3.8% in monetary terms. The generics market is growing steadily – it achieved a market share of 7.1% in volume terms and 4.6% in monetary terms in May 2004 – but it is still a long way from reaching the previous government's target for 2005, let alone the prescribing levels seen in mature generics markets.

A recent survey conducted by the market research company Teleperformance on behalf of the generics manufacturer Pliva may help to explain the continued underdevelopment of the generics market in Spain. In March and April 2004, Teleperformance interviewed 434 primary care physicians from across the country. The survey found that Spanish physicians are ambivalent about generics and often lack detailed knowledge of these drugs. Sixty-five percent of respondents believed generic prescribing was an important way to save the Spanish healthcare system money. However, 67.3% thought that pharmacists should not substitute lower-priced generics for drugs that exceed their reference prices.

Several factors influenced physicians' decisions whether to prescribe a brand or a generic: 41.2% cited time pressures, 34.6% quality issues, 23.5% cost considerations, and 18.4% pressure from generics manufacturers. The survey also found that many physicians were ill-informed about the Spanish generics market: almost half of respondents were under the misapprehension that generics were available in all therapeutic categories. Physicians identified cardiovascular medicine, antibiotics, and rheumatology as the main priority areas for the launch of new generics.

Survey participants believed that their patients lacked familiarity with generics but would generally be willing to accept a prescription for a generic. The survey found that 78.8% of primary care physicians thought their patients did not know enough about generics, but 52% believed that their patients would accept a switch from a familiar brand to a generic, whereas 26% expected their patients to reject such a change.

REIMBURSEMENT OF HOSPITAL MEDICINES

Drug prices to Spanish hospitals must not exceed maximum retail prices, but hospitals generally expect to receive very substantial discounts on these prices. The pharmacy service in each hospital is responsible for drug acquisition. In most cases, hospitals deal directly with manufacturers, but they occasionally use wholesalers or invite suppliers to bid for contracts for a particular drug, drug class, or therapeutic area. Purchasing groups are much less common in Spain than in some other European countries.

The social security system covers the full cost of all prescription medicines dispensed in Spain's public hospitals or private hospitals that have contracts with the SNS. However, patients who undergo private medical treatment have to pay for their medications unless they have private health insurance that provides comprehensive pharmaceutical coverage.

Spain has two categories of drugs that require a prescription from a hospital physician. Some medicines are restricted to *uso hospitalario* (hospital use, designated as category H products). Drugs that are subject to *diagnóstico hospitalario* (DH; hospital diagnosis) require an initial diagnosis and prescription from a hospital-based physician but may subsequently be dispensed by retail pharmacies.

Many pharmaceutical companies choose to launch innovative new drugs as hospital-only medicines or to market them exclusively for hospital use. This trend is in response to growing criticism of the rising demand for costly new therapies in the community, a market that tends to be subject to much closer scrutiny of pharmaceutical prices and spending than the hospital pharmacy market.

Recently, however, pharmaceutical expenditures in the hospital sector have attracted increasing attention. The Spanish government has encouraged the *Sociedad Española de Farmacia Hospitalaria* (SEFH; Spanish Society for Hospital Pharmacy) to find ways to reduce the country's expenditures on hospital pharmacy. One approach is GRDOSIS, a program to test the potential savings from introducing diagnosis-related groups (DRGs) in Spanish hospitals. Trials conducted in seven hospitals in 2001–2 showed savings of as much as 43% in pharmaceutical expenditures. Another study, Epimed 2001, found that formulary negotiations by pharmacists in 14 hospitals reduced pharmaceutical costs by an average of 20%. Pharmacists achieved savings of as much as 83% for omeprazole capsules but less than 6% for some antipsychotics – a drug class in which hospitals have much less bargaining power.

Every public hospital in Spain is required by law to have a multidisciplinary *comisión de farmacia y terapéutica* (CFT; pharmacy and therapeutics committee), a body that defines the criteria for including drugs in the hospital's formulary and decides which drugs meet these criteria. Although drug acquisition prices and daily-treatment costs remain crucial factors in formulary decision making, pharmacy and therapeutics committees pay increasing attention to a drug's cost–benefit ratio.

Toward the end of 2000, the European Association of Hospital Pharmacists (EAHP) conducted a survey of hospital pharmacists throughout Europe. A total of 2,825 questionnaires were sent to hospital pharmacists in 22 countries, and 748 pharmacists responded. This survey found that 99% of hospital pharmacists in Spain indicated that their hospitals had developed formularies – among the highest percentages in Europe. Spanish formularies comprised, on average, a total of 454 active ingredients (significantly higher than the European mean of 368 active ingredients) and 715 products (comparable with the European mean of 700 products). Spanish formularies therefore contained a mean of 1.57 products for each active ingredient, indicating that in many cases only one product was available for a given active ingredient and the range of generics tended to be limited.

The EAHP survey found that Spanish pharmacy and therapeutics committees tended to update their formularies less frequently than their counterparts in most other European countries. In Europe as a whole, 48% of hospitals updated their formularies annually, 35% biennially, and 17% less often than every two years. In Spain, by comparison, only 13% updated their formularies annually, 40% biennially, and 48% less frequently than every two years.

Hospitals set an annual pharmacy budget and then usually monitor their drug costs on a monthly basis. Physicians who deviate from hospital prescribing protocols or who are judged to be overspending may be asked to justify their prescribing decisions.

SALES AND PRESCRIBING TRENDS

The Spanish pharmaceutical market is the fifth-largest in Europe. IMS Health reports that 2003 pharmaceutical sales in Spain's retail pharmacies totaled \$8.8 billion at ex-manufacturer prices, a 34% increase over 2002 in US dollar terms. If the effect of the dollar's depreciation against the euro is excluded, the growth rate is smaller but still substantial at 11.7%. This growth rate was the fastest since 1996, when sales increased by 12.9%. Volume growth was the main contributor to the market's expansion, increasing sales by 7.85%. Structural change (the shift toward newer medications) boosted sales by 3.71%, and price increases increased sales by just 0.13%. Figure 13.1 traces the development of the Spanish pharmaceutical market since 2000, based on average exchange rates for each year.

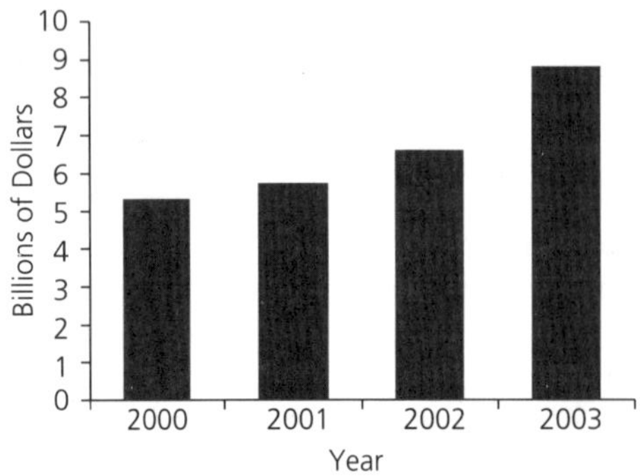

Figure 13.1 Evolution of the Spanish Retail Pharmacy Market at Exmanufacturer Prices, 2000–3

In 2003, government spending on pharmaceuticals in Spain increased by 11.7%. Reductions in the reference prices of 2,070 products in January 2004 slowed the growth of pharmaceutical expenditures in the first half of 2004. The Ministry of Health reports that spending increased by 7.02% in the first six months of the year.

As in the other major pharmaceutical markets, prescribing patterns in Spain have changed radically in recent years. Table 13.3 traces the sales evolution from 1997 to 2002 of the 30 best-selling drug classes in 2002. Antihyperlipidemics made the greatest advances over this period. In 1997, this drug class had total sales of €216 million ($244 million) and ranked fifth in the list of best-selling drug classes. By 2002, sales of antihyperlipidemics had increased to €600 million ($678 million), an increase of 178% in five years (equivalent to 22.7% per year). Neuroleptics, antiepileptics, nontricyclic antidepressants, antithrombotic agents, oral antidiabetics, antineoplastic hormone therapies, and bronchodilators and inhaled antiasthmatics were other drug classes that more than doubled their sales in five years.

Table 13.4 shows the sales evolution from 1997 to 2002 of the 20 best-selling compounds in 2002. Omeprazole remained the best-selling compound throughout that period, but atorvastatin closed the gap rapidly. Sales of the other two leading antihyperlipidemics, simvastatin and pravastatin, also grew vigorously. Paroxetine overtook fluoxetine as the best-selling antidepressant in Spain. The atypical antipsychotics olanzapine and risperidone also grew rapidly.

Older products dominate the Spanish pharmaceutical market in volume terms. Table 13.5 shows that products that have been on the market for more than 20 years consistently account for more than 45% of prescriptions, compared with a volume share of roughly 13% for products marketed for five years or less. In monetary terms, however, older medicines' market share is much more modest: products on the market for more than 20 years accounted for 18.7% in 2001, 18% in 2002, and 16.8% in 2003. Products marketed for less than five years also saw their market share in monetary terms decline, from 29.7% in 2001, to 25.1% in 2002, and 23.3% in 2003. Conversely, products marketed for 5–15 years experienced a significant increase in market share in both monetary and volume terms.

In proportion to the size of the overall Spanish pharmaceutical market, the Spanish hospital pharmacy market is among the largest in Europe. According to IMS Health, in 2002, ex-manufacturer sales of pharmaceuticals in Spanish hospitals totaled €1.9 billion ($2.1 billion), equivalent to 21.6% of the total Spanish pharmaceutical market (in monetary terms). Sales in the hospital sector grew by 8.9%, slightly slower than the 9.8% growth rate recorded in the retail pharmacy market in 2002.

The SEFH reports somewhat higher hospital pharmacy sales in 2002: €2.3 billion ($2.6 billion), equivalent to 25% of the total pharmaceutical market in Spain. Spending on medicines dispensed to inpatients totaled €1.4 billion ($1.6 billion), while the cost of drugs dispensed to outpatients amounted to €924 million ($1 billion). Overall, the market increased by 12.3% in 2002, but spending on outpatient medicines had a much higher growth rate (almost 23%) than spending on inpatient drugs (6%). According to the SEFH, the rapid growth in expenditures on outpatient medications is primarily

Table 13.3 Evolution, from 1997 to 2002, of SNS Spending on the 30 Best-Selling Drug Classes in 2002

Drug Class	*Sales (€ Million)*						*Change*	*Annual*
	1997	*1998*	*1999*	*2000*	*2001*	*2002*	*1997–2002(%)*	*Growth Rate (%)*
Antihyperlipidemics	216.0	290.3	374.0	429.1	507.4	600.1	177.8	22.7
H_2 antagonists and other antiulcerants	417.6	461.8	510.4	551.3	572.6	573.6	37.4	6.6
Other nontricyclic antidepressants	211.1	266.9	328.2	384.9	448.1	526.6	149.5	20.1
ACE inhibitors	319.3	353.4	409.0	454.1	469.5	514.7	61.2	10.0
Bronchodilators and inhaled antiasthmatics	229.2	287.1	332.8	382.0	435.6	487.3	112.6	16.3
Single NSAIDs	200.0	209.9	226.4	303.5	362.8	348.3	74.1	11.7
Calcium antagonists	261.6	268.7	274.5	272.8	276.4	283.1	8.2	1.6
Neuroleptics	83.2	131.1	168.4	192.6	224.6	271.5	226.5	26.7
Antihypertensives and diuretics associated with other substances (except beta blockers)	73.7	95.4	114.9	134.3	174.6	212.9	189.0	23.6
Antithrombotic agents	90.2	91.7	101.7	131.2	168.2	198.9	120.5	17.1
Antineoplastic hormone therapies	151.4	171.0	185.8	180.3	180.9	196.8	30.0	5.4
Other urologic agents (including antispasmodics)	83.4	103.2	119.3	138.2	159.4	179.1	114.6	16.5
Insulins	90.5	98.2	107.6	119.9	147.4	160.1	77.0	12.1
Antiepileptics	45.7	57.0	73.5	87.0	109.1	146.4	220.5	26.2
Oral antidiabetics	60.8	75.3	90.0	100.0	115.9	132.4	117.9	16.9
Other antipyretic analgesics	86.1	94.5	106.3	108.5	106.3	125.7	45.9	7.8
Peripheral and cerebral vasodilators	175.9	164.7	149.9	135.8	125.6	116.1	–34.0	–8.0
Macrolides	123.7	128.1	126.1	116.0	112.9	113.9	–7.9	–1.6
Immunosuppressants	59.5	72.8	87.2	91.6	95.2	108.0	81.4	12.7
Tranquilizers	80.1	87.3	93.6	100.3	102.5	106.3	32.7	5.8
Nitrates and analogues	N.A.	97.0	100.3	100.0	102.3	103.5	N.M.	N.M.
Topical glaucoma treatments	91.7	42.8	60.2	71.8	85.7	98.0	6.8	1.3
Other sex hormones and related substances	N.A.	N.A.	N.A.	50.9	75.1	93.4	N.M.	N.M.
Other products active on the CNS (including parasympathomimetics)	N.A.	N.A.	43.7	58.2	73.0	92.1	N.M.	N.M.
Cephalosporins	121.2	121.0	116.6	103.1	89.4	85.5	–29.4	–6.7
Capillary stabilizing agents	68.2	67.7	71.3	76.1	83.4	85.2	24.8	4.5
Quinolones and other antibiotics	82.0	82.8	88.6	88.3	86.6	84.9	3.5	0.7
Systemic antihistamines	59.6	62.2	65.6	70.0	80.1	84.0	40.8	7.1
Antibiotics containing other substances (except sulphonamides)	79.4	80.9	N.A.	77.1	76.0	82.1	3.5	0.7
Calcitonins	72.7	70.1	N.A.	82.9	83.5	78.2	7.5	1.5

ACE = Angiotensin-converting enzyme
ATC = Anatomical therapeutic chemical
CNS = Central nervous system
N.A. = Data not available
N.M. = Not meaningful
NSAID = Nonsteroidal anti-inflammatory drug
SNS = Sistema Nactional de Salud (National Healthcare System)

Note: Numbers reflect rounding

Table 13.4 Evolution, from 1997 to 2002, of SNS Spending on the 20 Best-Selling Compounds in 2002

Compound	*Sales (€ Million)*						*Change 1997–2002 (%)*	*Annual Growth Rate (%)*
	1997	*1998*	*1999*	*2000*	*2001*	*2002*		
Omeprazole	204.5	229.5	258.3	293.6	300.9	276.5	35.2	6.2
Atorvastatin	N.A.	64.9	99.6	122.2	161.3	230.4	N.M.	N.M.
Simvastatin	65.9	78.0	91.0	102.6	124.3	160.8	143.9	19.5
Paroxetine	61.7	80.7	103.6	119.5	129.9	156.5	153.6	20.5
Olanzapine	N.A.	54.0	77.5	86.2	99.6	124.1	N.M.	N.M.
Pravastatin	46.3	49.8	59.1	72.9	94.8	119.3	157.6	20.8
Clopidogrel	N.A.	N.A.	N.A.	45.6	77.1	109.8	N.M.	N.M.
Amlodipine	59.2	70.6	80.5	89.8	99.4	108.0	82.5	12.8
Risperidone	31.9	46.5	64.3	77.0	89.5	102.7	222.4	26.4
Enalapril	117.5	122.2	124.8	127.4	80.9	95.9	–18.4	–4.0
Sertraline	N.A.	N.A.	N.A.	N.A.	N.A.	93.0	N.M.	N.M.
Isophane insulin	60.5	66.0	72.5	77.7	74.9	88.9	47.0	8.0
Nitroglycerine	70.1	76.4	80.4	80.7	83.7	85.5	21.9	4.0
Pantoprazole	N.A.	N.A.	N.A.	44.8	61.9	83.4	N.M.	N.M.
Budesonide	93.5	94.4	96.2	94.0	90.3	82.3	–11.9	–2.5
Ranitidine	131.6	133.9	136.4	124.8	93.5	81.9	–37.8	–9.1
Diltiazem	85.6	87.2	88.0	85.0	75.6	81.0	–5.4	–1.1
Fluoxetine	88.5	93.7	96.0	94.4	81.8	80.3	–9.2	–1.9
Lansoprazole	N.A.	N.A.	N.A.	44.3	61.8	79.8	N.M.	N.M.
Venlafaxine	N.A.	N.A.	N.A.	42.5	58.3	78.8	N.M.	N.M.

N.A. = Data not available
N.M. = Not meaningful
SNS = Sistema Nacional de Salud (National Healthcare System)

Note: Numbers reflect rounding

Table 13.5 Monetary and Volume Market Shares of Medicines in Spain by Product Age, 2001–3

Years on the Market	*2001*		*2002*		*2003*	
	Monetary Share (%)	*Volume Share (%)*	*Monetary Share (%)*	*Volume Share (%)*	*Monetary Share (%)*	*Volume Share (%)*
<1	1.2	0.7	1.2	0.6	1.7	0.9
1–2	6.5	3.4	3.5	2.2	3.5	2.0
2–3	6.0	2.3	6.6	4.0	4.4	3.0
3–4	7.4	3.9	6.7	2.6	6.8	4.3
4–5	8.6	2.9	7.1	4.0	6.9	2.8
5–10	27.7	14.6	29.5	14.0	31.5	15.4
10–15	15.9	11.2	19.9	13.9	20.5	14.0
15–20	7.1	11.3	6.7	10.2	7.1	9.6
>20	18.7	46.5	18.0	45.6	16.8	45.2
Unknown	1.0	3.1	0.9	2.9	0.8	2.8

attributable to an increase in the number of outpatients and the growing use of complex and expensive therapies for diseases including cancers, AIDS, multiple sclerosis, and renal disorders. The SEFH reports that spending on rheumatoid arthritis therapies grew especially vigorously in 2002 and predicted that the increasing use of costly new treatment regimens for hepatitis C would stimulate hospital pharmacy expenditures in 2003.

By the SEFH's calculations, the Spanish hospital pharmacy market has grown faster than the retail pharmacy market in recent years. Since 1996, the overall annual growth rate of the hospital pharmacy market has ranged from 7.6% in 2001 to 17.7% in 1997. Total spending increased from €1.1 billion ($1.2 billion) in 1996 to €2.3 billion ($2.6 billion) in 2002.

OUTLOOK FOR THE SPANISH PHARMACEUTICAL MARKET

The pharmaceutical industry in Spain currently faces a more uncertain outlook than at any time in recent years. The new Socialist government has shown that it dislikes certain key elements of the previous administration's pharmaceutical policy but has not yet fully formulated an alternative strategy. In early August 2004, Elena Salgado, the new minister of health, announced that the government would not renew the stability pact that its predecessor had signed with the pharmaceutical industry in October 2001. Salgado told the pharmaceutical industry that this decision was "not a declaration of war but a new way of conducting relations."

The government's decision in early October 2004 to modify the reference-pricing system to make it less painful to domestic and generics manufacturers also portends a significant shift of direction. It is highly unlikely that the government will relax cost control simply to benefit Spanish companies and generics manufacturers. Rather, the expressions of concern for the welfare of these companies may signal the start of a cost-containment strategy that will focus more heavily on multinationals. The incremental sales tax is an early example of a policy that will hurt large multinationals more than small local companies.

Generics manufacturers will not lament the passing of the reference-pricing system. The AESEG criticized this initiative for prompting originator companies to slash their prices, thereby eroding generics' competitive advantage. It also accused the previous government of failing to explain the reference-pricing system adequately to physicians. The new government has indicated that it would like to stimulate substantially greater use of generics as a key element of its cost-control strategy.

On the other hand, the government wants to encourage innovation in the pharmaceutical market. In October 2004, José Martínez Olmos, the director general of the *Comisión de Farmacia* (Pharmacy Commission) noted that the SNS reimbursed 93% of new drugs launched in Spain in 2003 but asserted that 85% of these new medicines offered no real improvement over existing therapies. In the future, the new government intends to reimburse only drugs that are clearly superior to established treatments. To that end, the Ministry of Health has recently announced that it plans to introduce a pricing scale that will set the prices of new drugs according to their degree of therapeutic improvement.

The government dislikes pharmaceutical companies' influence over physicians' prescribing behavior. In October 2004, the minister of health criticized the pharmaceutical industry for exerting "pressure" on physicians to prescribe the most expensive medicines. To combat this influence, the government intends to introduce new controls on the industry. Physician detailing visits will be subject to strict regulations, manufacturers will have to follow guidelines on continuing education programs that they sponsor, and the Ministry of Health will provide physicians with independent information on medicines. All of these measures suggest that the government will take an increasingly critical view of industry efforts to promote drugs that are not deemed to be cost-effective.

A trend toward increasing decentralization of healthcare in Spain will also shape the evolution of the Spanish pharmaceutical market. Because regional governments are now responsible for their own healthcare budgets, many of them want to exercise greater control over pharmaceutical pricing and reimbursement decisions, prescribing guidelines, and cost-containment strategies. Over time, the Spanish market is likely to become increasingly fragmented along regional lines, presenting new challenges for pharmaceutical companies. Manufacturers will need to develop regional marketing strategies and may eventually even have to negotiate pricing and reimbursement terms region by region.

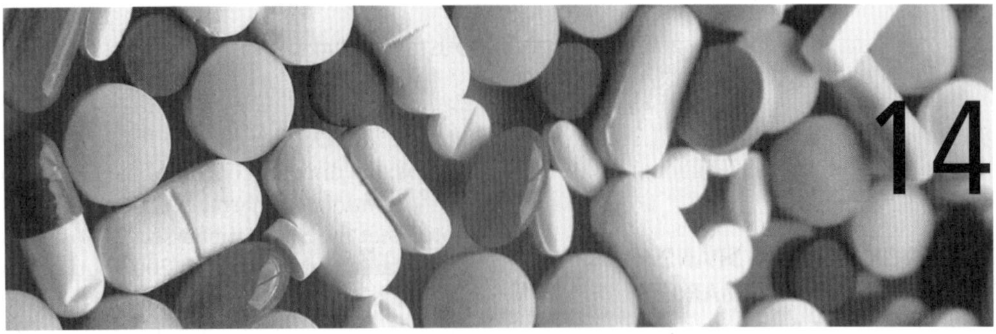

14

The Impact of German Reference Pricing on Statins

INTRODUCTION

Dyslipidemia is a largely asymptomatic disorder that seriously increases the cardiovascular risk of the majority of the adult population in Germany and other industrialized nations. Inadequate treatment of dyslipidemia can lead to coronary heart disease (CHD) or stroke, events that can have devastating or even fatal consequences.

The size of the dyslipidemic population and the severity of this disease and its complications make dyslipidemia a major public health issue for all industrialized nations. The German government is acutely conscious of the need to tackle this problem, but it has also been struggling for many years to slow down the relentless growth of public healthcare expenditures. The government has focused its cost-containment efforts primarily on pharmaceutical spending. This strategy is based on the contention that many of the best-selling drugs on the market lack innovation and are therefore overpriced, particularly in cases where other molecules from the same drug class are available as inexpensive generics. Pharmaceutical companies have a high degree of freedom in setting drug prices in Germany, but the government argues that they have too often abused this freedom.

In a bid to force manufacturers to lower their prices, the government recently began to extend reference pricing – a system that sets maximum reimbursement prices for medicines – to several major new drug classes. This action has proved extremely controversial because the affected drug classes are heavily prescribed and include best-selling drugs that are still patent protected. (From 1996 until the end of 2004, reference pricing was applied only to off-patent drugs.) The inclusion of the world's best-selling prescription drug, atorvastatin (Pfizer's Sortis [better known as Lipitor in many other markets]), in the same reference-pricing group as less-potent statins has been the most contentious step of all.

Pharmaceutical companies can respond to the imposition of reference pricing in two ways: they can accept this measure or fight it. Most manufacturers of branded drugs that have been subjected to reference pricing have complied by cutting their prices. Pfizer, however, has defied the reference pricing of atorvastatin and launched a counteroffensive on multiple fronts. The company's refusal to cut its prices has been costly in terms of lost sales and market share; it has also antagonized the government, the reimbursement authorities, the health insurance funds, and many physicians.

Reference pricing has had a seismic effect on the German statin market. Prescribing trends that began to emerge in 2003 have been greatly magnified in 2005. The impact of the reference pricing of statins in Germany is likely to have significant repercussions throughout the German pharmaceutical industry, and potentially far beyond Germany's borders. Governments in other countries observe Europe's largest pharmaceutical market very closely, and many (e.g., Belgium, Denmark, France, Italy, the Netherlands, Spain) have followed Germany's pioneering example in introducing reference pricing. Consequently, the international pharmaceutical industry cannot afford to ignore the implications of the reference pricing of statins in Germany.

OVERVIEW OF DYSLIPIDEMIA

Epidemiology

Based on data from the Bavarian Cholesterol Screening Project and the German National Health Interview and Examination Survey, it is estimated that 47.5 million Germans had dyslipidemia in 2004. Overall, approximately 34% of prevalent cases were diagnosed, but we believe that detection rates varied enormously according to disease severity. For example, we believe that the diagnosis rate was as high as 75% in the secondary prevention population (i.e., patients who have already had a cardiovascular event and need to control their dyslipidemia to prevent a recurrence) but only 25% in the low-risk primary prevention population (i.e., patients who have not had a cardiovascular event and have a limited risk). Similarly, drug treatment rates range from 60% of the diagnosed secondary prevention population to 20% of the diagnosed low-risk primary prevention population. We forecast that the overall prevalent population will increase to 49.4 million in 2014.

Current Medical Practice

Routine screening is recommended for adults every five years in Germany, but dyslipidemia is primarily determined through routine examinations by general practitioners (GPs) or internists. (See the Appendix for a glossary of German terms used in this chapter.) Total cholesterol, high-density lipoproteins (HDLs), and triglycerides (TGs) are measured. General practitioners (GPs) and internists begin treatment for approximately 80% of patients and refer the remaining patients, particularly those with complications, to specialists. Most German physicians follow the European Task Force guidelines, national recommendations, and National Cholesterol Education Program Expert Panel (NCEP) on Detection, Evaluation, and Treatment of High Blood Cholesterol in Adults (Adult Treatment Panel III [ATP III]) guidelines. The majority of experts agree that risk assessment through global risk calculation is a critical step in determining treatment.

Lifestyle modification is first-line treatment for all patients in Germany, although physicians report that only a few patients can adequately control their cholesterol levels exclusively with diet and exercise. Statins are by far the most common drug therapy used when pharmacotherapy is initiated; findings from one study show that approximately 95% of all drug-treated secondary prevention patients receive statin therapy.

The Role of Statins in the Management of Dyslipidemia

Although dyslipidemia encompasses a range of lipid abnormalities (i.e., raised low-density lipoprotein [LDL], raised TGs, low HDL), reducing LDL is the primary goal of therapy. Elevated LDL levels are strongly associated with progression of cardiovascular disease (CVD). Drug classes currently approved in Germany for the treatment of dyslipidemia include fibrates, cholesterol absorption inhibitors, and bile acid sequestrants, but therapy is dominated by the 3-hydroxy-3-methyl-glutaryl-CoA (HMG-CoA) reductase inhibitors, more commonly known as the statins. Statins lower serum LDL cholesterol concentrations by 20–65%, depending on the particular statin and the dosage used.

Major studies that have assessed the benefits of statins in primary prevention of CHD include the West of Scotland Coronary Prevention Study (WOSCOPS), the Air Force Texas Coronary Atherosclerosis Prevention Study (AFCAPS/TexCAPs), and the Heart Protection Study (HPS). Some physicians prescribe statins for primary prevention only in men aged 45–64 who are at a very high risk of acute myocardial infarction (AMI) or stroke. Others believe that the WOSCOPS and AFCAPS/TexCAPS results should encourage much more widespread use of statins in primary prevention, especially in elderly patients and patients with only moderately elevated lipids.

Much of the recent debate about statins centers on the optimal LDL threshold for high-risk patients. Several ongoing trials seek to determine whether lowering LDL levels below 100 mg/dL further reduces cardiovascular risk in patients with CHD or CHD-risk equivalents (the "lower is better" hypothesis). In addition to these trials, the 2004 updated NCEP ATP III guidelines are likely to influence prescribing behavior; physicians agree that their publication will result in greater statin use.

Although statins are generally well tolerated and cause few side effects, their safety profile has drawn increased scrutiny in recent years following the withdrawal of cerivastatin (Bayer's Lipobay) in August 2001 and more recent concerns about rosuvastatin (AstraZeneca's Crestor). Bayer withdrew cerivastatin after higher doses were linked to cases of life-threatening rhabdomyolysis (the destruction of skeletal muscle) that led to 31 deaths in the United States; 12 deaths occurred in patients who were receiving concomitant therapy with the fibrate gemfibrozil (Pfizer's Lopid, generics). Bayer's action resulted in a review of statins' safety and publication of new guidelines for their use by the key regulatory bodies in the major markets, including Germany. Because of rare but potentially serious hepatotoxicity, liver function monitoring is now recommended before and during treatment with statins.

The Statin Market in Germany

As noted earlier, statins overwhelmingly dominate dyslipidemia therapy in Germany. In 2004, ex-manufacturer sales of dyslipidemia therapies in Germany totaled $1.158 billion. Statins had sales of $1.04 billion, equivalent to 90% of the antihyperlipidemic market (in monetary terms). The other drug classes were cholesterol absorption inhibitors (with 2004 sales of $68.5 million), fibrates ($42.7 million), and bile acid sequestrants ($6.2 million). According to prescribing data from the Wissenschaftliches Institut der Allgemeinen Ortskrankenkassen (WidO; Scientific Institute of the Local General Health Insurance Funds), statins likewise accounted for 90% of all

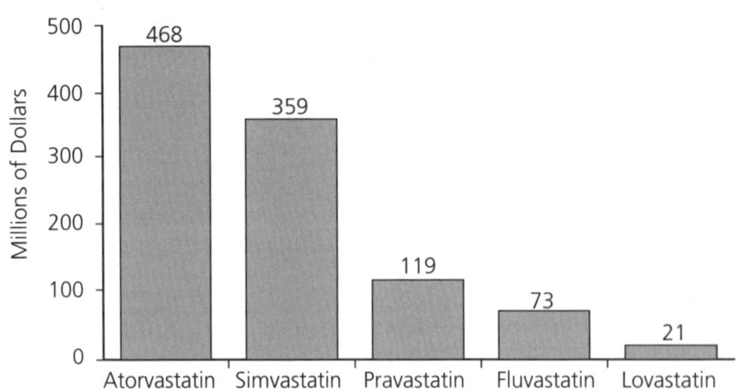

Figure 14.1 German Stain Market, 2004

antihyperlipidemic prescriptions dispensed within the Gesetzliche Krankenversicherung (GKV; statutory health insurance) system.

Figure 14.1 shows statin sales by molecule in 2004. Because atorvastatin is still patent protected, its sales came from a single product, namely Pfizer's Sortis. In contrast, approximately 30 companies marketed simvastatin products in Germany. The availability of inexpensive generic products enabled simvastatin to capture 52% of the statin market in unit terms in 2004.

ORGANIZATION AND FUNDING OF THE GERMAN HEALTHCARE SYSTEM

Germany has one of the highest levels of healthcare spending in the world. According to the Organization for Economic Cooperation and Development, Germany's expenditure on healthcare increased from 8.7% of its gross domestic product (GDP) in 1990 to 11.1% of its GDP in 2003. Among major economies, only the United States and Switzerland invested a larger proportion of their GDP in healthcare in 2003 (15% and 11.5%, respectively).

Although the federal government has ultimate control over healthcare policy in Germany, authorities in the country's 16 Länder (states) remain extremely influential. The regionalization of healthcare policy in Germany can prove complicated and sometimes slows down the decision-making process.

Most Germans rely on the GKV for their healthcare: approximately 90% of the population are enrolled in this program. Employers and employees share the cost of GKV premiums, which averaged 14.18% of gross income in 2005. The government pays the premiums of the unemployed, seniors, nonearning spouses, children, and civil servants. Self-employed workers and employees with annual incomes of more than €46,800 ($58,129) may opt for private Krankenversicherung (PKV; private health insurance) as an alternative to the GKV. The number of privately insured citizens has grown steadily, and approximately 8 million now rely exclusively on private insurance for their healthcare coverage. (In addition, some people use private insurance to supplement the GKV.) Private insurance typically offers more extensive benefits than the GKV.

The statutory health insurance system is administered by Krankenkassen (health insurance funds). Since 1993, everyone insured through the GKV system is free to choose their health insurance fund and to change this choice annually. Because of increasing competition, the number of GKV health insurance funds has been in decline for more than 30 years – a trend that has accelerated recently. The number of statutory health insurance funds fell from 1,146 in January 1994 to 267 in January 2005.

The annual GKV budget is set in the autumn of the preceding year. Funds are allocated to each of the main areas of expenditure, including pharmaceuticals. In theory, the maximum level of expenditure should not exceed the previous year's budget increased by the percentage growth in average wages. However, runaway costs have repeatedly frustrated the legal requirement for the GKV budget to balance.

In an effort to arrest the inexorable growth of GKV spending in general and pharmaceutical expenditures in particular, successive German governments have introduced a series of major healthcare reforms. Table 14.1 summarizes the key features of healthcare reforms introduced from 1988 to 2003 that are particularly significant to the pharmaceutical industry. The most recent of these laws – the Gesetz zur Modernisierung der Gesetzlichen Krankenversicherung (GMG; Statutory Health Insurance Modernization Act) – is also the most radical. The changes go far beyond the statutory health insurance system, affecting pharmaceutical companies, wholesalers, pharmacists, physicians, and patients, as well as health insurance funds. In a press release issued on October 17, 2003, Health Minister Ulla Schmidt stated, "This reform paves the way for a comprehensive structural renewal of the German healthcare system. We are freeing up rusted structures

Table 14.1 German Healthcare Reforms of Particular Significance to the Pharmaceutical Industry, 1988–2003

Year Enacted	*Law*	*Key Reforms for the Pharmaceutical Industry*[a]
1988	*Gesundheitsreformgesetz* (Healthcare Reform Act)	• Introduction of reference pricing • Increase in patient copayment for non-reference-priced drugs from DM2 to DM3 ($1.27-1.91) • Introduction of negative list
1992	*Gesundheitsstrukturgesetz* (Healthcare Structure Act)	• Strict budgetary control by area of expenditure (including medicines) • Introduction of copayments for all prescription medicines • Pharmaceutical prices cut and frozen
1997	*Zweites GKV-Neuordnungsgesetz* (Second Statutory Health Insurance Reorganization Act)	• Replacement of collective pharmaceutical budgets with indicative budgets • Increased patient copayments for prescription drugs
1998	*GKV-Solidaritätsstärkungsgesetz* (Act to Strengthen Solidarity in Statutory Health Insurance)	• Pharmaceutical budget for 1999 set at level of 1996 budget +7.5% • Reduction in patient copayments for prescription drugs • Reference prices to be set in bottom third of respective drug class
2000	*GKV-Gesundheitsreformgesetz 2000* (Statutory Health Insurance Healthcare Reform Act 2000)	• Groundwork laid for potential introduction of a positive list • Pharmacists required to meet quotas for dispensing parallel imports • Stricter monitoring and enforcement of physicians' indicative prescribing budgets
2001	*Festbetragsanpassungsgesetz* (Reference Pricing Adjustment Act)	• Reduction in reference prices until the end of 2003
2001	*Arzneimittelbudget-Ablösungsgesetz* (Pharmaceutical Budget Replacement Act)	• Regional drug budgets replaced by indicative prescribing volumes and regional targets • End of physicians' collective budgetary accountability
2001	*Gesetz zur Reform des Risikostrukturausgleichs* (Act to Reform the Risk Structure Equalization System)	• Promotion of disease management programs for select disorders
2002	*Arzneimittelausgaben-Begrenzungsgesetz* (Pharmaceutical Expenditure Limitation Act)	• Pharmaceutical industry pays government DM400 million ($254 million) to prevent imposition of price cuts/freeze • Introduction of generic substitution by pharmacists (*Aut idem* law) • Hospitals decide the drug therapy that patients receive after they are discharged • Pharmacy discounts to health insurance funds increased from 5% to 6% in 2002 and 2003
2002	*Fallpauschalengesetz* (Diagnosis-Related Groups Act)	• Diagnosis-related groups (DRGs) introduced as an option in public hospitals in 2003 • DRGs to become mandatory in public hospitals from 2004 onward
2002	*Beitragssatzsicherungsgesetz* (Contribution Guarantee Act)	• Imposition of increased rebates on manufacturers, wholesalers, and pharmacists
2003	*Gesetz zur Modernisierung der Gesetzlichen Krankenversicherung* (Statutory Health Insurance Modernization Act)	• Manufacturer rebate temporarily increased from 6% to 16% on many drugs that are not subject to reference pricing

Table 14.1 Continued

Year Enacted	*Law*	*Key Reforms for the Pharmaceutical Industry*[a]
		• Reference pricing to be progressively extended to many patent-protected drugs • Patient copayments changed from flat rates to 10% of a drug's retail price (with a minimum copayment of €5 [$6.21] and a maximum of €10 [$12.42]) • Patients must pay a quarterly practice fee of €10 ($12.42) to consult a physician • Changes to wholesalers' and pharmacists' margins. • Legalization of mail-order pharmacy • Modest relaxation of ban on ownership of multiple pharmacies

[a]This list focuses on reforms that are most relevant to the pharmaceutical industry
GKV = Gesetzliche Krankenversicherung (statutory health insurance)

and introducing more quality, consultation, and efficiency into the healthcare system. In addition, health insurance premiums will be reduced and the brakes will be applied to spending in the healthcare system. Every cent should be used as efficiently as possible."

PHARMACEUTICAL PRICING AND REIMBURSEMENT

Pricing

On average, pharmaceutical prices in Germany are higher than in most other European countries but much lower than those in the United States. Table 14.2 shows the results of an international price comparison conducted by the UK Department of Health, which monitors prices of the most frequently prescribed drugs in the United Kingdom, several other European markets, and the United States. (The analysis uses the United Kingdom as a benchmark for a multilateral comparison of average prices of branded prescription medicines in these markets. Fluctuations from year to year are attributable largely to exchange rate movements.)

During the 1990s, Germany had the highest average prices among the largest European markets. In 2000, however, the United Kingdom displaced Germany as the highest-priced of the major European markets. Unlike most other European countries, which regulate the prices of new drugs, Germany and the United Kingdom both allow pharmaceutical companies a high degree of freedom in setting the prices of innovative medicines. When setting prices, however, manufacturers in Germany and the United Kingdom inevitably have to take into account prevailing market prices (especially in competitive drug classes) if they want to capture a substantial share of the market.

Pharmaceutical companies in Germany are generally free to alter the prices of their products. At times, however, the government imposes comprehensive price cuts on prescription medicines. Prices take effect when they are published in the Lauer Taxe (the official list of pharmaceutical prices).

Retail prices for all pharmaceuticals sold in Germany include value added tax (a sales tax that is currently levied at 16%). Drugs that are prescribed and reimbursed by the GKV are subject to legally defined maximum margins for wholesalers and pharmacists, which are published in the Arzneimittelpreisverordnung (Pharmaceutical Price Ordinance). The 2003 Gesetz zur Modernisierung der Gesetzlichen Krankenversicherung (GMG; Statutory Health Insurance Modernization Act) made radical changes to these margins. Wholesalers' margins are degressive (i.e., they decline as baseline prices increase). Margins are calculated in bands that alternate between a percentage of the baseline price

Table 14.2 Multilateral Comparison of Average Exmanufacturer Prices of Branded Medicines in Select Markets as a Percentage of UK Average Exmanufacturer Prices, 1992–2003

Year (%)	*France (%)*	*Germany (%)*	*Italy (%)*	*Spain (%)*	*United States (%)*	*United Kingdom*
1992	93	158	108	95	172	100
1993	96	158	100	89	202	100
1994	100	143	90	88	192	100
1995	107	130	83	89	179	100
1996	105	125	93	89	191	100
1997	85	101	86	74	184	100
1998	85	109	88	77	188	100
1999	86	103	82	72	213	100
2000	83	94	82	70	241	100
2001	81	90	85	72	205	100
2002	83	94	86	77	194	100
2003	91	102	99	85	189	100
Average percentage, 1998–2003[a]	83	93	91	78	206	100

[a]Based on 2003 price data but converted to pounds sterling using average exchange rates for the period 1998–2002

and a fixed sum. The GMG introduced different methods of calculating pharmacists' margins depending on a drug's prescription status. For drugs that are not restricted to prescription-only status but that are prescribed and reimbursed by the GKV, the old system of degressive margins for pharmacists continues to apply. For prescription-only drugs, pharmacists now receive a fixed dispensing fee of €8.10 ($10.06) plus a payment equivalent to 3% of a product's pharmacy acquisition price. Pharmacists must pay the GKV a rebate of €2.00 ($2.48) for each item they dispense.

The GMG gives pharmacists in Germany the freedom to determine the retail price of drugs sold over the counter. This change is intended to reduce the prices for nonprescription medicines by promoting competition among pharmacies.

According to the Bundesvereinigung Deutscher Apothekerverbände (ABDA; Federal Union of German Pharmacists' Associations), in 2003, pharmaceutical manufacturers received on average 62.2% of the retail price of drugs prescribed in the GKV. This figure has risen from an average of 55.5% in 1990. Conversely, pharmacists' average share of the retail price of GKV-prescribed medicines has declined from 23.4% in 1990 to 17.3% in 2003. However, it is important to bear in mind that, in 2002 and 2003, manufacturers, wholesalers, and pharmacists were all required to pay substantial rebates to the GKV. In 2003, rebates accounted for 12.5% of the total retail sales of drugs reimbursed by the GKV.

Reimbursement

According to Article 12 of the Sozialgesetzbuch V (Social Code Book V), the GKV must provide coverage for "adequate, appropriate, and economical" healthcare services (including pharmaceuticals). However, these services must not exceed what is judged necessary.

Under the GMG, a powerful new body, the Gemeinsamer Bundesausschuß der Ärzte, Zahnärzte, Krankenhäuser und Krankenkassen (GBA; Joint Federal Committee of Physicians, Dentists, Hospitals, and Health Insurance Funds) is responsible for deciding whether a given therapy meets the criteria of Article 12 of the Sozialgesetzbuch V and, therefore, should be reimbursed by the GKV. The GBA's reimbursement decisions are binding on all physicians contracted to the GKV and on all statutory health insurance funds.

In practice, most registered medicines qualify for at least partial GKV reimbursement. However, the following drug categories are excluded from reimbursement:

- Drugs for the treatment of the common cold or influenza, drugs for the mouth or throat (except for antifungals), laxatives, and drugs for the treatment of motion sickness are not reimbursed for patients over age 18.
- Drugs deemed "inefficient" are added to the *negative list* of products that are ineligible for reimbursement.
- Drugs for "trivial" disorders that can generally be treated by other therapies may be excluded from reimbursement at the suggestion of the Minister of Health and the Finance Minister (subject to parliamentary approval).

Since the late 1980s, governments in Germany have tried to limit pharmaceutical spending by imposing a wide variety of cost-containment measures. The following chapters examine cost-containment measures of particular relevance to the statin market.

REFERENCE PRICING

Overview

Germany pioneered the concept of reference pricing in 1989, when the government implemented the *Gesundheitsreformgesetz* (Health Reform Act). A Festbetrag (reference price) is the maximum sum that the GKV system will reimburse for a drug that is subject to reference pricing. (Privately insured patients are not subject to reference prices on their prescription drugs.) If a drug is more expensive than its reference price, the patient must pay the excess. This charge is in addition to the standard coinsurance payment. Furthermore, there are no concessions on excess payments and no cap on these payments.

The objective of this cost-containment measure is to induce manufacturers to cut their prices to reference-price levels or lower. As of July 1, 2005, of a total of 27,908 reference-priced product presentations (i.e., individual dosages, dosage forms, and pack sizes of a product) in Germany, only 1,973 product presentations (7.1%) exceeded their reference price. The government's strategy has succeeded in curbing costs. From January 1, 1989, to December 31, 2003, the price index for reference-priced drugs declined by 33% (2.6% per year). Conversely, over the same period, the price index for drugs that were not subject to reference pricing increased by 27% (1.6% per year). Since its introduction, the reference-pricing system is estimated to have reduced pharmaceutical expenditures in Germany by an average of €1.2 billion ($1.5 billion) per year. Savings for 2004 are estimated at €2.5 billion ($3.1 billion).

Germany has three different levels of reference-pricing groups:

1. Level 1: Drugs that have the same active ingredient and bioavailability (if therapeutically relevant).
2. Level 2: Drugs that have pharmacologically and therapeutically comparable active ingredients (particularly chemically related agents).
3. Level 3: Drugs that have therapeutically comparable effects (particularly combination agents).

Level 1 groups are defined (and reference prices are set) when an originator product's patent has expired and several generic versions of the compound are on the market. Level 2 and 3 groups and reference prices for older drugs can be defined at any time. In 1996, the German government suspended level 2 and 3 reference pricing for all patent-protected drugs approved in Germany after December 31, 1995, and effectively restricted this cost-containment measure to off-patent medicines.

The Spitzenverbände der Krankenkassen (leading associations of the health insurance funds) are responsible for setting reference prices, which are generally reviewed annually. Not surprisingly, however, drug manufacturers have misgivings about the fact that health insurance funds, as principal payers for healthcare, are also responsible for setting reference prices for the products they reimburse.

Notwithstanding the use of reference pricing and other cost-containment measures for many years, spending on healthcare, including prescription drugs, has increased steadily – to the growing alarm of the German government. In an effort to curb expenditures, in October 2003, the government enacted the GMG, a major overhaul of healthcare funding in Germany. One of this law's most controversial measures is the gradual reintroduction of reference pricing for many patent-protected drugs. Under the new policy, an entire drug class can be subjected to reference pricing – even if all agents within the class are still patent protected – provided that the class comprises at least three compounds. For example, reference prices were imposed on the sartans and triptans despite the fact that all drugs in these two classes were still patent protected. Once a drug loses patent protection and generic versions are launched, these products will be added to the reference-pricing group. The much lower prices of generics will subsequently be taken into account in annual reviews of the reference prices for the drug class as a whole, leading to a reduction in reference prices within the class. The only products that will be safe from the threat of reference pricing will be those that have demonstrable therapeutic superiority over existing therapies. Speaking at a press conference in September 2003, Health Minister Ulla Schmidt justified this change as follows: "The healthcare system can no longer permit the reimbursement of high-priced sham innovations that have little benefit. Therefore, in future, patent-protected medicines that provide no significant therapeutic improvement will be included in the reference pricing regulation."

The GBA is now responsible for defining the new reference-pricing groups. It receives advice from another new organization, the Institut für Qualität und Wirtschaftlichkeit im Gesundheitswesen (IQWiG; Institute for Quality and Economy in the Healthcare System). Both organizations are the product of the GMG. In addition, another body, the Arzneimittelkommission der Deutschen Ärzteschaft (Pharmaceutical Commission of the German Medical Profession) has been given the task of identifying patent-protected medicines launched from 1996 onward that could be assigned to existing reference-pricing groups.

On January 1, 2005, new reference-pricing groups for proton-pump inhibitors, sartans, triptans, and statins took effect in Germany. The imposition in these four drug classes of reference prices that are, on average, 16.2% below 2004 retail prices is expected to save the statutory health insurance funds a total of €340 million ($422 million) in 2005. In July 2005, the GBA introduced another six new reference-pricing groups: antianemic agents, fluoroquinolones, heparins, macrolides, serotonin (5-HT3) receptor antagonists, and triazole antimycotics. The GBA is expected to introduce further waves of new reference-pricing groups in 2006 and 2007. Ultimately, the government hopes that new reference-pricing groups will save the German healthcare system approximately €1 billion ($1.2 billion) per year.

Table 14.3 summarizes reference-priced drugs' role in the German pharmaceutical market. As of July 1, 2005, a total of 436 active substances and combinations were subject to reference pricing. These drugs were available in 27,908 different product presentations. Level 1 products (i.e., drugs that have the same active substance and bioavailability) accounted for the majority of product presentations (15,429) subject to reference pricing and the greatest number of prescriptions (221.6 million). However, the number of level 2 products (i.e., drugs that have pharmacologically and therapeutically comparable active substances) subject to reference pricing increased substantially, and these products had the greatest sales as of July 1, 2005: €5.1 billion ($6.3 billion), equivalent to 24.1% of total pharmaceutical sales within the statutory health insurance system. This growth has been driven primarily by the new reference-pricing groups – including statins – implemented on January 1, 2005.

Table 14.3 Reference-Priced Drugs' Place in the German Pharmaceutical Market

	Level 1[a]	*Level 2*[b]	*Level 3*[c]	*Total*
Status as of July 1, 2004				
Active substances/combinations subject to reference pricing	189	174	28	391
Product groups subject to reference pricing	306	55	55	416
Packages subject to reference pricing	14,117	5,447	4,117	23,681
Sales (€ billion)	4.5	2.5	1.2	8.2
Share of total GKV drug sales (%)	19.7	10.9	5.2	35.8
Prescriptions (millions)	284.2	88.7	72	444.9
Share of total GKV prescriptions (%)	38.4	12.0	9.7	60.2
Status as of July 1, 2005				
Active substances/combinations subject to reference pricing	200	208	28	436
Product groups subject to reference pricing	326	65	59	450
Packages subject to reference pricing	15,429	8,304	4,175	27,908
Sales (€ billion)	4.1	5.1	1.0	10.2
Share of total GKV drug sales (%)	19.4	24.1	4.7	48.2
Prescriptions (millions)	221.6	120.1	46.2	387.9
Share of total GKV prescriptions (%)	39.4	21.3	8.2	68.9

[a]Drugs that have the same active substance and bioavailability (if therapeutically relevant)
[b]Drugs that have pharmacologically and therapeutically comparable active substances (particularly chemically related agents)
[c]Drugs that have therapeutically comparable effects (particularly combination agents)
GKV = Gesetzliche Krankenversicherung (statutory health insurance)

Reference Prices of Statins

On July 20, 2004, the GBA announced its decision to subject all statins to reference pricing. On October 29, 2004, the leading associations of the health insurance funds published the reference prices for each molecule, dosage, and pack size. The framework for setting reference prices is defined in the Arzneimittelpreisverordnung (Pharmaceutical Price Ordinance). Article 35 of this ordinance specifies that reference prices should be set in such a way that they generally ensure an adequate, appropriate, and economic pharmaceutical supply that is also of assured quality. Among other requirements, reference prices are meant to promote price competition and a therapeutically adequate range of medicines. Reference prices should be reviewed at least annually, and should be adjusted periodically to reflect changing market conditions.

Table 14.4 compares the reference prices and 2004 and 2005 retail prices of 100-tablet packs of a selection of statins. (We chose 100-tablet packs because patients with chronic disorders, such as dyslipidemia, generally prefer to obtain the largest pack size available.) The list includes branded products and, in the case of off-patent molecules, the most frequently prescribed generic product in 2004 and the lowest-priced generic product in 2005. It is apparent at a glance that reference prices were set substantially below the 2004 retail prices of branded statins but far above the 2004 retail prices of generic statins. The 2004 retail prices of 100-tablet packs of branded statins were, on average, 47.5% above their respective reference prices. By comparison, the 2004 retail prices of 100-tablet packs of the generics included in Table 14.4 were, on average, 50% below their respective reference prices. Therefore, generics companies, in contrast to manufacturers of branded drugs, did not need to cut their retail prices to ensure that they did not exceed the new reference prices for statins.

Table 14.4 Retail and Reference Prices of Select Statins, 2004 and 2005

Compound	*Brand/Product Name (Manufacturer)*	*Dosage*	*2004 Retail Price (€)*	*Reference Price (€)*	*2005 Retail Price (€)*	*2004 Retail Price as a Percentage of Reference Price (%)*	*2005 Retail Price as a Percentage of Reference Price (%)*	*Price Change 2004–5 (%)*
Atorvastatin	Sortis (Pfizer)	10 mg	102.00	67.36	102.61	151.4	152.3	0.6
		20 mg	150.12	93.04	149.73	161.3	160.9	(0.3)
		40 mg	178.62	130.11	180.11	137.3	138.4	0.8
		80 mg	—	183.59	233.43	—	127.1	N.M.
Simvastatin	Zocor (Dieckmann)	10 mg	94.37	60.90	60.90	155.0	100.0	(35.5)
		20 mg	154.21	84.13	84.13	183.3	100.0	(45.4)
		40 mg	183.51	116.95	116.95	156.9	100.0	(36.3)
		80 mg	218.31	164.63	164.63	132.6	100.0	(24.6)
Simvastatin	Simvahexal (Hexal)	10 mg	27.86	60.90	30.57	45.7	50.2	9.7
		20 mg	40.58	84.13	46.67	48.2	55.5	15.0
		40 mg	61.57	116.95	69.21	52.6	59.2	12.4
		80 mg	106.80	164.63	129.00	64.9	78.4	20.8
Simvastatin	Simvastatin Corax (Corax Pharma)	10 mg	27.81	60.90	27.38	45.7	45.0	(1.5)
		20 mg	40.53	84.13	41.56	48.2	49.4	2.5
		40 mg	61.49	116.95	62.08	52.6	53.1	1.0
Pravastatin	Pravasin (Bristol-Myers Squibb)	10 mg	93.06	59.17	59.17	157.3	100.0	(36.4)
		20 mg	136.13	80.79	80.79	168.5	100.0	(40.7)
		40 mg	197.19	112.76	112.76	174.9	100.0	(42.8)
Pravastatin	Mevalotin (Sankyo)	10 mg	93.06	59.17	59.17	157.3	100.0	(36.4)
		20 mg	136.13	80.79	80.79	168.5	100.0	(40.7)
		40 mg	197.19	112.76	112.76	174.9	100.0	(42.8)
Pravastatin	Pravastatin Ratiopharm (Ratiopharm)	10 mg	N.A	59.17	48.64	N.M.	82.2	N.M.
		20 mg	N.A.	80.79	68.10	N.M.	84.3	N.M.
		40 mg	N.A.	112.76	95.32	N.M.	84.5	N.M.
Pravastatin	Pravastatin Kwizda (Kwizda)	10 mg	N.A.	59.17	45.73	N.M.	77.3	N.M.
		20 mg	N.A.	80.79	63.97	N.M.	79.2	N.M.
		40 mg	N.A.	112.76	89.87	N.M.	79.7	N.M.
Fluvastatin	Locol (Novartis)	20 mg	84.38	60.33	60.33	139.9	100.0	(28.5)
		40 mg	101.87	83.31	83.31	122.3	100.0	(18.2)
		80 mg	122.50	116.07	116.07	105.5	100.0	(5.2)
Fluvastatin	Cranoc (Astellas)	20 mg	84.38	60.33	60.33	139.9	100.0	(28.5)
		40 mg	101.87	83.31	83.31	122.3	100.0	(18.2)
		80 mg	122.50	116.07	116.07	105.5	100.0	(5.2)
Lovastatin	Mevinacor (Merck Sharp & Dohme)	10 mg	81.43	57.99	57.99	140.4	100.0	(28.8)
		20 mg	110.29	79.52	79.52	138.7	100.0	(27.9)
		40 mg	166.59	110.59	110.59	150.6	100.0	(33.6)
Lovastatin	Lovahexal (Hexal)	10 mg	26.09	57.99	25.65	45.0	44.2	(1.7)
		20 mg	37.35	79.52	36.73	47.0	46.2	(1.7)
		40 mg	60.48	110.59	59.83	54.7	54.1	(1.1)
Lovastatin	Lovastatin 1A Pharma (1A Pharma)	10 mg	26.05	57.99	25.55	44.9	44.1	(1.9)
		20 mg	37.19	79.52	36.17	46.8	45.5	(2.7)
		40 mg	60.30	110.59	58.48	54.5	52.9	(3.0)

N.M. = Not meaningful

General Industry Response to Reference Pricing of Statins

The pharmaceutical industry is particularly critical of what it considers to be an unduly narrow definition of "therapeutic improvement" and the GBA's policy of combining patent-protected and off-patent medicines in "jumbo" reference-pricing groups (i.e., reference-pricing groups that include both patented and off-patent compounds). The *Verband Forschender Arzneimittelhersteller* (VFA; German Association of Research-Based Pharmaceutical Companies), the association that represents Germany's largest drug manufacturers, argues that the GBA should accept any of the following enhancements as evidence of therapeutic improvement:

- Superior efficacy with demonstrable effects.
- Less-severe side effects.
- Improved tolerability.
- Less-severe interactions with other drugs.
- A significant additional indication.
- More rapid effects.
- A new mechanism of action.
- A new dosage form.

The response of individual drug manufacturers to the reference pricing of statins depended largely on whether their products were branded or generic medicines. Because their 2004 retail prices for statins were already far below the reference-price levels, generics companies did not need to reduce their prices. Indeed, Table 14.4 shows that the prices of most of the generic statins included in our analysis remained stable, rising or falling by 3% or less. The one notable exception in our list is Simvahexal, which had price increases ranging from 9.7% for 10 mg tablets to 20.8% for 80 mg tablets. Simvahexal was the second-most-frequently prescribed statin product in the GKV market in 2004, surpassed only by Sortis. Moreover, in 2005, Simvahexal overtook Sortis as the best-selling and most frequently prescribed statin. In the first nine months of the year, 1.6 million GKV prescriptions for Simvahexal generated retail sales of €80.8 million ($100.3 million). This success is attributable in large measure to the fact that Hexal's product, as an authorized generic, was launched before the patent on simvastatin expired (see the Section Market Impact). Consequently, Hexal is better placed than smaller generics companies to increase its prices without losing market share. Moreover, Simvahexal's prices in 2005 are still far below reference-price levels.

The situation for manufacturers of branded medicines is very different: reference pricing has transformed the landscape of their market. Almost all companies responded by cutting the prices of branded statins to precisely the level of their reference prices – an average reduction of 26.2% for 100-tablet packs. Of course, aligning the retail prices of branded statins with their reference prices means that these products are still far more expensive than generic statins (in the case of molecules that are off patent [i.e., simvastatin, pravastatin, lovastatin]). However, by not exceeding reference prices, manufacturers of branded statins at least ensure that patients do not have to pay an excess to use their drugs. The only company not to adopt this strategy is Pfizer, which has defied the reference pricing of Sortis. (The following section discusses Pfizer's response.)

The extension of reference pricing to patent-protected medicines has had an additional consequence that the German government likely did not intend, namely deterring manufacturers from launching certain new drugs in Germany. In November 2004, AstraZeneca revealed that it had suspended its plans to launch Crestor (rosuvastatin) in Germany in 2005. The company was concerned that rosuvastatin would immediately be subject to reference pricing. The drug's price in countries in which it is already marketed is, on average, 40% higher than German reference prices. AstraZeneca warned that launching the drug in Germany at the same price as generic statins would deny it an adequate return on its investment and might open the door to massive parallel trade. Withholding a major new drug from the market to avoid the threat of reference pricing is without precedent in Germany and sends an ominous message on future access to innovative medicines in that country.

Pfizer's Response

Pfizer has been the most vociferous critic of the expansion of reference pricing in Germany, and the only manufacturer to refuse to comply with the reference pricing of statins. The company objects to the inclusion of Sortis in the same reference-pricing group as all other statins (including the three statins that are already off patent in Germany), arguing that clinical trials have demonstrated the superiority of atorvastatin.

Evidence of the Superiority of Atorvastatin

Pfizer asserts that atorvastatin's advantages over other statins are particularly pronounced in the case of five patient subpopulations:

1. Patients with acute coronary syndrome.
2. Patients with a family history of severe hypercholesterolemia.
3. Diabetics who have additional risk factors.
4. Patients who have an initial LDL cholesterol score so high that it cannot be reduced to therapeutically necessary levels by other statins, even if administered at their maximum dosage.
5. Patients who experience severe side effects (e.g., rhabdomyolysis) on the highest dosage of simvastatin.

Refusal to Cut the Price of Sortis

Table 14.4 shows that, in 2005, retail prices of Sortis remain far higher than the drug's reference price levels. The smallest percentage differential is for the 100-tablet pack of the 80 mg dosage (27.1% above its reference price), but the maximum dosage is prescribed relatively rarely. The much more frequently prescribed 20 mg dosage is priced 60.9% above its reference price. GKV patients who wish to obtain a 100-tablet pack of Sortis now have to pay the standard copayment of €10.00 ($12.42) plus an excess of €35.25 ($43.78) for the 10 mg dosage, €56.69 ($70.41) for 20 mg, €50.00 ($62.10) for 40 mg, and €49.84 ($61.90) for 80 mg. These sums are not excessive by US standards, but patients in Germany are unaccustomed to such substantial out-of-pocket payments. Indeed, until January 2004, the standard prescription charge for the largest packs of prescription drugs (e.g., 100 statin tablets) was just €5.00 ($6.21), and relatively few drugs that were subject to reference pricing exceeded their reference prices.

Open Letters to Decision-Making Bodies

In November 2004, Pfizer sent open letters challenging the reference pricing of Sortis to both IQWiG and the GBA. The letters, signed by Walter Köbele, the chairman of Pfizer Deutschland, and Friedemann Schwegler, the company's medical director, asked the two bodies to justify their decisions.

The open letter to IQWiG questioned the basis for the institute's recommendations and asked if all relevant scientific literature had been reviewed. Pfizer asked which alternatives to Sortis IQWiG would recommend for the five aforementioned subpopulations for whose treatment the company claims atorvastatin is superior to other drugs in its class. Other questions in the letter were as follows:

- Do you share the GBA's opinion that, among the statins, Sortis demonstrates the most potent cholesterol-lowering effects and rapidly reduces the risk of cardiovascular events, and that statins differ in many respects and therefore are not arbitrarily interchangeable?
- Which alternative statin and what dosage would you recommend to patients who are currently treated with 40 or 80 mg of Sortis?
- Are you of the opinion that patients can be switched from 40 mg of Sortis to 80 mg of simvastatin without any thought? If so, how do you support this view in the light of the results of the A-to-Z Study?

- Will you assume the legal responsibility for the patients (in the aforementioned subpopulations) who are switched by their physician to another statin on your recommendation?

The letter to IQWiG concluded with the comment that not only Pfizer, but also the public and the medical profession, would be interested in the answers to these questions.

In the open letter to the GBA, Köbele and Schwegler expressed the opinion that reference pricing atorvastatin was actually a contravention of the GMG, the very law that paved the way for expanded reference pricing. This contention was based on the belief that atorvastatin is a therapeutic improvement as defined in that law. The text of the letter reminded the GBA of the legal requirement for reference pricing to maintain a necessary, adequate, and appropriate pharmaceutical supply and to give physicians a choice of medicines that are available without the need for additional payments.

Pfizer stated that it would not yield to political pressure to cut the price of a drug that it considered to be a therapeutic improvement. The company criticized the GBA for following "short-term political savings targets" and ignoring expert opinion and new clinical trial results.

Advertising Campaign

Following the publication of the prospective new reference prices, Pfizer undertook a publicity campaign intended to highlight the potential impact of this cost-containment measure. The full-page newspaper and magazine advertisements carried the headline: "There'll be savings from January – on the heath of millions of patients with heart and circulatory problems." The text warned readers that "access to the best cholesterol-lowering drug will become more difficult for health insurance fund patients." The advertisement also asserted that atorvastatin is the drug that "lowers cholesterol amounts most effectively, reduces risk fastest, and is well tolerated even at the highest dosages. For many patients, there is no alternative to Sortis." Pfizer informed readers that approximately 1.5 million GKV patients would be affected by the reference pricing of Sortis.

Perhaps not surprisingly, this campaign provoked swift and sharp condemnation from the government, the GBA, the health insurance funds, and some physician organizations. (The response of these groups is discussed in the Section Reaction to Pfizer's Stance.) Unabashed by this criticism, Pfizer defended its right to free speech on a matter of public interest.

Patient Assistance Program

Notwithstanding its opposition to the reference pricing of atorvastatin, its criticism of the GBA and IQWiG, and its refusal to cut the price of Sortis, Pfizer understandably did not want to alienate patients who were taking Sortis. In an effort to help patients who could not afford the additional out-of-pocket payments for the drug, Pfizer established the Sortis-Partner-Programm – an initiative reminiscent of the patient assistance programs that are common in the United States. If patients could provide proof from their statutory health insurance fund that they had paid the equivalent of 2% of their annual income in copayments for prescription drugs and other healthcare services, and were exempt from copayments for the remainder of the calendar year, Pfizer would pay them the difference between the reference price and the retail price of their Sortis prescriptions.

This program attracted the attention of the regulatory authorities, and Pfizer was charged with violating the Heilmittelwerbegesetz (Healthcare Products Promotion Act). In June 2005, the Landgericht Karlsruhe (Karlsruhe State Court) ruled that the company had indeed committed an offense under this law. The court judged that payments of as much as €66 ($81.98) per prescription exceeded the minor payments permitted by this act. In addition, the court declared that the program impaired competition. Consequently, Pfizer was ordered to discontinue the Sortis-Partner-Programm.

The repercussions of this ruling are likely to be limited. Pfizer originally forecast that as many as 270,000 patients per year would qualify for the Sortis-Partner-Programm. However, at the time of the court's judgment, only approximately 800 patients had applied for the program, and just 120 had met the eligibility requirements.

Physician Support

To reinforce its campaign, Pfizer enlisted the help of 15,000 Germany physicians. They signed an open letter that supported Pfizer's claims for atorvastatin's superiority over other statins. The signatories stated that they knew, from their clinical practice, that "Sortis is indispensable for patients who have severely elevated cardiovascular risk." The letter also asserted that, "from a medical perspective, [atorvastatin] unequivocally fulfills the criteria for a therapeutic improvement and therefore, in line with the law, must not be subjected to the reference pricing rule."

Lawsuit

Pfizer's main hope of thwarting the reference pricing of atorvastatin was a lawsuit that challenged the legality of this action. On November 22, 2005, Pfizer lost this case in the Sozialgericht Berlin (Berlin Social Court) but immediately declared its intention to appeal against the court's decision.

The court rejected Pfizer's charge that proper procedure had not been followed in defining the reference-pricing group for statins. The GBA was deemed to have wide discretionary powers in its choice of expert advice and had been guided by the recommendations of the Arzneimittelkommission der deutschen Ärzteschaft (Pharmaceutical Commission of the German Medical Profession).

In particular reference to statins, the judge ruled that, because of their basic chemical structure, their mechanism of action, and their common applications, all drugs in this class are comparable; their effects do not differ. Drugs in this class can be considered interchangeable unless a particular agent has an officially approved indication that other statins lack.

In conclusion, the judge declared that atorvastatin is not innovative and does not offer demonstrable therapeutic improvements. The court based its opinion on IQWiG's assessment of the statins.

Not surprisingly, Pfizer was very disappointed with the verdict. A spokesman for the company commented: "We consider the Social Court's judgment to be legally and scientifically false, and we will appeal against it."

Reaction to Pfizer's Stance

The intensity and tone of Pfizer's protests against the reference pricing of atorvastatin has provoked a sharp backlash from many interested parties. For example, the Ministry of Health denounced Pfizer's press campaign: "From an ethical perspective, this campaign is reprehensible. It creates the impression, for reasons of pure profit, that the health of large numbers of people is in danger."

The *Kassenärztliche Bundesvereinigung* (KBV; Federal Union of Health Insurance Fund Physicians) and the Spitzenverbände der Krankenkassen (leading associations of health insurance funds) responded more vigorously to Pfizer's campaign, by printing flyers and posters for physicians' waiting rooms. The headline read: "Dear Patients: Don't Be Nervous." The text then explained that Pfizer's refusal to cut the price of Sortis might mean additional costs of more than €200 ($248.42) per year for patients prescribed this drug, rather than another statin. The text continued as follows:

> Do not be worried by the assertions made by the pharmaceutical company Pfizer. Your medical care is guaranteed. There are medically equivalent alternatives to Sortis, which are not more expensive than the so-called reference price. Take advice from your doctor. If you choose one of these other medicines, the official copayment is often less than €10. So, you can even save money. Doctors and health insurance funds ensure that you receive care with good medicines at reasonable prices.

The Sortis-Partner-Programm has also been widely criticized. Andreas Köhler, the head of the KBV, described this initiative as a "dubious customer loyalty program" that would make it more difficult for physicians to switch patients to "sensible but more reasonable alternatives." Leonhard Hansen, the head of the Kassenärztliche Vereinigung Nordrhein (North Rhine Union of Health Insurance Fund Physicians), was even more robust in his criticism, accusing Pfizer of fraud and condemning the company's demands for patient data as a condition of enrollment in its program. The Bayerischer Apothekerverband (Bavarian Pharmacists' Association) sent its members a circular warning that Pfizer's program does not contain adequate data protection measures. It suggested that the company might use the data it gathers to build a profile of the physicians who prescribe Sortis and the pharmacies that dispense the drug most frequently.

IQWiG Evaluation of Statins

Pfizer's criticisms of the reference pricing of atorvastatin prompted IQWiG to conduct a detailed literature analysis on statins. In September 2005, the institute published its Nutzenbewertung der Statine unter besonderer Berücksichtigung von Atorvastatin (Utility Assessment of Statins with Particular Reference to Atorvastatin), a 148-page evaluation of clinical trial data. The report contained the following key conclusions:

- The utility of statin therapy in reducing mortality in patients with stable CHD has been proved only for the active substances simvastatin and pravastatin. No such evidence of utility exists for atorvastatin, fluvastatin, and lovastatin.
- For patients with acute CHD, studies on utility to patients are available for the active substances atorvastatin, pravastatin, and simvastatin. Deficiencies in study design and reporting make it difficult to interpret the data in terms of comparing the active substances with each other. There is no proof that any particular active substance is superior to the other active substances in terms of patient-specific end points.
- Simvastatin is the only active substance that has proof of utility in reducing mortality in patients with diabetes mellitus. No such evidence of utility exists for atorvastatin, fluvastatin, lovastatin, and pravastatin.
- Discontinuation of therapy because of side effects is more common with the maximum approved dosage of atorvastatin than simvastatin. Elevated liver enzyme counts occur more frequently with the maximum dosage of atorvastatin than with either simvastatin or pravastatin.
- The available long-term interventional studies of various statins do not permit the conclusion that it is appropriate to use the degree of LDL cholesterol reduction as a means of generally proving or quantifying utility in regard to clinical end points.

IQWiG emphatically rejected Pfizer's claims of atorvastatin's superiority. Overall, the institute appeared to conclude that simvastatin is the statin that has the strongest body of evidence of clinical utility. The report does not mention that simvastatin (unlike atorvastatin) is available generically, but this fact is a further advantage of simvastatin's.

The report also contains some interesting comments on statins' mechanism of action. IQWiG notes that comparator-controlled studies have shown that drugs in this class have multiple effects, including an influence on blood coagulation and possible anti-inflammatory properties. The institute suggests that the clinical significance of each action is unclear and that it remains to be proved whether, and to what extent, LDL reduction is a positive influence on patients' health.

Market Impact

In 2004, the German statin market was dominated by Sortis and generic simvastatin products. Figure 14.2 shows each molecule's volume share of the GKV statin market in 2004. (Calculations are based on defined daily doses [DDDs], a measure of typical dosing per day.) With a total of 685.6 million DDDs, simvastatin products collectively accounted for 52% of the GKV market.

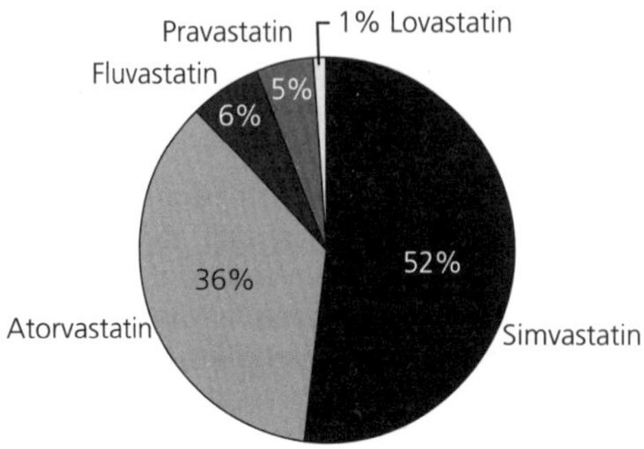

Figure 14.2 Composition of the German Statin Market in Volume Terms, 2004

However, the most frequently prescribed (and best-selling) individual product by far was Sortis: 475.3 million DDDs gave this drug 36% of the GKV market. The three other statins together accounted for only 12% of the market.

The introduction of reference pricing has dramatically altered the German statin market, and Sortis has been the main casualty. Pfizer's refusal to bow to reference pricing has proved very costly. In 2004, the drug's total sales in Germany amounted to approximately €400 million ($497 million). Pfizer reported that, in the first quarter of 2005, sales of Sortis in Germany totaled €24.2 million ($30.1 million), a decline of 68% over the first three months of 2004. This slump has been concentrated mainly in the GKV market. According to Pfizer, the drug's share of the GKV statin market declined from approximately 30% in the second half of 2004 to 7% in the first quarter of 2005. This decline accelerated in the second quarter of the year, and Sortis's volume share amounted to less than 5% in the first half of 2005. Sales and prescriptions plummeted by more than 90%. Patient out-of-pocket payments of €9.7 million ($12 million) reportedly accounted for 38% of Sortis's total sales in the first six months of the year. In contrast to its problems in the GKV market, Sortis reportedly maintained a market share of approximately 50% in the private sector (where reference pricing does not apply). As a result, Pfizer has condemned what it regards as the emergence of "Zweiklassenmedizin" ("two-class medicine") in Germany.

In marked contrast to the decline of Sortis, demand for simvastatin products has grown explosively. In the first half of 2005, simvastatin products' combined volume share of the market increased to 69%. The introduction of reference pricing of statins, combined with Pfizer's refusal to reduce the price of Sortis, has undoubtedly been the main stimulus for the growth of the simvastatin market in 2005. However, it is important to bear in mind that these factors have sharply accelerated, not caused, the rapid migration from atorvastatin to simvastatin. This trend began early in 2003, when the first generic simvastatin products were launched in Germany.

The German patent on simvastatin expired on May 6, 2003. Merck & Co.'s German subsidiary, Dieckmann, tried to defend its originator brand, Zocor, against the threat of generics competition by launching its own generic flanker brand, Zocor MSD, in January 2003. However, the prices of Zocor MSD were less than 10% lower than those of Zocor, a differential that generally did not impress the medical profession. In a further effort to limit generics erosion of Zocor's market, Dieckmann authorized Hexal and Betapharm to launch generic simvastatin products in March 2003 – two months before patent expiration. These generics were approximately 40% less expensive than the originator brand, a savings large enough to stimulate extensive prescribing. As soon as the patent on simvastatin expired, other companies entered the market, and approximately 25 generic products were available by August 2003. Within several weeks, generics prices declined to just 30% of the price of Zocor prior to its loss of patent protection. By the end of the third quarter of 2003, Dieckmann had just 20% of the German market for simvastatin. Simvahexal and Simvabeta have been the main beneficiaries of Dieckmann's defense strategy. In 2004, Simvahexal accounted for 32% of the

German simvastatin market in volume terms, and Simvabeta for 16%. By comparison, Zocor's market share in 2004 was just 3%, and Zocor MSD accounted for a mere 1% of the market.

The total number of DDDs of simvastatin dispensed in the GKV market increased by 68.9% in 2003, and growth was almost as strong (60.9%) in 2004. In contrast, demand for all other statins declined substantially in 2004. The fact that the GKV statin market grew by 12.8% in 2004 is attributable entirely to the rapid growth in the use of generic simvastatin products. Pfizer was already struggling to compete against the enormous price advantage of simvastatin products. The German simvastatin market is highly competitive, with at least 30 companies marketing products.

Seen against this backdrop, Pfizer's stubborn refusal to cut the price of atorvastatin is easier to understand. Aside from making a stand on a point of principle (i.e., the belief that therapeutic improvements should be rewarded by due respect for the rules of intellectual property protection), Pfizer evidently believes that capitulating to reference pricing of Sortis would effectively genericize the drug's market long before its patent expires. Furthermore, Pfizer is surely mindful of the dangers of setting a precedent by submitting to government pressure. Cutting the price of Sortis might encourage the German government, or other European administrations, to pursue the same aggressive strategy with some of the company's other patent-protected medicines. Arguably, very few companies are as well placed as Pfizer to resist government cost-containment pressures. The prospect of creating a potentially enormous reservoir for the parallel trade of atorvastatin must also deter Pfizer from cutting the drug's price in Germany. Finally, the company may be increasingly resigned to the fact that generic simvastatin products will continue to erode its share of the German statin market – with or without the complication of reference pricing.

OTHER COST-CONTAINMENT MEASURES

Reference pricing is undoubtedly the highest-profile cost-containment mechanism that currently affects the German statin market, but it is by no means the only strategy intended to curb expenditures. The government uses a variety of other cost-cutting measures, such as generics substitution, parallel imports, industry rebates, indicative prescribing amounts, and patient copayments.

Generics Substitution

Germany has the largest generics market in Europe and one of the highest rates of generics dispensing in Europe. According to Insight Health (formerly NDC Health), in 2004, the German generics market was worth €5.2 billion ($6.5 billion) at exmanufacturer prices. In 2004, generics accounted for 55.2% of the GKV pharmaceutical market in unit terms and 34.3% in terms of sales. In 2004, generics were actually dispensed in 74.1% of cases where a generic was available, and they accounted for 70.1% of sales in the potential GKV generics market (i.e., the market for all drugs that are available as generics).

Notwithstanding the size and steady growth of this market, the German government has tried to stimulate greater use of generics. In February 2002, the government introduced a controversial generics substitution requirement – commonly known as the *aut idem* rule (*aut idem* is a Latin term that means "or the same"). Where generics were available, pharmacists were henceforth required to substitute a product from the bottom third of the price range for the molecule in question – unless the physician had expressly forbidden substitution or had already chosen a bottom-third product. Data on the bottom third of the price range for generically available drugs were reviewed quarterly. However, the implementation of the *aut idem* system was beset by problems, including late publication of essential data and disagreements over how some aspects of the regulation should be interpreted.

Beginning January 1, 2004, the GMG simplified the *aut idem* rule by setting reference prices in the bottom third of the price range for products with equivalent active ingredients, so that pharmacists no longer need to calculate which products fall within the bottom third of the price range. Since April 2004, if a physician prescribes a drug by its generic name, the pharmacist must dispense one of the three lowest-priced products that conforms exactly to the prescription (in terms of formulation, dosage, pack size, indications, and dosage form). If a physician prescribes a drug by its brand name but does not forbid substitution, the pharmacist may dispense either the branded medicine or one of the three lowest-priced products that conforms exactly to the prescription. If the physician prescribes a branded drug and forbids substitution, the pharmacist must dispense the branded product. It is not known how often German physicians insist on having a branded medicine dispensed, but the Allgemeine Ortskrankenkasse Westfalen-Lippe (General Local Health Insurance Fund of Westphalia-Lippe) found in an analysis of a random sample of prescriptions dispensed to its members from September to November 2002 that substitution was prohibited on approximately 10% of prescriptions for drugs available generically.

Pharmaceutical companies in general, and generics manufacturers in particular, were initially concerned that this law would lead to a savage price war as producers of generically available drugs slashed their prices to ensure that they remained within the bottom third of the price range each quarter. However, the decline in prices was not as steep as some manufacturers had feared. From February 2002 to December 2003, prices of products subject to the *aut idem* rule declined by an average of 6.1%.

Critics have suggested that many manufacturers and pharmacists have exploited the system for their own gain. Some manufacturers reportedly circumvented the *aut idem* rule by making minor changes to their products (e.g., reducing a product's pack size from 100 tablets to 98) to preclude substitution. According to the Bundesverband der Betriebskrankenkassen (BKK; Federal Association of Occupational Health Insurance Funds) some generics manufacturers soon recognized the aut idem regulation as a new business opportunity. The BKK reports that the average price differential between new generics and their respective originator brands declined from an average of 40–50% before the introduction of generics substitution to an average of 20–25% after the implementation of the *aut idem* rule. Furthermore, the BKK asserts that the prices of generic products now typically vary by just a few cents, a situation that the association denounces as "cartel like."

Germany's new "grand coalition" government appears determined to curb what it regards as an abuse of rebates. In the first week of November 2005, the government announced its intention to outlaw manufacturer rebates in kind to pharmacists. In addition, the government plans to impose mandatory exmanufacturer price cuts for all medicines that are subject to reference prices, a step that will save approximately €300 million ($373 million) per year. Furthermore, the government plans to freeze the prices that health insurance funds pay for medicines. However, the Bundesverband der Pharmazeutischen Industrie (BPI; Federal Association of the Pharmaceutical Industry), an organization that represents many of Germany's midsize pharmaceutical companies, has pointed out that such action could be counterproductive, given that drug prices fell by an average of 0.4% in the preceding 12 months.

Some observers believe that the German healthcare system could do much better at cutting costs. For example, the 2005 edition of the Arzneiverordnungs-Report (an annual analysis of GKV prescribing data) calculated that, in 2004, the GKV could have saved an additional €2.9 billion ($3.6 billion) through more cost-effective prescribing – in most cases substituting the least expensive generic products on the market. This total consisted of the following potential savings: €1.1 billion ($1.4 billion) from using the lowest-priced generic versions of off-patent drugs, €1.2 billion ($1.5 billion) from switching patients to analogues within the same drug class (e.g., from atorvastatin [Pfizer's Sortis] to the lowest-priced generic simvastatin product), and €643 million ($799 million) from discontinuing the use of drugs of "disputed value" (so-called *umstrittene Arzneimittel*). A new feature of the 2005 edition of the Arzneiverordnungs-Report is a list of potential savings from drug substitution for each of the 50 pharmaceutical companies that had the greatest GKV sales in 2004. Pfizer would have been the main loser if physicians had followed the publishers' recommendations fully: the company's GKV sales would have been 31.4% lower than they were, largely as a consequence of patients' being switched to analogue drugs.

Parallel Imports

After several years of dynamic growth, the German market for parallel imports has fluctuated recently. According to the VFA, the organization that represents Germany's largest drug manufacturers, parallel imports' market share (in monetary terms) grew from 1.8% in 1998 to 6.8% in 2003. However, their market share declined to 6.8% in 2003 and 4.9% in 2004. Sales of parallel imports plummeted by 29.4% in 2004, but then increased by 21.6% in the first seven months of 2005.

Since June 2004, the government requires pharmacists to ensure that parallel imports account for at least 5.5% (in monetary terms) of the prescriptions they dispense each month. In addition, parallel imports must be at least 15% or €15.00 ($16.94), whichever is the smaller sum, less expensive than equivalent products sourced in Germany.

Industry Rebates

In January 2003, the German government imposed a 6% rebate on patent-protected drugs that were not subject to reference pricing. The rebate level for prescription-only drugs was increased to 16% from January 1, 2004. (The rebate remained at 6% for prescriptions of nonprescription medicines [i.e., drugs that are not restricted to prescription-only distribution].) In 2004, GKV pharmaceutical spending declined by 10.6%, and the volume of prescriptions fell by 23.4%.

From January 1, 2005, the rebate for prescription-only drugs returned to 6%, a change that triggered a substantial increase in pharmaceutical expenditures. According to the VFA, GKV spending increased by as much as 20% in the first few months of 2005, but the growth rate slowed to just 3.8% in July and averaged 10% in the first seven months of the year. In that period, the volume of prescriptions increased by 4.8% and the transfer of some patients to more expensive drugs (so-called structural change) boosted GKV spending by 5.9%. However, pharmaceutical prices fell by an average of 0.7%.

Indicative Prescribing Amounts

In 1993, the government introduced a national prescribing budget that threatened tough sanctions for physician overspending. Over the next eight years, the budget system was modified repeatedly. Toward the end of 2001, the Arzneimittelbudget-Ablösungsgesetz (Pharmaceutical Budget Replacement Act) abolished the pharmaceutical budget. Instead, associations representing health insurance funds and contracted physicians conclude Arzneimittelvereinbarungen (pharmaceutical agreements) for each state. These agreements include Richtgrößen (indicative prescribing amounts) – the maximum approved expenditure on medicines per patient per quarter. The Act does not define sanctions for exceeding these indicative prescribing amounts, but state authorities have the option of introducing penalties if they wish. State authorities may also choose to offer bonuses for complying with spending volumes.

According to the BKK, approximately 10% of physicians exceed their indicative prescribing amounts. However, only 2.5% overprescribe by such a margin that they face the threat of penalties, and only 0.4% actually incur penalties. The infrequency of penalties is a testament to the effectiveness of Richtgrößen as a means of controlling physicians' prescribing behavior.

Patient Copayments

The German government introduced copayments for prescription medicines in the 1980s. Until December 31, 2003, patient copayments for medicines depended on the size of the pack dispensed: €4.00 ($4.97) for small packs, €4.50 ($5.59) for medium-sized packs, and €5.00 ($6.21) for large packs. On January 1, 2004, the government replaced flat copayments with a percentage coinsurance payment. The standard coinsurance rate is 10% of the retail price, with a minimum payment of €5.00 ($6.21) and a maximum of €10.00 ($12.42). Factors such as the type of drug prescribed and its generic or branded status have no direct bearing on patients' payments.

Under the GMG, most patients are required to make significant out-of-pocket payments for their healthcare services. One of the most controversial innovations is a practice fee of €10.00 ($11.29) per quarter, which has reportedly deterred many patients from visiting their physicians.

OUTLOOK AND IMPLICATIONS

Outlook in Germany

Government Plans for Stricter Cost Containment

GKV pharmaceutical expenditures are expected to grow by €3.5 billion ($4.3 billion), a trend that has alarmed the German government. In December 2005, the new "grand coalition" government announced its intention to intensify pharmaceutical cost containment in Germany still further. The *Gesetzentwurf zur Verbesserung der Wirtschaftlichkeit in der Arzneimittelversorgung* (Improvement of Economy in the Pharmaceutical Supply Bill, abbreviated to *Arzneimittelversorgungs-Wirtschaftlichkeitsgesetz* [AVWG]) will introduce tough constraints on pharmaceutical prices and exert pressure on physicians to be economical in their prescribing practice. The objective is to save approximately €975 million ($1.2 billion) in 2006 and €1.3 billion ($1.6 billion) in 2007.

More-Aggressive Reference Prices At present, reference prices for level 1 reference pricing groups (i.e., drugs that have the same active ingredient and bioavailability [if therapeutically relevant]) are set at the upper end of the bottom third of the price range. From April 1, 2006, this method of calculating reference prices will be extended to level 2 reference pricing groups (i.e., drugs that have pharmacologically and therapeutically comparable active ingredients [particularly chemically related agents]) and level 3 reference pricing groups (i.e., drugs that have therapeutically comparable effects [particularly combination agents]). The only proviso is that the drugs that are used in setting reference prices must account for at least one-fifth of prescriptions and must comprise at least two comparable medicines. This change in the method of calculating reference prices is likely to result in substantially lower reference prices for statins.

On a more positive note for drug manufacturers, a change of one word in the existing law on reference pricing offers some encouragement to research-based pharmaceutical companies. At present, drugs must be innovative *and* offer a therapeutic improvement to be safe from the threat of reference pricing. Under the new law, drugs will have to be innovative *or* offer a therapeutic improvement to be guaranteed exemption from reference pricing. In other words, it will no longer be necessary to satisfy the dual requirements of innovation and therapeutic improvement. In Pfizer's recent lawsuit, Sortis was not judged to be innovative, given that its mechanism of action is common to all statins.

Price Freeze From April 1, 2006, to December 31, 2007, manufacturers will not be permitted to charge the health insurance funds more for medicines than the prices that prevailed on November 1, 2005. (The use of this historical benchmark will prevent manufacturers from circumventing the upcoming rule by increasing their prices between its announcement and implementation.) The government expects this measure to save the healthcare system approximately €700 million ($869 million) in 2007.

Price Cuts on Off-Patent Medicines and an End to Rebates in Kind The retail prices of drugs that are no longer patent protected will be reduced by the equivalent of 10% of the products' exmanufacturer prices. However, manufacturers can reduce the level of these price cuts by offering rebates to individual health insurance funds. In addition, off-patent drugs that have a retail price at least 30% below their respective reference prices will be exempt from this rule.

In addition, the government will outlaw the practice of *Naturalrabatte* (rebates in kind) – for example, providing pharmacists with one or more free packs of a medicine for each pack purchased. Pharmacists receive full reimbursement from the GKV when they dispense these free packs of medicine. The 2005 report of the *Sachverständigenrat zur Begutachtung der Entwicklung im Gesundheitswesen* (Expert Counsel for the Assessment of Progress in the Healthcare System) stated that "there can be no doubt that, in the German market for drugs that are available as generics, rebate competition for the benefit of pharmacists often takes the place of price competition for the benefit of health insurance funds and consumers." Together, the price cuts and the termination of rebates in kind are expected to save €375 million ($466 million) per year.

Daily Cost of Therapy Limits for Frequently Prescribed Medicines The health insurance funds will set daily cost of therapy limits (by indication) for drugs that are frequently prescribed. If physicians exceed these limits by 5–10% in a quarter, they will be liable to pay a fine equivalent to 20% of the excess. If physicians exceed these limits by 10–30% in a quarter, they will be required to pay a fine equivalent to 30% of the excess. If their spending is more than 30% over the limit, they will have to pay 50% of the excess as a penalty. This measure goes farther than the current indicative prescribing limits in that the fines will be mandatory (not left to the discretion of state governments) and will be indication specific. Health insurance funds may offer a bonus to physicians whose prescribing averages less than the daily cost of therapy. To promote compliance with this new rule, physicians will be required to use prescribing software that is approved by the KBV and that contains the GBA's therapeutic recommendations and prescribing guidelines.

Continued Pressure to Reduce Spending on Statins

Since the launch of the first generic simvastatin products in Germany in March 2003, pressure has been increasing on physicians to economize in their use of statins. The *Arzneiverordnungs-Report*, the annual review of GKV prescribing trends, has been one of the most prominent and forceful critics of spending on statins. The 2004 edition celebrated the fact that, in just the last nine months of 2003, the use of generics saved the GKV €220 million ($273 million) on simvastatin alone. The authors calculated that a further €107 million ($133 million) could have been saved in 2003 by substituting generic simvastatin for the remaining prescriptions for branded simvastatin products (i.e., Merck Sharp & Dohme's Zocor and Boehringer Ingelheim's Denan).

Not content with encouraging the use of generic simvastatin products in place of branded simvastatin, the *Arzneiverordnungs-Report 2004* called on physicians to prescribe the lowest-priced generic simvastatin products in place of all other statins in most cases. The only exception to this recommendation was the treatment of patients diagnosed with acute coronary syndrome, for which intensive therapy with high-dose atorvastatin should be prescribed. If physicians prescribed the least expensive generic simvastatin products wherever possible, the authors forecast potential savings of €583 million ($724 million) in 2004. Similarly, the *Arzneiverordnungs-Report 2005* calculated that maximizing the use of the lowest-priced simvastatin products would save the GKV €408 million ($507 million) in 2005. Figure 14.3 shows the potential savings by molecule in 2004 and 2005. The sharp fall from 2004 to 2005 in potential savings on pravastatin and simvastatin is attributable to the fact that inexpensive generic simvastatin largely replaced branded pravastatin and simvastatin products in 2004. According to GKV prescribing data, the number of DDDs of the two branded pravastatin products, Bristol-Myers Squibb's Pravasin and Sankyo's Mevalotin, each declined by 38% in 2004. The decline in branded simvastatin products was even more dramatic: the number of DDDs of Zocor declined by 70% and Denan by 80%. However, the explosion in the use of generic simvastatin boosted the total number of DDDs of simvastatin products by 61% in 2004. It will be interesting to see just how comprehensively generic simvastatin displaces atorvastatin over the course of 2005 as a whole. As noted previously, Pfizer's refusal to cut the retail price of Sortis to the reference price level has sharply accelerated the drug's loss of market share to generic simvastatin products.

Implications for Key Stakeholders

German Government

According to ABDA, pharmaceutical spending by the GKV amounted to €14.99 billion ($18.62 billion) in the first eight months of 2005. This sum was 18.7% higher than the €12.64 billion ($15.7 billion) spent in the first six months of 2004.

The VFA reports that GKV spending on pharmaceuticals totaled €14.57 billion ($18.1 billion) at retail prices in the first seven months of 2005, a 10% increase over the corresponding period in 2004. However, the association notes that spending in 2004 was depressed by the impact of the GMG, including the manufacturer rebate of 16% (now reduced to 6%) on medicines outside the reference-pricing system. In 2004 as a whole, GKV pharmaceutical spending declined by 10.6%, and the volume of prescriptions fell by 23.4%. According to the VFA, GKV spending increased by as much as 20% in the first few months of 2005, but the growth rate slowed to just 3.8% in July. In the first seven months of the year, the volume of prescriptions increased by 4.8% and the transfer of

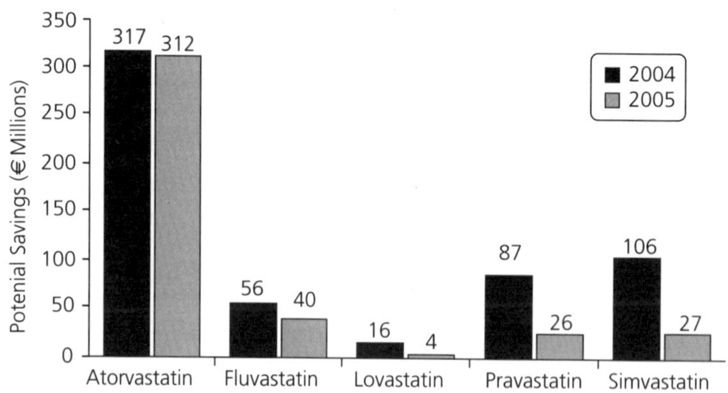

GKV = Gesetzliche Krankenversicherung (statutory health insurance)

Figure 14.3 Potential Savings to the GKV from Dispensing the Lowest-Priced Generic Simvastatin Products in Place of Other Statins, 2004 and 2005

some patients to more expensive drugs (so-called structural change) boosted GKV spending by 5.9%. However, pharmaceutical prices fell by an average of 0.7%.

The government has been quick to blame the pharmaceutical industry for the pronounced increase in pharmaceutical expenditures, but this charge ignores the impact of the mandatory rebate on spending in 2004. Drug manufacturers argue that an overall price reduction of 0.7% demonstrates exemplary self-restraint. However, the government is unlikely to be persuaded by the industry's protestations. Politically, it is much easier to target cost-containment measures at the pharmaceutical industry than physicians or patients. If implemented, the AVWG will increase the already enormous pressures on drug manufacturers in Germany. However, the government should be prepared for the possibility of unintended negative consequences of stricter cost containment.

If the pricing and reimbursement environment deteriorates further, manufacturers may become increasingly reluctant to invest in Germany. Some have already cut their spending on R&D in Germany. In addition, companies may decide they simply cannot afford to market new medicines in drug classes that are subject to level 2 or 3 references pricing in Germany. Launching a new drug into a market that is not only subject to reference pricing but that also caps reimbursement at the level of generics (as proposed in the AVWG) would be a most unattractive proposition. Aside from denying the manufacturer the opportunity of a reasonable return on investment in Germany, launching a new medicine at such low prices would expose the company to the threat of massive parallel trade. As a result, many more companies may follow AstraZeneca's lead in suspending the launch of rosuvastatin (Crestor) in Germany.

Even if new drugs reach the market in Germany, it is by no means certain that they will be widely prescribed. According to the VFA, in 2003, drugs launched in the preceding five years accounted for only 7.5% of total pharmaceutical sales in Germany. By comparison, medicines launched in the previous five years accounted for 20.5% of sales in Belgium and 23.3% in Spain.

The initial response to the AVWG suggests that this legislation will encounter stiff resistance from both the pharmaceutical industry and the medical profession. A backlash from patients can also be expected if the new law increases their out-of-pocket costs or reduces the quality of care they receive. The government may hesitate to incur the wrath of the electorate.

If stricter cost containment curbs the use of gold-standard therapies or impedes the launch of innovative medicines in Germany, public health could suffer. The idea of Germany as a country in which GKV patients are denied access to state-of-the art medicine would be anathema to the medical profession and patient organizations.

The future direction of German healthcare policy, including pharmaceutical cost containment, may ultimately depend on the durability of the new grand coalition government. The Ministry of Health is primarily under the control of the *Sozialdemokratische Partei Deutschlands* (SPD; Social Democratic Party of Germany), led by Ulla Schmidt, a fierce critic of the pharmaceutical industry. However, the media in Germany have suggested that attempts to pursue a very aggressive cost-cutting strategy might undermine the fragile coalition. For example, a consensus on the reforms contained in the AVWG was achieved only after the SPD's proposals were moderated.

Health Insurance Funds

The statutory health insurance funds have joined the government in criticizing the increase in pharmaceutical expenditures. Therefore, it is no surprise that the health insurance funds are generally very supportive of the proposed new cost-containment measures.

Independently of the government's initiatives, health insurance funds have begun to explore opportunities to reduce their spending on medicines. For example, the Barmer Ersatzkasse has negotiated rebates for certain products from eight generics companies and one manufacturer of branded medicines (Merck KGaA). These savings apply to approximately 1.5 million members (out of Barmer's total enrollment of 7.5 million) who have signed up to receive primary care through a designated family physician.

Future funding of medicines may also be affected by the growth of disease management programs in Germany. Breast cancer and type 2 diabetes were the first indications covered in this government-endorsed initiative, but programs on CHD have recently been added. It remains to be seen whether these programs will promote increased use of statins in primary and secondary prevention.

Physicians

Physicians generally like to have the widest possible choice of drugs at their disposal, and often resent measures that restrict their clinical freedom, particularly on economic grounds. In the statin market, however, they have the consolation of a selection of highly effective agents. Physicians' high opinion of atorvastatin is confirmed by the fact that most continue to favor this agent for their privately insured patients, who are subject to comparatively few cost constraints. However, the enormous gulf in prices that has developed between Sortis and the least expensive generic simvastatin products has prompted physicians largely to abandon the use of Sortis for their GKV patients.

Drugs' efficacy and side-effect profile remain physicians' most important criteria in prescribing decisions, but retail price, the availability of generics, and patient copayments are also significant. It is now difficult for physicians to prescribe atorvastatin to most of their GKV patients without strong justification. Physicians are required to inform patients about the reference pricing of atorvastatin, the need to pay the excess for this drug, and the availability of less expensive options. In these circumstances, it is hardly surprising that the number of prescriptions for atorvastatin has collapsed in 2005.

Aside from their concerns about the cost of atorvastatin to their patients, physicians are understandably also worried about the potential personal costs of prescribing this drug extensively. The prospect of facing financial penalties for exceeding their indicative prescribing amounts is daunting. By prescribing the least expensive appropriate drugs, they minimize their risk of exceeding their indicative prescribing amounts.

The prospective new daily cost of therapy limits, if implemented, will be much tougher. The limits for statins will presumably be based on low-priced simvastatin products. The possible promise of bonuses for prescribing below daily cost of therapy limits would offer physicians another powerful incentive to favor the least expensive statins.

In this increasingly price-sensitive environment, German physicians are likely to revert to the widespread use of atorvastatin for their GKV patients only if its retail price is cut to the reference price (or lower). In the future, however, that reference price will probably drop to the level of generics.

Patients

Unlike the pharmaceutical industry and physicians, patients will not be directly penalized by the more stringent cost-cutting measures contained in the AVWG. On the contrary, they stand to benefit in at least two ways from lower statin prices. First, physicians may be more inclined to prescribe statins if these drugs are less expensive. Second, patients' copayments are likely to decline. However, much lower prices could ultimately restrict patients' choice if they drive some companies out of the German statin market.

Pharmaceutical Industry

In July 2005, the BPI published the Studie der Aktuellen Situation der Pharmazeutischen

Industrie in Deutschland 2005 (Study of the Current Situation of the Pharmaceutical Industry in Germany 2005). Between mid-March and mid-April 2005, 275 BPI member companies responded to a detailed survey on the impact of the GMG. The results made gloomy reading for the pharmaceutical industry.

Fifty-four percent of participating companies believed that the GMG's impact on drug manufacturers had been bad, and 30% considered the effects to be very bad. An analysis of data from IMS Health found that, among Germany's 100 largest manufacturers of prescription and over-the-counter (OTC) medicines (as defined by sales), 31% of leading prescription drug manufacturers had seen their sales decline by as much as 30% following the implementation of the GMG. Therefore, it is not surprising that the BPI survey found that 55% of respondents considered the financial environment in Germany to be bad or very bad for prescription drugs, and 51% judged the financial environment bad or very bad for OTC medicines. In contrast, only 28% of respondents thought the financial environment was bad or very bad for generic drugs, whereas 52% believed conditions to be good or very good for generics.

Many companies have reacted to the deteriorating commercial environment in Germany by reducing their workforce or cutting R&D investment. The BPI survey found that 38% had reduced their number of employees: the median decrease was 10%. In addition, 33% of companies indicated that they had cut their spending on R&D: the median decrease was 20%, but some companies reported that they had discontinued R&D entirely.

Generics Companies The reference pricing of statins has been an enormous boon to the generics industry. Even before the imposition of reference prices, generics had rapidly achieved a dominant position in the simvastatin market and had seriously eroded branded products' share of the pravastatin and lovastatin markets. More significantly, atorvastatin had begun to lose prescriptions to generic simvastatin. The trickle of 2003 turned into a steady flow in 2004, and the introduction of reference prices in January 2005 breached the dam. However, the potential for switching patients from atorvastatin to generic simvastatin has now been almost fully exploited.

Not surprisingly, more generics companies have launched simvastatin products than pravastatin or lovastatin products. Official guidelines have almost universally adopted simvastatin as their benchmark, and our survey confirms that physicians share the view that simvastatin is the best available alternative to atorvastatin.

It will be interesting to see how generics companies respond to the more aggressive reference prices threatened in the AVWG. Price is generally the primary selling point of generics, but as discussed previously in this chapter, generics manufacturers in Germany have been criticized for a lack of competition. The BKK found that the average price differential between new generics and their respective originator brands declined from an average of 40–50% before the introduction of generics substitution to an average of 20–25% after the implementation of this rule. Furthermore, the BKK condemned the fact that the prices of generic products now typically vary by just a few cents.

Pfizer Events in 2005 have been extremely challenging for Pfizer, and the outlook appears even bleaker. The company certainly cannot be accused of a lack of vigor in its defense of Sortis: it has fought reference pricing on multiple fronts. However, its efforts have failed dismally to arrest the slump in the brand's sales.

The appeal against the Berliner Sozialgericht's recent verdict in its lawsuit may offer Pfizer some hope. The AVWG's proposal to end the requirement for a drug to be deemed both innovative and a therapeutic improvement as grounds for exemption from reference pricing may help

Pfizer's cause. The fact that atorvastatin shared the same mechanism of action as the other statins was judged a barrier to innovative status, but the company may yet be able to provide persuasive evidence of therapeutic improvement. However, the general climate of opinion does not appear favorable for Pfizer.

An unsuccessful appeal would certainly be bad news for Pfizer. If the company still refused to cut the price of Sortis, criticism of its stance would likely intensify. However, it would be difficult and risky for Pfizer to cut its prices to reference price levels, particularly if the AVWG reduces reference prices to the level of the least expensive generic statins. If the company took that course, it would likely regain much of its lost market share, but sales would be much lower than before the imposition of reference pricing. Furthermore, an abundant supply of atorvastatin priced at or near the level of generics would create an enormous reservoir for parallel trade (see the discussion on Parallel Trade later in this chapter).

Whatever the outcome of Pfizer's appeal and its ultimate response to the reference pricing of atorvastatin, the company will have to deal with the legacy of its robust campaign against this cost-containment measure. Pfizer's actions have antagonized the German government and health insurance funds, and alienated many physicians. It will take time to restore good relations with these stakeholder groups.

Other Manufacturers of Branded Statins
The manufacturers of other branded statins – Dieckmann (Zocor), Merck Sharp & Dohme (Zocor MSD and Mevinacor), Bristol-Myers Squibb (Pravasin), Sankyo (Mevalotin), Novartis (Locol), Astellas (Cranoc) – have also faced the challenge of reference pricing, but they have responded differently from Pfizer. Without exception, they have aligned their retail prices with the respective reference prices for each dosage and pack size of their products. However, these prices are still much higher than generics prices, and the branded statins have lost ground to generic simvastatin.

The prospect of lower reference prices under the AVWG will present a new challenge for these companies. They will have to decide if they are willing to cut their prices further. Alternatively, they might decide to follow Pfizer's example and defy reference pricing. However, it would be difficult for manufacturers of drugs that are already off patent to pursue this strategy: their market would be almost entirely lost to generic versions of the molecules they developed.

A display of solidarity by manufacturers of branded statins might prompt the German government to reconsider this policy, but such an outcome appears highly improbable. The genericization of the German statin market is now virtually complete, and it is difficult to see any way back to the market conditions that prevailed before simvastatin lost patent protection.

Outlook in Other European Markets

France, Italy, and Spain are among the many other European countries that have followed Germany's lead in introducing reference pricing. These countries will certainly observe the impact of reference pricing on the market for statins and other drug classes that include patent-protected medicines. If they judge this latest German experiment to be a success, they will likely follow suit again.

The United Kingdom is the one major European market that has not adopted reference pricing. The UK government has devised other highly effective methods to curb prescribing costs, but it has generally been more relaxed than most of its European neighbors about the steady growth in spending on statins.

France

On October 1, 2003, *tarifs forfaitaires de responsabilité* (reference prices) were introduced in France. The government had hoped to implement this new cost-containment measure on July 1, 2003, but postponed the start date to give manufacturers ample time to reduce their prices to reference price levels if they wished to do so. Any product that is subject to reference pricing but does not show its reference price on its label is not reimbursed by the social security system.

The first wave of products to undergo reference pricing comprised all substances that were available as generics but that had a generics substitution rate in April 2003 of 10–45%. Products containing a total of 29 substances, divided into 72 generics groups, fell within the government's target range in that month and therefore became subject to reference pricing from October 1, 2003. Before that deadline, many manufacturers reduced their prices to reference price levels to ensure that patients would not have to pay the excess or accept an alternative product. On June 1, 2005, the *Comité Economique des Produits de Santé* (CEPS; Economic Committee for Healthcare Products) implemented France's second wave of reference prices, which comprised 11 compounds and 17 product presentations.

In July 2004, the French Parliament passed the *Projet de Loi Relatif à l'Assurance Maladie* (the Health Insurance Bill), a bill that introduced radical reforms in the funding of healthcare in France. Among its many measures, this bill made the reference-pricing system much more aggressive: The *Comité de Suivi des Génériques* (Generics Monitoring Committee) meets monthly to review the generics dispensing rates of drugs that have been off patent for a year or longer. Reference prices are imposed if a drug's generics dispensing rate does not reach 50% (60% in the case of drugs with substantial sales) within one year of patent expiration and 70% (80% in the case of drugs with substantial sales) within two years of patent expiration. These conditions may be relaxed if generics dispensing is growing strongly but has not reached the targeted rates, or if the range of generics on the market is limited.

In early October 2005, however, the government published the *Projet de Loi de Financement de la Sécurité Sociale* (PLFSS) 2006 (Social Security Finance Bill 2006). In an effort to reduce the deficit in the healthcare budget from an estimated €8.3 billion ($10.3 billion) in 2005 to €6.1 billion ($7.6 billion) in 2006, the government announced plans to impose a wide range of stringent cost-cutting measures, including the automatic imposition of reference pricing two years after the patent on a compound expires. French pharmacists were so indignant at the proposed reform that they threatened to boycott generics substitution as a protest. In December 2005, the government relented and abandoned the proposal for automatic reference pricing. Instead, the government will continue to impose reference prices on molecules that do not attain a generics dispensing rate of 50% (60% in the case of drugs with substantial sales) within one year of patent expiration.

The introduction of reference pricing in France has helped to moderate the prices of off-patent medicines. The CEPS reports that, in 70% of cases, manufacturers of branded medicines that were subjected to reference pricing reduced their prices to the level of the reference prices. Overall, very few drugs have not had their prices aligned with their respective reference prices. Of 541 reference-priced products, only 34 (6.3%) exceeded their reference prices. The mean price difference between the reference prices and retail prices of these drugs was 41.5%, a surprisingly large margin. Manufacturers of these products presumably concluded that the potential loss of sales from refusing to cut their prices was greater than the reduction in revenues that would result from lower prices. These companies may have hoped that established patients would remain loyal to familiar brands, even if they had to pay a premium to continue taking them.

In November 2004, *Les entreprises du médicament* (Leem; Pharmaceutical Companies), the association that represents French drug manufacturers, estimated that the first wave of reference pricing in France had saved the social security system approximately €115 million ($143 million) to date. Most of this savings (€95 million

[$118 million]) came from manufacturers' price cuts, while increased use of generics saved €20 million ($25 million). Figure 14.4 shows that, from 2003 to 2004, generics' share of the market for off-patent drugs increased among both reference-priced and nonreference-priced drugs, but the growth rate was much faster among reference-priced drugs. In 2004, generics accounted for 49% of prescriptions for reference-priced drugs, compared with only 34% of prescriptions for off-patent drugs that were not subject to reference pricing.

The French government has also sought to cut pharmaceutical expenditures by actively encouraging a reduction in the use of three very widely prescribed drug classes: statins, antibiotics, and anxiolytics/hypnotics. The government set a target of a 12.5% reduction in reimbursement spending on statins in 2005. The focus on statins is not surprising, given that, in 2004, the health insurance system spent €1.1 billion ($1.4 billion) on more than 46 million packs of statins – higher spending than on any other drug class.

Besides encouraging physicians to prescribe statins more abstemiously, the French government hopes to reduce spending on this drug class by other means. It recently imposed price cuts of 7–15% on two pravastatin products: Bristol-Myers Squibb's Elisor and Sanofi-Aventis's Vasten. Beginning June 2005, the *Caisse Nationale de l'Assurance Maladie* (CNAM; National Health Insurance Fund) is checking that prescriptions for rosuvastatin (AstraZeneca's Crestor) and ezetimibe (Merck Sharp & Dohme-Chibret's Ezétrol) observe the strict conditions for reimbursement. (Both these drugs are approved only for second-line therapy in patients whose elevated LDL count has failed to respond to another agent.) A study conducted by CNAM in February 2005 found that 27.6% of all prescriptions for Crestor were issued to patients who had not been taking another statin throughout the six preceding months. If widespread violation of reimbursement conditions persists, CNAM might suspend reimbursement. This threat would apply equally to other drugs that are prescribed outside their respective reimbursement conditions.

Spending on statins will also be reduced by the growth of generics. The first generic simvastatin products were launched early in May 2005 and achieved a 13% market share (in monetary terms) that same month; by September 2005, this share had increased to 45%, according to IMS Health. The expected launch of the first generic pravastatin products in August 2006 will likely stimulate demand for generic statins still further.

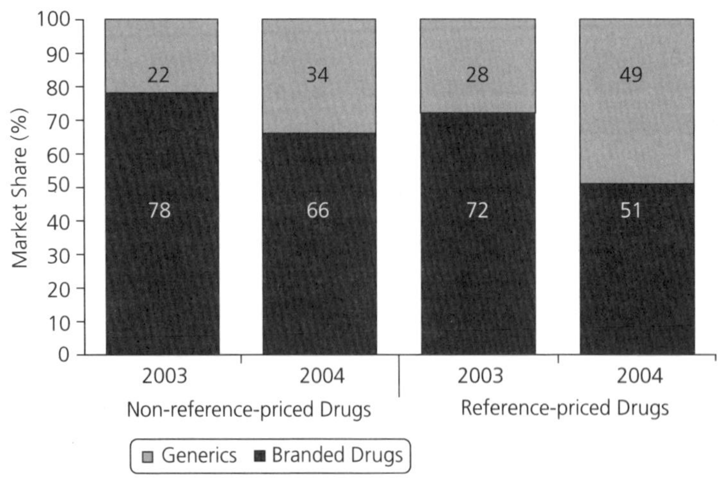

Figure 14.4 Generic and Branded Medicines' Share of Prescriptions for Off-Patent Drugs in France, 2003–4

Italy

Italy's 1994 Finance Act made provision for reference pricing, but the system was not actually established until September 2001. The program initially covered approximately 1,000 patent-expired products containing 38 multisource substances categorized by anatomic therapeutic chemical (ATC) classifications. The price ceiling was set as the weighted average of all products in the group that are at least 20% less expensive than the originator product. The *Servizio Sanitario Nazionale* (SSN; National Health Service) reimbursed the full cost of drugs that did not exceed the reference price, but patients had to pay the excess for drugs that were priced above the reference price.

Just weeks after the program was inaugurated, the government adopted a decree law that radically changed the system. Since November 1, 2001, reference prices are set at the level of the least expensive available generic rather than based on a weighted average. In addition, if a prescribed drug appears on the reference list, pharmacists are authorized to substitute the least expensive generic equivalent unless the prescribing physician explicitly forbids substitution. Furthermore, physicians who prescribe products that exceed reference prices must inform their patients about the excess they would have to pay and advise them if less expensive options are available. As of May 2005, 138 compounds are included in the Italian reference pricing list. Regional governments have some discretion in deciding reimbursement terms in their territories for reference-priced medicines.

In addition to reference pricing for off-patent medicines, Italy imposes strict reimbursement ceilings on patent-protected drugs. The *Prontuario Farmaceutico Nazionale* (PFN; national formulary) determines reimbursement status on the basis of a drug's cost effectiveness. Drugs dispensed by retail pharmacies are assigned to *categorie terapeutiche omogenee* (homogeneous therapeutic categories) based on ATC fourth-level classification. A homogeneous therapeutic category is defined as "a group of drugs that, in relation to the main therapeutic indication, share the same mechanism of action and are characterized by similar clinical efficacy and profile of undesired side effects. Individual drugs, however, may differ in terms of additional therapeutic indications." For example, in the antiulcerants drug class, H_2 antagonists and proton pump inhibitors are assigned to different homogeneous therapeutic categories as a result of their different mechanisms of action.

Products that do not exceed their price ceilings in the PFN are included in reimbursement class A (100% reimbursement), but products that are priced above this level are assigned to class C (no reimbursement at all). The threat of dereimbursement is a powerful incentive for manufacturers to cut their prices. In January 2003, when the government introduced its reform of the PFN, only 21 product presentations (out of a total of 4,039 that were eligible for class A status) were assigned to class C because their manufacturers refused to reduce their prices to the level of the reimbursement ceiling.

Spain

Reference pricing was introduced in Spain on December 1, 2000, and soon became the mainstay of the government's cost-containment strategy. Drugs within the system were assigned to "homogeneous groups" – medicines that were therapeutically equivalent and had the same qualitative and quantitative composition, pharmaceutical form, dosage form, and route of administration. All homogeneous groups had to contain at least one generic drug. The *Sistema Nacional de Salud* (SNS; National Health System) reimbursed reference-priced drugs only to the level of the reference price for the respective homogeneous group.

Originally, the reference price was the average of the prices of the least expensive drugs that collectively accounted for 20% of sales within each homogeneous group. In May 2003, however, the *Ley de Cohesión y Calidad del Sistema Nacional de Salud* (Law on the Coherence and Quality of the National

Healthcare System) changed the method for calculating reference prices: reference prices were thereafter based on the average price of the three products in a homogeneous group that have the lowest daily treatment costs. Each of the three products used in setting a reference price had to be marketed by a different manufacturer. Products that had an exmanufacturer price of less than €2.00 ($2.48) were excluded from these calculations. Prices for generics were not allowed to exceed the group's reference price.

If pharmacists received a prescription for a product that was in a generics group but exceeded its reference price, they were required to substitute a product that did not exceed the reference price. In the event that a product less expensive than the reference price was not available, the pharmacist dispensed the prescribed product but charged the patient the reference price. The manufacturer was then required to reimburse the pharmacist the difference between the reference price and the retail price of its drug.

In October 2003, the government published the new *Orden de Precios de Referencia de Medicamentos* (Pharmaceutical Reference Pricing Order). On January 1, 2004, the reference prices of 2,070 different presentations of 62 frequently prescribed compounds were reduced by an average of 28%, but some products were subjected to cuts of as much as 80%. In 2002, SNS spending on the targeted drugs totaled €1.64 billion ($2.04 billion), a sum that the government hoped to reduce by €463 million ($575 million) per year.

In March 2004, the *Federación Empresarial de Farmaceúticos Españoles* (FEFE; Business Federation of Spanish Pharmacists) suggested that reference pricing was not achieving the level of savings that the government had expected. FEFE attributed this situation to the fact that many physicians were prescribing more-expensive innovative therapies in place of drugs that are subject to reference pricing. A study conducted by IMS Health on behalf of the Ministry of Health supported the belief that Spanish physicians often avoided prescribing reference-priced drugs. For example, sales of simvastatin, a drug that was subject to reference pricing, grew by 4.6% in 2003 as a whole but declined by 14.3% in December 2003, shortly after reference price cuts were announced. Conversely, sales of atorvastatin, a drug that was excluded from reference pricing, increased by 13.1% in December 2003 and by 23% in the year as a whole. Similarly, sales of the proton pump inhibitor pantoprazole, which was not subject to reference pricing, grew much faster than sales of omeprazole, a drug that was reference priced.

In early October 2004, the Spanish Ministry of Health surprised observers by announcing plans for radical changes to the reference-pricing system. Since coming to power in March 2004, the new Socialist government has been disappointed by the savings achieved by the reference-pricing system – €210 million ($261 million) instead of the €430 million ($534 million) forecasted in 2003. Furthermore, the government is concerned that the reference-pricing system causes what it describes as "collateral damage." Some domestic manufacturers and generics companies have lost as much as 25% of their sales as a result of reference pricing, whereas the impact on multinationals has been much smaller (0.5–3.0%). The government stated that it wanted to save money "without suffocating pharmaceutical companies." Pending reforms, the government suspended the reference-pricing system, on the grounds that this system was unpredictable and arbitrary – penalizing some companies but largely excluding the manufacturers of certain drugs that were judged to be innovative.

In December 2005, the Spanish government passed the *Ley de Garantías y Uso Racional de los Medicamentos y Productos Sanitarios* (Law on the Security and Rational Use of Medicines and Medical Devices). A Ministry of Health press release explained that "the objective is to ensure quality, security, transparency, and universality in pharmaceutical services, driving the rational use of medicines and the financial sustainability of the system." Among many other reforms, this law establishes a new reference-pricing system. According to the Ministry of Health, the new system will "generate greater savings for the National Health System, will be predictable, objective, and stable, will have a gradual impact on the pharmaceutical industry, will make it possible to keep generics as the most economical option, and will affect all drugs that are in a mature stage of market development." The reference-pricing system will have the following key features:

- All drugs reimbursed by the SNS that cost €2 ($2.48) or more, that have been marketed in Spain for more than 10 years (or 11 years in the case of drugs that have been approved for an additional indication), that have the same active substances and dosage forms, and that are available as generics will be assigned to reference pricing groups. In contrast to current practice, the government will no longer be able to exclude any such drugs from reference pricing on the grounds that certain products that meet these conditions are "innovative." Reference prices will be the average of the three lowest-priced versions of compounds.
- In the event that a reference price is more than 30% below a drug's retail price, the manufacturer may either reduce the price in one step or in stages of at least 30% per year until the reference price is reached. If the manufacturer opts for staged price cuts, the drug will not be formally added to the reference-pricing system until its price falls to the reference price level.
- In exceptional cases, new reference price groups and reference prices will be set immediately (in agreement with the *Comisión Interministerial de Precios de los Medicamentos* [CIPM; Interdepartmental Commission on Drug Pricing]) when three generic versions of a compound are approved. This provision will expedite the reference pricing process.
- Reference-priced drugs will be dispensed in the following circumstances:

  1. When a physician prescribes a drug that belongs to a reference-pricing group and that has a price equal to or less than its reference price, the pharmacist will dispense the prescribed drug.
  2. When a physician prescribes a drug that belongs to a reference-pricing group and that has a price higher than its reference price, the pharmacist must substitute the lowest-priced generic of identical composition.
  3. When a physician prescribes, by its international nonproprietary name, an active substance that is subject to reference pricing, the pharmacist will dispense the lowest-priced generic.

Products that offer useful "incremental innovations" (e.g., a beneficial new formulation) may qualify for a temporary premium 25% above the relevant reference price. This premium will then be reduced to 15% after one year, 10% after two years, and 5% after three years. Thereafter, the prices of these products will be aligned with their reference prices.

United Kingdom

The UK government has considered following most other European countries in adopting a reference-pricing system but ultimately rejected the idea. The Pharmaceutical Price Regulation Scheme, the system that regulates prices by limiting the profits that manufacturers make from the sale of patent-protected drugs to the National Health Service (NHS), allows pharmaceutical companies relative freedom in setting their prices. However, pharmaceutical spending is controlled by prescribing restrictions (primarily guidance from the National Institute for Health and Clinical Excellence [NICE]) and a strong culture of generics prescribing and dispensing.

The UK generics market is the second largest in Europe. The Department of Health reports that in 2004 net ingredient costs for generics dispensed in England totaled £2 billion ($3.7 billion), equivalent in monetary terms to 25% of the total pharmaceutical market. Generics penetration rates are also among the highest in Europe. (The dollar-to-pound-sterling exchange rate used in this chapter is the 2004 average rate: $1 = £0.54604.) In 1991, 41% of prescriptions in England were written generically, and 35% were dispensed generically. By 2004, the generics prescribing rate in England had risen to 79%, and the generics dispensing rate had risen to 58%.

The NHS encourages rather than compels physicians and pharmacists to use generics whenever possible. Trainee physicians are taught to prescribe drugs using their international, nonproprietary name, even if products are still patent protected. Computerized prescribing systems notify physicians of generic alternatives to drugs they propose to prescribe. In addition, pharmacists have financial incentives to source the lowest-priced generics available.

Price differentials between originator drugs and generics tend to be much greater in the United Kingdom than in other European countries. The extremely low prices in the United Kingdom are attributable in part to the dominance of unbranded generics in this market. Exmanufacturer prices in the United Kingdom often drop by 70–80% within four years of a drug's patent expiration, but price erosion is sometimes far more dramatic. For instance, the day after captopril's UK patent expired, competition from 13 generics reduced prices by 50–60%. Within a week of patent expiration, generic captopril was available at just 20% of the original branded price. Similarly, the price of fluoxetine declined by 77% within nine months of that molecule's patent expiration. The price of generic simvastatin has also plummeted. For example, the reimbursement price of a 28-tablet pack of simvastatin 20 mg has declined from £16.00 ($29.30) in July 2004 to £2.26 ($4.14) in April 2005, a decrease of 86% in less than a year.

The UK government has promoted increased use of statins in recent years. From 1999 to 2004, the use of lipid-regulating drugs (overwhelmingly statins) increased by 250% in unit terms and 170% in sales terms. A total of 28.1 million statin prescriptions were dispensed in England in 2004, with atorvastatin and simvastatin dominating the market. In 2004, atorvastatin accounted for 39.9% of statin prescriptions and 48.7% of statin sales in England; simvastatin's market share was 45.2% in unit terms and 34% in sales terms. Support for extensive use of statins in the NHS received a further boost in November 2005, when NICE issued guidelines that recommended much wider use of statins in primary prevention of heart attacks and stroke. If fully implemented, this guidance would increase the number of patients in England who take statins from 2.3 million to 5.6 million, an increase of 143%. However, NICE presumes that only 50–75% of the 3.3 million additional patients who are now eligible for statin therapy will actually receive this treatment. If these patients receive prescriptions for generic simvastatin (NICE's recommendation), the additional cost to the NHS will total £55–82 million ($101–150 million) per year.

Parallel Trade

Germany is the second-largest parallel import market in Europe, surpassed in the total volume of parallel imports only by the United Kingdom. The importance of parallel imports in both these countries is attributable to two main factors: prescription drug prices that are typically much higher than in the other major European pharmaceutical markets, and government policy that pressures pharmacists to dispense parallel imports. Parallel traders generally buy medicines in low-priced European Union member states (e.g., France, Italy, Spain, Greece) for export to higher-priced markets (e.g., the United Kingdom, Germany, Denmark, and Sweden).

The extension of reference pricing to patent-protected medicines in Germany could alter parallel trade patterns, or conceivably even reverse the direction of trade in some cases. In other words, Germany could become a significant source of parallel exports, and the size of the German market (Europe's largest) would also make it easier for parallel traders to locate substantial stocks of medicines than in small markets such as Greece and Portugal.

In the statin market, atorvastatin would undoubtedly be the prime target for parallel export from Germany to other European markets if Pfizer cut the German price to reference price levels. Molecules that are already available generically in most markets (e.g., simvastatin) are generally not very attractive to parallel traders, given that it is difficult to undercut the prices of generics. At present, the retail price of atorvastatin is higher than in most other major European markets, and the drug's reference prices are comparable with retail prices elsewhere in Europe. However, if the drug's reference prices were cut substantially and Pfizer complied with those prices, substantial price differentials between Germany and other countries would probably emerge, creating a powerful incentive for parallel trade in atorvastatin. European governments that have hitherto ignored parallel importation might then be motivated to encourage this trade as a way of curbing their pharmaceutical expenditures. This threat is undoubtedly an important factor in Pfizer's continued refusal to cut the price of atorvastatin in Germany to reference pricing levels.

Conclusion

The consensus in the research-based pharmaceutical industry is that German reference pricing of statins has been bad news for manufacturers, but this cloud does have a silver lining of a sort. Forty-four percent of the GPs and internists who participated in our survey indicated that the introduction of reference pricing for statins has led them to prescribe drugs from this class more frequently than in 2004. The estimated mean increase in the number of prescriptions was 16% (median 13%, mode 20%). This finding suggests that lower prices may have encouraged physicians to make more extensive use of statins. Prescribing data from Insight Health confirm increased use of statins: the volume of prescriptions for this drug class grew by 13.7% in the first quarter of 2005. However, this trend is probably of limited comfort to manufacturers of branded statins, given that generics companies stand to gain most from increased statin prescribing.

The German government's ultimate objective is to include 70–80% of all medicines marketed in Germany in the reference-pricing system. Indeed, this cost-containment mechanism is the German government's main weapon in the war it has declared on "sham innovations" in the pharmaceutical market. This weapon is undeniably potent: it will likely succeed in its aim of eliminating "sham innovations," but the government may find that it also inflicts substantial collateral damage. Companies may decide not to launch new drugs in Germany unless these products offer an unequivocal therapeutic improvement over agents within an established drug class or have a completely new mechanism of action. AstraZeneca's decision to suspend the launch of Crestor may set an ominous precedent for the German pharmaceutical market. The government, and many physicians, may not be unduly disturbed by the loss of what they regard as a "me-too" drug in a very mature drug class, but if many companies follow suit, therapeutic choice could become much narrower in Germany than elsewhere in Europe.

Just as other European countries took their time – more than a decade in some cases – to study reference pricing in Germany before adopting and adapting the system, so these countries will closely observe the impact of reference pricing of statins and other major drug classes that include patent-protected medicines. If they judge this strategy to be an effective way to contain costs without harming the quality of care, they will likely embrace it themselves. The research-based pharmaceutical industry should therefore be on its guard.

GLOSSARY, IMPACT OF GERMAN REFERENCE PRICING ON STATINS

Glossary of Abbreviations and Foreign-Language Terms Used in This Report

Abbreviation/Foreign-language Term	*Translation*
AFCAPS/TexCAPs	Air Force Texas Coronary Atherosclerosis Prevention Study
Arzneimittelbudget-Ablösungsgesetz	Pharmaceutical Budget Replacement Act
Arzneimittelkommission der Deutschen Ärzteschaft	Pharmaceutical Commission of the German Medical Profession
Arzneimittelpreisverordnung	Pharmaceutical Price Ordinance
Arzneimittelvereinbarungen	Pharmaceutical Agreements
Bayerischer Apothekerverband	Bavarian Pharmacists' Association
Bundesverband der Betriebskrankenkassen (BKK)	Federal Association of Occupational Health Insurance Funds
Bundesverband der Pharmazeutischen Industrie (BPI)	Federal Association of the Pharmaceutical Industry
Bundesvereinigung Deutscher Apothekerverbände (ABDA)	Federal Union of German Pharmacists' Associations
Categorie terapeutiche omogenee	Homogeneous Therapeutic Categories [Italy]
CHD	Coronary Heart Disease
Comisión Interministerial de Precios de los Medicamentos (CIPM)	Interdepartmental Commission on Drug Pricing [Spain]
Comité de Suivi des Génériques	Generics Monitoring Committee [France]
Comité Economique des Produits de Santé (CEPS)	Economic Committee for Healthcare Products [France]
Federación Empresarial de Farmaceúticos Españoles (FEFE)	Business Federation of Spanish Pharmacists [Spain]
Festbetrag	Reference Price
Gemeinsamer Bundesausschuß der Ärzte, Zahnärzte, Krankenhäuser und Krankenkassen (GBA)	Joint Federal Committee of Physicians, Dentists, Hospitals and Health Insurance Funds
Gesetzentwurf zur Verbesserung der Wirtschaftlichkeit in der Arzneimittelversorgung (AVWG)	Improvement of Economy in the Pharmaceutical Supply Bill
Gesetzliche Krankenversicherung (GKV)	Statutory Health Insurance
Gesetz zur Modernisierung der Gesetzlichen Krankenversicherung (GMG)	Statutory Health Insurance Modernization Act
GP	General Practitioner
HDL	High-density Lipoprotein
Heilmittelwerbegesetz	Healthcare Products Promotion Act
Institut für Qualität und Wirtschaftlichkeit im Gesundheitswesen (IQWiG)	Institute for Quality and Economy in the Healthcare System
Kassenärztliche Bundesvereinigung (KBV)	Federal Union of Health Insurance Fund Physicians

Abbreviation/Foreign-language Term	*Translation*
Kassenärztliche Vereinigung Nordrhein	North Rhine Union of Health Insurance Fund Physicians
Krankenkasse(n)	Health Insurance Fund(s)
Länder	States
LDL	Low-density Lipoprotein
Les entreprises du médicament (Leem)	Pharmaceutical Companies [the French Pharmaceutical Industry Association]
Ley de Cohesión y Calidad del Sistema Nacional de Salud	Law on the Coherence and Quality of the National Healthcare System [Spain]
Ley de Garantías y Uso Racional de los Medicamentos y Productos Sanitarios	Law on the Security and Rational Use of Medicines and Medical Devices [Spain]
Naturalrabatte	Rebates in Kind
Orden de Precios de Referencia de Medicamentos	Pharmaceutical Reference Pricing Order [Spain]
Projet de Loi de Financement de la Sécurité Sociale (PLFSS) 2006	Social Security Finance Bill 2006
Projet de Loi Relatif à l'Assurance Maladie	Health Insurance Bill [France]
Prontuario Farmaceutico Nazionale (PFN)	National Formulary [Italy]
Richtgröße(n)	Indicative Prescribing Amount(s)
Sachverständigenrat zur Begutachtung der Entwicklung im Gesundheitswesen	Expert Counsel for the Assessment of Progress in the Healthcare System
Servizio Sanitario Nazionale (SSN)	National Health Service [Italy]
Sistema Nacional de Salud (SNS)	National Health System [Spain]
Sozialdemokratische Partei Deutschlands (SPD)	Social Democratic Party of Germany
Sozialgesetzbuch V	Social Code Book V
Spitzenverbände der Krankenkassen	Leading Associations of the Health Insurance Funds
Tarif forfaitaire de responsabilité	Reference Price [France]
TG	Triglyceride
Umstrittene Arzneimittel	Medicines of Disputed Value
Verband Forschender Arzneimittelhersteller (VFA)	German Association of Research-based Pharmaceutical Companies
Wissenschaftliches Institut der Allgemeinen Ortskrankenkassen (WidO)	Scientific Institute of the Local General Health Insurance Funds
WOSCOPS	West of Scotland Coronary Prevention Study

Unless otherwise indicated, terms in this list relate to Germany

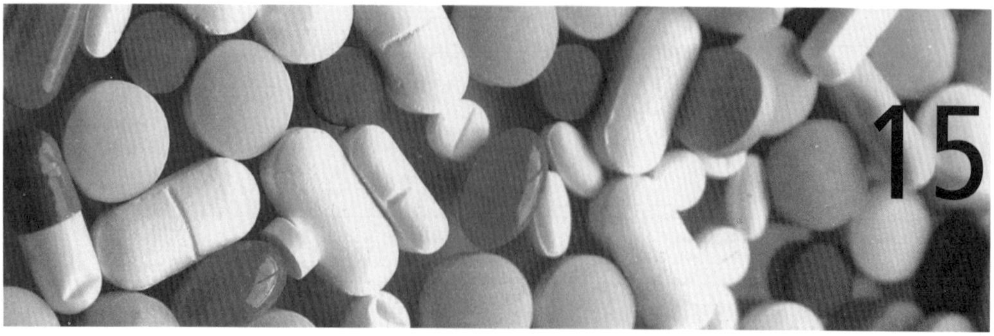

15

Opportunities and Challenges in the Japanese Market for Cancer Therapies

OVERVIEW

Since 1981, cancer has been the leading cause of death in Japan, and cancer mortality in that country has grown rapidly. Table 15.1 shows that the number of recorded deaths from cancers in Japan increased from 217,413 in 1990 to 320,358 in 2004, an increase of 47.3% in 14 years. In 2004, the death rate per 100,000 of population was 253.9, equivalent to 31.1% of the total number of deaths. According to the Ministry of Health, Labor, and Welfare (MHLW), cancers of the respiratory system (i.e., trachea, bronchus, lungs) were the most common causes of cancer-related mortality, followed by stomach and colorectal cancer.

The aging of the Japanese population is expected to contribute to a continued increase in cancer mortality. Table 15.2 shows that the number of people aged 65 and older increased from 10.7 million (9.1% of the total population) in 1980 to 24.9 million (19.5% of the total population) in 2004. By 2015, the elderly are projected to account for approximately 26% of the total Japanese population.

Given the increase in cancer incidence and mortality in the aging Japanese population, it is not surprising that the market for oncology drugs has grown vigorously – from $2.1 billion in 2000 to $3.6 billion in 2004. The market has the potential for further dynamic growth, but pharmaceutical companies face considerable challenges.

We begin this chapter by reviewing a recent government initiative to expedite access to international gold-standard cancer therapies in Japan and an additional measure to broaden the range of approved indications for oncology drugs. We then analyze the consequences of the shortage of chemotherapy specialists in Japan and recent steps to tackle this deficit. Further, we examine changes in the procedures for clinical development and drug approval, and consider economic issues in cancer treatment. We conclude with a brief assessment of the outlook and implications for the pharmaceutical industry.

UNAVAILABILITY OF GOLD-STANDARD THERAPIES

Lack of access to international gold-standard cancer therapies has long been one of the main deficiencies of the Japanese oncology system. Novel anticancer drugs generally

Table 15.1 Deaths From Cancer in Japan, 1990–2004

Year	*Deaths*	*Index (%)*[a]
1990	217,413	100.0
1991	223,727	102.9
1992	231,917	106.7
1993	235,707	108.4
1994	243,670	112.1
1995	263,022	121.0
1996	271,183	124.7
1997	275,413	126.7
1998	283,921	130.6
1999	290,556	133.6
2000	295,484	135.9
2001	300,658	138.3
2002	304,586	140.1
2003	309,543	142.4
2004	320,358	147.3

[a]Number of deaths each year expressed as a percentage of number of deaths in 1990

Table 15.2 Growth of the Elderly Population in Japan, 1980–2004

	Total Population (millions)	*Elderly Population (millions)*	*Elderly as a Share of Total Population (%)*
1980	117.1	10.7	9.1
1990	123.6	14.9	12.1
2000	126.9	22.0	17.3
2004	127.7	24.9	19.5

reach the market in Japan several years after their launch in other major pharmaceutical markets. The inadequate clinical development infrastructure of many pharmaceutical companies and a shortage of qualified reviewers have been major factors in the delayed launch of oncology drugs in Japan.

In an effort to accelerate the launch of important new drugs in Japan, in January 2005, the MHLW established an expert panel called the Mishoninyaku Shiyo Mondai Kentokaigi (Study Council on the Use of Unapproved Drugs). Drugs nominated for review by this council are assigned to one of three categories:

1. Drugs approved in one or more of four major Western markets (i.e., France, Germany, the United Kingdom, and the United States) after April 2005.
2. Drugs requested by academic societies and/or patient groups in the past five years and that are approved in any of the aforementioned Western markets.
3. Drugs whose approval has not been requested by academic societies and/or patient groups, but that have been approved in any of the aforementioned Western markets in the past two years and are regarded as highly useful.

Drugs that meet these criteria do not automatically qualify for review by the council: preference is given to medicines that are regarded as innovative and/or first-in-class in Japan. As of October 2005, oncology drugs accounted for the majority of unapproved drugs on the agenda (Table 15.3).

Council members evaluate the clinical need for and scientific evidence in support of each candidate drug, and the details of these discussions (including the outcomes) are published on the Internet. The manufacturers of drugs recommended by the council are then petitioned by the MHLW either to begin clinical trials on these compounds or to conduct supplementary trials that would allow wider access to these agents before they are formally approved. A provision known as *tsuikateki shiken* (additional trials) allows patients who are not enrolled in regular clinical trials to use an unapproved drug in specific circumstances. Another type of supplementary trial – *anzensei kakunin shiken* (safety confirmation trials) – may be added to postapproval Phase III study. (In Japan, oncology drugs are generally approved on the basis of evidence of tumor shrinkage from Phase II clinical trials, but manufacturers of these agents must submit plans for postapproval Phase III studies [see further on].) Additional trials and safety confirmation trials are conducted in the following circumstances:

- The diagnosed disease is life-threatening, irreversible, and seriously damages patients' quality of life.
- No alternative therapy is available in Japan.
- The drug's efficacy and side-effect profiles are proven to be clinically superior to existing therapies.
- The drug is used as standard therapy in the United States and the major European countries.

Table 15.3 Cancer Therapies Reviewed by the Study Council on the Use of Unapproved Drugs

Drug	*Status*	*Indication*	*Developer*
Oxaliplatin	Approved in March 2005	Colorectal cancer	Yakult
Thalidomide	Preclinical	Multiple myeloma	Fujimoto
Bortezomib	Phase II	Multiple myeloma	Janssen
Pemetrexed	Phase II/II	Non-small-cell lung cancer/mesothelioma	Eli Lilly
Bevacizumab	Phase II	Colorectal cancer	Chugai
Cetuximab	Phase II	Colorectal cancer	Bristol-Myers Squibb/Merck & Co.
Erlotinib	Phase II	Non-small-cell lung cancer	Chugai
Temozolomide	Preparation for application	Malignant glioma	Schering-Plough
Streptozocin	None	Pancreatic islet cell carcinoma	Not yet determined

Note: Status as of October 2005

Patients enrolled in these additional clinical trials can take advantage of a provision known as *tokutei-ryoyohi* (specified medical care coverage), whereby the public health insurance system covers all treatment costs except the cost of the product itself, which patients have to pay out of pocket. AstraZeneca took advantage of this provision when reimbursement terms were not settled in time for the launch of gefitinib (Iressa). Japanese physicians were eager to use the drug, and *tokutei-ryoyohi* enabled them to prescribe it without imposing an excessive financial burden on patients.

Not all medicines on the council's agenda are selected for clinical development with additional clinical trials. Drugs are prioritized according to their potential degree of novelty to the Japanese market. For example, the council recommended that the clinical development of the vascular endothelial growth factor inhibitor bevacizumab should be prioritized and an application submitted based on Phase I studies in Japan and foreign Phase II/III data. The council also called for safety confirmation trials to be conducted during the review period.

By comparison, the council did not recommend prioritizing the clinical development of the epidermal growth factor receptor inhibitor erlotinib, and additional trials will not be conducted until after approval is granted. This decision was based on erlotinib's second-to-market status (after getfinib) in Japan. Moreover, Phase I trial data suggest that erlotinib has no advantages over gefitinib in terms of the occurrence of adverse events (notably interstitial pneumonia).

Most pharmaceutical companies that receive a request from the MHLW to begin clinical trials with a view to the approval of a drug in Japan, or to conduct additional trials, comply with the request. In the event that a chosen drug does not already have a developer in Japan, the compound may be assigned to investigator-initiated trials (i.e., trials that are conducted under the auspices of medical researchers, rather than manufacturers). However, given that Japan's infrastructure for investigator-initiated trials remains underdeveloped, this option may not prove to be workable until the infrastructure for such trials improves significantly.

The creation of the new framework for drug approval is an attempt by the Japanese government to reconcile two opposing imperatives: patients' desire to have access to the international gold-standard therapies as soon as possible and the need to maintain the safeguards provided by Japan's existing clinical trial system. The new framework has the potential to reduce the current substantial delay between the launch of innovative cancer therapies in other major pharmaceutical markets and Japan. However, the impact of the new framework in practice will depend largely on how effectively individual pharmaceutical companies conduct clinical development and submit applications in Japan. Given that the deliberations of the Study Council on the Use of Unapproved Drugs are published, pharmaceutical companies are likely to face vocal criticism from interested parties (especially patient organizations) if they do not expedite the development of drugs recommended by the council. To avoid such pressure, drug manufacturers need to strengthen their drug development capabilities in Japan.

OFF-LABEL USE OF ONCOLOGY DRUGS

Because the public health insurance system reimburses medicines only if they are prescribed for approved indications, Japanese physicians tend to avoid off-label use of oncology drugs – including some treatment options that are accepted as standard practice in the United States and Europe. In fact, patients in Japan who receive off-label therapy or treatment with drugs that are not yet approved in Japan may forfeit their right to reimbursement for all treatments for the prescribed indication, not just for the off-label or unregistered therapy. This forfeiture can impose a heavy financial burden on patients.

Given these tough reimbursement restrictions, manufacturers of cancer therapies might be expected to pursue approval for additional indications for their drugs, but many companies appear content with the status quo. Although the public health insurance system forbids off-label reimbursement, individual institutions or payers may cover off-label prescribing to cancer patients on an ad hoc basis. Consequently, manufacturers have not been strongly motivated to spend time, energy, and money on pursuing additional indications for their oncology drugs.

To promote the approval of oncology drugs for broader indications, the MHLW established the Koganzai Heiyo Ryohoni Kansuru Kentokai (Committee for Combination Therapy with Anticancer Drugs) in December 2003. Considering suggestions from academic societies and/or patients' groups, a working group identifies drugs that could be used in additional indications and gathers evidence on the efficacy and safety of these drugs from the literature and other sources. The group then discusses the data with the relevant company. The Yakuji Shokuhin Eisei Shingikai (Council on Drugs and Food Sanitation [CDFS]) also evaluates the data that have been gathered; if it decides in favor of additional indications, the MHLW asks the manufacturer to submit an application for the new indications.

These applications receive priority review, which takes approximately four months. Approval, if granted, is conditional on postmarketing safety measures. Drugs approved by this procedure are eligible for reimbursement under the aforementioned specified medical care coverage provision that covers all medical costs except the cost of drug itself. This coverage is available from the time a candidate drug receives its preliminary evaluation from the CDFS.

Of 61 therapies that have been reviewed for use in additional indications, seven proposed therapies had already reached an advanced stage in the regular approval process and therefore completed that process, and 21 therapies in great demand have undergone the new procedure for approval of additional indications. Table 15.4 lists therapies approved for additional indications as of September 2005. The remaining therapies were not judged to be in great demand and therefore were not approved through this framework. After completing its evaluation of the 21 therapies in great demand, the committee was dissolved in February 2005.

The committee is generally considered to have fulfilled its role to improve the status of off-label use of anticancer drugs. Some officers of the MHLW have suggested that the framework for off-label use drugs could continue after the dissolution of the committee, but no official announcement on future policy for off-label use of oncology agents has been made. Based on the perceived

Table 15.4 Oncology Drugs Approved for Additional Indications in Japan

Drug	*Additional Indication*	*Date of Approval*
Doxorubicin/cyclophosphamide (AC)	Breast cancer	February 2005/September 2005
Pamidoronate	Breast cancer	November 2004
Ifosfamide	Soft tissue and bone sarcomas	February 2005
Doxorubicin	Soft tissue and bone sarcomas	February 2005
Doxorubicin	Solid tumors of childhood	February 2005
Etoposide	Solid tumors of childhood	February 2005
Cisplatin	Osteosarcoma	February 2005
Doxorubicin/cisplatin (AP)	Endometrial cancer	February 2005
Cisplatin	Malignant lymphoma	September 2005
Vincristine, doxorubicin, dexamethazone (VAD)	Multiple myeloma	February 2005
5-Fluorouracil infusion	Head and neck cancer	February 2005
Procarbazine	Malignant astrocytoma/oligodendroglioma	February 2005
Vincristine	Malignant astrocytoma/oligodendroglioma	February 2005
Infusional 5-FU/ l-LV	Colorectal cancer	February 2005
Cisplatin	Solid tumors of childhood	September 2005
Carboplatin	Solid tumors of childhood	September 2005
Actinomycin-D	Solid tumors of childhood	September 2005
Epirubicin/cyclophosphamide (EC, CEF)	Breast cancer	September 2005
Dexamethasone	Chemotherapy-induced nausea and vomiting	September 2005

success of the Committee for Combination Therapy With Anticancer Drugs, we believe that the MHLW could set up a similar ad hoc committee in the future to handle off-label issues as they arise.

LACK OF MEDICAL ONCOLOGISTS

A chronic shortage of chemotherapy specialists has constrained the development of the Japanese market for oncology drugs. Historically, surgeons have played the dominant role in the overall treatment of solid cancers in Japan – indeed, Japan probably has the highest frequency of surgical oncology in the world. Conversely, Japanese physicians have attached less importance to the contribution of chemotherapy in improving the survival rate of cancer patients. Internists' role in the management of cancer has generally been limited to the diagnosis of the disease. Few medical schools in Japan have incorporated medical or clinical oncology into their educational programs. The number of Japanese physicians who can conduct high-level chemotherapy is therefore very limited, and the majority of chemotherapy specialists are surgeons, internists, and hematologists. Most of these specialists are employed in university and cancer hospitals.

In Japan, oncology training for both surgeons and nonsurgical practitioners has traditionally focused on individual organs of the body, and clinical practice reflects this training. Unlike their counterparts in the United States, Japanese cancer specialists are not accustomed to treating patients with different cancer indications.

The standard of cancer therapy, especially chemotherapy, varies significantly from one region of the country to another, and even from one institution to another. Because some physicians (mainly surgeons) prescribe chemotherapeutic agents without a full understanding of these drugs, subtherapeutic dosing is relatively common. Physicians who have received only limited training in chemotherapy tend to favor the use of oral fluoropyrimidines (e.g., tegafur/uracil, doxifluridine, fluorouracil) rather than standard therapeutic regimens. Indeed, tegafur has become one of the best-selling oncology drugs in Japan, with sales of $490 million in 2004.

The lack of widespread experience in advanced chemotherapy may have contributed to a significant adverse event problem in Japan. As of April 2005, interstitial pneumonia and acute lung injury had been reported in 1,555 patients treated with gefitinib, of which 607 had died. An ethnic predisposition may have been a factor in the unusually high incidence and mortality of these adverse events, but thought leaders believe that Japan's lack of training in chemotherapy also contributed to this problem.

Initiatives to Raise Oncology Standards

The Japanese Society of Medical Oncology (JSMO), an organization composed mainly of chemotherapy specialists, has sought to raise the standard of chemotherapy in Japan. In 2002, the JSMO announced plans to establish a certification system for chemotherapy specialists, with a view to promoting multi-departmental management of cancers in Japan. The essential requirements for JSMO certification as a chemotherapy specialist are as follows:

- Membership in the JSMO for two years or longer.
- Five or more years of clinical experience in cancer treatment (with adequate achievements).
- Completion of more than two years of training based on a specified curriculum in an institution certified by the JSMO.

In July 2005, the JSMO announced plans to offer advanced training in cancer chemotherapy. The curriculum is based on the guidelines of the American Society of Clinical Oncology (ASCO) and the European Society for Medical Oncology (ESMO). Initially, 110 JSMO-certified medical institutions will participate in this program, but the number is expected to increase in the next few years. The JSMO has provisionally assigned 1,124 experienced physicians as *zantei shidoi* (instructor physicians). The first examination of chemotherapy specialists took place in November 2005, and the first specialists received their certification in April 2006. The JSMO expects to certify approximately 500 medical oncologists each year. Within 10 years, the JSMO hopes that Japan will have a total of 3,000–4,000 certified medical oncologists, which the society considers the minimum necessary to maintain an acceptable level of chemotherapy across the country.

In a move to further improve oncology practice in Japan, the JSMO, the Japanese Society of Clinical Oncology (an organization comprised mainly of surgical oncologists), and the Japan Cancer Association (a body that promotes basic cancer research) recently agreed to establish a collaborative certification system for overall cancer treatment. A joint committee will determine the curriculum and certification method, but details have not yet been published.

Furthermore, in August 2005, the MHLW unveiled plans to work with the Japanese Society of Hospital Pharmacists (JSHP) on developing a certified training program for oncology pharmacists. Initially, around 10 medical institutions, including the National Cancer Center Hospital, will be designated training institutions. The three-month course will include both lectures and practical training. The first students started their training in 2006. The MHLW expects to certify approximately 300 oncology pharmacists each year (1,500 in the first five years of the program).

These recent reforms should gradually improve the quality of cancer treatment in Japan in general and chemotherapy in particular. Disparities among regions and medical institutions are also likely to diminish gradually, but in the short-to-medium term, Japanese physicians will remain generally cautious in their use of chemotherapy. In the wake of the aforementioned gefitinib side-effect problem, the Japanese media have been quick to report news of major adverse events – a situation that has heightened physicians' inhibitions about practicing aggressive chemotherapy. Until large numbers of physicians and pharmacists trained in the new oncology programs are working in institutions across the country, the use of innovative cancer drugs in Japan is likely to remain somewhat limited.

CLINICAL DEVELOPMENT AND DRUG APPROVAL

As noted previously, approval of oncology drugs in Japan has generally been based on evidence of tumor shrinkage from Phase II clinical trials. Companies usually conduct several early Phase II studies and more than two independent late Phase II studies for approval. This system is similar to the accelerated approval system in the United States. Before a cancer drug is approved, the applicant is required to submit its plans for postapproval Phase III studies. Companies are required to conduct a minimum of one – and in most cases at least two – independent, randomized comparative Phase III studies in the postmarketing setting in Japan.

In November 2005, the MHLW announced plans to implement new guidelines for clinical evaluation of oncology drugs starting in April 2006. A key change is the added requirement that applications for therapies for common cancers (e.g., colorectal cancer, stomach cancer, breast cancer, non-small-cell lung cancer) include data from a Phase III study that uses survival rate and survival period as primary end points. Provided they comply with the revised guidelines, these Phase III trials may be conducted in Japan or overseas. Oncology drugs that are judged to be clearly innovative on the basis of solid clinical data may be approved prior to completion of a Phase III clinical trial (as is currently the case), an attempt on the part of the MHLW to discourage the commercialization of "me-too" drugs in Japan.

The impact of this new rule will depend on how innovation in the Japanese market is interpreted in practice. Drugs that would be the first in a new class in Japan and/or that are clearly superior to existing therapies will probably not be affected by this reform and will continue to be prioritized for approval before Phase III. On the other hand, manufacturers of oncology drugs that are not novel may have to invest more time and money in launching their products in Japan. The additional burden should be limited if companies have already completed Phase III trials overseas that meet the requirements of the new guidelines. As noted previously, most cancer therapies reach the Japanese market several years after they have been launched in the United States and Europe, so Phase III data will be readily available in many cases. Multinationals that plan to launch oncology drugs in Japan should consider the MHLW's new requirements when designing their clinical trials, to ensure that Phase III data can be extrapolated to the Japanese population.

ECONOMIC ISSUES

Newer oncology drugs have been launched in Japan at prices much higher than those of conventional cytotoxic drugs, whose prices have been eroded in the biennial price revisions that are a distinguishing feature of the Japanese pharmaceutical market. Table 15.5 shows the initial prices of the five molecular-targeted cancer therapies that are currently available in Japan. These drugs were all priced by a method known as *genka keisan hoshiki* (cost calculation), a procedure that is used if no comparable drug is available in Japan. Cost calculation adds sales and administrative costs, operating profit, production costs, distribution costs, and other costs to the cost of manufacturing or importing the raw material. Japan is one of the last major pharmaceutical markets to employ cost-plus methodology in drug pricing. This procedure actually gives companies greater flexibility than the MHLW's preferred pricing method, *ruiji*

Table 15.5 Initial Prices of Molecular-Targeted Oncology Drugs Marketed in Japan

Drug	*Indication*	*Dosage*	*Price (¥)*	*Price ($)*
Trastuzumab	Metastatic breast cancer	60 mg	31,674	292.80
		150 mg	80,879	747.67
Imatinib	Chronic myelogenous leukemia	100 mg	3,474.40	32.12
Gefitinib	Non-small-cell lung cancer	250 mg	7,216.10	66.71
Rituximab	Non-Hodgkin's lymphoma	100 mg	54,424	503.11
		500 mg	266,134	2,460.23
Gemtuzumab	Acute myelogenous leukemia	5 mg	241,154	2,229.31

yakko hikaku hoshiki (similar efficacy comparison), which benchmarks a new drug against an established therapy. The complex formula for cost calculation allows companies considerable flexibility, but the MHLW tends to scrutinize transfer prices very closely.

Because new cancer therapies are generally already available in other major pharmaceutical markets, the prices settled on by the MHLW are then modified under the "foreign price adjustment rule." Once a new drug's proposed price has been calculated, the MHLW determines the product's average public price in four reference markets – France, Germany, the United Kingdom, and the United States. If a drug's initial reimbursement price falls outside the range of 75–150% of the average foreign price, it is subject to the foreign-price adjustment rule. For example, if the drug's initial reimbursement price is 151% of the average foreign price or greater, its price is reduced. Conversely, if its initial reimbursement price is 74% of the average foreign price or less, its price is increased. If a drug is already marketed in the United States, an upward adjustment in its Japanese reimbursement price is not uncommon. The higher prices of new cancer therapies (compared with older agents) will boost the size of the Japanese market for oncology drugs in monetary terms.

The increasing cost of innovative cancer therapies will present the universal health insurance system with serious challenges. For example, in the case of colorectal cancer, oxaliplatin therapy costs the equivalent of ¥ 6,747 ($62.37) per day – substantially more than its comparator drug, irinotecan, which costs the equivalent of¥ 3,720 ($34.39) per day. Oxaliplatin is currently prescribed with 5-fluorouracil and leucovorin in the FOLFOX 4 regimen, a therapeutic option that is considered costly. The potential addition of monoclonal antibodies such as bevacizumab and cetuximab (both currently in Phase II in Japan) to the armamentarium could substantially increase the economic burden on the universal health insurance system.

In a bid to reduce spending on high-priced therapies, the government has begun to implement diagnosis procedure combinations (DPCs), a flat-sum reimbursement system for the acute care of inpatients. In fiscal year 2005, 144 Japanese hospitals have adopted the DPC system and 145 other hospitals have introduced it on a trial basis, with more expected to follow in the future. The MHLW has ruled that, from July 2005, some expensive therapies (e.g., rituximab for non-Hodgkin's lymphoma) must be excluded from the DPC system and reimbursed on a fee-for-service basis. This decision was prompted by a sizable gap between the treatment costs as calculated in the DPC and fee-for-service systems. Drugs that are more expensive than the DPC cost are funded by medical institutions, a situation that defeats the objective of the DPC system (i.e., cutting the costs of acute inpatient care). The MHLW suggests that such a situation is exceptional and transient, but it has not offered a clear solution to this problem. Therefore, it may be necessary to reserve expensive cancer therapies for the outpatient setting (where the DPC system is not used).

OUTLOOK AND IMPLICATIONS FOR THE PHARMACEUTICAL INDUSTRY

The research-based pharmaceutical industry can take encouragement from recent government actions to reduce the delay between the launch of new gold-standard therapies in other major pharmaceutical markets and their launch in Japan. In addition, the training of more medical oncologists and oncology pharmacists should improve the routine practice of chemotherapy in Japan. Demand for innovative oncology drugs will increase, and subtherapeutic dosing will become less common as physicians become more familiar with international standards of treatment. Inequalities in the standard of cancer care across Japan should gradually diminish. These trends will present commercial opportunities for manufacturers of oncology drugs.

On the other hand, pharmaceutical companies will also face some significant challenges. Innovation will become increasingly critical to the success of new cancer therapies in Japan. The government has clearly signaled its determination to favor oncology therapies that it considers to be novel; drugs that are not the first in a new class in Japan or that do not have demonstrable evidence of clinical superiority over existing treatments will face increased obstacles. For example, the new requirement for the submission of Phase III trial data for therapies for common cancers is likely to impact drugs that are not judged to be innovative, potentially increasing the time and money required to launch these medicines in Japan.

The growing influence of patient organizations in Japan has been a major factor in the recent changes in the government's position on unapproved drugs and off-label prescribing. Use of the Internet has heightened awareness of Japan's belated access to modern cancer therapies and intensified lobbying activity. For instance, in May 2005, more than 20 organizations representing cancer patients held a rally in Osaka. They called for the creation of a cancer information center to standardize access to therapies across the country and submitted a petition to the minister of health. In August 2005, the MHLW responded by including the establishment of a consultation/support center and an anticancer information center in the Anti-Cancer Measures Promotion Action Plan. This response from the government will encourage further lobbying by patient organizations in the future.

The aging of the population and the steady rise in the incidence of many cancers will pose increasing challenges for the Japanese healthcare system in the next decade and beyond. State-of-the-art chemotherapy will offer an increasing array of treatment options, but the costs will be substantial. Healthcare reforms in Japan tend to occur in small steps, but the government may have to face the need for radical change to ensure that the universal public health insurance system does not collapse under the steadily growing burden of demand for treatment of a range of costly diseases, including cancers.

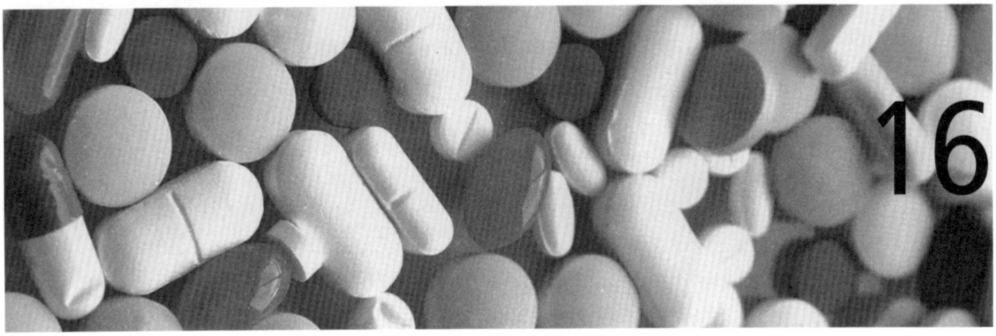

16

Cancer Therapies Face Increasing Reimbursement Pressures in Europe and Japan

INTRODUCTION

According to a recent report published by the Karolinska Institutet in Stockholm, Sweden, approximately 3 million residents of the 25 member states of the European Union (EU) were diagnosed with cancer in 2004. In that same year, approximately 1.7 million EU residents died from this disease. Since 1981, cancer has been the leading cause of death in Japan, and cancer mortality in that country has grown rapidly – from 217,413 recorded deaths in 1990 to 320,358 in 2004.

These figures graphically demonstrate the dreadful social cost of cancer. The economic burden imposed by this disease – in terms of both the direct costs of treatment and the indirect costs of disability, lost income and taxation, and premature death – is also terrible. Innovative cancer therapies can play an important role in mitigating the impact of cancer, but these drugs are often expensive. Consequently, government agencies have the unenviable task of determining how best to stretch finite resources to cover these treatments.

In this chapter, we provide a detailed overview of the current reimbursement environment for cancer therapies in the five largest European markets (France, Germany, Italy, Spain, and the United Kingdom) and Japan. In addition, we assess the outlook and implications for the pharmaceutical industry in terms of the coverage of oncology drugs.

FRANCE

Both the public and private sectors play an important role in cancer care in France, and patients frequently move between the two sectors during the course of their treatment. For example, patients may undergo surgery in a public hospital but then receive chemotherapy in a private clinic. Figure 16.1 shows the distribution of cancer chemotherapy by type of institution in 2002. Overall, 45% of patients received chemotherapy in general, teaching, or regional hospitals, 36.3% in private for-profit clinics, and 14.2% in *centres de lutte contre le cancer* (CLCC; cancer centers). More recently, a small but increasing number of patients have received chemotherapy in their own homes (see further on).

Pharmaceutical Pricing and Reimbursement

Most cancer therapies on the market in France are classified as *médicaments à*

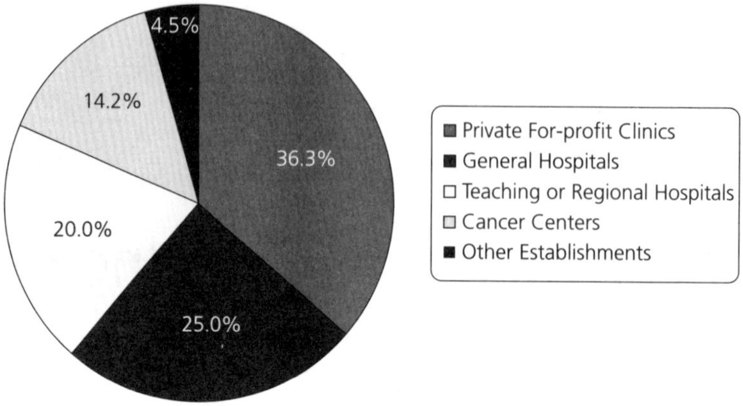

Figure 16.1 Distribution of Cancer Chemotherapy in France by Type of Institution, 2002

prescription restreinte (drugs subject to prescribing restrictions). Whereas prescription medicines dispensed by retail pharmacies undergo protracted pricing and reimbursement procedures, drugs dispensed in hospitals have traditionally been priced freely. Manufacturers that wish to market a hospital-only medicine must apply to the *Commission de la Transparence* (CT; Transparency Commission) for inclusion in the *liste des médicaments agréés aux collectivités et divers services publics* (list of authorized drugs for institutions and miscellaneous public services).

The CT judges each new therapy by two distinct measures: its *service médical rendu* (SMR; medical benefit) and its *amélioration du service médical rendu* (ASMR; improvement in medical benefit). Based on its degree of clinical utility, a drug is given an SMR rating of major, important, moderate, weak, or insufficient. The ASMR rating compares a drug's therapeutic benefit with that of competing therapies. A new drug's degree of improvement is measured on a six-point scale, from I (major improvement) to VI (unfavorable opinion). The ASMR is a major influence on a new drug's price in community pharmacies, but is less significant in the hospital sector. In the community, a rating of I or II offers the potential of price premiums and concessions on sales volume restrictions. Conversely, a rating of V necessitates lower prices and a rating of VI precludes reimbursement. Very few drugs qualify for an ASMR rating of I or II; a score of V is common. Cancer therapies have generally fared well in CT evaluations: most have received an SMR rating of "important" and an ASMR score of I or II. However, a few agents (e.g., AstraZeneca's Arimidex [anastrozole], Schering-Plough's Caelyx and Elan's Myocet [doxorubicin]) have received ASMR scores as low as V. Table 16.1 summarizes the CT's evaluation of a selection of innovative cancer therapies.

In March 2004, *Les Entreprises du Médicament* (Leem; Pharmaceutical Companies), the association that represents the French pharmaceutical industry, signed a framework agreement with the government for a new pricing procedure for the hospital pharmacy market. Under the terms of this agreement, a manufacturer notifies the *Comité Economique des Produits de Santé* (CEPS; Economic Committee for Healthcare Products), the organization responsible for setting reimbursement prices in France, of the price it plans to charge for a medicine. The company then has to provide the CEPS with documentation to justify its proposed price, including the product's price and

Table 16.1 Evaluation of Select Cancer Therapies by France's Transparency Commission

Drug	*Date of Appraisal*	*Indication*	*SMR*	*ASMR*	*Target Population*
Arimidex (anastrozole)	January 2001	Advanced hormone-dependent breast cancer in postmenopausal women	Important	V	10,900–12,200
	May 2004	Adjuvant treatment of hormone-receptor-positive breast cancer in postmenopausal women	Important	III	24,000–27,000
Avastin (bevacizumab)	June 2005	Metastatic colorectal cancer	Important	II	18,000
Caelyx (doxorubicin)	March 2001	Advanced ovarian cancer	Moderate	V	—
	December 2003	Monotherapy of metastatic breast cancer	Important	III	4,000–6,000
Eloxatin (oxaliplatin)	November 2005	Adjuvant treatment of stage III colon cancer (Dukes' C)	Important	III	7,500–10,000
Erbitux (cetuximab)	March 2005	Metastatic colorectal cancer	Important	V	8,600
Gemzar (gemcitabine)	November 2004	Recurrent metastatic breast cancer	Important	V	6,000
Glivec (imatinib)	June 2002	Chronic myeloid leukemia Ph+	Important	I	390–465 adults; 11–18 children
	December 2002	Gastrointestinal stromal tumors	Important	I	300–360
Herceptin (trastuzumab)	March 2001	Metastatic HER2-positive breast cancer	Important	—	—
	July 2005	In combination with docetaxel, treatment of metastatic HER2-positive breast cancer	Important	II	6,000
MabCampath (alemtuzumab)	January 2002	Treatment-resistant chronic lymphoid leukemia	Important	—	300–500
MabThera (rituximab)	October 2003	In combination with CHOP, treatment of aggressive diffuse large B-cell non-Hodgkin's lymphoma	Important	I	3,300
	June 2005	In combination with CVP, treatment of previously untreated stage III–IV follicular lymphoma	Important	II	2,600
Myocet (doxorubicin)	September 2001	Metastatic breast cancer	Important	V[a] III[b]	—
Navelbine (vinorelbine)	May 2001	Non-small-cell lung cancer	Important	II	—
	December 2005	Metastatic breast cancer	Important	V	15,300
Tarceva (erlotinib)	March 2006	Locally advanced or metastatic non-small-cell lung cancer	Important	IV[c] V[d]	9,800–10,500
UFT (tegafur uracil)	July 2001	Metastatic colorectal cancer	Important	II	—
Xeloda (capecitabine)	February 2003	Treatment-resistant metastatic or locally advanced breast cancer	Important	II	22,300
	March 2005	Metastatic colorectal cancer	Important	II	15,000
	April 2006	Adjuvant treatment of stage III colon cancer (Dukes' C)	Important	V	—

[a]Relative to epirubicin
[b]Relative to other doxorubicin products
[c]Third-line therapy
[d]Second-line therapy

reimbursement status in other major European markets. If the product has been marketed elsewhere in the EU for more than a year, the company is also required to provide details of its annual sales in each market. In addition, the dossier must include the CT's assessment of the product (if completed), a three-year sales forecast, and a commitment to notify the CEPS of the product's price, sales volume, and any price changes in the major European markets. If the CEPS accepts the proposed price, it publishes the information immediately. If the CEPS disagrees with the price, it has 15 days to reject it. The CEPS is entitled to reject a proposed price for several reasons – for example, if the price is higher than that of the same product or similar products in other European countries or if the price would likely lead to exceptionally high spending in France. Following a rejection of its proposed price, the manufacturer has 15 days to propose a new price. The CEPS's second decision is final. The list price is a ceiling price, and hospitals generally expect manufacturers and wholesalers to offer them substantial discounts.

Prospective Payment

France has historically operated a bimodal system of hospital funding. Public hospitals and private hospitals working in the public sector receive a *dotation globale* (global budget) that is divided among various areas of expenditure, whereas private hospitals receive *per diem* or activity-based payment. However, as part of its *Plan Hôpital 2007* (Hospital Plan, 2007) reform program, the French government wants all hospitals engaged in medicine, surgery, or obstetrics to adopt a system known as *tarification à l'activité* (T2A; activity-based pricing). This new approach to hospital funding in France is based on *groupes homogènes de séjour* (GHSs; uniform hospitalization groups), a system similar to the diagnosis-related groups (DRGs) used in many other countries. (Governments in many countries have begun to move from cost-based reimbursement for services rendered to prospective payment systems that pay providers a predetermined amount according to specific definitions. Prospective payment systems are typically based on DRGs, a system that groups patients on the basis of factors such as their primary or secondary diagnosis, complications and comorbidities, procedures, age, and sex.) The French government expects to realize the following key benefits from the T2A system:

- Greater role for clinical factors in funding.
- More responsible behavior by leading stakeholders and an incentive for them to change.
- Greater equality of treatment between the (public and private) sectors.
- The development of health economic steering mechanisms (management controls) at the heart of public and private hospitals.

The timetable for the T2A program calls for a steady migration from cost-based reimbursement to activity-based funding. Figure 16.2 shows the government's targets for the percentage of total spending in public hospitals and private hospitals working in the public sector that will be derived from activity-based funding in select years from 2004 to 2010, the year when the transition is scheduled for completion.

As a general rule, medicines are included in the GHSs. However, the French government recognizes that certain drugs and other technologies (notably medical devices) are too expensive to fit within the GHSs; therefore, these products will be funded separately. The Ministry of Health and the *Agence Technique de l'Information sur l'Hospitalisation* (ATIH; Technical Agency for Information on Hospitalization) have compiled a list of approximately 80 products that qualify for supplementary reimbursement. About half of these products are oncology-related medicines (Table 16.2). The Ministry of Health will update the list annually.

To control spending on drugs that qualify for supplementary reimbursement, ceiling prices will be determined either through negotiations between the manufacturers and the CEPS or through a decree from the ministers of health and social security. Manufacturers will also be subject to price/volume constraints, whereby they will have to reduce their prices if sales volume is judged to have grown excessively.

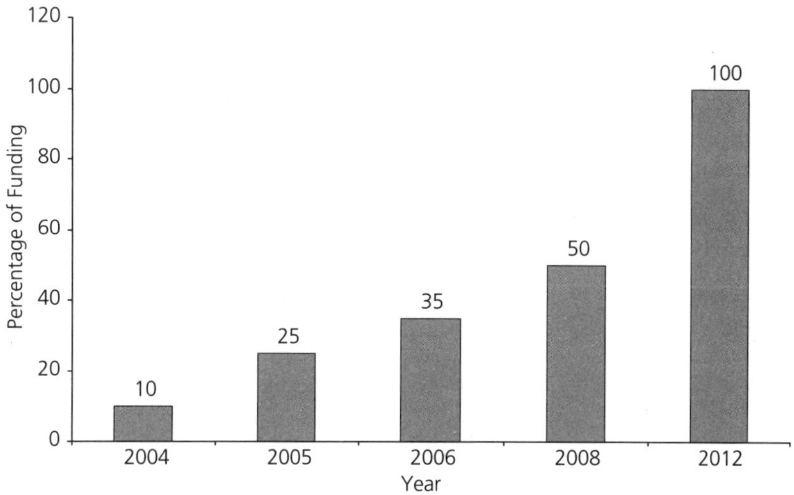

Figure 16.2 Activity-Based Funding in France: Projected Share of Total Budget for Public Hospitals and Private Hospitals Working in the Public Sector in Select Years, 2004–12

High-priced new drugs can be added to this list as soon as they receive marketing authorization in France. After 12 months on the market, a drug will either be approved to remain on this list, in which case it will become subject to a ceiling price, or it will be removed from the supplementary reimbursement list and covered by the relevant GHS tariff.

Hospitals will be reimbursed for medicines on the supplementary reimbursement list at the level of a drug's ceiling price. To encourage hospital pharmacies to negotiate manufacturer discounts on these medicines, hospitals will be permitted to keep a proportion of any price difference they secure between the ceiling price and their actual purchase price.

Hospitals will also be required to sign a contract for the good use of medicines. This contract permits prescribing only if it satisfies one of the following conditions:

- A drug's licensed indications.
- Therapeutic protocols jointly defined by the *Institut National du Cancer* (INCa;National Cancer Institute), the *Agence Française de Sécurité Sanitaire des Produits de Santé* (AFSSAPS; French Agency for the Safety of Healthcare Products), and the Haute Autorité de la Santé (HAS; National Health Authority). The first such *protocole temporaire de traitement* (PTT; temporary treatment protocol) – for the adjuvant use of Roche's Herceptin (trastuzumab) in breast cancer – was issued in October 2005.
- Uses supported by international literature or the work of academic societies.

Institutions that fail to sign this contract will have their reimbursement rate for drugs on the supplementary reimbursement list reduced to just 70%, leaving them out-of-pocket. Similarly, if a hospital fails to comply with the terms of its contract for the good use of medicines, the local *agence régionale d'hospitalisation* (ARH; regional hospitalization agency) can call on the health insurance funds to cut the reimbursement rate to 70%.

Pharmacy Decision Making

Most hospitals in France operate strict formularies and use formulary inclusion as a bargaining token with manufacturers. Since January 2002, all hospitals are legally required to operate a *commission du médicament et des dispositifs médicaux stériles* (COMEDIMS; pharmaceutical and sterile medical devices commission). COMEDIMS' responsibilities include

Table 16.2 Oncology Drugs Eligible for Supplementary Reimbursement in France, 2006

Drug Class/International Nonproprietary Name	*Brand Name*	*Manufacturer*
Antineoplastic drugs		
Aldesleukin	Proleukin	Chiron
Alemtuzumab	Mabcampath	Schering AG
Arsenic trioxide	Trisenox	Cell Therapeutics
Bevacizumab	Avastin	Roche
Bortezomib	Velcade	Janssen-Cilag
Busulfan	Busilvex	Pierre Fabre
Carmustine	Bicnu	Bristol-Myers Squibb
Cetuximab	Erbitux	Merck Lipha Santé
Cladribine	Leustatin	Janssen-Cilag
Cytarabine	Depocyte	Mundipharma
Daunorubicin	Daunoxome	Gilead Sciences
Docetaxel	Taxotère	Sanofi-Aventis
Doxorubicin	Caelyx, Myocet	Schering-Plough, Elan Pharma
Epirubicin	Farmorubicin	Pharmacia (Pfizer)
Fludarabine	Fludara	Schering AG
Fotemustine	Muphoran	Servier
Fulvestrant	Faslodex	AstraZeneca
Gemcitabine	Gemzar	Lilly France
Ibritumomab-tiuxetan	Zevalin	Schering AG
Idarubicin	Zavedos	Pfizer
Irinotecan	Campto	Sanofi-Aventis
Oxaliplatin	Eloxatin	Sanofi-Aventis
Paclitaxel	Taxol	Bristol-Myers Squibb
Pemetrexed	Alimta	Lilly France
Pentostatin	Nipent	Wyeth-Lederle
Pirarubicin	Theprubicine	Sanofi-Aventis
Raltitrexed	Tomudex	AstraZeneca
Rituximab	MabThera	Roche
Tasonermine	Beromun	Boehringer Ingelheim
Topotecan	Hycamtin	GlaxoSmithkline
Trastuzumab	Herceptin	Roche
Vinorelbine	Navelbine	Pierre Fabre
Other oncology-related drugs		
153Sm-samarium-acid	Quadramet	Cis Bio International
89Sr-strontium chlorure	Metastron	Amersham Health
Amifostine	Ethyol	Schering-Plough
Darbepoetin alfa	Aranesp	Amgen
Dexrazoxane	Cardioxane	Chiron France
Erythropoietin alfa	Eprex	Janssen-Cilag
Erythropoietin beta	Neorecormon	Roche
Iodine-131 lipiodil	Lipiocis	Cis Bio International
Rasburicase	Fasturtec	Sanofi-Aventis
Sodium porfimer	Photofrin	Isotec
Thyrotrophine	Thyrogen	Genzyme
Yttrium chloride	Ytracis	Cis Bio International

the following tasks:

- Choosing economic medicines and evaluating, monitoring, and analyzing their use.
- Tracking technological and therapeutic developments to anticipate innovations.
- Tracking regulatory developments.

Le Médicament à l'Hôpital (Pharmaceuticals in Hospitals), a government-commissioned study published in May 2003, found that COMEDIMS often did little more than develop formularies. Shortages in the number of physicians and pressure on them to participate in many other hospital commissions and committees reduced physicians' influence in COMEDIMS and weakened the decision-making process. In addition, the fact that COMEDIMS typically included only one specialist in a given field limited the impact of the specialist's expert opinion. Not surprisingly, the authors found that COMEDIMS were most active in larger hospitals – *centres hospitaliers universitaires* (teaching hospitals) and *centres hospitaliers* (hospital centers). Many of these institutions had developed strong pharmacoeconomic programs that focused particularly on costly new drugs.

Among several examples of particularly active COMEDIMS, *Le Médicament à l'Hôpital* reported that the CLCCs had established a federal observatory of innovation to anticipate the launch of expensive new therapies in order to measure the potential impact of these treatments on budgetary and strategic plans. The observatory also aims to propose a coordinated preliminary policy for the centers within the CLCC network. A committee of expert oncologists defined pharmacoeconomic recommendations that influenced the group's pharmacists in their purchasing decisions.

Hospital Prescribing to Outpatients

The French government has become increasingly concerned by the growth of a prescribing practice known as *rétrocession hospitalière* (hospital sale to the public), whereby hospital pharmacies dispense drugs that are reserved for hospital use to outpatients. In 2005, this practice cost the French social security system more than €1.1 billion ($1.4 billion), equivalent to 6.6% of total pharmaceutical expenditures. (The US dollar-to-euro exchange rate used in this chapter is the 2005 average rate [i.e., $1 = €0.80453].)

To reduce the cost of hospital prescribing to outpatients, in June 2004, the government issued a decree that revised the rules governing the prescribing of restricted medicines. This decree increased the number of categories of restricted medicines from three to five:

A. *Médicaments réservés à l'usage hospitalier* (RH; hospital-only medicines). These drugs may be prescribed only by a hospital-based physician and dispensed only by a hospital pharmacy for patients receiving hospital treatment.
B. *Médicaments à prescription hospitalière* (PH; hospital-prescribed medicines). These drugs may be prescribed only by a hospital-based physician but may be dispensed by either a hospital pharmacy or a retail pharmacy.
C. *Médicaments à prescription initiale hospitalière* (PIH; hospital-initiated medicines). The initial prescription for these drugs must be written by a hospital-based physician, but primary care physicians may renew the prescription.
D. *Médicaments à prescription réservée à certains médecins spécialistes* (PRS; medicines that may be prescribed only by certain specialists). The initial prescription for these drugs must always be written by a specialist, but some medicines in this category may subsequently be prescribed by nonspecialists.
E. *Médicaments nécessitant une surveillance particulière pendant le traitement* (SP; medicines that require special monitoring during treatment). Patients must comply with periodic monitoring requirements as specified in a drug's marketing authorization.

Categories B and D are new. Category D drugs may also belong to category E and/or to one of categories A, B, or C. Category E drugs may also belong to category D and/or to one of categories A, B, or C. Table 16.3 shows the classification of oncology drugs.

Hospital-only medicines (category A above) are now excluded from *rétrocession hospitalière* (i.e., hospital pharmacies may no longer dispense these drugs to outpatients). Outpatients who require drugs that belong to one of the other restricted categories listed above may no longer obtain their medications from a hospital pharmacy but have to visit a community pharmacy.

Cost Sharing

The French social security system covers the full cost of drugs that are dispensed in public hospitals; funding comes from hospitals' global budgets. If they are prescribed medicines in the community, French cancer

Table 16.3 Prescribing Restrictions on Oncology Drugs in France

INN	*Brand Name*	*ATC Code*	*Marketing Company*	*Prescribable Only by Specialists (Category D)*	*Special Monitoring Required (Category E)*	*May Be Sold to the Public with a Prescription*
Hospital-only medicines (Category A)						
Aldesleukin	Proleukin	L03AC 01	Chiron France	√	√	
Antilymphocyte immunoglobulin (equine)	Globulines Antilympho-cytaires Fresenius	L04AA 03	Fresenius Hemocare Immune Therapy			
Arsenic trioxide	Trisenox	L01XX 27	Cell Therapeutics	√	√	
Azathioprine	Imurel	L04AX 01	GlaxoSmith Kline			
Basiliximab	Simulect	L04AA 09	Novartis Europharm			
Busulfan	Busilvex	L01AB 01	Pierre Fabre	√	√	
Carmustine	Gliadel	L01AD 01	Guilford Pharmaceuticals	√	√	
Cytarabine	Aracytine	L01BC 01	Pfizer	√	√	
Cytarabine	Cytarbel	L01BC 01	Aventis	√	√	
Cytarabine	Depocyte	L01BC 01	Skyepharma	√	√	
Daclizumab	Zenapax	L04AA 08	Roche			
Infliximab	Remicade	L04AA 12	Centocor	√		
Methotrexate	Multisource	L01BA 01	Wyeth Lederle	√	√	
Mitoxantrone	Elsep	L01DB 07	Wyeth Lederle	√	√	
Muromonab-cd3	Orthoclone	L04AA 02	Janssen-Cilag			
Mycophenolic acid	Cellcept	L04AA 06	Roche			
Pemetrexed	Alimta	L01BA 04	Lilly France	√	√	
Plicamycin	Mithracine	L01DC 02	Pfizer	√	√	
Porfimer sodium	Photofrin	L01XD 01	Axcan Pharma International	√	√	
Tacrolimus	Prograf	L04AA 05	Fujisawa			
Tasonermine	Beromun	L03AX 11	Boehringer Ingelheim	√	√	
Temoporfine	Foscan	L01XX	Biolitec Pharma	√	√	
Hospital-prescribed medicines (Category B)						
Aldesleukin	Proleukin	L03AC 01	Chiron France	√	√	√
Alemtuzumab	Mabcampath	L01XC 04	Ilex Pharmaceuticals	√	√	√

Table 16.3 Continued

INN	*Brand Name*	*ATC Code*	*Marketing Company*	*Prescribable Only by Specialists (Category D)*	*Special Monitoring Required (Category E)*	*May Be Sold to the Public with a Prescription*
Amifostine	Ethyol	V03AF 05	Medimmune Oncology	√	√	√
Amsacrine	Amsalyo	L01XX 01	OTL Pharma	√	√	√
Amsacrine	Amsidine	L01XX 01	OTL Pharma	√	√	
Bexarotene	Targretin	L01XX 25	Ligand Pharmaceuticals	√	√	
Busulfan	Myleran	L01AB 01	GlaxoSmith-Kline	√	√	
Capecitabine	Xeloda	L01BC 06	Roche	√	√	
Carboplatin	Multisource	L01XA 02	Aguettant	√	√	√
Carboplatin	Paraplatine	L01XA 02	Bristol-Myers Squibb	√	√	
Carmustine	Bicnu	L01AD 01	Bristol-Myers Squibb	√	√	√
Cisplatin	Multisource	L01XA 01	Baxter	√	√	√
Cladribine	Cladribine Janssen-Cilag	L01BB 04	Janssen-Cilag	√	√	√
Cladribine	Leustatine	L01BB 04	Janssen-Cilag	√	√	
Cyclophosphamide	Endoxan	L01AA 01	Baxter	√	√	√
Dacarbazine	Dacarbazine Faulding	L01AX 04	Faulding Pharmaceuticals	√	√	
Dacarbazine	Deticene	L01AX 04	Aventis	√	√	√
Dactinomycin	Cosmegen	L01DA 01	Merck Sharp & Dohme Chibret	√	√	√
Daunorubicin	Cerubidine	L01DB 02	Aventis	√	√	
Daunorubicin	Daunoxome	L01DB 02	Gilead Sciences	√	√	√
Dexrazoxane	Cardioxane	V03AF 02	Chiron	√	√	√
Docetaxel	Taxotere	L01CD 02	Aventis Pharma	√	√	√
Doxorubicin	Caelyx	L01DB 01	Schering-Plough	√	√	
Doxorubicin	Multisource	L01DB 01	Pierre Fabre	√	√	√
Doxorubicin	Myocet	L01DB 01	Elan Pharma International	√	√	
Epirubicin	Farmorubicine	L01DB 03	Pfizer	√	√	√

(continued)

Table 16.3 Continued

INN	*Brand Name*	*ATC Code*	*Marketing Company*	*Prescribable Only by Specialists (Category D)*	*Special Monitoring Required (Category E)*	*May Be Sold to the Public with a Prescription*
Etoposide	Celltop	L01CB 01	Baxter	√	√	
Etoposide	Multisource	L01CB 01	Pharmache-mie Bv	√	√	√
Etoposide	Vepeside	L01CB 01	Pharminvest Patrimonial	√	√	
Fludarabine	Fludara	L01BB 05	Schering AG	√	√	√
Fluorouracil	Multisource	L01BC 02	Dakota Pharm	√	√	√
Gemcitabine	Gemzar	L01BC 05	Lilly	√	√	√
Idarubicin	Zavedos	L01DB 06	Pfizer	√	√	√
Ifosfamide	Holoxan	L01AA 06	Baxter	√	√	√
Irinotecan	Campto	L01XX 19	Pfizer	√	√	
Mesna	Uromitexan	V03AF 01	Baxter	√	√	√
Mitotane	Lysodren	L01XX 03	HRA Pharma	√		
Mitoxantrone	Novantrone	L01DB 07	Wyeth Lederle	√	√	
Mitoxantrone	Onkotrone	L01DB 07	Baxter	√	√	√
Oxaliplatin	Dacplat	L01XA 03	Debioclinic	√	√	
Oxaliplatin	Eloxatine	L01XA 03	Sanofi-Aventis	√	√	√
Paclitaxel	Paclitaxel Bristol-Myers Squibb	L01CD 01	Bristol-Myers Squibb	√	√	
Paclitaxel	Paxene	L01CD 01	Norton Healthcare	√	√	
Paclitaxel	Taxol	L01CD 01	Bristol-Myers Squibb	√	√	√
Pentostatin	Nipent	L01XX 08	Pfizer	√	√	
Raltitrexed	Tomudex	L01BA 03	AstraZeneca	√	√	√
Rasburicase	Fasturtec	V03AF 07	Sanofi-Aventis	√	√	√
Rituximab	MabThera	L01XC 02	Roche	√	√	√
Sargramostim	Sargramo-stim Lederle	L03AA 09	Wyeth Lederle	√	√	
Streptozosin	Zanosar	L01AD 04	Pfizer	√	√	
Tegafur in combination	UFT	L01BC 53	Merck Santé	√	√	

Table 16.3 Continued

INN	*Brand Name*	*ATC Code*	*Marketing Company*	*Prescribable Only by Specialists (Category D)*	*Special Monitoring Required (Category E)*	*May Be Sold to the Public with a Prescription*
Temozolomide	Temodal	L01AX 03	Schering-Plough	√	√	
Thiotepa	Thiotepa Genopharm	L01AC 01	Pharminvest Patrimonial	√	√	
Tioguanine	Lanvis	L01BB 03	GlaxoSmith Kline	√	√	
Topotecan	Hycamtin	L01XX 17	GlaxoSmith Kline	√	√	√
Trastuzumab	Herceptin	L01XC 03	Roche	√	√	√
Tretinoin	Vesanoid	L01XX 14	Roche	√	√	
Vindesine	Eldisine	L01CA 03	EG Labo-Laboratoires Eurogenerics	√	√	√
Vinorelbine	Navelbine	L01CA 04	Pierre Fabre	√	√	√
Hospital-initiated medicines (Category C)						
Miltefosine	Miltex	L01XX 09	Baxter	√	√	

patients do not have to worry about out-of-pocket payments for essential drugs. Because they treat life-threatening diseases, oncology drugs are generally fully reimbursed. Moreover, patients diagnosed with cancer, or any of 29 other *affections de longue durée* (ALD; chronic disorders), are exempt from copayments for drugs dispensed in the community. At the end of 2004, approximately 6.6 million members of the healthcare system's *régime général* (general program) had a chronic disorder. The number of patients diagnosed with a cancer-related ALD totaled 1.3 million, an increase of 84% from 1994.

In April 2006, the *Caisse Nationale de l'Assurance Maladie* (CNAM; National Health Insurance Fund) published new data on the management of ALDs. Drugs used specifically to treat any ALD itself are fully reimbursed, but all other drugs prescribed to patients registered as having a chronic disorder should be written in a separate section of the prescription form for reimbursement at the standard rate for each drug (i.e., 35%, 65%, or 100%). However, many physicians continue to prescribe all drugs to ALD patients at the 100% reimbursement rate.

In an attempt to improve the management of chronic disorders in France, the HAS plans to publish physician guides for each ALD. The first two such guides, covering diabetes (type 1 and 2) and hepatitis C, were published on May 31, 2006. The HAS hopes to publish guides for the remaining ALD indications by the end of 2007. These guides are intended to standardize the products and procedures that are included in the *protocoles de soins* (treatment protocols) that are now required for each ALD patient.

Off-label Prescribing

Physicians are permitted to prescribe off-label in France but must overcome some substantial hurdles. Clinicians must assume responsibility for the medical consequences of prescribing a drug for an unlicensed indication and could face criminal charges in the event that such a decision is judged to have harmed a patient. Prescribers must also inform the patient of the risks of using the proposed drug. Outpatient prescriptions for off-label indications are generally not reimbursed by the French social security system – a significant deterrent to this practice. Consequently, physicians must also notify their patients that they (the patients) would have to pay the full cost of medications prescribed off-label. The letters "NR," for *nonremboursable* (not reimbursable), must be written on all off-label prescriptions.

National Cancer Plan

In March 2003, the French government unveiled the *Plan Cancer*, a radical new program for the management of cancer in France. The plan proposed 70 measures – including the creation of the *Institut National du Cancer* (INCa; National Cancer Institute) – to raise standards of cancer care across the country. These measures have been supported by increased funding, beginning with an additional investment of €100 million ($124 million) in 2003 and projected to reach a cumulative total of €640 million ($795 million) by 2007. The plan envisages that 32% of the increased funding (i.e., €205 million [$255 million] by 2007) is allocated to improving access to innovative treatments. In the cancer plan, the government identified a need to harmonize the funding of costly and innovative drugs as well as devices in the public and private sectors in order to ensure uniform access to these treatments.

The government recognizes the value of France's accelerated marketing authorization procedure for cancer therapies and other treatments for life-threatening diseases but notes that the evidence submitted in these applications is insufficient for the purposes of pharmacoeconomic evaluation of these agents. The cancer plan therefore proposed two new measures:

- Establishing a system for public monitoring of postmarketing studies for new cancer therapies. The CT and INCa share responsibility for this program.
- Giving INCa an independent mission to evaluate new cancer therapies while these agents have an *autorisation temporaire d'utilisation* (authorization for temporary use) or after they have received full marketing authorization. Working closely with AFSSAPS and pharmaceutical companies, INCa can propose studies and seek expert opinion on affected patients and a therapy's conditions of use.

The cancer plan also expressed the government's intention to increase investment in *hospitalisation à domicile* (home hospitalization), a system that allows certain patients to receive care in their own homes. Key objectives included expanding access to home hospitalization, defining clear rules for the administration of cancer chemotherapy in patients' homes, guaranteeing adequate funding for home administration of costly chemotherapeutics, and facilitating the involvement of hospital pharmacies in the supply of medicines for this service. As of December 1, 2005, 6,826 patients were undergoing home hospitalization (for all indications), a 44% increase over the total in 2002. Cancer patients account for the majority of cases of home hospitalization.

GERMANY

Approximately 90% of the German population is enrolled in the country's *Gesetzliche Krankenversicherung* (GKV; statutory health insurance) system. Approximately 8 million now rely exclusively on private insurance for their healthcare coverage. (In addition, some people use private insurance to supplement the GKV.) Private insurance typically offers more extensive benefits than the GKV.

Unlike the practice in most other European countries, cancer patients in Germany are frequently treated by office-based physicians – oncologists or other specialists (e.g., internists, gynecologists, pulmonologists, gastroenterologists, dermatologists). Indeed, economic pressures have deterred some hospitals from accepting cancer patients. In April 2002, the *Gesellschaft zur Förderung der Ambulanten Krebstherapie* (GEFAK; Society for the Promotion of Ambulatory Cancer Therapy) reported that many hospitals that were unwilling or unable to pay for costly cancer therapies were referring patients to office-based practices for treatment.

Pharmaceutical Pricing and Reimbursement

Pharmaceutical companies are theoretically free to set ex-manufacturer drug prices in Germany. Retail prices are then determined by adding strictly controlled wholesale and pharmacy margins and value added tax (a sales tax). In the hospital sector, drug prices are usually set by negotiations between hospital pharmacists and manufacturers' sales representatives. In return for including a manufacturer's drugs in their formularies, hospitals expect to receive substantial discounts or rebates on the list prices of these products. Savings in excess of 50% on retail prices are reportedly common, and some manufacturers even supply hospitals with certain drugs virtually free of charge. The incentive for such generosity is the influence that hospitals have on outpatient prescribing. Primary care physicians tend to continue the therapy initiated in hospital (unless it proves ineffective or inappropriate). This influence will increase in the future. Under the *Arzneimittelausgaben-Begrenzungsgesetz* (Pharmaceutical Expenditure Limitation Act), hospitals are required to determine the therapy patients receive when they are discharged and to advise them on generic drug options.

Prospective Payment

In April 2002, the German Parliament passed the *Gesetz zur Einführung des diagnoseorientierten Fallpauschalensystems* (Act for the Introduction of a Diagnosis-Related Group System). The introduction of this new DRG system began in 2004 and was originally scheduled for completion in 2007, but the government was persuaded that this timetable was too aggressive. The *Zweites Fallpauschalenänderungsgesetz* (Second Diagnosis-Related Group Modification Act), enacted in December 2004, extended the deadline for the full implementation of the DRG system to January 1, 2009, with the possibility of a further one-year extension, if necessary. As of October 2005, approximately 1,720 acute care hospitals (94% of the national total) had begun the process of implementing the new DRG system. These hospitals had a total of 494,000 beds, managed 15.3 million cases, and had combined expenditures of €45 billion ($56 billion).

DRG rates vary from state to state. By 2009, payments to all hospitals must converge on the rate for their particular state. High-priced hospitals will lose from this exercise, whereas low-priced hospitals will gain.

A key objective of DRG-based reimbursement is to shorten the length of hospital stays. New cost management systems will measure how effectively a given treatment reduces overall therapy costs while achieving the same clinical outcomes. Product evaluations will need to take account of the following factors:

- Therapy costs that correlate duration of treatment with length of stay.
- Cost of managing side effects.
- Administration and disposal costs.
- Cost of treating therapy failures.

At present, DRGs apply only to inpatient procedures, with the exception of two semiambulatory groups related to renal dialysis. Beginning in 2007, however, the government plans to introduce DRGs for office-based specialists.

In a position statement published in March 2004, the *Verband Forschender Arzneimittelhersteller* (VFA; German Association of Research-Based Pharmaceutical Companies) described the introduction of the new DRG system as "the greatest structural reform in the [German] hospital sector in the last 30 years." The new system presents the pharmaceutical industry with both opportunities and challenges. Drug costs are generally included in the standard DRG rates, but additional funding is available for new therapies in specific circumstances. Hospitals can apply for a *Zusatzentgelt* (supplementary payment) for drugs or devices that are not yet covered by

DRGs. Supplementary payments are available for technologies that meet any of the following conditions:

- Insufficient data available for inclusion in a DRG.
- Use in multiple DRGs.
- Potentially significant impact on the cost of a given DRG or on the hospital's overall expenditures.

Table 16.4 lists the drugs that are eligible for supplementary payments in 2006. Payments are dose-dependent.

Supplementary payments, along with DRGs and days of treatment, are used to set a hospital's revenue budget. The full amount of the supplementary payment is available if hospitals submit their applications to statutory health insurance funds in advance of treatment, but retroactive submissions qualify for only 75% reimbursement. If a hospital exceeds its revenue budget, it must generally repay 65% of the surplus to the statutory health insurance funds, but this rate is reduced to 25% for excess revenues derived from supplementary payments for drugs and devices. On the other hand, if a hospital earns less than its revenue budget, it generally receives 40% of the shortfall from the statutory health insurance funds – but nothing for a shortfall in revenues from supplementary payments for drugs and devices. Supplementary payments are a budget-neutral measure – in other words, monies allocated to supplementary payments reduce funding for other areas of the overall budget.

Table 16.4 Drugs Eligible for Supplementary Payments in Germany, 2006

Code	*Drug*
ZE13	Alemtuzumab
ZE15	Docetaxel
ZE17	Gemcitabine
ZE19	Irinotecan
ZE23	Oxaliplatin
ZE24	Paclitaxel
ZE25	Rituximab
ZE27	Trastuzumab
ZE30	Prothrombin complex
ZE38	Human immunoglobulin for cytomegalovirus
ZE39	Caspofungin
ZE40	Filgrastim
ZE41	Polyvalent human immunoglobulin
ZE42	Lenograstim
ZE43	Liposomal amphotericin B
ZE44	Topotecan
ZE45	Voriconazole (oral)
ZE46	Voriconazole
ZE47	Antithrombin III
ZE48	Aldesleukin
ZE49	Bortezomib
ZE50	Cetuximab
ZE51	Human immunoglobulin for hepatitis B surface antigen
ZE52	Liposomal doxorubicin
ZE53	Pemetrexed

Note: Unless otherwise indicated, coverage relates to parenteral administration

Integrated Care

The government wants to improve the coordination of medical services in Germany. To that end, the 2003 *Gesetz zur Modernisierung der Gesetzlichen Krankenversicherung* (GMG; Statutory Health Insurance Modernization Act) removed legal barriers and provided financial incentives for the development of *integrierte Versorgung* (integrated care). Family physicians, specialists, and medical and nonmedical healthcare practitioners in both the primary care and hospital sectors are encouraged to work together to improve the quality of patient care. In some cases, pharmacists may also be invited to participate in integrated care initiatives. Statutory health insurance funds may invest up to 1% of their total revenues in the development of integrated care.

The GMG also enables hospitals to offer ambulatory care for certain indications and highly specialized services. In addition, hospitals may become involved in the provision of ambulatory care where there is a shortage of office-based specialists. However, integrated care has been slow to take off in oncology in Germany.

Disease Management

In July 2002, the German government launched a new healthcare strategy: *strukturierte Behandlungsprogramme für chronische Krankheiten* (structured treatment programs for chronic illnesses), more commonly known as disease management (DM) programs. Breast cancer and type 2 diabetes were the first diseases to be covered by a DM program. As an incentive to participate in these programs, health insurance funds offer a reduction in out-of-pocket payments for treatments related to the given disease.

On March 28, 2003, the *Bundesversicher-sicherungsamt* (BVA; Federal Insurance Office) approved Germany's first DM program – a breast cancer program in the state of North Rhine Westphalia. By June 2006, a total of 2,447 programs had been registered throughout Germany. Enrollment in these programs has grown steadily and totaled 36,874 in February 2006.

Prescribing Budgets

Since the early 1990s, the German government has tried to curb pharmaceutical spending by a succession of budgetary limits on physicians working outside the hospital sector. Office-based physicians are currently subject to *Richtgrößen* – indicative prescribing amounts that determine the maximum expenditure on medicines per patient per quarter. Clinicians who exceed these amounts by more than 25% face the prospect of heavy fines. Indicative prescribing amounts are set at state level and vary substantially by physician specialty. The allowances are much higher for senior citizens than for nonelderly patients. For example, in Berlin, general practitioners' indicative prescribing amounts in 2006 are €39.46 ($49.05) per quarter for each nonelderly patient and €112.83 ($140.24) for senior citizens. By comparison, indicative prescribing amounts for specialist internists are €91.30 ($113.48) per quarter for each nonelderly patient and €133.21 ($165.57) for senior citizens. These amounts are averages for all patients who visit physicians within a quarter. Concessions are granted to practices that have a disproportionately large number of patients who require costly treatments, and some expensive therapies are excluded from indicative prescribing amounts. For example, some states include cancer therapies in the list of *Praxisbesonderheiten* (practice special cases) that are exempt from indicative prescribing amounts.

Cost Sharing

Under the GMG, patients pay a flat sum of €10.00 ($12.43) per day for inpatient treatment (for a maximum of 28 days). The GKV covers the full cost of medicines dispensed in the hospital.

Patients are also required to pay a *Praxisgebühr* (practice fee) of €10.00 ($12.43) for the first visit in a calendar quarter to any office-based physician. This fee covers all visits to the chosen practice in that quarter, as well as referrals to other physicians during that period. Drugs dispensed by retail pharmacies are generally subject to a 10% coinsurance payment, with a minimum payment of €5.00 ($6.21) and a maximum of €10.00 ($12.43).

The GMG requires almost all patients to make out-of-pocket contributions toward the cost of their healthcare. For most patients, annual out-of-pocket payments are capped at the equivalent of 2% of their gross income. Patients with severe chronic illnesses are required to pay a maximum of 1% of their gross income each year; previously they were exempt from out-of-pocket payments after the first year of their illness. However, cancer is not automatically classified as a severe chronic illness. Moreover, many health insurance funds reportedly use patients' gross income in the preceding year as the basis for their calculations. In addition, some funds levy out-of-pocket payments throughout the year and then refund excess payments.

Oncologists note that cancer patients frequently have out-of-pocket costs of €50–€70 ($62.15–$87.00) per week – relatively modest sums compared with the copayments required of some US cancer patients, but a substantial amount by European standards. In an article published in the newspaper *Die Tageszeitung* on May 20, 2005, Peter Borchmann, an oncologist at the university clinic in Cologne, reported that a growing number of his patients indicated that they had not filled certain prescriptions "because they could not afford the copayment." In the same article, Marion Weyl, the head of patient management at the Berliner Charité hospital stated that ambulatory cancer therapy caused "considerable financial difficulties" for 70–80% of patients.

The German government has plans to introduce a package of reforms that would, among numerous other measures, mean higher copayments for cancer patients who had previously failed to take advantage of screening provisions or who did not comply with their prescribed regimen of therapy in a DM program. Patients who had not undergone screening for a given cancer when offered and who subsequently developed that particular disease would not be eligible for the reduced annual cap on out-of-pocket payments (i.e., 1% of annual gross income) that is available to chronically ill GKV beneficiaries. Similarly, patients enrolled in DM programs who did not comply with their prescribed treatment would risk losing reductions in their out-of-pocket payments. The government hopes to implement the new healthcare reform package early in 2007.

Off-label Prescribing

Off-label prescribing has been the subject of considerable controversy in Germany in recent years. Several landmark court cases, together with decisions from official bodies that formulate national healthcare policy, have progressively defined the circumstances in which it is acceptable for physicians to prescribe off-label.

A judgment by the *Bundessozialgericht* (Federal Social Court) on March 19, 2002, first focused attention on the issue of off-label prescribing. The case concerned the use of intravenous immunoglobulin to treat visual impairment suffered by a female patient as a side effect of cortisone therapy for multiple sclerosis. The woman's health insurance fund had refused to reimburse the immunoglobulin therapy, arguing that the efficacy of this treatment was unproven. The court ruled that the health insurance fund was not obliged to cover off-label prescribing in this case but defined three circumstances in which statutory health insurance funds should be required to reimburse off-label therapy:

- The disease to be treated is a condition that is life-threatening or causes chronic impairment of quality of life.
- No other therapy is available.
- There is reasonable evidence that the treatment in question could achieve therapeutic success (remedial or palliative). Such evidence could take one of the two forms listed below:
  1. The manufacturer has already applied for an extension of the drug's label for the intended indication and the results of a controlled Phase III clinical trial (using standard therapy or placebo as the comparator) have been published and have demonstrated clinically relevant efficacy and acceptable risks.
  2. Published data, gathered outside the scope of a licensing application, provide reliable, scientifically verifiable evidence of the quality and efficacy of the drug in its new indication, thereby creating a consensus in the relevant community of experts on the proposed new usage.

If all three of these conditions are satisfied, health insurance funds are obliged to reimburse off-label prescribing.

In December 2005, the *Bundesverfassungsgericht* (Federal Constitutional Court) strengthened the grounds for off-label prescribing. The court ruled that it is unlawful to refuse patients – who have a life-threatening disease for which no approved treatments are available – reimbursement for an alternative therapy, as long as the alternative offers at least some prospect of a cure or an appreciable effect on the course of the disease. Given that the overwhelming majority of German residents are legally obliged to enroll in – and contribute to – the statutory heath insurance system, the court reasoned that the government should not force patients to fund their own treatment if they develop a serious disease. This ruling is likely to have an impact not only on physicians' freedom to prescribe off-label but also on the future development of treatment guidelines and on the composition of reference-pricing groups. Disease severity and the range of available therapies will exercise an increased influence on decision making in the future.

The German government has sought to rationalize off-label prescribing. In September 2002, the Ministry of Health established the *Expertengruppe Off-Label* (Off-Label Expert Group) within the *Bundesinstitut für Arzneimittel und Medizinprodukte* (BfArM; Federal Institute for Medicines and Medical Devices), with a brief to focus on oncology. In August 2005, the ministry created additional expert groups to evaluate off-label prescribing in neurology/psychiatry and infectious disease (with an emphasis on HIV/AIDS). The original group has been criticized for being too slow in its deliberations, but it has recently published decisions on the off-label use of six cancer therapies. With the exception of the use of inhaled interleukin-2 in the treatment of metastatic renal cell carcinoma, the group has approved all proposed off-label uses reviewed to date (Table 16.5). Not surprisingly, however, the judgments generally subject the off-label use of these therapies to strict conditions (e.g., eligibility of patients, duration of treatment, monitoring).

Since 2004, the *Gemeinsamer Bundesausschuß der Ärzte, Zahnärzte, Krankenhäuser und Krankenkassen* (GBA; Joint Federal Committee of Physicians, Dentists, Hospitals, and Health Insurance Funds) has been responsible for deciding whether a given therapy should be reimbursed by the GKV (statutory health insurance) system. The GBA's reimbursement decisions are binding on all physicians contracted to the GKV and on all statutory health insurance funds. In April 2006, the GBA identified the following prerequisites for off-label prescribing:

- An off-label indication should be positively assessed by one of the aforementioned expert groups. Their evaluations form the basis for the GBA's subsequent appraisal of drugs.
- The manufacturer should confirm the appropriateness of off-label usage of a drug.

Drugs that meet these requirements will be added to a new Appendix (9A) to the official pharmaceutical guidelines. Medicines that are not judged suitable for the off-label usage – on clinical or economic grounds – will be added to Appendix 9B of the official pharmaceutical guidelines.

Physicians can face substantial fines for improper off-label prescribing. For example, in July 2005, the *Sozialgericht Berlin* (Berlin Social Court) ordered a cardiothoracic surgeon to refund a sum of €53,000 ($65,877) to a statutory health insurance fund as a penalty for improper off-label prescribing of iloprost (Schering AG's Ilomedin). This ruling is likely to be a powerful deterrent to unrestrained off-label prescribing in Germany.

Table 16.5 Judgments of Germany's Off-label Expert Group

Drug	*Off-label Use*	*Outcome*
Carboplatin	Palliative chemotherapy of advanced non-small-cell lung cancer	Approved
Disodium cromoglycate	Treatment of systemic mastocytosis	Approved
Fluorouracil	Adjuvant therapy in breast cancer	Approved
Fluorouracil	Use without a combination with folic acid in (neo-) adjuvant therapy of colorectal cancer	Approved
Irinotecan	Small-cell lung cancer	Approved
Interleukin-2 (inhaled)	Metastatic renal cell carcinoma	Rejected

ITALY

The publicly funded *Servizio Sanitario Nazionale* (SSN; National Health Service) is the dominant source of funding for cancer therapy in Italy. Approximately 60% of cancer patients receive their chemotherapy in the hospital outpatient setting, a system known as *ospedale di giorno* (day hospital).

Pharmaceutical Pricing and Reimbursement

The setting of pharmaceutical prices in Italy is a complex exercise in which national regulatory authorities play a prominent role. The *Agenzia Italiana del Farmaco* (AIFA; Italian Pharmaceutical Agency), works with a group of government-appointed experts in evaluating all new drugs and determining acceptable prices for inclusion in the *Prontuario Terapeutico Nazionale* (PTN; national formulary). The PTN also assigns drugs to one of three categories: class A (drugs that are available in retail pharmacies and are fully reimbursed by the SSN), class C (drugs that are available in retail pharmacies and excluded from SSN reimbursement), or class H (hospital-only drugs that are fully reimbursed by the SSN). A fourth category – class B (drugs that were available in retail pharmacies and reimbursed by the SSN at 50% of their retail price) – was abolished in January 2001. Cancer drugs are generally categorized as class H medicines.

Pricing decisions are based on the following factors:

- Comparative efficacy and price of any competing or similar drugs.
- Degree of innovation and therapeutic value.
- Prices of the same or similar products in other European Union countries.
- Market forecasts, including sales, market share, number of patients treated, and number of prescriptions.

Representatives of AIFA and several government ministries review this evidence, taking into account the drug's likely impact on SSN pharmaceutical spending (except in the case of orphan drugs). Innovative compounds are frequently compared with existing therapies for the same indication. Pharmacoeconomic data are required for orphan drugs or highly innovative pharmaceuticals, but manufacturers have the option of including cost-effectiveness, cost-utility, or cost-benefit data in their applications for other kinds of drugs.

In many European countries, manufacturers are allowed much greater freedom in setting drug prices in the hospital sector than in retail pharmacies. Italy is an exception to this rule. In the Italian hospital pharmacy market, manufacturers are legally obliged to offer substantial discounts relative to the retail prices of drugs in classes A and H. In the case of drugs registered through Italy's national registration procedure, manufacturers must reduce their prices to hospitals by at least 50% of the retail prices (net of value added tax). In the case of hospital-only drugs approved by the European Medicines Evaluation Agency (EMEA), manufacturers must reduce their prices to hospitals by at least 40% of the retail prices (net of value added tax).

Inpatients in Italian public hospitals benefit from full reimbursement of the cost of their medicines. Funding for hospital medicines comes from *aziende sanitarie locali* (ASLs; local health authorities) and *aziende ospedaliere* (AOs; hospital authorities).

Prospective Payment

Italy was one of the first countries in Europe to introduce a prospective payment system, in January 1995. Most hospital services are now subject to DRG-based reimbursement, and a *scheda di dimissione ospedaliera* (hospital discharge form) must be completed when a patient is discharged. Maximum reimbursement rates are defined nationally, but regional authorities may choose to set lower rates within their territories.

The DRG system has promoted the growth of day hospital care in Italy. The system offers financial incentives to hospitals to treat patients in the outpatient setting, rather than in acute inpatient beds, wherever possible.

Many physicians express concern that DRG payments are inadequate to cover the cost of the most innovative oncology drugs and may therefore impair the quality of cancer care provided in Italian hospitals. A 2004 survey of 500 oncologists commissioned by the *Associazione Italiana di Oncologia Medica* (AIOM; Italian Association for Medical Oncology) found that 95% of respondents believed that the DRG system was inadequate to meet the demands of innovative oncology and therefore needed to be changed.

Exceptional Reimbursement

The Ministry of Health controls the use of certain drugs by a procedure known as *File F*, a mechanism for financing certain hospital medicines from ASL funds rather than from hospital budgets. For example, File F provides ASL funding for expensive inpatient therapies that would not be covered by hospital budgets, drugs administered in hospital outpatient clinics, and hospital drugs that are dispensed for administration in patients' homes.

Pharmacy Decision Making

Hospitals favor the prescribing of drugs listed in their own *prontuario terapeutico ospedaliero* (PTO; hospital formulary). The addition of new drugs to a formulary often takes 12–18 months, but innovative therapies with exceptional clinical value tend to achieve much faster formulary inclusion. In addition, hospitals may sometimes allow the use of new drugs before they are listed in their formularies – especially if these drugs appear to be superior to more established therapies.

In addition to local hospital formularies, many of Italy's regions have introduced a *prontuario terapeutico ospedaliero regionale* (regional hospital formulary) for all public hospitals within their territories. Cost containment is an important objective of such regional formularies. For example, the *Bolletino Ufficiale della Regione Campania* (Official Bulletin of the Region of Campania) states that "over the years, publishing a formulary has become not just a choice of medical specialties and diagnostics but also a task of great political and social responsibility because the scarcity of financial resources dedicated to healthcare demands that [these resources] are used in the most rational way possible."

Off-label Prescribing

Off-label prescribing is subject to strict regulatory controls in Italy. The following conditions must be satisfied before a drug is prescribed for any use other than its licensed indication:

- The physician assumes direct responsibility for prescribing the drug for an unlicensed use.
- The drug is prescribed to an individual patient and only in the absence of therapeutic alternatives.
- Usage is outside clinical trials or for a patient who is not eligible for a trial.
- Off-label usage is supported by evidence published in accredited international scientific journals.
- The patient is provided with detailed information on the off-label usage and gives informed consent to the treatment.
- The method of prescription allows for the identification of the prescribing physician.

The SSN generally reimburses off-label prescriptions only if they are provided by means of a clinical trial.

Financial Constraints

As noted earlier, the overwhelming majority of Italian oncologists believe that the country's DRG system is a significant obstacle to the practice of innovative cancer therapy. Specialists also express more general concern about the financial constraints imposed by the SSN. The aforementioned survey conducted by AIOM found that 9% of oncologists reported that they were very much subject to financial constraints, 42% considered themselves somewhat restricted, 37% indicated that they were a little restricted, and only 12% stated that they were not at all restricted.

In another survey published by AIOM in October 2005, 83% of oncologists agreed with the statement that some financial aspects of the Italian healthcare system could pose a problem for access to new cancer therapies. In addition, 89% of respondents expressed that the existing rules were inadequate to support off-label prescribing based on strong clinical evidence.

SPAIN

The *Sistema Nacional de Salud* (SNS; National Health System) covers 98.5% of the Spanish population. Regional governments are now responsible for determining and implementing healthcare policy within their territories, but the national Ministry of Health retains ultimate authority in strategic matters such as cost containment, product approvals, drug safety, implementing EU directives, and drug pricing and reimbursement.

According to the *Sociedad Española de Oncología Medica* (SEOM; Spanish Society for Medical Oncology), 85% of cancer treatments in Spain are now administered in the outpatient setting – mainly in *hospitales de día oncológicos* (oncology day hospitals). This approach to cancer therapy offers patients greater convenience and reduces costs for the SNS.

Pharmaceutical Pricing and Reimbursement

Retail prices for drugs reimbursed by the SNS are determined by negotiations between manufacturers and the *Comisión Interministerial de Precios de los Medicamentos* (CIPM; Interdepartmental Committee on Pharmaceutical Prices). Drug prices to hospitals must not exceed maximum retail prices, but hospitals generally expect to receive very substantial discounts on these prices.

In addition to prescription medicines that are available in retail pharmacies, Spain has two categories of drugs that require a prescription from a hospital physician. Some medicines are restricted to *uso hospitalario* (hospital use, designated as category H products). Drugs that are subject to *diagnóstico hospitalario* (DH; hospital diagnosis) require an initial diagnosis and prescription from a hospital-based physician but may subsequently be dispensed by retail pharmacies.

The social security system covers the full cost of all prescription medicines dispensed in Spain's public hospitals or private hospitals that have contracts with the SNS. However, patients who undergo private medical treatment have to pay for their medications unless they have private health insurance that provides comprehensive pharmaceutical coverage.

Pharmacy Decision Making

Every public hospital in Spain is required by law to have a multidisciplinary *comisión de farmacia y terapéutica* (CFT; pharmacy and therapeutics committee), the body that defines the criteria for including drugs in the hospital's formulary and decides which drugs meet these criteria. Although drug acquisition prices and daily treatment costs remain crucial factors in formulary decision making, pharmacy and therapeutics committees are paying increasing attention to a drug's cost-benefit ratio.

Hospitals set an annual pharmacy budget and then usually monitor their drug costs on a monthly basis. Physicians who deviate from hospital prescribing protocols or who are judged to be overspending may be asked to justify their prescribing decisions.

Access to Innovative Therapies

The aforementioned study by the Karolinska Institutet found that Spain ranked with Austria and Switzerland as the countries that offered the best overall access to innovative cancer drugs in Europe. The fact that Spain has the lowest drug prices – overall and for cancer therapies – among the major pharmaceutical markets is undoubtedly a significant factor in that country's rapid adoption of innovative medicines.

UNITED KINGDOM

The National Health Service (NHS) is the dominant source of healthcare financing and provision in the United Kingdom. Private healthcare focuses primarily on areas where waiting times for NHS interventions are long (e.g., elective surgery for conditions that are not life-threatening) and areas where NHS-funded services are severely restricted (e.g., optical and dental care). Pharmaceutical sales to the private sector are small compared with sales to the NHS.

The UK government has identified the improvement of cancer care as a priority in its healthcare strategy. In September 2000, the Department of Health (DH) unveiled the NHS Cancer Plan, described by the then Health Secretary as "a national strategy to prevent, diagnose, and treat cancer; to reform the way cancer services are delivered; to standardize care and improve patient experience; to coordinate research and to invest in equipment and the cancer workforce." This mission statement implicitly acknowledged the necessity to overcome structural flaws in the UK oncology system (e.g., the need for a substantial increase in the number of medical oncologists and oncology pharmacists in the NHS to improve the quality of oncology prescribing).

The government has established a system of 34 cancer networks consisting of regional cancer centers and smaller satellite cancer units. Because NHS specialists are hospital based, general practitioners (GPs) (the gatekeepers to the UK healthcare system) invariably refer cancer patients to a hospital for diagnosis and treatment. Patients are often admitted to a hospital for initial treatment (e.g., surgery) and then receive follow-up treatment (e.g., radiotherapy, chemotherapy) as outpatients. However, the dominance of the hospital sector in UK cancer care is likely to wane in coming years. Primary care trusts (PCTs) – 152 functionally autonomous groups of primary care practices – now control 80% of the NHS budget and therefore have a significant influence on the treatment that their patients receive. PCTs qualify for a payment of £5,000 ($9,090) if they appoint a lead clinician in cancer care to coordinate the provision of oncology services. (The US dollar-to-pound sterling exchange rate used in this chapter is the 2005 average rate [i.e., $1 = £0.55004].)

Since April 1, 2004, GPs are subject to a new contract for general medical services (GMS). This agreement is intended to increase the level of support for the primary care sector and thereby improve the quality of patient care. One element of this contract is "a quality and outcomes framework which [provides] resources and rewards GPs on the basis of how well they care for patients rather than simply the number of patients they treat, leading to good chronic DM in the community and relieving pressures on hospitals." The quality and outcomes framework covers 10 common disorders, including cancer.

Pharmaceutical Pricing and Reimbursement

The United Kingdom offers pharmaceutical companies a high degree of freedom in setting the prices of new drugs. The government controls prices indirectly by means of the Pharmaceutical Price Regulation Scheme (PPRS), a system that (contrary to its name) regulates manufacturers' overall profits, not their prices. Admission of a product to reimbursement in the United Kingdom is generally straightforward. Manufacturers advise the DH of their intention to launch a product and request that it be added to the official Drug Tariff. The drug is added automatically unless the DH objects. The Drug Tariff states the price of the product, which may be subject to periodic variations. Products used exclusively in hospitals are not subject to Drug Tariff listing and therefore benefit from automatic admission to reimbursement.

The NHS covers the full cost of drugs dispensed to patients in public hospitals in the United Kingdom. Funding has historically come from hospitals' pharmaceutical budgets, but the following section discusses changes that are in progress.

Prospective Payment

Until very recently, hospital budgets were set on the basis of historical expenditures. In October 2002, however, the DH published *Reforming NHS Financial Flows*, a blueprint for a new patient-centered funding system known as Payment by Results (PbR). This system gives NHS patients the freedom to choose when and where they receive hospital treatment, a right they had never previously enjoyed. The mechanism has been summarized with the motto "the money follows the patient." Specifically, PbR has the following key objectives:

- Promoting choice and competition.
- Increasing efficiency and value for money.
- Facilitating therapeutic innovation.
- Cutting waiting times and inpatient length of stay.
- Improving equity and transparency in the healthcare system.

The implementation of this new system began on a limited scale in 2004 and was then expanded in 2005 to include all elective inpatients. From 2006 to 2008, the system will be extended to nonelective inpatients, emergency room admissions, and outpatients. Beginning in 2008, PbR will be introduced into the primary care sector.

PbR is based on healthcare resource groups (HRGs), a form of DRG that groups patients who have similar clinical conditions and similar consumption of healthcare resources. The HRG system has been refined repeatedly to make it more discriminating, and a further review is in progress, with the objective of identifying all disease complications and comorbidities. HRGs provide the data that underpin the national tariff for services provided within the PbR system. Efficient hospitals that can provide services for less than national tariff prices will be permitted to keep the surplus. By reinvesting the money saved in their organizations, these hospitals can improve the quality of their services and attract patients away from less-efficient hospitals.

The national tariff does not include procedures that are highly specialized, rarely performed, or subject to price volatility. Furthermore, high-cost drugs (including some chemotherapy drugs) and devices are excluded from the PbR national tariff. Hospitals that wish to use these drugs have to commission supplementary funding from local PCTs. In addition, new technologies, as well as some existing drugs and devices that have a high price or uneven distribution, may qualify for pass-through status for a maximum of two years. PCTs must notify the DH if they grant pass-through status to drugs used by hospitals in their respective catchment areas.

Pharmacy Decision Making

The drug and therapeutics committee (DTC) in each hospital is usually responsible for deciding the composition of the formulary. A subcommittee, the new drugs committee, may assess novel therapies in some institutions. In some hospitals, a committee of senior managers makes formulary decisions based on the DTC's evidence-based recommendations.

Not surprisingly, DTCs' primary considerations tend to be a drug's clinical value and its cost to the hospital. But they also take account of a drug's potential economic impact in the local primary care sector. Representatives of NHS trusts and local PCTs meet together regularly to discuss matters of common interest, including prescribing patterns and the formulary status of costly drugs. In addition, hospital DTCs are responsible for ensuring that NICE guidelines are fully implemented within their institutions.

National Institute for Health and Clinical Excellence

In April 1999, the UK government established the National Institute for Health and Clinical Excellence (NICE) to guide the NHS in England and Wales on the optimal use of medical technologies. (Scotland and Northern Ireland have their own advisory bodies.) NICE appraises the clinical and cost-effectiveness of health technologies, including pharmaceuticals, medical devices, and medical procedures. Its stated goals include promoting the faster uptake of new interventions and eliminating inequalities in patient access to healthcare.

NICE issues two main forms of guidance: technology appraisals (i.e., evaluations of the clinical-effectiveness and cost-effectiveness of specific drugs, devices, and procedures) and broader clinical guidelines (i.e., recommendations on best practice in the management of particular disorders). To date, NICE has published 10 sets of clinical guidelines in oncology:

- Breast cancer (August 2002).
- Urological cancers (September 2002).
- Hemato-oncology (October 2003).
- Supportive and palliative care (March 2004).
- Colorectal cancer (June 2004).
- Head and neck cancer (November 2004).
- Cancers in children and young people (August 2005).
- Skin tumors, including melanoma (February 2006).
- Sarcoma (March 2006).
- Brain tumors (June 2006).

However, technology appraisals account for most of NICE's output to date. As of October 2006, NICE had completed a total of 110 technology appraisals, including approximately 20 reviews of earlier appraisals. The institute's Web site lists 24 current appraisals of oncology drugs (more than for any other therapeutic area). Table 16.6 summarizes key findings of NICE appraisals of cancer therapies. Three clinical guidelines and 14 technology appraisals in the field of oncology are currently in progress.

One of the government's key objectives in establishing NICE was to eliminate "postcode prescribing" (also known as "postcode rationing" or the "postcode lottery"), whereby patients' access to innovative medicines depends on the reimbursement policy of their local strategic health authority or PCT. To that end, in January 2002, the government imposed a statutory obligation on all health authorities and PCTs to provide funding for NICE-approved therapies within three months of NICE's publication of its decision.

To provide funding for NICE-approved treatments, the PbR budget was increased by £304 million ($553 million [0.7%]) in financial year 2004–5 and by £328 million ($596 million [0.7%]) in financial year 2005–6. The 0.7% increase was based on national averages and may not have been sufficient to cover increased expenditures in hospitals that had an above-average usage of NICE-endorsed technologies.

A performance assessment known as the annual health check will determine whether hospitals and PCTs are meeting their PbR obligations. These organizations will be required to declare whether they are conforming to NICE's technology appraisals and taking the institute's clinical guidelines into account in the delivery of healthcare. To make such a declaration, hospitals and PCTs must have robust systems to assess, plan for, and monitor the financial impact of implementing NICE's guidance.

Review of Variations in the Use of NICE-approved Cancer Drugs

In 2003, several pharmaceutical companies expressed concerns about disparities in the uptake of NICE-approved cancer therapies in the United Kingdom. For instance, in September 2003, Roche published the results of a survey that found persistent inequalities in access to Herceptin (trastuzumab), a treatment for advanced human epidermal growth factor receptor 2 (HER2)-positive breast cancer. Notwithstanding a positive appraisal from NICE in March 2002, only 33% of eligible patients in England, Scotland, and Wales had access to the drug 18 months later. Penetration rates ranged from just 14.1% of eligible patients in the Midlands to 61% in southwest England.

Disturbed by such reports, in October 2003, the government commissioned Professor Mike Richards, the national cancer director, to work with strategic health authorities, cancer networks, and the pharmaceutical industry to investigate reported prescribing variations, determine the reasons for these disparities, and recommend measures to achieve more-uniform access to NICE-approved cancer drugs. The results of this investigation were

Table 16.6 Summary of NICE Technology Appraisals of Cancer Therapies, April 2001 to October 2006

Drug/Drug Class	*Issue Date*	*Key Judgment*	*Projected Population*	*Projected Annual Cost to the NHS (£ MM)*	*Projected Annual Cost to the NHS ($ MM)*
Temozolomide	April 2001	Patients with recurrent malignant glioma (brain cancer) who have failed first-line chemotherapy treatment with other agents (either because of lack of efficacy or because of side effects) may be considered for treatment with temozolomide	150	1	1.8
Gemcitabine	May 2001	May be considered as a treatment option for patients with advanced or metastatic adenocarcinoma of the pancreas and a Karnofsky performance score of 50 or more, where first-line chemotherapy is to be used	600–840	0.8–3	1.5–5.5
Fludarabine	September 2001	Recommended as second-line therapy for B-cell chronic lymphocytic leukemia (CLL) for patients who have either failed, or are intolerant of, first-line chemotherapy, and who would otherwise have received combination chemotherapy of CHOP, CAP, or CVP			
Taxanes	September 2001[a]	The use of docetaxel in combination with an anthracycline in first-line treatment of advanced breast cancer is not currently recommended. As paclitaxel is not licensed for first-line use with anthracycline, its use was not considered in this indication			
		Docetaxel and paclitaxel should be available for the treatment of advanced breast cancer where initial cytotoxic chemotherapy (including anthracycline) has failed or is inappropriate	5,000	20	36.4
Trastuzumab	March 2002	Trastuzumab in combination with paclitaxel is recommended as an option for people with tumors expressing human epidermal growth factor receptor 2 (HER2) at levels of 3+ who have not received	450	17	30.9

Table 16.6 Continued

Drug/Drug Class	*Issue Date*	*Key Judgment*	*Projected Population*	*Projected Annual Cost to the NHS (£ MM)*	*Projected Annual Cost to the NHS ($ MM)*
		chemotherapy for metastatic breast cancer and in whom anthracycline treatment is inappropriate. Trastuzumab monotherapy is recommended as an option for people with tumors expressing HER2 at levels of 3+ who have received at least two chemotherapy regimens for metastatic breast cancer			
Rituximab	March 2002	Not recommended for third-line or subsequent treatment of patients with recurrent or refractory stage III or IV follicular lymphoma. For "last-line" treatment, rituximab is recommended only in the context of a prospective case series	9,000		
Vinorelbine	December 2002	Vinorelbine monotherapy should not be first-line treatment for advanced breast cancer. Monotherapy should be an option for treating advanced breast cancer when initial anthracycline therapy has failed or is unsuitable for the patient. Routine use of vinorelbine as an element in combination therapy is not recommended	5,000	(13.5)[b]	(24.5)[b]
Paclitaxel	January 2003[c]	A platinum-based drug, alone or in combination with paclitaxel, should be first-line chemotherapy (usually postoperative) for ovarian cancer. In the event of recurrence, "re-challenge therapy" (i.e., repetition of a successful first-line therapy) should be considered. If the patient's response to the first-line therapy was inadequate, a different treatment regimen should be considered for second-line therapy Paclitaxel should be considered as an element of second-line therapy if it was not used in first-line treatment but should not be prescribed in second-line treatment if it	4,000	28	50.9

(continued)

Table 16.6 Continued

Drug/Drug Class	*Issue Date*	*Key Judgment*	*Projected Population*	*Projected Annual Cost to the NHS (£ MM)*	*Projected Annual Cost to the NHS ($ MM)*
		was previously used in initial therapy			
Capecitabine	May 2003	For locally advanced or metastatic breast cancer, capecitabine in combination with docetaxel is preferable to docetaxel monotherapy if anthracycline-based regimens are unsuitable or have failed.	7,500	(1.2)[b]	(2.2)[b]
Capecitabine and tegafur with uracil	May 2003	Oral therapy with either capecitabine or tegafur with uracil (in combination with folinic acid) is recommended as an option for the first-line treatment of metastatic colorectal cancer	7,000	(10.5)[b]	(19.1)[b]
Rituximab	September 2003	Recommended for use in combination with CHOP for the first-line treatment of people with CD20-positive diffuse large-B-cell lymphoma at clinical stage II, III, or IV. Not recommended for use when CHOP is contraindicated	750–1,425	9.1–17.2	16.5–31.3
Imatinib	October 2003	Recommended as first-line treatment for patients with Philadelphia-chromosome-positive chronic myeloid leukemia (CML) in the chronic phase		4–6 in first year, rising to 16–20	7.3–10.9 in first year, rising to 29.1–36.4
Imatinib	October 2004	Recommended as first-line therapy for unresectable or metastatic KIT-positive gastro-intestinal stromal tumors. Treatment should be reviewed every 12 weeks and discontinued if no further benefits are discernible. The dosage of 400 mg per day should not be increased	240	1.7–6.8	3.1–12.4
Paclitaxel, PLDH, and topotecan	May 2005[c]	Paclitaxel in combination with carboplatin or cisplatin is recommended as an option for second-line (or subsequent) therapy of advanced ovarian cancer in suitable patients. Paclitaxel monotherapy or PLDH are recommended as alternative second-line (or subsequent) therapy for patients not suited		0.1–4.4	0.2–8

Table 16.6 Continued

Drug/Drug Class	*Issue Date*	*Key Judgment*	*Projected Population*	*Projected Annual Cost to the NHS (£ MM)*	*Projected Annual Cost to the NHS ($ MM)*
		to platinum-based therapy. Topotecan is recommended as a second-line (or subsequent) treatment only for patients who are not suited to the aforementioned therapeutic options			
Irinotecan, oxaliplatin, and raltitrexed	August 2005[c]	Irinotecan or oxaliplatin is recommended in combination with 5-FU/FA as first-line treatment for advanced colorectal cancer. Irinotecan monotherapy is recommended for subsequent therapy Raltitrexed is not recommended for the treatment of advanced colorectal cancer		64–128	116.4–232.7
Capecitabine and oxaliplatin	April 2006	Capecitabine monotherapy or oxaliplatin in combination with 5-FU/FA is the recommended adjuvant treatment of stage III (Dukes' C) colon cancer	3,100	10.3	18.7
Docetaxel	June 2006	Recommended as a treatment option for hormone-refractory metastatic prostate cancer. Treatment should not exceed 10 cycles and should not be repeated if the disease recurs	4,700	20	36.4
Trastuzumab	August 2006	Trastuzumab should be offered as a treatment option to women with early-stage HER2-positive breast cancer after surgery and chemotherapy (and sometimes radiotherapy). The drug should be administered every 3 weeks for 12 months, or until the breast cancer recurs, whichever is sooner.	4,273	99.9	181.6
Docetaxel	September 2006	Docetaxel in combination with doxorubicin and cyclophosphamide is recommended as a possible adjuvant therapy for early node-positive breast cancer	1,589	8.8	16.0
Rituximab	September 2006	Rituximab in combination with cyclophosphamide, vincristine, and prednisolone is recommended as a possible first-line therapy for	374	3.5	6.4

(continued)

Table 16.6 Continued

Drug/Drug Class	Issue Date	Key Judgment	Projected Population	Projected Annual Cost to the NHS (£ MM)	Projected Annual Cost to the NHS ($ MM)
		symptomatic stage III or IV follicular lymphoma			
Paclitaxel	September 2006	Not recommended for adjuvant treatment of early node-positive breast cancer			

[a]Review of earlier appraisal: no material changes to original judgment
[b]Projected annual savings to the National Health Service
[c]Review of earlier appraisal: material changes to original judgment
5-FU/FA = 5 fluorouracil plus folinic acid; CAP = Cyclophosphamide, doxorubicin, and prednisolone; CHOP = Cyclophosphamide, doxorubicin, vincristine, and prednisolone; CVP = Cyclophosphamide, vincristine, and prednisolone; HER2 = Human epidermal growth factor receptor 2; NHS = National Health Service; NSCLC = Non-small-cell lung cancer; and PLDH = Pegylated liposomal doxorubicin hydrochloride

Note: The US dollar-to-pound sterling exchange rate used is the 2005 average rate (i.e., $1 = £0.55004)

published in June 2004. The key findings were as follows:

- Overall usage of cancer drugs generally increases following positive appraisals from NICE.
- Variation in usage does exist across the country and cannot be accounted for by differences in case-mix and, for most drugs, is unlikely to be accounted for by cross-boundary flows alone. However, variation does appear to lessen over time once a positive appraisal from NICE has been published.
- Reasons for variations are complex but do not appear to be associated with direct funding restrictions on the use of these drugs. Instead, the main impact on usage seems to be constraints in service capacity and differences in clinical practice.

For the period July to December 2003, the authors analyzed hospital sales data from IMS Health and prescribing data from the 34 cancer networks. Researchers favored data from the cancer networks, when available, because these data reflected local knowledge about the reasons for variations. The study covered the 16 cancer therapies that had been approved by NICE as well as four comparator drugs that NICE had not appraised. Prescribing rates for NICE-approved treatments typically showed a three- or four-fold variation. Roche's MabThera (rituximab) had the narrowest variation in uptake (2.6-fold). At the other end of the spectrum, penetration rates for Schering-Plough's Temodal (temozolomide) varied 11.6-fold. Prescribing rates for the four comparator drugs had much smaller variations (2.3- to 2.7-fold).

The study investigated the reasons for these variations in prescribing rates. Survey responses from the 34 cancer networks suggested that direct-funding restrictions were not the reason for limited prescribing in certain areas. Rather, researchers identified several other limiting factors:

- *Limited capacity*. The rapid growth in the use of chemotherapy in recent years has exceeded treatment capacity in some areas. The use of certain drugs may be hindered by a lack of suitable facilities in which to prepare toxic drugs or shortages of specialist physicians, nurses, and pharmacists.
- *Clinician preferences*. Some physicians continue to prescribe their favored therapies in preference to drugs recommended by NICE.
- *Participation in clinical trials*. Some trusts may be involved in clinical trials that use alternatives to NICE-endorsed therapies. In addition, drugs used in clinical trials may be omitted from prescribing audits.

Survey respondents from pharmaceutical companies echoed the first two of these points. However, they suggested that funding restrictions may sometimes be a barrier to the uptake of NICE-approved cancer therapies. Pharmaceutical companies also identified variations in the effectiveness of local NHS leadership, particularly differences in the degree to which PCTs, NHS trusts, and cancer networks work together to plan for the impact of therapies that are undergoing NICE appraisal.

The authors offered suggestions on how to widen the uptake of NICE-approved cancer therapies. Key recommendations were as follows:

- NICE appraisals should include an assessment of the resources required to implement the institute's recommendations. This assessment, which could take the form of an "implementation toolkit," should provide guidance on nonpharmacological costs and other implementation issues. This document could be tailored to the needs of local health economies.
- The DH, in partnership with the NHS, should develop a capacity planning model for cancer chemotherapy. This exercise should be included within the wider chemotherapy review that has recently been commissioned by the national cancer director.
- Given that good information is the key to altering clinical practice, a system should be developed to audit physicians' prescribing behavior in relation to national benchmarks and to provide prompt feedback to networks and individual physicians. The feedback should include data on "the number of patients treated and the indications for treatment, so that the appropriateness of treatment can be assessed against NICE guidance" (i.e., whether the number of patients treated with particular drugs matches NICE's projections). Experience in other areas of healthcare suggests that providing such feedback could make a major contribution toward achieving more-uniform prescribing patterns across the country.

In September 2006, the national cancer director published an updated review of the use of NICE-approved cancer drugs. The methodology for the analysis of prescribing data was the same as for the study conducted in 2003, but the period covered was January to June 2005. The review found that geographic variations in the level of usage had diminished for all of the NICE-approved drugs included in the study – most dramatically in the case of Pierre Fabre's Navelbine (vinorelbine), down from an 8.1-fold variation to a 3.1-fold difference. However, the level of variation remained disturbingly large in some cases: 9.5-fold for Temodal and 5.8-fold for Schering-Plough's

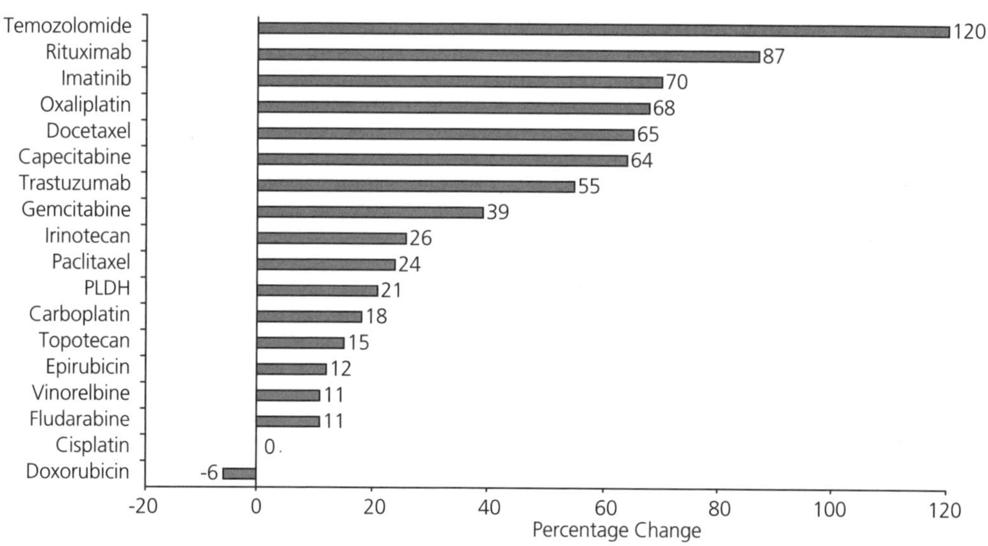

PLDH = Pegylated liposomal doxorubicin hydrochloride
Note: Consumption was calculated on the basis of prescribed milligrams of each drug per 1,000 population

Figure 16.3 Percentage Change in Median Usage Rates of Select Oncology Drugs in England, July–December 2003 Versus January–June 2005

Caelyx (pegylated liposomal doxorubicin). The study also found substantial increases in the median usage rates (measured in terms of prescribed mg per 1,000 population) of all of the NICE-approved drugs under review. Figure 16.3 shows the percentage change in median usage rates of the drugs under review from the first study period (July to December 2003) to the second study period (January to June 2005). The percentage increases in the use of Temodal (temozolomide) (120%) and MabThera (rituximab) (87%) are particularly striking, but because of very limited usage in the first study period, the growth in consumption in absolute terms was relatively modest.

Government Agency Criticizes Inadequate Implementation of NICE Guidance

In September 2005, the Audit Commission published *Managing the Financial Implications of NICE Guidance*, a report based on research conducted in conjunction with the NICE. Data were gathered from site visits and from questionnaires sent to a range of bodies in the catchment areas of 10 strategic health authorities.

The review found that NICE's technology appraisals were generally implemented more consistently than the institute's clinical guidelines. The Audit Commission attributed the disappointing implementation of NICE's clinical guidelines to the difficulties of making the necessary "substantial changes to local care pathways, often involving both primary and secondary care" and to the fact that NHS bodies are not required to implement these guidelines.

The Audit Commission predicted that the implementation of the PbR system would improve compliance with NICE technology appraisals. PCTs will have incentives to comply with technology appraisals that are covered by the national tariff. As noted earlier, the annual health check will determine whether NHS bodies are meeting their PbR obligations – including implementation of NICE's technology appraisals and clinical guidelines.

The authors identified a number of areas that require attention to ensure that NICE guidance is fully implemented in the changing NHS. The report made the following key recommendations:

- Horizon scanning of NICE guidance should be undertaken systematically by NHS bodies. Draft guidance should be consulted to assess the current level of compliance and likely financial impact of implementation. This function can be shared across NHS bodies locally.
- NHS bodies should develop a clear understanding of what guidance is inside and outside the tariff and ensure that this understanding is consistent with that of other local bodies. Where guidance falls outside the PbR tariff, NHS bodies should undertake the appropriate negotiations to ensure that funds are provided to implement the guidance. These negotiations should cover all costs associated with implementation of the guidance, including capital costs.
- NICE, in conjunction with the [DH] PbR team, should indicate at draft stage whether guidance is likely to be inside or outside of the tariff, which will help with financial planning for the implementation of guidance.
- Cost templates should be used where available to estimate the costs of NICE guidance to the local health community.
- NICE should undertake activities to raise the awareness of cost templates and promote their use within NHS bodies.

PCTs should develop a system of monitoring to ensure that services paid for under PbR are provided, with individual treatment that conforms to NICE guidance.

Patient Action Against Lack of Access to Certain Drugs

In the short term, the creation of NICE has, paradoxically, hindered access to new drugs in parts of England and Wales. Many PCTs refuse to cover medicines that have not yet been reviewed by NICE – a phenomenon known as "NICE blight." In November 2005, NICE reported that "both patients and primary care trusts tell us PCTs will not pay until they have seen our guidance." Some patients afflicted with serious, or even life-threatening, diseases have protested against this situation by taking legal action against their local PCTs. Several lawsuits initiated by patients who were denied access to

Herceptin for the treatment of early-stage breast cancer have received particularly extensive media coverage in recent months.

Notwithstanding the fact that Herceptin was not yet approved for early-stage HER2-positive breast cancer, in November 2005, the DH indicated that PCTs should fund the drug for this indication on a case-by-case basis. Jane Kennedy, a junior health minister, went even further, suggesting that patients denied access to new cancer therapies should consider legal action against their PCTs if the patients believed the refusal of treatment to be "inappropriate."

Accelerated NICE Appraisal Process

The controversy over access to Herceptin likely played a role in the UK government's decision to implement measures to expedite NICE's appraisal of important new drugs. In November 2005, the DH and NICE announced the introduction of the single technology appraisal (STA) process to complement the standard NICE appraisal process in England and Wales. In the new procedure, manufacturers will submit a combined dossier for the purposes of registration and NICE appraisal, and these two processes will be conducted simultaneously. In addition, when comparing new drugs with established therapies, NICE will omit some of the usual consultations. NICE expects that the STA process should take an average of six months – far less than the current average of 18 months (and as much as three years in some cases) required for a conventional appraisal. As a result, it should generally be possible to publish a NICE appraisal based on the STA process within approximately eight weeks of a product's registration. Fourteen drugs – all but one of them cancer therapies – were nominated to be the first agents to undergo the STA process, but EuroGen Pharmaceuticals has subsequently withdrawn its licensing application for Orathecin (rubitecan). Table 16.7 lists the 13 remaining candidates for the STA process.

In February 2006, Roche submitted a dossier to NICE for appraisal of Herceptin in early-stage HER2-positive breast cancer even before it submitted its application for marketing authorization to the EMEA. NICE published the appraisal in August 2006 – six months after the submission of the dossier.

Off-label Prescribing

Prescribing medicines off label is, in theory, relatively straightforward in the United Kingdom. The *British National Formulary* (BNF) states that "unlicensed use of medicines becomes necessary if the clinical need cannot be met by licensed medicines; such use should be supported by appropriate evidence and experience." The BNF warns physicians that "prescribing medicines outside the recommendations of their marketing authorization alters (and probably increases) the doctor's professional responsibility."

In practice, however, off-label prescribing can be extremely difficult and inconsistent in the United Kingdom. As exemplified by the use of Herceptin in early-stage breast cancer, many PCTs refuse to fund off-label treatment, especially for new or risky therapeutic approaches. The typical rationale for such decisions is that it would be unethical to endorse unlicensed drug usage, but critics suggest that PCT decision makers are motivated more by financial than ethical considerations. PCTs' varying policies on off-label prescribing have contributed to the postcode lottery.

JAPAN

Enrollment in a social health insurance program is mandatory in Japan. Workers at large companies are covered by employee health insurance, while employees of small or midsize companies are covered by government-managed health insurance programs. Mutual aid associations insure government employees, and national health insurance (NHI) covers all other groups (e.g., the self-employed, farmers, the unemployed). Because of the rapid growth in the number of senior citizens in Japan, the government has made special provision for citizens aged 70 or older (health insurance for the elderly) and

Table 16.7 Candidates for Single Technology Appraisal in the United Kingdom

INN	*Brand Name*	*Marketing Companies*	*Indication*	*Original Publication Schedule*	*New Publication Schedule*
Atrasentan[a]	Xinlay	Abbott Laboratories	Hormone-refractory prostate cancer	N.A.	N.A.
Bortezomib	Velcade	Ortho-Biotech	Multiple myeloma	N.A.	July 2006
Cetuximab[a]	Erbitux	ImClone Systems/Merck KGaA	Locally advanced recurrent metastatic head and neck cancer	N.A.	N.A.
Docetaxel	Taxotere	Sanofi-Aventis	Early-stage breast cancer	February 2007	June 2006
Erlotinib	Tarceva	Roche/OSI Pharmaceuticals/ Genentech	Non-small-cell lung cancer	N.A.	N.A.
Ezetimibe	Ezetrol	Merck & Co./ Schering-Plough	Hyperlipidemia	N.A.	N.A.
Fludarabine	Fludara	Schering AG	Lymphocytic leukemia	June 2007	September 2006
Gemcitabine	Gemzar	Eli Lilly	Advanced metastatic breast cancer	April 2007	September 2006
Irinotecan[a]	Campto	Sanofi-Aventis	Pancreatic cancer	N.A.	N.A.
Paclitaxel	Taxol	Bristol-Myers Squibb	Early-stage breast cancer	February 2007	June 2006
Pemetrexed	Alimta	Eli Lilly	Non-small-cell lung cancer	N.A.	N.A.
Rituximab	MabThera	Roche	Non-Hodgkin's lymphoma	February 2007	June 2006
Trastuzumab	Herceptin	Roche	Early-stage breast cancer	N.A.	September 2006

[a]Subject to marketing authorization
INN = International nonproprietary name
N.A. = Data not available

Note: Rubitecan (EuroGen Pharmaceuticals' Orathecin) for pancreatic cancer was included in this list, but the manufacturer has subsequently withdrawn its licensing application

for families that care for elderly relatives at home (nursing care insurance).

All insured patients and their dependents are free to consult any physicians and to attend any type of medical facility; referral by a GP is not necessary. Many people prefer to seek treatment from a consultant at an outpatient department of a hospital rather than to visit their local primary care practice.

Cancer care in Japan is administered predominantly in the inpatient setting. A November 2002 survey of 1,635 Japanese hospitals found that only 16% had outpatient chemotherapy facilities at that time. A further 21% of surveyed hospitals had plans to establish outpatient chemotherapy facilities, but 63% of hospitals did not intend to introduce ambulatory care for cancer patients.

Pharmaceutical Pricing and Reimbursement

Japan's NHI system employs several different procedures for setting reimbursement prices for prescription drugs. Most new medicines in Japan are priced using a method known as *ruiji yakko hikaku hoshiki* (similar efficacy comparison method) in which a comparable drug that is already on the market is used as a pricing benchmark. Two forms of this method are used in setting prices. Similar efficacy comparison method I is used for drugs that are novel or at least have limited competition from existing therapies. Similar efficacy comparison method II is reserved for products that are deemed to lack novelty; this method is intended to set prices at a lower level than would be the case if similar efficacy comparison method I were used. Drugs priced by similar efficacy comparison method I may be granted price premiums if they are judged to be innovative or useful.

New oncology drugs are often priced by a method known as *genka keisan hoshiki* (cost calculation), a procedure that is used if no comparable drug is available in Japan. Cost calculation adds sales and administrative costs, operating profit, production costs, distribution costs, and other costs to the cost of manufacturing or importing the raw material. This procedure gives companies greater flexibility than the similar efficacy comparison.

Because new cancer therapies are generally already available in other major pharmaceutical markets, the prices settled on by the Ministry of Health, Labor, and Welfare (MHLW) are then modified under the "foreign price adjustment rule." Once a new drug's proposed price has been calculated, the MHLW determines the product's average public price in four reference markets – France, Germany, the United Kingdom, and the United States. If a drug's initial reimbursement price falls outside the range of 75–150% of the average foreign price, it is subject to the foreign price adjustment rule. For example, if the drug's initial reimbursement price is 151% of the average foreign price or greater, its price is reduced. Conversely, if its initial reimbursement price is 74% of the average foreign price or less, its price is increased. If a drug is already marketed in the United States, an upward adjustment in its Japanese reimbursement price is not uncommon.

Prospective Payment

In April 2003, the Japanese government introduced a new flat-sum reimbursement system – based on diagnosis-procedure combinations (DPCs) – for acute care of inpatients at 82 special function hospitals and other hospitals that provide advanced medical treatment. The mean fee-per-day determined for each diagnosis group is adjusted according to the mean length of stay at individual hospitals. The MHLW forecasts that, by the end of fiscal year 2006, 360 hospitals will have adopted the DPC system, with more expected to follow in the future. The pharmaceutical industry is concerned that DPC reimbursement might lead to inappropriate prescribing behavior. In an analysis published in June 2004, the Healthcare System Subcommittee of the Federation of Pharmaceutical Manufacturers' Associations of Japan (FPMAJ) suggested that "the expansion of the DPC system is acceptable only to the extent that it does not affect the proper use of drugs." The authors predicted that the DPC system will expand and warned that this trend "will necessarily make medical institutions more strongly concerned about the use of drugs." The DPC system is likely to prompt hospitals to increase their use of generics in order to reduce their drug acquisition costs. To this end, hospitals are introducing electronic prescribing systems that facilitate prescribing by international nonproprietary names.

The MHLW has ruled that, from July 2005, some expensive therapies (e.g., rituximab for non-Hodgkin's lymphoma) must be excluded from the DPC system and reimbursed on a fee-for-service basis. This decision was prompted by a sizable gap between the treatment costs as calculated in the DPC and the fee-for-service systems. Drugs that are more expensive than the DPC cost are funded by medical institutions, a situation that defeats the objective of the DPC system (i.e., cutting the costs of acute inpatient care). The MHLW suggests that such a situation is exceptional and transient, but it has not offered a clear solution to this problem. Therefore, it may be necessary to reserve some expensive therapies for use in the outpatient setting (where the DPC system is not used).

Unavailability of Gold-standard Therapies

Lack of access to international gold-standard cancer therapies has long been one of the main deficiencies of the Japanese oncology system. Novel anticancer drugs generally reach the market in Japan several years after their launch in other major pharmaceutical markets. The inadequate clinical development infrastructure of many pharmaceutical companies and a shortage of qualified reviewers have been major factors in the delayed launch of oncology drugs in Japan.

In an effort to accelerate the launch of important new drugs in Japan, in January 2005, the MHLW established an expert panel called the Mishoninyaku Shiyo Mondai Kentokaigi (Study Council on the Use of Unapproved Drugs). Drugs nominated for review by this council are assigned to one of three categories:

- Drugs approved in one or more of four major Western markets (i.e., France, Germany, the United Kingdom, and the United States) after April 2005.
- Drugs requested by academic societies and/or patient groups in the past five years and that are approved in any of the aforementioned Western markets.
- Drugs whose approval has not been requested by academic societies and/or patient groups, but that have been approved in any of the aforementioned Western markets in the last two years and are regarded as highly useful.

Drugs that meet these criteria do not automatically qualify for review by the council: preference is given to medicines that are regarded as innovative and/or first-in-class in Japan. As of July 2006, oncology drugs accounted for the majority of unapproved drugs on the agenda (Table 16.8).

Council members evaluate the clinical need for and scientific evidence in support of each candidate drug, and the details of these discussions (including the outcomes) are published on the Internet. The manufacturers of drugs recommended by the council are then petitioned by the MHLW either to begin clinical trials on these compounds or to conduct supplementary trials that would allow wider

Table 16.8 Cancer Therapies Reviewed by Japan's Study Council on the Use of Unapproved Drugs

Drug	*Status*	*Indication*	*Developer*
Oxaliplatin	Approved	Colorectal cancer	Yakult
Thalidomide	Application pending	Multiple myeloma	Fujimoto
Bortezomib	Preregistered	Multiple myeloma	Janssen
Pemetrexed	Preregistered	Non-small-cell lung cancer/mesothelioma	Eli Lilly
Bevacizumab	Preregistered	Metastatic colorectal cancer	Chugai
Cetuximab	Phase II	Metastatic colorectal cancer	Bristol-Myers Squibb/Merck &Co.
Erlotinib	Preregistered	Non-small-cell lung cancer	Chugai
Temozolomide	Approved	Malignant glioma	Schering-Plough
Streptozocin	None	Pancreatic islet cell carcinoma	Not yet determined
Ibritumomab tiuxetan	Preregistered	B-cell non-Hodgkin's lymphoma	Nihon Schering
Liposomal doxorubicin	Preparation for application	Ovarian cancer/AIDS-related Kaposi's sarcoma	Janssen
Clofarabine	None	Acute lymphoid leukemia (pediatric)	Not yet determined
Nelarabine	Preregistered	T-cell acute lymphoblastic leukemia, T-cell lymphoma	GlaxoSmithKline
Pegaspargase	None	Acute lymphoid leukemia	Not yet determined

Note: Status as of July 28, 2006

access to these agents before they are formally approved. A provision known as *tsuikateki shiken* (additional trials) allows patients who are not enrolled in regular clinical trials to use an unapproved drug in specific circumstances. Another type of supplementary trial – *anzensei kakunin shiken* (safety confirmation trials) – may be added to postapproval Phase III study. (In Japan, oncology drugs are generally approved on the basis of evidence of tumor shrinkage from Phase II clinical trials, but manufacturers of these agents must submit plans for postapproval Phase III studies.) Additional trials and safety confirmation trials are conducted in the following circumstances:

- The diagnosed disease is life-threatening, irreversible, and seriously damages patients' quality of life.
- No alternative therapy is available in Japan.
- The drug's efficacy and side-effect profiles are proven to be clinically superior to existing therapies.
- The drug is used as standard therapy in the United States and the major European countries.

Patients enrolled in these additional clinical trials can take advantage of a provision known as *tokutei-ryoyohi* (specified medical care coverage), whereby the public health insurance system covers all treatment costs except the cost of the product itself, which patients have to pay out of pocket. AstraZeneca took advantage of this provision when reimbursement terms were not settled in time for the launch of Iressa (gefitinib). Japanese physicians were eager to use the drug, and *tokutei-ryoyohi* enabled them to prescribe it without imposing an excessive financial burden on patients.

Not all medicines on the council's agenda are selected for clinical development with additional clinical trials. Drugs are prioritized according to their potential degree of novelty to the Japanese market. For example, the council recommended that the clinical development of the vascular endothelial growth factor inhibitor bevacizumab should be prioritized and an application submitted based on Phase I studies in Japan and foreign Phase II/III data. The council also called for safety confirmation trials to be conducted during the review period. As of July 2006, bevacizumab is in preregistration for metastatic colorectal cancer, with safety confirmation under way.

By comparison, the council did not recommend prioritizing the clinical development of Chugai's epidermal growth factor receptor inhibitor Tarceva (erlotinib), and additional trials will not be conducted until after approval is granted. This decision was based on erlotinib's second-to-market status (after gefitinib) in Japan. Moreover, Phase I trial data suggest that erlotinib has no advantages over gefitinib in terms of the occurrence of adverse events (notably interstitial pneumonia).

Most pharmaceutical companies that receive a request from the MHLW to begin clinical trials with a view to the approval of a drug in Japan, or to conduct additional trials, comply with the request. In the event that a chosen drug does not already have a developer in Japan, the compound may be assigned to investigator-initiated trials (i.e., trials that are conducted under the auspices of medical researchers, rather than manufacturers). However, given that Japan's infrastructure for the investigator-initiated trials remains underdeveloped, this option may not prove to be workable until the infrastructure for such trials improves significantly.

The creation of a new framework for drug approval is an attempt by the Japanese government to reconcile two opposing imperatives: patients' desire to have access to international gold-standard therapies as soon as possible and the need to maintain the safeguards provided by Japan's existing clinical trial system. The new framework has the potential to reduce the current substantial delay between the launch of innovative cancer therapies in other major pharmaceutical markets and Japan. However, the impact of the new framework in practice will depend largely on how effectively individual pharmaceutical companies conduct clinical development and submit applications in Japan. Given that the deliberations of the Study Council on the Use of Unapproved Drugs are published, pharmaceutical companies are likely to face vocal criticism from interested parties (especially patient organizations) if they do not expedite the development of drugs recommended by the council. To avoid such pressure, drug manufacturers need to strengthen their drug development capabilities in Japan.

Off-label Prescribing

Because the public health insurance system reimburses medicines only if they are prescribed for approved indications, Japanese physicians tend to avoid off-label use of oncology drugs – including some treatment options that are accepted as standard practice in the United States and Europe. In fact, patients in Japan who receive off-label therapy or treatment with drugs that are not yet approved in Japan may forfeit their right to reimbursement for all treatments for the prescribed indication, not just for the off-label or unregistered therapy. This can impose a heavy financial burden on patients.

Given these tough reimbursement restrictions, manufacturers of cancer therapies might pursue approval for additional indications for their drugs, but many companies appear content with the status quo. Although the public health insurance system forbids off-label reimbursement, individual institutions or payers may cover off-label prescribing to cancer patients on an ad hoc basis. Consequently, manufacturers have not been strongly motivated to spend time, energy, and money on pursuing additional indications for their oncology drugs.

To promote the approval of oncology drugs for broader indications, the MHLW established the Koganzai Heiyo Ryohoni Kansuru Kentokai (Committee for Combination Therapy With Anticancer Drugs) in December 2003. Considering suggestions from academic societies and/or patients' groups, a working group identifies drugs that could be used in additional indications and gathers evidence on the efficacy and safety of these drugs from the literature and other sources. The group then discusses the data with the relevant company. The Yakuji Shokuhin Eisei Shingikai (Council on Drugs and Food Sanitation [CDFS]) also evaluates the data that have been gathered; if it decides in favor of the additional indications, the MHLW asks the manufacturer to submit an application for the new indications.

These applications receive priority review, which takes approximately four months. Approval, if granted, is conditional on post-marketing safety measures. Drugs approved by this procedure are eligible for reimbursement under the aforementioned specified medical care coverage provision that covers all medical costs except the cost of the drug itself. This coverage is available from the time a candidate drug receives its preliminary evaluation from the CDFS.

Of the 61 therapies that the committee reviewed for use in additional indications, 7 proposed therapies had already reached an advanced stage in the regular approval process and therefore completed that process, and 21 therapies in great demand have undergone the new procedure for approval of additional indications. Table 16.9 shows that, by September 2005, all 21 of these therapies had been approved for additional indication(s). The remaining therapies were not judged to be in great demand and therefore were not approved through this framework. After completing its evaluation of the 21 therapies in great demand, the committee was dissolved in February 2005.

The committee is generally considered to have fulfilled its role to improve the status of off-label use of anticancer drugs. Some officers of the MHLW have suggested that the framework for off-label use drugs could continue after the dissolution of the committee, but no official announcement on future policy for off-label use of oncology agents has been made. Based on the perceived success of the Committee for Combination Therapy with Anticancer Drugs, we believe that the MHLW could set up a similar ad hoc committee in the future to handle off-label issues as they arise.

OUTLOOK AND IMPLICATIONS FOR THE PHARMACEUTICAL INDUSTRY

The enormous economic and social burden of cancer will continue to grow in line with

Table 16.9 Oncology Drugs Approved for Additional Indications in Japan

Drug	*Additional Indication*	*Date of Approval*
Doxorubicin/ cyclophosphamide (AC)	Breast cancer	February 2005/September 2005
Pamidronate	Breast cancer	November 2004
Ifosfamide	Soft tissue and bone sarcomas	February 2005
Doxorubicin	Soft tissue and bone sarcomas	February 2005
Ifosfamide/doxorubicin	Soft tissue and bone sarcomas	February 2005
Doxorubicin	Solid tumors of childhood	February 2005
Etoposide	Solid tumors of childhood	February 2005
Ifosfamide	Solid tumors of childhood	February 2005
Cisplatin	Osteosarcoma	February 2005
Doxorubicin/cisplatin (AP)	Endometrial cancer	February 2005
Cisplatin	Malignant lymphoma	September 2005
Vincristine, doxorubicin, dexamethazone (VAD)	Multiple myeloma	February 2005
5-Fluorouracil infusion	Head and neck cancer	February 2005
Procarbazine	Malignant astrocytoma/oligodendroglioma	February 2005
Vincristine	Malignant astrocytoma/oligodendroglioma	February 2005
Infusional 5-FU/l-LV	Colorectal cancer	February 2005
Cisplatin	Solid tumors of childhood	September 2005
Carboplatin	Solid tumors of childhood	September 2005
Actinomycin-D	Solid tumors of childhood	September 2005
Epirubicin (EC, CEF)	Breast cancer	September 2005
Dexamethasone	Chemotherapy-induced nausea and vomiting	September 2005

the increasing prevalence of this disease in the aging societies of Europe and Japan. Cancer patients in Europe and Japan have been largely insulated from the high costs of treating cancer, but national healthcare systems have had to bear this expense and will face difficult choices in the future. With manufacturers' pipelines bulging with new cancer therapies, including many potentially expensive biologic agents, controlling drug costs will undoubtedly be a high priority for national governments. In its analysis of patient access to cancer drugs, the Karolinska Institutet offered the following assessment of healthcare policy in Europe: "Although drug costs account for less than 10% of the total health care expenditure for cancer, it can be argued that because drug acquisition costs can be easier to identify and calculate, they become a greater focus for cost control than some of the more general (and more difficult to calculate) costs of cancer health care."

The implementation of prospective payment systems is a key element in many governments' cost-containment strategies. At present, the impact of this measure is largely limited to inpatient treatment, but some governments have declared their intent to expand this initiative to hospital outpatient treatment and even to the primary care sector. The expansion of prospective payment systems could present manufacturers with an awkward dilemma: should they price new drugs on a par with established therapies to ensure that they do not exceed DRG reimbursement rates or risk limiting the uptake of their products by setting higher prices? In theory, most prospective payment systems offer additional payments for costly new therapies until DRGs are adjusted to take account of increased costs, but securing such funding may prove difficult in practice.

Accommodating a host of new oncology drugs in relatively rigid prospective payment systems will be a challenging task. Targeted therapies are likely to be particularly expensive, but overall costs will be limited by the restricted populations in which these agents will be used. Horizon scanning and advance budgetary planning at national and local levels will become increasingly important. The biopharmaceutical industry must recognize this need and find ways to support this process.

The prospect of extensive off-label prescribing of a multitude of new therapies would worry all payers. Governments in Europe and Japan have acknowledged a valuable role for appropriate off-label use, but they are likely to intensify restrictions on prescribing that is deemed to be unsuitable. Manufacturers will play an important part in providing evidence to support the use of their drugs for indications that are not yet licensed.

Biopharmaceutical companies will need to adjust to an environment that places growing emphasis on the use of health economics and health technology assessment (HTA) in reimbursement decision making. The United Kingdom has been a pioneer in this field, but other countries are following suit. France's HAS and Germany's Institut für Qualität und Wirtschaftlichkeit im Gesundheitswesen (IQWiG; Institute for Quality and Economy in the Healthcare System) have recently agreed on a collaboration with NICE, and Italy's AIFA publicizes NICE judgments.

The recent decline in the role of inpatient cancer care will continue, and probably accelerate. Increasingly, patients will receive chemotherapy in hospital outpatient departments, specialist oncology centers, and office-based chemotherapy facilities. Other countries may also follow the French example in supporting home hospitalization. In addition, the launch of growing numbers of drugs that have self-injectable or oral dosage forms will greatly facilitate the administration of treatments by patients or their relatives.

The promotion of integrated care will stimulate closer collaboration between primary and secondary care sectors. A growing range of healthcare professionals will be involved in treating cancer patients. In some countries (e.g., Germany and the United Kingdom), DM programs will be used to coordinate the care provided by multiple practitioners. If other countries perceive this policy to be successful, they will likely follow suit.

In all of the countries under review, more extensive and effective screening programs will result in earlier detection and treatment of cancer. This trend will offer a valuable opportunity for the biopharmaceutical industry. Drug therapy will make an essential contribution to the treatment of early-stage cancer.

In the future, manufacturers may have to reconcile themselves to lower prices for new cancer drugs. Until recently, innovative treatments for particular cancers have faced little competition, but the launch of additional drugs for the same indications will profoundly alter the dynamics of the market. In the United States, Amgen recently decided to launch Vectibix (panitumumab), a treatment for colorectal cancer, at a price approximately 20% below that of ImClone Systems' more established Erbitux (cetuximab). Similarly, Genentech has decided to cap the annual cost of Avastin (bevacizumab).

In the longer term, the launch of biosimilar versions of cancer biologics will accelerate price erosion. Physicians may have certain reservations about the bioequivalence of these products, but payers will strongly promote their use. It will be interesting to see if Germany – and possibly some other European countries – considers including oncology biosimilars in reference-pricing systems.

Cancer will be an increasing public health priority in Europe and Japan, and national cancer plans demonstrate the importance that governments attach to tackling this politically sensitive disease. Lobbying by patient organizations and medical societies could help to improve access to innovative therapies. Given the wealth of new treatments in development, the biopharmaceutical industry has the opportunity to be seen as the patients' champion. However, if companies seriously misjudge their pricing and reimbursement strategies in this therapeutic area, the industry could easily be cast as the villain of the piece.

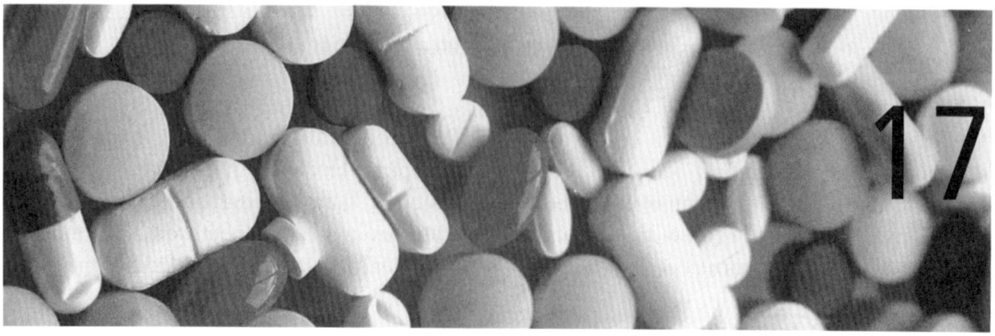

17

The Pharmaceutical Pricing and Reimbursement Environment in China

INTRODUCTION

Given its sizeable population and rapid urbanization, China represents a potentially lucrative market for drug manufacturers. The size of the country makes its position in the worldwide pharmaceutical market difficult to gauge. Currently the ninth largest pharmaceutical market in the world, China's pharmaceutical market is valued at $12 billion, while the Chinese government claims the number is $55 billion. But, among other factors, the lure of marketing drugs in China is tempered by China's pharmaceutical pricing and reimbursement system. Drug prices are largely controlled by the Chinese government, and mark-ups on drug prices at the retail level threaten to make some drugs unaffordable. Insurance schemes as they currently exist vary greatly by location. These differences vary from province to province, but also within provinces, as urban health insurance schemes find themselves better funded than the options given to rural residents. In this chapter, we begin with a brief overview of China's current healthcare system. We then look at the rules and regulations governing the pricing of pharmaceuticals in China, the insurance schemes currently in place to cover drugs marketed in China, and assess the major issues going forward that will affect the pricing and reimbursement of drugs in China.

OVERVIEW OF CHINA'S HEALTHCARE SYSTEM

Providing healthcare to more than 1 billion people living in widely divergent regions, both geographically and economically, is a constant challenge in China. The country's current healthcare system is characterized by huge disparities in the availability and quality of healthcare services between the towns and cities of the more affluent east coast, south-central, and capital region and the largely agrarian rural areas. Government funding of healthcare in China is among the lowest of any nation in the world; the patient pays for most of his or her healthcare costs. Even though China has approximately 300,000 hospitals, clinics, and health centers, these institutions are largely self-funded and earn a high percentage of their income through fees paid by patients for services and treatments. This funding structure is a barrier to medical care for many people because approximately 45% of the urban population and 80% of the rural population do not have health insurance and must pay for medical services out of pocket.

When the People's Republic of China was formed in 1949, the government instituted a public healthcare system modeled on that of the Soviet Union. This three-tier system provided healthcare services at the provincial, city or prefecture, and county levels. All hospitals were publicly funded and physicians were employees of the state, resulting in the dissolution of private hospitals and private practices. In rural areas, the Cooperative Medical System, managed and funded by the communes that owned and operated the farms and supplied social services, was established to provide basic healthcare to the rural population, many of whom were extremely poor.

Although urban areas still had higher-quality care and more highly trained healthcare providers on a per-capita basis than did the rural areas, the rural population did have medical coverage through the Cooperative Medical System, which offered prevention, treatment, and health maintenance through the use of "barefoot physicians," local residents (often farmers) who were given one to two years of training in basic medical procedures. These physicians provided Western and Chinese medicine and administered basic public health service. Barefoot physicians were poorly paid and supplemented their income through the sales of drugs to their patients. As a result, many of these providers overprescribed medicines, and it was quite common, for example, for children to receive an injection for something as simple as a cold.

From the 1950s through the early 1980s, China made tremendous progress in healthcare services through this highly centralized system of administration. The "Chinese model" made gains in controlling infectious diseases such as malaria and schistosomiasis and earned the praise of both the World Health Organization and the World Bank.

A series of reforms begun in the 1980s focused on the privatization of China's economy and decentralization of government. These reforms diverted government spending from healthcare to programs designed to stimulate the economy, which largely benefited urban areas. From 1978 to 1999, the central government's share of healthcare spending dropped from 32% to 15%, and the emphasis for funding shifted to taxes levied by provincial and local authorities. Health centers and hospitals were given a fixed subsidy from taxes but were free to generate additional revenue by charging fees for services and high-tech healthcare and by earning a profit on drug prescriptions. This system favored the wealthier eastern coastal towns and provinces over less-affluent rural areas and incentivized hospitals to provide profitable services and prescribe drugs that were often not necessary to cover their costs. Hence, public hospitals came to function akin to that of profit making, privatized units.

As China privatized its economy, it dismantled the agricultural communes and forced rural villages to fund their own services. Because the rural economy was in no position to fund healthcare, the Cooperative Medical System rapidly dissolved, resulting in 900 million rural and mostly peasant Chinese having no medical coverage because healthcare expenses were too costly. Many barefoot physicians became unemployed and were forced to become private healthcare practitioners, providing a service for which they had very little training. Selling drugs became a more lucrative means of support and resulted in steadily increasing drug prices in rural China, further diminishing the rural population's access to healthcare.

Also during the 1980s, in order to stimulate a profit-driven healthcare structure, the government revised the price system of health services. While continuing tight controls on hospital and clinic charges for routine visits, services, and commonplace pharmaceuticals, facilities were permitted to earn profits from new drugs, new tests, and high technology; profit margins were 15% and above. In addition, hospital physicians' salaries were modified to include bonuses linked to revenue they generated within their hospitals. This new structure resulted in a massive increase in the sale of expensive pharmaceuticals and high-tech services and increases in healthcare spending and prices, particularly in urban areas, where a portion of the population could afford such services. Unfortunately, funding the acquisition of the most recent technology often occurred at the expense of reducing funding for the expansion of basic preventive medical services.

In 2000, the Healthcare Reform Act established a two-tier system of healthcare delivery, creating a distinction between private (for-profit) and public (nonprofit) hospitals. In 2005, for-profit institutions made up about 10% of all healthcare establishments; most of these large, well-equipped hospitals are in cities such as Beijing, Jiangsu, Zheijiang, and Shanghai. These cities, home to more than 10% of the nation's population, account for 25% of total national health expenditures.

Despite these changes, disparities still exist between urban and rural communities and between those who can afford private health insurance and those who cannot. Certain government agencies and private entities offer employee-based medical insurance, and the government funds a basic medical insurance program for the urban poor. Together, these programs cover approximately 45% of the urban population, and an additional 10% purchase private insurance. In the rural areas, only 20% of the population has health insurance, and half of that group is insured through private or other forms of insurance. In spite of increasing insurance levels, though, responsibility for healthcare funding still lies inordinately with the individual. In comparison, governments in developed countries typically fund more than 70% of the healthcare spending in their country.

OVERVIEW OF PHARMACEUTICAL PRICING AND REIMBURSEMENT IN CHINA

Current Pharmaceutical Pricing Regulations in China

The two decades between 1980 and 2000 – a time of great economic and healthcare reform in China – saw the Chinese government controlling the prices of drugs from manufacturer to retailer. The government followed a basic formula when calculating the prices of pharmaceutical products: ex-manufacturer prices were determined by taking the production costs of a drug and adding a 5% markup; the wholesale price was determined by adding a 15% markup to the ex-manufacturer price; and the retail price was calculated by adding 15% to the wholesale price.

During the same time period, the costs for medical services were reduced, yet the government expected hospitals to remain profitable. The main avenue for hospital profitability then became the dispensing of pharmaceuticals (approximately 85% of pharmaceutical dispensing occurs at hospitals rather than independent retailers). Because both retailers (including hospitals) and wholesalers made their profits on pharmaceuticals from a fixed percentage allowed by the government, these two parties began to favor higher-priced products. Manufacturers, hoping to capitalize on this preference, pressured the government to increase prices for their products to attract the attention of wholesalers and retailers. Some observers speculate that physicians also overprescribed drugs to increase hospital profits, a trend that drained the government-funded insurance schemes that covered urban workers' medical costs.

To help curb the problem of soaring pharmaceutical prices, the Chinese government changed its pricing policy at the end of 2000 from absolute control over the pricing of pharmaceutical products at every level to setting retail prices for certain cost-effective, commonly prescribed drugs.

The current rules governing the pricing of pharmaceutical products in China can be found in two publications: the "Drug Administration Law of the People's Republic of China" and the "Regulations for the Implementation of the Drug Administration Law of the People's Republic of China."

Article 48 of "Regulations for the Implementation of the Drug Administration Law of the People's Republic of China" stipulates the three ways in which drugs are priced in China:

- Fixed by the government.
- Guided by the government.
- Regulated by the market.

The National Development and Reform Commission (formerly known as the State Commission of Development and Planning) used the National Essential Drug List (NEDL) (which includes the drugs for which government reimbursement is available) when deciding which drugs it would set prices for.

The NEDL has two groups of drugs. Type A drugs have prices fixed by the central government. These retail prices are the highest prices a retailer may charge for the drug. The prices of Type B drugs are not "fixed" by the central government but rather "guided" by the government. These guiding prices set by the central government are used by the provincial governments, which are allowed to adjust the guiding retail prices 5% higher or lower.

Drugs for which the prices are neither set nor guided by the government must comply with Article 56 of the drug administration law, which states that drug prices must be established "on the principles of fairness, rationality, good faith, and commensuration of price with quality, in order to provide the users with drugs of reasonable prices." The article also prohibits "usurious profits and fraud in pricing" in its guidance.

For drugs subject to governmental pricing, the retail price of a drug is determined using the following formula: retail price = ex-manufacturer price (or, in the case of an imported drug, the port price) inclusive of taxes × (1 + distribution price differential). The distribution price differential takes into account costs and profits of wholesalers and retailers; drugs with higher prices use differentials on the low end of the scale, and drugs with lower prices use a higher rate.

Regarding premium pricing in China, if the manufacturer of a drug subject to governmental pricing believes that its drug is more efficacious, safer, or more cost effective than other drugs in its class, the manufacturer can apply for special pricing with the Chinese government.

Until recently, retailers have been allowed to mark up the price of pharmaceuticals 15% from the wholesale price. As of June 2006, however, the government forbids public hospitals from selling pharmaceuticals at prices above 15% of the ex-manufacturer price.

Comparison of Pharmaceutical Prices per Pill in China versus G7 Prices per Pill

It is important to note that China's currency, the renminbi (RMB), is considered by many economists and governments to be undervalued. Although the RMB was once fixed to the US dollar – meaning it did not appreciate or depreciate in response to market forces – on July 21, 2005, the RMB became "adjustable," although the Chinese government set the maximum amount the RMB can raise or fall each day at 0.3%. The inflexibility of the RMB means that exports from China will be less expensive and imports into the country (including pharmaceuticals) will be more expensive. In August 2005, Bloomberg reported that US legislators believed that the RMB was undervalued by 40% (Bloomberg.com, August 4, 2005).

Figures 17.1–17.3 express exmanufacturer prices of select brand-name drugs used to treat type 2 diabetes, hypertension, and dyslipidemia in China and the seven major pharmaceutical markets (United States, France, Germany, Italy, Spain, United Kingdom, and Japan) as percentages of US prices. Where applicable in China, we

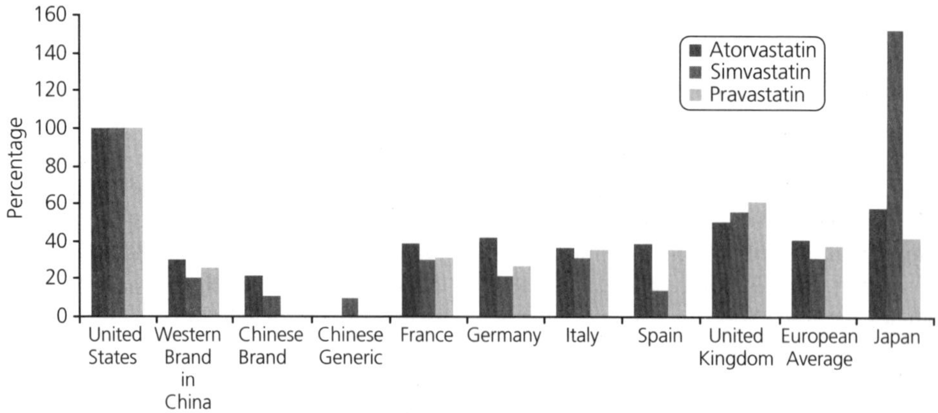

Notes: Strengths priced: atorvastatin (10 mg); simvastatin (20 mg); pravastatin (20 mg). Generic Chinese versions of atorvastatin and pravastatin not available in our data. Chinese brand version of pravastatin not available in our data. European average equals the average price of a molecule in France, Germany, Italy, Spain, and the United Kingdom

Figure 17.1 Average Exmanufacturer Prices of Three Leading Statins as a Percentage of US Prices in the United States, China, Europe, and Japan

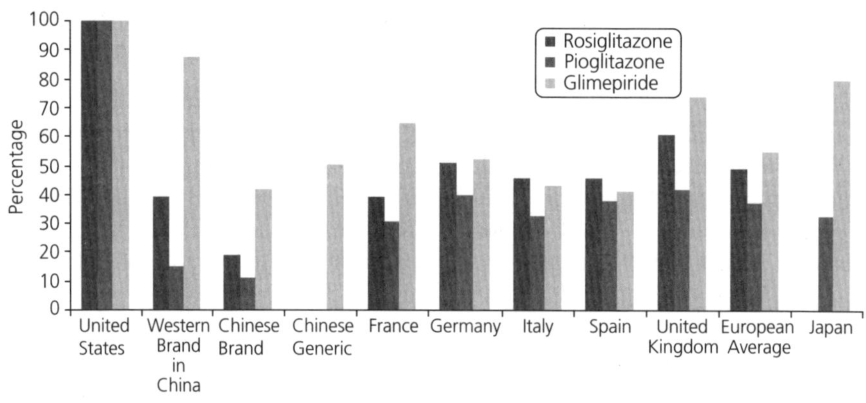

Notes: Strengths priced: rosiglitazone (4 mg); pioglitazone (30 mg); glimepiride (2 mg). Variation in dosing: 15 mg pioglitazone priced for Western brand in China and Chinese brand. Generic Chinese versions of rosiglitazone and pioglitazone not available in our data. Rosiglitazone not available in Japan. European average equals the average price of a molecule in France, Germany, Italy, Spain, and the United Kingdom

Figure 17.2 Average Exmanufacturer Prices of Three Leading Oral Antidiabetics as a Percentage of US Prices in the United States, China, Europe, and Japan

compared the prices of Western brands marketed in China, Chinese brands, and Chinese generics. While not every drug examined has a Western brand in China, a Chinese brand, or a Chinese generic, this does not mean that such drugs are not available in China, but rather may indicate a lack of available data. The Chinese brand prices and Chinese generic prices are averages of the prices of the drug at identical strengths but produced by different manufacturers.

Figures 17.1–17.3 cover three types of drugs: oral antidiabetics to treat type 2 diabetes; statins to treat dyslipidemia; and

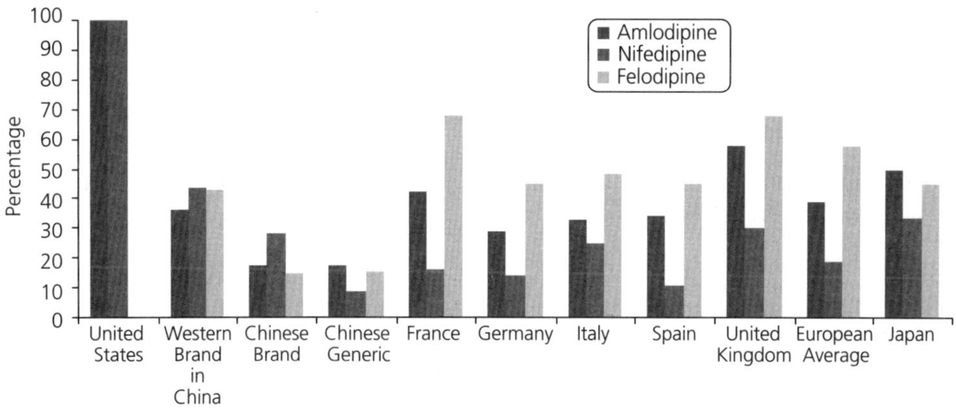

Notes: Strengths priced: amlodipine (5 mg); nifedipine (20 mg); felodipine (5 mg). Variations in strength priced: nifepidine (30 mg) priced for Western and Chinese brands in China. European average equals the average price of a molecule in France, Germany, Italy, Spain, and the United Kingdom

Figure 17.3 Average Exmanufacturer Prices of Three Leading Calcium-Channel Blockers as a Percentage of US Prices in the United States, China, Europe, and Japan

calcium-channel blockers to treat hypertension. In each drug type, we chose three drugs to compare, based on the prescribing patterns of interviewed Chinese physicians.

While, on average, the ex-manufacturer prices of Western brand pharmaceuticals marketed in China were lower than the prices in the United States, Europe, and Japan, European countries whose drug prices are typically lower when compared to the other major markets (e.g., Italy and Spain) occasionally saw the ex-manufacturer prices of Western brand pharmaceuticals at lower levels than in China. Also, the prices of Western brand pharmaceuticals in China occasionally surpass the average price of the same drugs in the five European countries under study (e.g., nifedipine in Figure 17.3).

Also of note is the fact that in the markets in which multiple versions of a drug exist in China, significant price competition exists among the Western brand, the Chinese brand, and the Chinese generic. In fact, in most cases, the Chinese generic price is equal to or greater than the Chinese brand price. In contrast, in the United States, generic prices are usually significantly lower than their brand-name counterparts. One possible explanation for this phenomenon could be the fact that hospitals – the main dispensers of prescription drugs in China – need to be profitable. Because prescription drugs are an area in which high margins can be made, physicians may prescribe a more expensive drug in order to gain a higher profit on the sale. In this case, in order to be competitive in the market, generic drugs may be priced closer to brand-name drugs to gain more market share. This pricing pattern was confirmed by our interviews with physicians, who stated that in some cases the price differential between branded drugs and generics was not sufficient incentive to prescribe the generic drug.

Drug Class Price Comparisons from Exmanufacturer to Retail Level in China

In order to examine whether any manufacturers have a pharmaceutical pricing strategy in China, we examined the prices of leading drugs in various classes at both the ex-manufacturer and retail levels. Our retail prices were obtained from the published prices of one of China's largest hospitals, Peking Union Medical College (PUMC) Hospital. To compare the prices of the drugs, and elicit any manufacturer pricing strategy, we expressed the drugs in each class as a percentage of the highest-priced drug in each class (hence, the highest-priced therapy in each category is invariably 100%). Some drugs for which ex-manufacturer prices were available were not available at PUMC hospital, so comparisons between ex-manufacturer and retail prices were not possible for certain drugs.

Table 17.1 compares exmanufacturer prices of drugs in different classes, expressed as percentages of the highest-priced drugs in each respective class. Table 17.2 compares retail prices of drugs in different classes,

Table 17.1 Exmanufacturer Prices in China as a Percentage of Leading Drug in Each Class

Class/Product	*Strength*	*Price per Pill (%)*
Angiotensin II receptor antagonists (fixed-dose combinations)		
Merck's Hyzaar	Combo	100
Sanofi-Aventis's Coaprovel	Combo	79
Angiotensin II receptor antagonists		
Merck's Cozaar	50 mg	100
Novartis's Diovan	80 mg	96
Takeda's Blopress	8 mg	87
Boehringer Ingelheim's Micardis	80 mg	80
Sanofi-Aventis's Aprove!	150 mg	74
Cholesterol and triglyceride reducers		
Pfizer's Lipitor	20 mg	100
Bristol-Myers Squibb's Pravachol	20 mg	80
Merck's Zocor	20 mg	70
Novartis's Lescol	40 mg	45
Fournier's Lipanthyl	200 mg	42
Calcium-channel blockers		
Pfizer's Norvasc	5 mg	100
Bayer's Adalat	30 mg	90
AstraZeneca's Plendil	5 mg	67
Angiotensin-converting enzyme inhibitors		
Bristol-Myers Squibb's Monopril	10 mg	100
Novartis's Lotensin	10 mg	100
Merck's Renitec	5 mg	94
AstraZeneca's Zestril	10 mg	90
Sanofi-Aventis's Tritace	2.5 mg	67
Oral antidiabetics		
GlaxoSmithKline's Avandia	4 mg	100
Takeda's Actos	15 mg	74
Novartis's Starlix	120 mg	32
Sanofi-Aventis's Amaryl	1 mg	30
Bayer's Glucobay	50 mg	22
Takeda's Basen	0.2 mg	19
Bristol-Myers Squibb's Glucophage	500 mg	14
Pfizer's Minidiab	5 mg	8
Beta blockers		
Roche's Dilatrend	6.25 mg	100
Sumitomo's Almarl	10 mg	81
Merck KGaA's Concor	5 mg	70
Bristol-Myers Squibb's Sotacor	80 mg	37
AstraZeneca's Betaloc	50 mg	13
Recombinant human insulins		
Novo Nordisk's Novolin	All strengths	100
Eli Lilly's Humulin	All strengths	92

Table 17.2 Retail Prices in China's PUMC Hospital as a Percentage of Leading Drug in Each Class

Class/Product	*Strength*	*Retail Price per Pill (%)*
Angiotensin II receptor antagonists		
Merck's Cozaar	50 mg	100
Novartis's Diovan	80 mg	94
Boehringer Ingelheim's Micardis	80 mg	79
Sanofi-Aventis's Aprovel	150 mg	74
Cholesterol and triglyceride reducers		
Pfizer's Lipitor	20 mg	100
Bristol-Myers Squibb's Pravachol	20 mg	84
Merck's Zocor	20 mg	74
Novartis's Lescol	40 mg	48
Fournier's Lipanthyl	200 mg	45
Calcium-channel blockers		
Pfizer's Norvasc	5 mg	100
Bayer's Adalat	30 mg	94
AstraZeneca's Plendil	5 mg	68
Angiotensin-converting enzyme inhibitors		
Novartis's Lotensin	10 mg	100
Bristol-Myers Squibb's Monopril	10 mg	99
Merck's Renitec	5 mg	92
Sanofi-Aventis's Tritace	2.5 mg	90
Oral antidiabetics		
GlaxoSmithKline's Avandia	4 mg	100
Sanofi-Aventis's Amaryl	1 mg	31
Bayer's Glucobay	50 mg	22
Takeda's Basen	0.2 mg	20
Bristol-Myers Squibb's Glucophage	500 mg	14
Pfizer's Minidiab	5 mg	6
Beta blockers		
Roche's Dilatrend	6.25 mg	100
Sumitomo's Almarl	10 mg	84
Merck KGaA's Concor	5 mg	69
Bristol-Myers Squibb's Sotacor	80 mg	37
AstraZeneca's Betaloc	50 mg	13
Recombinant human insulins		
Novo Nordisk's Novolin	All strengths	100
Eli Lilly's Humulin	All strengths	100

Note: Some drugs from Table 17.1 are not included here because they are not available at PUMC Hospital

expressed as percentages of the highest-priced drugs in each respective class. Table 17.3 presents the price mark-up that each drug underwent from the ex-manufacturer level to retail level.

Of note, the leading ex-manufacturer drug prices in Table 17.1 were predominantly the same as the leading retail drug prices in Table 17.2. This suggests that price mark-ups throughout the distribution of drugs from the manufacturer to the retailer were applied in a uniform manner to all drugs, regardless of initial price. Additionally, as seen in Tables 17.1 and 17.2, price differences between drugs in each class were roughly the same in nearly every case at both the ex-manufacturer and the retail level, implying even more uniformity of mark-ups, since percentages of the differential remained basically constant.

Table 17.3 shows that mark-ups to drug prices from the exmanufacturer level to the retail level ranged from 14% to 127%; however, mark-up percentages predominantly were increases between 65% and 80%. In the coming months, it will be of interest to note if the Chinese government's recent declaration that public hospitals can no

Table 17.3 Percentage Mark-up in China from Exmanufacturer to Retail Prices

Class/Product	*Strength*	*Price Increase, per Pill (%)*
Angiotensin II receptor antagonists		
Merck's Cozaar	50 mg	73
Sanofi-Aventis's Aprovel	150 mg	73
Novartis's Diovan	80 mg	70
Cholesterol and triglyceride reducers		
Fournier's Lipanthyl	200 mg	76
Novartis's Lescol	40 mg	74
Bristol-Myers Squibb's Pravachol	20 mg	73
Merck's Zocor	20 mg	72
Pfizer's Lipitor	20 mg	64
Calcium-channel blockers		
Bayer's Adalat	30 mg	83
AstraZeneca's Plendil	5 mg	77
Pfizer's Norvasc	5 mg	74
Angiotensin-converting enzyme inhibitors		
Sanofi-Aventis's Tritace	2.5 mg	127
Novartis's Lotensin	10 mg	71
Bristol-Myers Squibb's Monopril	10 mg	69
Merck's Renitec	5 mg	67
Oral antidiabetics		
Bristol-Myers Squibb's Glucophage	500 mg	75
Takeda's Basen	0.2 mg	73
Bayer's Glucobay	50 mg	70
Sanofi-Aventis's Amaryl	1 mg	70
GlaxoSmithKline's Avandia	4 mg	67
Pfizer's Minidiab	5 mg	14
Beta blockers		
Sumitomo's Almarl	10 mg	76
AstraZeneca's Betaloc	50 mg	74
Roche's Dilatrend	6.25 mg	71
Bristol-Myers Squibb's Sotacor	80 mg	70
Merck KGaA's Concor	5 mg	68
Recombinant human insulins		
Eli Lilly's Humulin	All strengths	86
Novo Nordisk's Novolin	All strengths	71

longer charge over 15% of the ex-manufacturer price will drive down the mark-up percentages shown here.

Looking at Tables 17.1–17.3, no manufacturer has a clear pricing strategy in China. No single manufacturer is consistently pricing its products the highest or the lowest in the drug classes represented, although Merck placed in the top-three highest-priced drugs in three of the drug classes in Tables 17.1–17.3.

National Essential Drug List

The basis for pharmaceutical reimbursement in China is the NEDL. The first version of the NEDL was approved in China in 1982 (Hu S, 2001). It was created as a cost-containment measure for government insurance schemes (GISs).

The NEDL is organized by China's Ministry of Labor and Social Security (MOLSS) and is updated biennially. The last update occurred in 2004; it expanded the list to include more than 1,000 Western drugs and more than 800 traditional Chinese medicines. A product must meet five criteria to be included in the list: clinical need, safety, efficacy, whether the product is "reasonable" as a therapy, and availability. As mentioned previously, the NEDL is divided into two categories: Type A products and Type B products.

In terms of reimbursement, Type A products are products for which greater reimbursement is given and are chosen on the basis of three characteristics: efficacy, lower prices, and safety profile. On the national level, Type A drugs are typically reimbursed 100%. Type B products do not allow full reimbursement. Agents are placed in this category because although they are clinically effective, less-expensive alternatives are available.

In addition, although the list of drugs in the Type A category is set by the central government and cannot be removed, the Type B drugs on a particular province's drug list can be substituted by the provincial government. Local governments cannot have Type B drug lists where more than 15% of the drugs included in the list vary from the list provided by the central government. Provincial governments can adjust reimbursement amounts for products in the list, provided they do not stray too far from the central government recommendations. Ultimately, reimbursement levels likely vary based on how well a particular health plan is funded.

The government has a three-stage process when updating the drug list every two years. Stage 1 is a preliminary stage in which a search for panel members occurs, new products and therapies are selected for consideration, and the process by which the previous list was selected is reviewed. Private entities, including members of the pharmaceutical industry, are also allowed to give input at this stage.

Stage 2 brings together the central panel – consisting of health officials from various ministries and scientists – to come up with a draft, which is then reviewed by the Ministry of Health, National Development and Reform Commission, and TCM Administration for approval. Provincial governments also review the draft for comment and submit changes to the central government.

Step 3 is the final step, in which the list is published and provincial governments are trained in how to enforce the list. Inclusion in the NEDL is very important for pharmaceutical companies because exclusion from the list means health insurance plans will not reimburse a drug. It is also important to note that even if a drug has been through clinical trials in markets outside of China, the drug must undergo clinical trials in China before it can be added to the NEDL; this rule applies to both branded drugs and generics. In addition, a drug must meet the requirement of being a cost-effective product in the Chinese market for two years before it is eligible for addition to the NEDL.

Health Insurance Plans in China

The landscape of healthcare reimbursement in China has changed dramatically in the past few decades. The former rural cooperative medical system collapsed as a result of China's transition from a fixed market to a free market, leaving millions of rural Chinese without reimbursement for their medical costs. In addition, as a result of rising medical costs and expenditures, China's urban health insurance mainstays – the GIS and the Labor Insurance Scheme (LIS) – have introduced more cost-sharing measures, and some have neglected to provide promised reimbursement for medical treatment at all owing to a lack of funds. In this section, we examine the key payers in the Chinese market today – both urban and rural – and briefly conclude with some projections on coverage in the future.

Urban Health Insurance

There are three major types of health insurance in urban China today: the GIS, the LIS, and the Urban Basic Medical Insurance (BMI) System.

The beneficiaries of the GIS are government employees and retirees, disabled veterans, teachers, and university students. Dependents of GIS beneficiaries do not receive benefits under the program. Prior to 1980, the central government controlled the entire GIS budget. After 1980, individual government agencies managed the budget given to them by the central government. If an individual agency goes over its allotted healthcare budget, it is responsible for making up the deficit through its own operating budget or it must raise the funds in some other way. Traditionally, the GIS offers the best reimbursement rates, which can vary by the individual agency.

The LIS is an insurance system for the employees and retirees of state-owned enterprises (SOEs). Limited coverage is offered to the dependents of beneficiaries. SOEs with at least 100 employees are required to offer LIS to their employees, and the system is a voluntary offering for SOEs with fewer than 100 employees and some collective-owned industries. Each SOE finances its own insurance plan by setting aside a pretax amount equaling 11–14% of the SOE's total wages, and SOEs incurring more health costs than the money they put aside pay the difference themselves out of after-tax profits.

The GIS and LIS systems traditionally offered very comprehensive coverage with minimal cost-sharing requirements; therefore, when healthcare costs began to rise in a freer market, employees did not feel the sting of high costs, continued to overuse medical services, and felt no need to find the most cost-effective resources. However, rising healthcare costs caused many enterprises and agencies to run deficits, and they became unable to pay for employees' medical costs. In addition, dwindling funds due to increased spending on healthcare prevented many enterprises and agencies from effectively operating in a more competitive environment as profits dwindled. Many reforms were enacted as early as the 1980s to rework the urban insurance market to compensate for rising medical expenditure.

Many GIS and LIS reforms tried to stop rising medical costs through cost-sharing initiatives. The most significant to date was announced by the State Council in 1998, which introduced the BMI. The goal of the government is to replace the GIS and LIS with this new system in major cities.

Under the BMI, instead of government agencies and SOEs assuming all the costs and risks associated with healthcare, employees of governmental agencies and SOEs are responsible for the partial funding of their own healthcare costs. And for the first time, private sector employees in urban areas are covered. Under the BMI, each eligible employee contributes 2% of his or her salary to a personal medical savings account (MSA). The employer then divides 6% of the employee's wages into two accounts: 1.8% goes into the employee's MSA and 4.2% goes into a social risk pool (SRP) fund that is funded by all employees of that particular company/agency/enterprise. Although there is some variation as to how the benefits of each BMI plan are structured, a typical plan uses the employee's MSA to cover the employee's own outpatient medical service costs. Once the MSA is depleted, the employee pays the remainder of his/her outpatient services for the year out-of-pocket, although if the employee has remaining funds in the MSA at the end of the year, the balance can be carried over to the next year. The SRP fund is used by employees for inpatient services only after a deductible (10% of the employee's yearly wages) is reached; the SRP covers an employee up to four times the average wage of an employee in their city. After the employee pays the deductible and is drawing from the SRP, the employee is often required to pay some sort of coinsurance as well. After coverage is maxed out, the employee either must pay expenses out of pocket or through a supplementary insurance plan offered by his/her employer or private insurance.

Although the GIS and LIS systems are proposed to be phased out in favor of BMI, they are still in existence. In addition to these three systems, supplemental medical insurance is available for urban residents.

A medical subsidy for civil servants is offered so that their benefits under the BMI system will not be less than the benefits they obtained under the GIS system. A civil servant's subsidy is financed by the level of government in which he or she works.

The medical financial assistance (MFA) program is an early-stage program available to urban and rural poor residents in China who meet certain criteria in their respective geographic areas. There is no national policy on the implementation of MFA, so different cities and counties run their own programs. In addition to helping the urban poor, MFA covers the employees of urban enterprises who are not, by definition, poor but whose current financial standing prevents an employee from contributing to the BMI.

There is also a growing market for private insurance in China in both urban and rural areas. Private insurance has enjoyed a rise in popularity because of the declining coverage under the GIS, LIS, and BMI, as well as the collapse of the old rural cooperative medical system. Private insurance offers an option other than out-of-pocket spending for urban citizens not covered under the three main urban plans, and it can act as a supplement to cover medical expenses not covered by these plans. Private insurance coverage varies from policy to policy, but some provide services such as a free physical examination every year, coverage into retirement, and coverage outside of one's province given that government insurance generally covers a citizen only in his or her own province. Some private plans offer better coverage and reimbursement than the government-sponsored plans, but the drawback is often their more expensive premiums.

Rural Health Insurance

Rural areas have yet to recover from the collapse of the rural cooperative medical scheme (RCMS) that provided approximately 90% of the rural population with healthcare coverage in the 1970s. The former RCMS was financed from a communal fund in each village. The village would place a percentage of its revenues from local enterprises into this fund, and the fund was supplemented by contributions from individuals. In some cases, governmental support for equipment and the salaries of medical personnel was provided. After economic reforms of the 1980s brought about the collapse of the RCMS, the 90% coverage of the rural population by RCMS dropped to 10%, forcing 90% of the population to pay for all healthcare-related costs out of pocket.

Although several initiatives tried to revive healthcare in rural China, a new RCMS rose out of the China National Rural Health Conference on October 9, 2002. The new RCMS, rolled out in select counties in each province, is a system partially financed by the local government and partly by the individual joining the plan. Although the government describes the RCMS as a voluntary system, in practice, it is largely compulsory as organized and enforced by local governments. Each participant contributes 10 RMB (approximately US $1.25) annually, which is matched by a 10 RMB yearly contribution from the local government (in the poorer central and western rural areas, the central government contributes an additional 10 RMB yearly). The structure of the RCMS encourages the local government to assist those unable to afford their 10 RMB contribution in these poorer regions. If an individual cannot contribute the required portion of the premium, the local government does not contribute its portion. In turn, the central government does not provide its contribution until the local government has paid its portion of the premium. Because the local government does not want to lose the financial contribution of the central government, if the individual cannot afford the 10 RMB, the local government steps in and provides financial assistance.

The Ministry of Health anticipates that the new RCMS will cover all rural inhabitants by 2010. The Ministry of Health also announced yearly projections for coverage under the new RCMS: 40% of cities/towns covered in 2006; 60% covered in 2007; and 100% of cities/towns in 2008 (although 100% of cities/towns are anticipated to be covered by 2008, the Ministry of Health projects that not everyone within the cities and towns will be covered until 2010). As of the end of September 2005, 671 cities/towns have joined the new RCMS. Of the 233 million inhabitants of these cities/towns, 177 million have joined the RCMS. This figure represents nearly 20% of all rural inhabitants in China, nearly double the 9.5% of rural inhabitants covered by this program in 2003.

OUTLOOK

The pharmaceutical pricing and reimbursement rules in China indicate an environment that – while freer than in the recent past – is still not a free market. In this section we discuss current practices and statistics that China has in place to curb spiraling drug prices and show the extent to which the population of China is covered by some form of insurance. Based on these practices and statements from the Chinese government, we discuss their likely future impact on this market.

Pricing

One of the major influencing factors is the Chinese government's reduction of retail prices over the past eight years. As a measure of cost-control policy, since 1998, the government has cut the retail prices of drugs 19 times, most recently in August 2006. Figure 17.4 shows the annual growth rate of Western pharmaceutical prices at the retail level over 1995–2004. Prior to 1998, although Western pharmaceutical retail prices were still increasing, the rate of growth was steadily declining. In 1998, the retail prices of Western pharmaceuticals showed a decline, and the rate of decline has remained fairly constant over 2001–4.

The 17th price cut, which occurred in late 2005, affected 22 types of medicines – although this cut mainly targeted antibiotics. The price cut was initially scheduled for the first half of 2005, but the National Development and Reform Commission postponed the price cut amid outcry from local antibiotics manufacturers who were worried that the cuts would render their businesses unprofitable and run them out of business. When the price cut finally occurred in September 2005, it was estimated that the retail prices of the affected pharmaceuticals would drop as much as 40%.

The 18th round of price cuts occurred in June 2006 and primarily affected 62 cancer drugs. In August 2006, the National Development and Reform Commission announced the most recent price cuts, considered the 19th round, affecting 99 antibiotics.

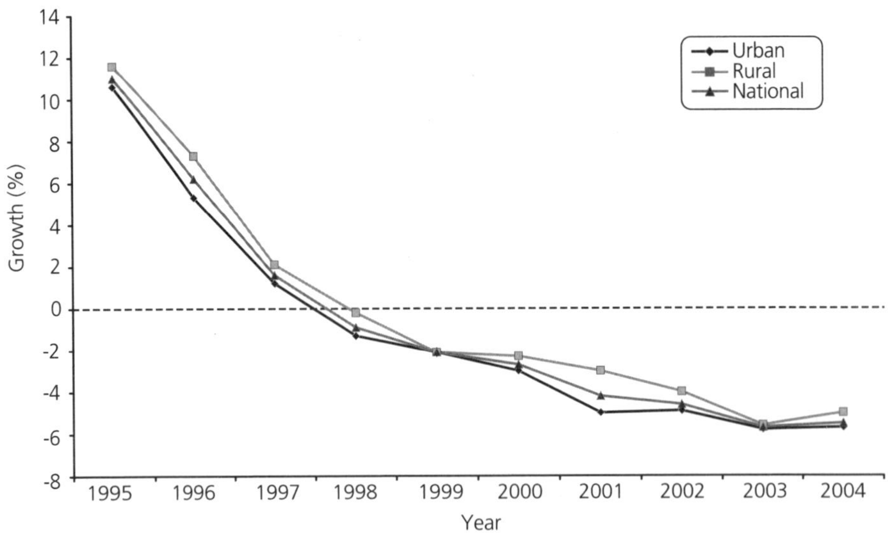

Figure 17.4 Annual Growth of Western Medicine Retail Prices in China, 1995–2004

The government has indicated that price cuts are unlikely to stop anytime soon. The National Development and Reform Commission and Ministry of Health have also hinted that more pricing and reimbursement regulations are forthcoming, including increased vigilance in the monitoring of general pricing and an experiment to control exmanufacturer prices.

The retail price cuts are closely related to the mark-ups of pharmaceuticals at the retail level. When the government slashes the price of a drug, profit the hospital or other retailers makes from the sale of the drug is lower. On paper, retailers are not allowed to mark up the price of a drug by more than 15% of the ex-manufacturer price, but in practice, retailers routinely do so in order to keep the hospitals afloat. If the retail price of a drug is cut, the mark-up may increase, or doctors may prescribe a higher-priced drug in its place to make up for the difference without relying on raising the mark-up. As a result, drug manufacturers are adversely affected by these retail price cuts.

The Chinese government's announcement of a watchdog group to ensure mark-ups are regulated may help to curb high mark-ups, but it cannot stop doctors from prescribing higher-priced medicines. In addition, because China has no formal history of regulating and enforcing proper mark-ups of pharmaceuticals, no procedures are in place to ensure that this new group will be efficient and able to produce immediate results for patients. Until mark-ups are properly controlled, retail price cuts will continue to be the best solution for the government to keep medical spending costs down.

Reimbursement

Table 17.4 compares health insurance coverage in China according to data gathered in the 1998 and 2003 National Surveys on Health Services. Although the Chinese government has made strides to increase insurance coverage over the past few decades, the most informative numbers on the current status of medical insurance are the percentages of people paying for medical costs out-of-pocket in urban and rural areas. Although the number of self-paying individuals declined overall and in rural areas (there was a slight increase in urban areas), the overall number of self-paying individuals in China still remained at slightly above 70% in 2003. Nearly 80% of the rural population was self-paying.

Also of note in Table 17.4 is the increase in private (commercial) insurance in China over 1998–2003. Rural residents especially seem to have taken advantage of private insurance, likely owing to the fact that the new RCMS program was not yet available, and private insurance offered some coverage in an area with few other options.

With many new initiatives in place for urban and rural health insurance, it remains to be seen how China will handle the challenges ahead. For the BMI plan set to replace the GIS and LIS in urban areas, projections for maximum coverage in urban areas average in the low 50% range given that the new

Table 17.4 Health Insurance Coverage in China, 1998 and 2003

	Total (%)		*Urban (%)*		*Rural (%)*	
	1998	*2003*	*1998*	*2003*	*1998*	*2003*
Basic insurance	—	8.9	—	30.4	—	1.5
Government insurance	4.9	1.2	16	4	1.2	0.2
Labor insurance	6.2	1.3	22.9	4.6	0.5	0.1
Cooperative insurance	5.6	8.8	2.7	6.6	6.6	9.5
Others	5	2	10.9	4	3	1.3
Commercial insurance	1.9	7.6	3.3	5.6	1.4	8.3
Self payment	76.4	70.3	44.1	44.8	87.3	79

plan does not cover dependents, students, the self-employed, or rural residents who work in urban areas. It should be noted, however, that in our discussions with insurance officials in Shanghai and Beijing, some form of coverage was offered to the self-employed and rural residents, although the services were limited. There is also variance in the level of coverage offered to current and former employees. Also, although private insurance has been gaining share in the Chinese health insurance market, private insurance may not be an affordable option for students and dependents, who will need coverage once the GIS and LIS plans are dissolved.

Although coverage estimates for rural plans were initially pessimistic – because affordability of the individual contribution of 10 RMB per year in the poorer regions was seen as an unlikely possibility – the government's willingness to help those who cannot afford the monthly premium indicates that the government's goal of covering all rural residents under the new RCMS is feasible. But given the size of the population, the government's goal of covering all residents by 2010 may still be too aggressive to achieve. There also appears to be provincial variance in coverage under rural health plans. Wealthier provinces, such as Jiangsu, have essential drug lists. The wealth of a province is likely to have a significant impact on whether a local RCMS plan can afford an essential drug list and, if it can, what level of reimbursement it will offer.

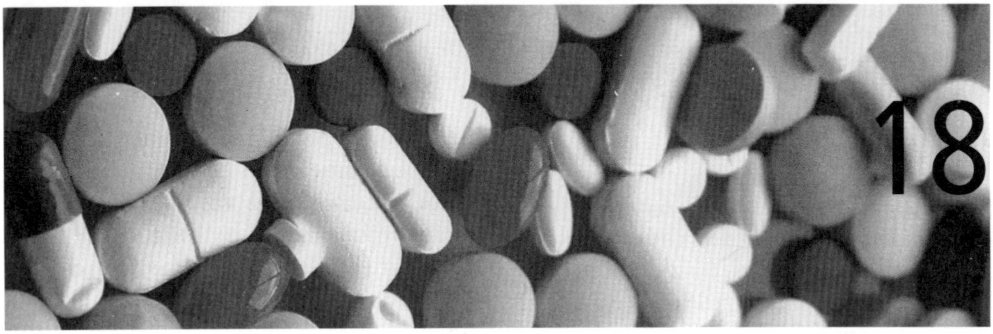

Will Point of Care Come of Age by 2010?

INTRODUCTION

In 2010, the point of care (POC) testing market is expected to achieve $6 billion in worldwide sales, or approximately twice its 2003 sales levels. Recent industry reports describe developments and projected growth in a bullish light and suggest that by 2010, POC products will be well on the way to becoming standard tools for primary healthcare. However, the POC industry faces several challenges that may retard its growth rate. Although the industry is technology savvy and the Food and Drug Administration (FDA) and third-party payers increasingly favor POC testing, the industry needs greater financial support and stronger sales and marketing initiatives in order to realize its projected $6 billion market potential by 2010.

Two high-value, over-the-counter (OTC) segments (pregnancy testing and home glucose monitoring) account for 43% of the global POC market. Sales in South America, Southeast Asia, and Europe of low-priced, rapid, non-OTC diagnostic tests make up another 34% of the POC market. The remaining 23% is the non-OTC POC market in the United States; sales to hospitals or laboratories account for 90% of that market; sales to physician offices account for only 10%. Tapping the remaining US physician and patient market – through improved marketing, technology development, regulatory change, and collaboration with the managed care industry – will be a key driver of future growth.

A shift in customer focus to physicians and patients must be accompanied by a corresponding shift in sales and marketing approaches; in this effort, the POC industry can learn from other industries that have demonstrated success in consumer sales and marketing, particularly the pharmaceutical industry. Above all, the POC industry needs leadership that can address the multiple challenges it faces and trigger the changes in corporate thinking that will enable the industry to realize its full market potential.

As the world's largest POC market, the United States is the focus of this chapter. The historic, erratic 5–10% growth rate and lackluster corporate performance in this market is surprising for an industry that has long been expected to command 20–25% growth rates. This chapter looks strategically at the multiple influences on the POC market growth in the United States and considers their influence on the market growth through 2010, when the POC market has been projected to double in size.

AN IDENTITY CRISIS

The definition of the POC industry, with respect to its function and its customer, is not clear because companies, financial investors, and technology transfer institutes have different perceptions of what it should be. Lack of a single strategic definition does not by itself cause industrial turmoil, but it does reflect the evolutionary fits and starts and restricted technology horizons that are impeding the POC industry's evolution.

Function and customer are adequately defined in other fast-moving industrial subsegments that can provide lessons for the POC companies. For example, pharmaceutical generics manufacturers have a function of low cost and a customer base of discount pharmacists. With function and customer thus defined, generics manufacturers can include a wide array of new and unlikely products within generic pharmaceuticals – everything from intravenous drugs to multivitamins.

Before the POC industry can effectively communicate its strategy to potential financiers and customers and design products that further its ability to revolutionize diagnostic testing, it must establish a clear strategic identity based on definitions of its function and customer.

POC's Function

The College of American Pathologists (CAP) defines POC technology as "those analytical patient-testing activities provided within the institution, but performed outside the physical facilities of the clinical laboratories. The central criterion of POC technology is that it does not require permanent dedicated space." This definition commonly embraces everything from lateral flow rapid tests through biochips, but it excludes some important gray areas, particularly telemedicine and medical diagnostic decision support tools.

Take, for example, software-only products like Promedas (a large Bayesian network for diagnosis in internal medicine) for lipid control and Isabel (an online clinical decision support and information system that covers the whole spectrum of pediatrics and is designed particularly to help doctors make quick, accurate diagnoses and select appropriate treatments) for pediatric management. Both are based on extensive research programs, are used outside of clinical laboratories, do not require dedicated space, and deliver results rapidly. Yet these software-only diagnostic products are generally regarded as non-POC tools. Admittedly, software-only diagnostic tests require a fundamentally different regulatory and reimbursement approach and perhaps even electronic distribution. However, their exclusion appears to be based on the fact that POC has evolved from a culture that is more comfortable with chemical- or signal-based technologies than, for example, the psychological metric of a software-driven rapid test to diagnose clinical depression.

Such restrictive thinking is central in preventing POC from realizing its potential, for it is in the eventual marriage of software, hardware, chemistry, and genetic technologies that POC will eventually find its greatest utility as well as its killer applications. If POC is to double its size by 2010, its funders and regulators must embrace POC in all current and future forms and rethink the current criteria underpinning approval and commercialization.

POC's Customers

The overall laboratory diagnostics market, generally thought to consist of major distributors selling automated or semiautomated tests to high-volume hospital or private laboratory services organizations, grows at only 4–5% annually. The POC market is commercially embedded in the overall laboratory market, and its market growth rate remains in the range of 5–10%.

If the POC industry is to increase its growth rate, it must consider the needs of the customer base for which it was originally designed: the physician and the consumer. Currently, physicians and consumers accept the fact that POC technology is used predominantly in hospital and laboratory settings, and consequently, communication of test results to patients is slow (Saxena, 1993). As in all industries, attracting new customers for established products requires new ways of selling, pricing, marketing, and distributing. As we examine each of the influences that impede or advance the POC industry's future, it is essential to examine both the customers that the industry satisfies today and the customers for whom the POC products were originally intended. These customers fundamentally differ in their training, influences, and motives when it comes to choosing a technology. Targeting physicians and consumers requires a shift in thinking about the marketing spend and the capital structure, but companies that are successful in doing so will achieve the first billion-dollar POC brands.

THE TECHNOLOGY TRAJECTORY

Over the past 10 years, we have seen a long list of failures among the POC-focused companies or divisions whose technology platforms promised to take premier positions in the market. For example, Cambridge Biotech (Rockville, Maryland) and Saliva Diagnostics (Vancouver, Washington) invested heavily in rapid HIV testing, and Careside (Culver City, California) invested in a multi-analyte POC instrument. Although these companies were positioning themselves with leading POC technologies, they fell short of the cost of market entry or failed to overcome the regulatory hurdles.

In that same time frame, however, several technology platforms or enabling technologies have moved forward, creating great potential for the industry's growth. Rapid immunoassay test platforms use dry imprinted reagents, and flow-through devices are developed to a point where their accuracy is equal to and sometimes better than that of their equivalent laboratory tests. Simple OTC pregnancy and ovulation tests and glucose-monitoring products have become a standard of sorts, and leading brand names such as Pfizer's e.p.t, Clear Blue, and Predictor make up at least a quarter of the global $3 billion industry. We can certainly anticipate the launch of new tests for different disease areas on rapid immunoassay test platforms over the next five to six years.

Instrumented readers have been developed that surpass Roche's Accutest or Johnson & Johnson's Lifescan, both used for glucose monitoring. Companies like Cholestech and Metrika are already commercializing products for cholesterol and Hba1C monitoring. The development of advanced readers is an important step and signals the need for POC technology to connect remote tests to centralized systems that facilitate the multiple administrative activities in physicians' offices that are involved in managing a patient's diagnosis.

Microfluidics technology is producing platforms that miniaturize big laboratory analyzer functionality to microchip or desktop scale. In an effort to replicate laboratory testing, companies like Qualigen and Becton Dickinson have broken into the market with benchtop analyzers and disposable packs. With the ability to perform more robust quantitative tests, this technology will be further simplified, conform to higher quality control (QC) requirements, and include broad test menus. One particular challenge for microfluidics technology is that physicians are unlikely to want four or five desktop instruments, each running different yet overlapping tests; such multiple platforms are unlikely to reduce physician workloads or costs. Without a major collaborative marketing investment to promote a single microfluidics platform, penetration of the physician market will be challenging, even though the technology holds great promise for POC diagnosis.

Biochips are expected to increase the quantitative capability of POC testing. Biochip technology is still in an embryonic stage. Its maturation depends on the clarification of genetic intellectual property (IP) rights and resolution of regulatory and reimbursement issues that will arise. Affymetrix, Agilent, and Motorola are among the many companies that have a major investment in biochips. Despite the extent of investment and the potential of this technology, a major breakthrough is unlikely to occur by 2010.

The success of the technology platforms we have discussed in the physician market depends not just on their ability to deliver immediate, onsite test results but also on their ability to increase the productivity of physicians' office processes. Wireless connectivity and patient management interfaces will be key to physicians' acceptance of POC technology in the next six years. Industry expert James Nichols, in his review of POC testing, said that integration of POC testing devices with information systems is critical to acceptance of POC technology. Wireless communication and patient management interfaces are now inexpensive enough and are also robust enough to be applied to POC tests for direct transmission of results to patient record and billing software. Such integration of technology will eliminate steps that are a direct cost to physicians.

While the accuracy, quantification, and connectivity capabilities essential to a killer technology platform for POC already exist, they will not suffice to fulfill the potential of POC technology by 2010 unless the market agrees on standards defined for instruments, QC requirements, result reporting, and connectivity. Unlike telecommunications, software development, or automotive manufacture, where industry incumbents have led standards development to ensure the long-term well-being of those industries, the POC industry is still too fragmented to follow suit. It will be up to the market forces and, possibly, to new, deep-pocketed software and telecommunications providers to establish the standards.

However, many key POC companies will include multiple disciplines in their design and technical support teams by 2010. By marrying chemistry, molecular science, electronics, and software in easy-to-use devices, these companies will be able to ease customers into POC use with novel tests and further enhance the reputation of POC technology.

REGULATORY ISSUES

Since 1999, the FDA has united the various parts of the regulatory machine – including the Clinical Laboratory Improvement Amendments (CLIA) certification process – under one umbrella to address the increased complexity arising from miniaturization and molecular testing and the potential for a shift of diagnosis from expert pathologists to diagnostically untrained doctors, nurses, and patients.

To educate these new test users, the FDA published new guidelines in April 2003 to clarify the rules for QC in physician-office labs, effectively doing away with the *moderate complexity* rating for tests and reducing specific requirements to *waived* and *highly complex*. (To date, the moderate complexity rating for simple rapid tests appears to have nothing to do with test complexity; many of these tests are extremely simple to operate. Rather, it has been an FDA classification for markers that have not had sufficient real-life experience in the hands of nonpathologists.)

Although this modification of the rating system for tests appears to be a simplification, it imposes increased regulation (and increased cost) on some 30,000 physicians who currently use moderately complex tests in their own offices because tests originally rated as moderately complex will now be rated as highly complex. For example, tests like Gryphus's BV Blue and Xenotopes Trichomonas for vaginitis, which are simple to use, started their lives with a moderate complexity rating. Under the new rules, these tests must conform to high-complexity QC requirements similar to those imposed on hospital laboratories, thus limiting their ability to move into the physician marketplace. The new rating system may also stifle the growth of several new, easy-to-use, rapid tests that would likely have been categorized as moderately complex under the old system.

The process for achieving a CLIA waiver, which enables the shift of tests into the hands of the majority of physicians, is not much clearer. Although the FDA has consulted with the industry and promised a much-vaunted simplification of rules for the CLIA waiver, simplified rules have not yet been published. Test manufacturers therefore must consider the implications of the rules on a case-by-case basis. Because the FDA's rationale with regard to the new marker and the CLIA waiver approval is not clear, the case-by-case approach is indeed confusing for an industry that is trying to design products for the physician office or consumer market.

Changes to the CLIA classification, coupled with the shift of POC tests from hospital laboratories to physicians and consumers, call for a dialogue between the FDA and key stakeholders that revisits the fundamentals of POC testing, as it exists today, and seeks new regulatory pathways – but it is not clear who can lead this dialogue. The CAP has addressed POC testing in terms of definition and guidelines, but CAP's POC committee is only one of 50 or so committees and does not command the college's primary focus. Furthermore, CAP's definition of POC is outmoded in the context of an industry that has advanced well beyond the devolved testing of miniaturized ELISA plates. Neither a widely accepted industry body nor a strong market leader stands ready to take the leadership role in the necessary dialogue between the FDA and POC technology stakeholders.

Without pressure from POC stakeholders or a political mandate (e.g., widespread deployment of antibioterrorism tests), we can expect additional rules from the FDA as it reacts to profound shifts in diagnostic management driven by new technology and markers. Given that historically these policies have often forced abrupt market readjustment and suppressed growth (Figure 18.1), they are more likely to hinder than to promote the growth of the POC industry.

MANAGED CARE

As a driver of cost efficiency in the market, the managed care industry should embrace many aspects of POC testing. POC testing reduces the number of physician visits required, the number of wrong treatment answers, and the incidence of antibiotic resistance, which can occur when treatment is given empirically while physicians await lab results. POC testing also supports managed care's long-term goal of forcing as much care as possible to the gatekeepers and away from expensive specialty care providers. Improved patient satisfaction emanating from on-the-spot care at a time of poor consumer relations could be a side effect. Nevertheless, the managed care industry seems ambivalent about POC testing.

Managed care organizations (MCOs) focus on some five to ten diseases that are high-cost conditions, such as diabetes. By doing so, MCOs can control 80% of their

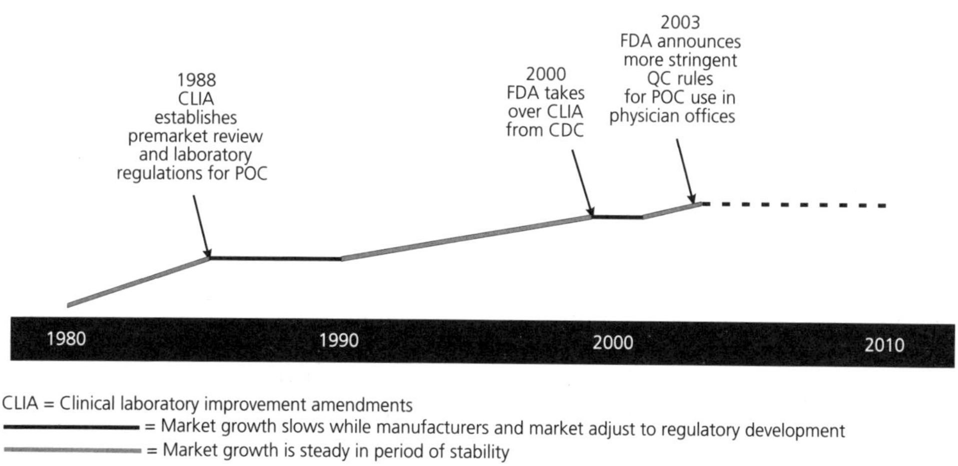

Figure 18.1 Regulatory Policies of Care and Their Impact on Market Growth in the United States

disease management costs. Therefore, MCOs will evaluate POC tests for these five to ten diseases according to their ability to reduce downstream healthcare costs. Invariably, the onus is on the POC manufacturer to convince the MCO that the benefits of the POC test justify reimbursement, particularly when tests do not address these five to ten diseases that are most costly to treat. Because of the high cost of educating physicians in new diagnostic methods and the uncertain impact of yet another decentralized cost, the top-10 MCOs have not initiated any proactive programs to promote POC testing.

Instead, the transparency created by centralizing laboratory-testing costs has prevailed over POC education programs. Paradoxically, users continue to seek and receive reimbursement for individual POC tests under their respective current procedural terminology (CPT) codes, but this practice appears to be just a holding position until the strength of the centralizing bias is truly tested by, for example, a novel POC screening test. Until then, it appears that the impact of the managed care industry on the POC market of 2010 will be neutral at best.

FINANCIAL INVESTMENT

Because today's start-ups may be commercializing products in 2010, it is important to reflect on the future availability – or unavailability – of financial resources for the development of this market. Unfortunately, venture capital (VC) investors have been disappointed by the POC industry's turbulent past. Consequently, projects that involve diagnostic start-ups are not likely to top the business plans of most venture financiers.

However, the blame for past corporate failures could be shared with many of these same VC investors, who have shown their naïveté in funding POC companies. Specifically, VC investors have failed to support good management teams with enough funding to enable early commercialization of their products, development of sales lines and marketing programs, and continued development of their cutting-edge technologies.

For the VC investors, the average waiting period of four years for a POC product to become commercialized is often too long. As a result, by the time POC companies are ready to market their tests and need commercialization money, the original investors have long since lost interest in the project's original vision. The result is a large number of cash-hungry companies whose products are undermarketed. It is possible that deep-pocketed investors will attempt consolidation between now and 2010, taking advantage of the myriad small, cash-hungry companies; however, because such a consolidation would require dedicated POC management expertise, it is unlikely to be driven by VC alone.

Even though much of the technology pain is past, the recent history of failed POC companies will induce venture capitalists to financially underfeed new start-ups or market development. This process will weed out financially weak companies and only keep those that survive, which would be in a very small number. Also, the number of start-up companies that could have emerged after 2010 will be reduced.

DEVELOPMENT AND PROTECTION

Intellectual property development and protection have not been the strong points of the POC industry. An endemic practice of avoiding, ignoring, or engineering around diagnostic technology patents has added to the industry's poor reputation among funders and partners.

The emergence of a whole subspecies of low-cost generics manufacturers, from China to California, has marked the development of the three biggest product areas: pregnancy testing, ovulation testing, and glucose monitoring. Hundreds of companies are developing and manufacturing these tests for marginal profits, and few are investing in the serious IP programs that distinguish other segments of the healthcare industry.

In the pharmaceutical industry, a recognized measure of innovative strength is the number of new chemical entities (NCEs) that are approved annually in the United States and are aimed at the same physician audience that the POC industry targets (Figure 18.2). Consider, by contrast, the number of new diagnostic entities (NDEs) approved by the FDA (excluding generic versions): currently, approximately thirty CLIA-waived NDEs are registered in the United States.

Multiple variations of already approved tests are granted approval annually, but the number of novel tests approved for use in physician offices remains abysmally small – just two or three annually. Part of the problem clearly lies with the POC industry's comparative underinvestment in seeking approval for existing tests and marketing them appropriately in the US physician-office market. However, it appears too that the costs associated with ongoing regulatory uncertainty and the slow pace of physician and consumer market approvals, combined with a low threshold for competitor entry, tend to justify the original underinvestment.

Slowly, companies are making efforts to improve the current state of POC IP. Several developments promise to have a profound impact on diagnostic IP over the next five to six years.

First, companies such as Inverness Medical Innovations are moving to protect existing IP. The company's recent acquisition and enforcement of its lateral flow device patents against Pfizer, Acon Laboratories, Qualis, and Princeton BioMeditech attacks the manufacturers of generic pregnancy and ovulation tests. Provided Inverness is not allowed to become monopolistic in its approach to these primary patents and actively license them into areas that do not interest Inverness, its aggression through the courts will help to tidy up IP across the whole sector.

Second, several new forces will raise barriers to the development of a new core IP for POC. The POC industry is relying on the pharmaceutical industry to develop substantially more biomarkers (often discovered during the drug development process) for

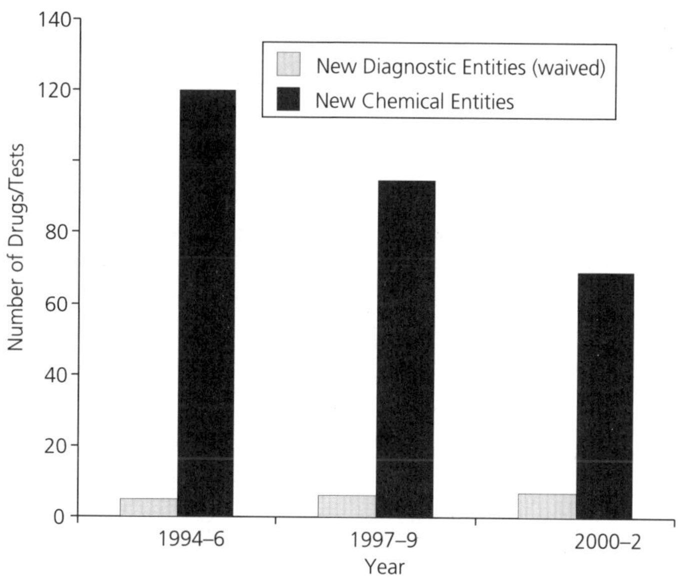

Figure 18.2 Number of Novel Drugs and Novel Waived Rapid Tests Approrved by the FDA, 1994–2002

commercialization. Such biomarkers are not necessarily automatic candidates for POC tests, but POC tests make the most sense to an industry whose business is based on empowering physicians to prescribe its products (see Section Theranostics). Any drive to commercialize biomarkers discovered within the pharmaceutical industry is likely to be accompanied by high levels of IP investment.

Another example of new core IP for the POC industry involves molecular research, where gene sequences are being patented for both their diagnostic and therapeutic applications. In contrast to the low-cost generics companies' frequent disregard for IP, Oxford Gene Technologies, Affymetrics, and Incyte Genomics are involved in IP disputes over original rights to POC technology. Although no products have reached the POC market, these examples serve as a backdrop to the market in 2010 and beyond.

A third development that promises to have a profound impact on POC diagnostic IP over the next five to six years is the introduction of the new supporting technologies for telecommunication and software interfaces. The companies behind these technologies have invested several million dollars in their development and have a culture of building and defending their IP. As these technologies become embedded in POC tests, the companies that developed them will seek to defend their technology positions.

In sum, a small revolution in POC IP is unfolding, with new incentives, new companies, and aggressive litigation around existing IP all contributing greatly to support the growth of technology in the POC market in 2010. Although disruptive in the short term for companies that develop and sell generic POC tests, ultimately this new IP environment will incentivize innovative companies to build and protect their own IP. Barriers to entry will be important if innovative companies are to end the downward price spiral resulting from a disorderly IP culture (particularly in the pregnancy and ovulation markets) and establish prices and reimbursements that reflect the clinical value inherent in POC tests.

THERANOSTICS

The growth of the *theranostics* concept – that is, developing and marketing tests for specific treatment – has been much discussed in recent industry reports. There are obvious synergies between the pharmaceutical industry, which seeks to treat more people, and the POC industry, which identifies people who need treatment. Industry observers frequently cite deals between big pharmaceutical companies and diagnostics companies as indication of the synergies between these two industries.

FDA initiatives support the synergy between testing and treatment. A recent FDA goal is to monitor blood test results that could signal a potential problem with a new medication in real time. In addition, the FDA has suggested the need for genetic tests to precede approval of genetic therapy. Both initiatives will incentivize the pharmaceutical industry to work more closely with manufacturers of real-time diagnostics.

The concept of theranostics is not new. Glucose testing and insulin treatment and anticoagulation therapy and home coagulation monitors are now intimately linked test-and-treatment regimens. In the early 1990s, some companies attempted to launch high-profile campaigns that joined their own diagnostic and therapeutic products – for example, Cortecs (now Provalis) attempted joint campaigns for its therapies and diagnostics in diabetes and osteoporosis, but the company could not sustain investors' interest. However, theranostics is attracting greater interest now, when the pharmaceutical industry is under shareholder fire to continue growing the blockbuster brands, and the POC industry sees hope for growth in synergistic diagnostic/therapeutic products.

Admittedly, the test/treat concept is not wholly about POC, but ultimately, the concept is most effectively realized in a POC setting – when there is an on-the-spot alternative, treatment that depends on a delayed laboratory response makes no sense. However, the momentum for POC that could be sparked by this new cross-industry approach is far from certain.

Richard Sykes, recently retired CEO of GlaxoSmithKline (GSK), was a major proponent of joint pharmaceutical and diagnostic programs, building the Glaxo Predictive Medicine Unit to further his vision (shortly after Sykes retired, GSK shut down the Predictive Medicine Unit). He recently speculated that a key barrier to melding these two industries would be pharmaceutical companies' fear that use of a diagnostic test as a prerequisite to therapy would restrict a therapy's market share by removing it from the current, predominantly empirical treatment paradigm.

This is a valid concern for the pharmaceutical industry. For example, if a mandatory test for erectile dysfunction (ED) assessed a patient's likely response to therapy, ED drugs probably would not be the several-billion-dollar market that they are today. A mandatory test might exclude patients with marginal or temporary ED function loss or the substantial social use population; currently, these two groups do receive treatment.

Another issue is the unequal expectations of alliance partners regarding development timelines and sales and marketing copromotions in primary or specialist care markets. For example, PharmaNetics recently filed a lawsuit against Aventis Pharmaceuticals, alleging that Aventis has engaged in false and misleading advertising of its drug Lovenox by failing to copromote the PharmaNetics Enox test. (The Enox test is a rapid POC test used to detect any anticoagulant effects of enoxaparin [Lovenox].) The lawsuit is based on the fact that Aventis helped PharmaNetics to develop the Enox test and, according to PharmaNetics, was supposed to promote the test together with Lovenox.

Nevertheless, several companies – Prometheus and Genaissance, for example – are basing their business models on joint pharmaceutical/diagnostic test and treat programs. This development is encouraging because POC diagnostics companies have not been willing in the past to mount major, joint, direct-selling campaigns on their own dime. POC companies that base their business models on physicians' test and treat needs or on the brand share needs of pharmaceutical companies will understand and perfect the construction of test-and-treat marketing campaigns.

SALES AND MARKETING

Sales and marketing are central to changing the perception and stimulating growth of this market. As previously discussed, current POC revenue in the United States emanates predominantly from hospitals and laboratories. In the United States, less than 10% of all diagnosis (excluding pregnancy and glucose testing) is conducted by physicians and consumers, the markets where POC tests have the greatest value. The POC industry has had little experience in selling and marketing directly to this sophisticated healthcare audience.

Companies that claim to have a presence in the US physician office predominantly use national physician distributors, such as Physician Sales and Service or McKesson. These large selling organizations are experienced in taking and delivering orders, but by their own admission, their representatives are not equipped to explain the technical and clinical merits of a test or able to spend the necessary 15–30 minutes, let alone take the time to help clinics set up new testing techniques. A five-minute visit and a catalogue of other products is insufficient to inform a user of a POC product's capabilities.

Consider the pharmaceutical industry's methods in selling novel products to the same target audience. Big pharmaceutical companies employ direct salesforces that number in the thousands. They allot sufficient money to prelaunch promotion, brand development, cost-effectiveness studies, and development of high-quality clinical literature. More recently, leading companies have been conducting direct-to-consumer (DTC) advertising campaigns to drive brand awareness. Their reward for this leadership is billion-dollar brand equity.

To launch a new product, a pharmaceutical company will spend upwards of $300 million while a POC company will spend on average approximately $300 thousand. The POC industry does not need to match pharmaceutical product spend, but the difference demonstrates the profound gap in thinking between these two industries.

Why does the pharmaceutical industry spend so much on sales and marketing and the diagnostic industry spend so little? One argument has been cost versus return. Considering the low barriers to competitor market entry, the high cost of direct sales and brand marketing is one that the POC industry and its financiers have been unwilling or unable to bear. The industry has chosen instead to sell rapid tests to medium-sized laboratories, hospitals, and out-of-country distributors, all areas where pricing pressures are intense. This choice is equivalent to a pharmaceutical company's choosing to drop a drug at the end of its patent life because the switch to the OTC market will mean new competition and increased TV advertising expense. In competitive markets, branding produces sales.

Instead, the predominant POC culture measures market leadership in numbers of products and size of revenues, not on the pharmaceutical paradigm of building brand equity. Figure 18.3 shows the brand spend of several POC companies and their revenue. POC industry spend does not line up against the pharmaceutical industry's spend; consequently, its revenue suffers.

This difference in paradigm is the greatest of the POC industry's shortcomings; a new paradigm is a prerequisite to an industrial coming-of-age for POC. Defining the POC industry and its ability to realize the original estimates of its worth depend on a refocus toward the billion-dollar customers: physicians and consumers. If the development of billion-dollar brands in POC diagnostics seems doubtful, put aside the history of the POC industry in selling to the laboratory market; instead, consider the behavior of physicians and consumers and their tried and tested ability to drive major healthcare brand revenues.

Even though an individual POC test may not reach the heights of Lipitor or Prilosec, a test family that has good reimbursement and a broad customer base in the primary care market could, in theory, reach the billion-dollar mark. For an example, see the sidebar, "The Revenue Potential Model."

The Revenue Potential Model: Applying POC Diagnostics to Sexually Transmitted Diseases

Our revenue model is based on initial diagnosis of a sexually transmitted disease (STD) by means of a hypothetical, accurate, DNA-based, three-minute chlamydia test (chlamydia has huge downstream costs associated with missed diagnosis – for example, infertility and cancer). Such a test might cost $40 and be a valid test for primary care providers, including family and general physicians, urologists, planned parenthood clinics, gynecologists, and emergency care units. Collectively, these potential customers number more than 65,000 in the United States.

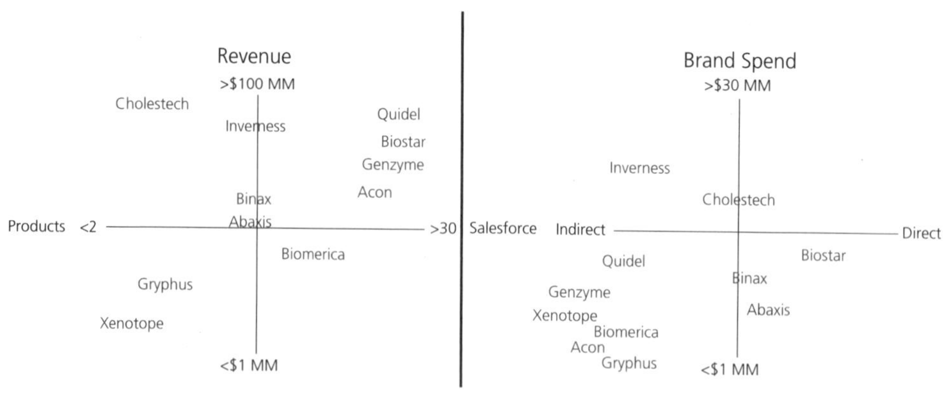

Figure 18.3 Point of Care Companies Based on Revenue and Brand Spend

Our revenue model assumes a lead market share of 40% of the target audience (based on a successful pharmaceutical first-mover advantage). The test could be used for populations that are at high risk for infection; the U.S. Preventive Services Taskforce recommends screening of all sexually active women under the age of 25. A positive test might lead to subsequent testing for related STDs (e.g., herpes, human papillomavirus (HPV), bacterial vaginitis, trichomonas) in 25% of patients tested with the chlamydia test.

Our revenue model shows how a related brand family for STD testing might generate $1.2 billion yearly from physicians alone:

Chlamydia Test Price	*Average Patients per Month per Clinic for Whom Testing Is Appropriate*	*Revenue per Physician*	*Revenue from 40% of (or 25,000) Primary Care Physicians*	*Additional Revenue from Four Related Tests in the Same Brand Family Used on 25% of Chlamydia-tested Patients to Identify Likely Co-infections or Resolve Nonchlamydia Symptoms*
$40	50	$2,000 per month; $24,000 per year	$600 million per year	$600 million per year

REVIEWING INFLUENCES ON THE POC MARKET

The faculty of the Sloan School of Management at MIT study the trajectories of new markets and technologies. They have observed that all new technologies have a similar life cycle, known as the S-curve. Initially, the S-curve describes a period of slow market growth (often 15–20 years in length) that parallels the development of other, prerequisite influences on long-term market adoption. At some point along this initial trajectory, all the key components of rapid growth align, enabling a strong growth period followed by an acceleration of growth to the zenith of market acceptance.

POC technology fits this model well. In its initial phase, it enjoyed growth but suffered financing, regulatory, and other setbacks that kept it from achieving its market potential. The industry still faces downward pressures, but they are evenly matched by factors that promote its long-term success. As we look forward to 2010, the projected development of the POC marketplace suggests that the POC industry could successfully address its shortcomings over the next five to six years and achieve its market potential of $6 billion.

However, MIT thought leaders will also tell you that most often, change in market growth is led by a single new product or an entrepreneur who takes advantage of all the positive influences and ably manages the negative ones to create major corporate growth. What is arguably a state of flux in the industry could be a springboard to success for a new leader.

So, where is the POC market leader? Recently, Roche and Abbott have both accomplished a departure from a pure focus on developing their POC segments by selling their product suites. The traditional leadership of dominant players, therefore, is unlikely to come from the big pharmaceutical companies. Among the much smaller enterprises that specialize in POC technology – such as Quidel and Biostar – none appear prepared or able to lead the development of the POC market, judging from their corporate responses to date and their financing operations during the past 10 years.

And yet – POC visionaries backed by smart capital could, within the next 24 months, produce an array of innovative, complementary products; invest heavily in establishing their clinical value to physicians and consumers and their cost benefit to payers; and promote them with the branding techniques established by the pharmaceutical industry. Products would likely be sold directly by a direct salesforce dedicated to building long-term customer relationships. Regulatory and reimbursement tasks would be embraced rather than ignored, and the importance of IP in maintaining leadership would be given paramount importance. A complementary strategy might be to build valuable alliances with the synergistic pharmaceutical and managed care industries, ultimately embedding their products and services in the very relationships that can direct and finance their future innovation.

REFERENCE

Saxena, S. Does the emergency department need a dedicated stat laboratory? Continuous quality improvement as a management tool for the clinical laboratory. *American Journal of Clinical Pathology.* 1993;100(6):606–10.

PART II

Pharmacogenomics

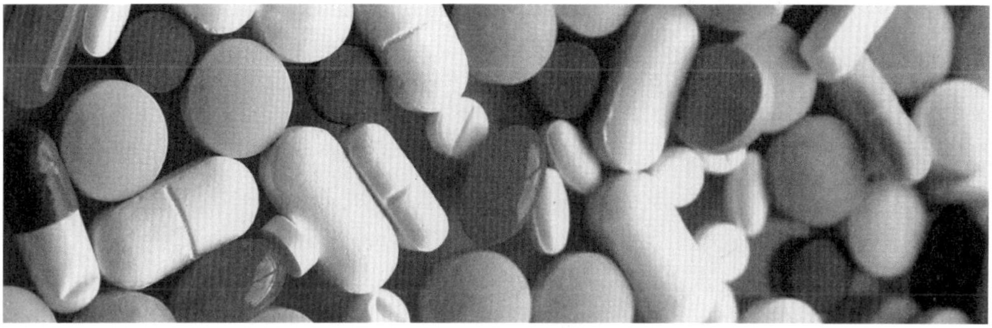

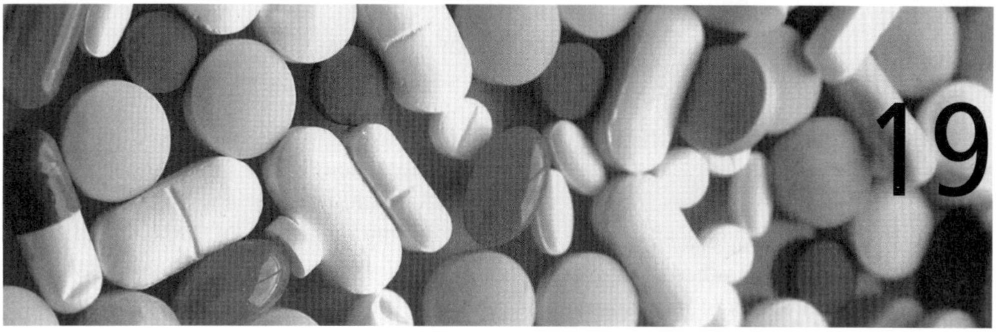

Has Genomics Failed to Deliver?

THE EARLY PROMISE OF GENOMICS

By 2000, the human genome had largely been sequenced, and by 2001, the first human genome map had been generated. The science and medical communities were very excited about the possibility of thousands of new genomics-derived drugs entering product development pipelines.

One of the key goals of early genomics companies was to quickly transform into pharmaceutical concerns. The founders of these companies argued that thanks to the high-throughput genomics and bioinformatics tools that could be used to analyze huge stretches of DNA or masses of proteins, they would be able to identify completely novel targets and leap ahead of their competitors in the race to cure many diseases. Most of these companies set their sites on a wide range of targets; rather than focusing on specific indications, they planned to use their tools to examine hundreds, or even thousands, of potential targets. From that huge pool, they would pick the ones that seemed most lucrative.

To date, no genomics-derived product has passed the juncture of Phase III trials. Indeed, it will still be another two to four years before a significant number of the genomics compounds, which are now in early-stage development, reach this critical juncture. In the meantime, genomics companies face a continuing challenge in supporting the cost of their clinical development.

The last couple of years have been notable for the genomics industry. Human Genome Sciences (HGS) and CuraGen replaced their CEOs, as did Millennium (an early genomics pioneer that has changed its business focus to developing personalized medicines), and several early genomics companies have restructured their business strategies significantly. Although these events gained a lot of attention, the most important development has been the slow and steady progress of a handful of companies that are still moving genomics-based products through to clinical trials.

Given the high expectations for genomics at the turn of the last decade, we ask, "Has genomics failed to deliver?" In this chapter, we review the ever-changing fortunes of the genomic drug discovery and development industry, focusing on the strategies that companies are using to stay competitive and, in many cases, solvent. We present a SWOT (strengths, weaknesses, opportunities, and threats) analysis that assesses the current strengths and weaknesses of this industry sector, and we identify those opportunities and threats that are likely to shape the future of genomics, and predict how that future will look.

GENOMICS PALES COMPARED WITH BIOTECH

2005 was a banner year for biotechnology, and it serves to remind other developers of drug discovery platforms of the rich rewards that await those that can successfully find faster and/or better ways of making new drugs. Genomics companies will launch their protein-based products in many of the same therapeutic markets as those of biotechnology and monoclonal antibody (MAb) companies. All these companies exploit the information about a gene or genes to produce different types of drugs, including proteins, MAbs, small molecules that target the proteins, genes for gene therapy, and oligonucleotides for expression-disruption technologies, such as RNA interference.

As Figure 19.1 depicts, the past 25 years have brought a steady succession of therapeutic proteins to the marketplace. Protein products fall into three categories:

1. Recombinant proteins.
2. Protein extracts.
3. MAbs.

The majority of proteins are made from the expression of genes through recombinant DNA techniques. In fact, recombinant proteins represent 59% of the 143 approved proteins; insulin is the first recombinant product, approved in 1982. Prior to the advent of recombinant DNA, most protein products were painstakingly purified from protein extracts. Some proteins are still made in this fashion, and the protein extract group constitutes 28% of approved proteins. The remaining 13% of approved proteins are MAbs.

The path to the approval for these breakthrough products was not easy. One of the first technologies for producing MAbs was invented by Kohler & Milstein in 1975, more than 30 years ago. It took 10 years for the first therapeutic antibody to enter the marketplace – OKT3 was approved in 1986 for preventing kidney-transplant rejection. The next eight years (1986–94) saw a succession of clinical failures, stemming in part from human immune responses to mouse antibodies (e.g., human antimouse antibody [HAMA] responses).

In the early 1990s, the MAb companies Centocor (now Johnson & Johnson) and

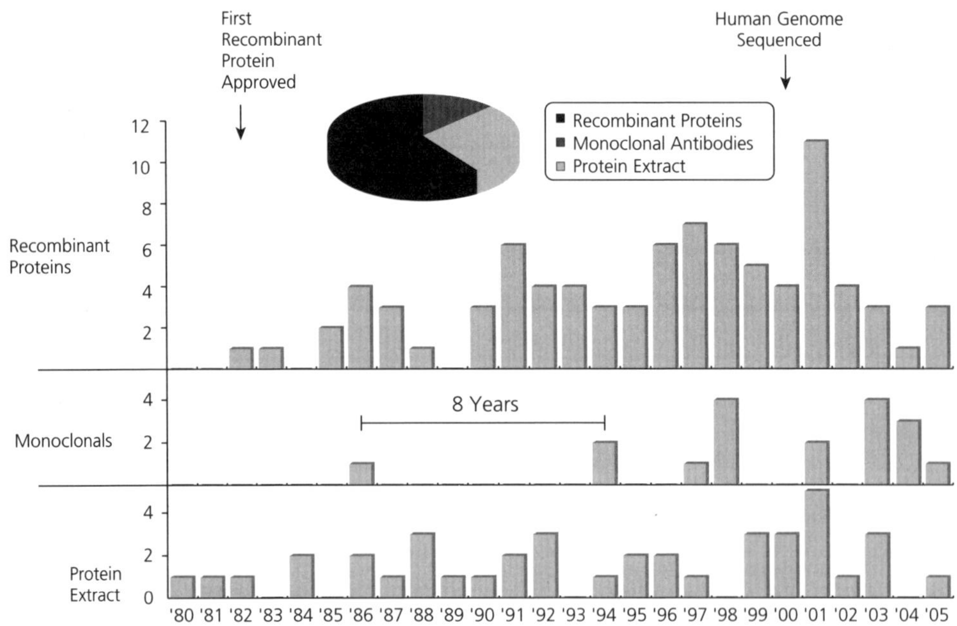

Figure 19.1 Year of Introduction of 143 Approved Protein Drugs, 1980–2005

Xoma both experienced high-profile failures of their MAbs in Phase III trials for sepsis. This drought of MAb approvals finally ended in 1994, when Centocor obtained approval to market abciximab (ReoPro) for patients at high risk for complications from coronary angioplasty. By the end of 2005, 18 MAbs had been approved, representing 12% of the approved therapeutic proteins. Many people compare the present-day struggles of genomics companies to bring products to market with the difficulties experienced by these early MAb companies.

Biotech products – recombinant proteins and MAbs alike – have enjoyed substantial market success. In fact, many of these therapeutic proteins have achieved blockbuster status (sales exceeding $1 billion a year) (Table 19.1). Markets for protein drugs have expanded rapidly; in 2005, worldwide sales totaled more than $62 billion (Figure 19.2). From 2002 to 2005, sales of MAbs increased 179%, reaching $14 billion worldwide. Recombinant protein sales increased 54%, to $44 billion worldwide, and the protein-extract group increased 25%, totaling $3.9 billion in worldwide sales. The US market is the largest; in 2005, it represented 61% of the worldwide MAb market, 51% of the worldwide recombinant protein market, and 44% of the worldwide protein-extract market.

Table 19.1 Best-selling Protein-based Products, 2005

Generic Name	*Product*	*Company*	*First Introduced*	*Worldwide (millions of US dollars)*	*United States (millions of US dollars)*
Monoclonal antibodies					
Infliximab	Remicade	Johnson & Johnson, Schering-Plough, Tanabe	1998	3,592	2,065
Rituximab	Rituxan, MabThera	Genentech, Roche	1997	3,244	1,832
Trastuzumab	Herceptin	Genentech, Roche	1998	1,723	747
Adalimumab	Humira	Abbott Laboratories	2003	1,400	849
Bevacizumab	Avastin	Genentech, Roche	2004	1,337	1,133
Palivizumab	Synagis	Abbott Laboratories, Dainippon, MedImmune	1998	1,118	905
Recombinant proteins[a]					
Epoetin alfa	Epogen, Procrit, Eprex, ESPO	Amgen, Johnson & Johnson, Kirin	1988	6,171	4,701
Insulin	Humulin R, human insulin, devices, and analogues	Eli Lilly, Novo Nordisk	1983	4,646	1,035
Etanercept	Enbrel	Amgen, Wyeth, Takeda	1998	3,682	2,470
Darbepoetin alfa	Aranesp	Amgen	2001	3,273	2,104
Interferon-beta-1a	Avonex, Rebif	Biogen Idec, Serono	1996	2,813	1,329
Somatropin	Many brands	Many companies	1987	2,333	857
Pegfilgrastim	Neulasta	Amgen	2002	2,288	1,900
Epoetin-beta	Epogin, EPOCH, NeoRecormon	Chugai, Roche	1986	1,810	—
Antihemophilic factor	Recombinate	Baxter International	1992	1,527	653
Insulin glargine	Lantus	Sanofi-Aventis	2000	1,510	892
Interferon-alpha-2a	Pegasys	Roche	2001	1,454	545
Filgrastim	Neupogen, GRAN	Amgen, Kirin	1991	1,362	805
Insulin lispro	Humalog	Eli Lilly	1996	1,198	740
Interferon-beta-1b	Betaferon, Betaseron	Schering AG	1993	1,079	372
Interferon-alpha-2b	Intron A, PEG-Intron	Schering-Plough	1986	1,038	320
Protein extracts					
Botulinum toxin type A	Botox	Allergan	1989	831	614

[a]Several of these proteins face "biogeneric" competition as early as 2009 when key patents begin to expire. This includes protein classes for interferon-alpha, insulin, erythropoietin, colony-stimulating factor, human growth factor, and interferon-beta

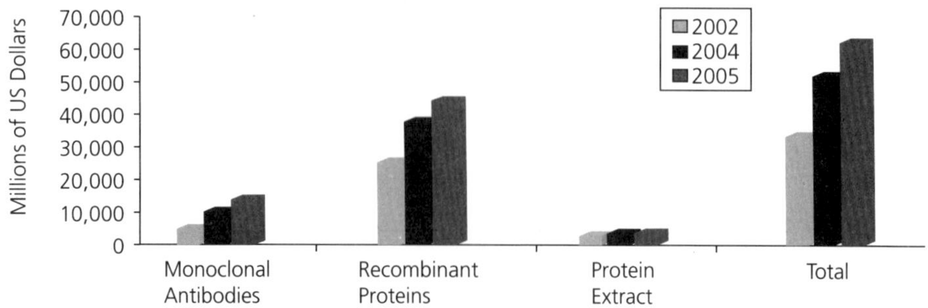

Figure 19.2 Worldwide Protein-based Product Sales, 2002, 2004, and 2005

Against this backdrop of extraordinary success for biotech proteins and MAbs, genomics companies have no sales to date and continue to struggle to bring their first products to market.

CAN GENOMICS JUMPSTART A BROAD PORTFOLIO?

Many start-up genomics firms of the late 1990s and 2000 were hoping to set up revenue streams based on their ability to generate valuable preclinical candidates. Initial optimism about genomics led to some mammoth deals, such as CuraGen's record-breaking $1.5 billion agreement with Bayer (discussed further in this chapter, under section "Genomics-Derived Clinical Pipelines under CuraGen").

A number of companies managed to raise significant cash during that heyday, and several companies, including Celera Genomics, CuraGen, deCode Genetics, Human Genome Sciences, Exelixis, Lexicon Genetics, Millennium Pharmaceuticals, Rigel, and ZymoGenetics, made a serious effort to build real portfolios with a wide range of genomics-derived drugs.

The first wave of products into clinical development largely failed, prompting skepticism regarding the value of these targets and the ability of genomics companies to bring many new drug candidates to market. Is it the product, technology, or company management that is failing to deliver? The industry has responded by replacing many of the early CEOs and sharply refocusing its business strategies (discussed further in this chapter, under section "Evolving Business Strategies").

The tide has clearly shifted, and now that the later-stage product pool is drying up, many pharmaceutical companies are looking for early-stage deals. Because most genomics products in the "first wave" of clinical candidates have failed, genomics companies are working on producing a second wave of genomics-derived drug candidates to help them make some early-stage deals. As can be seen in Table 19.2, a significant number of deals for early-stage compounds have been made, and the value of these deals is high – $147–$800 million. Genomics companies thus see an opportunity for a second chance at big collaborations, and several have already signed deals. This development shows that large pharmaceutical companies are still open to deals with genomics-based companies. However, if this field is to stay active, these second-wave compounds will need to perform far better than their first-wave counterparts.

GENOMICS-DERIVED CLINICAL PIPELINES

One thing that is clear from comparing the present genomics industry pipeline with the one from just two years ago is that several

Table 19.2 Select Deals for Early-stage Compounds and Their Targets, Late 2005 to Early 2006

Pharmaceutical Partner/Developer (date announced)	*Compound(s)/Target (indication)*	*Phase of Development*	*Potential Deal Value/Upfront Payment[a] (millions of dollars)*
Sankyo (Daiichi Sankyo)/ KAI (01-09-06)	KAI-9803/delta protein kinase C inhibitor (cardiovascular disease)	Phase I/II	$300/$20
Wyeth/Trubion (01-03-06)	TRU-015 and others[b]/CD-20 (rheumatoid arthritis)	Phase II	$800/$40
AstraZeneca/Targacept (12-28-05)	TC-1734/neuronal nicotinic receptors (Alzheimer's disease, cognitive deficits in schizophrenia and other cognitive disorders)	Phase II	$300/$10
Wyeth/Exelixis (12-22-05)	Farnesoid X receptor (metabolic and liver disorders)	Preclinical	$147.5/$10
Novartis/Astex[c] (12-6-05)	Cell-cycle-targeting compounds: AT-9311 and AT-7519 (cancer and other diseases)	Preclinical (AT-9311) Phase I (AT-7519)	$520/$25
Roche/BioCryst Pharmaceuticals (11-30-05)	BCX-4208/purine nucleoside phosphorylase inhibitor (transplant rejection and autoimmune diseases)	Phase I	$530/$25
Genentech/Piramed (11-30-05)	PI-3 kinase-targeting compounds (cancer)	Preclinical	$230/not disclosed
Pfizer/Incyte (11-21-05)	INCB-3284 and other CCR2 antagonists (multiple indications including rheumatoid arthritis)	Phase IIa and preclinical	$803/$40
Serono/Rigel (10-25-05)	Aurora kinase inhibitors, including R-763 (cancer)	Preclinical	$160/$25

[a]Potential deal value includes milestone payments, funded research, and upfront fees but not royalties
[b]These compounds are small modular immunopharmaceuticals, which are single-chain polypeptides that are one-third to one-half the size of monoclonal antibodies
[c]Over the last two years, Astex claims a deal flow of more than $1 billion based on small-molecule drug candidates identified using drug fragments that bind to specific target proteins. Partners include Astellas Pharma, AstraZeneca, Berlex, Boehringer Ingelheim, Mitsubishi Pharma, Novartis, Sanofi-Aventis, and Schering AG

drugs that were leading products have dropped out altogether. Most importantly, many of these drugs, such as Rigel's R-112 and ExonHit's Ikomio (EHT-0201), failed during the later stages of their clinical development, after a great deal of money had been spent on them. This result suggests that their targets may simply not have been the key players in the disease process and that better validation may be warranted.

At the World Health Congress in 2005, William Haseltine, who by then had left his position as CEO at HGS, stated that a major challenge for a company is to be able to continue to shift resources away from projects that are likely to fail to projects that seem to be better bets for the money ploughed into them. If the new projects are substantially different from their predecessors, the company's structure will also need to change substantially. It is difficult enough to build a good team once, but when major reorganizations occur over and over again, the company loses momentum, and morale takes a beating. This effect can be enormous even when the shifts are taking place in the early-stage pipeline, but once a project is in later-stage clinical trials, a single failure can have a huge impact, leading to greater delays as new teams are assembled and the appropriate processes are put into place. As a result, companies trying to bring products into multiple clinical areas have been at a disadvantage overall.

In the following sections, we profile some of the leading companies still working to generate robust pipelines derived mainly from genomics- and/or proteomics-based

Table 19.3 Genomics-derived Drugs in Clinical Development from Select Companies, 2006

Company	*Product Name*	*Compound*	*Phase of Development*	*Indication*
CuraGen	Velafermin (CG-53135)	Fibroblast growth factor-20 (FGF-20)	Phase I (treatment) Phase II (prevention)	Oral mucositis
CuraGen	CR-002	Fully human monoclonal antibody (MAb) to platelet-derived growth factor-D (PDGF-D)	Phase I	Kidney inflammation
CuraGen	PXD-101	Small-molecule inhibitor of histone deacetylase (HDAC)	Phase II	Multiple myeloma and T-cell lymphomas[a]
			Phase I	Ovarian and colorectal cancers
deCode Genetics	DG-031	Small molecule that binds 5-lipoxygenase-activating protein (FLAP)[b]	Phase II	Myocardial infarction
deCode Genetics	DG-041	Small molecule that binds EP3 receptor for PGE2	Phase I	Atherosclerosis of the extremities (peripheral arterial disease)
deCode Genetics		Mitogen-activated protein kinase (MAPK) inhibitor	Phase II	Asthma
deCode Genetics	DG-061	Small molecule that binds EP3 receptor for PGE2	Preclinical	Inflammatory pain
Exelixis	Becatecarin (XL-119)[c]	Small molecule	Phase III	Bile duct cancer
Exelixis	XL-999	Small-molecule inhibitor of FGFR, VEGFR, and PDGFR	Phase II	Various cancers
Exelixis	XL-647	Small-molecule inhibitor of EGFR, HER2, VEGFR, and FLT3	Phase I	Non-small-cell lung and breast cancers
Exelixis	XL-784	Small-molecule inhibitor of ADAM-10 metalloprotease	Phase I	Diabetic nephropathy
Exelixis	XL-880	Small-molecule inhibitor of c-Met and VEGFR2	Phase I	Cancer
Exelixis	XL-820	Small-molecule inhibitor of VEGFR2, KIT, and PDGFR	Phase I	Cancer
Exelixis	XL-844	Small-molecule inhibitor of CHK1 and CHK2 kinases that control the cell cycle	Phase I	Chronic lymphocytic leukemia
Exelixis	XL-184	Small-molecule inhibitor of VEGFR2 and MET	Phase I	Cancer
ExonHit	EHT-0202	Small molecule	Phase I	Parkinson's disease and Alzheimer's disease
GlaxoSmithKline	Darapladib (GSK-480848)	Small-molecule inhibitor of Lp-PLA2	Phase III	Atherosclerosis
GlaxoSmithKline	GSK-716155 (formerly HGS's Albugon)	Long-acting form of glucagon-like peptide-1 (GLP-1)	Phase I	Diabetes
GlaxoSmithKline	Relacatib (GSK-462795)	Small-molecule inhibitor of cathepsin K	Phase II	Bone metastases
Human Genome Sciences	Raxibacumab (ABthrax)	Human MAb to *Bacillus anthracis* protective antigen	Phase I	Anthrax
Human Genome Sciences	Albuferon	Albumin-interferon-alpha-2b	Phase II	Hepatitis C
Human Genome Sciences	Belimumab (LymphoStat-B)	Human MAb to B-lymphocyte stimulator (BLyS)	Phase II Phase II	Rheumatoid arthritis Systemic lupus erythematosus (SLE)

Table 19.3 Continued

Company	*Product Name*	*Compound*	*Phase of Development*	*Indication*
Human Genome Sciences	Mapatumumab (HGS-ETR1)	Human MAb to TRAIL receptor 1	Phase II	Hematopoietic cancers, colorectal cancer, and non-small-cell lung cancer
Human Genome Sciences	HGS-ETR2 and HGS-TR2J	Human MAbs to TRAIL receptor 2	Phase I	Cancer
Human Genome Sciences	CCR5 MAb	Human MAb to the CCR5 receptor	Phase I	HIV/AIDS
Millennium	MLN-8054	Small-molecule aurora kinase inhibitor	Phase I	Solid tumors
Rigel	R-788[d]	Inhibitor of spleen tyrosine kinase (SYK)	Phase I	Rheumatoid arthritis
Rigel	R-763	Multiaurora kinase inhibitor	Preclinical	Cancer
ZymoGenetics	IL-29	Recombinant interleukin-29	Preclinical	Hepatitis C
ZymoGenetics	IL-21	Recombinant interleukin-21	Phase I	Metastatic melanoma and renal cell carcinoma
ZymoGenetics	TACI-Ig	Soluble receptor that binds BLyS and aproliferation-inducing ligand (APRIL)	Phase I	SLE, rheumatoid arthritis, and advanced B-cell malignancies

[a]Cutaneous T-cell lymphoma, peripheral T-cell lymphoma, and T-cell non-Hodgkin's lymphoma
[b]Licensed from Bayer, the compound binds to FLAP and inhibits leukotriene synthesis
[c]Licensed exclusively to Helsinn Healthcare. The other Exelixis compounds may be optioned by GlaxoSmithKline following a clinical proof-of-concept by Exelixis
[d]R-788 is an oral, solid-dose formulation of R-406

EGFR = Epidermal growth factor receptor; FGFR = Fibroblast growth factor receptor; FLT3 = Fms-like tyrosine kinase 3, a tyrosine kinase oncoprotein; HER2 = A receptor tyrosine kinase in the EGFR family; KIT = A membrane receptor for stem-cell factor; MET = An oncogene encoding hepatocyte growth factor receptor; PDGFR = Platelet-derived growth factor receptor; PGE2 = Prostaglandin E2; SLE = Systemic lupus erythematosus; SSKI = Spectrum selective kinase inhibitor that targets multiple receptor tyrosine kinases; TACI-Ig = A soluble fusion protein that links the Fc portion of immunoglobulin (Ig) with a portion of transmembrane systemic lupus activator (TACI); and VEGFR = Vascular endothelial growth factor receptor

drug discovery and research. Table 19.3 lists select protein, MAb, and small-molecule drugs from their pipelines. These companies, overall, seem to be making progress, though the biggest challenges in late-stage clinical development still lie ahead. It is not surprising that genomics can produce interesting clinical candidates, and it is reassuring that some drug candidates are still in Phase II and seem to be headed for Phase III trials.

Celera Genomics

In January 2006, Celera Genomics acquired full ownership of Celera Diagnostics. At the Biotechnology Industry Organization's CEO & Investor Conference in February, President Kathy Ordoñez described the focus of the newly merged company as one that will discover, develop, manufacture, and register molecular diagnostic products that can be used in targeted medicine. From this point forward, the company plans to partner its therapeutic development activities and to concentrate on diagnostic opportunities internally.

The Human Genome Project led to the complete sequencing of the human genome by 2000. It took Celera another five years to develop the tools to correlate gene sequences with disease. For instance, Celera uses a functional genomics screen that employs 30,000 single nucleotide polymorphisms (SNPs) to identify gene variants associated with a disease. Celera has identified multiple SNPs for coronary heart disease and is generating "genetic risk scores" for testing or making predictions on hepatitis C treatment modalities, liver fibrosis, and breast cancer and determining which patients may benefit the most from statin therapy. The company routinely validates drug targets and, from

2003 to 2005, generated 32 fully validated targets from its proteomics program. In February 2006, Abbott selected four additional targets for MAb development, and it now has six Celera targets under development. Seattle Genomics has one cancer antigen under development with Celera, and Merck has a cathepsin K inhibitor in Phase I trials for osteoporosis.

Through its partnership with Abbott, Celera has developed diagnostic products for testing for cystic fibrosis and genotyping HIV to detect mutations in the virus that make it resistant to drugs. Genetic tests for thrombosis risk using factor 2, factor V Leiden, and MTHFR are under way with Abbott. A second diagnostic collaboration with LabCorp is developing analyte-specific reagents (ASRs) that can detect fragile X syndrome, the leading cause of inherited mental retardation.

CuraGen

CuraGen built one of the first and highest-profile genomic drug discovery and development "engines" in the mid-1990s. CuraGen also scored one of the biggest pharmaceutical deals of the century with Bayer: a $1.5 billion agreement centered on 80 gene and protein targets for obesity and adult-onset diabetes and the use of CuraGen's functional genomic and pharmacogenomic technologies to assess Bayer's drug candidates. That collaboration was built largely around milestones. Since then, CuraGen has found collaborators relatively scarce and has had difficulty pushing its own drugs forward, although it has several in development (Table 19.3).

CuraGen's genomics research programs have identified 8,000 potential targets, which have given rise to a set of 500 qualified targets associated with disease. The company has five products in preclinical and clinical development. The lead product, velafermin (CG-53135), was one of the first genomics-derived products to enter clinical trials. In December 2005, CuraGen announced that velafermin failed to meet its primary goal in Phase II trials in mucositis patients taking high-dose chemotherapy in preparation for bone marrow transplantation. The drug, a recombinant human fibroblast growth factor-20 (rhFGF-20), did show some efficacy in one subgroup of patients, but the trial as a whole was a setback. CuraGen is initiating another Phase II trial of the drug, to which the FDA has given orphan drug status and designated fast-track development.

CuraGen has a small-molecule product, PXD-101, in Phase II trials for multiple myeloma and T-cell lymphoma. This drug is a histone deacetylase (HDAC) inhibitor licensed from TopoTarget. CuraGen's CR-002 product is a fully human MAb against platelet-derived growth factor-D (PDGF-D) in Phase I trials for kidney inflammation. The company has three MAbs (CR-O11, CR-O12, and CR-O14) in preclinical development for cancer indications. CR-O11 and CR-O14 are antibody-drug conjugates, and CR-O12 is a naked antibody.

deCode Genetics

deCode's core area of expertise is genetic variation. Much of the research in this field has been based on inexact tools and approaches or too few data samples, but with exclusive access to data on many patients in Iceland, where deCode is located, the company has what could be a very important strategic advantage. Experts agree that, if done correctly, genetic variation studies should reveal important new information about potential drug targets and patients' responses to particular types of drugs.

deCode uses its population genetics approach to identify variants in human genes that give rise to disease. A person who inherits one of these disease-associated variants can have a significantly higher risk of developing that disease. To date, deCode has mapped 30 genes and identified 15 targets of interest. It has nine products in drug development and three products in clinical trials for myocardial infarction, peripheral arterial disease, and asthma.

Several of deCode's drug candidates affect the arachidonic and leukotriene pathways

(Figure 19.3). DG-041 is a small-molecule inhibitor to prostaglandin E2 receptor 3 (EP3). The company identified the target EP3 and brought DG-041 into a Phase I clinical trial in less than three years, a very short time frame. The drug inhibits platelet aggregation and is under development for peripheral arterial disease. deCode has 140 EP3 inhibitors in its small-molecule library. When rofecoxib (Merck's Vioxx) was withdrawn in September 2004 for risks associated with cardiovascular events, deCode saw an immediate opportunity for its EP3 inhibitors and chose DG-061 for development to treat

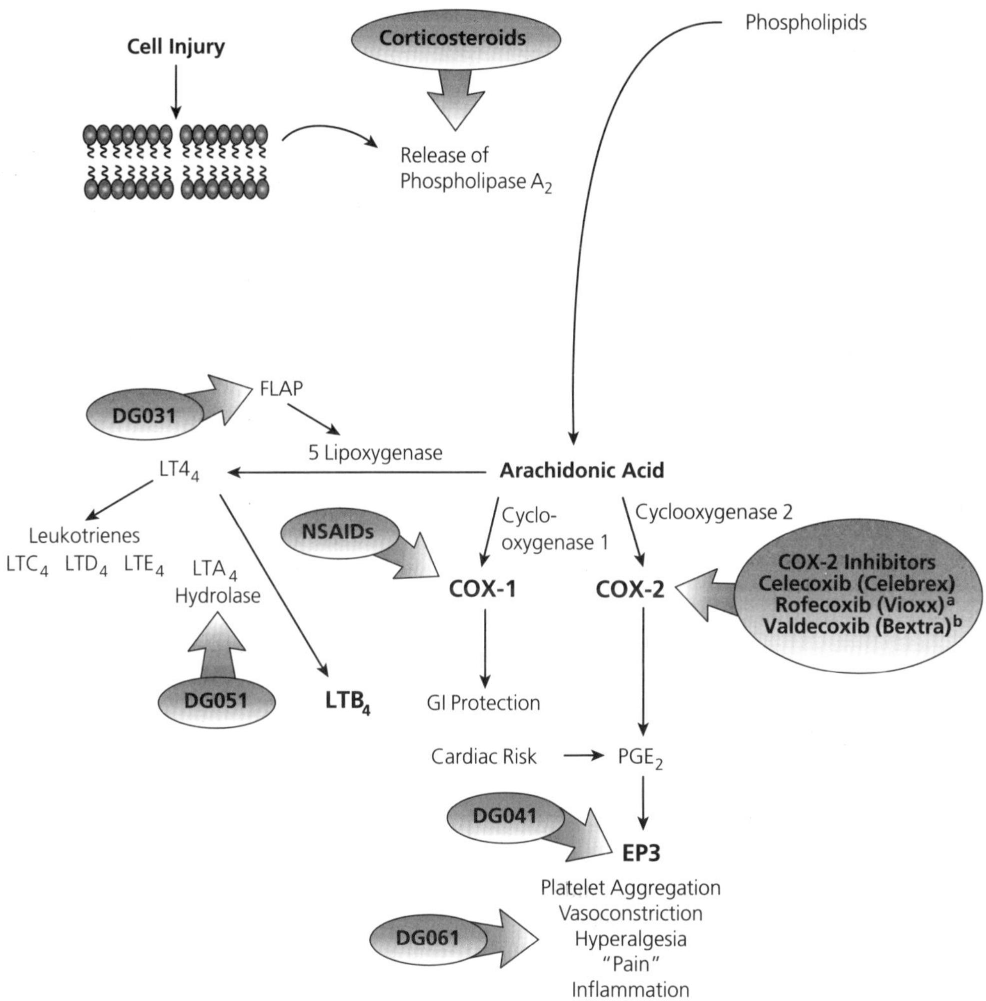

[a]Rofecoxib (Vioxx) was withdrawn September 2004
[b]Valdecoxib (Bextra) was withdrawn April 2005

COX = Cyclooxygenase
EP3 = Receptor for prostaglandin E_2
FLAP = 5-lipoxygenase activating protein
GI = Gastrointestinal
LT = Leukotriene
NSAIDs = Nonsteroidal anti-inflammatory drugs
PGE_2 = Prostaglandin E_2

Figure 19.3 Drugs in Development by deCode Genetics in the Arachidonic Acid and Leukotriene Pathways

pain caused by inflammation. This drug acts downstream of prostaglandin E2 production, so it is not expected to trigger the gastrointestinal bleeding and cardiovascular side effects associated with cyclooxygenase-2 (COX-2) inhibitors.

deCode has two compounds under development for myocardial infarction: DG-031 in Phase II trials and DG-051 in preclinical studies. These compounds inhibit two different targets in the leukotriene pathway (Figure 19.3). deCode has found that the presence of an at-risk variant of the *LTA4 hydrolase* gene increased the risk of heart attack in 16% of Caucasian Americans but in 250% of African-Americans (Helgadottir et al., 2006).

In January 2006, deCode announced that it had discovered a variant of the gene for transcription factor 7-like 2 (TCF7L2) that is a major risk factor for type 2 diabetes, a long-hoped-for discovery (Grant et al., 2006). People having one copy of the variant had a 45% increased risk of disease, while people with two copies of the variant had a 141% increased risk. Patients carrying one or two copies of the disease variant account for 20% of type 2 diabetics.

Exelixis

Exelixis has stayed close to its functional genomic roots. The company has more than 4 million compounds and expertise in structure-based design, pharmacodynamics, and pharmacokinetics that it uses to identify, screen, and develop promising lead candidates. Several years ago, the company inlicensed a compound then in Phase I/II clinical trials from Bristol-Myers Squibb. That compound, becatecarin (XL-119), is now entering Phase III trials for bile duct tumors, a step that suggests a potential revenue stream is on the horizon.

The company has made lucrative deals on a steady basis, including deals in 2005 with the following companies: Bristol-Myers Squibb ($38 million), Genentech ($16 million), Genoptera ($14 million), GlaxoSmithKline (GSK) ($35 million), Helsinn ($4 million), Wyeth ($10 million), and Symphony ($80 million), as well as an equity offering ($50 million). In March 2006, the company signed a deal with Sankyo that includes $20 million in upfront payments.

At the J.P. Morgan Conference in January 2006, Exelixis stated that in addition to the aforementioned $250 million in funding, it has the potential for another $1 billion in funding contingent on meeting development milestones. For instance, late 2006, Exelixis licensed compounds targeting the farnesoid X receptor (FXR), a nuclear hormone receptor implicated in a variety of metabolic and liver disorders, to Wyeth. Exelixis received a $10 million upfront payment and will receive up to an additional $147.5 million in development and commercialization milestone payments as well as royalties on the sale of products commercialized under the collaboration. This steady stream of revenue is one reason that Exelixis is aggressively moving compounds into clinical trials.

Except for becatecarin and XL-844, all of Exelixis's cancer compounds are spectrum-selective kinase inhibitors (SSKIs), which are kinase inhibitors acting on multiple kinases. This class of drugs is particularly intriguing because Pfizer and Bayer have similar compounds that have shown remarkable efficacy in hard-to-treat cancers, such as kidney cancer and gastrointestinal stromal tumors (GIST), that are resistant to imatinib (Novartis's Gleevec). Following a clinical proof-of-concept by Exelixis, GSK has the option to develop seven of the Exelixis compounds listed in Table 19.3, not including becatecarin, which has been exclusively licensed to Helsinn Healthcare. It is unlikely that this relatively small company can pursue all the drug candidates in its internal pipeline through clinical development, so it will continue its aggressive licensing strategies.

ExonHit

ExonHit has unique expertise in the study of splice variants, which are RNA transcripts that are assembled in various, slightly altered forms. Its lead product was ikomio

(EHT-0201), which could have been the first genomics-based drug to be approved had it not failed during a pivotal Phase III trial in 2004 as a result of lack of efficacy. The drug, which was being tested for amyotrophic lateral sclerosis (ALS), did not demonstrate any benefit in survival compared with placebo. The company's lead product is now EHT-0202 for Alzheimer's disease and Parkinson's disease. ExonHit has also taken major steps in applying its technology to diagnostics and has key partnerships in that field, including agreements with Agilent and Affymetrix relating to the manufacture and distribution of microarray products and with bioMérieux to develop blood-based diagnostics for cancer.

Human Genome Sciences and GlaxoSmithKline

Having started out with one of the best cash cushions in the field (more than \$1.5 billion), HGS was able to quickly launch multiple drug projects. In fact, the company claimed to have set a record for getting biotechnology products into clinical trials. Unfortunately, those projects suffered many setbacks, making it unclear whether this strategy was wise after all. Over the years, drugs – including a myeloid progenitor inhibitory factor drug (Mirostipen); a keratinocyte growth factor-2 drug (Repifermin); an interleukin-2 albumin-fusion protein (Albuleukin); a growth hormone-albumin fusion protein (Albutropin); and a B-lymphocyte stimulator (LymphoRad) – all dropped out of the pipeline.

HGS has a very strong partner in GSK. The two companies have several different drugs in development based upon HGS's genomics technology (see Table 19.3) including several in Phase II and III trials. The company's most advanced drug is LymphoStat-B, a human MAb to B lymphocyte stimulator, which is in Phase II for both rheumatoid arthritis and systemic lupus erythematosus. The FDA designated LymphoStat-B for fast-track status for systemic lupus erythematosus (SLE) and selected it for inclusion in the Continuous Marketing Application Pilot 2 Program, which provides for frequent scientific feedback and interactions. As a result, this drug could be one of the first genomics-based products to reach the market.

In mid-2005, GSK opted to codevelop and co-commercialize both LymphoStat-B and mapatumumab, a human MAb to TRAIL receptor 1. In addition, GSK acquired exclusive worldwide rights to Albugon (now GSK-716155) in October 2004 and paid HGS \$12 million in milestone payments in 2005 in a deal worth up to \$183 million. GSK is also developing several drugs on its own that were discovered using HGS's technology and patents. They include darapladib, rilapladib, and goxalapladib, all inhibitors of lipoprotein-associated phospholipase A2 (Lp-PLA2). Darapladib is believed to be the first genomics-derived small molecule to enter clinical trials. It is now in Phase III trials for atherosclerosis, and GSK expects to file an NDA in 2008. Rilapladib and goxalapladib are in Phase I trials for atherosclerosis. GSK has a cathepsin K inhibitor, relacatib, in Phase II trials for bone metastases with a potential NDA filing in 2008. Over time, HGS will receive payments and royalties on various GSK drugs as development milestones are met.

HGS has several drugs in development independent of GSK. They include drugs for anthrax prevention (ABthrax), cancer (MAbs to TRAIL receptor 2), HIV/AIDS (MAb to CCR5), and hepatitis C (albumin-interferon-alpha-2b [Albuferon]). The most advanced of these drugs is Albuferon, which is in multicenter Phase II trials in combination with ribavirin versus Roche's peginterferon-alfa-2a (PEGASYS) with ribavirin. HGS plans to look for a development partner before commencing Phase III trials for Albuferon. In March 2006, HGS reported interim clinical trials results from two trials: one in patients who had failed conventional interferon-alfa therapy and one in patients with no prior therapy. Although the results from both trials were encouraging, questions remain over the ability of Albuferon, if approved by the FDA, to break into the market long established by PEGASYS and Schering's peginterferon-alfa-2b (PEG-INTRON).

In October 2005, HGS entered into a contract with the US government regarding raxibacumab (ABthrax). If the government exercises its option to purchase 100,000 doses of ABtrax for the Strategic National Stockpile, HGS could achieve its very first product sales 18–24 months later – a major milestone for a 14-year-old genomics company.

Rigel

Rigel has also seen prized drug candidates fail because of lack of efficacy. In December 2005, the company announced that what was then its lead drug candidate, R-112, failed in a comparative Phase II clinical study with beclomethasone (GSK's Beconase) for treating nasal allergy symptoms. The company's next leading drug, a novel oral hepatitis C RNA polymerase inhibitor known as R-803, had already dropped out. In November 2004, Rigel announced that although R-803 was well tolerated in hepatitis C patients, it was present in the bloodstream at sufficient levels for only a limited number of hours during the course of each dosing day. Although viral levels in these patients did decline, the decline was not statistically significant or clinically meaningful.

To replace these two lead candidates, Rigel advanced clinical development programs for R-788 for the treatment of inflammatory diseases and for R-763, a multi-Aurora kinase inhibitor, for the treatment of cancer. The company initiated a Phase I trial to investigate the safety and pharmacokinetics of R-788 in combination with methotrexate in the treatment of rheumatoid arthritis patients. It also filed an investigational new drug application (IND) with the Food and Drug Administration (FDA) for R-763, triggering a $5 million milestone payment from Serono in January 2006.

ZymoGenetics

Founded as Zymos in 1981, ZymoGenetics had the unique early experience of collaborating with Novo Nordisk to develop recombinant human insulin in 1982 and cloning human factor VII. Renamed ZymoGenetics in 1983, it was acquired by Novo in 1988 and continued to develop novel protein therapeutics and methods for manufacturing several major protein drugs, including factor VIIa and PDGF. In 1994, the company became the first to clone thrombopoeitin (TPO). Currently, ZymoGenetics reports that it has a stake in the following five recombinant protein products being marketed by third parties and with annual aggregate sales exceeding $3 billion: Novolin and NovoRapid (two forms of insulin from Novo), NovoSeven (Novo's factor VIIa), Regranex (Johnson & Johnson's PDGF), and GlucaGen (Novo, Bedford, and Eisai's glucagon).

ZymoGenetics chose to capitalize upon its expertise in protein therapeutics by building a bioinformatics driven, genomics discovery research effort, and in 2000, it reestablished itself as an independent company at the peak of the genomics boom. The company had the advantage of already having some products and thus a cash flow.

ZymoGenetics' genomics-based product candidates are TACI-IG, IL-21 (interleukin-21), and IL-29. TACI-IG is a soluble fusion protein that links the Fc portion of immunoglobulin (Ig) with a portion of transmembrane activator (TACI) and has potential applications for the treatment of autoimmune diseases, including systemic lupus erythematosus and rheumatoid arthritis. The product, which is being codeveloped by ZymoGenetics and Serono, entered Phase I trials in 2003. In January 2006, promising preliminary results from the RA trial were announced, including dose-dependent reductions of IgM, IgA, and IgG and of rheumatoid factor, a biologic marker of disease.

IL-21 is a novel protein that regulates natural killer cells and cytotoxic T cells. ZymoGenetics is studying it in a Phase I trial for metastatic melanoma and renal cell carcinoma. IL-21 is licensed to Novo Nordisk for commercialization outside of North America, while ZymoGenetics retained commercialization rights within North America. The company's IL-29 is in preclinical development for the treatment of hepatitis C.

ZymoGenetics had a fourth product in development – recombinant factor XIII (rFactor XIII) – but licensed it to Novo Nordisk in 2004 so that the company could focus on the development of recombinant human thrombin (a biological coagulant now in Phase III) and its three newer genomics-based drugs. ZymoGenetics also licensed alpha-1-antitrypsin (AAT) to Arriva Pharmaceuticals. It is in Phase II trials for emphysema.

SWOT ANALYSIS

The genomics sector is now more than a dozen years old. In view of the billions of dollars that have been spent, has genomics lived up to its early promises of generating numerous new candidates for drug development? In the following sections, we present a SWOT – strengths, weaknesses, opportunities, threats – analysis of this sector.

Strengths

The genomics sector holds significant assets and strengths, including the following:

- The human genome and several other genomes have been sequenced, thereby generating a stockpile of genes and SNPs that can be used for drug discovery and development. In addition to the 25,000 or so human genes, recent studies have identified important regulatory elements in other parts of the genome that may be implicated in the disease process.
- Genomics has given rise to a number of different "omic" technologies that have been integrated into pharmaceutical companies' Research and Development (R&D) programs. Proteomics, toxicogenomics, and metabolomics all provide valuable information in identifying and validating targets for drug development.
- Even with no products yet in the marketplace, genomics remains a major tool in drug discovery and development. The most dramatic results from genomics might one day be seen in the pipelines of such companies as Genentech, Novartis, and Vertex, which have long integrated genomics with a host of other established technologies.
- Having a stockpile of gene sequences has enabled population genetics. Different people can now be screened to identify gene mutations, and those mutations correlated with disease. Biomarkers are finding use throughout drug development, from the identification of disease-causing genes to better selection of patients to take part in clinical trials.

Weaknesses

In view of the amount of money that has been invested in genomics, it is reasonable to expect new genomics-derived products already in the marketplace and full product development pipelines. However, hard-learned experience over the last decade has identified the following weaknesses in the genomics sector:

- Having a gene sequence in hand does not easily translate into identifying useful drug targets or new drug candidates for development. There are many steps between the expression of a gene and the development of a disease process, which often involves complex pathways of proteins and numerous points for drug intervention. Bioinformatics and high-throughput tools have not solved the basic problem that the science behind disease is very complex.
- Understanding and manipulating the underlying biology are essential to choosing good drug targets. The first wave of genomics-derived drugs to enter clinical pipelines was largely unsuccessful. A much better validation of potential targets is of vital importance.
- The cost of clinical development, especially in late-stage trials, is large. Genomics companies today are rapidly burning through their assets (cash and outlicensing intellectual property) in attempts to bring products through successful Phase III clinical trials and beyond. Continued failures in Phase III trials could be devastating.
- Many genomics companies are suffering from a credibility issue because of their inability to bring products to market and to produce product sales. The sector recently responded by replacing CEOs, many of whom had been with the company since its founding. For example, in the last year, HGS and CuraGen replaced their CEOs, as did Millennium, an early genomics pioneer that has changed its business focus to developing personalized medicines.

Opportunities

In spite of the money that has been spent and the many product failures, the future of the genomics sector remains very encouraging.

Among the numerous opportunities are the following:

- A second wave of genomics-derived products has entered early-stage development; several early-stage deals have already taken place (Table 19.2). Because of the pharmaceutical industry's need to enhance its product development pipeline, genomics companies are hoping to obtain much-needed revenue through such deals. However, the trend is toward lower, upfront payments in these deals and, larger, milestone payments when specific product development hurdles have been circumvented.
- The integration of "omics" technologies into the process that pharmaceutical companies use to develop drugs has improved the understanding of disease processes and helps identify and validate targets for further development. Pharmacogenomics is a major driving force toward the establishment of personalized medicine. The paradigm is changing from an one-drug-fits-all approach to a which-drug-fits-which-patient approach. The knowledge created from genomics is the key to this shift.
- Significant amounts of information are being derived from comparative genomics, a field in which scientists compare regions of the human genome with similar regions of the genomes of other species. This method has resulted in the identification of many functional elements that are involved in regulating genes. The Encyclopedia of DNA Elements (ENCODE) project of the National Human Genome Research Institute is one repository of these elements.
- Several genomics companies own extensive patent estates based on gene and protein information. For instance, the US Patent and Trademark Office database from 1973 to the present day contains the following numbers of patents issued for these companies:

  1. *Human Genome Sciences*: 459 patents.
  2. *Millennium*: 431 patents.
  3. *ZymoGenetics*: 345 patents.
  4. *Applera (parent corporation of Celera Genomics and Applied Biosystems)*: 263 patents.
  5. *Incyte Genomics*: 162 patents.
  6. *Curagen*: 73 patents.

Although not itemized on a company's financial statement, these patent estates confer significant opportunities to a company for future revenues either from direct product sales or from outlicensed royalties and license fees. Much of the value of this asset is yet to be realized.

Threats

The genomics sector faces significant threats. Many early companies have either gone out of business or those that still exist are forced to drastically alter their business strategies. The following threats will continue to haunt this sector:

- Companies must manage cash burn and devise a faster means to reach profitability than they have done to date. Public markets have been depressed for a couple of years and are likely to stay stagnant for the foreseeable future. Several companies have licensed away assets, down-sized, and restructured in an attempt to stem the cash burn (discussed further in this chapter, under section "Evolving Business Strategies"). Product sales are critical to turning this situation around.
- For the next three to five years, revenue streams into genomics companies will come not from product sales but from license fees, pharma-supported drug development and clinical trials, milestone payments, and perhaps some royalty income as the first genomics-derived products reach the market. Genomics companies have begun to aggressively seek collaborators and outlicense genes and targets to generate revenues. This activity must be balanced with retaining sufficient drug candidates in-house to meet a company's independent product development goals.
- The patent estates of several genomics companies will steadily erode over time as effective patent terms run out. The threat of biogeneric legislation and regulations is on the horizon as several key biotech patents expire for drugs in protein classes for interferon-alpha, insulin, erythropoietin, colony-stimulating factor, human growth factor, and interferon-beta.
- Significant amounts of money are required to prosecute and defend large patent estates around the world. Obtaining and maintaining a global patent estate is a great expense, given that opposition, interference, and litigation proceedings will surely arise for numerous gene and protein sequences, many of which were sequenced in government-funded programs.

Funding these worldwide patent costs further drains revenue away from clinical development programs.

- Lastly, the discovery of "dark DNA" and small RNA molecules, such as microRNAs, has added another level of complexity to understanding the gene regulation and to identifying the disease-causing agents. The human genome comprises about 25,000 genes representing only 1.5% of its 3 billion bases. The other 98.5% of the genome that does not code for proteins is known as dark DNA or "junk DNA." It has long been thought that these noncoding regions were inert and had no function (e.g., dark or evolutionary junk). However, it is now thought that elements in the dark DNA are, in fact, remote control elements that can turn regular genes on or off. It may turn out that many elements involved in causing diseases are not in the gene or protein sequences themselves but in this dark DNA. For example, microRNAs, which turn off other genes, have already been implicated in diabetes, hepatitis C, and various cancers. The paradigm of one gene, one protein, and one disease may be the exception rather than the rule.

EVOLVING BUSINESS STRATEGIES

Genomics companies have employed multiple tactics in an effort to remain competitive or even solvent. The year 2005 has been a pivotal year in evolving business strategies. Companies have chosen a variety of approaches to improve their financial situation and get their products to the market. Among these strategies:

- Refocusing drug development activities on a limited number of disease indications.
- Restructuring programs to improve flexibility in order to make decisions in a timely fashion.
- Leveraging assets to concentrate on internal diagnostic, pharmacogenomic, or therapeutic development programs but not on all of them.
- Reducing cash consumption/burn and laying off employees.
- Focusing on faster paths to profitability.
- Bringing in new leadership.
- Aggressively seeking out collaborations and licensing technology.
- Monetized assets by spinning out technology and patents.

Several very high-profile companies have extensively refocused the goals of their genomics-based drug discovery and development programs, as we discuss in the following sections.

Celera Genomics

In January 2006, Celera Genomics, the former "king" of selling genomic information, announced that it had acquired full ownership of Celera Diagnostics. The company has shifted its focus to molecular diagnostics and personalized medicine. Its small-molecule programs were all in early stages of development and will be partnered or sold. The merged company will have 180 fewer employees and anticipates $75 million in cost savings from the closing of its small-molecule programs. Celera plans to use its extensive expertise in genomics, proteomics, and bioinformatics to develop diagnostic products internally and to partner out therapeutic programs. The net result is a leaner, more flexible company that has a much reduced cash burn. Celera is hoping that by focusing on diagnostics and partnering out therapeutic programs, it will be able to grow faster and become profitable much sooner than it would have before the merger and restructuring.

Millennium Pharmaceuticals

Millennium dropped out of the gene-sequencing race early and focused its efforts on pharmacogenomics. In 2005, the company brought in Deborah Dunsire as CEO to replace Mark Levin, who had been with Millennium since the company began. In addition to changing CEOs, the company is also being restructured; it reduced its workforce from about 1,500 employees in 2004 to 1,142 employees (as of February 28, 2006) and hopes to be profitable for the first time in its 12-year history by achieving a net income of $5 million in 2006 (a nongenerally accepted accounting practice [non-GAAP] estimate). In 2006, Millennium is expecting revenues of $225–250 million from sales of bortezomib

(Velcade), the company's small-molecule proteasome inhibitor for cancer, and of \$115–\$125 million in royalty income.

Millennium's expertise is in pharmacogenomics and understanding disease pathways. In an effort to leverage these assets effectively, the company decided in 2005 to focus its efforts on oncology and not to work on multiple disease indications. This strategy includes development of bortezomib for additional cancer indications, of MLN-518 for acute myeloid leukemia, and of MLN-8054 for advanced malignancies.

In mid-2005, Schering-Plough acquired the balance of US rights for the product eptifibatide (Integrilin), an inhibitor of gpIIb/IIIa under development for cardiovascular indications, and will pay royalties to Millennium. Millennium obtained rights to eptifibatide when it acquired COR Therapeutics in 2002 and had been copromoting the product in the United States with Schering. Millennium is no longer involved in inflammation at the discovery level but does have MLN-1202 in Phase II trials for multiple sclerosis and atherosclerosis, though it dropped development of this drug for rheumatoid arthritis. As Millennium has narrowed its development focus, it has also begun to position itself to become a major player in translational medicine and to use its pathway and biomarker expertise to develop personalized medicines.

HGS-CoGenesys

HGS underwent a restructuring in early 2004 when it laid off 20% of its workforce, reprioritized its pipeline, and brought in new leadership. After 12 years, CEO William A. Haseltine left the company and was replaced by H. Thomas Watkins, who had 20 years of experience at Abbott Laboratories and had been the president of TAP Pharmaceutical Products. HGS refocused its efforts on specific drug candidates in later-stage development and concentrated on bringing its first products to market, while managing a cash burn that generated \$239.4 million in losses in 2005.

In December 2005, HGS announced plans to spin off its CoGenesys division as a means to "monetize its less critical assets." The strategy is to license early-stage drug candidates that do not qualify for HGS's development pipeline and to seek private-equity funding to finance CoGenesys. In January 2006, HGS licensed an undisclosed gene to Amgen and an undisclosed target to PDL BioPharma in exchange for upfront licensing fees, milestone payments, and royalties. In a similar fashion, CoGenesys will receive rights to a body, but not all, of early-stage HGS genes and targets. HGS will transfer a team of 60 employees, including 20 PhD-level scientists, to CoGenesys and seed it with a \$10 million loan to be repaid in equity or cash at a future date. HGS will receive a portion of the revenues that CoGenesys generates and will retain the right of first refusal for specific products and the option to have CoGenesys perform preclinical research and development for as many as two products a year for HGS.

The goal is for CoGenesys to obtain enough independent funding that it can become a separate company. This strategy has two immediate ramifications. The first is that HGS has amassed a patent estate covering thousands of human genes and cannot possibly develop all of the antibody, protein, and small-molecule drugs that could be generated for each gene. A broad-based licensing strategy could get more genomics-derived products into development, return revenues to HGS, and create value before the usefulness of many of these patents expire. With nearly \$250 million in losses last year based on only \$19.1 million in revenues, HGS is in critical need of a strong revenue stream.

The second ramification is that HGS's fortunes are very tightly bound to GSK through its many collaborative agreements, licenses, and shared products under development. GSK could well acquire HGS in the near future. By spinning out certain technology and patents into an independent CoGenesys, HGS may be separating those assets so that they would remain outside a future acquisition. In May, HGS announced that it has entered into an agreement with a real estate investment trust (REIT), BioMed Realty Trust, on the sale/leaseback of its 290,000-square-foot manufacturing facility that can be used for the production of mammalian proteins. HGS will receive $220 million in cash along with a 20-year lease for renting the facility with options to renew and rights to repurchase.

Nuvelo

Nuvelo began essentially as a genomics tool maker called Hyseq, which was founded by two Yugoslavian scientists who had developed a process called signature-by-hybridization (SBH). With the help of venture funding, Hyseq became a tools and drug discovery company focusing on the collection of novel and rarely expressed genes identified through SBH. When George Rathmann joined the company's board in the spring of 2000, the business strategy changed to that of creating a biopharmaceutical company. Following Hyseq's merger with Variagenics in 2002, the combined company changed its name to Nuvelo. Within two years, the company had spun off its tool business into a subsidiary called Callida Genomics, launched its first clinical trial, and acquired another genomics pioneer – Variagenics, an early pharmacogenomics company.

Rathmann used his considerable influence to help Nuvelo acquire a compound (alfimeprase) from the biotech pioneer Amgen, which he cofounded in 1980. Although alfimeprase seemed promising, Amgen's leaders did not believe that it fit in with their company's portfolio: alfimeprase was an ideal prospect for a firm that needed its first product.

That gamble paid off early in 2006 when Bayer Healthcare (BHC) agreed to pay up to $385 million for the non-US rights to develop and commercialize alfimeprase. Alfimeprase is a first-in-class thrombolytic that directly degrades fibrin. Clinical trials to date show that the drug triggers rapid clot dissolution and has a well-tolerated safety profile. Under the terms of the agreement, Nuvelo will retain all commercialization rights and profits from alfimeprase sales in the United States, while BHC will commercialize alfimeprase in all territories outside the United States. Over the course of the agreement, Nuvelo is eligible to receive up to $385 million in milestone payments, including a $50 million upfront cash payment, up to $165 million in development milestones, and $170 million in sales and commercialization milestones. Nuvelo's current strategy is to use revenues from its collaboration with Bayer to become a fully integrated biopharmaceutical company.

In general, Nuvelo has turned away from genomics, but it retains a research focus on secreted proteins and antibodies. The company is developing NU-206, a growth factor that stimulates the gastrointestinal tract to regenerate. It is in preclinical development with Kirin for cancer-therapy-induced mucositis. NU-206 is one of a number of novel secreted proteins that Nuvelo attributes to its genomics research. Callida Genomics, meanwhile, continues to develop its DNA sequence analysis products, which are based on its ProbeUniverse technology. Callida Genomics' stated long-term strategy is to use those tools to discover genetic variants that can be used in new DNA diagnostic tests for personalized and preventive medicine.

Incyte Pharmaceuticals

Incyte was initially a very high-profile seller of genomics information and one of the fastest runners in the race to patent genes. Incyte's expertise included functional genomic technologies, proteomic databases, and protein therapeutics. When the market for genomics data completely dried up, partly as a result of public competition, the company underwent a dramatic restructuring, basically dropping databases and devoting itself to pharmaceutical development in 2004.

Incyte's CEO, Paul A. Friedman, had been the president of DuPont Pharmaceuticals Research Laboratories until DuPont sold its pharmaceutical division to Bristol-Myers Squibb in 2001. When Friedman moved to Incyte, he brought in many former colleagues from the anti-inflammatory program at

DuPont and helped Incyte make a total transition, away from protein therapeutics, and toward small-molecule drug discovery and development.

Incyte was able to identify a CCR2 antagonist for clinical development within 12 months of screening. Its most advanced CCR2 antagonist is INCB-3284, which is in Phase IIa clinical trials for rheumatoid arthritis and insulin-resistant obesity. In November 2005, Incyte entered into a deal with Pfizer, whereby the latter has worldwide development and commercialization rights to Incyte's CCR2 antagonists for all indications except multiple sclerosis and one additional (undisclosed) indication. Incyte retained the rights to certain compounds. Pfizer agreed to pay Incyte an upfront payment of $40 million, milestone payments of up to $743 million, and royalties on sales. Pfizer also agreed to purchase $20 million in convertible subordinated notes and another $10 million in notes after Incyte files an IND for a retained Incyte indication.

In addition to INCB-3284 and related CCR2 antagonists, Incyte has other products in development, including a sheddase inhibitor in Phase II trials for cancer. A newly identified compound, a small-molecule inhibitor of 11-beta hydroxysteroid dehydrogenase type 1 called INCB-13739, is expected to begin Phase I trials in the first half of 2006 for type 2 diabetes. In April, the company discontinued development of dexelvucitabine (DFC), which was in Phase II trials for HIV, due to possible complications from pancreatic inflammation.

OUTLOOK

All in all, the year 2005 was one of discontent for genomics companies and their investors. The genomics industry has spent billions of dollars and needs to bring products to market soon to continue funding product development. That said, genomics has spawned the creation of dozens of new tools that can be used to discover and develop new drugs. Each new tool can be used to investigate a different part of the disease process and thus contribute a new piece of information to the mix. The key for pharma companies is to use the data generated by the different tools to determine a pathway to drug development and to market. This process will take time to develop into a coherent clinical program. To date, the industry has been frustrated by genomics' failure to rapidly fill clinical pipelines. The reality is that genomics may or may not be able to shorten development timelines. However, genomics-derived tools have been widely integrated into the drug development process, and many are uniquely suited to identify drugs to treat those patients who can most benefit from them.

How genomics companies fare in the near term will depend largely on how much cash they have and how far they can go with it. Most of these companies generate very little in revenues but are dealing with large losses in the range of $60 million to more than $200 million per year; the exception is Millennium, which is now focusing on traditional products and pharmacogenomics rather than on genomics and which had revenues exceeding $500 million in 2005 (Table 19.4). Based on the cash in hand and the current level of operating expenses, genomics companies have two to three years before their current cash reserve runs out. Managing cash burn continues to be of vital importance to these companies and undoubtedly contributed to the strategic refocusing that occurred in 2004 and 2005.

Personalized Medicine

Genomics has long been hailed as the "future" of pharmaceuticals. Many enthusiasts believe that, through genomics, drug discovery and development will become faster and more precise. Currently, drugs are designed to treat all patient groups in a single, large market, even though subgroups of these patients may not benefit from the treatment. Eventually, though, drugs will be individualized based on patients' genetic makeup and the specific characteristics of their disease (e.g., subtype

Table 19.4 Financial Profile of Select Companies, Year-End 2005

Company	*Founded*	*Cash and Investments (millions of dollars)*	*Revenues (millions of dollars)*	*Net Loss (millions of dollars)*	*Market Cap[a] (millions of dollars)*
CuraGen	1991	226.5	23.5	73.2	273
deCode	1996	155.6	44.0	62.8	536
Exelixis	1994	210.5	76	84.4	932
Human Genome Sciences	1992	646.2	19.1	239.4	1,808
Incyte	1991	345.0	7.8	103.0	501
Millennium	1993	645.6	558.3	198.2	3,257
ZymoGenetics	1981	366.3	42.9	78.0	1,442

[a]Determined March 6, 2006

of cancer). This field is known as personalized medicine. Many of the predicted developments are taking place but not at the pace, or in the order, anticipated.

Rather than an ever-growing stream of genomics drugs, a new tool kit is evolving. The key elements of this kit, and their applications, are first being demonstrated in oncology, where the new paradigm for molecular drug development is being established. The current model is not driven by quantities of data but rather by a focus on the quality of data. Instead of generating zillions of data points with gene arrays and then sifting through those with bioinformatics, researchers are finding the most success when they look deeply into individual targets, which they study in a range of models using a variety of tools. The key is not having a magic application that can pick targets out of databases but truly understanding a single target and using the tools appropriately to test compounds against it.

A dramatic example of this approach comes from one of the first targeted therapies developed for the treatment of breast cancer – trastuzumab (Genentech/Roche/Chugai's Herceptin) (see the sidebar, "Targeted Therapy in Breast Cancer," for more information). Trastuzumab demonstrates the brilliant use of molecular information for rapid advancement of medicine. Such advances become more common as more biomarkers are validated, many of them perhaps through genomics and proteomics. deCode Genetics is especially well positioned to make a major impact in this area through its expertise in population genetics and in correlating gene variants with disease.

Companies that are rapidly positioning themselves to be leaders in personalized medicine include Celera and Millennium. The past 18 months have witnessed a major restructuring of Celera, for example, to focus on diagnostics and pharmacogenomics and to partner out therapeutic advances. Both Millennium and Celera are well ahead of pharma companies in developing strategies designed to treat specific patient groups and thereby segment a disease market.

Targeted Therapy in Breast Cancer

Many proponents of genomics suggest that as the field matures, it will drive personalized medicine, which is becoming increasingly common in targeted therapies in oncology. Trastuzumab (Genentech/Roche/Chugai's Herceptin) is one of the first targeted therapies, and oncology is one of the first therapeutic areas to benefit from targeted therapies. A recombinant humanized monoclonal antibody (MAb), trastuzumab binds to the extracellular domain of the human epidermal growth factor receptor 2 (EGFR2), also known as the *HER2* receptor. Trastuzumab was developed after scientists determined that the *HER2/neu* amplification, a genetic alternation found in 20–25% of patients, leads to an aggressive form of breast cancer. By inhibiting *HER2*, physicians greatly improve these women's prognosis. Patients who do not overexpress *HER2* do not benefit from treatment with trastuzumab. Decision Resources predicts that sales of trastuzumab will nearly triple over 2004–2014, from $795 million in 2004 to more than $2.0 billion in 2009 and more than $2.5 billion in 2014.

Recently, at a meeting of the American Association for Clinical Cancer Research, UCLA researcher Dennis Slamon, who led key early work on *HER2*, described a small set of early results from trials combining trastuzumab and bevacizumab (Genentech's Avastin) in breast cancer patients who had no prior chemotherapy. Of nine patients, two experienced complete remission, and several more showed measurable responses. Slamon pointed out that his group selected this particular drug combination based on studies showing that *HER2*-positive patients, who are the women eligible for trastuzumab treatment, also have elevated levels of vascular endothelial growth factor (VEGF), which bevacizumab targets. Larger-scale clinical trials are under way. This compelling evidence suggests that well-chosen combinations of targeted drugs can be very effective.

Information about additional molecular markers may further improve treatment. For example, women whose tumors show amplification of topo II are more likely to respond to the chemotherapy doxorubicin (Pfizer's Adriamycin), which targets that protein.

Genomics-derived Therapeutics

Although genomics obviously generates a wealth of important tools and potentially valuable information, no convincing evidence suggests that expertise in genomics can generate a broad range of drug candidates in a shorter-than-usual time. One unanticipated problem, in fact, is that a number of genomic candidates have simply proved ineffective. These drugs sail through Phase I trials, generating high hopes, but then stall at Phase II or III – siphoning off huge amounts of capital before they are deemed failed projects. The industry is still in the middle stages of understanding how best to use all the tools it has spawned. Enabling developments continue to occur, such as the availability of RNAi for target validation, the revelation that microRNAs also play critical roles in health and disease, improvements in pathways analysis, and new imaging tools that allow proof-of-concept studies early in the development process. Genentech, GSK, Novartis, and Vertex Pharmaceuticals are just a few of the companies that have either integrated many genomics tools in their drug discovery and development platforms or are working closely with partners with a strong expertise in genomics.

In the meantime, the second wave of genomics-based drugs is beginning to move through company pipelines, and several of these drugs could conceivably complete Phase III over the next one to four years. GSK's darapladib (480848) and HGS's Lymphostat B currently have the best chances of being first-to-market genomics-based drugs. Phase III is a crucial testing ground for any product, and these trials will play a big role in the fortunes of genomics companies. GSK is very active in genomics-based drugs and has high hopes for darapladib in particular. The drug inhibits Lp-PLA2, an enzyme associated with the formation of atherosclerotic plaques. GSK expects to submit an NDA for the drug, which is in Phase III, in 2008. Given the fact that GSK has launched two other Lp-PLA2 compounds into Phase I trials, the company apparently has confidence in this drug target.

In addition to its agreements with HGS (discussed earlier in this chapter, under Section Human Genome Sciences and GlaxoSmithKline), GSK has agreements with Exelixis, including rights to option the majority of drug candidates that Exelixis has under development. Exelixis has leveraged its lead identification and pharmacodynamics-screening platforms into alliances with numerous pharma companies. This aggressive licensing strategy may provide the company with the revenues needed to develop products on its own, as long as it retains sufficient rights over its own products and potential markets. The combined assets that GSK has amassed with HGS and Exelixis could make it the leading beneficiary of genomics-derived products in the foreseeable future.

HGS remains the leader in bringing genomics-based drugs into clinical development, and it has the fullest pipeline. Its fortunes are very much tied to its collaborations with GSK, a situation that raises the question of how much longer HGS will function as an independent company. Though some of the HGS patents and drug targets may be spun off into its recently created CoGenesys vehicle, there is still a significant patent estate including claims to genes, proteins, and their uses in discovering drugs.

Genomics-derived Diagnostics

It is not just drug discovery that stands to gain from genomics but diagnostics as well. DiaDexus, for example, is a diagnostic firm trying to exploit Lp-PLA2. That company's Plac test, which measures the enzyme, is already on the market and is used to predict the risk for ischemic stroke associated with atherosclerosis. It is also telling that Celera Genomics has refocused its efforts in drug discovery on the pursuit of diagnostics, and ExonHit, one of the smallest genomics firms, has expanded its diagnostics business. Genomics research approaches nicely integrate these two fields because gene expression can be a marker as well as a target. Given that it will take a lot of time and money to bring genomics-derived drugs to market, some companies are hoping it will be quicker to turn some of the biological markers discovered along the way into diagnostics. Celera, in particular, is trying to leverage its broad genomics-derived assets into creating diagnostic value as a faster means to generate revenue streams and reach profitability.

REFERENCES

Grant, S.F., et al. Variant of transcription factor 7-like 2 (TCF7l2) gene confers risk of type 2 diabetes. *Nature Genetics.* 2006; 38: 320–3.

Helgadottir, A., et al. A variant of the gene encoding leukotriene A4 hydrolase confers ethnicity-specific risk of myocardial infarction. *Nature Genetics.* 2006; 38: 68–74.

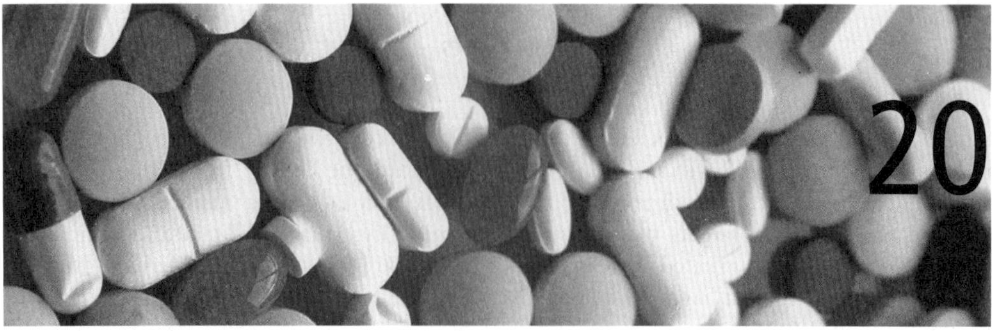

The Role of Pharmacogenomics in Personalized Medicine

THE PERSONALIZATION OF MEDICINE

In the 21st century, personalized medicine is a growing trend. The pharmaceutical industry is very gradually moving away from the blockbuster model of drug development, which is based on the theory that "one drug treats most patients most of the time," to a model whereby medicines are designed to treat the specific patient, not the population as a whole. Pharmaceutical companies that are able to navigate the path from the blockbuster to the personalized medicine model of drug development will become early leaders in this new era of medicine.

Several new technologies will facilitate the development of personalized medicine; key among them is pharmacogenomics, which determines how genomic variations in people modify the behavior of drugs. Pharmacogenomics combines pharmacology with genomic information and can be used during the development of new drugs to identify the most appropriate drug to treat an individual based on that person's genomic makeup.

Pharmacogenomics has built on information generated by the Human Genome Project and the SNP Consortium. The Human Genome Project determined the sequence of all human genes; the consortium is a public/private collaboration established to discover and characterize single nucleotide polymorphisms (SNPs) that represent common DNA sequence variations in different individuals. These polymorphisms and other biomarkers are needed not only to correlate a particular genetic variation with a disease but also to develop a diagnostic test to screen for the presence or absence of that genetic variation. A person's genetic profile ultimately determines how that person will respond to a drug.

In this chapter, we examine the role of pharmacogenomics in personalized medicine and how it will affect today's drug development strategies. We explain how pharmacogenomics works and discuss how regulatory authorities are addressing pharmacogenomics and its role in the drug development process.

PHARMACOGENOMICS DEFINED

Pharmacogenomics should help create better medicines because it addresses the underlying genetics involved in causing a disease rather than just the symptoms of the disease. Pharmacogenomics has the potential to provide more-effective drug treatment by addressing the individual patient's response to drugs based on his or her genomic makeup. By integrating pharmacogenomics into clinical development, the pharmaceutical industry may be able to enhance its overall efficiency by improving the design and outcomes of late-stage clinical trials. However, any potential savings from increased clinical-trial success will be offset by the additional costs incurred in the early stages of drug development to determine patients' genomic profiles. Likewise, drug sales will likely be lower because of the segmentation of the overall disease market into smaller patient subpopulations based on genomic makeup. In cases of small disease populations segmented by genomics, it is questionable whether sufficient reimbursement will be available to provide the commercial incentives necessary to develop drugs to treat these diseases.

The traditional approach to drug development has been to develop drugs that are effective in animal models, almost all of which use inbred (nonhuman) animal strains that display a high degree of genomic uniformity. Populations of human patients are less genomically homogeneous and therefore often display pronounced variations in response when treated with a particular drug. A schematic representation of these variations is shown in Figure 20.1. Before the advent of genomics, one drug (Drug A) treated a heterogeneous patient population; the result was groups of people who responded well to the drug, those who did not respond, and those who suffered adverse reactions to the drug. By applying pharmacogenomic profiling to the same patient population, the opportunity exists to develop different drugs (Drug A, Drug B, and Drug C) that are effective in the different groups of patients.

In the following sections, we discuss the potential impact of pharmacogenomics on drug efficacy and drug metabolism and give examples of products that demonstrate the effectiveness of pharmacogenomics in drug development.

Drug Efficacy

The existence of genomic variations in different people means that different people may respond differently to the same drug. The variable drug responses can be attributed to the following:

- Different levels of expression of the drug target.
- The existence of rare isoforms of a drug target that are not commonly expressed.

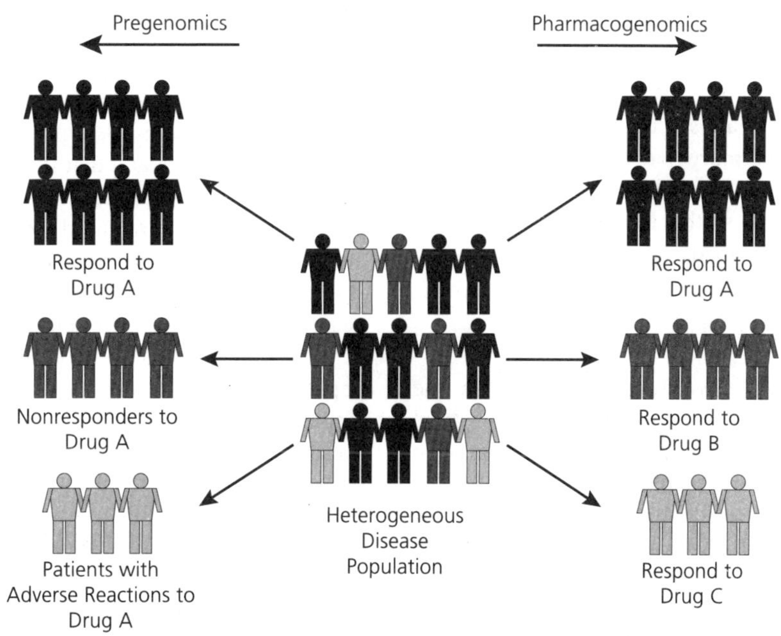

Figure 20.1 Application of Pharmacogenomics and Effects on Drug Responses

- The existence of different forms of the target that vary in their response to the drug.
- The existence of genomic variations in pivotal enzymes that metabolize drugs.

This last variation is perhaps the most readily addressed. Different people metabolize drugs in various ways depending on the genes they carry for enzymes that either metabolize drugs or transport them. It is increasingly recognized that genomic profiling of these enzymes should be done in patients selected for inclusion in late-stage clinical trials, even if the patients who will subsequently be treated with an approved drug will not be profiled in a similar fashion. This metabolic screening may improve the effectiveness of clinical-trial results by enabling the stratification of people into different groups.

In the following sections, we cite examples of genomic variations in target proteins that can affect responses to drugs. Some of these examples provide clear evidence of ways in which pharmacogenomics can benefit patients (by ensuring that only those in whom the treatment is likely to be effective are treated), healthcare payers (by reducing costs), and pharmaceutical suppliers (by enhancing the reputation of the product). These examples also highlight the fact that problems may not become apparent until the late-stage clinical development, thereby underscoring the need for pharmaceutical companies to use tools such as pharmacogenomics to ascertain as early as possible why clinical results are disappointing so that the late-stage trials can be better designed.

Bronchodilators

Most of the bronchodilators used in the treatment of respiratory diseases are partial agonists of the β_2 receptor, and many genomic polymorphisms in this receptor have been identified. Some polymorphisms reduce the efficacy of a fixed dose of drug while others enhance the patient's response to the drug. These effects are often similar for the whole drug class and specifically affect responses to drugs such as salmeterol (GlaxoSmithKline's Serevent) and albuterol (GlaxoSmithKline's Ventolin, Schering's Proventil). There has not yet been a systematic pharmacogenomic mapping of these variations, probably because these drugs are well established and generally effective and dosing is readily altered. The role of pharmacogenomics is less important in such situations, where several different products exist and can be substituted for one another.

Gefitinib and Erlotinib

By contrast, the variable and generally poor efficacy of gefitinib (AstraZeneca's Iressa) in the treatment of non-small-cell lung cancer (NSCLC) led to its withdrawal from general use in the United States in June 2005. Gefitinib is an inhibitor of epidermal growth factor receptor (EGFR) tyrosine kinase. It was developed to treat refractory NSCLC and showed considerable promise in Phase II studies but little benefit in the larger Phase III studies. It was still approved for use because of its potential to be effective in some patients. The drug has been approved in many countries worldwide but not in Europe. In January 2005, AstraZeneca withdrew its European marketing authorization application (MAA). In Japan, gefitinib appeared to be more effective for NSCLC. The differences in observed response rates in the United States (10%) and Japan (25%) suggested that genomic variations might account for the different responses.

Subsequent studies determined that this was indeed the case and that the presence of specific mutations in the tyrosine kinase domain of EGFR is required for gefitinib to be efficacious (Lynch et al., 2004). Other studies have suggested that there is a high degree of correlation between the frequency of these mutations in both US and Japanese populations and the observed responses to the drug. Therefore, there is little point in prescribing gefitinib treatment unless the patient has been shown to express a sensitive EGFR mutation. The complexity of such factors in affecting drug responses is further illustrated by the superior response rates seen in patients treated with erlotinib (OSI/Genentech's Tarceva). In preclinical models, erlotinib was very similar to gefitinib in both chemical structure and profile of activity, yet it appears to be more efficacious than gefitinib in treating patients with NSCLC.

Trastuzumab

The best example to date of integrating pharmacogenomics into drug treatment strategies is trastuzumab (Genentech/ Roche's Herceptin). This anti-HER-2 antibody is highly effective in the treatment of breast cancer, but only in the subset of patients (approximately 20%) who express significant levels of human epidermal growth factor receptor 2 (HER-2). Because the cost of the treatment is \$40,000–\$50,000 per patient per year, it was obviously beneficial to develop a screening test to identify the patients who would benefit from trastuzumab. The FDA approved trastuzumab in September 1998 at the same time it approved DAKO's HercepTest, a screening test to identify women with elevated levels of HER-2. A second, more precise test (PathVysion) was subsequently developed by Vysis and is now marketed by Abbott.

Drug Metabolism

Genomic variability in pivotal enzymes involved in the metabolism of drugs and/or variations in transporter proteins such as P-glycoprotein are a fundamental cause of variations in drug response or lack thereof. Metabolic variations pose problems in a number of ways because they can affect the absorption, distribution, and excretion of drugs and their metabolites. For example, if a drug is not absorbed efficiently in a patient, low levels of the drug will result in poor therapeutic activity. If the drug is metabolized and generates a toxic metabolite (or prodrug), high concentrations of the metabolite can produce adverse effects. Likewise, too rapid excretion of a drug can result in too short a duration of action.

Using metabolic information to genotype patients for variations in relevant enzymes should result in more-effective titration of drug doses. Alternatively, a different drug could be used based on specific issue(s) that arise due to the presence of particular genomic variations. Although some 30 families of enzymes are involved in the metabolism of drugs, the most pertinent for most drugs are certain isoforms of cytochrome P450 (CYP). These isoforms have been studied in great detail at the genomic level and can be assessed in early-stage drug discovery to minimize issues of P450 liabilities in the clinical development of drug candidates.

Four of the most critical isoforms of P450 are CYP2D6, CYP2C9, CYP2C19, and CYP3A4. CYP3A4 metabolizes about 50% of marketed drugs; CYP2D6 metabolizes about 20% of marketed drugs. The effects of CYP2D6 and CYP2C19 tend to be more class specific. CYP2D6, for example, metabolizes beta blockers and antidepressants, while CYP2C19 metabolizes anticonvulsants and oral contraceptives.

Genetic variations in CYP2D6 and CYP2C19 differ among geographical and racial populations. Scientists have identified a plethora of functional isoforms of CYP2D6. Roche's AmpliChip Cytochrome P450 Genotyping Test, approved by the FDA in December 2004, identifies 29 known variants of the *CYP2D6* gene and two major variants of the *CYP2C19* gene. A small percentage of patients (typically 7% of Caucasians, 1–2% of Asians, and 2–4% of African-Americans) metabolize drugs poorly because of different genotypic expression of CYP2D6. This difference dramatically affects drugs' plasma concentrations. Therefore, profiling clinical trial patients for variations in CYP2D6 provides an opportunity to identify those patients who may have ultrarapid metabolism (because of the multiple gene expression), normal metabolism, or varying degrees of reduced metabolism, depending on the functional activity of the expressed genotype.

It has been well documented that unwanted inhibition of P450 metabolism can give rise to toxic side effects. Some of the best-known cases are associated with the inhibition of CYP3A4. The well-known cardiac side effects associated with terfenadine (Hoechst Marion Roussel's Seldane), astemizole (Janssen Pharmaceutica's Hismanal), and cisapride (Janssen Pharmaceutica's Propulsid), which, in each case, resulted in the withdrawal of the drug from the market, were due to inhibition of CYP3A4 in combination with other drugs or, in some cases, in combination with grapefruit juice. In the case of terfenadine, these effects were directly attributed to preventing the conversion of the administered drug to its active metabolite, fexofenadine. This metabolite is the active ingredient in the allergy drug fexofenadine (Sanofi-Aventis's Allegra).

Pharmacogenomic interactions in vivo can be complex, as illustrated by the presence of varying plasma concentrations of the antihistamine fexofenadine in different people. These differences are attributable to a single polymorphism in the P-glycoprotein transporter that can reduce the drug's peak plasma concentration by nearly twofold. The fact that multiple enzymes and proteins can affect a drug's pharmacogenomics emphasizes the need to determine the genotype of transporter proteins as well as the metabolic enzymes. It further highlights the multiplicity of factors that need to be considered in the pharmacogenomic profiling of a patient population.

THE ECONOMICS OF PERSONALIZED MEDICINE

From the patient's point of view, it is clear that pharmacogenomics offers the potential to develop better medicines. The pharmaceutical industry, on the other hand, has spent decades of time and significant resources optimizing its business strategies to develop blockbuster drugs to treat whole populations of patients. Restructuring these business processes and their associated markets to successfully produce and sell personalized medicines will be expensive. In the following sections, we discuss the effect of pharmacogenomics on clinical trial costs, drug revenues and markets, the blockbuster model of development, and other commercial strategies.

Pharmacogenomics' Impact on Clinical Trial Costs

The Tufts Center for the Study of Drug Development (TCSDD) estimates that the cost of bringing a new chemical entity (NCE) to market has escalated in recent years to $897 million. This cost encompasses both the costs directly attributable to developing an approved drug as well as all the lost costs attributable to the many drug candidates that fail. The cost of late-stage clinical trials is the largest contributor to the cost of drug development. In some cases, a single Phase III study may cost as much as $100 million, which is the estimated cost of the Omapatrilat Cardiovascular Treatment Assessment Versus Enalapril (OCTAVE) study used to evaluate the angioedema side effects of omapatrilat (Bristol-Myers Squibb's Vanlev). In 1995, TCSDD estimated that the failure rate of late-stage studies was 80%. Any measures to reduce costs and/or improve success rates would be extremely valuable. Pharmacogenomics has the potential to achieve these goals if it is integrated early into drug development strategies.

As discussed earlier, problems can arise in the clinical evaluation of new drugs when they are tested in a heterogeneous population. Side effects (serious or relatively minor) may be observed in some patients while differences stemming from genomic influences on the action, uptake, or metabolism of the drug may limit efficacy in other patients. Given these variable responses in different people, larger trials must be performed to demonstrate that the drug has significantly better efficacy than a placebo.

Pharmacogenomic profiling of relevant genotypes in patients who will take part in clinical studies should provide a more homogeneous population for analysis. Those patients who should be more responsive to the drug could be selected for later-stage clinical trials. Figure 20.1 depicts examples of patient stratification. Through pharmacogenomic profiling, a heterogeneous population of patients may be stratified into groups so that those groups of people likely to respond can be further studied in clinical trials designed to test the hypothesis. Ideally, patient stratification should be done before the initiation of late-stage clinical trials, but it can also be applied retrospectively to identify subsets of patients who experience a significant response. The sidebar "Case History: deCODE Genetics' Use of Pharmacogenomics in Heart Attack Trails" discusses the use of pharamacogenomics in patient recruitment.

Applying pharmacogenomic profiling to clinical trials offers at least three potential advantages. The first is the ability to perform smaller late-stage trials; the second is the likelihood that such trials will fail less often (provided that the chosen target is sufficiently relevant to the disease under study). Both advantages can help reduce the costs of late-stage clinical development and thus the overall cost of successfully developing a drug. The third advantage is that the number of NCEs that reach the market may increase.

On the other hand, adopting pharmacogenomic strategies in the development of new drugs has disadvantages too. It necessitates the identification of pharmacogenomic markers at an early stage in the development process, preferably some time before starting work on the design of the trials. Doing so requires the investigators to determine the genomic profile of all relevant biomarkers in each of the potential participants in the trial. This extra effort in assay development and genetic screening will increase the costs of setting up trials, but the increased cost should be offset by cost reductions resulting from the use of smaller trials. Pharmacogenomic profiling may also hamper patient recruitment because it may prove difficult to identify and recruit a sufficient number of patients who possess the desired genomic profile.

Some level of pharmacogenomic profiling is likely to be used for indications such as cancer, a disease in which it has become apparent that specific genomic variations are directly linked to cancer phenotypes. For instance, profiling cancers for expression of oncogenic products such as Ras or p53 and then optimizing treatment based on such results should have clear cost benefits. The cost of such profiling should be relatively small because of the limited number of markers that must be evaluated. Likewise, the increasing availability of low-cost assays for profiling P450 isoforms and their general applicability to most drug-treated patients are likely to boost the use of such methods to provide a more scientific basis for dose titration in low responders and high responders.

Genomic profiling is likely to be extensively applied to patients involved in clinical trials, provided that the time and cost of developing and using such assays do not impose too great a burden. For disease indications that affect small numbers of patients, the burden may be too large to make drug development economically feasible. However, the alternative is the potential failure of expensive late-stage trials and the consequent loss of development costs when the drug candidate cannot be successfully brought to market.

Case History: deCODE Genetics' Use of Pharmacogenomics in Heart Attack Trials

Based on genetic studies of patients and their families, deCODE Genetics has determined that the risk for heart attack doubles for people carrying certain variations in the gene encoding 5-lipoxygenase-activating protein (FLAP). The gene variations appear to increase production of pro-inflammatory leukotrienes, which precede the development of atherosclerotic plaques.

Several FLAP inhibitors were previously evaluated as potential treatments for asthma, but none progressed beyond Phase III clinical development. deCODE inlicensed one such inhibitor – DG-031 (previously known as BAY-x1005) – from Bayer that had already been shown to be safe. deCODE is evaluating it in genomically stratified groups of patients at risk of heart attack. In a Phase IIa trial, DG-031 inhibited the production of LTB4 in patients at risk of coronary events.

Patient recruitment for a multicenter Phase III study is ongoing; the two-year study will assess the value of DG-031 in protecting patients from a second heart attack. This trial will be performed in genotyped patients and therefore should substantially reduce the cost of the trial and improve the chances of a positive outcome.

Three key aspects of genomic profiling of patients for clinical trials are as follows:

- The profiling of key metabolic enzymes and transporter proteins, such as CYP enzymes, in patients expected to take part in the trial.
- The identification of genomic variations in the chosen drug target that may affect patients' response to the drug.
- The identification of specific biomarkers in patients that may be modulated by the drug's action.

Because genomic profiling of metabolic enzymes and transporter proteins is applicable to all studies and the marginal cost of such profiling is relatively low (aided by the availability of devices such as AmpliChip), it is likely to be widely applied in all phases of clinical development.

The other two factors are less easily addressed because of their specificity to a drug's mechanism of action and to the disease targeted. Accordingly, pharmaceutical companies will need to establish novel, validated protocols for such studies. It is preferable for target variations and biomarker data to be available before efficacy studies begin because of the value of the genomic data in influencing trial design. The major impact of such studies on costs will result from the costs of the research required to establish and validate assays rather than the costs of using the assays. The likely impact of adopting such a strategy will be a shifting of costs (expenditure) to an earlier stage in the development process, which will increase the demand that development projects place on preclinical resources. This approach should have little impact on large pharma, but it is a significant issue for smaller biotechnology companies.

Pharmacogenomics' Impact on Drug Revenues and Markets

The implementation of pharmacogenomics will greatly affect drug revenues and markets. The cost of pharmacogenomic tests will determine whether they are prescribed by physicians and reimbursed by payers; the potential use of pharmacogenomics information will affect marketing strategies in competitive markets; and pharmacogenomics testing will break up existing markets into smaller ones.

If the costs of pharmacogenomic tests are set too high, their routine application in the clinic may be prohibited because of the reimbursement issues. As the cost of testing falls, it may become the standard procedure to apply pharmacogenomics to determine which drug(s) to prescribe.

Pharmacogenomic screening will increase the medical treatment costs, but the effects on drug development costs will vary. Screening for polymorphisms of P450 isoforms and transporters could well become ubiquitous. Screening for specific polymorphisms in drug targets will probably require the codevelopment of a screening assay together with the new drug development, which should lead to simultaneous regulatory approval. This codevelopment pathway will significantly affect the cost of drug development.

For the most part, there will be little incentive to develop pharmacogenomic tests for currently approved drugs, unless those drugs have been withdrawn from the market and are being rehabilitated. Sufficient advantage is likely to accrue in only a few cases, for example, companies that successfully develop tests to augment the prescription and especially the marketing of their products. One context in which this situation may occur is when several drugs are competing in a relatively high-value market segment. The company marketing a second-place or a third-place drug may seek to enhance its market share by showing that its drug is better suited to treating a readily defined group of people through the application of genomic screening. This strategy may prompt physicians to switch to this drug. For example, prior to the application of pharmacogenomic screening, Drug A has the largest share of the market. When the maker of Drug B introduces a value-added pharmacogenomics approach, its market share increases to the detriment of the market shares of Drugs A and C. The overall size of the combined market will remain unchanged unless the value added by the pharmacogenomic screening is sufficient to support a price increase for Drug B.

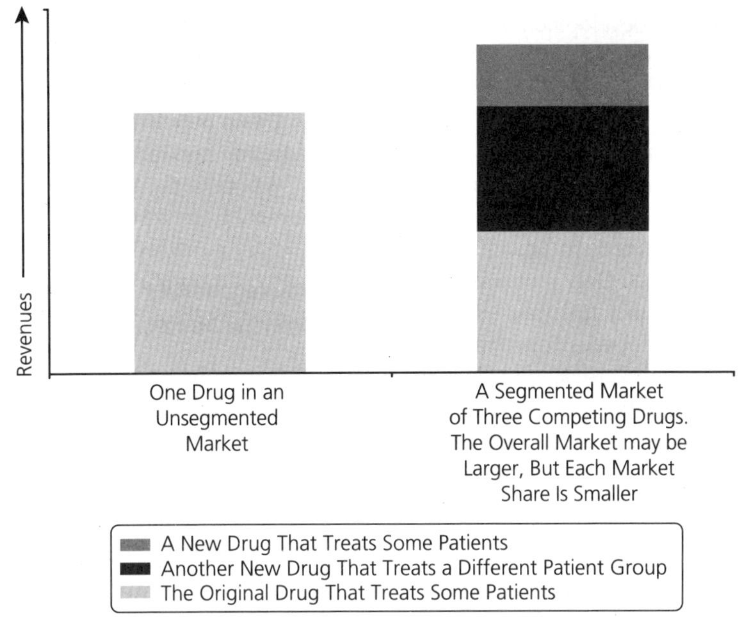

Figure 20.2 Potential Impact of Pharmacogenomics on Drug Revenues, Gains, and Losses

Another application of pharmacogenomic screening and its potential effect on market segments for drugs and drug sales is shown in Figure 20.2. In the absence of pharmacogenomics, one drug captures all revenues for the treatment of a specific condition. In this instance, it is assumed that different dosages of the drug are used to treat high responders and poor responders. With the application of pharmacogenomic screening, new drugs can be used to treat different groups of people and each will obtain a share of the overall market. Under this scenario, it is possible that differential pricing could be used for the new drugs thanks to their effective targeting of patient groups. The result would be a larger total market for all three drugs combined, but a considerably smaller market share for the original drug.

Although pharmacogenomics offers the potential to develop more NCEs for each targeted patient group, the segmentation of the overall market and the smaller size of each market segment pose several problems that major pharmaceutical companies will need to address. Virtually all pharmaceutical companies have adopted an internal hurdle for minimum predicted annual revenue, which a drug candidate must exceed in order to be developed and marketed. The level at which this hurdle is set varies from company to company, but it is probable that most major companies set this level at or above $500 million. Drug candidates that would produce lower sales are not developed under this model because it is not cost-effective for the company. Increased market segmentation driven by the application of pharmacogenomics means that this strategy will need to be reevaluated. Pharmacogenomics is expected to result in companies having larger portfolios of modestly successful drugs rather than a small number of blockbuster drugs. Many more opportunities will exist for biotechnology companies or companies that can quickly adapt their strategy to development and marketing of products for a segmented market.

Pharmacogenomics' Impact on the Blockbuster Model of Drug Development

Widespread application of pharmacogenomics will reduce the number of potential blockbusters. As we stated earlier, the blockbuster model of drug development is based on the theory that "one drug treats most patients most of the time." Because of the increased market segmentation resulting from the use of pharmacogenomics and therefore the smaller size of each market segment, opportunities to successfully develop new blockbuster products will be limited, at least for non-biotechnology products. Only premium-priced products, a category that few small-molecule drugs fit, will enjoy blockbuster revenues. The exceptions will be market-leading agents that are developed for highly prevalent conditions, agents that are shown to be effective in the treatment of multiple conditions, and agents that can be used by most of the potential patient populations for diseases with moderately high prevalence.

At the present time, the focus of all major pharmaceutical companies is to develop blockbusters and sustain revenues by replacing blockbusters that go off-patent with new blockbusters. This strategy has several pitfalls. Prominent among them is the fact that side effects seen in a small number of patients can force the withdrawal of a blockbuster product with potentially catastrophic effects on the company's revenues and share prices. Recent examples include the withdrawal of cerivastatin (Bayer's Lipobay/ Baycol) and rofecoxib (Merck's Vioxx). (Sales of rofecoxib – $2.55 billion – accounted for 11.3% of Merck's revenues in 2003; sales of cerivastatin were expected to exceed $1 billion when Bayer withdrew the drug from the market in 2001 and then initiated a major restructuring of the company.) Although not all instances of drug withdrawals are the result of adverse effects in a genomically defined subset of patients, more-comprehensive pharmacogenomic profiling of patients should reduce the number of blockbuster withdrawals.

The increasing application of pharmacogenomics will also impinge on the development of global brands. In recent years, there has been a steady transition toward use of global brand names as well as attempts to synchronize global regulatory filings. Genomic profiling of patient populations will almost certainly disrupt these strategies because it will reveal that different drugs should be the agents of choice in the different major markets. The effect will be most pronounced in Japan because its population is more genomically distinct than populations in Western countries. In certain disease indications, there will also be clear genomic distinctions between populations in the United States and Western Europe.

Pharmacogenomics' Impact on Other Commercial Strategies

A decline in the number of blockbuster drugs and lower revenues generated by new NCEs as a result of the market segmentation will necessitate changes in strategies for developing and marketing new products. Although significant benefits should accrue to patients from the widespread adoption of pharmacogenomic technologies, there are pitfalls for the industry.

First, the pharmaceutical industry will have to adjust its thinking about medium-revenue drugs ($250–$999 million per year) and, most importantly, readdress its internal hurdle rates. This strategic change poses further problems. If the blockbuster revenues become generally unachievable, it will be necessary to bring many more NCEs successfully to the market in order to achieve comparable revenues (Figure 20.3). Replacing a single blockbuster that had sales of $2.5 billion in 2004 may require the launch of many new products. In this hypothetical scenario, for example, revenues from the single blockbuster could have grown from $2.5 billion in 2004 to $4.1 billion by 2014, representing a compound annual growth rate of 6%. This figure is well below the double-digit growth that has been prevalent in the industry until recently. To achieve $4.1 billion in sales by 2014 in the absence of such a blockbuster drug, several new products (six are shown in Figure 20.3) would have to be successfully developed during the same 10-year period.

Second, the development of so many new agents will give rise to capacity problems, which could further reduce the number of new NCEs launched each year. Declining NCE launches in the pharmaceutical industry have been attributed, in part, to the "innovation deficit" described by Juergen Drews

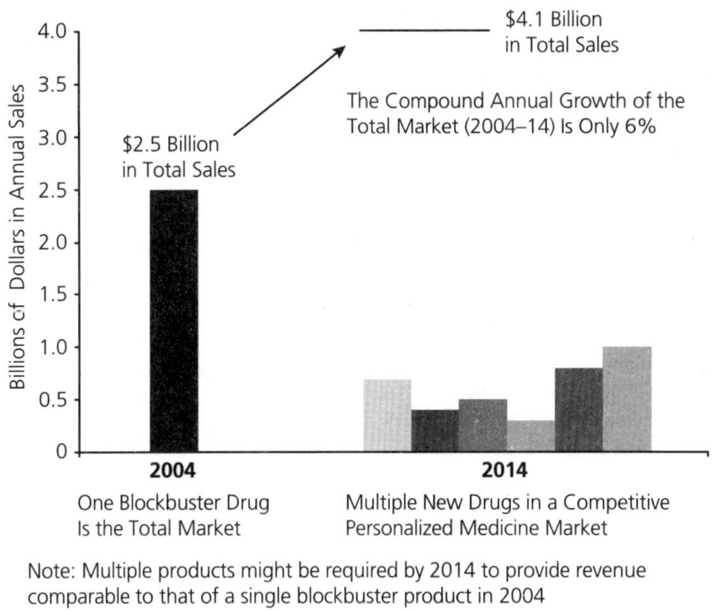

Figure 20.3 Maintaining Revenues in a Pharmacogenomic Era

(Drews and Ryser, 1996). This deficit stems from the fact that fewer products are coming out of drug discovery that can be used for drug development. Through the application of pharmacogenomics, the innovation deficit could be exacerbated by a "resource deficit." Potential resource limitations may not be as onerous as Figure 20.3 implies because the application of pharmacogenomics should also result in much lower attrition rates in a late-stage development than has been the case.

The development of many more NCEs will inevitably lead to many more regulatory filings each year, which could create significant congestion at regulatory authorities due to lack of review capacity. A serious result of a capacity shortfall would be substantially longer approval times, which was typical in the late 1980s and early 1990s. The delay would offset much of the temporal gain achieved by more-efficient clinical studies.

Another problem will be the increased costs associated with bringing more agents to the market. On the one hand, the cost of late-stage clinical trials is a significant factor in the overall cost of drug development, and pharmacogenomics has the potential to significantly reduce these costs. On the other hand, drug development of a single NCE is costly, and these costs are additive when more than one NCE must be developed. Hence, the combined cost of bringing multiple NCEs to the market to treat different patient groups will be large. Overall development costs will increase and corporate profitability will decline. The expense of parallel development of multiple NCEs may be offset if drugs can be codeveloped with their respective diagnostic tests in a cost-effective manner. Although the Food and Drug Administration (FDA) is encouraging such drug-diagnostic codevelopment, whether it will be routinely adopted and integrated into big pharma's drug development practices remains to be seen. The following are examples of drug-diagnostic codevelopment:

- Trastuzumab (Genentech/Roche's Herceptin) was developed for advanced breast cancer based on the Her2/neu biomarker.
- Imatinib (Novartis's Gleevec) was developed for chronic myeloid leukemia based on the Philadelphia chromosome of Bcr-abl biomarker and for gastrointestinal stromal tumors (GIST) based on the *c-kit* oncogene (*CD117*).

- Cetuximab (ImClone/Merck KgaA/Bristol-Myers Squibb's Erbitux) was developed for advanced colorectal cancer based on the EGFR biomarker.

Overall, this analysis would suggest that larger companies will be less interested in developing products whose revenues will likely fall below a certain threshold figure. Only if the application of pharmacogenomics can result in a significant drop in development costs is this threshold figure likely to be as low as $250 million.

Some companies may try to offset drug development costs by exploiting orphan- drug legislation. Pharmacogenomics can be used to scientifically identify segments of a patient population that are small enough to qualify drugs developed for that segment as orphan drugs. The criteria for such designation differ in the United States, Europe, and Japan. The major pharmaceutical companies will likely seek orphan drug designations more often for initial approvals and then request additional approvals for other indications that would not meet orphan-drug requirements.

Although pharmacogenomics should provide many commercial opportunities for emerging companies, it will affect their commercial and financial strategies. Many smaller companies will lack the financial and personnel resources to pursue extensive pharmacogenomic profiling at an early stage of a project. Yet, as shown in Figure 20.4, pharmacogenomics will push the cost burden of developing a drug to an earlier stage of development. This temporal shift will increase the financial pressure on smaller companies and will prompt them to outlicense or partner a drug candidate at an earlier stage of development than has been the case. Major pharmaceutical companies will likely reap the benefit of having more early-stage licensing and partnering deals available to them.

Case Study: Treatment of Ten Hypothetical Patients with and without Pharmacogenomic Testing

The extent to which pharmacogenomic profiling will be implemented in the pharmaceutical industry depends on a number of factors, including strategies for setting prices of drugs and diagnostic tests

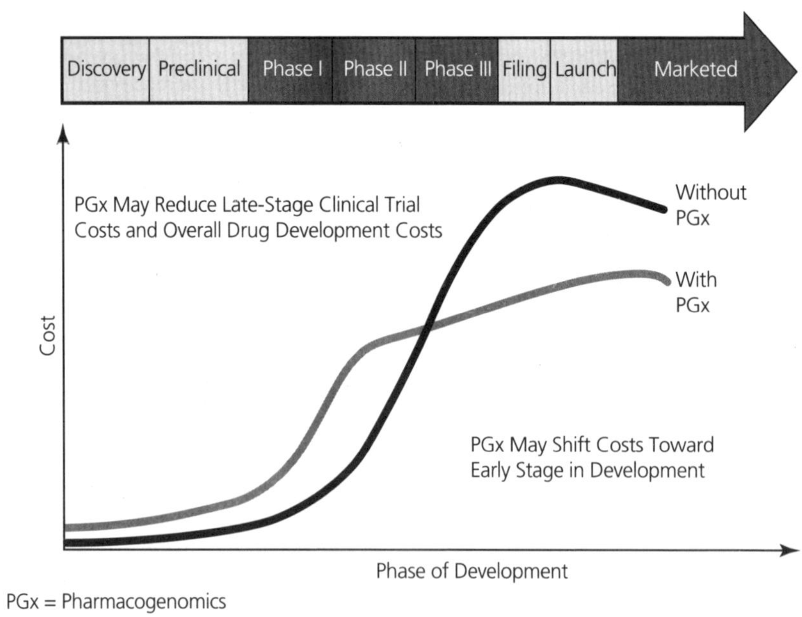

Figure 20.4 Pharmacogenomics: Potential Effect on Drug Development Costs

Table 20.1 Diagnosis and Treatment Revenues for 10 Patients with and without Genomic Testing

Scenario	*Tx only No PGx No Dx*	*Therapy with Preselection of Patients Based on PGx*				
		Tx Component	*Dx Component*	*Combined Tx + Dx*	*Savings with PGx*	*Savings with PGx (%)*
Treatment costs $24,000; 10% of patients respond Diagnostic test costs $1,000	240,000	24,000	10,000	34,000	206,000	86
Treatment costs $24,000; 40% of patients respond Diagnostic test costs $1,000	240,000	96,000	10,000	106,000	134,000	56
Treatment costs $10,000; 10% of patients respond Diagnostic test costs $500	100,000	10,000	5,000	15,000	85,000	85

Dx = Diagnostic; PGx = Pharmacogenomics; and Tx = Treatment

and strategies for optimizing revenues and determining reimbursement by payers. We provide a case study of the diagnosis and treatment of 10 hypothetical patients being treated with a drug with and without the use of pharmacogenomics profiling (Table 20.1). We discuss the effect of different pricing strategies and their ramifications on market dynamics.

Our 10 hypothetical patients are treated (Tx) at an annual cost of either $10,000 or $24,000 per patient, representing $100,000 or $240,000 in annual drug revenues in the absence of pharmacogenomics (PGx). If a diagnostic (Dx) test is available ($500 or $1,000 per test), then all 10 patients are screened in order to identify the patients who are likely to respond to treatment and therefore will be treated. We consider different scenarios in which 10% or 40% of patients are responders. Although real-life markets will involve more complex analyses, our simple scenarios highlight a number of important considerations for the industry, including the following:

- In the absence of pharmacogenomics and diagnostic testing, a pharmaceutical company receives the maximum amount of revenues ($100,000 or $240,000). To generate total sales of more than $1 billion a year (i.e., a blockbuster), 100,000 patients must be treated ($10,000 per patient). This number drops to 42,000 patients if the cost of treatment is increased to $24,000 per patient, thereby underscoring the close correlation between setting a drug's price and achieving the blockbuster status for that drug.
- When pharmacogenomics is available to preselect patients, treatment revenues decline significantly ($10,000, $24,000, or $96,000) compared with revenues in the absence of pharmacogenomics ($100,000 or $240,000). This loss in revenue is a major negative factor in a company's decision to switch from a blockbuster to a personalized-medicine model of drug development. With pharmacogenomics screening, the therapeutic market is smaller, making it 2.5–10 times more difficult for a pharmaceutical company to achieve blockbuster status with a new drug.
- With pharmacogenomics, revenues from the diagnostic component ($5,000 or $10,000), though smaller, become more significant compared with those of the therapeutic component ($10,000, $24,000, or $96,000). This increase represents the creation of a new diagnostic market (e.g., $50–$100 million when 100,000 patients need to be prescreened).
- The combined revenues of treatment and diagnosis ($15,000, $34,000, or $106,000) vary considerably depending on the number of responders. Pharmaceutical companies will have more incentive to develop personalized medicines for disease indications for which a significant number of responders can still be treated with one drug.
- If a company controls both the therapeutic drug and the diagnostic test used for pharmacogenomics preselection, then combined revenues ($15,000, $34,000, or $106,000) improve compared with therapeutic revenues alone ($10,000, $24,000, or $96,000). Creating a combined Tx/Dx market represents a potential new opportunity when pharmacogenomics

information is available: it provides the potential to set prices for both Tx and Dx components in order to maximize revenues. This advantage is lost if Tx and Dx products are developed and marketed by independent companies.

- In the presence of pharmacogenomics, the payer gains significant savings ($85,000, $134,000, or $206,000) compared with its costs for treating patients in the absence of pharmacogenomics (either $100,000 or $240,000). The gain to the payer (56–86%) comes at direct loss to the pharmaceutical company. However, the payer can enjoy this advantage only if it refuses the reimbursement of treatment costs to patients who, based on pharmacogenomics screening, will not benefit from the treatment.

This gain/loss is the crux of the problem now facing the industry in deciding whether to embrace the development of personalized medicines. If the pharmaceutical companies continue to promote drugs to treat everyone in the population, regardless of their ability to respond to treatment, physicians will be under considerable pressure to prescribe the treatment – everyone will want it, even though many patients may not benefit. More often than not, the payer will become the gatekeeper, deciding whom to "treat" by refusing to reimburse treatments for patients based on pharmacogenomics tests.

This example illustrates how strong the link will be between diagnostic testing and drug treatment in personalized medicine. There are advantages in codeveloping diagnostic and therapeutic products because the pricing of one will affect the other. Drug development, pricing, and marketing strategies will differ depending on whether one company attempts to develop and sell both products, whether a pharma company partners with a diagnostic company to develop and price the products together, or whether two independent companies are involved in separate diagnostic and therapeutic product development and pricing.

RECENT PHARMACOGENOMIC DEALS AND ALLIANCES

Pharmaceutical companies will have to develop new strategies in order to apply pharmacogenomics to drug discovery and development. These strategies must address the issues discussed earlier in this chapter relating to the replacement of the blockbuster drug model with the development of multiple NCEs for segmented markets, the effective allocation of resources, and the management of overall development costs. Some of these issues may be addressed through the utilization and exploitation of internal resources; others may be better addressed by external partnerships or acquisitions. Partnerships provide an opportunity for major companies to enhance their pharmacogenomic programs and extend the sales of drugs into specialized markets that have been defined by partner companies.

Clinical Data has been especially active in acquiring other companies in order to create a leadership position in providing clinical diagnostic, pharmacogenomic, and metabolomic services to clients worldwide. Table 20.2 lists some of its recent acquisitions. In March 2006, the company established two new business units for therapeutic

Table 20.2 Clinical Data's Acquisitions in the Fields of Pharmacogenomics and Molecular Diagnostics, 2005–6

Company Acquired	*Benefit from the Acquisition*	*Acquisition Cost ($MM)*	*Acquisition Date*
Genome Express	For expansion into European pharmacogenomics and molecular services markets	3.16	March 2006
Icoria	Biomarker discovery, metabolomics, and RNA profiling	12.5	December 2005
Electa Lab	Immunochemistry, erythrocyte sedimentation rate, and coagulation products	1.8	December 2005
Genaissance Pharmaceuticals	Target identification, pharmacogenomics, and therapeutic diagnostics	56	October 2005

diagnostics and biomarkers (PGxHealth) and for pharmacogenomics and molecular services (Cogenics) in addition to its third business unit (Vital Diagnostics), which is engaged in clinical in vitro diagnostics (IVDs).

Gene Logic and deCODE Genetics are just two of the companies that have entered into pharmacogenomics-based collaborations with several pharmaceutical partners. (Table 20.3 lists select Gene Logic collaborations in the pharmacogenomics field.) Gene Logic functions primarily as a service company, providing genomic and toxicogenomic profiling services to major pharmaceutical companies. In September 2005, Gene Logic entered into a different type of collaboration with Pfizer; through this collaboration, the companies hope to rehabilitate clinical drug candidates that were discontinued. The company signed a second "drug-repositioning" agreement with Roche relating to several Roche candidates that were successful in Phase I but were discontinued in Phase II and Phase III. Such an approach provides an opportunity for a pharmaceutical company to salvage the drug candidates on which considerable sums of time and money have already been expended.

deCODE Genetics has a distinct business model; it uses population genetics to identify genetic markers that can be correlated with specific diseases. The company has compiled an extensive database containing genomic and genealogical data from the generally homogeneous population of Iceland. The company uses population genetics to identify markers of genetic disease and to validate disease-specific targets. This approach has attracted the interest of several major companies (Table 20.4). Roche recently expanded its partnership with deCODE to include the discovery and development of inhibitors of phosphodiesterase 4 enzyme for the treatment of vascular diseases such as stroke. deCODE has identified at least three genes that are linked to obesity and is working with Merck to screen Merck's compounds against validated obesity targets. deCODE is also working with an unidentified company on the clinical development of a compound against MAP3K9 kinase that is predictive of increased risk of developing asthma.

Table 20.3 Gene Logic: Select Pharmacogenomics Collaborations

Partner	*Date of Collaboration*	*Scope of Collaboration*
Pfizer	September 2005	Drug repositioning agreement for multiple drug candidates from different therapeutic areas whose development had been discontinued
Roche	December 2005	Drug repositioning agreement for multiple Roche drug candidates that were discontinued during Phase II and III clinical development
Millennium	July 2004	Gene Logic acquired imaging, screening, ADME, and metabolomic technologies to be used to establish its Drug Repositioning Division

ADME = Absorption, distribution, metabolism, excretion

Table 20.4 deCODE Genetics: Select Pharmacogenomic Collaborations

Partner	*Date of Collaboration*	*Scope of Collaboration*
Roche	November 2004	Agreement to codevelop inhibitors of PDE4 for treatment and prevention of vascular indications, including stroke
NIAID	September 2004	Contract to discover genetic factors for infectious diseases and predicting responses to vaccines
Merck	February 2004	Collaboration to apply pharmacogenomics to create "info-rich" clinical trials for Merck compounds
Bayer Healthcare	November 2003	Agreement for DG-031, a compound previously in development by Bayer for asthma that deCODE found was associated with myocardial infarction.
Merck	September 2002	Alliance to identify genes linked to obesity and then to screen Merck compounds against validated obesity targets
Roche	June 2001	DNA-based diagnostics for predisposition to disease and predicting therapeutic responses

NIAID = National Institute of Allergy and Infectious Diseases and PDE4 = Phosphodiesterase 4 enzyme

In its own product development pipeline, deCODE's most-advanced lead candidate is DG-031, which is in Phase III trials for heart attack. Rights to this compound were acquired from Bayer. In January 2006, deCODE acquired a privately held Icelandic company, Urdur Verdandi Skuld (UVS), for $5.5 million in stock. UVS has the research and clinical data from cancer patients in Iceland since 1998 that deCODE will use to develop products for cancer diagnosis and treatment.

REGULATORY INITIATIVES TO SUPPORT THE USE OF PHARMACOGENOMICS IN DRUG DEVELOPMENT

Regulatory agencies worldwide are collaborating to promote the use of pharmacogenomics in drug discovery and development to create safer and more effective drugs. The use of pharmacogenomic data in regulatory submissions preceded the development of official regulations defining its role. As of 2005, 121 labels contain pharmacogenomic information, and almost 40% of all new labels in 2005 contained genomic information. This upward trend is expected to continue as the industry more routinely applies pharmacogenomics to the clinical development of NCEs.

The increasing use of pharmacogenomics data in regulatory submissions has prompted the European Medicines Agency (EMEA), the FDA, and Japan's Ministry of Health, Labor, and Welfare to develop formal guidelines. In March 2005, all three regulatory authorities produced preliminary documents that addressed pharmacogenomics, though not yet regulating it. To what extent the regulatory position will differ among these three authorities remains to be seen. The US and European authorities may adopt similar guidelines, but the Japanese guidelines may be different because the population there is more genetically distinct from Western populations. Privacy issues, such as protecting the confidentiality of genetic test data, are also a major concern in Japan, Europe, and the United States.

In general, any differences in Japanese regulations may not be a major factor in the development of most products. One potential exception is the development of global brands, which could be adversely affected, for example, by labeling requirements that are specific to a particular group of patients or by clinical trial results that are produced in a group of patients who are not well represented in the Japanese population. Should the Japanese guidelines be substantially different from those in Western markets, the time lag between the introduction of products in Europe and the United States and their introduction in Japan will likely expand.

United States

In March 2004, the FDA issued a white paper outlining its views on pipeline problems faced by the pharmaceutical industry and the slowdown in the number of innovative medical therapies reaching patients. The paper included the FDA's perception that genomic technologies could accelerate drug development and approval, but it did not attempt to address the regulatory issues that these technologies raise (FDA, 2004).

In March 2005, the FDA issued further guidance on pharmacogenomics based on a draft document first published in 2003 (FDA, 2005). This document outlines the agency's current thinking regarding the use of pharmacogenomics to support the clinical trial process. The FDA has established an Interdisciplinary Pharmacogenomics Review Group (IPRG) and procedures for voluntary pharmacogenomics data submissions (VGDS) and required pharmacogenomics data submission (RGDSs). These procedures are designed to collect voluntary, recommended, or required information on biomarkers and their uses in IND, biologics license application (BLA), or NDA submissions (Table 20.5). As of March 2006, the FDA has received 25 different VGDSs.

Table 20.5 FDA Guidance for Pharmacogenomic Data Submissions, March 2005

	IND	*New (Unapproved) NDA, BLA, or Supplement*	*Previously Approved NDA or BLA*
Known valid biomarker	RGDS	RGDS	RGDS
Probable valid biomarker	Submission is not required, but the FDA welcomes a VGDS	The FDA recommends submission	RGDS
Exploratory pharmacogenomic data	The FDA welcomes a VGDS	The FDA recommends submission but also welcomes a VGDS	The FDA welcomes a VGDS

BLA = Biologics license application; IND = Investigational new drug application; NDA = New drug application; RGDS = Required pharmacogenomics data submission; and VGDS = Voluntary pharmacogenomics data submission

The draft document recommends procedures for dealing with the design and performance of clinical studies within an IND. In particular, it stresses that in cases where pharmacogenomic data are used to define dosing schedules or distinguish specific patient groups, then the "FDA recommends codevelopment of the drug and the pharmacogenomic tests, if they are not currently available, and submission of complete information on the test/drug combination to the agency."

In February 2006, the FDA released a draft guidance document that contains nonbinding recommendations for nucleic-acid-based tests that are submitted for premarket approval (PMA) and premarket notification (510[k]) applications for genetics-based diagnostic devices (FDA 2006). These tests include the use of single markers, such as SNPs, or multiple markers/multiplex tests, such as those that use microarrays. The document suggests the "least burdensome" way to design and develop tests to obtain the information preferred for regulatory submissions.

Europe

Because all significant European applications are now filed through the central recognition procedure, rather than via national routes, the EMEA's position on pharmacogenomics is most relevant.

In February 2005, the EMEA's Committee for Medicinal Products for Human Use (CHMP) established a Pharmacogenetics Working Party to develop guidelines for the use of pharmacogenomic data (an initial concept paper was produced in 2003). In March 2005, a draft was issued with comments to be accepted on these proposals until September 30, 2005 (European Medicines Agency, Committee for Medicinal Products for Human Use 2005). One goal of the guidelines, which are expected to be finalized in the second quarter of 2006, is to establish a framework within which regulators and industry can discuss the use of pharmacogenomic data in support of drug submissions. This document does not address the incorporation of such data into formal regulatory submissions.

No position paper has yet been issued seeking to formalize the use of pharmacogenomic data in submissions of MAAs, so it will probably be 2008 at the earliest before a legal framework for the use of such data can be established in Europe.

Japan

In Japan, the MHLW issued final guidance on pharmacogenomics on March 18, 2005 (Yoshiaki Uyama, 2006). As in Europe and the United States, the Pharmaceuticals and Medical Devices Agency (PMDA) established a Pharmacogenomics Discussion Group to encourage the sharing of information and inclusion of pharmacogenomics data in regulatory submissions. The guidance requests that pharmaceutical companies submit validated pharmacogenomics data that have implications for drug indication, dosage, and safety. These guidelines were based on a draft document published in June 2004. These guidelines will likely differ from those in other markets because of Japanese legal requirements relating to the protection of personal information.

OUTLOOK

The widespread application of pharmacogenomics has clear benefits for patients. By enabling personalized medicine, it should become possible to provide better treatment for patients and therefore better disease control. According to a report released by Business Communications in May 2005, the worldwide pharmacogenomics market will increase, at an average annual growth rate of 24.5%, from $1.24 billion in 2004 to $3.7 billion in 2009. The 2009 total encompasses $1.66 billion for genotyping, $1.65 billion for diagnostics, and $397 million for SNP identification. Life science companies that develop the diagnostic tests and companies that provide genetic testing services should benefit from these increased revenue streams.

The benefits to biotechnology companies are less substantial. Although pharmacogenomics may improve patient selection in clinical trials – an advantage that should reduce the overall cost of developing a new drug – it may well hamper the ability of smaller companies to progress NCEs through the early-stage clinical development and may force them to consider earlier partnering arrangements.

The Public's Perspective

Overall, Americans favor the use of genomics in the development of new medicines to treat disease. Many Americans also have strong reservations relating to the privacy of genomics data and to the future insurability of patients who have been identified as carrying high-risk genes. In the United States, the Genetic Information Nondiscrimination Act of 2005 is wending its way through Congress. It seeks to prohibit discrimination based on genetic information and to extend medical privacy and confidentiality rules in the workplace and in the health insurance market. The confidentiality of genomic data is also a key issue in Japan and the European Union.

Pricing and Reimbursement

Although the widespread application of pharmacogenomic screening to the diagnosis and treatment of disease will benefit patients, immediate benefits to pharmaceutical companies and healthcare payers are more difficult to ascertain. The application of pharmacogenomics will increase the costs to develop drugs in the near term, and new genetic testing may be necessary, which will increase medical costs. The likely segmentation of therapeutic markets could significantly reduce annual revenues from most new drugs. However, mid-level therapeutics that are not initially blockbusters may still be quite successful, as exemplified by Genentech/Roche's trastuzumab. In 2005, this drug had worldwide revenues of more than $1.7 billion, even though only about 20% of breast cancer patients benefit from its treatment. Although the industry is quite concerned with the potential of pharmacogenomics to segment markets, strong markets may be created for products that are known to be effective in definable patient groups.

For their part, healthcare payers may be reluctant to reimburse expensive new screening tests. As determined in the 2005 CGAT survey by Cogent Research, a large majority of Americans (68%) believe that insurance companies will do everything possible to use genetic information to deny health coverage and to deny coverage for drugs people need if their genetic profiles indicate a low chance of responding (69%). This concern is not unfounded. In June 2005, Cigna Healthcare released a Coverage Position paper (#0381) that stated that it "does not cover the AmpliChip Cytochrome P450 Genotyping test because its use in clinical practice is considered experimental, investigational, or unproven." This test has been approved in the United States and Europe, but the company is asking for more studies demonstrating that the test can help improve health outcomes. Meanwhile, in the United Kingdom, a woman is suing for the right to receive the drug trastuzumab to treat her breast cancer with the costs to be paid by a primary care trust. The woman had met the eligibility requirements for Herceptin treatment, but the primary care trust refused to pay, citing its policy of funding Herceptin treatment only in exceptional circumstances. The Court of Appeals will soon weigh in, at least in this case, on legal issues relating to access to this new type of healthcare and who qualifies for reimbursed care and when.

Development of Diagnostic Tests

In the near term at least, the application of pharmacogenomics will make it more difficult for pharmaceutical companies to develop and market drugs. The need to develop many more NCEs, perhaps in combination with a diagnostic test, and the potential impact of these developments on corporate revenues and profitability are causes of concern. The decision on how to deal with the diagnostic part of product development will be a key strategic decision.

Major pharmaceutical companies are unlikely to be the first to employ widespread application of pharmacogenomics in the diagnosis and treatment of patients unless they have significant diagnostic divisions. Larger diagnostic companies will more likely be the first to devote significant resources to developing pharmacogenomic tests, instruments, and screening methods. Roche, Abbott, and Johnson & Johnson have all demonstrated interest in pharmacogenomics. Celera Genomics may well jump ahead of these companies following its repositioning of its business strategy in 2005 to concentrate on diagnostics and personalized medicine.

Most pharmaceutical companies are not well-versed in IVD (in vitro diagnostic) test development and will most likely seek a diagnostic partner. The FDA's new pathway for the codevelopment of a diagnostic test/drug is logically correct but logistically difficult to deploy. Much will depend on a company's ability to identify and validate an appropriate biomarker, to coordinate use of the biomarker to identify select patient groups, and to cocoordinate clinical trials for both diagnostic and therapeutic agents.

The development of pharmacogenomics to enhance the marketing of the established drugs, as part of a strategy of life-cycle management, may become an attractive option for many pharmaceutical companies. When a drug is facing generics competition, for example, the company may gain a marketing advantage by using diagnostic tests to identify the groups of patients who would or would not benefit most from treatment with that drug.

The era of personalized medicine will bring about a great change in the pharmaceutical industry and the treatment of diseases in general. Despite the challenges, it behooves the industry to move as quickly as possible to exploit the tools, such as pharmacogenomics, that will help it develop drugs that can better treat patients.

REFERENCES

Drews, J., Ryser, S. Innovation deficit in the pharmaceutical industry. *Drug Information Journal.* 1996; 30: 97–107.

European Medicines Agency, Committee for Medicinal Products for Human Use. Guideline on pharmacogenetics briefing meetings. March 2005. www.emea.eu.int/pdfs/human/pharmacogenetics/2022704en.pdf

FDA. Stagnation or innovation – challenge and opportunity on the critical path to new medical products. March 2004. www.fda.gov/oc/initiatives/criticalpath/whitepaper.pdf

FDA. Guidance for industry – pharmacogenomic data submissions. March 2005. www.fda.gov/cber/gdlns/pharmdtasub.pdf

FDA. Draft guidance for industry and FDA staff: pharmacogenetic tests and genetic tests for heritable markers. February 2006. www.fda.gov/cdrh/oivd/guidance/1549.pdf

Lynch, T.J. et al. Activating mutations in the epidermal growth factor receptor underlying responsiveness of non-small-cell lung cancer to gefitinib. *NEJM.* 2004; 350(21): 2129–39.

Yoshiaki Uyama. Office of New Drug III Pharmaceuticals and Medical Devices Agency at BIO Japan, Yokohama. Pharmacogenomics relating to drug evaluation. September 9, 2005. www.jhsf.or.jp/intro/BioJapan/Biojapan_A10–3.pdf. Accessed April 4, 2006.

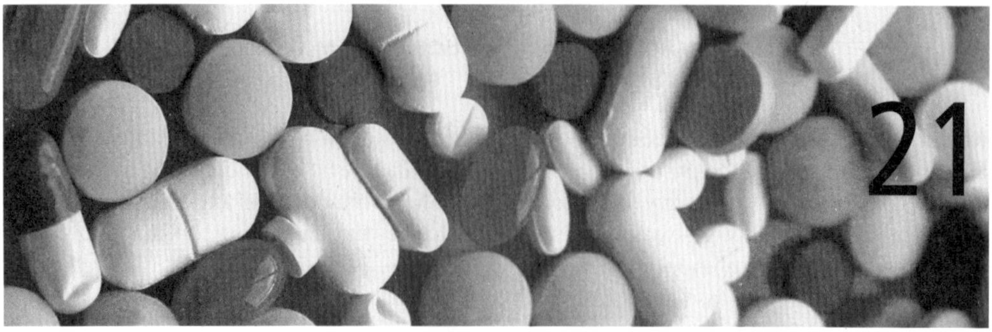

Cell Therapy: A Decade of Opportunity

CELL THERAPY'S POTENTIAL

Tissue engineering uses cells to regenerate, repair, or replace tissue lost as a result of disease, trauma, or congenital disorders. The three segments of tissue engineering are the ex vivo growth of tissue using cell-seeded matrices, the in vivo promotion of tissue growth stimulated by the implantation of biomaterials, and the transplantation of living cells, known as *cell therapy.* In cell therapy, which is the focus of this report, scientists engineer cells to accomplish specific therapeutic tasks as well as repair tissue in the body. Cell therapy has applications in the treatment of a variety of disorders, including oncological, musculoskeletal, metabolic, infectious, and autoimmune diseases.

Market opportunities for cell therapy applications are substantial. In 2001, for example, the market for chronic congestive heart failure therapies was valued at $2.7 billion in the seven major pharmaceutical markets (United States, France, Germany, Italy, Spain, United Kingdom, and Japan). The major-market total for breast cancer therapeutics reached $2.5 billion that year. Cell therapy will potentially expand the cardiovascular and oncology sectors even further by offering treatment options in cases in which no therapy is currently available or the unmet therapeutic need is high. Although cell therapy may replace the need for certain pharmaceuticals, it will more likely be used in conjunction with pharmaceuticals.

Large market segments that have a medical device component (e.g., cardiovascular disease) are also expected to benefit from the adoption of cell therapies. In certain segments, cell therapies will replace surgeries or other procedures that involve medical equipment and devices. Thus, cell therapy presents a cannibalization threat to both pharmaceutical and medical device companies.

We expect the cell therapy market to grow from about $500 million in 2002 to $30 billion in 2010. Currently marketed therapies include cartilage repair and reconstitution of the bone marrow for cancer patients. Therapies for cartilage, bone, and cardiovascular repair are in various stages of development; they will begin to affect the market in 2006.

In this chapter, we investigate the application of cell therapy to various patient populations, including musculoskeletal disorders, cardiovascular disease, central nervous system (CNS) disorders, and metabolic diseases. We analyze how cell therapies will fuel market expansions for these indications; we explore the various business models used in cell therapy companies; and we speculate on the future of companies in this industry.

KEY CELL THERAPY SEGMENTS

Cell therapy will be adopted rapidly when the products and services are easy to use and reimbursed by major healthcare payers. The most significant treatment impact will be on diseases of aging such as osteoarthritis, cardiovascular disease, and cancer. The primary driver for cell therapy in each of the segments is the same – the promise of providing successful therapies for the diseases and disorders that currently lack either treatment options or have only unsatisfactory treatments available.

Musculoskeletal Disorders

Articular cartilage covers the ends of bones at the joint interface and allows bones to move easily. Over time, injury and use can damage the cartilage, causing the bones to rub against each other, resulting in pain and immobility. To treat cartilage injury and chronic osteoarthritis, physicians perform approximately 1 million arthroscopic procedures and 350,000 knee and hip replacement surgeries in the United States each year. These costly surgeries, about $25,000 each, often result in significant morbidity. Joint replacement is considered a poor choice for people younger than age 50 because of the relatively short life of the replacements, about 10–15 years. Alternative treatments for joint disorders, particularly cartilage repair and replacement, represent a growing market opportunity for cell therapies, with little, if any, competition from other types of products.

Several companies market cartilage cell therapy, and more products are in various stages of development. In 1997, Genzyme Biosurgery introduced the first cell therapy product in the United States – Carticel autologous chondrocytes. Verigen, co.don, and Fidia market cell-based therapies for cartilage repair in Europe. The companies listed in Table 21.1 are developing cartilage and other cell therapies for joint and bone repair.

Cardiovascular Disease

Accounting for more than 40% of deaths each year, cardiovascular disease remains the leading cause of mortality in the United States. Contributing to this mortality are two key conditions: myocardial infarction and congestive heart failure. Myocardial infarction triggers the formation of scar tissue, which is one of the causes of congestive heart failure.

Ironically, the recent improvements in treating ischemic disease have increased the number of patients living with congestive heart failure, the fastest-growing segment of cardiovascular disease. Current treatments for congestive heart failure provide a limited palliative outcome; therefore, myocardial infarction and congestive heart failure could benefit substantially from cell therapies. Such therapies could benefit not only patients but also the healthcare system in terms of burden of resources and financing.

Several companies, including Bioheart, Genzyme Biosurgery, Osiris Therapeutics, and Kourion, are researching a variety of approaches involving cell therapy to treat cardiovascular disease. These methods include heart muscle regeneration using autologous skeletal muscle cells, autologous bone marrow cells derived from stromal cells, and embryonic stem cells (ESCs). Table 21.2 lists select companies and their programs or products for cardiovascular conditions.

Central Nervous System Disorders

The various diseases and disorders of the CNS represent a broad market opportunity for cell therapies. Today, patients suffering from Alzheimer's disease (AD), Parkinson's disease, Huntington's disease, and stroke have few, if any, effective treatment options. Moreover, as the elderly population in the seven major markets continues to expand, the burden on the healthcare system to provide costly long-term care for patients afflicted with CNS disorders will increase.

Table 21.1 Companies with Cartilage and Bone Cell Therapy Programs and Products

Company	*Programs/Products*
Aastrom	• AastromReplicell System to produce TRCs and TCs • OC-I for severe osteoporosis • OCG-I for bone grafting in fusions and nonunion fractures
BioTissue Technologies	• Osteochondral construct for joint defects • BioSeed-Oral Bone to treat receded jawbones • BioSeed-C for autologous cartilage replacement
CellFactors	• Skeletex is a bone repair product composed of hypertrophic chondrocytes that produce a matrix for bone regeneration and replacement • Skeletex has applications in bone reconstruction, dentistry, spine fusion, and bonding of prostheses
co.don	• Chondrotransplant for autologous cartilage cell transplants • Osteotransplant for autologous bone cell transplants
Fidia	• Products are based on modified forms of the naturally occurring polymer hyaluronic acid • Hyalograft 3D for dermal replacement • Laserskin autograft is a biodegradable membrane that allows for rapid reepithelialization • Hyalograft C is a cartilage substitute for the treatment of femoral chondyle, knee cap, and tibial plate defects
Genzyme Biosurgery	• Carticel service to repair cartilage • Synvisc, an intra-articular treatment for osteoarthritis
IsoTis	• Replacement tissues using hybrid technologies that incorporate cell therapy, biomaterials, and biotechnology with programs in tissue-engineered bone and cartilage
Isto Technologies	• IstoCyte Chondral Allograft, ex vivo cultured human articular cartilage • IstoCyte Osteochondral Allograft, ex vivo human articular cartilage cultured on bone substrate • IstoGen Bone Graft Matrix, an osteoconductive and osteoinductive bone graft substitute
Kourion	• Developing its Unrestricted Somatic Stem Cell (USSC) using placental cord blood stem cells • The goal is to create off-the-shelf cell therapies to treat heart and bone disorders
Osiris Therapeutics	• Developing technologies where adult stem cells are used in the functional restoration of tissues • OTI-050 to treat bone disorders • OTI-030 for meniscal regeneration
Tigenix	• ChondroCelect is based on proprietary genetic marker technology to improve the selection, characterization, and expansion of stable hyaline cartilage-forming cell populations to repair cartilage defects • ChondroCelect-P uses adult stem-cell technology
Verigen	• Specializes in the field of tissue engineering and orthopedic applications through Autologous Chondrocyte Implantation (ACI) • Matrix-induced Autologous Chondrocyte Implantation (MACI) technology renders excision of a periosteal graft unnecessary; instead, a reabsorbable porcine Collagen I/III membrane is used to cover defect

Table 21.2 Companies with Cardiovascular Cell Therapy Programs and Products

Company	*Programs/Products*
Bioheart	• MyoCell is a tissue-regeneration product comprising autologous myoblasts for the treatment of myocardial infarction and congestive heart failure • Phase I/II trials are under way in Europe and a Phase I trial was authorized in the United States in September 2002
Genzyme Biosurgery	• Cardiovascular program includes combinations of technologies involving gene therapy, cell therapy, biomaterials, and devices that address both ischemic heart disease and congestive heart failure • A Phase II trial began in December 2002 to test the safety and efficacy of cardiac myoblast cell transplantation for the treatment of myocardial infarction and congestive heart failure
Kourion	• Developing its Unrestricted Somatic Stem Cell (USSC) using placental cord blood stem cells • The goal is to create off-the-shelf cell therapies to treat heart and bone disorders
Neuronyx	• Developing human adult bone-marrow-derived stem cells (hABM-SCs) • For the treatment of cardiovascular disorders
Osiris Therapeutics	• Developing technologies in which adult stem cells are used in the functional restoration of diseased tissues • OTI-020 to treat acute myocardial infarction • OTI-021 to treat chronic heart failure

The most common cause of dementia in the elderly is the neurodegenerative condition AD. Approximately 4 million people in the United States are affected by AD, which is responsible for 100,000 deaths a year.

Parkinson's disease is estimated to affect between 500,000 and 1 million people in the United States. Approximately 150,000 people in the United States are in the late stages of the disease.

Huntington's disease affects about 25,000 people in the United States. Each year, an additional 1,500 patients are diagnosed with the disease. Currently, about 20,000 patients are in the late stages of the disease.

Stroke is the third-leading cause of death in the United States and the leading cause of long-term disability. Each year, some 600,000 people experience a new or recurrent stroke.

Tissue regeneration in the nervous system is particularly challenging. The opportunity to introduce cell therapy products to the large population of individuals with CNS disorders (who have unmet treatment needs that otherwise result in significant morbidity and mortality) has many companies working on products in this field (Table 21.3).

Cancer

Cell therapy's applications in the treatment of cancer rest on its ability to help stimulate the immune system to eradicate the disease. Gamida-Cell, for example, is developing an expanded cord blood stem-cell product for the treatment of leukemia and lymphoma. Advances in cell therapy technology may also help regenerate the blood cells and

Table 21.3 Companies with Neurological Cell Therapy Programs and Products

Company	*Programs/Products*
BresaGen	• Human embryonic stem-cell (hESC) implantation to treat Parkinson's disease • Company's cell therapy division focuses on cell differentiation, human stem cells, and catheters and imaging
CellFactors	• Neucell comprises immortalized neural cell lines for in vitro use • Human whole-cell therapy targets Parkinson's disease and other neurodegenerative diseases
CyThera	• Cell replacement therapies use its proprietary stem-cell technology that enables expansion of undifferentiated stem cells • Developing treatments for Parkinson's disease, macular degeneration, and stroke
IsoTis	• Developing replacement tissues and organs using hybrid technologies that incorporate cell therapy, biomaterials, and biotechnology with programs in tissue-engineered nerves
Kourion	• Developing cell therapies for the treatment of bone defects and for myocardial regeneration • Developing novel, off-the-shelf cell therapy products for disease indications for which no adequate treatment is available
Layton Bioscience	• Developing LBS-Neurons to treat chronic and subacute stroke • The LBS-Neurons may also be used to treat spinal cord injury, Huntington's disease, and Parkinson's disease
Macropore	• Acquired StemSource in November 2002 • Developing an internal program focused on stem-cell applications to treat spinal cord injuries
Neuralstem	• Developing neural stem cells for neurodegenerative disorders • Potential applications include Parkinson's disease, Huntington's disease, Alzheimer's disease, epilepsy, spinal cord injury, and multiple sclerosis
Neuronyx	• Developing hABM-SCs • For the treatment of central nervous system disorders
Osiris Therapeutics	• Developing its proprietary adult, human MSCs • For the treatment of stroke and spinal cord injury
Proneuron	• Developing activated macrophages for immune modulation • Cell therapy targeting incomplete spinal cord injury
StemCells	• Developing human neural stem cells for neurodegenerative disorders • Potential applications include Parkinson's disease, Huntington's disease, AD, epilepsy, spinal cord injury, stroke, and multiple sclerosis

bone marrow following chemotherapy or chemoradiotherapy.

Cell therapy involving dendritic cells that function as antigen-presenting cells can be manipulated ex vivo to upregulate the immune response to disease. T cells can also be collected and expanded ex vivo with disease specificity to increase the immune system's defenses. Stem cells from both autologous (self) and allogeneic (other) sources can be collected and expanded for use in repopulating the immune and blood system following myeloablative or myelo-suppressive cancer treatments.

Many companies in this field, including those listed in Table 21.4, are developing stem-cell transplant therapies based on cell-separation and/or cell-expansion devices.

Metabolic Diseases

Both chronic liver disease and diabetes are potentially lucrative areas for cell therapies. Table 21.5 lists select cell therapy programs and products used to treat these diseases.

Chronic Liver Disease

In the United States, chronic liver disease is the 10th most common cause of death. Viral hepatitis is the most common cause of chronic liver disease. An estimated 1.3 million people suffer from chronic hepatitis B virus (HBV), another 2.7 million people are diagnosed with hepatitis C virus (HCV), and 70,000 individuals have hepatitis D virus (HDV) infections. Each year, liver insufficiency

Table 21.4 Companies with Cancer Cell Therapy Programs and Products

Company	*Programs/Products*
Aastrom	• AastromReplicell System to produce TRCs and TCs • SC-I (bone marrow stem cells) to treat solid cancers • CB-I (cord blood) to treat leukemia and genetic blood diseases
Gamida-Cell	• Develops products based on proprietary stem-/progenitor-cell-expansion technology • StemEx is an expanded cord blood stem-cell product to treat leukemia and lymphoma
Baxter	• Isolex 300i Magnetic Cell Selection System is used in stem-cell selection to separate stem cells from other cells in a bone marrow or blood sample
Osiris Therapeutics	• Developing technologies where adult stem cells are used in the functional restoration of diseased tissues • OTI-010 for use in bone marrow transplant support (peripheral blood stem cells) • OTI-011 for use in bone marrow transplant support (cord blood)

Table 21.5 Companies with Liver and Pancreas Cell Therapy Programs and Products

Company	*Programs/Products*
CyThera	• Cell replacement therapies using its proprietary stem-cell technology that enables expansion of undifferentiated stem cells • Developing treatments for diabetes and liver disease
DeveloGen	• Program based on proprietary phenotype-first technology and stem-cell expertise • Targeting metabolic diseases such as diabetes and obesity
ES Cell International	• Human embryonic stem (hES) cell technology platform • Developing treatments for Parkinson's disease, diabetes, cardiovascular disease, and hematology indications such as leukemia
Geron	• Combining human pluripotent stem cells, telomerase expression, and nuclear transfer technology • Developing a universal source of replacement cells for transplantation and cell therapies for restoring the function of degenerating organs
StemCells	• Characterizing and isolating liver stem cells from human tissue to restore liver function due to colorectal cancer, liver cancer, chronic liver disease, acute liver failure, and metabolic disorders • Characterizing and isolating pancreatic stem cells from human tissue and transplanting them into the pancreas of individuals with diabetes to restore organ function
VitaGen	• Extracorporeal Liver Assist Device (ELAD) – an artificial liver containing a cultured human liver cell line (C3A) to treat fulminant hepatic failure

results in 300,000 hospitalizations, and liver failure causes 30,000 deaths.

Currently, the only treatment option for patients with acute insufficiency of the liver is an organ transplant. Of the 17,500 people awaiting liver transplants annually, only about 5,000 donor livers become available. The cost of a liver transplant is approximately $150,000. The complication and difficulties that result from liver transplantation include lifelong immunosuppression, potential for rejection, long hospitalization, and lack of organ availability. Cell therapy could present patients with a much more attractive treatment option: the implantation of non-immunogenic liver cells which, in turn, would reduce the cost to the patient and increase the number of patients who can be successfully treated.

Diabetes

In the United States, the Centers for Disease Control estimates that 16 million people have diabetes, of whom some 50% are undiagnosed. Worldwide, more than 135 million people are affected by this disease, and that number is escalating rapidly. By the year 2025, the World Health Organization calculates, more than 300 million people will have diabetes.

Non-insulin-dependent (type 2) diabetes is the most common, affecting approximately 90% of the diabetic population. In aggregate, type 2 diabetics represent the majority of the insulin market in the United States because so many people are affected, despite the fact that most of these patients do not currently use insulin as part of their therapy.

In the United States, more than $45 billion in direct costs is spent on treating diabetes each year. Indirect costs, which include medical costs, disability, work loss, and premature mortality, bring the total to an estimated $92 billion a year.

Diabetes is also associated with numerous complications, such as heart disease, stroke, hypertension, blindness, kidney diseases, and CNS diseases. Two-thirds of people with diabetes die of some form of cardiovascular disease. Given the lifelong effects of diabetes and the costly and painful management of the disease, cell therapy is expected to be highly successful in this market with patients receiving nonimmunogenic insulin-producing pancreatic islet cell implants that will provide pancreatic function and preclude the need for insulin injections.

DESIGNING A CELL THERAPY

Companies may undertake any one of the two general strategies in designing a cell therapy, which are as follows:

- Infusing or implanting tissue-restricted stem cells or progenitors that will differentiate after transplantation.
- Predifferentiating the stem cells prior to transplantation.

The method used will depend on whether the tissue niche in which the cells are implanted has the capacity to induce appropriate differentiation. This environment may be present in the case of traumatic or ischemic disorders such as myocardial infarction, stroke, and spinal cord damage. However, slow degenerative diseases such as Parkinson's disease will probably require cells that were previously differentiated in vitro and more likely are off-the-shelf products. The key near-term challenge for off-the-shelf products remains the development of reliable and well-characterized immortalized cell lines.

The use of uncommitted stem cells also remains uncertain because of the issue of plasticity, or the triggering of cells to migrate and differentiate appropriately. Plasticity is a significant concern because uncommitted stem-cell therapy relies on the principle that cell phenotype is determined by both the starting-cell population and the environment into which the cells are seeded. Therefore, the effective use of uncommitted stem-cell therapies rests upon the characterization and optimization of these combined determinants.

Autologous Cell Therapy

Near-term cell therapy opportunities will rely on autologous adult stem cells. They will include treatments for cartilage, bone, and cardiac muscle. Neurological cell therapy and cell therapy for metabolic diseases, which will primarily involve the use of off-the-shelf cell products, are expected to reach the market closer to 2010. Cell therapies that can utilize autologous adult stem cells such as bone, cartilage, and heart muscle offer the following advantages:

- No ethical issues.
- Accessibility.
- Fewer technological hurdles.
- Fewer regulatory hurdles.
- Currently marketed autologous products.
- Unlikely to trigger immune reaction.

Allegeneic Cell Therapy

An alternative approach to using autologous cells for cell therapies is developing off-the-shelf therapies that provide a more "drug-like" product model. Off-the-shelf cell therapies will be important for treating diseases and conditions for which collecting autologous cells is either impossible or unfeasible. Essentially, the off-the-shelf cell therapies must meet regulatory requirements (yet to be determined) that are equivalent to those of a drug and will therefore have higher upfront costs and risks.

Three critical factors must be resolved before substantial monetary investments will become available to companies primarily involved in developing off-the-shelf cell therapy products:

- Global patent protection, particularly in key markets like Europe, must be secured.
- A clear and harmonized regulatory path must be devised.
- The companies must be assured they will receive reimbursement from third-party-payer organizations.

Regulatory Issues

Demonstration of clinical efficacy remains a major hurdle in obtaining cell therapy approval. In May 1996, autologous cell therapy came under the auspices of the FDA and companies planning to market autologous cell therapies had to begin registering their production facilities and complying with good manufacturing practice (GMP). As a result, clinical studies may take up to eight years.

In Europe, autologous products are exempt from the European Device Directive and Pharmaceutical Directive of the European Union. Therefore, marketing approval must be obtained separately in each country.

Genzyme Biosurgery, along with tissue-engineering companies like Advanced Tissue Sciences, Organogenesis, and Ortec, has cleared the regulatory and reimbursement paths that most cell therapy companies will utilize. Genzyme Biosurgery, the first company to introduce cell therapy products, is the only company with an approved autologous chondrocyte product in the United States. The FDA approved this product, Carticel, in 1997. It is used to repair damaged knee cartilage in patients who have had an unsatisfactory response to surgery.

The confirmatory postmarketing long-term studies that Genzyme is conducting will have a significant impact on the cell therapy market. The company completed its first study in 2000; that study compared patient outcomes before and after Carticel implants and showed positive results from treatment. The long-term data obtained through these studies will be important to both clinicians and third-party payers. Outcomes that affirm the long-term safety of using Carticel and lasting patient improvements in function will provide the first time-tested evidence to support the use and reimbursement of cell therapy.

Cell Therapy Business Models

As illustrated in the previous sections, cell therapy is applicable to a wide spectrum of diseases. The type of therapy most likely to be adopted will vary from segment to segment. For diseases and disorders in which acquiring autologous cells is problematic (e.g., Parkinson's disease), cord blood or stem-cell cultures will be useful alternatives. Cell therapy companies tend to focus on several segments that utilize cells from the same stem-cell origin so the segment focus tends to drive the business model. Companies developing cell therapies for the CNS will more likely use stem cells and an off-the-shelf or cell-bank approach. When autologous cells are available, this approach offers a lower product risk for near-term products and a means of entering the market sooner.

The restrictions associated with creating products in a specific segment drive the cell therapy business model. The business models among cell therapy companies are to a significant degree driven by the cell source used in the products. The costs associated with developing cell therapies vary widely, depending upon the type of off-the-shelf product being created.

Table 21.6 summarizes the cell therapy business models and lists the companies within each category. As we stated before, those using autologous cells will introduce products as early as 2006 and companies using an off-the-shelf cell therapy approach will enter the market closer to 2010. All of these business models are expected to be valid throughout the decade unless one particular approach results in unequivocal failure, in which case the model could quickly vanish.

Device Driven

Device-driven companies (e.g., Aastrom, Baxter, Eligix, and CellExsys) develop tools to isolate, separate, and, in some cases, expand stem cells. The first cell therapy business model was device driven. To create the cell therapy industry, companies focused on the identification, separation, and isolation of cells. The last key factor for success – cell population expansion – was ignored by most of the early players. Aastrom, the exception

Table 21.6 Cell Therapy Business Models

Model Type	*Key Characteristics*	*Examples*
Device driven	Develops devices to isolate, separate, and possibly expand stem cells	Aastrom, Baxter, Eligix, and CellExsys
Adult autologous committed therapy	Uses a proprietary process to generally isolate, characterize, and expand adult stem cells	Bioheart, Verigen, and co.don
Adult allogeneic uncommitted therapy	Uses a proprietary process to generally isolate, characterize, and expand adult stem cells that differentiate following implantation or injection in vivo	Osiris Therapeutics
Committed off-the-shelf therapy	Uses a proprietary process to generally isolate, characterize, and expand fetal or adult stem cells. Committed cells are derived from the specific tissue and are immortalized to create cell lines or "drugs"	Stemcells, CellFactors, Neuronyx, and Neuralstem
Uncommitted off-the-shelf therapy	Uses a proprietary process to isolate, characterize, and expand embryonic or neonatal stem cells. The cell population immortalized is then stimulated to differentiate and cell lines are created	Kourion, ES Cell International, and BresaGen
Cell banking	Banks placental and cord blood stem cells to produce a reservoir of stem cells for autologous and possibly allogeneic use in the future	Anthrogenesis, Netcord, and ViaCord
Multitechnology	Applies a portfolio of cell therapy and related platforms to treat diseases or disorders	Genzyme Biosurgery and Celgene

to this early trend, had developed and now markets its cell-expansion system in Europe: the Aastrom Replicell System is based on a multiuse instrumentation platform that incorporates single use, therapy-specific kits for each application to produce patient-specific cell treatments.

Adult Autologous Committed Therapy

Companies that focus on adult autologous committed cell therapies (e.g., Bioheart, Verigen, and co.don) use a proprietary process to generally isolate, characterize, and expand adult stem cells. The expanded cell population is either injected at the organ site via catheter or implanted via an opened or closed surgical procedure.

Adult Allogeneic Uncommitted Therapy

Companies following the adult allogeneic uncommitted cell therapy business model (e.g., Osiris Therapeutics) generally perform the same process as the previously mentioned companies but they use undifferentiated cells that are either implanted or infused and then migrate to where they are needed. At the site of treatment, responding to local environmental cues, these stem cells will differentiate accordingly.

Committed Off-the-shelf Therapy

Companies that develop committed off-the-shelf cell therapies (e.g., Stemcells, CellFactors, Neuronyx, and Neuralstem) generally isolate, characterize, and expand fetal or adult stem cells using a proprietary process. Committed cells are derived from the specific tissue and are immortalized to create cell lines. These cells lines can essentially be viewed as "drugs," and the processes used to create them can be considered the manufacturing process. This approach will require characterization, assay development, and long-term testing to demonstrate the reliability and purity of the cell lines used.

Uncommitted Off-the-shelf Therapy

Companies that develop uncommitted off-the-shelf therapies (e.g., Kourion, ES Cell International, and BresaGen) generally isolate, characterize, and expand embryonic or neonatal stem cells using a proprietary process. By immortalizing the cell population and stimulating it to differentiate, the companies create cell lines.

Cell Banking

Companies that focus on banking placental and cord blood stem cells (e.g., Anthrogenesis, Netcord, and ViaCord) collect the samples at birth to produce a reservoir of stem cells for autologous and possibly allogeneic use in the future. Cord blood stem cells are considered immunologically naïve so fewer problems are caused by type mismatching. Some compatibility markers are more important than others – the important ones must be identified for systematic use in typing and cross-matching.

Using neonatal stem cells from cord blood offer the following advantages:

- No ethical issues as compared with ESCs.
- Cell acquisition is safe from cord blood, and there is no risk to the donor compared with adult stem-cell collection.
- Safety data have been collected for more than eight years on the use of cord blood versus ESCs.
- The expansion capacity of cord blood stem cells is excellent.
- Many disease indications can be treated because of the multilineage potential of cord blood stem cells.
- Allogeneic cord blood banks offer access to GMP-grade, diverse starting material.

Multitechnology

Multitechnology companies (e.g., Genzyme Biosurgery, Celgene) apply a portfolio of platforms in the treatment of diseases. These companies are pursuing the development of several types of therapies such as small-molecule therapeutics, gene therapy, and cell therapy – all for treating the same or similar conditions.

MARKET ENTRY CHALLENGES

Cautious Investment Environment

Given the unclear regulatory pathway, the challenging reimbursement environment, and inherent product development risks, the overall risk for a return on cell therapy investment is perceived as high. The level of uncertainty in combination with the need for new skill sets and intellectual property creates an environment that deters near-term investment. Only when later-stage clinical trial data show promise will more companies want to enter the market.

Of course, following the release of positive late-stage trial data, the problem will then be that fewer companies will be available for partnering and acquisition, resulting in a more competitive environment with higher acquisition costs. But for some companies, this scenario is preferable to acquisitions today when technology and product risk are significantly higher.

The problem with this wait-and-see attitude is that corporate cultures need time to adjust and people need firsthand experience to build corporate knowhow. Although a wait-and-see attitude will certainly lower the risk of failure, it could increase the risk of poor performance. Allowing early players to absorb the initial product development risks and market missionary work makes sense, but now, the market is already beginning to weed out the companies with problematic products and business models. Fewer companies will remain in the market and the cost of developing a multitech approach will continue to climb.

Determining Market Strategy

The bankruptcies of several leading tissue engineering/cell therapy companies in the United States, and the absence of such bankruptcies in Europe highlight a key difference in their respective strategies. In the United States, the failed or reorganizing companies' approach was to develop off-the-shelf products requiring substantial financing of research, development, clinical testing, and new facilities. Extensive research created significant debt, and problems developed because immediate market success did not follow. By contrast, many European companies grew out of medical university clinical research programs that offered autologous cell therapies – a cost structure with a lower initial investment hurdle.

With ready access to public equity markets and solid big medical device partnerships in place, and by investing in broader pipelines and building programs necessary to avoid becoming a single-product company, the early cell therapy companies seemed poised for growth and expansion. Companies like Advanced Tissue Sciences and Organogenesis had numerous product development programs, while companies like Ortec focused on a single product. In the aftermath of the market downturn and slow sales, Ortec's conservative strategy has proven the more successful.

In February 2002, Organogenesis announced that it would refocus its business on two core areas: living wound-healing products and bioengineered surgical products. In the course of restructuring, Organogenesis reduced its workforce by 16%, yielding a net annualized savings of $5 million. The company formed its own sales and marketing group in fall 2001 and launched its first product, FortaPerm, in October 2001. FortaGen, the company's second tissue repair product, was launched in January 2002. However, in October 2002, the company filed for Chapter 11 bankruptcy protection.

Throughout late 2001 and 2002, the number of cell therapy and tissue-engineering companies undergoing restructuring continued to grow. Several companies emerged stronger from this process. Stemcells repositioned itself beginning in January 2001 by recapitalizing and cleaning up its balance sheet. Through a series of financial moves that included selling its Modex shares, establishing a $30 million equity credit line, and bringing in $20 million in equity before the events of September 11, 2001, the company has been able to maintain its mission focus. Stem cells has resisted the temptation to begin building out its organization and continues its lean approach by advancing its most near-market programs only to further reduce the company's burn rate.

Another company that has successfully survived multiple traumas is Aastrom. At Aastrom, the stability and tenacity of its leadership represent a sharp contrast to the revolving-door management approach of many companies undergoing dramatic downturns. Aastrom's ability to retrench after the market for its bone marrow transplant market disappeared in 1997, it lost its partner Cobe (now Gambro) in 1999, and the market for its peripheral blood stem-cell breast cancer cell therapy disappeared in 2000 highlights again the success of building a single product focus during early company development. Today, Aastrom has leveraged its platform technology – the AastromReplicell System to produce tissue-repair cells (TRCs) and therapeutic cells (TCs) – across several product segments that have emerged during the time the company spent refining its products.

The Partnering Vacuum

Partnerships between small cell therapy companies and pharmaceutical, large biotechnology, or medical device companies have not provided much support for the industry. For medical device companies in particular, the transition from open procedures to closed procedures and mechanical solutions to biological solutions – as represented by cell therapy – place many of these companies at market risk. These companies could see product cannibalization from new biological approaches, yet few have made substantial commitments to cell therapy. This resistance may be due to the difficulty of rapidly acquiring the core competencies needed to operate in the cell therapy field and/or a combination of unanswered science, regulatory obstacles, and reimbursement hurdles.

Few major companies have made a commitment to cell therapy. An exception is Novartis, a company that apparently remains undeterred despite its three unsuccessful attempts to create marketable cell therapy products. Novartis's acquisition of Systemix and its programs for bone marrow stromal cell (BMSC) expansion came to a halt in the mid-1990s. In 1999, Novartis canceled an alliance with Osiris for the development of treatments using mesenchymal stem cells (MSCs). More recently, Novartis's problems in its relationship with Organogenesis resulted in another exit from the cell therapy/tissue-engineering segment.

Other companies have also tried to enter the cell therapy market in the past including AstraZeneca through an alliance with CytoTherapeutics for the development of encapsulated bovine adrenal cells to treat chronic pain. The alliance was discontinued in 1999, leading to the restructuring of CytoTherapeutics and a narrowing of its focus to stem-cell technologies. Cobe canceled its agreement with Aastrom when the market opportunity declined. Other companies include Smith & Nephew, a company which will ultimately receive the products from its joint venture with Advanced Tissue Sciences after the company was liquidated in late 2002. Finally, Baxter now owns the cell separation system developed by Nexell Therapeutics which was also liquidated in late 2002.

Despite the technology, regulatory, reimbursement, and market hurdles, cell therapies remain compelling technologies for many key therapeutic areas. Cell therapics that work when no other treatments are available or that offer improved outcomes are sought after by physicians and patients. While pharmaceutical partnering has been, and continues to be, a major source of funding for both R&D and the commercialization of new biotechnology-based treatments; this is not the case for cell therapy.

If the autologous product can be infused into the patient, then a pharmaceutical company would be a logical partner for an autologous cell therapy company. Other types of partners could also be used in this approach, such as combination service and equipment providers like Fresenius and Cobe. However, if the autologous product requires a surgeon to learn a new or special procedure, then the selling process would be much closer to a medical device sale so a medical device partner would be more appropriate from a distribution standpoint. The problem to overcome here is that most medical device companies have R&D departments that are geared toward devices and cannot provide assistance in cell therapy development. In fact, they are often trying to avoid getting involved in pharmaceuticals and biologicals. The list of exceptions to this pattern is growing and now includes Johnson & Johnson's Mitek leap into cell therapy via its partnership with Verigen. Also, in March 2003, Boston Scientific entered into an alliance with Osiris Therapeutics to develop and commercialize a cardiovascular cell therapy to treat patients following myocardial infarctions using Osiris' MSC technology.

This partnering vacuum could end up being filled by companies that provide cell culture and manufacturing, such as Cambrex/Biowhitaker. Perhaps having a development partner and a different marketing and distribution partner is one way to solve the financing dilemma as well as offer the expertise and endorsement that cell therapy companies need from major established medical companies.

Many pharmaceutical companies could use cell therapies to create broader-based therapeutic franchises. Here, the type of selling is very different, and in this case, if the pharmaceutical companies could convert portions of their salesforce to hands-on selling, they could reap big rewards with increased physician loyalty that would support their franchises. On the other hand, biotechnology companies have an understanding of cell therapy and are culturally suited to a match. But with so many projects and so little funding to go around, and much of that funding coming from pharmaceutical companies, biotech is too focused on what they have already to invest in cell therapy.

The obstacles to partnering remain large. With controversy continuing to cloud the science of cell therapy and robust proofs of principle often lacking, the risk of investing in cell therapy may be perceived as higher by pharmaceutical companies than it is by medical device companies. However, when the treatment benefits of cell therapies are proven in substantial markets, both biotechs and pharmaceutical companies may be more comfortable with investing in the cell therapy segment.

OUTLOOK FOR THE CELL THERAPY MARKET

Market Expansion Factors

Sales of cell therapy and tissue-engineering products in the 1990s were lackluster. This poor sales performance can be attributed to product-use problems and delays in obtaining product reimbursement codes. These problems will ease as product performance improves and market acceptance increases. Several therapeutic markets will undergo rapid expansion as cell therapies are introduced to treat heretofore untreatable conditions. Surgical procedures will decline in parallel, primarily in the treatment of joint disorders and cardiovascular disease. By 2010, we anticipate, the market for cell therapies will be robust – in the $30 billion range.

The growth will come from cord blood, mesenchymal cells, and autologous adult stem cells. These three segments will provide the first rapidly accepted products. The technological, ethical, and financial problems associated with the use of ESCs will prevent ESC technology from contributing to market growth during the first decade of cell therapy use. However, following the recognition of the benefits achieved using adult and cord blood stem cells and the continued research and development of ESCs, use of ESC-based therapies could become prominent after 2010. Table 21.7 discusses developing technologies in this field.

Currently, the rapidly organizing and growing cord blood segment offers tremendous stability to the cell therapy market as a whole. Banking of cord blood is an outgrowth of blood banking. Essentially, the groundwork has already been laid for the banking of blood and other tissues, both

Table 21.7 Companies with Embryonic Stem-Cell Therapy Programs and Products

Company	Programs/Products
Advanced Cell Technology	• Developing technology to produce primitive human embryonic stem cells using nuclear transfer and parthenogenesis • Donor cells are taken from the patient to develop cells for cloning and tissues for cell and organ transplantation
BresaGen	• hESC implantation to treat Parkinson's disease • Company's cell therapy division focuses on cell differentiation, human stem cells, and catheters and imaging
ES Cell International	• hES cell technology platform • Developing treatments for Parkinson's disease, cardiovascular disease, and hematology indications such as leukemia
Geron	• Combining human pluripotent stem cells, telomerase expression, and nuclear transfer technology • Developing a universal source of replacement cells for transplantation and cell therapies for restoring the function of degenerating organs

allogeneic and autologous. The use of blood and tissue banks can provide a reservoir for the future. Despite the interest in the use of ESC clones to create replacement tissue in the future, it is likely that in the long term, newborns will all have their cord blood banked and available for use in any personalized medicine required during childhood or adulthood. The advantage of this approach is that the tissue, a universal, off-the-shelf product, is available quickly and can be used for emergency procedures. However, for the treatment of chronic conditions, autologous banked tissue may be preferred. Much depends on the technology applied and how quickly tissues can be grown and made available for use.

Industry Consolidation

Poor capitalization and a lack of financial options are driving rapid consolidation of the cell therapy segment. When financing opportunities reappear, the new cell therapy companies will be positioned to advance programs that are now on hold, contributing to a range of product introductions by 2010.

During 2001 and 2002, most cell therapy companies restructured their businesses at least once. The restructurings involved focusing resources on product candidates and products with near-term profit potential. The objectives of this process are cost reduction, and refocusing and repositioning the company for potential product commercialization. For example, Genzyme Tissue Repair, the predecessor company of Genzyme Biosurgery, acquired Biosurface Technologies in 1995 and established its position in the tissue-engineering arena. Genzyme Biosurgery was formed when Genzyme Tissue Repair was combined with BioMatrix in 2000. Genzyme Biosurgery went on to acquire Focal as well. The resulting company has core competencies in biomaterials, gene therapy, and cell therapy. Complementary strengths provide a broad technology platform from which Genzyme Biosurgery can treat both joint conditions and cardiovascular diseases.

Future Partnerships

The Macropore acquisition is a sign of what is to come in the cell therapy market. In November 2002, Macropore acquired StemSource, thereby making a commitment to developing an internal program focused on stem-cell applications to treat spinal cord injuries. Some companies, like Johnson & Johnson's Mitek and Macropore, are positioning for future market dominance through efforts to create a new generation of products based on breakthrough cell therapy technologies, while competitors continue to maintain their more narrow focus on mechanical-based medical devices.

Cellgene's acquisition of Anthrogenesis, completed in January 2002, is the first major move into cell therapy by a biopharmaceutical company. Eventually, in each segment where cell therapy will have an impact, acquisitions and partnerships fueled by successful clinical trials, anticipated product dominance, and increasing competition will level the playing field.

In the next few years, partnering will focus on near-term commercial opportunities that involve lower-risk scenarios. Therefore, autologous cell therapy companies with successful Phase II clinical trials will be highly sought after, particularly by medical device companies.

Many of the newer partnerships involve personalized medicine cell therapy products rather than off-the-shelf products. On June 14, 2002, Johnson & Johnson's Mitek Worldwide and Verigen announced an agreement to market an advanced, minimally invasive articular cartilage-repair system throughout the United States and Canada. Verigen is a company specializing in autologous cell therapies for cartilage repair, with products currently marketed in Europe and Australia. Mitek will conduct US clinical trials and file for the regulatory approval.

Unlike many of the equipment-driven cell therapy partnerships of the 1990s (e.g., Aastrom and COBE, Nexell with Baxter), newer partnerships will use cell therapy products as the core of their deals. For example, in October 2002, Targeted Genetics' cell therapy spin-off company, CellExSys, formed a strategic alliance with Itochu to launch a cell therapy business in Japan focused on the treatment of infectious diseases and cancer. The approach will involve clinical applications developed using CellExSys's proprietary Rapid Expansion Method (REM) to generate antigen-specific T cells. Following the acquisition of GMP facilities in Japan, Itochu and CellExSys will develop and manufacture antigen-specific T cells for use as therapeutic agents.

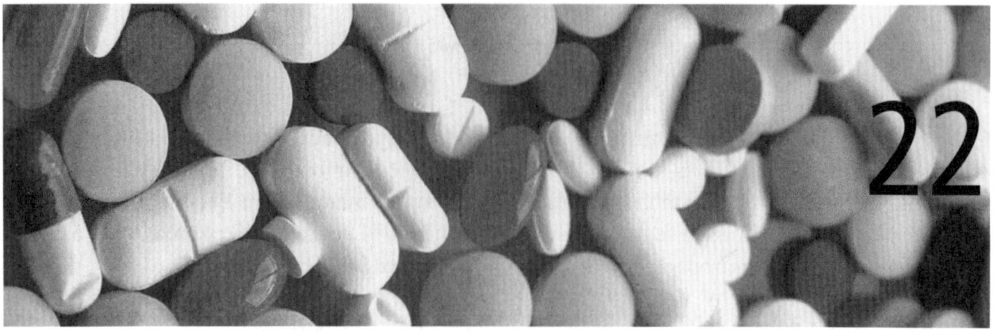

Nanotechnology in Medicine: Its Time Has Come

MOMENTUM IS STEADILY BUILDING

Nanotechnology has been likened to a modern-day "industrial revolution" that is expected to have a major influence on industry, science, global economies, and society in general. Its presence is already felt in the miniaturization that is occurring across all fields of science. Nanotechnology has applications in a broad range of industries including electronics, materials sciences, chemical manufacturing, and pharmaceuticals. In fact, nanomedicine's time has come; at least 12 products have already been approved, and many more are in the pipeline.

The term *nanotechnology* encompasses a spectrum of applications and products that are defined by their very small size, which is measured in nanometers (nm). The National Nanotechnology Initiative defines nanotechnology as the understanding and control of matter at dimensions of roughly 1–100 nm. This small size enables nanotech structures to interact at the atomic, molecular, and macromolecular levels.

To put the nanometer size in perspective, there are 1 million nanometers in a millimeter or 1 billion nanometers in a meter. The diameter of DNA is approximately 2.5 nm, while red blood cells are about 1,000 times larger at 2,500 nm. Still larger is a human hair at 60,000–120,000 nm in diameter. In comparison, a nanotube, which is a tubular structure with either open or closed ends, is about 100,000 times smaller than a human hair and has a diameter of approximately 1.3 nm.

Nanoparticles derive specific properties from their minuscule size. First, particles of this size are no longer subject to the laws of classical physics but of quantum physics. This feature of nanoparticles provides them with unique optical, magnetic, and electrical properties. Second, their exceptionally large surface area to mass ratio allows them to exert a strong influence over their environment.

Nanotechnology has become a global phenomenon. It continues to receive worldwide attention and unprecedented levels of government funding. In December 2005, the European Science Foundation released the results of a two-year study that concluded nanomedicines are already "contributing to improved healthcare in the 21st century" and recommended that Europe devise strategies to stay competitive in this rapidly evolving area. In the United States, Lux Capital reported that nanotech will most likely become the largest government-funded science initiative since the space race, exceeding even the level of funding spent on the Human Genome Project. Nanotechnology is still a conundrum, however; on the one hand, it has been overhyped, yet on the other, its potential to fundamentally change our world cannot be underestimated.

Nanotechnology touches on many aspects of medicine, including drug delivery, diagnostic imaging, clinical diagnostics, nanomedicines, and the use of nanomaterials in medical devices. Interestingly, many nanotechnology products will likely be combination products as defined by the Food and Drug Administration (FDA) (21 CFR 3.2 (e)), combining drug-device, drug-biologic, device-biologic, or drug-device-biologic. (We discuss these products later in this chapter.)

Momentum is steadily building for the successful development of products based on nanotechnology to diagnose and treat disease, and the next five years should see a steady succession of new nanomedicines entering the marketplace.

In this chapter, we cover recent developments in nanotechnology as well as general trends in the industry. We explore the nanotechnology industry that is involved in developing medical products and procedures, the corresponding therapeutic and diagnostic markets, products under development, the current investment climate, challenging patent and business strategies, and the outlook for nanotechnology in medicine.

WORLDWIDE LANDSCAPE

Nanotechnology has already become a worldwide phenomenon. Roughly 700 private companies and 200 public companies are involved in various fields of nanotech research and development; 77 of them are large, listed corporations. The portion of these companies involved in developing nanomedicines is approximately 17%.

Countries worldwide have recognized the potential of nanotechnology. From 2005 to 2008, the US government will spend $3.7 billion on nanotech as part of the 21st century Nanotechnology Research & Development Act; Japan will spend $3 billion. The European Commission funded a pilot project called Project NanoRoadSME as part of the Sixth Framework Program and authorized $1.7 billion for the time period from 2002 to 2006. The commission is expected to authorize another $7.5 billion for 2007–13. China is another large player; it now ranks third behind the United States and Japan in numbers of nanotech patents (Hassan, 2005).

This trend in government-funding initiatives is likely to continue for the foreseeable future. It is matched, in part, by the billions of dollars that corporations spend on R&D programs and, to a much lesser extent, by venture capital and public markets, which are discussed later in this chapter.

MARKETS

From a commercial perspective, nanotechnology has gained the attention of everyone from academics and entrepreneurs to governments and venture capitalists, and it is expected to influence worldwide markets in many different health-related sectors.

Distinct market segments for nanotechnology products are developing. For the purpose of this report, the nanomedicine market segments to be addressed include drug delivery/nanodrugs, in vivo imaging/molecular diagnostics, and nanoenabled devices.

The National Science Foundation predicts that the global nanotechnology market for all industries, including chemicals, pharmaceuticals, and electronics, will reach $1 trillion within five years. For nanomedicine markets, Freedonia has made the following predictions:

- Nanotech-enabled drug delivery will grow from $406 million in 2004 to $3 billion by 2009 and $16.6 billion by 2014.
- Nanodiagnostics, including in vivo imaging and in vitro diagnostic testing, will grow to $1.1 billion in 2009 and to $4 billion by 2020.
- Nanoenabled medical supplies and devices will grow from a $35 million market in 2004 to $2.4 billion in 2009 and to $8.9 billion by 2014.

- When combined, these collective nanomedicine markets will grow 48% per year from 2005 to 2009 to reach a total of $6.5 billion in 2009.

As more nanotech products reach the market and revenues grow, there should be more active investment into funding nanomedicine development. The trigger points for this investment will most likely come from a significant product breakthrough or the convincing demonstration of the superiority of one nanoparticle technology over another one.

The number of nanoparticle compositions, sizes, and shapes that were under development at the end of 2005 is somewhat daunting. A company cannot invest in them all, so which one(s) does it choose? One positive indicator is that investors often look for commercially validated markets, and medical nanotech market segments are quickly becoming populated with new products.

PRODUCTS

The field of nanotech-enabled medicine has steadily matured during the past five years. Several medical products have been approved, and many others are in late-stage development, as we will discuss.

Nanomedicines

Drug delivery currently represents the major medical use of nanotechnology. The global drug delivery market is large (more than $66 billion) and highly competitive. The industry is turning to nanotechnology to reformulate drugs in order to improve poor bioavailability as well as to extend market life after the original drug patents expire.

In addition to drug formulations, nanomedicines also include new agents, such as microbubbles. These nanoparticles have the potential either to become drug-free therapeutic agents or to be used in combination with other drugs (discussed later in this chapter).

Nanoformulations and Drug Delivery

The news is good and looking better every day for the use of nanotech to enhance drug delivery and create new medicines. At least seven nanoenabled drugs have been approved, and many more are in the pipeline. (See Table 22.1 for approved drugs and Table 22.2 for drugs in late-stage clinical trials.)

Nanoformulations help solve an unmet need in the pharma industry relating to solubility, toxicity, dose, and bioavailability. Nanotechnology can make drugs more soluble by drastically reducing particle size and increasing surface area (a process called "nanosizing"). This process is especially important for drug candidates that have low water solubility, require high doses to be effective, or demonstrate unwanted toxicity profiles.

The first nanoformulated drugs to be approved used Elan's nanocrystal technology. Nanocrystals are very small particles of drugs that are milled to a diameter of less than 1,000 nm. For instance, sirolimus (Rapamune) was approved in August 2000 as an immunosuppressant to prevent organ rejection in kidney-transplant patients. It was a solid-dose reformulation of a drug already marketed by Wyeth (American Home Products) as an oral solution. Aprepitant (Emend) was approved in March 2003 to prevent nausea and vomiting during cancer chemotherapy. It was developed in collaboration with Merck as a new chemical entity in a nanocrystal formulation. Abbott received approval for its cholesterol-lowering agent, fenofibrate (Tricor), in November 2004.

These drug approvals represent the first proof-of-principle for the use of nanotechnology in drug delivery. Elan has drug delivery agreements with Bristol-Myers Squibb (initiated in 2003), Janssen (2003), Aventis, now Sanofi-Aventis, (2004), Roche (2005), Johnson & Johnson Pharmaceutical Research & Development (2004), and MAP Pharmaceuticals (2005). It is the most successful nanoformulation company to date.

Table 22.1 Approved Drugs Developed with Nanotechnology-based Formulations

Brand (Compound)	*Company*	*Indication*	*FDA Approval Date*	*Comments*
Estrasorb (17β-estradiol)[a]	Novavax	Estrogen therapy in menopause	October 2003	Micellar nanoparticles
Emend (aprepitant)	Merck	Chemotherapy-induced nausea and vomiting	March 2003	Developed as a new chemical entity in a nanocrystal[b] formulation
Tricor (fenofibrate)	Abbott	Lipid and cholesterol disorders	November 2004	Nanocrystal formulation dissolved faster, was absorbed easier, required a lower dose, and could be taken with or without food
Triglide (fenofibrate)[c]	SkyePharma	Lipid and cholesterol disorders	May 2005	Water-insoluble drug core stabilized with phospholipids in a nanoparticle
Megace (megestrol acetate)	Par Pharmaceuticals	Anorexia or cachexia in AIDS	July 2005	Nanocrystal drug particles
Abraxane (paclitaxel)[d]	American Pharmaceutical Partners	Metastatic breast cancer	January 2005	Albumin-bound paclitaxel nanoparticle
Rapamune (sirolimus)	Wyeth	Prevention of renal transplant rejection	August 2000	Nanocrystal drug particles; reformulation of already marketed drug

[a]Novavax has received payments of $10.0 million to date from Esprit Pharma for the North American marketing rights
[b]Nanocrystals are nanometer-sized particles that are up to 50 times smaller than particles manufactured by conventional pharmaceutical milling techniques
[c]First Horizon Pharmaceuticals licensed US rights from SkyePharma in May 2004
[d]Abraxane is under development by Abraxis Oncology, a subsidiary of American Pharmaceutical Partners. In November 2005, American Pharmaceutical Partners announced plans to merge with its parent company, American Bioscience, to create Abraxis Bioscience. As of November 2005, there were 74 clinical trials including 20 Phase II and 7 Phase III trials for breast, lung, ovarian, prostate, melanoma, and head and neck cancers

Nanoformulations also can be used to successfully target specific tissues and to release the drug at that site. Abraxane, a controlled-release formulation of the chemotherapeutic agent paclitaxel, comprises nanoparticles having a mean particle size of 130 nm. Many tumors express the SPARC protein, which, in turn, has an affinity for albumin bound on Abraxane nanoparticles. Because of the SPARC-albumin interaction, nanoparticles congregate at the site of the tumor and slowly release paclitaxel to kill tumor cells.

In January 2005, Abraxane was approved in the United States for metastatic breast cancer. When compared side by side with Bristol-Myers Squibb's Taxol (paclitaxel) in a randomized, multicenter trial, Abraxane required one-sixth the infusion time and produced almost double the tumor-response rate. American Pharmaceutical Partners says that it is conducting more than 74 Abraxane clinical trials, including seven Phase III studies.

Other nanodrug approvals include SkyePharma's Triglide (fenofibrate) for cholesterol disorders and Novavax's Estrasorb (17β-estradiol), a topical emulsion for estrogen therapy. Triglide was approved by the FDA in May 2005 and launched in the United States in July 2005. Estrasorb is a micellar nanoparticle formulation of 17β-estradiol that received FDA approval in October 2003 and was launched in June 2004.

It is evident from these nanodrug approvals and the pipeline of nanodrugs in later-stage clinical trials that nanotechnology has already entered the drug delivery marketplace. Many more nanoformulated drugs are expected to enter the marketplace in the next five years. What remains unclear is whether any particular type of nanoparticle will be significantly superior to another type, or whether many different types of nanoformulated drugs

Table 22.2 Nanomedicines Under Development in Later-stage Clinical Trials

Drug	*Company/Brand*	*Indication*	*Development Status*	*Comments*
Paliperidone palmitate	Johnson & Johnson Pharmaceutical Research & Development/Paliperidone	Schizophrenia	Phase III complete; NDA submitted November 2005[a]	Extended-release nanoparticles using Elan nanocrystal technology
Propofol[b]	SkyePharma/Propofol IDD-D	Anesthetic and sedative	Phase III	Nanoparticle stabilized with phospholipids
Bioavailable iron	Advanced Magnetics/Ferumoxytol	Iron replacement therapy in anemic conditions, such as chronic kidney disease	Phase III multicenter trials	Iron oxide nanoparticles
Paclitaxel	American Pharmaceutical Partners/ Coroxane	Peripheral arterial disease	Phase II/III	Controlled-release formulation of albumin-bound nanoparticles
Paclitaxel	American Pharmaceutical Partners/ Coroxane	Coronary artery disease using bare metal stents	Phase II	Controlled-release formulation of albumin-bound nanoparticles
Human recombinant insulin	Flamel Technologies/Basulin[c]	Type I diabetes	Phase IIa complete	Controlled-release formulation using nanoparticles made of a leucine-glutamate co-polymer
NB-001	NanoBio/NanoHPX	Herpes labialis (cold sores)	Phase II	Water/oil emulsions using uniformly sized droplets in the nanometer range
NPI-32101	Nucryst Pharmaceuticals	Atopic Dermatitis	Phase II completed in adults; Phase II initiated October 2005 in children and adolescents	Silver nanocrystal-based topical cream
32-P BioSilicon	pSivida/BrachySil[d]	Liver cancer	Phase II	The radioisotope ^{32}P is embedded in porous silicon and delivered via a fine-gauge needle directly into a tumor

Interleukin-2	Flamel Technologies/IL-2 XL	Cancer	Phase I/II[e] initiated December 2004	Controlled-release formulation of IL-2 using poly-amino acid nanoparticles
Recombinant interferon alpha-2b	Flamel Technologies/IFN-alpha-XL	Hepatitis B and hepatitis C	Phase I/II[f] initiated December 2004	Controlled-release formulation of interferon-alpha 2b using poly-amino acid nanoparticles
Doxorubicin	BioAlliance Pharma/Transdrug	Hepatocellular carcinoma	Phase I/II	Nanoformulation of chemotherapy agent based on the polymer PIHCA (poly-iso-hexyl-cyanoacrylate)
DNAs	Copernicus Therapeutics[g]	Nonviral gene replacement in cystic fibrosis	Phase I/II	Compacted DNA nanoparticles formulated as aerosol mists
2-Methoxy-estradiol	Entremed/Panzem	Advanced cancer	Phase I	Uses Elan's nanocrystal technology

[a]If approved, will be marketed in the United States by Janssen, L.P., a wholly owned subsidiary of Johnson & Johnson. The new drug application (NDA) filing is based on a global clinical program that involved more than 1,600 patients in 23 countries. Potential US launch in late 2006 or early 2007

[b]North American rights licensed to Endo Pharmaceuticals in 2002

[c]Bristol-Myers Squibb terminated its Basulin development agreement in September 2004 citing a reprioritization of its pipeline and a recent restructuring

[d]pSivida, an Australian company, merged with Control Delivery Systems in Boston late in 2005

[e]Will compare a long-acting nanoformulation of interleukin-2 with Proleukin, an interleukin-2 product sold by Chiron to treat renal cancer

[f]Will compare a long-acting nanoformulation of interferon-alpha with an immediate-release interferon-alpha (Viraferon) by Schering-Plough

[g]Received $1 million from Cystic Fibrosis Foundation Therapeutics in 2005 to support Phase II development of nanoparticle-delivered gene therapy treatment for cystic fibrosis

IFN = Interferon; IL = Interleukin

will compete against one another for market share in an already competitive drug delivery market. Nanoformulated drugs that should be able to compete successfully will be those that confer an added benefit, such as that observed for Abraxane over Taxol.

The use of nanoformulated drugs in cancer treatment is a very active area of drug delivery; several Phase II trials are ongoing. In the next few years, it should become possible, for the first time, to compare different nanoparticles side by side in drug delivery and efficacy applications in order to determine which types of nanoparticle are likely to be most effective in which disease applications.

Microbubbles

Microbubbles are small gas-filled particles or "bubbles" that are smaller than red blood cells and can easily travel through the smallest of capillaries. They are under development as therapeutics and as imaging agents (discussed further in the next section). A unique advantage of microbubbles is that they can be designed to encapsulate specific drugs inside the bubble or shell. This process may eventually lead to targeted drug therapy, whereby microbubbles travel to the site of disease and the encapsulated drug is released with the local application of ultrasound.

For example, in acute ischemic stroke, thrombolytic agents often fail to completely lyse blood clots, resulting in the reocclusion of blood vessels. For more effective clot lysis, there must be maximum exposure of both the surface and interior of a clot to the thrombolytic agent. Nanotechnology is emerging as a promising means of accomplishing this task. When microbubbles are injected, they travel through the bloodstream and congregate at the location of a clot. When ultrasound is applied locally, the microbubbles vibrate, burst, and produce bubbles at the vicinity of the clot. The result is a mechanical disruption of the clot and drug-free thrombolysis. When used in combination with a thrombolytic agent, the thrombolytic is able to penetrate the clot more deeply, an advantage that may, in turn, result in faster and more effective clot lysis.

ImaRx Therapeutics is developing microbubble technology under the trade name SonoLysis. Microbubbles and ultrasound alone, or in combination with a thrombolytic agent, are being tested in two Phase II clinical trials in ischemic stroke. The combination of microbubbles and ultrasound is also in a Phase I/II clinical trial for peripheral arterial occlusions.

ImaRx is pursuing the use of microbubbles to deliver oxygen in emergency situations, such as in hemorrhagic shock caused by traumatic blood loss. Microbubbles, under the trade name NanO2, are in a preclinical stage of development.

Nanodiagnostics

Another active field of development for medical nanotechnology is nanoenabled diagnostics. This sector includes nanoformulations for use as in vivo imaging agents as well as the in vitro use of nanoparticles in diagnostic tests.

In Vivo Imaging

The use of nanotech-enhanced imaging agents is a rapidly growing field for medical nanodiagnostics. One example is ImaRx Therapeutics' injectable microbubbles for cardiac imaging. These microbubbles encapsulate perfluoropropane (an inert, biocompatible gas) inside a sphere made of naturally occurring phospholipids. ImaRx licensed diagnostic rights to the microbubbles to DuPont but retained all therapeutic rights (see previous section for ImaRx's ongoing therapeutic trials).

Bristol-Myers Squibb Medical Imaging acquired the technology when it acquired DuPont and further developed microbubbles as ultrasound-imaging agents sold under the trade name Definity. In 2001, the FDA approved Definity, which is now a leading contrast agent used in echocardiography in the United States.

Nanotechnology is also employed in the creation of superparamagnetic contrast agents used in magnetic resonance imaging (MRI). These nanoparticles contain an organic nucleus and a thick shell of magnetite that can be coated with protein ligands for tissue-specific imaging.

In December 2004, ImaRx entered into a collaboration with Guerbet (France) to develop imaging agents to target cancer cells. Nanoformulations will be developed combining ImaRx's microbubbles with Guerbet's magnetic resonance contrast agents and targeting ligands.

Other nanotech-derived MRI agents already on the market include Advanced Magnetics' Feridex I.V. and GastroMark products. These products combine superparamagnetic iron oxide nanoparticles with the MRI agents ferumoxides and ferumoxsil, respectively. Feridex is used to image liver lesions and is approved and marketed in the United States, Europe, and elsewhere. GastroMark is a gastrointestinal imaging agent used to delineate the bowel. It is approved and marketed in the United States by Mallinckrodt and in Western Europe and Brazil by Guerbet S.A. under the trade name Lumirem. A third Advanced Magnetics' product, Combinex, uses nanoparticle technology in combination with the MRI agent ferumoxtran-10 to distinguish cancerous lymph nodes from normal ones. The company received an approvable letter from the FDA in March 2005.

Schering has a contrast-enhanced MRI product on the market that is a colloidal solution of the contrast agent ferucarbotran and superparamagnetic iron oxide nanoparticles. It is marketed in Europe and Japan under the trade name Resovist and is in Phase III trials in the United States for imaging liver lesions.

In Vitro Clinical Diagnostics

Many nano-based clinical diagnostic products are in early development, and a handful are already on the market. This sector is an emerging market segment for nanomedicines.

Immunicon and Veridex (a Johnson & Johnson company) entered into an agreement in 2000 to develop Immunicon's magnetic nanoparticle technology. Since July 2004, Veridex has received three 501(K) clearances from the FDA to market an automated instrument and two specific reagent kits. These products are for in vitro diagnostic use to capture and detect rare cells, such as circulating tumor cells. Sold under the trade name CellTracks, the system uses magnetic nanoparticles consisting of a magnetic core that are conjugated with antibodies to target cells. When the antibodies bind to their target, such as a breast cancer antigen, the resulting complex can be isolated with a magnetic field.

Another nanodiagnostic product for in vitro use is the automated system produced by Nanogen for molecular diagnostics. This system is an electronic microarray that is sold under the trade name NanoChip. In 2004 and 2005, Nanogen entered into many agreements designed to consolidate its position in molecular diagnostics, including the following:

- An equity position in Jurilab, with an option to acquire the company, for diagnostic rights to gene marker technology.
- A merger with Epoch Biosciences for genomic testing products.
- The acquisition of Synx for point-of-care diagnostics products, such as a diagnostic test for congestive heart failure.

In September 2005, Nanogen completed a $20 million private placement to help fund these merger and acquisition activities. The company is one of the most active players in the development of nanodiagnostics for in vitro use.

Nanomaterials in Medical Devices

Nanotechnology helps solve several unmet needs in the medical device industry. One example is the use of nanomaterials to produce antimicrobial coatings on medical devices. Another example is the use of nanocoatings on medical implants (e.g., stents) to add function, such as improving MRI. Without these coatings, the metal in the stent or other metal implants interferes with the image that is produced by the powerful MRI magnets. Drug-eluting stents represent yet another type of nanocoated medical device that has added functionality; we discuss them in more detail later.

The nanocrystalline silver technology (Silcryst) of Nucryst Pharmaceuticals is an example of using nanomaterials to coat medical devices in order to prevent bacterial infection. Smith & Nephew incorporated this technology into wound dressings sold under the trade name Acticoat. Silver ions in the coating act as the antimicrobial agent. These barrier dressings have been approved in the United States and in more than 30 countries worldwide. In 2004, Nucryst received $24.7 million in revenues from wound care products.

The ON-Q SilverSoaker catheters developed by I-Flow and AcryMed are coated with SilvaGard silver nanocrystals and were approved by the FDA in December 2005.

In the field of drug-eluting stents, Nanocopoeia announced in January 2006 that it had received $361,000 in grants from the US government to further develop and scale up its manufacturing process for coating medical devices with nanoparticle-based coatings of drugs and polymers. The company's ElectroNanoSpray technology produces drug particles in a size range of 2–200 nm, which may or may not prove to be an advantage over the polymer-encapsulated drug-eluting stents already on the market. These products include a sirolimus-eluting stent sold by Cordis under the trade name Cypher and a paclitaxel-eluting stent sold by Boston Scientific under the trade name Taxus. In the third quarter of 2005, Taxus sales were $601 million versus $656 million for Cypher in this very competitive and dynamic market.

Additional examples of nanotechnology in medical devices include its use in tooth and bone implants and, in the longer term, the use of nanotech to improve scaffolding matrices required for tissue-engineering products.

INVESTMENT CLIMATE

Not surprisingly, many nanotechnology companies have been seeking funding from private and public markets and from Big Pharma and Big Biotech. In recent years, there has been a lot of hype surrounding the new enabling technologies, such as systems biology, stem-cell biology, RNA interference, and nanotechnology. Although no one denies the ultimate potential of these technologies to do great things over time, private investors and Big Pharma alike have become selective in their investments. In public markets, investors are more sophisticated; they are interested in what a technology can do today and what products and revenues will be available in the near term.

For the most part, recent funding and investment activity has been very slow, a situation that has certainly had a dampening effect on the ongoing development efforts. Even so, many significant industry-related events have occurred during the past 18 months.

Launch of the Nanotech Stock Index

In 2004 and 2005, the investment community launched no fewer than six stock indices to track the nanotechnology sector (Table 22.3). On a positive note, the creation of these indices underscores the importance of emerging nanotechnologies to investors. On the downside, the new nanotech indices generally track with overall stock market performance, an occurrence that, in turn, mutes their relative significance for nanotech.

This tracking phenomenon has been attributed to two factors. The first is the broad range of nanotech companies included in the indices. Companies listed in an index are involved in nanotech, but they actually operate in disparate fields of electronics, material sciences, drugs, energy, and chemistry. The second factor is that several indices list large companies alongside smaller, emerging companies. Larger companies are engaged in multiple business interests, overshadowing the contribution of nanotech to their stock values. For instance, Hewlett-Packard,

Table 22.3 Nanotechnology Stock Indices

Nanotechnology Stock Index	*Exchange Symbol*	*Description*
Global Crown Capital Nanotechnology Index	To be listed soon	An index of 19 companies launched December 2005; describes itself as the first "pure play" nanotech that does not include large "blue chip" companies
Innovest Strategic Value Advisors Nanotech Index	Not traded	An index of 15 companies launched September 2005; companies in the index are selected from 200 public and 100 private companies
Lux Nanotech Index	AMEX-LUXNI	An index of 26 nanotechnology companies launched March 2004
Merrill Lynch Nanotech Index	AMEX-NNZ	An index of 27 nanotechnology companies launched April 2004, 9 of which are nanobiotech companies
Newbridge Nanotechnology Index	PSE-NNIX	An index of 24 companies launched June 2004
PowerShares Lux Nanotech EFT	AMEX-PXN	An ETF launched October 2005
Punk Ziegel Nanotech Index	Not traded	An index of 19 publicly traded companies launched March 2004

AMEX = American Stock Exchange; ETF = Exchange traded funds (index funds that trade like stocks); PSE = Pacific Stock Exchange

Note: Nanomedicine-related companies and venture capital firms that are listed in various indices include Altair Nanotechnologies, American Pharmaceuticals, Arrowhead Research, BASF, BioDelivery Sciences, Biosante Pharmaceuticals, Combimatrix, Elan, Flamel Technologies, Harris & Harris, Immunicon, Nanogen, Novavax, Orthovita, Pharmacopeia, pSivida, SkyePharma, Starpharma, Symyx Technologies, and Westaim

BASF, IBM, NEC, General Electric, General Motors, 3M, and EI DuPont de Nemours are included in the Lux Nanotech Index. These companies represent approximately 25% of the index and have large market capitalizations.

In December 2005, Global Crown Capital launched a new nanotech index it describes as the "first pure play nanotechnology index." Large blue-chip companies are not included in this index, which concentrates on companies that obtain a significant amount of their revenues from nanotech activities. Global Crown hopes this index will better track the success of the emerging nanotech sector.

In 2005, several nanotech indices performed worse than the NASDAQ or Standard & Poors (S&P) 500 markets. The Lux Nanotech Index, Merrill Lynch Nanotech Index, and Punk Ziegel Nanotech Index were all down for the year, at approximately 8%, 14%, and 13%, respectively. In comparison, NASDAQ was up approximately 3.3% for the year, and S&P 500 was up about 4.6%.

This performance reflects a rather lackluster investment environment for nanotech – in part because of general market conditions but also, in large part, because of the need for the industry to break through with additional products and revenues that will help drive up values.

Initial Public Offering Environment

In 2005, US markets continued to be unfavorable for initial public offerings (IPOs) in many industry sectors, including nanotechnology. Burrill and Company reported that only 17 biotech IPOs were completed, raising approximately $809 million. In 2004 and 2005 combined, nanotech companies completed only four IPOs (Table 22.4).

Nucryst Pharmaceuticals is one of the nanomedicine-related companies that went public. It registered its IPO in December 2005, at a price 23% below its anticipated range. Nucryst is developing nanocrystalline silver coatings for use in wound care. It is one of two major investments for Westaim, which still owned about 65% of Nucryst following its IPO.

The National Venture Capital Association, a trade association representing the US venture capital industry, forecasts that the IPO market will not rebound significantly in 2006.

Venture Capital Environment

Some companies, such as Nanosys, which pulled back an IPO in 2004 because of unfavorable market conditions, were able to obtain additional venture funding in 2005. Table 22.4 lists some nanotech investment

Table 22.4 Money Raised in the Nanotech Sector, 2004–5 (millions of US dollars)

Company/Exchange-Stock Symbol	*Date*	*Amount Raised*	*Comment*
Acrongenomics/OTCBB-AGNM	December 2005	4	Private placement
Advanced Nanotechnology/ASX-ANO	February 2005	9	IPO[a]
ImaRx Therapeutics/private	December 2005	15	Private placement
Immunicon/NASDAQ-IMMC	April 2004	48	IPO[b]
Lumera/NASDAQ-LMRA	July 2004	42	IPO
Nanogen/NASDAQ-NGEN	September 2005	20	Equity placement
NanoHorizons/private	December 2005	2.2	Round A funding
Nanosys/private	November 2005	40	Private placement[c]
Novavax/NASDAQ-NVAX	November 2005	18	Public offering[d]
Nucryst Pharmaceuticals/NASDAQ-NCST	December 2005	45	IPO[e]
pSividia/NASDAQ-PSDV	October 2005	15	Private placement
Starpharma/ASX-SPL	December 2005	11	Private placement

[a]Spin-out from a Western Australian university; the IPO values the eight-year-old company at $33 million

[b]The offering price dropped from $12 to $14 per share for 6 billion shares down to $9–11 per share. It then settled at $8 a share, the price of the final offering

[c]Withdrew its planned $100 million IPO on August 5, 2004, citing "adverse market conditions"

[d]Filed a $100 million self-registration statement on December 22, 2005

[e]Priced 4.5 million shares (1.27 million shares less than expected) at $10 per share, a 23% discount to its proposed $12–$14 range

ASX = Australian Stock Exchange; NASDAQ = National Association of Securities Dealers Automated Quotation; and OTCBB = Over-the-counter bulletin board

activity that occurred in 2004 and 2005. Although several investments were made, venture funding for nanotech was depressed relative to the huge investments made earlier in the decade.

Lux Research, a firm dedicated to nanotechnology research and analysis, estimates that from 1995 to 2005, venture capital firms made 258 investments in 143 nanotech start-ups. During this 10-year period, venture capital investments in nanotech reached a combined total of $2 billion. In 2004, total venture capital investment in all industries in the United States exceeded $21 billion, only $200 million of which was invested in nanotechnology.

In comparison, Burrill and Company reported that the US biotech industry raised a record $32 billion in 2005 alone: $17 billion from financings (public and private) and $15 billion from partnering activities. At the end of November 2005, the market cap of the biotech industry also hit an all-time high of $488 billion, surpassing its previous high of $475 billion in the summer of 2000. The market cap of the biotech giants, Amgen and Genentech, both hit the $100 billion mark for the first time in 2005.

For comparison, Table 22.5 lists the market caps of several companies involved in nanomedicine and nanodiagnostics. Most have market caps considerably less than $1 billion. Many of the nanotech companies have a small market cap (less than $200 million), reflecting their relative youth, the small number of products they have under development, their continuing search for Big Pharma and Big Biotech partners to help fund research and product development, and stagnant public markets.

The drug delivery companies (e.g., American Pharmaceutical Partners, SkyePharma, Flamel Technologies), which engage in several types of drug delivery technology, including nanotech, have much larger market caps in the range of $0.5 billion to more than $2 billion. These higher market caps underscore the fact that nanotech-enabled drug delivery is but one of the many choices available to deliver a drug and that drug delivery will be a very competitive market for small nanotech companies seeking to break into the sector.

An interesting trend in the venture capital industry is the creation of venture firms that specialize in nanotechnology and are publicly traded (Table 22.6). Harris & Harris Group and Westaim have market caps of $290 million and $334 million, respectively. Both firms are listed on most nanotech stock

Table 22.5 Market Capitalization of Select Nanomedicine-related Companies (millions of US dollars at year-end 2005)

Company/Exchange-Stock Symbol	*Market Capitalization*	*Comments*
American Pharmaceutical Partners/NASDAQ-APPX	2,799	Specializes in injectable drugs; Abraxis Oncology is a division focusing on cancer
Symyx Technologies/ NASDAQ-SMMX	924	Develops high-throughput robotics, software, and tools to optimize drug formulations
SkyePharma/NASDAQ-SKYE	558	Specializes in drug delivery with oral, injectable, topical, inhalation, and enhanced solubility technologies
Flamel Technologies/ NASDAQ-FLML	404	Specializes in controlled-release drug delivery, including nanoparticle formulations for the delivery of therapeutic proteins drugs
Novavax/NASDAQ-NVAX	195	Specializes in drug delivery using micellar nanoparticles
Orthovita/NASDAQ-VITA	186	Develops biomaterials for tissue engineering and restoration of the human skeleton
Nucryst Pharmaceuticals/ NASDAQ-NCST	165	Develops products to treat infection and inflammation based on nanocrystalline silver technology
Nanogen/NASDAQ-NGEN	154	Develops medical diagnostics, arrays, and chips; SynX, a subsidiary, creates point-of-care diagnostic tests
Altair Nanotechnologies/ NASDAQ-ALTI	124	Specializes in controlled release of drugs using ceramic nanomaterials
Biophan Technologies/ OTCBB-BIPH	119	Specializes in controlled drug delivery by bonding drugs to nanomagnetic materials that respond to externally applied magnetic fields
pSivida/NASDAQ-PSDV	117	Specializes in controlled drug delivery based on biodegradable silicon-based nanostructures
Immunicon/NASDAQ-IMMC	101	Develops magnetic nanoparticles used to isolate circulating tumor cells or circulating endothelial cells in order to detect disease
Acrongenomics/OTCBB-AGNM	79	Develops nanotechnology platforms to detect biomarkers useful for molecular diagnostics
Acacia Research-CombiMatrix/ NASDAQ-CBMX,	53	Develops custom arrays for molecular diagnostics including cancer diagnostics
Biodelivery Sciences International/ NASDAQ-BDSI	30	Specializes in drug delivery using nanocrystalline "cochleate" cylinder technology
Royal Bodycare/OTCBB-ROBE	15	Develops nutritional and skin care supplements based on nano-sized powder that combines with the supplements

NASDAQ = National Association of Securities Dealers Automated Quotation and OTCBB = Over-the-counter bulletin board

Table 22.6 Publicly Traded Venture Capital Firms Specializing in Nanotechnology (millions of US dollars at year-end 2005)

Firm/Exchange-Stock Symbol	*Market Capitalization*	*Comments*
Westaim/NASDAQ-WEDX	334	Two technology investments: Nucryst Pharmaceuticals (nanocrystalline silver technology) and iFire Technology (flat panel displays)
Harris & Harris Group/ NASDAQ-TINY	290	Has invested more than $41 million in nanotechnology since 2001, with approximately $16 million of this amount invested in 2005
Arrowhead Research/ NASDAQ-ARWR	87	Two drug delivery subsidiaries: Insert Therapeutics (cyclodextrin-containing polymer delivery) and Calando (nanostructure-based delivery for RNA interference)
Advance Nanotech/ OTCBB-AVNA	67	Currently funding 21 portfolio companies in nanoelectronics, biopharma, and nanomaterials

indices, illustrating their relative importance in the nanotech industry. Westaim (WEDX) did well during 2005, ending the year up approximately 40%. Harris & Harris stock (TINY) ended the year down about 13%.

In summary, investments in nanotech are depressed, in part because of flat public markets and lackluster IPO windows. The venture capital industry is under pressure to develop an exit strategy for nanotech investments it has made in past years. As Table 22.4 shows, several additional rounds of venture financing occurred late in 2005 to help keep various nanotech companies operating. The general consensus is that venture capital firms will look for merger and acquisition opportunities in the near future as a means to cash out of their early investments.

With investments from venture capital and public markets all down, federal government initiatives currently represent a major source of nanotech funding and will likely continue to do so well into 2006. The investment climate is further exacerbated by additional impediments to commercialization, including intellectual property uncertainties and potential health, safety, and environmental issues.

A CHALLENGING PATENT CLIMATE

The number of nanotech-based patent applications has soared during the past 10 years. Applicants have blanketed worldwide patent offices with thousands of claims for nanotech compositions and their uses. Biomedical claims include nanotech uses in drug delivery, molecular diagnostics, medical implants, biosensors, tissue regeneration, nanomedicines, and in vivo imaging. This deluge of patent applications has been likened to a "gold rush," as companies hurry to stake their claims.

Patent offices have had to wrestle with brand-new technologies and new jargon as they interpret prior art, compare similar inventions, and determine patentability. The result has been the issuance of some early, probably overly broad patent rights as well as a steady stream of overlapping patent rights for different types of nanoparticles.

The immediate challenge confronting Big Pharma and Big Biotech is to dissect this mosaic of intellectual property rights to determine which ones might stand the test of time and which ones will be necessary for freedom to operate in any particular nanotechnology application. As with most complicated patent situations, companies need to have a compelling reason to spend the time and money to do this analysis, which is not a trivial undertaking. It is far easier for the industry to sit back and take a "wait and see" approach.

This state of affairs has left many smaller nanotechnology companies starving for corporate alliances and funding because their patent strengths and weaknesses may not be readily obvious.

To help make nanotech patent examinations more consistent, patent offices worldwide have created expanded classification systems. In the US Patent and Trademark Office, class 977 is now devoted to nanotechnology. In May 2005, there were 1,348 patents in this class with 271 patents in technology center 1600, which covers biotechnology and organic chemistry. Class 977 includes a new list of 263 subclasses for use in categorizing nanotech inventions. In the World Intellectual Property Organization, the new nanotechnology class is IPC Class B82B, while in the Japanese Patent Office, nanotechnology falls under the new "Micro-Structural Technology; Nanotechnology" classification.

For the foreseeable future, the landscape for nanotechnology patents will remain complicated. In March 2005, Lux Research and Foley & Lardner attempted to decipher the maze of intertwining patent claims relating to several different types of nanoparticles. They identified approximately 3,818 US nanotech patents issued since 1985 and another 1,777 patent applications filed since 2001. The authors then analyzed 19,485 patent claims from 1,084 of the issued US patents. They concluded that patent claims in the areas of dendrimers and quantum dots are already quite crowded with little ability for companies to operate without becoming ensnared in another party's patent rights. The situation may be less crowded for carbon nanotubes, fullerenes, or nanowire patent claims, but each of these technologies still has at least one or more dominant patent holders. Some dominant patent rights holders include the following:

- *Nanotubes:* NEC Corp (Tokyo), Carbon Nanotechnologies, and Arrowhead Research.
- *Dendrimers:* Dendritic NanoTechnologies under agreement from Dow Chemical.
- *Fullerenes:* Mitsubishi.
- *Nanowires:* Nanosys.
- *Nanocrystals:* Nanosystems, the drug delivery business unit of Elan.
- *Quantum dots:* Nanosys, Quantum Dot, Evident Technologies, and Ultratech.

Some nanoparticles have quite complicated structures (see Figure 22.1), and the underlying patent situation is equally complicated.

It will take many years to unravel nanomedicine-related claims through patent proceedings and in the courts. Numerous challenges will undoubtedly be launched and appealed, including reexamination, interference or opposition proceedings, and infringement lawsuits. This process costs considerable amounts of money, time, and effort – important resources that leave smaller nanotech companies and universities at a disadvantage.

Considering the high costs of prosecuting and defending nanopatent rights worldwide, it may be more palatable for a pharma partner to obtain multiple nonexclusive licenses to nanotechnologies whose worth

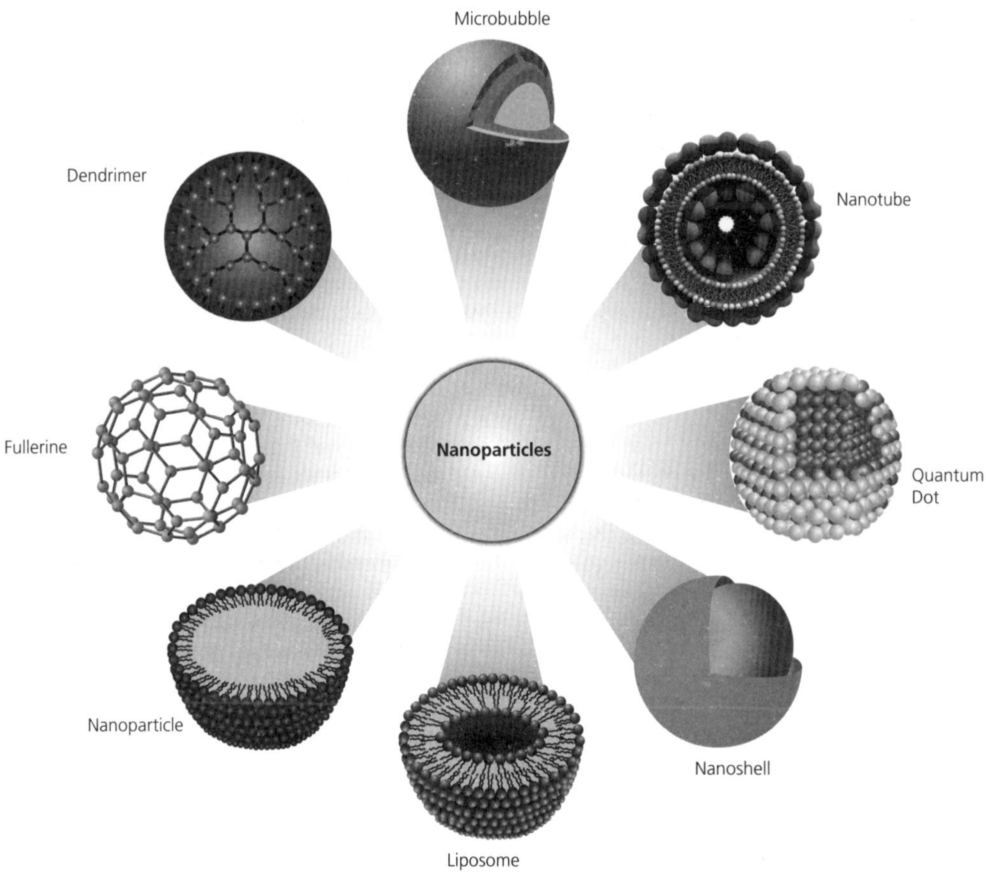

Figure 22.1 Different Types of Nanoparticles

and value have not yet been proved, as opposed to paying much more for carefully selected exclusive patent rights.

Nonexclusive access to specific patent rights solves a fundamental problem relating to the intrinsic value of nanotechnology. Is it a product in its own right, or is it an enabling technology or "platform technology" that helps create a product? Much like the genetic engineering, genomics, and bioinformatics technologies of the recent past, nanotechnology may well be an enabling technology that is best to license broadly for maximum success.

Genomics companies of the 1990s illustrate this concept. Many companies, such as Human Genome Sciences (HGS), were actively involved in cloning and sequencing every gene of the human genome. They amassed correspondingly large patent estates protecting these sequences and their uses. Yet, neither HGS nor its select partners could ever possibly have created the many therapeutic and diagnostic products relating to each of these genes. As a result, the patent term of the corresponding patents has slowly been eroding, reducing the value of this costly asset. The intrinsic value of nanotechnology patent rights may similarly be squandered if not managed and licensed effectively.

BUSINESS STRATEGIES

Cross-licensing

The general consensus is that the complicated patent situation for nanotech will be resolved, in part, by a series of cross-licensing activities as players come together to share patent protection under their collective patent rights. This activity has already begun in the nanotechnology industry as exemplified by the 2004 cross-licensing agreement between BioCrystal and Crystalplex. These companies had complementary nanocrystal technologies that should be useful in clinical diagnostics. They decided to work together rather than compete.

Another example is the January 2005 agreement between Starpharma, Dendritic NanoTechnologies, and Dow Chemical. Dow Chemical assigned its entire dendrimer patent estate (196 patents in 41 patent families) to Dendritic NanoTechnologies. Starpharma, an Australian company with a large equity holding in Dendritic, obtained rights under the three-way agreement to develop polyvalent, dendrimer-based pharmaceuticals. In October 2005, Starpharma received $20.3 million in funding from the National Institute of Allergy and Infectious Diseases (NIAID) to develop VivaGel, a dendrimer-based, vaginal microbiocide to prevent infection with HIV. In January 2006, the FDA designated VivaGel for fast-track status.

Mergers and Acquisitions

Another anticipated outcome of the challenging patent climate is that companies may pursue mergers and acquisitions as a way of consolidating their patent estates and acquiring missing pieces. For example, in October 2005, Invitrogen announced that it had acquired Quantum Dot as well as the BioPixels business unit of BioCrystal. The nanocrystal technologies of these companies will augment Invitrogen's biomolecular-labeling business.

Other recent mergers and acquisitions include the following:

- In January 2006, pSivida acquired Control Delivery Systems (CDS) for $104 million. This merger united the drug delivery technologies of both companies, including CDS's implantable and controlled-release technologies and pSivida's nanosilicon-based technology.
- In November 2005, American Pharmaceutical Partners announced that it would merge with its parent company, American Bioscience, to create a new company called Abraxis Bioscience. The combined company will have a market value of approximately $7 billion. Also in November, American Bioscience licensed rights to Abraxane to Taiho Pharmaceutical of Japan for more than $50 million in up-front and milestone payments, as well as royalty payments.
- The Molecular Profiling Institute acquired NanoBiomics, a molecular diagnostics company, in June 2005 for an undisclosed amount.

Molecular Profiling is a reference laboratory focusing on cancer.

- Solvay announced in March 2005 that it would acquire Fournier Pharma, a leader in fenofibrate products for treating high lipid levels. Fournier Pharma has an agreement with Abbott Laboratories covering fenofibrate-products (brand name Tricor) that will continue after the acquisition.
- Nanogen acquired Epoch Biosciences (point-of-care market) in December 2004 and SynX Pharma (real-time polymerase chain reaction [PCR] market) in April 2004 to consolidate its position in clinical diagnostics.

Research and Product Development Collaborations

The most widely anticipated trend will be the entry of Big Pharma and Big Biotech into collaborations with nanotech companies to fund research and product development. Although some alliances exist today, recent activity in this arena has been frustratingly slow. With so many different types of nanoparticles from which to choose and with so little known about their relative merits, pharma and biotech companies appear to be very selective about which companies they partner with and how much they spend. Collaborations that have taken place recently are as follows:

- In October 2005, pSivida and Cirrus Pharmaceuticals entered into an agreement to reformulate generic and proprietary drugs using pSivida's nanosilicon drug delivery technology.
- Debiopharm and NanoCarrier began a collaboration in April 2005 to develop a platinum anticancer compound based on NanoCarrier's micelle drug delivery system.
- Roche broadened its license agreement with Elan in January 2005 for nanocrystal technology to be used to formulate a number of different Roche drug candidates. In July 2005, MAP Pharmaceuticals also expanded its agreement with Elan to employ nanocrystal technology in multiple respiratory diseases, including asthma.
- In January 2005, Altair Nanotechnologies, a nanomaterials company, licensed its lanthanum-based phosphate-binding agent to Spectrum Pharmaceuticals. The product is a nonaluminum, noncalcium-based drug that binds excess phosphate in chronic kidney disease.
- NanoPass Technologies and GlaxoSmithKline entered into an agreement in February 2004 to use NanoPass's nanoneedle technology to deliver vaccines. Nanoneedles are being developed to effectively inject large molecules, such as the antigens used in vaccines, into the epidermis layer of skin.

On the downside, Bristol-Myers Squibb terminated its $165 million agreement with Flamel Technologies in September 2004. The agreement involved the development of a long-acting human insulin (Basulin) using Flamel's nanoparticle delivery system. In 2002, Novo Nordisk terminated a similar insulin development agreement with Flamel worth approximately $42 million.

SAFETY, NANOTOXICOLOGY, AND BIOETHICAL ISSUES

Nanotechnology is steadily fulfilling its potential to create new medicines and diagnostics to improve human health, yet, at the same time, very little is known about the possible risks to people or to the environment. Questions about health, safety, and environmental impact are all valid. More information is needed on the risk benefit of different types of nanoparticles, and a framework must be created to manage and communicate risk effectively. Several initiatives to address the issues of regulation, safety, and environmental risk are under way, as shown in Table 22.7.

In a June issue of the *Wall Street Journal*, Fred Krupp, president of Environmental Defense, and Chad Holliday, chairman and CEO of DuPont, stated, "An early and open examination of the potential risks of a new product or technology is not just good common sense – it's good business strategy." Indeed, the consequences of not managing risk benefits effectively can lead to significant problems for an industry, including damage in reputation and public trust.

Currently, the FDA believes that its existing policies and procedures are adequate to

Table 22.7 Select Recent Activities Relating to Issues on the Environment, Health, and Safety Impacts of Nanotechnology

In 2005, the Woodrow Wilson International Center for Scholars and the Pew Charitable Trusts launched the Project on Emerging Nanotechnologies to assess EH&S impacts.
The National Nanotechnology Initiative will fund $39 million to study EH&S issues.
The National Institutes of Health and National Institute of Environmental Health Sciences oversee the National Toxicology Program, which looks at hazards associated with nanomaterials, such as potential skin absorption of quantum dots of titanium dioxide and zinc oxides in sunscreen products.
The Nanotechnology Interest Group (NTIG), created by the FDA, coordinates the approval of nanotechnology products across its centers.
In December 2005, the US Environmental Protection Agency released a "Nanotechnology White Paper" for external review.
The UK government released a December 2005 report addressing sources of human exposure, minimizing workplace exposure, human toxicokinetics, and testing strategies, among other topics.
DuPont and Environmental Defense are working on a framework to address "the responsible development, production, use, and disposal" of nanomaterials.
Rice University's Center for Biological and Environmental Nanotechnology (CBEN) created a database that catalogs studies on the risks and benefits of nanoparticles.

EH&S = Environmental, health, and safety

cover nanotech applications, yet the door is open to new regulations as the field and/or need develops. The FDA approves products on a product-by-product basis, not on whether the product involves a particular type of technology, such as nanotechnology. Although the regulatory pathways for nanotechnology products remain to be fully determined, it seems likely that many nanoproducts will be combination products (e.g., drug-device, drug-biologic, device-biologic, drug-device-biologic). Consider, for example, a "drug delivery device." Several different FDA centers may be involved in approving such a device.

The Office of Combination Products is intended to streamline the approval process and thus eliminate overlaps and delayed approval times. A single marketing application should be sufficient to obtain the necessary clearance, approval, or licensure needed for most combination products. An assessment of the primary mode of action (PMOA) of a nanotech combination product will be used to determine which FDA center will act as the lead in the overall approval process.

The FDA is currently examining the effects of nanoparticles, such as quantum dots, on skin absorption. Some nanotech products are already on the market in sunscreens, for example. One concern is that the metallic atoms in the titanium dioxide or zinc oxide nanoparticles used in these products could enter the body to create free radicals. These free radicals have the potential to destroy cells in a fashion similar to the way in which alcohol and cigarette smoke destroy cells. Studies are under way to better understand these types of issues.

The Environmental Protection Agency (EPA) is especially interested in the potential impact of nanoparticles released into the environment. In December 2005, the agency released a "Nanotechnology White Paper" for external review and comment that addresses issues of risk assessment, controlling production and release of nanomaterials, and the best means to protect human health and safeguard the environment. Voluntary regulations are also under discussion. The EPA believes that the greatest risk to exposure from nanoparticles is in workplaces where these particles are manufactured and used.

Nanotechnology has recently been likened to the splitting of the atom – it holds tremendous potential for good but at the same time could lead to horrific, unintended consequences. Stakeholders in this industry – nanotech companies, government, academia, and the general public alike – must all commit the time and effort to better understand the potential risks and benefits of nanotech, to enact appropriate safeguards, and to communicate effectively with a worldwide audience.

OUTLOOK FOR NANOTECHNOLOGY IN MEDICINE

The outlook for nanotechnology in medicine remains positive. In the first 11 months of 2005, the FDA approved 70 new drug applications, three of which employed nanotechnology (paclitaxel-protein-bound particles [Abraxane], fenofibrate [Triglide], and megestrol acetate [Megace ES]). Many more nanomedicines are in the pipeline, and this field should develop rapidly over the next five years.

The marketplace for nanomedicines will be competitive, and nano-based products will have to battle for market share. For instance, in 2004, Abbott's fenofibrate product, Tricor, had sales of $779 million. In the past 16 months, the FDA has approved six more fenofibrates:

- *Reliant's Antara*, approved November 30, 2004.
- *SkyePharma's Triglide*, approved May 7, 2005.
- *Teva's generic*, approved May 13, 2005.
- *Ranbaxy's generic*, approved October 31, 2005.
- *Par Pharmaceuticals' generic*, approved December 29, 2005.
- *Cipher's Lipofen*, approved January 13, 2006.

These recent drug approvals will create a complex market, composed of competing generic and branded fenofibrates, including two formulations based on unique nanotechnologies (Triglide and Tricor).

The pharma industry is actively using nanotechnology in its strategies to extend the patent term, exclusivity, and market life of existing products. We expect this trend to continue for the foreseeable future. For instance, to protect its fenofibrate market, Abbott employed two market conversions of Tricor: first from capsules to tablets in 2001 and then to a nanoformulated product in November 2004. At the same time, Teva launched a paragraph IV challenge under the Hatch-Waxman Act in an attempt to bring a generic fenofibrate to market. As Abbott's strategies evolved, Teva filed two abbreviated new drug applications (ANDAs), resulting in two 30-month stays and a finding of noninfringement of some of Abbott's patent claims. In response to Abbott's second market conversion, Teva alleged that Abbott had violated antitrust laws in an attempt to continually thwart generic competition. Abbott responded that it had continuously and lawfully made improvements to its product.

Ultimately, the true value of nanomedicines will be that they are not simply a different way to formulate a product, but they are a better way. For example, nanoformulated fenofibrates may become dominant in the market not because they are different but because they can be taken without food or because they produce the same effect at a lower dosage – a clear improvement.

We project that nanotechnology will continue to steadily improve drugs and solve unmet needs in the pharma industry concerning solubility, bioavailability, and the better targeting of medicines to sites of disease. Nanoformulation companies such as Elan and companies such as Nanogen that are consolidating positions in diagnostic tests and instruments should become early leaders in this field.

REFERENCE

Hassan, M.H.A. Policy forum: Nanotechnology: Small things and big changes in the developing world. *Science*. 2005; 309: 65–6.

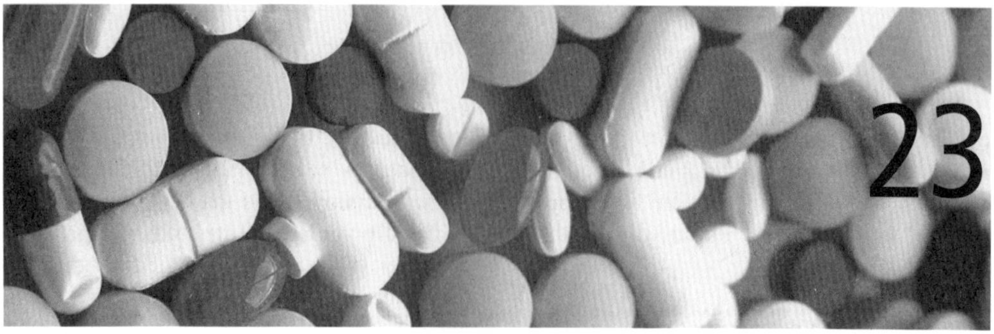

23

Clinical Proteomics: An Engine for *In vitro* Diagnostics Growth?

INTRODUCTION

Use of proteomics as a tool to discover new diagnostic markers is drawing significant interest, despite the emphasis on genomics. Whereas genomics provides a basis for the development of new nucleic-acid-based diagnostic tests, proteomics focuses on proteins for the development of new protein-based diagnostics and expression proteomics focuses on determining the quantitative differences in expression of proteins characteristic of normal and pathological states. A number of clinical proteomics business models exist, including tools companies, service companies, companies developing diagnostic assays based upon proprietary technology, and hybrid companies. We review companies pursuing these various models in this chapter, which also provides an explanation of the potential value of proteomics, a review of technology developments and challenges, and a report on ongoing research.

The expression of proteins is a complex, dynamic process influenced by cellular interactions, states of cellular differentiation, environmental conditions, and pathological states. Various national and international collaborations are addressing issues important to the use of proteomics to develop new diagnostic tests. Included in the international effort is the Plasma Proteome Project (PPP), which is focused on using serum or plasma as the source of proteins.

Two-dimensional polyacrylamide gel electrophoresis (2D-PAGE) and mass spectroscopy (MS) are two key technologies for proteomics. Surface-enhanced laser desorption/ionization (SELDI) MS is becoming widely used in diagnostic marker discovery as well as the development of new assay formats such as proteome patterns (groups of proteins that correlate with normal or disease states). Traditionally, in vitro diagnostics (IVDs) have relied upon individual, identified proteins as assays. In contrast, proteome pattern analysis relies upon the overall pattern, or footprint, made up of large numbers of unidentified proteins. Carefully controlled MS experiments, combined with sophisticated statistical techniques, enable the simultaneous determination of a large number of proteins that can be correlated with healthy or disease states. The individual proteins that characterize a proteome pattern do not have to be identified because it is the pattern of the expression of the proteins that is important, not the individual protein identities.

Although regulatory hurdles must be overcome, ultimately diagnostic tests will emerge that will quantify multiple proteins simultaneously, either identified on an individual basis or perhaps using proteome pattern analysis. Major IVD manufacturers will undoubtedly utilize new markers derived from proteomic studies, which will most likely come about through licensing arrangements.

THE VALUE OF PROTEOMICS IN DEFINING NEW DIAGNOSTIC AND THERAPEUTIC PROTEINS

Having determined the sequence of the human genome, attention has now turned to an even more complicated task: the elucidation of the human proteome. The human proteome is the protein complement of the genome – the set of proteins expressed by a cell or organ at a particular time and under specific conditions. Proteins ultimately carry out all the functions of the body. The sequence of the genes provides a template, defining the potentialities for protein expression, but it does not explain why different cells express different proteins, why different proteins are expressed in normal versus diseased tissue, and how the various proteins interact with one another in complicated biochemical and metabolic pathways. Proteomics is the discipline that attempts to answer these questions, and proteomics will provide exciting new opportunities for diagnostic and therapeutic intervention and consequent advances in healthcare.

Many challenges face proteomics researchers. The human genome sequence consists of 20,000–25,000 genes, and the number of proteins that can be produced from those genes is much greater. Messenger RNA (mRNA) molecules transcribed from the genes can be put together in different ways by alternative splicing. This alternative splicing can result in multiple amino acid sequences for the protein. As many as a half a million proteins may be expressed from the 20,000–25,000 human genes. In addition, proteins can be further modified by various posttranslational mechanisms, including proteolysis (chopping into smaller pieces), phosphorylation (adding phosphate groups), and glycosylation (adding carbohydrate molecules). These posttranslational modifications are functionally important. The phosphorylation state of proteins is known to produce altered function. Glycosylation is functionally important for incorporating proteins on the surface of cells and also for yielding proteins that will be secreted from cells. Proteolysis can produce multiple biologically active peptides from the same protein. Although genomic sequences are important for both diagnostics and therapeutics, proteins ultimately determine the various metabolic functions that yield a normal or pathological status of various physiological systems. Proteins are thus most useful as diagnostic markers and therapeutic targets.

The broadest definition of the field of proteomics encompasses the efforts to establish the identities, quantities, structures, and biochemical and cellular functions of all proteins in an organism, organ, or organelle and how these properties vary in space, time, and physiological state. The primary goal for proteomics is to determine the quantitative differences in the expression of different cell types and variations in these cell types, depending on their normal or pathological status. The expression and the modification of proteins is a dynamic process influenced by cellular interactions, state of differentiation, environmental conditions, and pathological states and is often referred to as expression proteomics. This aspect is most important to IVDs, focusing on differences between normal and disease states. The three-dimensional structure of proteins and the interactions of proteins are areas of proteomics that are of more interest to pharmaceutical and biotechnology companies because they help to define specific therapeutic targets for drug development.

The concept of biomarkers has been widely discussed, and the terms *biomarkers* and *diagnostic markers* have been used interchangeably. A biomarker is a molecule that indicates a change in the physiological state of an individual in relation to a health or disease state, or drug treatment. Biomarkers can be based on RNA or proteins. Biomarkers are not static – they change over time. Biomarkers have received much attention from the pharmaceutical industry because of their potential for facilitating drug discovery and development, particularly with regard to targeted therapeutics. The earliest efforts using biomarkers to guide drug discovery and development focus on biomarkers that predict the safety of the drug candidate. Proteins can be very useful as biomarkers for the discovery of new drugs and also to potentially combine the diagnostic tests for these biomarkers with targeted therapeutics (theranostics).

However, there are differences between biomarkers useful for drug discovery and diagnostic functions. Diagnostic markers are correlated with disease states. A diagnostic marker may also be a biomarker, but not all biomarkers meet the requirements of sensitivity and specificity for diagnostic markers and, thus, not all biomarkers useful to the pharmaceutical industry will necessarily prove useful for commercialization as a diagnostic marker. Researchers at Roche Diagnostics have provided a useful classification of diagnostic markers (Zolg and Langen, 2004). They have defined "disease specific proteins" (DSPs) as a protein or group of proteins whose type and concentration can vary and correlate with the disease state as compared with the healthy state. These diagnostic markers fall into four classifications: screening, prognostic, stratification, and efficacy markers:

- Screening markers can discriminate the healthy state from a beginning disease state, preferably before other symptoms have appeared. These markers would be used to test populations of people at regular intervals for the first appearance of a disease state. Early cancer detection markers would fall into this class.
- Prognostic markers can predict the likely course of a disease after a disease state is established.
- Stratification markers can predict the likely response to a drug before starting treatment. These markers can classify individuals as likely "responders" or "nonresponders."
- Efficacy markers can be used to monitor the efficacy of drug treatment once the responder status is established.

TECHNOLOGY OVERVIEW

Challenges

The challenges in elucidating the human proteome are significant:

- The differences between abundant proteins and rare proteins are 1,000-fold.
- Proteins are present in many different cellular organelles and structures including the cytoplasm, nucleus, microsomes, and nucleus.
- Proteins can undergo many different types of posttranslational modifications that may be important for differential function.
- Many different cell types express both common and specialized proteins.
- The expression of proteins within a cell is constantly in flux because of changes in environmental conditions, communications with other cells, stage of differentiation, and pathological conditions that may involve all of the above as well as the interaction of genetic factors.

Expression proteomics involves three basic tasks:

1. The proteins to be analyzed must be separated.
2. The separated proteins must be identified.
3. The proteins must be quantified to allow comparison between multiple states (e.g., healthy versus diseased).

Advances in analytical sciences – especially MS, separation sciences, and bioinformatics – have fueled the increased interest and progress in clinical proteomics.

Separation

The separation of proteins can be accomplished in several ways. Because of the large number of proteins to be separated, separation is performed on the basis of multiple properties. Proteins, composed of amino acids and modified by various posttranslational mechanisms, have an inherent electrical charge. Based on their amino acid composition, they have a characteristic size (molecular weight) and solubility (hydrophobicity). These properties are used to separate proteins in an orthogonal manner and thus provide resolution of as many different protein forms as possible.

Two-dimensional Polyacrylamide Gel Electrophoresis

Proteomics began with and continues to use two-dimensional polyacrylamide gel electrophoresis (2D PAGE). This technique, first described 30 years ago, separates proteins based on their isoelectric point (pI; the pH at which the positive and negative charges in a protein molecule cancel each other out) and their denatured subunit molecular weight. In the first step of 2D-PAGE, called isoelectric focusing (IEF; the first dimension), researchers load protein mixtures at one end of a polyacrylamide gel strip that contains a pH gradient. An electric field migration of charged molecules, known as ampholytes, is used to measure the solubilization of proteins and establish their separation in a pH gradient. These ampholytes can be obtained for narrow or broad pH ranges; consequently, they enable increased resolution over narrow pH ranges (for more detailed examination of specific proteins) and over a broad pH range (providing a more complete picture). Proteins composed of amino acids have a characteristic pH at which the protein bears no net charge and will thus remain stationary in an electric field. When isoelectric focusing (IEF) is complete, protein gels containing proteins separated on the basis of their inherent charge are rotated 90 degrees and placed at one edge of a slab of sodium dodecyl sulfate (SDS) polyacrylamide. An electric field is applied to the gel, and the proteins migrate toward the other end of the slab according to their molecular weight. Proteins are detected using radioactive labels or various types of protein stains. This process allows for an orthogonal separation based on pI (molecular charge) and denatured subunit molecular weight (Figure 23.1).

2D-PAGE also allows for the detection of multiple forms of the same protein that differ

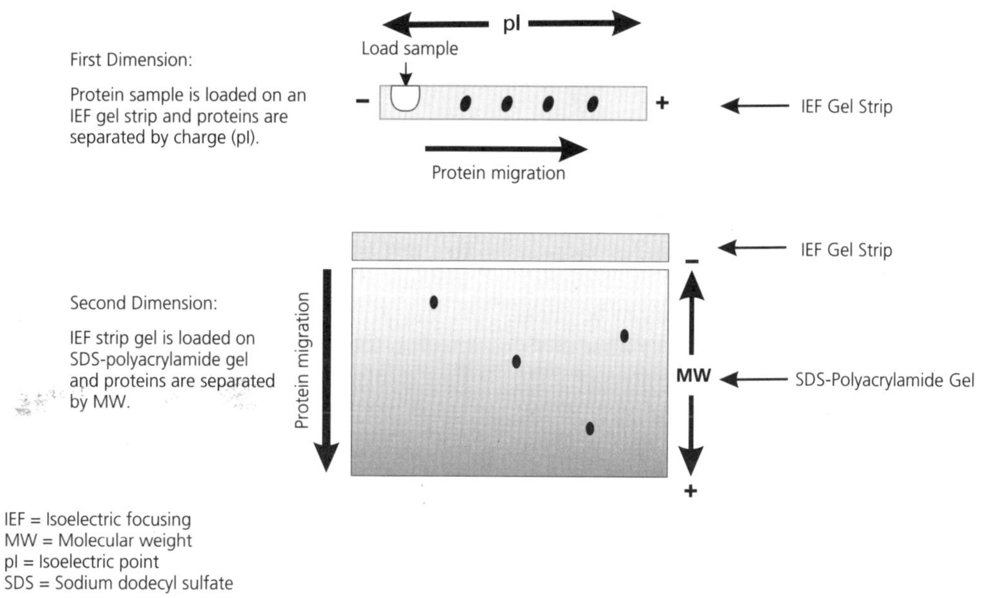

Figure 23.1 Two-dimensional Gel Electrophoresis

by charge because of posttranslational modifications. In addition, these gels often allow for the detection of products resulting from the cleavage of specific proteins. After proteins are separated by 2D-PAGE, proteins from the gels are excised and digested with proteases, and the peptides then identified by mass spectroscopy (MS), usually matrix-assisted laser desorption/ionization (MALDI) (discussed further on), and compared with databases of known peptides and the proteins from which they are derived.

2D-PAGE is still the most widely used means of separation for expression proteomics. Despite limitations, the technology provides a picture of the separated proteins from samples obtained under different conditions. The limitations associated with 2D-PAGE involve limits to the hydrophobicity, isoelectric point (pI), and molecular weight range of proteins resolvable using conventional two-dimensional gels. Conventional two-dimensional gels can separate on the order of a few thousand proteins during a single separation; however, incomplete separation of proteins on the gel can lead to overlapping spots and, subsequently, to problems with protein identification using the MALDI-MS peptide mass-mapping approach.

Multidimensional Protein Identification Technology

Rather than using 2D-PAGE for separation of the protein sample, multidimensional protein identification technology (MUDPIT) consists of a two-dimensional chromatography separation of proteolytic peptides directly coupled to electrospray mass spectrometry. Complex mixtures of peptides can be separated based upon each peptide's unique physical properties of charge and hydrophobicity. The first dimension is normally a strong cation exchange (SCX) column, as these columns have high loading capacities. The second dimension is reverse phase (RP) chromatography, which complements the SCX as it is efficient at removing salts and has the added advantage of being compatible with electrospray mass spectrometry.

Typically, a denatured protein complex is digested with trypsin. The acidified peptide mixture is loaded onto the SCX column. A discrete fraction of peptides is displaced from the SCX by a step elution and automatically transferred to the RP column. This fraction is eluted from the RP column using a slow reversed-phase solvent gradient, and a mass spectrometer analyzes the peptides. This iterative process elution (10–15 cycles) is repeated, allowing for the determination of the fragmentation patterns of peptides in the original peptide mixture.

Identification of Proteins/Peptides

Mass Spectroscopy

Advances in mass spectroscopy (MS) have fueled the rapid advances being made in clinical proteomics. These advances in MS and analytical tests are too complex to discuss here, but it is useful to understand some of the basic principles most relevant to clinical proteomics.

The instruments are made up of three primary components:

1. A source, which produces ions for analysis.
2. A mass analyzer, which identifies the ions based on their mass-to-charge ratios (*m*/*z*).
3. A detector, which quantifies the ions resolved by the analyzer.

Many different types of ion sources, analyzers, and detectors have been developed, and different components can be combined in a myriad of ways to create many different instrument types, but the basic principle is the same in each case: a spectrometer creates ion mixtures from a sample and then resolves them into their component ions based on their *m*/*z* values. Improvements now allow for gentler precision analysis of biomolecules that were too fragile to survive earlier instrumentation.

The three ionization methods most commonly used for analysis of peptides and proteins are MALDI, surface-enhanced laser desorption/ionization (SELDI), and electrospray ionization (ESI); these ionization sources are often coupled to time-of-flight (TOF) or quadrupole analyzers, or some combination of these analyzers. These ionization methods utilize soft ionization and allow the analysis of a wide variety of biomolecules in the picomole to femtomole concentration range.

MALDI and SELDI are similar in that each depends upon the spotting of a biological sample on a solid substrate and subsequent ionization by a high-energy source. MALDI samples are deposited on a solid substrate in a chemical matrix containing chemicals that absorb light at specific wavelengths, and the matrix and the sample are vaporized into a gas cloud. Protons are ejected from matrix molecules and transferred to nearby proteins and peptides, resulting in positive ions. Although the matrix molecules will absorb most of the energy from the photons, minimizing the amount of energy absorbed and damage incurred by the biomolecules, there is still some fragmentation of peptides and proteins. The ion gas cloud is subsequently accelerated into the mass analyzer electrostatically.

In contrast to MALDI, SELDI employs selective surfaces of a ProteinChip probe (Ciphergen Biosystems, Fremont, California) to capture some subset of proteins from a complex mixture in biological samples. The surfaces of the ProteinChip are coated with various chromatographic ligands that allow for different proteins of interest to be separated on the basis of cation/anion exchange, RP (for hydrophobic interactions), and metal affinity chromatography. After the sample is applied to the ProteinChip, the surface is washed to remove unbound proteins and impurities, and a photoactive matrix is then applied to the chip surface. This technique has been modified so that laser desorption can be carried out without the addition of a chemical matrix. The various coatings allow for the selection of different subsets of the protein sample. The technique is sensitive to the femtomole range.

ESI can observe larger biomolecules than SELDI or MALDI because the ionization is gentler. ESI does not require spotting of a sample on a solid substrate; instead, it creates an ion-gas cloud in the source directly from the sample solution. A stream of the aqueous sample is directed through an electrified needle held at a high voltage, producing a fine mist of highly charged droplets. These droplets, which contain the proteins and peptides of interest, are electrostatically driven through nitrogen gas, air, heat, solvents, or other drying agents to evaporate water and solvents from the surface. As the droplets decrease in size, the surface charges are deposited onto the peptides and proteins.

The MALDI and SELDI ionization approaches are often connected to TOF analyzers. TOF analyzers have a practical mass limit between 150,000 and 300,000 daltons (Da). ESI instruments have a mass limit of 70 kDa and are most commonly paired with quadrupole and other analyzers. TOF analyzers are more simply designed than other instruments and rely on calculations of mass from the time required for ions to travel to the detector from the ionization source. Quadrupole analyzers consist of four parallel metal rods to which is applied direct current (DC) and radiofrequency (RF) voltages. These voltages create selective magnetic fields that control which ions pass through to the detector.

In those cases where liquid separations are used online, such as the MUDPIT technique described previously, tandem mass spectrometry (MS/MS) can be used to induce fragmentation of individual tryptic peptides after online liquid phase separation. Tandem mass analyzer instruments are often made from combinations of analyzers. An example is Applied Biosystems' QSTAR, a hybrid system that joins two quadrupoles in tandem with a TOF analyzer. Low-energy collision-induced dissociation (CID) fragmentation of peptides provides useful information for identification related to the amino acid sequence. In high-throughput proteome analyses, this information becomes valuable for searching constrained protein databases with defined protease digest and peptide CID fragmentation rules. Some of the more advanced tandem mass analyzers, such as Applied Biosystems' QSTAR, can select particular tryptic peptide fragments to be subfragmented sequentially and then measured in the TOF analyzer, allowing for the direct determination of the peptide sequence.

Quantitation and Comparison of Proteins

To compare different states of cells, tissues, or body fluids such as plasma or serum, it is necessary to be able to compare and quantitate different samples. This comparison is difficult with any of the technologies described. 2D-PAGE allows for semiquantitative comparisons using various stains or isotopic labeling followed by autoradiography of dried gels, but it is still difficult to compare samples representing different states. The highest precision of quantitation is based, in part, on improved methods for chemical and metabolic stable isotope labeling of proteins and peptides. Protein labeling can be accomplished using one of the various chemical or metabolic samples, depending on the sample.

For noncellular body fluid samples such as plasma, serum, or urine, chemical methods are required. One of the most important chemical methods is the use of a chemical group or label made in two different isotopic forms. These two forms can be distinguished by MS on the basis of their small mass differences, but their incorporation into proteins or peptides does not affect their separation. These labels, termed *isotope-coded affinity tags* (ICAT) can be coupled to all the proteins in a sample that contain the amino acid cysteine (free sulphydryl groups). The ICAT labels come in pairs, with one labeled with the normal isotope and the other with a heavier isotope. For example, heavy isotope is added to a sample characteristic of the diseased state and the normal light isotope is used to label the corresponding sample characteristic of the normal state. The samples are then combined and, after the proteins are digested, the peptides are analyzed by MS. The mass spectrometer is then able to determine the relative abundance of each of the paired peptides, which differ only very slightly in mass.

In those cases where actively metabolizing tissue or cells are available, metabolic labeling can be used to differentially label the cells with heavy and light isotope-containing amino acids. Normal cells versus diseased cells can be compared using this methodology.

RECENT PROGRESS IN CLINICAL PROTEOMICS

Two current lines of research are particularly relevant to clinical diagnostics. The first area is the long-term and far-reaching PPP being conducted by an international consortium, the Human Proteome Organization (HUPO). The second area of research is the use of SELDI-MS-defined patterns of multiple unidentified proteins (proteome patterns) as a standalone diagnostic test.

The Plasma Proteome Project

HUPO's initial efforts are focused on the plasma proteome (proteins present in plasma and/or serum). The PPP is extremely important to clinical diagnostics because serum/plasma is the primary sampling source. Blood is a highly accessible human tissue, and it is straightforward to get samples and informed consent. Also, many stored specimen banks are available.

The challenges of elucidating the plasma proteome are formidable. Although only about 500 genes appear to generate blood components, researchers estimate that plasma contains as many as 40,000 forms of secreted proteins. The task is further complicated by 500,000 forms of tissue proteins and 10 million clonal forms of immunoglobulins. In addition to the difficulty of analyzing the large number of proteins present, the concentration of the most abundant proteins is more than 10 orders of magnitude greater than the concentrations of the least abundant proteins (Anderson and Anderson, 2002). Revealing the plasma proteome requires removal of the most abundant proteins so that the other less-abundant proteins may be observed. Albumin by itself makes up nearly 50% of the plasma proteome on a mass basis. Immunodepletion of the most abundant proteins is often used for minimizing the concentration of these abundant proteins prior to separation.

In the pilot phase of the PPP, scientists from 50 labs in 13 countries are using various technology platforms to analyze common reference specimens of serum and plasma. The plasma specimens have been assembled from populations in the United States, the United Kingdom, and China. The wide variety of technologies being used include 2D-PAGE, 3D liquid phase separation, MALDI-MS, tandem MS/MS, SELDI-MS, microarrays, and combinations of fractiona-tion and analytical techniques. The University of Michigan is performing extensive bioin-formatics analyses, and this information about the identity of peptides and proteins in the reference samples will be stored in a freely accessible master database at the European Bioinformatics Institute (EBI) in Cambridge, England. Gilbert S. Omenn of the University of Michigan, director of the PPP, believes that, because all the laboratories will be studying the same reference samples with different technologies, the answers to the following key questions should be answered:

- How can the confirmation rate of protein identifications be improved in the same speci-mens after analysis by different laboratories?
- Depending on the technology, which works better: serum or plasma?
- If plasma is the preferred sample source, what anticoagulant (e.g., ethylenediaminetetraacetic acid [EDTA], heparin, or citrate) should be used?
- How many freeze/thaw cycles can proteins in plasma tolerate?
- What are the advantages and disadvantages of each technology platform?
- Is it necessary to remove the most abundant proteins to detect the lower-abundance proteins?
- What database search engines are most reliable for identifying proteins?

Leigh Anderson is a pioneer in the analy-sis of the plasma proteome by 2D PAGE and is the head of the Plasma Proteome Institute (PPI) (www.plasmaproteome.org), a research institute that is also a major participant in the PPP. PPI, together with its collaborators, has compiled a database of identified proteins of the plasma proteome (Anderson et al., 2004). These proteins have been identified from several different laboratories using different technologies, as well as from previously published data in the scientific literature. The group has identified 1,175 nonredundant proteins. There are clear source-related differences associated with the different sources. These differences are significant because they illustrate the need to use multiple technologies in defining the plasma proteome, but also emphasize the necessity of using the same technologies for compar-ing the results. At the 15th meeting of Methods in Protein Structure Analysis, August 29 to September 2, 2004, Dr. Richard Smith of the Pacific Northwest National Lab (PNNL) reported that PNNL has identified nearly 4,000 nonredundant proteins of the plasma proteome. This group uses Fourier transform ion cyclotron resonance (FTICR), a unique, highly advanced form of MS. With this methodology, the group is able to detect approximately 10 zmol (about 6,000 molecules), far exceeding other existing technologies.

Anderson has suggested a new functional classification for the various proteins when cataloging the plasma proteome. This classi-fication provides an excellent overview of the potential of the plasma proteome for defining new diagnostic markers. Many of these protein classes – such as secreted proteins, tissue leakage products, and aberrant secretions – are likely to be informative regarding tissue status and are excellent candidates for diagnostic markers.

Use of SELDI-MS for Pattern Diagnostic Markers

SELDI-MS has received significant attention because of its versatility, ease of use, and relatively low cost. As noted previously, the versatility of the technology lies in its ability to utilize a variety of affinity surfaces to separate proteins by virtue of different molecular properties of the proteins. SELDI-MS is not a high-resolution separation as is the case for 2D-PAGE, MUDPIT, or other techniques, but it is very straightforward in applying serum or plasma, washing, and performing MS using a relatively simple MS system.

A number of studies by E.F. Petricoin (of the FDA's Center for Biologics Evaluation and Research [CBER]) and L.A. Liotta (of the National Cancer Institute's [NCI's] Center for Cancer Research) and their collaborators have used this technology for discovery of proteome patterns for the early detection of various types of cancer, most notably ovarian cancer. Proteome patterns do not represent individual identified proteins, but rather a subset of the proteome analyzed by SELDI-MS and interpreted by very sophisticated artificial intelligence algorithms. Most of the proteins and peptides that constitute the proteome pattern are uncharacterized and unidentified. The often-cited study published in the *Lancet* in 2002 (Petricoin et al., 2002) used MS to analyze blood proteins to provide a snapshot of thousands of proteins. A new computer-based artificial intelligence algorithm was used to identify diagnostic patterns. Serum samples from 50 women with known ovarian cancer and 50 women without disease-defined distinct proteomic patterns that distinguished cancerous from noncancerous samples. When these patterns were used to analyze an independent set of blinded samples, 50 from women with ovarian cancer and 66 from unaffected women or those with nonmalignant disorders, the investigators were able to correctly identify all 50 ovarian cancer cases, including all 18 stage I cases. Of the 66 nonmalignant cases, 63 were identified as not being cancer. This result yielded a sensitivity of 100% and a specificity of 95%. These results are impressive and have been further extended in additional studies with improved MS instrumentation and data interpretation.

Petricoin et al. focus their analysis on smaller peptides and proteins (<15,000 Da). They believe that these molecules represent naturally occurring small-molecular-weight biomolecules as well as cascades of enzymatically and proteolytically clipped biomarker fragments. These small enzymatically generated peptides may arise from the diseased tissue, or they may arise indirectly from the diseased tissue microenvironment. In any event, they argue that these patterns are characteristic of normal or diseased tissue and can thus be used for diagnosing disease. Critics have suggested that the patterns observed by Petricoin and Liotta may represent "epiphenomena" that accompany disease, but do not specifically define it.

These researchers have shown that low-molecular-weight proteins, metabolites, and peptides that define the proteomic pattern for early detection of ovarian cancer accumulate on larger, highly abundant carrier proteins in the blood such as albumin. They believe that low-molecular-weight peptide fragments, produced within the unique tissue microenvironment and generated as a consequence of the disease process, permeate the endothelial cell-wall barrier and trickle into the circulation. These fragments are immediately bound with circulating high-abundance carrier proteins, such as albumin, and protected from kidney clearance. The resultant amplification of the biomarker fragments enables these low-abundance entities to be seen by MS-based detection and profiling. This inclusion of albumin in the samples is in contrast to the methods of most other researchers, who selectively remove major plasma proteins such as albumin before analyzing plasma or serum so that they do not obscure the detection of lower-abundance proteins. As noted earlier, this obscuration is especially a problem for 2D-PAGE analysis.

Proteome patterns have also been applied in the diagnosis of breast, prostate, and bladder cancer. Based on results of these experiments, the concept of using proteome patterns rather than specifically identified proteins has received much positive attention in the scientific literature and in the popular press. Reproducing the results of different laboratories has been difficult because the process does not identify individual proteins but rather a large group of proteins. There is considerable skepticism about the feasibility of using complicated MS profiles rather than the identified proteins that have served as traditional diagnostic markers. Dr Eleftherios P. Diamandis of the University of Toronto has been the most outspoken skeptic, and there have been a series of point-counterpoint discussions in the scientific literature. Diamandis acknowledges that the results for ovarian cancer are impressive but suggests caution and that much more research must be done to validate the approach. Diamandis (2004) notes that the differences in proteome patterns observed and correlated with cancer versus noncancer may represent differences in (1) variability in sample collection, processing, and storage; (2) baseline characteristics of study subjects (e.g., sex, age, ethnicity, level of exercise, menopausal status, nutritional habits, drug use); (3) inappropriate statistical design; and (4) variations in mass spectrometer stability and protein chip performance. Diamandis suggests, and many others concur, that identification of key discriminatory proteins/peptides would facilitate the validation of the discrimination and could demonstrate unequivocally that proteome pattern technology is a viable diagnostic paradigm.

These issues will receive further debate and scrutiny because of the 2004 announcement that the OvaCheck test is being developed by Correlogic Systems (Bethesda, Maryland) in collaboration with LabCorp and Quest Diagnostics, the two major national reference laboratories.

On July 12, 2004, the Office of In Vitro Diagnostic Device Evaluation and Safety (OIVD) at the FDA informed Correlogic and the two reference labs that, although the OvaCheck test is proposed to be conducted by the reference laboratories, the FDA will require premarket approval for the software being used to determine the proteome patterns and final results. The FDA does not intend to regulate the activities of Correlogic's reference laboratory (CSIRL) or its laboratory partners, LabCorp and Quest, in the ongoing provision of the OvaCheck testing service. The FDA will not regulate these activities because the trials would be done under Clinical Laboratory Improvement Amendments (CLIA) of 1988 supervision of reference laboratories at LabCorp, Quest Diagnostics, and Correlogic. On July 14, Correlogic responded and indicated it would remove the installed software at Quest and LabCorp, which would then use their own equipment and related software to extract data from patient blood specimens. Quest and LabCorp would then send the data to Correlogic's CLIA-certified lab in Bethesda, Maryland, to be analyzed by Correlogic, which then would provide a written report to Quest and LabCorp. The FDA has not yet publicly responded.

The OvaCheck test employs three elements in common with the NCI/FDA Clinical Proteomics Program: the "hidden patterns" concept and process, the same mass spectrometer, and the same software (Proteome Quest), which builds the computational models. The OvaCheck test does, however, utilize a different chip; an electrospray (nESI) chip is used to introduce the serum into the mass spectrometer. The class of molecules analyzed by these two approaches, and thus the molecules that constitute the diagnostic patterns, would be expected to be different from those data previously published.

Not all of the work with SELDI is using proteome patterns. The technology is also being used to first profile serum samples and then identify specific protein biomarkers that distinguish samples from normal and disease states. This work is less controversial because it uses the SELDI technology as a discovery tool. Analytes could be detected using SELDI, but this detection would be of specific protein/peptides and not a very complex overall pattern.

PROTEOMICS BUSINESSES

Companies with significant interests in clinical proteomics have adopted a variety of business models, including tools companies, service companies, and assay companies. Tools companies provide the tools for clinical proteomics research and development.

These companies include manufacturers and vendors of equipment for 2D-PAGE and MS, as well as imaging software and robotic instruments for automating proteomics. Service companies offer complete packages of proteomic analysis for pharmaceutical, biotechnology, and (more rarely) diagnostic companies. Assay companies provide complete assays based upon the use of proteomic technology. In contrast to current IVD assays, these companies focus on the use of multiple diagnostic markers, most commonly in the form of proteome patterns.

Many companies, however, have business models that combine various aspects. Tools companies and service companies, of course, are always interested in a piece of the final product; if their proprietary technologies bring sufficient value to the users of their tools and services, they are sometimes able to negotiate financial participation in resulting products. This interest in the final product is especially true for diagnostic products that may result from services offered to pharmaceutical and biotechnology customers who themselves do not have a direct business interest in diagnostic products.

Service and Hybrid Companies

A number of service companies offer proteomic services. The proteomics service sector has been a difficult area to survive in, and as a result, a number of companies have gone out of business or significantly redirected their business models. Of those companies remaining in the proteomics service sector, a few have research contracts/collaborations that contain provisions for the proteomics service provider to receive milestone and royalty payments for their participation.

SurroMed

SurroMed (Menlo Park, California) combines proteomics, metabolomics (MS profiling of metabolites), and cell detection technology for biomarkers. The company reports that it has developed a panel of more than 100 validated immunoassays in various research areas. The company's cell detection technology, SurroScan cytometry, is a proprietary, micro-volume laser-scanning cytometry system that can analyze and profile hundreds of different cell populations and cell-surface markers in small volumes of whole blood and other biofluids. Information from all these analyses together with clinical data is accessible for data mining through SurroMed's integrated informatics suite. The company has research contracts/collaborations with a variety of companies including PPD Discovery, Biogen Idec, UC Davis MIND Institute, Eli Lilly, Intermune, Wyeth, Merck, Bruker Daltonics, Palo Alto Medical Foundation (PAMF), and Eunoe.

GeneProt

In 2000, a group of Swiss scientists who are pioneers in proteomics and protein databases founded GeneProt (formerly Geneva Proteomics) (Geneva, Switzerland). The company has an integrated set of capabilities spanning sample collection, protein separation and identification, bioinformatics, and chemical synthesis of specific proteins.

GeneProt's facility in Geneva is the world's first protein discovery and production site capable of handling very large sample volumes (up to 2,500 mL). This capability to process large amounts of plasma is critical to identifying low-abundance proteins.

GeneProt has collaborations and alliances with several companies including Novartis and Serono. The partnership with Novartis is for analyzing the protein profile (proteome) of three human diseased tissues or body fluids and their healthy counterparts. Novartis made a total equity investment of $43 million and became GeneProt's preferred pharmaceutical partner. The collaboration with Serono relates to a set of novel polypeptides and proteins discovered through data mining. These novel polypeptides and proteins will be synthesized chemically by GeneProt and will be tested by Serono, which under the agreement has an option to obtain an exclusive license to any of polypeptides and proteins supplied by GeneProt.

Proteome Systems

As is the case for GeneProt, Proteome Systems (Sydney, Australia) was founded by well-respected pioneers in proteomics research. The two halves of this business qualify it as a hybrid tools/assay business. Proteome Systems is organized into two distinct but complementary businesses: Technology and Discovery & Diagnostics. The Technology business is a tools business and includes bioinformatics, MS, robotic equipment, and an inkjet printer for transferring proteins from gels to membranes for immunoblotting.

The Discovery & Diagnostics business uses its expertise in proteomics for discovery and development together with DiagnostIQ, a rapid and quantitative test format for the commercialization of diagnostic markers. The Discovery business has both partnered and internal programs. The DiagnostIQ tests are point-of-care, lateral-flow membrane devices that can be quantitatively read in an accompanying bench-top reader. The test device can be read in less than five minutes and can assay multiple analytes at one time.

Using its rapid diagnostic test format, the company is working on programs for sports-drug monitoring, tuberculosis, cystic fibrosis, and an agricultural marker for testing wheat quality. The company has ongoing collaborations with a number of academic and clinical institutions worldwide including Sigma-Aldrich and Millipore. The agreement with Sigma-Aldrich is for the codevelopment and distribution of consumables for proteomics, and the collaboration with Millipore is for the development and distribution of consumables and kits for proteomics.

Ciphergen

Ciphergen (Fremont, California) is also a hybrid company with tools, services, and a newly formed diagnostic assay business. The company's base technology is SELDI-MS and all its equipment is associated with that technology. Its tools division, the Biosystems Division, develops, manufactures, and markets ProteinChip Systems. These products are turnkey systems consisting of various proprietary ProteinChip arrays for affinity separations of proteins, the SELDI-MS TOF spectrometer, and associated software for analysis. As noted previously, this system is being widely used by research laboratories engaged in biomarker discovery as well as the development of diagnostic assays based upon individual biomarkers or proteome patterns.

The company also provides contract services for clinical, research, and process proteomics applications though its Biomarker Discovery Center laboratories. Ciphergen's Diagnostics Division has undertaken its own discovery and development efforts as well as a number of external collaborations. These external collaborations involve a variety of potential licensing agreements ranging from Ciphergen receiving first rights for exclusive licenses to the company retaining all rights with royalties to be paid to collaborators. The company's external partners include Aaron Diamond AIDS Research (ADARC), The Johns Hopkins University School of Medicine, and the Eastern Virginia Medical School (EVMS)/Virginia Prostate Center (VPC).

Assay Companies

Correlogic Systems

Correlogic Systems (Bethesda, Maryland) is a clinical proteomics company focused on developing proteomic and genomics-based clinical diagnostic systems and new drug discovery. As noted previously, Correlogic has developed OvaCheck, a protein-pattern proteomics blood test for ovarian cancer, and is collaborating with the reference laboratories LabCorp and Quest Diagnostics to perform product testing. Correlogic's core technology is its proprietary pattern-recognition and pattern-discovery software, the Knowledge Discovery Engine (KDE). The software uses genetic or evolutionary algorithms to generate and compare a large number (15,000–20,000+) of candidate biomarkers through a very large number of iterations until it finds a set that optimally segments diseased from healthy samples. Another Correlogic product, Proteome Quest, is a specialized research application software derived from the KDE that is designed specifically for the creation of computational biological state models.

The company has research collaborations with the University of North Carolina for using MS-based proteome pattern detection for prostate cancer, with Johns Hopkins University for the study of inflammatory vascular disease, and with the Windber Research Institute and Walter Reed Army Medical Center Clinical Breast Cure Project for the application of Correlogic's technology to the early detection of breast cancer. In addition to its proteome pattern MS-based test for ovarian cancer, the company also is offering its KDE technology through software licensing and in-house bioinformatics analytical services. Correlogic also has a clinical laboratory that is regulated under the CLIA of 1988 and that is designated to perform high-complexity testing using the company's proteomics tools.

Matritech

Matritech (Newton, Massachusetts) develops proteomics-based diagnostic products specifically for the detection of cancer. The company's first two products, the NMP22 Test Kit and the NMP22 BladderChek Test, have been approved for both the monitoring and diagnosis of bladder cancer. The NMP22 products are based on Matritech's proprietary nuclear matrix protein (NMP) technology, exclusively licensed from the Massachusetts Institute of Technology, which correlates levels of NMPs in body fluids to the presence of cancer. BladderChek is a point-of-care, CLIA-waived test for screening and monitoring for bladder cancer.

The company is also using MS to discover new biomarkers for other types of cancer. It has discovered certain proteins (NMP66) in the blood of breast cancer patients that were generally not present in the blood of women without detectable breast malignancy. Matritech has also described NMPs found in blood that it claims are characteristic of individuals with known prostate malignancies (NMP48) or in the blood of individuals with colon cancer (NMP35). Matritech is investigating opportunities to utilize these various proteins in a proprietary laboratory procedure using MALDI-MS, which it would license to laboratories.

The company has also identified a NMP associated with cervical cancer and cervical precancerous conditions (NMP179) and has conducted preclinical studies investigating the utility of using this protein in conjunction with routine and follow-up cervical testing. Matritech granted an exclusive worldwide license for the use of NMP179 technology for automated, nonslide-based laboratory instruments to Sysmex, a leading manufacturer of automated laboratory instruments based in Kobe, Japan.

Predictive Diagnostics

Predictive Diagnostics (Vacaville, California), a wholly owned subsidiary of Large Scale Biology, is a diagnostics company that has developed a comprehensive technology platform for identifying biomarker fingerprints from a simple blood test for use in diagnosing diseases such as cancer. Biomarker Amplifier Filter (BAMF) technology is the company's proprietary pattern-recognition engine and discovery platform, whose primary purpose is to find disparate features in the blood. The BAMF technology suite comprises many highly specialized discovery and classification methodologies. Because of the medical risks and expense associated with invasive diagnostic biopsies for cancer detection, a serum test that could distinguish patients with benign disease from those with malignant disease would be of great clinical value. Analytical MS combined with pattern recognition has been shown to detect unique fingerprints for biologic states. Using BAMF technology, Predictive Diagnostics analyzes high-resolution MS data to generate discriminatory proteomic profiles in human blood. Based on the publicly available datasets from the NCI/FDA Clinical Proteomics Program described previously, the BAMF technology has been used in research studies to diagnose ovarian cancer. The company has also studied several other cancers, including lung, breast, prostate, and pancreatic. Predictive Diagnostics has also used its BAMF technology to perform research studies for the diagnosis of multiple sclerosis. The company has an exclusive comarketing agreement with PerkinElmer for the use of its BAMF technology with PerkinElmer's high-sensitivity MS instruments.

Power3 Medical Products

Power3 Medical Products (The Woodlands, Texas) is also developing assays based on proteome patterns, but rather than using SELDI-MS, it uses 2D-PAGE and MS identification to identify the patterns, which it calls "footprints." The company is developing a breast cancer test (Breast Cancer NAFTest) based on 2D-PAGE patterns of nipple aspirate fluid. The collection of the nipple aspirate fluid is a noninvasive procedure utilizing a modified breast pump to obtain a drop of fluid from the nipple. The aspirate is analyzed to identify the specific breast cancer protein footprints. The test is being developed in collaboration with the University of Texas M.D. Anderson Cancer Center. The company is also developing a test that it claims can detect and distinguish various neurodegenerative diseases, such as Alzheimer's, Parkinson's, and amyotrophic lateral sclerosis (ALS).

Tools Companies

Although tools companies generate significant proteomics sales, they are of minimal importance in understanding how clinical proteomics relates to the IVD industry. Therefore, we do not provide a detailed description of these tools companies. Table 23.1 shows many of the major tool suppliers.

Table 23.1 Proteomic Tool Suppliers

Company	*Tools*			
	2D-PAGE	*LC and MS*	*Software*	*Other*
Agilent	—	LC and MS (separate and combined)	—	—
Amersham	Gels, IEF, SDS systems	—	Image analysis	Spot picker
Applied Biosystems	—	Wide variety of MS	—	Protein sequencer, ICAT reagents
Biometra	IEF and SDS systems	—	—	—
Bio-Rad	Gels, IEF, and SDS systems	—	Image analysis	Spot picker
Bruker Daltonics	—	Wide variety of MS	—	—
Cambrex	Gels	—	—	—
C.B.S. Scientific	IEF and SDS systems	—	—	—
Compugen	—	—	Image analysis	—
Decodon	—	—	Image analysis	—
Geneva Bioinformatics	—	—	Image analysis	—
Genomic Solutions	Gels, IEF, and SDS systems	—	Image analysis	Spot picker robot
Invitrogen	Gels	—	—	—
Jule Biotechnologies	SDS gels and systems	—	—	—
Nonlinear Dynamics	—	—	Image analysis	—
R. Shadel	IEF system	—	—	—
Scimagix	—	—	Image analysis	—
Sigma	Gel systems	—	—	Sample prep kits
Stratagene	SDS gels and system	—	—	—
Thermo Electron	—	MS and LC	—	—
Waters	—	LC and MS	—	—
Wita	SDS system	—	—	—
Zaxis	SDS gels, IEF, and SDS systems	—	—	—

ICAT = Isotope-coded affinity tag; IEF = Isoelectric focusing; LC = Liquid chromatography; MS = Mass spectroscopy; PAGE = Polyacrylamide gel electrophoresis; SDS = Sodium dodecyl sulfate

Start-up and Emerging Clinical Proteomics Companies

Similar to any other area of biotechnology, the landscape of clinical proteomics is always changing, with some companies exiting and new companies emerging. In this section, we describe select new and emerging companies.

ProteinLogic

ProteinLogic (Cambridge, United Kingdom) has developed a multianalyte testing technology that measures 200–300 proteins in bodily fluids, providing a pattern or "fingerprint" that the company says can reflect a variety of pathological states. The technology is based on monoclonal antibodies and, although not described, is probably a protein chip of some type. The company expects to produce a prototype diagnostic kit within the next 12–18 months, and it will initially market a blood test for appendicitis – an indication for which the company believes 20% of operations are unnecessary.

SynX Pharma

SynX Pharma's research focuses on diagnosing a disease in its earliest stages, monitoring disease progression and treatment effectiveness, and significantly shortening the drug discovery and development process. In April 2004, the company became a wholly owned subsidiary of Nanogen (San Diego, California), a microfluidics-based lab-on-a-chip development company. SynX Pharma (Toronto, Canada) uses its Proteomics Discovery Platform (PDP) to discover new biomarkers for point-of-care and rapid format assays. Nanogen hopes that SynX Pharma's clinical proteomics program will be synergistic with its microfluidics-based platform technology, allowing for microfluidics-based diagnostic devices.

The first products to emerge from SynX Pharma's PDP include point-of-care diagnostic tests for congestive heart failure, stroke, traumatic brain injury, Alzheimer's disease, and insulin resistance. Some of these tests are marketed in Canada and Europe. The company had a research agreement with Ortho Clinical Diagnostics (Johnson & Johnson) for an Alzheimer's test, but this agreement has now been terminated. SynX Pharma has current strategic partnerships with genOway, University of Ottawa Heart Institute Research Corporation, National Research Council of Canada, and University of Liege in Belgium.

Caprion Pharmaceuticals

Caprion (Montreal, Canada) has developed a proprietary platform technology, CellCarta, that incorporates quantitative MS (without the need for peptide labeling), subcellular fractionation, and advanced bioinformatic tools that employ robust nonlinear peptide alignments. One of the components of its CellCarta technology, Constellation Mapping, identifies and locates individual peptides within highly complex samples by using each peptide's signature and its proximity to neighboring peptides. The company claims to be able to do quantitative comparison of samples without having to resort to any of the isotope-labeling technologies described earlier. The company has drug and/or biomarker discovery programs with Wyeth, Abbott, AstraZeneca, and Idec Pharmaceuticals (now Biogen Idec).

Europroteome

Europroteome (Hennigsdorf/Berlin, Germany) combines a proteomics research laboratory, a bioinformatics program, and an extremely broad access to clinical samples and expertise through the Clinical Cancer Network (CCN), which it founded and now operates. The network consists of experts from approximately 20 European institutions. The company's goals include the discovery and development of novel cancer molecular diagnostics suitable for screening and early disease detection, monitoring, and prognostics, including both single and combination markers. Europroteome has discovery programs in colorectal, stomach, lung, and pancreatic cancer. The company also has an exclusive partnership with Abbott Diagnostics for breast cancer markers. In this partnership, Europroteome uses its advanced proteomic and bioinformatic technologies to analyze serum samples from women with breast cancer. Data will be aligned with a panel of cancer markers from Abbott, and markers or combinations of markers will be selected for further development and integration into Abbott's instrument platforms.

OUTLOOK FOR CLINICAL DIAGNOSTICS

As noted previously, few new diagnostic markers have been commercialized in the past 10 years. This rarity is due in large part to the elimination, or severe reduction, of discovery research at most of the IVD manufacturers. The extreme price pressure that the industry has endured in recent years has not allowed for the levels of investment seen in earlier eras. R&D efforts of the major IVD companies are now focused on cost reduction for its customers, the clinical laboratories, through laboratory automation – particularly workstation consolidation – and expansion of the test menu of already commercialized analytes on these consolidated workstations. The prevailing paradigm of many IVD manufacturers is to license new, validated markers from academic sources and smaller specialty diagnostic or biotechnology companies. Thus far, this strategy has produced few commercialized markers, although it could be argued that clinical proteomics has not yet produced any candidates, and that this model will work once candidate markers begin to appear.

All the major IVD companies have publicly embraced the long-term potential of proteomics. However, few companies have actually made investments in the technology. Among the major IVD players, Roche Diagnostics has been the most forward-looking in terms of collaborations, both in its internal efforts and externally with other groups. Roche's success in molecular diagnostics, in large part owing to its proprietary position in polymerase chain reaction (PCR), has shown the value of and contributed financially to promoting genomics and proteomics efforts. In 2003, the company indicated that it spent 25–30% of its $550 million annual R&D budget on discovering new biomarkers via genomics and proteomics. Roche Diagnostics has initiated a program within its Integrated Cancer Care Unit (ICCU) to identify new diagnostic markers or marker profiles with a focus on developing screening tests for early cancer detection. Abbott Diagnostics and Europroteome have the previously described proteomics program for breast cancer.

Smaller diagnostic and biotechnology companies will continue to drive the discovery phase for new diagnostic markers. The discovery phase for biomarkers that can be used as diagnostic markers is well under way; there are, however, multiple steps between the discovery of a diagnostic marker and its commercialization. Commercialization of a newly discovered potential marker requires early development, validation, and clinical trials. These efforts generally require investment by the major IVD manufacturers, because it is still extremely difficult for small diagnostics and biotechnology companies without competitively distinct platform technology to raise the necessary capital. These agreements would have to pass rigorous financial and market screens before the IVD manufacturers would invest significant funds to codevelop potential markers.

Cancer will continue to be a very attractive area for the discovery and development of new diagnostic tests. New tests that provide early detection so as to guide therapeutic intervention and significantly increase overall survival are urgently needed. This need is the driving force for the Early Detection Research Network (EDRN) of the NCI. Ovarian cancer and prostate cancer are also the focus of many clinical proteomics programs. With the increasing skepticism regarding the clinical utility of PSA, it seems likely that even more emphasis will be placed on more reliable diagnosis of prostate cancer to distinguish more benign states from truly life-threatening disease. Cardiovascular disease, with an emphasis on congestive heart failure, is also being studied using proteomics and continues to be increasingly relevant to an aging population.

The progress of the Plasma Proteome Project of the Human Proteome Organization is extremely important to the IVD industry. Its progress in standardizing sample preparation and storage, provision of universal standards, and cataloging the various proteins that constitute the plasma proteome is a key first step in accelerating progress in clinical proteomics. The IVD industry should publicly support, monitor, and participate in this effort.

A paradigm shift will occur in diagnostics toward multiplex testing for certain disease states such as cancer. It is very unlikely that single markers will describe the biological and pathological processes that underlie these complex diseases. It can be argued that a complete understanding of these processes is not necessary to provide useful diagnostic tools, but some understanding will be required. Molecular diagnostics is already beginning to deal with the complexities of multiplex testing as developers negotiate with the FDA about DNA-based microarrays. Roche Diagnostics and the FDA have talked about the requirements for manufacturing and performance controls as well as the validation of the algorithms and associated software for detecting multiple analytes versus the usual single analyte. Correlogic is beginning a similar dialogue with the FDA concerning its OvaCheck protein-based assay.

There are many challenges to translating proteomics discovery research into commercial diagnostic tests. Because of the expense, it is difficult to validate tests that rely on high-cost equipment and that are very labor intensive to perform. Validation also requires access to large, well-organized sample sets. Prospective tests must address significant healthcare areas for which some preventive or therapeutic intervention is possible. The intellectual property issues for individual markers, as well as proteome-pattern approaches, will most likely be complicated because multiple licenses are required for testing.

Despite the challenges, the long-term potential for new diagnostic markers derived from proteomics is exciting. Rapid evolution of technology, especially in MS, is providing increasing amounts of information on proteins present in the plasma proteome. An open-source database of these proteins is being developed. The potential for multiplex testing and testing of patients over time is likely to increase the availability of useful diagnostic information and enable more-informed healthcare decisions. The commercialization of proteomics-based diagnostics will not be easy, or quick, but in the long term, this approach will significantly improve the ability to diagnose and monitor disease.

REFERENCES

Anderson, N.L. and Anderson, N.G. The human plasma proteome: history, character, and diagnostic prospects. *Molecular and Cellular Proteomics.* 2002; 111: 845–67.

Anderson, L. et al. The human plasma proteome: a nonredundant list developed by combination of four separate sources. *Molecular and Cellular Proteomics.* 2004; 3: 311–26.

Diamandis, E.P. Analysis of serum proteomic patterns for early cancer diagnosis: drawing attention to potential problems. *Journal of National Cancer Institute.* 2004; 96: 353–6.

Petricoin, E.F. et al. Use of proteomic patterns in serum to identify ovarian cancer. *Lancet.* 2002; 359: 572–7.

Zolg, J.W. and Langen, H. How industry is approaching the search for new diagnostic and biomarkers. *Molecular and Cellular Proteomics.* 2004; 3(4): 345–54.

PART III

Therapeutics

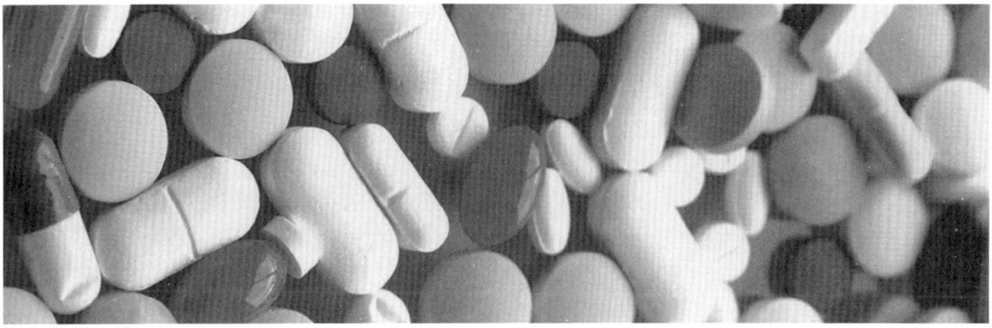

SECTION A

Oncology

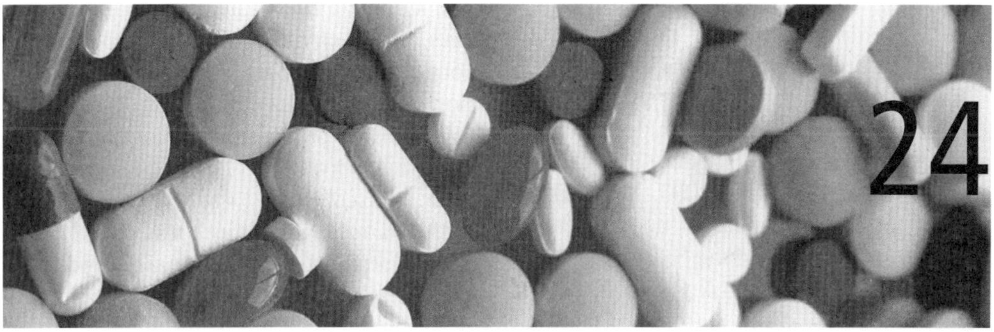

24

Novel Strategies in Oncology Clinical Trials: The Use of Biological and Imaging Biomarkers

IMPROVING CANCER THERAPIES: GOING BEYOND SURVIVAL

The gold standard for evaluating an oncology drug candidate's effectiveness is survival. However, the emergence of biotherapeutics for use in oncology has shifted attention to intermediate indicators of progress in patient-treatment evaluations. By evaluating immunological responses to biotherapeutics, insight may be gained into potential therapeutic improvements to optimize dosage, delivery, and combinations with other therapeutics. Evaluation of the immune response requires quantifying the biological changes, or creating "biomarkers," that can be related to clinical outcomes. As we discuss, both biological biomarkers and imaging biomarkers are emerging to fill this role.

The development and application of these biomarkers for use in evaluating oncology biotherapeutics and other drugs has the potential to simplify the arduous drug development pathway. Potential applications of biomarkers include a role in the decision whether to continue development of particular products and in the selection of appropriate patients for therapy, as well as the clinical monitoring of progress during and following the treatment. Considerable cost savings can be realized during clinical trials by preselecting patients who exhibit the genetic patterns that correlate with responsiveness to treatment. Experts are optimistic that biomarkers can contribute to improvements in oncology therapeutics. To this end, the National Cancer Institute (NCI) announced in November 2004 that it had earmarked $9.8 million in funding for 17 laboratories that are pursuing cancer biomarkers.

The Food and Drug Administration (FDA) is also committed to the development and application of biomarkers for use in oncology clinical trials. In early 2003, the FDA's Center for Drug Evaluation and Research (CDER), in concert with the NCI, formed the Interagency Oncology Task Force (IOTF) to achieve the FDA's stated objective of increasing availability and use of safe and effective treatments for cancer as well as the NCI's stated challenge goal of eliminating suffering and death from cancer by 2015. The IOTF will leverage the expertise and capabilities of both agencies to streamline and accelerate the development of diagnostic, preventive, and therapeutic interventions for cancer. Within its plan, the IOTF has objectives including the development of biomarkers of clinical benefit (including the use of biological and imaging biomarkers) in oncology drug development and the collaborative development of the scientific data needed to establish improved surrogate end points for cancer clinical trials.

To accomplish the goal of improving the development process, both biological and imaging biomarkers are being incorporated into clinical trials. This chapter provides a definition of biomarkers and describes how they are developed. In particular, we focus on how biomarkers have been used in clinical trials to date. We discuss some of the challenges in the development and use of assay-based biomarkers and examine how biomarkers may impact oncology clinical development strategies, particularly as the number of targeted therapeutics in development continues to rise. Finally, we detail the regulatory response to the use of biomarkers and provide insight into the future of oncology clinical development.

BIOMARKERS DEFINED

According to the Biomarkers Definitions Working Group, established by the National Institutes of Health (NIH) to study biomarkers and surrogate end points, a biomarker measures a characteristic using objective criteria for its evaluation and use as an indicator of normal biological processes, pathogenic processes, or pharmacological responses to a therapeutic intervention The biomarker can then be used either to supplement the data gathered through clinical trials or, if it is determined that it can accurately predict the benefit of a drug, as a surrogate for a clinical end point, which measures how a patient feels, functions, or survives.

Biomarkers are based on the pathophysiology of cancer and fall into one of four categories: biochemical, anatomical or morphological, histological, or a biomarker that measures symptoms or other clinical responses. Each type of biomarker provides data about the treatment through a different measure:

- An in vivo biochemical marker might measure CD4+ levels, for example.
- An anatomical or morphological biomarker can measure (using magnetic resonance imaging [MRI], computed tomography [CT] scans, or positron emission tomography [PET] scans) the tumor size prior to, during, and following treatment.
- Histological biomarkers involve obtaining data from biopsy tissue.
- Clinical biomarkers of symptoms and other signs include markers such as blood pressure, genetic status, and pain relief.

In most cases, a biomarker should satisfy the following two criteria:

1. The biomarker must be associated with the biological mechanisms of a disease or its treatment.
2. A statistical correlation must exist between the biomarker and the clinical outcomes.

By satisfying these two critical criteria, a biomarker can accurately represent the molecular action or a biological effect of a drug. For a biomarker to be useful in treatment decisions, a rationale or hypothesis of why the biomarker observations accurately reflect or predict these changes must be developed, even when the precise pathways of the drug action remain unknown.

DEVELOPING AND EVALUATING NEW BIOMARKERS

Most oncology product portfolios incorporate drugs and drug candidates that address the following six acquired capabilities of cancer cells (Hanahan and Weinberg, 2000):

1. A self-sufficiency with respect to growth signals.
2. Antigrowth or insensitivity to inhibitory growth signals.
3. The ability to evade apoptosis (programmed cell death).
4. An unlimited ability to replicate.
5. Continual angiogenesis.
6. The capabilities of tissue invasion and metastasis.

Drug candidates block these functions by disrupting the signal pathways associated with the capabilities, resulting in the inability of the tumor to survive. Each pathway also has the potential for biomarker identification. For example, biomarkers have been identified for several tyrosine kinase receptors, including epithelial growth factor receptor (EGFR) related to colon cancer, human epidermal growth factor receptor 2 (Her-2) related to breast cancer, and c-Kit related to gastrointestinal stromal tumors (GISTs). Each of these disease pathways is switched off by monoclonal antibodies (MAbs) that target these receptors (cetuximab, trastuzumab, and imatinib, respectively).

Biomarker development is progressive and iterative. To identify biomarkers, a subset of samples is used to identify the measurable biological changes that occur during the drug treatment and these changes are correlated to the clinical outcomes. This process is initiated during the preclinical phases when the identification of biomarkers begins in the model system used to evaluate the drug candidate. The process is repeated and refined during the course of early clinical studies in humans.

The determination of the biomarker's utility is made based on its statistical correlation with clinical events and whether it can be used to monitor, diagnose, or predict the outcome of disease progression and/or treatment. Evaluating the correlation between the biomarker and the drug's biological mechanism of action or progression of disease is crucial to determining the marker's usefulness. Once a biomarker is identified, an assay must be developed that will accurately measure it.

Confirming the relevance, utility, and robustness of a biomarker will increase the likelihood that it will be used. The NCI's Early Detection Research Network (EDRN) has developed a process for biomarker validation. The process involves a series of steps and bears a resemblance to the clinical trial phases that are used in the drug-approval process. To ensure that the biomarker has clinical relevance and utility, the process will involves a more stringent approach than is often seen in drug discovery and will ensure that the biomarker is robust by testing it in multiple laboratories. These laboratories will be required to use identical methods and carefully calibrate the instruments used in the validation process.

In the following sections, we discuss the development of two types of oncology biomarkers: tumor marker assays and imaging biomarkers.

Tumor Marker Assays

Tumor markers are substances that, in the presence of malignant tumors, can be found in increased concentration in tumor tissues and/or body fluids. They are either formed by a tumor cell and found on its surface or formed by the body as a reaction to the presence of a tumor. Tumor marker assays are laboratory tests that measure changes in the level of these substances. They can be used for diagnosing, determining a patient's prognosis, and monitoring the progression of malignant tumors as well as the effectiveness of treatment.

Tumors are generally clonal – that is, they develop from a single cell. This cell acquires a series of genetic mutations or epigenetic changes that influence cellular pathways and processes, including signal transmission and DNA repair. These genetic or epigenetic changes that interfere with certain cellular processes are also called pathway events and include changes in the base sequence of DNA and methylation (modification of a molecule by the addition of a methyl group) of DNA bases in the promoter regions of the genes. The occurrence of a pathway event in a normal cell can confer a growth advantage on the resulting cell clone. After expansion of the clone, another pathway event occurs in another of the clone's cells, once again conferring a growth advantage; this process can continue indefinitely. This model of tumor development via a series of pathway events in a specific sequence is known as the multistage model of carcinogenesis. According to this model, a tumor goes through a series of stages before becoming manifestly malignant, and transition from each stage to the next is associated with a specific new pathway event. Whereas promoter methylation generally inactivates cellular processes, mutations may, depending on their type, either activate or inactivate cellular processes.

Imaging Biomarkers

Imaging biomarkers are characteristics associated with a disease – tumor size, bone marrow density, the presence of metastases – that are measured using imaging methods such as X-rays, MRI, or molecular imaging. These markers all have the potential to be correlated with the disease progress and the treatment effectiveness. The Massachusetts General Hospital (MGH) Center for Biomarkers in Imaging examines the use of biomarkers in both preclinical and clinical development stages to verify a drug candidate's potential usefulness in achieving the treatment objective. The center, which serves as an access point for the extensive imaging and research resources of the MGH Department of Radiology, maintains one of the largest imaging research infrastructures in the world. The center has worked with more than 35 drug and device companies and over 30 discrete biomarkers in preclinical and clinical trials.

APPLICATION TO ONCOLOGY CLINICAL TRIALS

Incorporating biomarkers into oncology clinical trials and therapy regimens can provide enhanced and more accurate information on precisely how a drug or bio-therapeutic performs. Using biomarkers can improve the dosing range of a therapeutic by relating the symptom or clinical sign to indications such as pain relief, reversal of disease, or disease halting. The value of biomarkers includes their use in identifying the new patient populations that might benefit from existing drugs, improving dosing regimens, and altering the delivery routes to adjust responses.

Increasingly, clinical trial designers see the biomarkers as useful clinical indicators, and these markers will gain importance as continuing developments in genomics, genetics, and proteomics enable researchers to map pathways and identify markers of disease. Biomarkers that precisely link drug performance to clinical outcomes have the potential to streamline drug development by enabling the markers to be used as surrogate end points in clinical evaluations, improving patient selection, helping to determine dose response and formulation selection, and reducing the necessary development time.

Surrogate End Points in Clinical Trials

Traditional clinical end points for oncology trials are mortality and morbidity; however, increasingly, drug developers are looking for other discrete, measurable end points that are sensitive as well as relevant to the clinical outcome of disease-related symptoms and overall survival.

Incorporating the use of surrogate end points into clinical trials can be challenging. While some biomarkers can be used to establish biological activity, this measurement may not always correlate to clinical efficacy. The following list highlights some of the reasons why a biomarker may not be an appropriate surrogate end point:

- The biomarker is not in the causal pathway of the disease process.
- The disease has multiple causal pathways, and the treatment has an effect on only one pathway that is measured by the surrogate. In this case, the treatment may have little or no impact on the disease; however, the assay will show a change.
- Conversely, if the surrogate is not in the pathway of the treatment's effect, or is insensitive to its effect, then the biomarker will not correlate to any treatment of the disease.
- If the drug functions via mechanisms of action that are independent of the disease process, the drug may prove useful in achieving patient benefit; however, the surrogate biomarker would not be useful in measuring that benefit.

To use biomarkers effectively as surrogate end points in clinical trials, they must be validated; that is, they must be able to be consistently and accurately measured and be meaningful to the clinical end point. The effect of the treatment on the surrogate end point must reliably predict the effect of the treatment on the clinical end point (i.e., overall survival). Therefore, the effect of the treatment must be captured in the surrogate end point or biomarker.

A surrogate end point can be validated statistically by analyzing the clinical trial data or validated clinically through an understanding of the disease pathways and the agent's mechanisms of action. With this knowledge, it is possible to determine the true clinical efficacy using a biomarker as a surrogate end point in clinical trials.

The FDA is now showing an increased willingness to consider the use of biomarker imaging as a primary end point in determining a drug candidate's effect. During the trials for trastuzumab (Genentech's Herceptin), for example, the MGH Center for Biomarkers in Imaging used CT scans to measure tumor volume. The tumor-volume data generated by the CT scans were included in the decision to approve trastuzumab for the treatment of metastatic breast cancer. (We discuss the trastuzumab trials in greater detail later in this report.)

Patient Selection

Increasingly, companies developing oncology treatments are incorporating the use of assays to screen potential patients. Screening patients using biomarkers to determine the patient's potential response to treatment can significantly improve the effectiveness of a clinical trial. Further, by examining population heterogeneity using biomarkers, the patient population can be segmented into subgroups that incorporate the likelihood of response to a given drug candidate.

Diagnostic tests used in combination with cancer therapies (biotherapeutics, in particular) will become increasingly important. The ability to identify patients who will respond to treatment with the biotherapeutic is vital in developing the market for a given biotherapy. As a result, we expect the use of biomarkers to identify potentially responsive patients to become a routine part of product development.

The following subsections examine the use of biomarkers in patient screening for trials of specific drugs from three companies: Genentech, ImClone, and Novartis. We then discuss AstraZeneca, which notably did not use such screening during the development of one of its agents and suffered significant setbacks as a result.

Trastuzumab (Genentech's Herceptin)

The association between the *Her-2/neu* (*c-erb-B2*) gene and HER-2/neu (c-erb-B2) protein and their correlation with adverse outcome in breast cancer was discovered in the mid-1980s. Researchers discovered that overexpression of the HER-2 protein correlated with a more aggressive disease and a poorer outcome.

The overexpression of Her-2/neu occurs in approximately one-fourth of breast cancer patients. The new biomarker was incorporated into the patient-screening process for the development of trastuzumab, Genentech's humanized MAb indicated for the treatment of advanced metastatic breast cancer in patients who had failed first- and second-line chemotherapy. Trastuzumab was initially approved in 1998 for use in patients with metastatic breast cancer who were found to overexpress the Her-2 protein. The clinical trials used Her-2 protein expression levels as the key selection criteria for the study of trastuzumab. The Phase III clinical trials of trastuzumab in Her-2-positive patients with earlier-stage disease were recently halted because of the demonstrated improvement in both primary and secondary end points (disease-free survival and overall survival, respectively). Trastuzumab was tested in the adjuvant setting with and without chemotherapy, and the data further show that the genetic tumor mutation that results in Her-2 overexpression correlates with a positive treatment outcome.

DakoCytomation developed HercepTest, the first test for the Her-2/neu protein biomarker, which was approved by the FDA and launched in 1998. Subsequently, Abbott/Vysis developed the first genomic Her-2/neu test, PathVysion, which has been available since January 2002. The accuracy of the genomic test is considered to be higher than that of the protein-based test for determining patient benefit from trastuzumab.

Cetuximab (ImClone's Erbitux)

Cetuximab, a chimeric antibody, is indicated for use in combination with CPT-11 (irinotecan [Pfizer's Camptosar]) for the treatment of advanced and refractory metastatic colorectal cancer (CRC). DakoCytomation introduced the biomarker genomic test called EGFR pharmaDx, which detects EGFR in tumor cells from CRC patients, in conjunction with the launch of cetuximab in February 2004. As with trastuzumab patient selection using the Her-2/neu biomarker, the clinical development of cetuximab incorporated DakoCytomation's immunohistochemical test for determining EGFR overexpression to define patient eligibility for clinical trial participation.

Cetuximab works by preventing the signals that trigger colorectal tumor growth via blocking the extracellular ligand-binding domain of EGFR. Blocking this signal inhibits metastasis, angiogenesis, and resistance to chemotherapy and radiotherapy. Using EGFR pharmDx, EGFR-positive tumors can be identified. Upregulation of the expression of EGFR occurs in many epithelial tumors including colorectal and non-small-cell lung cancer. However, the cetuximab/EGFR pharmaDx combination also highlights one of the potential risks of using this method of patient selection: the elimination of patients who may derive benefit from the treatment based on their screening results. A percentage of patients have EGFR-positive tumors that do not express EGFR at detectable levels. In a recent pilot study conducted by ImClone and Bristol-Myers Squibb, patients who had tested negative for EGFR expression using the current immunohistochemistry test were retested. Approximately 80% of these patients tested positive. This discrepancy may be due to the use of what may now be considered antiquated technology in conjunction with reader variability. Further, new data are pointing to a lack of correlation between the EGFR expression and the benefit from cetuximab treatment. Emerging screening criteria may better identify patients who will benefit from cetuximab.

Imatinib Mesylate (Novartis's Gleevec/Glivec)

The development of Novartis's imatinib is a demonstration of the company's focus on using molecular pathways that may be shared by various diseases as a strategy for its research and development programs. Imatinib was first approved in May 2001 for patients with chronic myelogenous leukemia

(CML). Imatinib is a protein-tyrosine kinase inhibitor of *bcr-abl* tyrosine kinase, which plays a crucial role in CML pathogenesis. The Philadelphia chromosome abnormality in CML produces this abnormal tyrosine kinase. Imatinib targets this *bcr-abl*-positive tumor-cell line to decrease proliferation and cause apoptosis. In the early chronic phase of CML, imatinib administration can result in complete, durable hematologic and cytogenetic remissions while causing minimal toxic effects.

Novartis continues to study imatinib and presented data at the American Society of Hematology (ASH) annual meeting in December 2004 from the International Randomized Interferon versus STI571 (IRIS) study demonstrating a link between the complete cytogenetic response (CCR) and clinical outcome. In another imatinib study presented at the ASH meeting, patients taking a higher dose were found to have a major molecular response (MMR) defined as a thousand-fold reduction in levels of Bcr-Abl, the tyrosine kinase responsible for stimulating the proliferation of white blood cells that is characteristic of CML. It was suggested that monitoring Bcr-Abl levels could be used as a surrogate to predict long-term outcomes. Patients who achieved a CCR and had a MMR at 12 months can be expected to remain disease-free for another 12 months. These clinical studies help to demonstrate the process involved in linking biomarkers to clinical outcomes in order to develop meaningful and reliable benchmarks for evaluating drug effectiveness and disease progression.

Imatinib also inhibits other receptor tyrosine kinases including platelet-derived growth factor (PDGF), stem cell factor (SCF), and c-Kit. In addition, imatinib has been found to cause apoptosis of GIST cells that express the activating c-Kit protein mutation. c-Kit or KIT (CD117) is a cellular enzyme or tyrosine kinase that, when activated, results in growth, proliferation, and survival. In February 2002, imatinib also received regulatory approval for the treatment of relapsed and metastatic KIT (CD117)-positive GISTs. These tumors involve the activation of a mutation in the c-Kit receptor tyrosine kinase (*RTK*) gene.

The location of the c-Kit mutation can be used to predict treatment response. To identify patients likely to respond to treatment, immunohistochemically based detection of c-Kit overexpression is used. Although c-Kit overexpression indicates that imatinib may provide a benefit for treating GISTs, not all patients exhibiting an overexpression of c-Kit derive a response from imatinib. The antibodies used to detect c-Kit currently do not distinguish the activated or phosphorylated version, and, therefore, the response to imatinib may not be fully appreciated. Researchers have found that patients with tumors expressing exon 11 mutant KIT protein are more responsive to imatinib than those expressing exon 9 mutant KIT protein, with responsiveness rates of 83.5% and 47.8%, respectively. It has been suggested that mutations in PDGF receptor-alpha (PDGFRA) may explain these variations in responsiveness (Heinrich et al., 2003). DakoCytomation has filed for FDA approval of its c-Kit marker to predict patient responsiveness to imatinib in treating GISTs.

Gefitinib (AstraZeneca's Iressa)

Since its approval to treat non-small-cell lung cancer in Japan in 2002 and the United States in 2003, the tyrosine kinase inhibitor gefitinib has not achieved its clinical or commercial expectations. This disappointing performance is due solely to the lack of patient selection in its clinical trials and subsequent clinical use. By year end 2002, gefitinib was implicated in 81 deaths in lung cancer patients in Japan, and by December 2003, gefitinib-associated deaths in that country rose to approximately 160 treated patients. Despite these growing mortality statistics, AstraZeneca posted 2004 sales in the United States of $176 million and sales in Japan of $136 million. Following a May 3, 2004 report published in the *New England Journal of Medicine* that elaborated on the important genomic discovery of the molecular mechanism underlying gefitinib sensitivity, gefitinib sales rose. However, since then, sales have declined as continued morbidity and mortality associated with gefitinib have been reported.

Gefitinib was approved under accelerated approval regulations as a third-line treatment in the United States based on a 10% response rate. These regulations enabled approval based on surrogate end points (50% tumor shrinkage lasting at least one month) expected to predict clinical outcomes that must subsequently be proved in ongoing trials. The response rate to gefitinib treatment was dramatic for some patients; the median duration of response was seven months. Differences in activity have been identified among groups of patients in the United States including a low response rate in men and smokers (5%) and a higher response rate in women and patients with adenocarcinoma (17%).

Despite some high response rates (25–30% in Japan), the consequences of gefitinib treatment are significant for nonresponders. The overall incidence of interstitial lung disease associated with gefitinib use is approximately 2% in Japanese patients, 1% overall, and 0.3% in US patients participating in the expanded access program (a Phase III study for non-small-cell lung cancer patients who have failed or are ineligible for other treatments and were either ineligible or unavailable for earlier gefitinib trials). Of the patients contracting interstitial lung disease, one-third have died. A genomic study to identify responders versus nonresponders to gefitinib, which targets the tumor protein EGFR, identified specific mutations on the *EGFR* gene that correlated with clinical response. Deletions or amino acid substitutions around the adenosine triphosphate (ATP) binding site of gefitinib increased EGFR signaling and susceptibility to inhibition. These mutations were identified in eight of nine responders but not in any of the nonresponders. Lung cancer cells with mutations are 10 times more responsive than normal cells; these mutations are much more common in tumor cells from Japanese patients, a factor that may account for the higher response rate among Japanese patients treated with gefitinib.

In December 2004, AstraZeneca released its preliminary analysis of the Iressa Survival Evaluation in Lung Cancer (ISEL) trial. The results did not show a statistically significant increase in survival, although a statistically significant improvement in tumor shrinkage and time to treatment failure was seen. After the release of this analysis, AstraZeneca decided to suspend promotion of gefitinib in the United States, but the drug remains available for patients deriving benefit from the treatment. Sales continue in Japan with regulatory consent. AstraZeneca is continuing all ongoing gefitinib studies in other cancer types, while its use in non-small-cell lung cancer is under review by the FDA, Japan's Ministry of Health, Labor, and Welfare (MHLW), and other regulatory authorities. Sales of gefitinib in the first quarter of 2005 were $81 million worldwide. Sales in the United States for that quarter were $30 million, a decline of 41%.

AstraZeneca announced the withdrawal of its marketing authorization application (MMA) to the European Medicines Agency (EMEA) for gefitinib in January 2005 following the release of the ISEL trial data. The EMEA had advised AstraZeneca that gefitinib would meet the approval requirements, and the company will consider submitting a new MMA based upon the results of the full ISEL data analysis.

AstraZeneca entered into an agreement involving gefitinib biomarkers with ViroLogic in early March 2005. ViroLogic will test tumor samples from the gefitinib-treated lung cancer patients to evaluate the use of its proprietary eTag assays for patient screening. AstraZeneca plans to provide ViroLogic with more than 100 tumor samples from its Phase IV clinical trial of gefitinib. ViroLogic will use eTag assays to identify specific protein biomarkers that are indicative of activated cancer growth signaling pathways in cells. The eTag assays examine functional proteins and may be predictive of gefitinib's ability to modulate disease progression and therefore a patient's likelihood of response to treatment.

In the case of gefitinib, the failure to identify biomarkers for diagnostic tests that could have been used for patient selection in clinical trials and subsequently in clinical use will continue to be extremely costly to AstraZeneca in terms of lost sales, unrecouped research and development expenses, and a potentially tarnished image. By developing an assay for patient screening, gefitinib could have been administered to appropriate patients to slow disease progression while excluding nonresponders, eliminating their exposure to gefitinib's toxic effects. In addition, screening biomarkers would eliminate the financial burden for nonresponders – in this case approximately $2,000 per month – of using a drug that will not provide any benefit to them. Ultimately, the clinical trials could have been enriched or stratified, perhaps at an early date, with a greater number of patients who respond to tyrosine kinase inhibitors creating a more efficient development process.

Dose Response and Formulation Selection

Selecting the appropriate drug dose for cancer treatment can be challenging, and finding clinical measures of dose response remains a key element of this challenge. In addition, a drug's formulation can significantly affect the bioavailability and metabolism of a drug candidate, which could affect the pharmacodynamic properties of the drug. Drug developers must accurately measure the effects that dose and formulation have on a treatment's efficacy. In certain therapeutic indications, clinical end points of morbidity and mortality are highly variable and may require large sample sizes to confirm that the dose–response and formulation relationships are accurately modeled. In these cases, trials large enough to provide statistical confidence may be impractical because of cost.

Identifying biomarkers that can be correlated with drug mechanism, therapeutic benefit, and toxicity significantly adds to the pharmacokinetic/pharmacodynamic (PK/PD) modeling of therapeutic intervention. In turn, an improved PK/PD modeling at the earlier stages of clinical development leads to a more rational and appropriate selection of dose, timing, and formulation when moving to pivotal trials. Ultimately, the improved accuracy of these selections can reduce the number and length of the late-stage trials, saving companies money and development time.

Reducing Development Time

It is beneficial for companies to identify indications that might have a greater probability of success and that may shorten a drug's development path to market. By determining the therapeutic indications for which the drug candidate will have the most utility as early as possible during the development process, companies can identify the nearest-term commercial opportunity for pivotal trials. Biomarkers that monitor the response of various patient groups help scientists design pivotal trials by identifying the patient sets that have the best therapeutic indices and by providing information that can help further development in other indications.

Biomarkers can also be used to gather additional data regarding a drug's efficacy, potentially allowing for considerable savings in time and resources. For example, Novartis recently engaged the MGH Center for Biomarkers in Imaging to measure tumor uptake of the radiotracer 18F-fluoro-deoxy-glucose (18F-FDG) by PET scanning. The company used these data as an internal decision-making tool while evaluating imatinib for the treatment of GISTs, noting the close correlation between uptake and a formal study end point: tumor regression by CT or MRI scanning.

REGULATORY RESPONSE

As already discussed, although the trastuzumab and cetuximab clinical trials successfully integrated patient selection biomarkers, AstraZeneca's gefitinib received

FDA approval without the benefit of biomarker screening. Ensuing problems with this drug have, in part, focused the FDA's attention on the critical importance of incorporating biomarkers into clinical development. The problems with gefitinib, along with pressure from the public and politicians to expedite drug approvals while maintaining a stringent safety-review process, is driving the agency toward incorporating new technological screening and end points in clinical trial designs. The FDA's white paper, "Innovation or Stagnation: Challenge and Opportunity on the Critical Path to New Medical Products," initially released in March 2004, focuses on how the agency can work together with industry and academia to solve the "pipeline problem" (the reduced rate of medical innovations reaching patients) and increase the efficiency of drug development.

The FDA has initiated guidance for drug developers on pharmacogenomics (the use of detailed genetic information to predict an individual patient's response to therapy) and genomic data submissions, including data on drug/test combinations. The white paper on increasing efficiency in drug development also highlights the use of imaging biomarkers for guiding dose selection and as surrogate end points. Programs are evolving to incorporate biosimulation (computer-based models that integrate relevant biological data to reproduce a system's control principles and that can be used to simulate a system's future biological behavior), which uses quantitative methods of presenting disease progression. Although the FDA has not set policy and standards regarding the use of pharmacogenomics in drug development, the agency is encouraging companies to submit the data with their filings. Following the close of its commentary period on pharmacogenomics in early 2004, the FDA issued its final pharmacogenomic guidance in early 2005 on when and how pharmacogenomic data should be filed.

With this guidance, the FDA has created a regulatory path for the voluntary submission of pharmacogenomic data. These data can be submitted even without a clear understanding of the pathophysiology involved or when the submitter does not expect that the data will impact the clinical outcome. In addition, the agency is developing an advisory committee that will recommend how genomic biomarkers can be incorporated into clinical trials.

Currently, the FDA expects information that can influence dose response to be included in a product's label. For instance, genotype (the genetic makeup of an individual) can be an important intrinsic factor to dose response. The question that arises is whether drugs with known relationships between genotype and dose response should be required to be relabeled and whether an assay to determine genotype should be required before prescribing. For example, irinotecan was approved for the treatment of refractory metastatic CRC patients in 1996. At the approved dose range, irinotecan prolongs survival but can have side effects including severe diarrhea and neutropenia. A recent study of 63 patients with known genotypes showed that grade 4 neutropenia occurred exclusively in two genotypes (Innocenti et al., 2004). Requiring that this information be added to the irinotecan label and that all patients be genotyped prior to treatment with the agent would potentially reduce the number of patients who develop this severe side effect. Should the FDA decide to implement these types of requirements, it would set a major precedent that could essentially require the use of genotype data for patient selection for all drugs, regardless of whether the drug is a candidate or marketed product. However, it is more likely that relabeling would be initiated by individual pharmaceutical companies, with or without prodding by the FDA.

THE FUTURE OF ONCOLOGY CLINICAL DEVELOPMENT

Incorporating biomarkers into cancer drug development poses both benefits and risks (Table 24.1). The identification of biomarkers can aid in the understanding of mechanisms

Table 24.1 Benefits and Risks of Biomarker Use in Drug Development

Benefits	*Risks*
For NMEs with a novel mechanism of action, clinical biomarker evaluations are key to understanding the mechanism of action and establishing proof of concept	A biomarker that is nonspecific and does not correlate with clinical outcome may lead to incorrect conclusions
Biomarker evaluations should help contain the cost of drug development by allowing early termination of NMEs that may have a low likelihood of success	If a biomarker is associated with only a portion of the clinical outcome, it may not identify all of the relevant effects of the therapy, including adverse effects
If successful, biomarkers may help preselect patient populations that are most likely to benefit	Biomarker analysis is expensive and time consuming
Biomarkers that predict the course of disease may serve as a useful tool for clinicians	Biomarker-based decisions could become biased unless a priori criteria are set up for decision-making in addition to biomarker data
Diagnostic kits could be developed where appropriate to aid in patient selection	Patient preselection may reduce the potential market size

NME = New molecular entity

of action and assist in establishing proof of concept. Biomarkers can also reduce the time and cost of drug development by providing data to determine a therapy's likelihood of success and by identifying patient populations most likely to benefit from new therapies. On the other hand, if care is not taken in correlating the marker with clinical outcome, the behavior of the marker may not indicate a benefit for the patient. Also, identifying and developing biomarkers as well as assays to measure them is costly and time-consuming. In addition, the possibility always exists that a company is unnecessarily limiting its market by eliminating potential patients who may derive benefit from the drug but do not exhibit the characteristic that is identified through screening.

Despite these drawbacks, we believe that developing and commercializing drugs based on pharmacogenomics could become efficient and cost-effective for many drugs in the future. However, this movement will require a paradigm shift in the way clinical studies are conducted. While changes that incorporate genomic studies into clinical development are certainly well under way, this process will continue to be an evolutionary one. Yet the pressure to couple biomarkers with biotherapeutics will continue to increase as the treatment focus for cancer shifts in favor of targeted biologic therapies. Biomarkers will become central in selecting the drug, dose, and administration route and will also be used for monitoring the ongoing treatment of cancer patients.

To this end, Novartis has already revamped its research and development process to reflect the importance of incorporating the biomarkers into drug development. Novartis has moved away from the traditional development model – research, development, and preclinical followed by clinical development – to a model the company calls translational medicine. During the discovery phase, the translational medicine model incorporates human genetics, transgenic models, PK/PD modeling, pathway analysis, biomarker development, and molecular toxicology. This stage is followed by an exploratory phase, during which target discovery and validation occur followed by proof of concept clinical trials. If the drug candidate is successful at this point, it enters clinical development (also called the confirmatory phase); otherwise, the project is discontinued.

While the industry, FDA, payers, and the public certainly want the variability associated with drug activity and any potential for injury to be understood and mitigated prior to drug launch, at this stage, many clinical development programs are still utilizing a trial-and-error approach. In the future, we believe, pharmaceutical and diagnostics companies will increasingly work in tandem to develop predictive diagnostic tests and drugs, as already evidenced in the trials for trastuzumab and cetuximab.

For drug/test combinations to succeed, however, they must receive a level of reimbursement that will motivate their use. For example, since the PathVysion Her-2/neu test was approved, Medicare payments for its use have been low, resulting in difficulties for clinical laboratories because their costs may not be reimbursed and placing patients at risk for losing access to the test. Although the Centers for Medicaid and Medicare Services (CMS) covers and pays for genomic tests, the reimbursement does not always cover the full cost. CMS agreed to amend the pricing of the PathVysion Her-2/neu test effective January 2005.

Clearly, it is in payers' best interests to support advances in the application of pharmacogenomics. Targeting treatments to patients more likely to benefit results in both a cost-savings for the payer and a reduction in wasted time in treatment and risk for the patient. It is important to remember, however, that it may not be completely possible to preselect all patient responders for a given therapy. As the biomarkers become available for targeted therapies, their success will depend on how companies that develop them balance the benefits, risks, and costs.

REFERENCES

Hanahan, D. and Weinberg, R.A. The hallmarks of cancer. *Cell.* 2000; 100: 57–70.

Heinrich, M., et al. Kinase mutations imatinib response in patients with metastatic gastrointestinal stromal tumour. *Journal of Clinical Oncology.* 2003; 21: 4342–9.

Innocenti, F., et al. Genetic variants in the UDP-glucuronosyltransferase 1A1 gene predict the risk of severe neutropenia of irinotecan. *Journal of Clinical Oncology.* 2004; 22: 1382–8.

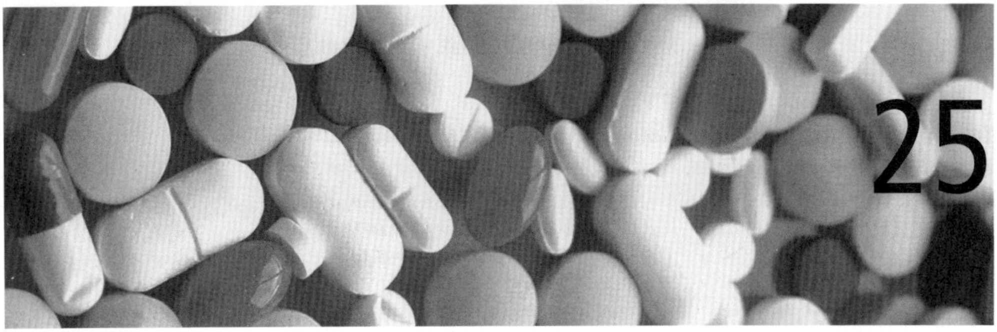

Antitumor Biologics: Strategies for Success in an Expanding Market

INTRODUCTION

The development of biological products, specifically protein drugs, has been a cornerstone of the biotechnology industry, and it has played a key role in the advancement of cancer treatments over the past 15 years. Biotechnology researchers and companies have used major protein drug technologies – namely, recombinant DNA and monoclonal antibody (MAb) technologies – to design and produce protein drugs directed against cancer. Development of anticancer biological agents has spanned more than three decades, from the overblown excitement over interferons as cancer treatments in the late 1970s and early 1980s (which proved to be largely unfounded) to the marketed drugs of the 1990s and early 21st century. The market for biological anticancer agents exceeded $9.5 billion worldwide in 2005 and has grown at a rate of 20% annually since 2000.

Biological anticancer agents can be subdivided into two categories: agents that directly attack tumors, and agents that serve as adjunct therapies designed to ameliorate the side effects of chemotherapy. Although the latter category contains a number of highly successful agents, including the recombinant protein drugs Johnson & Johnson's Procrit (epoetin alfa), Amgen's Aranesp (darbepoetin alfa), Amgen's Neupogen (filgastrim), and Amgen's Neulasta (pegfilgrastim), the majority of new development in this therapeutic area focuses on antitumor agents. Therefore, this report discusses the major classes of antitumor agents, including recombinant cytokines, MAbs, other recombinant proteins, targeted cytotoxins, and radiological agents.

In this chapter, we provide an overview of biological antitumor agents; we describe classes of biologics launched or in development, including an examination of some of the best-selling available therapies. We then discuss emerging agents, highlighting how they differ from existing agents and whether these differences are likely to give these new agents a competitive advantage in the marketplace. Next, we present a case study of Genentech/Roche/Chugai's Herceptin (trastuzumab), a highly successful MAb that is increasing its market potential through further clinical study. We address some of the concerns associated with reimbursement of these agents, particularly regarding the off-label prescribing of expensive MAbs.

Table 25.1 Select Antitumor Biologic Therapeutic Approaches

Therapeutic Approach	*Comments*
Monoclonal antibodies (MAbs)	The most successful class of antitumor biologicals Made using recombinant DNA technology The majority of emerging agents in development are MAbs
Cytokines	Recombinant versions of human cytokines, such as interferons or interleukins
Targeted cytotoxins and radiological agents	Products in which a recombinant protein or MAb moiety is used to target a cytotoxic or radiological moiety specifically to a tumor cell

Finally, we present our outlook for the biological antitumor market. Table 25.1 lists select antitumor biological therapeutic approaches.

EXISTING BIOLOGIC ANTITUMOR AGENTS

The mainstay treatments for most cancers are cytotoxic agents. Although cancer cells are more sensitive to cytotoxic drugs than most normal cells (usually because of their rapid proliferation), these drugs are also toxic for normal cells, especially those with proliferative activity (e.g., immune cells, blood-forming cells, intestinal cells, hair-follicle cells). As such, treatment with these agents causes severe side effects, and doses must be limited to ensure the safety of the patient, limiting the ability of chemotherapy to completely knock out the patient's tumors.

Driving the development of biological agents is the hope that they can be more-specific therapies (targeting cancer cells and not normal cells) and/or harness the body's own defenses (especially the immune system) in fighting cancer. Additionally, there is the possibility of developing less-toxic drugs with wider therapeutic indices (the therapeutic index is the ratio of the toxic dose to the therapeutic dose of a drug) than are typical for cytotoxic drugs. Efforts have also been made to develop protein drugs that can be combined with cytotoxic drugs, creating a combination therapy that will be more effective than cytotoxic monotherapy, with the same or lesser levels of toxicity. Table 25.2 details specific agents that are currently available.

Monoclonal Antibodies

MAbs are the most successful class of antitumor agent in terms of sales, applicability to the largest number of cancers, and number of agents in development. All MAbs used as antitumor therapeutics are produced using recombinant DNA technology. The antibody binding sites for antigens on these agents are derived from mouse MAbs, linked to amino-acid sequences derived from human antibody (Ab) molecules. The structure of an antibody (and its antigen binding site) is shown in Figure 25.1.

The first type of mouse–human hybrid MAb molecule, known as a chimeric Ab, is a recombinant molecule that consists of the variable region of a mouse MAb (selected for antigen specificity) grafted onto the constant sequences of a human Ab. As MAb technology has progressed, the amount of human sequence contained in the molecule has increased. Humanized MAbs consist of a construct containing mouse MAb hypervariable (HV) regions and human framework regions (FR) and constant regions. Most recently, researchers have developed fully human MAbs, which contain no mouse sequences. (While fully human MAbs have reached the market – for example, Cambridge Antibody Technology/Roche's Humira (adalimumab) – no fully human MAbs are approved for the treatment of cancer.) In general, MAbs with a greater amount of human sequences have a lesser chance of triggering antimouse Ab immune responses in patients, which can result in the neutralization and clearance of the MAb drug – diminishing the therapeutic effect – or infusion and allergic reactions, including anaphylaxis.

Table 25.2 Current Antitumor Protein Drugs, 2006

Generic Name	*Company/Brand*	*Description*	*Approved Cancer Indications*	*2005 Worldwide Sales ($MM)*
Monoclonal antibodies				
Rituximab	Biogen Idec/Genentech/ Roche's Rituxan/MabThera	Chimeric MAb; anti-CD20	CD20-positive B-cell non-Hodgkins lymphoma (NHL)	3,244
Trastuzumab	Genentech/Roche/ Chugai's Herceptin	Humanized MAb, anti-Her2	Her2-overexpressing metastatic breast cancer	1,723
Bevacizumab	Genentech's Avastin	Humanized MAb, anti-VEGF	Colorectal cancer	1,337
Cetuximab	ImClone/Merck KGaA/ Bristol-Myers Squibb's Erbitux	Chimeric MAb, anti-EGFR	Metastatic colorectal cancer Head and neck cancer	684
Alemtuzumab	Genzyme/Berlex's Campath	Humanized MAb, anti-CD52	B-cell chronic lymphocytic leukemia (CLL)	82
Cytokines				
Aldesleukin (interleukin-2)	Chiron's Proleukin	Recombinant interleukin-2	Metastatic renal carcinoma Metastatic melanoma	124
Interferon-alfa-2a	Roche's Roferon-A	Recombinant interferon-alpha-2a	Hairy cell leukemia Chronic myelogenous leukemia (CML)	104
Interferon-alfa-2b	Schering's Intron A	Recombinant interferon-alpha-2b	Melanoma Hairy cell leukemia Follicular (non-Hodgkin's) lymphoma AIDS-related Kaposi's sarcoma	287
Targeted cytotoxins and radiological agents				
Denileukin difitox	Ligand's Ontak	Recombinant fusion protein containing sequences of interleukin-2 linked to diphtheria toxin sequences	Persistent or recurring cutaneous T-cell lymphoma (CTCL) positive for the CD25 component of the IL-2 receptor	31
Gemtuzumab ozogamicin	UCB/Wyeth's Mylotarg	Humanized MAb, anti-CD33, linked to the cytotoxic antibiotic calicheamicin	CD33-postitive acute myelogenous leukemia (AML)	95
Ibritumomab tiuxetan	Biogen Idec's Zevalin	Humanized MAb, anti-CD20, linked to the radioisotope indium-111 or yttrium-90 via the linker tiuxetan	Rituximab-refractory CD20-positive B-cell non-Hodgkin's lymphoma (NHL)	51

EGFR = Epidermal growth factor receptor; VEGF = Vascular endothelial growth factor

Rituxan

According to the data of 2005, Biogen Idec/Genentech/Roche's Rituxan/MabThera (rituximab) was the highest-selling antitumor MAb, with that year's worldwide sales of more than \$3.2 billion. Rituxan targets the cell surface protein CD20 and is currently indicated for treatment of CD20-positive B-cell non-Hodgkin's lymphoma (NHL). In February 2006, the FDA approved

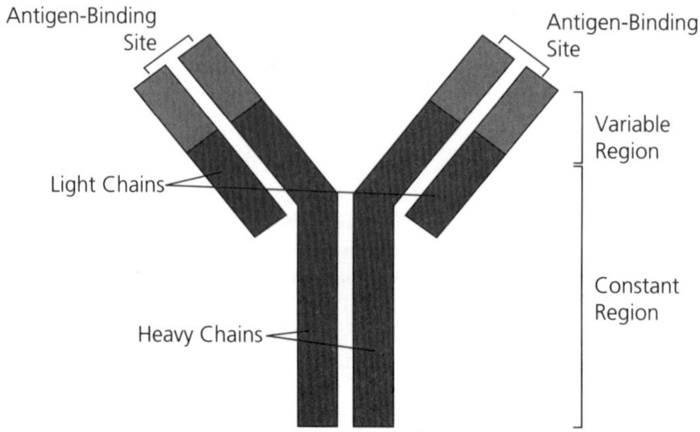

Note: Antibodies consist of two light chains and two heavy chains that are joined to form a "Y" shaped molecule. The light and heavy chains consist of two domains – the variable and the constant region. Within each variable region, there are three hypervariable (HV) regions (also referred to as complementarity determining regions [CDRs]), which are brought together by the framework regions (FR) and which, together with the CDRs on the other chain, form the antigen-binding site

Figure 25.1 Antibody Structure

Rituxan for treatment of rheumatoid arthritis in certain patients with inadequate responses to other therapeutics. In addition, Rituxan is being developed by Genentech for first-line treatment of indolent (i.e., slow-growing) NHL, relapsed chronic lymphocytic leukemia, and various immunologic diseases, including multiple sclerosis.

Herceptin

Genentech/Roche/Chugai's Herceptin (trastuzumab) targets the cell surface protein Her2, which is overexpressed in approximately 25% of breast cancers. It is indicated as a monotherapy for patients with metastatic Her2-positive breast cancer who have failed at least one round of chemotherapy and in combination with paclitaxel in patients with Her2-positive metastatic breast cancer who are chemotherapy naive. Herceptin is also being developed by Genentech for adjuvant therapy (i.e., therapy after surgery) of Her2-positive early-stage breast cancer.

For the same year of 2005, worldwide sales of Herceptin exceeded $1.7 billion, making it the second highest-selling antitumor MAb, after Rituxan. The development life cycle of Herceptin provides insight into the potential expansion strategies of an agent with an initially small target patient population, and we discuss this in detail later in this report.

Avastin

Genentech's Avastin (bevacizumab) is a MAb approved for the treatment of cancer in February 2004. Avastin targets the angiogenic growth factor vascular endothelial growth factor (VEGF). It attacks tumors indirectly by inhibiting angiogenesis (the formation of new blood vessels), and thus the blood supply that solid tumors require for their growth and survival. The role of angiogenesis in cancer was first hypothesized by Judah Folkman (Harvard Medical School) approximately 40 years ago, and many antiangiogenic drug candidates have been tested in the laboratory and the clinic since that time. However, many have failed in the clinic, and Avastin is the first antiangiogenic drug to reach the market.

Avastin was initially approved for the treatment of metastatic colorectal cancer in combination with a standard cytotoxic chemotherapy, 5-fluorouracil. In theory, however, an antiangiogenic therapeutic that has proven to be safe and efficacious in one solid tumor indication in humans should also be applicable to other solid tumor indications, and Genentech is developing the agent for many other cancers, including lung, breast, ovarian, and prostate. In all cases, Avastin should be especially efficacious in combination therapies with cytotoxic agents and/or targeted drugs that attack tumor cells directly. Such combinations would attack both a tumor's blood supply and the ability of tumor cells to proliferate and/or survive.

Avastin has been widely adopted since its 2004 launch, including a significant amount of off-label prescribing for treatment of other solid tumor indications. Worldwide sales of the agent reached $1.3 billion in 2005.

Recombinant Cytokines

With the introduction of interferon-alpha in 1986, recombinant cytokines became the first antitumor biologics to reach the market. Cytokines are secreted proteins that regulate immunity, inflammation, and hematopoiesis. Recombinant cytokines used as antitumor drugs include interferons and interleukin-2 (IL-2). Both of these agents address small markets, which is reflected in their modest sales: $124 million for IL-2 and $415 million for interferons.

IL-2 (aldesleukin, Chiron's Proleukin) is indicated for metastatic melanoma and metastatic renal carcinoma. It is thought to work by stimulating immune cells that target immunogenic tumors, especially melanoma and renal carcinoma. High-dose recombinant IL-2 is the only agent that has been shown to produce any durable responses in patients with these diseases, despite the development of new targeted therapies for RCC, and despite the designation of the cytotoxic agent dacarbazine as the gold-standard treatment for metastatic melanoma (Hutson and Quinn, 2005; Tarhini and Agarwala, 2005). However, the numbers of durable responses are small, representing just a few percent of treated patients. Moreover, systemic high-dose IL-2 therapy induces severe acute toxicities, especially pulmonary edema; these generally reverse rapidly after therapy is completed.

In antitumor therapy, interferons are used principally in treating certain hematological cancers. The mechanisms by which interferons produce antitumor effects are not well understood. They exhibit direct antiproliferative effects against target tumor cells, and they may also work by modulating the host immune system. Interferon-alfa-2a (Roche's Roferon-A) is approved for treatment of hairy cell leukemia and chronic myelogenous leukemia (CML). Interferon-alfa-2b (Schering's Intron A) is approved for treatment of hairy cell leukemia, follicular (non-Hodgkin's) lymphoma, melanoma, and AIDS-related Kaposi's sarcoma. In addition to their uses in oncology, these two products are also approved for treatment of hepatitis C.

Targeted Cytotoxins and Radiological Agents

The therapeutic strategy behind targeted cytotoxins and targeted radiological agents is to target a toxin or a radionuclide directly to tumors, not to the entire body. Theoretically, this should give a better therapeutic index than toxins or radiological agents that are given systemically, and it should even allow the use of compounds that are too toxic to give systemically. Targeted cytotoxins link a targeting moiety (i.e., a MAb) to a natural toxin, such as diphtheria toxin; targeted radiological agents link a targeting moiety with a radioactive isotope.

Ligand's targeted cytotoxin Ontak (denileukin difitox) is a fusion protein between a portion of the IL-2 molecule and diphtheria toxin sequences. It is designed to target diphtheria toxin to T-cell tumors that are positive for the CD25 protein chain of the IL-2 receptor. Ontak is approved for treatment of cutaneous T-cell lymphoma (CTCL). UCB/Wyeth's Mylotarg (gemtuzumab ozogamicin) is a MAb linked to the cytotoxic antibiotic calicheamicin that targets CD33-positive cells; it is indicated for treatment of CD33-positive acute myleogenous leukemia (AML).

Biogen Idec's Zevalin (ibritumomab tiuxetan) is a targeted radiological agent that targets the radioisotopes indium-111 and yttrium-90 to CD20-positive B-cell NHL that is refractory to Rituxan. It is supplied as a kit and is used to produce one dose each of Zevalin-indium-111 and Zevalin-yttrium-90, which are used together with Rituxan in a therapeutic regimen.

EMERGING ANTITUMOR BIOLOGICS

Biological antitumor agents in development are listed in Table 25.3; agents that have reached Phase II or later are described in detail in the following sections. The majority of these agents are MAbs; however, several employ novel mechanisms of action, including the induction of apoptosis.

Although this chapter focuses on protein biologics, there are several other approaches to antitumor biologics, listed in Table 25.4. Most of these approaches are in the early stages of development, although one gene therapy, Introgen's Advexin, has reached Phase II and III clinical trials in various cancers. Advexin is designed to deliver the tumor suppressor gene *p53* (via an adenoviral vector) to cancers that lack a functional version of this gene. The FDA has designated Advexin as a fast-track development program for recurrent, unresectable squamous-cell carcinoma of the head and neck; the agency has also designated Advexin as an orphan drug for this indication.

Panitumumab

Amgen is developing the MAb panitumumab for the treatment of metastatic colorectal cancer, non-small-cell lung cancer (NSCLC), and renal-cell carcinoma. Unlike currently marketed MAbs, panitumumab is a fully human MAb specific for epidermal growth factor receptor (EGFR), a cell surface protein implicated in several different forms of cancer. In March 2006, Amgen filed a Biologics License Agreement (BLA) for metastatic colorectal cancer with the FDA, and in April it filed a Market Authorization Application (MAA) with the European Medicines Agency (EMEA). The FDA accepted the BLA in June, and the agent was granted priority review.

The results of a multinational open-label Phase III trial of panitumumab were reported in April 2006 at the 97th Annual Meeting of the American Association for Cancer Research (AACR). In this trial, 463 metastatic colorectal cancer patients who had failed standard chemotherapy were randomized to receive either panitumumab plus best supportive care (BSC) every two weeks or BSC alone. Patients in the panitumumab group had a 46% decrease in the rate of tumor progression as compared with the BSC group. Panitumumab also demonstrated a survival advantage; at week 24, 18% of patients on panitumumab were alive and progression-free, compared with 5% of patients on BSC alone. At week 32, 10% of patients treated with panitumumab were alive and progression-free, compared with 4% in the BSC group.

Treatment with panitumumab gave only a 1% rate of infusion reactions, none severe. No antihuman Ab or antipanitumumab Abs were formed as the result of panitumumab treatment. Adverse effects that were seen more in the panitumumab group than in the BSC group were skin reactions, fatigue, abdominal pain, nausea, diarrhea, and hypomagnesemia (low blood magnesium).

Cetuximab (ImClone/Merck KgaA/Bristol-Myers Squibb's Erbitux), a MAb approved for the treatment of metastatic colorectal cancer and head and neck cancer, also targets EGFR; however, panitumumab appears to have several advantages over the existing agent. As a fully human MAb, panitumumab has the potential for a better safety profile than the chimeric cetuximab. Moreover, in colorectal cancer, panitumumab shows a major survival advantage, which has not been seen with cetuximab. Panitumumab, which is given every two weeks (the dosing schedule for many cytotoxic chemotherapy regimens), is more convenient than cetuximab, which

Table 25.3 Select Emerging Antitumor Biologic Agents, 2006

Drug	*Company*	*Description*	*Stage*
Panitumumab	Amgen (formerly Abgenix)	Fully human MAb; anti-EGFR	Preregistration
Pertuzumab (Omnitarg)	Genentech/Roche	Humanized MAb; anti-Her2 First in class of Her dimerization inhibitors, which block the ability of Her2 to dimerize with other HER family receptors and thus block cell signaling	Phase II, platinum-resistant ovarian cancer, in combination with chemotherapy
Galiximab	Biogen Idec	Primatized MAb; anti-CD80, B-cell specific cell surface protein	P hase II, relapsed or refractory follicular non-Hodgkin's lymphoma (NHL), in combination with rituximab
Volociximab	PDL BioPharma/Biogen Idec	Chimeric MAb; anti-alpha5 beta1 integrin Antiangiogenic	Phase II; renal cell carcinoma, melanoma, pancreatic cancer, and NSCLC
Mapatumumab	Cambridge Antibody Technology/Human Genome Sciences/ GlaxoSmithKline	Fully human MAb; anti-TRAIL receptor-1 Designed to induce apoptosis in tumor cells that express the receptor.	Phase II, NSCLC; relapsed or refractory NHL, colorectal cancer Phase I, in combination with chemotherapy, various solid tumors
CAT-3888	Cambridge Antibody Technology	Fusion protein between a murine anti-CD22 disulfide-linked Fv antibody fragment, and the modified *Pseudomonas* exotoxin CD22 is a cell surface receptor expressed on many B-cell cancers	Phase II, hairy cell leukemia Phase I, chronic lymphocytic leukemia (CLL) and pediatric acute lymphoblastic leukemia (pALL)
CDP-791	UCB/ImClone	Pegylated humanized MAb fragment; anti-VEGFR2 Antiangiogenic	Phase II, NSCLC, in combination with carboplatin and paclitaxel
IMC-11F8	ImClone	Fully human MAb, anti-EGFR	Phase I, solid tumors
IMC-A12	ImClone	Fully human MAb, anti-insulin-like growth factor 1 receptor (IGF-1R)	Phase I, solid tumors
IMC-1121B	ImClone	Fully human MAb; anti-VEGFR-2 Antiangiogenic	Phase I, solid tumors
HGS-ETR2	Cambridge Antibody Technology/Human Genome Sciences	Fully human MAb; anti-TRAIL receptor-2 Designed to induce apoptosis in tumor cells that express the receptor	Phase I, advanced solid tumors
AMG-102	Amgen	Fully human MAb; antihepatocyte growth factor (HGF) HGF signaling via its receptor c-Met is implicated in many cancers	Phase I, cancer
AMG-479	Amgen	Fully human MAb; insulin-like growth factor 1 receptor (IGF-1R)	Phase I, cancer
AMG-655	Amgen	Fully human MAb; anti-TRAIL receptor-2 Designed to induce apoptosis	Phase I, cancer
Apo2L/TRAIL	Genentech/Amgen/ Immunex	Recombinant form of a human protein that regulates apoptosis	Phase I, in a variety of solid tumors and hematological malignancies
AMG-386	Amgen	A recombinant Fc fusion protein with a synthetic peptide that targets angiopoeitins Antiangiogenic	Phase I, cancer

Note: AstraZeneca acquired Cambridge Antibody Technology in May 2006

Table 25.4 Early-stage Approaches to Biological Cancer Treatment

Therapeutic Approach	*Comments*
Recombinant proteins	Recombinant proteins other than cytokines or MAbs
Tumor vaccines	Immunotherapeutic products designed to induce an immune reaction to a tumor. All in early-stage development
Cellular immunotherapies	Immunotherapies that consist of autologous immune cells (e.g., T cells or natural killer cells), usually activated in vitro by a cytokine. Research in this area is 20 years old, but there are no approved products
Viral therapies	Therapies based on using a virus designed to specifically kill tumor cells. All in early-stage development, including agents being developed by Introgen and Onyx
Gene therapies	One gene therapy, Introgen's Advexin, in late-stage development

requires weekly dosing. Moreover, patient doses of panitumumab require significantly less drug by weight (in terms of grams per square meter) than cetuximab. This gives Amgen the option of pricing panitumumab lower than cetuximab, without hurting its profit margin.

Pertuzumab

Roche and Genentech are developing the humanized MAb pertuzumab (Omnitarg) for the treatment of breast, ovarian, and NSCLC cancers. Pertuzumab is the first in a class of agents known as Her dimerization inhibitors. Similar to Herceptin, pertuzumab targets Her2; however, it has a different mechanism of action than the marketed agent.

The polypeptide chains of Her family receptors must dimerize to initiate signal transduction. Binding of epidermal growth factor (EGF) to its receptor, EGFR, initiates dimerization and leads to normal intracellular signaling. Her2, however, has no known ligand, and it can dimerize with itself or other Her family members (especially Her3), particularly in situations where Her2 is overexpressed (Burgess et al., 2003). This dimerization results in constitutive intracellular signaling and stimulation of uncontrolled cell proliferation. Pertuzumab binds to Her2 and blocks the binding pocket that is essential for receptor dimerization and signaling (Franklin et al., 2004).

In May 2005, Genentech presented results from Phase II clinical trials of pertuzumab at the 41st Annual Meeting of the American Society of Clinical Oncology (ASCO) (Orlando, Florida). These were studies of pertuzumab as a single agent in patients with ovarian, breast, and prostate cancer. The studies suggested that pertuzumab may have limited efficacy as a single agent in these cancers, but that further studies were warranted.

Galiximab

Biogen Idec's galiximab is a primatized MAb that targets CD80, a cell surface protein that is expressed specifically in B cells and B-cell leukemia. Primatization is an alternative to Ab humanization, where the variable regions of a MAb contain macaque Ab sequences instead of human sequences. This technology was developed by Idec prior to its 2004 merger with Biogen. Galiximab is currently in Phase II clinical trials in combination with Rituxan for treatment of relapsed or refractory follicular NHL.

The combination of galiximab and Rituxan targets two proteins specific to B cells: CD80 and CD20. In June 2005, Biogen Idec reported at the International Conference on Malignant Lymphoma (Lugano, Switzerland) that in a Phase II clinical trial, the combination prolonged event-free survival in patients with relapsed or refractory follicular NHL in comparison with the previous results with Rituxan monotherapy. In the study, 73 patients were treated with escalating doses of galiximab in combination with a standard therapeutic course of Rituxan. In the 64 patients who received the highest dose of galiximab (500 mg/m^2 weekly for four weeks), the combination therapy produced a 64% overall response rate; 31% of the patients achieved a compete response, and 33% achieved a partial response. This treatment achieved an increase in event-free survival without increased toxicity compared with reported historic data with Rituxan alone. (Note that there was no side-by-side comparison in this trial.) The median event-free survival for patients treated with galiximab plus Rituxan was 12.1 months.

Volociximab

PDL BioPharma/Biogen Idec's volociximab is a mouse/human chimeric MAb that interacts with the α5β1 integrin, a cell surface molecule involved in cell adhesion critical to the migration and survival of the endothelial cells involved in the formation of new blood vessels in angiogenesis. The integrins α5β1and αvβ3, and their extracellular matrix substrate, fibronectin, are centrally involved in cellular adhesion in angiogenic endothelial cells. These two integrins are poorly expressed in endothelial cells in quiescent blood vessels and are coordinately upregulated during angiogenesis, making them potential anticancer targets (Boudreau and Varner, 2004).

Volociximab is designed to inhibit adhesion mediated by α5β1. Although there is currently an antiangiogenic cancer therapeutic on the market, Avastin, and several more in development, these agents target VEGF or its receptors. However, there are several known growth factors that stimulate tumor angiogenesis, and drugs that modulate only the VEGF/VEGFR system may not inhibit tumor angiogenesis that is stimulated by other factors. PDL BioPharma and Biogen Idec are hoping volociximab may inhibit tumor angiogenesis regardless of which growth factors stimulated new blood vessel growth.

Volociximab is being developed for melanoma, NSCLC, pancreatic cancer, and renal cancer. In June 2006, interim results from three Phase II open-label clinical trials of volociximab were presented at the 2006 ASCO meeting in Atlanta. In trials in patients with refractory metastatic clear cell renal cell cancer (RCC), metastatic pancreatic adenocarcinoma, and metastatic melanoma, the agent was generally well tolerated. The companies will be conducting further Phase II studies using higher doses of volociximab.

Mapatumumab

Cambridge Antibody Technology (a subsidiary of AstraZeneca since May 2006), Human Genome Sciences, and GlaxoSmithKline are developing the fully human MAb mapatumumab. Mapatumumab is designed to stimulate apoptosis (the major pathway of programmed cell death) in cancer cells. In healthy cells, apoptosis is induced by p53; however, this protein is either mutated or otherwise inactivated in the majority of human cancers. Mapatumumab targets TNF-related apoptosis-inducing ligand (TRAIL) receptor-1, which has been found to selectively induce apoptosis in cancer cells independent of the tumor suppressor p53.

In 2005, Human Genome Sciences (HGS) reported the results of clinical trials of mapatumumab as a monotherapy in NHL, NSCLC, and colorectal cancer. In NSCLC and colorectal cancer, the drug was well tolerated, and stable disease was observed in several of the patients who were treated with the drug. HGS concluded that further tests, in combination with chemotherapy, were warranted.

The results of Phase II clinical trials of mapatumumab as a monotherapy in advanced NHL were reported in December 2005, at the 47th Annual Meeting of the American Society of Hematology in Atlanta. The drug was well tolerated and showed a clinical response in patients with follicular lymphomas who had been heavily treated with other agents and had relapsed or refractory disease. Among these patients, clinical responses (one complete response and two partial responses) were seen in 3 of 17 patients (18%), and 11 of 17 patients (65%) with follicular lymphomas showed either a clinical response or stable disease. Of all the patients (i.e., with follicular lymphomas or other classes of relapsed or refractory NHL) treated with mapatumumab, 3 of 40 (8%) patients showed clinical responses, and 12 of 40 patients (30%) showed stable disease. HGS plans to initiate follow-on Phase II studies of mapatumumab in hematological malignancies, in combination with chemotherapy.

CAT-3888

Cambridge Antibody Technologies is developing the targeted cytotoxin CAT-3888 for multiple forms of B-cell cancer. A disulphide group links a toxin to a murine Ab fragment (i.e., a fragment that contains the combining region of an Ab), which is specific for CD22, a cell surface receptor that is expressed on many B-cell cancers. The cytotoxin moiety of this fusion protein is a modified *Pseudomonas* exotoxin. Data from a Phase II trial in patients with hairy-cell leukemia was presented at the AACR meeting in April 2006 (Washington, D.C.). In this trial of 25 chemotherapy-resistant patients who received CAT-3888, 44% showed a complete response and an additional 32% showed a partial response to the therapy.

CDP-791

UCB/ImClone's CDP-791 is a pegylated humanized MAb fragment being developed for the treatment of NSCLC. CDP-791 inhibits the VEGF2 pathway, which, as discussed previously, stimulates angiogenesis in the blood vasculature cells that feed tumor cells. Pegylation is the addition of a long-chain PEG group to the antibody fragment, which enhances its half-life in the patient's bloodstream. This process enables the Ab fragment to be expressed and manufactured in bacteria, which is not possible with full-length Abs. UCB developed CDP-791 in collaboration with Nektar, a leading company in pegylation technology.

HERCEPTIN: A MODEL FOR EXPANDING AN AGENT'S REACH

The development of therapies to treat cancer has been an iterative process. Traditional cytotoxic chemotherapies usually provide advanced cancer patients with only a slightly longer survival prognosis, and their quality of life is often negatively impacted. However, combination approaches, which utilize chemotherapy, surgery, and radiotherapy, have improved upon early monotherapy approaches, in some cases providing a cure, as with the majority of childhood acute lymphoblastic leukemia (ALL) and Hodgkin's lymphoma cases.

The development of targeted therapies, including antitumor biologics, generated the hope that more-specific therapies would provide dramatic improvement, including long-term remissions, possible cures, and significantly less toxicity than traditional cytotoxic drugs. However, the reality thus far is that our limited knowledge of cancer disease pathways has resulted in new classes of targeted antitumor drugs that provide only marginally improved benefit, with the likelihood of eventual drug resistance.

However, the availability of these agents offers the potential that they may be either combined with other treatments (similar to the development of combination therapies using cytotoxic drugs) or expanded to new patient populations to provide greater efficacy. Additionally, the study of these agents can lead to greater understanding of disease pathways, leading to more rational development of second-generation agents and/or combination therapies. The development history of Genentech's Herceptin provides an excellent model for how drug developers can expand a targeted drug to reach a greater patient population and improve both the survival benefit for the patient and the overall potential of the drug. Results of critical clinical trials for Herceptin can be seen in Table 25.5.

Herceptin was first approved in 1998 for treatment of Her2-overepressing metastatic breast cancer. The agent was approved as

Table 25.5 Critical Clinical Trial Results for Trastuzumab

Indication/Study	*Percentage Long-term Survivors*		*Percentage Long-term Progression-free or Disease-free Survivors*	
	Trastuzumab plus Chemo	*Chemo Only*	*Trastuzumab plus Chemo*	*Chemo Only*
Metastatic Her2-positive breast cancer				
Study 1[a]	35	20	18	2
Study 2[b]	33	16	–	–
Early-stage Her2-positive breast cancer, adjuvant therapy				
Study 3[c]	91.4	86	85.3	67.1

[a]Slamon, D.J., et al. Use of chemotherapy plus a monoclonal antibody against HER2 for metastatic breast cancer that overexpresses HER2. *New England Journal of Medicine*. 2001;344:783–92
[b]Extra, J.M., et al. Long-term survival demonstrated with trastuzumab plus docetaxel: 24-month data from a randomized trial (M77001) in HER2-positive metastatic breast cancer. ASCO Annual Meeting, 2005. Abstract 555
[c]Romond, E.H., et al. Trastuzumab plus adjuvant chemotherapy for operable HER2-positve breast cancer. *New England Journal of Medicine*. 2005;353:1673–84

a monotherapy in patients who have received one or more courses of chemotherapy and in combination with paclitaxel in patients who are chemotherapy naive. The approval was based on Phase III data that showed Herceptin plus standard chemotherapy gave a 25.1-month median survival compared with a 20.3-month median survival with chemotherapy alone. Median progression-free survival was 4.6 months on chemotherapy alone and 7.4 months on chemotherapy plus Herceptin. Addition of Herceptin to standard chemotherapy regimens reduced the relative risk of death by 20% at a median follow-up of 30 months. The percentage of survivors at 50 months after enrollment was approximately 35% of patients treated with paclitaxel plus Herceptin, compared with approximately 20% of patients on paclitaxel alone (Slamon et al., 2001). Data from an additional study, reported in May 2005, show that 33% patients who received Herceptin plus docetaxel (Sanofi-Aventis's Taxotere, another taxane drug) survived after three years, compared with 16% on docetaxel alone (Extra et al., 2005).

These data showed that the addition of Herceptin to chemotherapy (taxanes) resulted in a larger number of long-term survivors. The median overall and progression-free survival rate improvements were modest, however, and the agent was indicated only for a small percentage of patients. As mentioned earlier, only about 25% of breast cancers are Her2-overexpressing, and Herceptin is indicated only for patients with metastatic cancers, a condition for which the prognosis remains very poor.

In 2001, Genentech sponsored two trials investigating the efficacy of Herceptin as an adjuvant therapy for operable, earlier-stage Her2-positive breast cancer. The trials were conducted by collaborative groups of academic researchers, and major funding was provided by the National Cancer Institute (although Genentech provided the supply of Herceptin and some funding, the company did not participate in the trial design, data collection, or analysis). In October 2005, interim results from two Phase III trials with women with early-stage node-positive or high-risk node-negative Her2-positive operable breast cancer were published in the *New England Journal of Medicine* (Romond et al., 2005).

The patients in these studies, who were followed for a median of two years, received surgery to remove the tumors, followed by adjuvant chemotherapy (initial treatment was with doxorubicin and cyclophosphamide), followed by paclitaxel with or without Herceptin. The study showed that addition of Herceptin gave a 49% improvement in overall survival and reduced the risk of recurrence of breast cancer by 52%. After four years of the study, 33% of women treated with chemotherapy alone had a recurrence of breast cancer, compared with 15% of women treated with Herceptin plus chemotherapy (i.e., 85.3% disease-free survival with the combination therapy and 67.1% with chemotherapy alone). In terms of overall survival, 91.4% of women treated with Herceptin plus chemotherapy were still alive after four years of the study, compared with 86% of women treated with chemotherapy alone. The lead author of the study, Dr Edward H. Romond (University of Kentucky), said that these results represent the largest improvement in outcome for any group of breast cancer patients in 25 years. He further stated that if the results from ongoing follow-up studies are similarly positive, the prognosis of women with early-stage Her2-positive breast cancer may change from poor to good.

The study indicates that using Herceptin early in the course of disease, as part of adjuvant chemotherapy, will provide the best chance of long-term survival for women with Her2-positive breast cancer. As a result of this study, in February 2006, Genentech applied to the FDA and the EMEA for approval to expand use of Herceptin to the new early-stage breast cancer indication. In May 2006, Herceptin was approved for this indication in the European Union (EU); however, in August 2006, the FDA requested further information, delaying approval. This expansion into early-stage treatment will significantly increase the patient base for Herceptin, and its efficacy in this treatment indicates it may see strong adoption.

Researchers continue to investigate ways to increase the usefulness of Herceptin. Recent studies of signaling pathways in breast cancer may offer some hope in decreasing the likelihood of resistance to the agent. The tumor suppressor gene *PTEN* (phosphatase and tensin homolog deleted on chromosome ten) inhibits key pathways involved in cell growth and survival of cancer cells, which become activated when *PTEN* function is lost. A deficiency in *PTEN* was discovered to be a strong predictor of resistance to Herceptin therapy, indicating that signaling pathways controlled by *PTEN* are important in the antitumor activity of Herceptin. Moreover, inhibitors of phosphoinositol-3-kinase (PI3K), a signaling molecule whose effects are reversed by *PTEN*, reversed trastumzumab resistance caused by *PTEN* deficiency in animal models. This suggests the possibility that small-molecule inhibitors of PI3K, or perhaps of signaling molecules that are downstream of PI3K and *PTEN*, may reverse those cases of Herceptin resistance in human patients that are caused by *PTEN* loss (Nagata et al., 2004).

As seen with Herceptin, companies very often test approved biological products in new settings and as part of new combination therapies, largely in order to increase the market for their drugs. Even in situations where companies are slow to sponsor new studies, oncologists will often prescribe these agents off-label in new settings. This expansion strategy may, in some cases, enable drug developers to find settings in which drugs that initially give modest results now give more dramatic results. Given the demand for more-effective therapies and even cures by the cancer patient community, and the pressure from third-party payers to justify the high prices of antitumor biological drugs (as discussed in the next section, where Herceptin again serves as an example), this strategy may well increase in importance.

REIMBURSEMENT CONCERNS WITH ANTICANCER BIOLOGICS

Cancer biologics are some of the highest-priced drugs available, a reality that drug developers state is necessary for numerous reasons: the high degree of risk and high cost of the R&D needed to discover and develop these drugs, their high manufacturing costs, the capital needed to continue R&D into new antitumor drugs, and the value to society in having effective – and eventually curative – treatments for cancer. However, as the number of approved anticancer biologics increases and more patients become candidates for their use, both third-party payers and patients are increasingly expressing concern over the cost of these treatments. Many third-party payers are re-examining their policies regarding off-label use of these agents, in some cases refusing or delaying payment. Patients, faced with out-of-pocket copayments that can cost $10,000 to $20,000 per year, are considering forgoing these treatments, particularly in cases where the benefit of treatment is marginal.

This growing concern is well illustrated by a UK court battle regarding Herceptin treatment. Ann Marie Rogers, a UK citizen in her early 50s, was diagnosed with early-stage, operable breast cancer in late 2004. In May 2005, after surgery and a three-month course of chemotherapy, it was determined that the cancer was Her2-positive, prompting the oncologist to prescribe Herceptin. At the time, Herceptin was an off-label treatment for early-stage breast cancer (the agent has since been approved for this indication), and the local National Health Service (NHS) Primary Care Trust (PCT) refused to pay for Herceptin treatment based on the agent's lack of approval and exceptional circumstances that would justify the use of the drug.

Ms. Rogers borrowed money to begin treatment at a private hospital and pursued relief in the courts. Although a judge ordered the PCT to pay for the drug while the court case was pending, in February 2006 the court ruled in favor of the PCT, a decision that was later overturned on appeal. In May 2006, the EU approved Herceptin for use in adjuvant therapy of Her2-positive early-stage breast cancer, and in June the United Kingdom's National Institute for Health and Clinical Excellence (NICE) recommended that the drug be covered by the NHS for the new indication.

A *New York Times* article illustrates how some of these same issues are playing out in the United States (*New York Times*, 2006). Avastin, the first approved antiangiogenesis drug, is currently used to treat metastatic colorectal cancer in combination with 5-fluorouracil. For this indication, the cost of the drug is approximately $50,000 per year. Genentech has also been testing the drug, in combination with standard chemotherapies, for use in late-stage breast and lung cancer. The company applied for sBLAs in NSCLC in April 2006 and breast cancer in May 2006. The trials for these two new indications involve higher doses of bevacizumab than are used for colorectal cancer, raising the cost of treatment to what some analysts speculate could be twice the cost of treating colorectal cancer. Currently, health insurers generally pay for the approved use of Avastin in colorectal cancer but decide on a case-by-case basis on whether to pay for off-label use of the drug for breast or lung cancer. According to the *New York Times* article, third-party payers are often choosing not to cover the off-label use of the drug.

The cost-effectiveness of an agent is one of the primary factors in a third-party payer's decision whether to cover the cost of a treatment. An economic analysis of the use of Herceptin for early-stage breast cancer, carried out in Belgium and published in 2005, illustrates some of the issues involved in determining the cost-effectiveness of biological treatments for cancer (Neyt et al., 2006). According to this analysis, addition of Herceptin to adjuvant therapy for early-stage Her2-positive breast cancer more than doubled the cost of adjuvant treatment per patient. Additionally, the available patient population increases with the expansion into earlier stage treatment, further increasing the cost to the healthcare system. However, the agent may still be considered cost-effective if the use of the drug in the early stages of the disease prevents the development of metastases, significantly reducing the costs of treating metastatic disease.

Nevertheless, the high cost of the drug, its relatively long period of use per patient (up to one year), and the large patient populations can impose a large financial burden on healthcare systems such as Medicare and European national health agencies, and there is no clear answer on what long-term policies these agencies will adopt in regard to these agents. Currently, companies that develop breakthrough cancer biologics have commanded premium prices for these agents, with the expectation that payers will cover the cost. However, there are a few cases of antitumor biologics in development that may offer lower treatment costs than current agents. For example, panitumumab, which requires lower, less-frequent doses, may be an acceptable substitute for cetuximab in treatment of EGFR-dependent cancers. The antiangiogenic agent CDP-791, which has lower manufacturing costs than most MAb drugs, may replace more-expensive antiangiogenic agents to treat NSCLC. Emerging small-molecule agents, not discussed in detail in this chapter, may also replace higher-priced biologics. Some of them, if approved, may be used as a potentially less-expensive, orally delivered alternative to Herceptin. Nonetheless, drug price is determined in large part by the market (Cox et al., 2004), and there is no guarantee that these agents that require lower dosing or that have lower manufacturing costs will be priced lower than existing biologics. However, issues of reimbursement are likely to affect the pricing decisions regarding emerging agents, and manufacturers of current therapies will need to respond accordingly.

OUTLOOK

Over the past 15 years or so, the field of antitumor protein drugs has advanced considerably, as evidenced by the steady growth of anticancer biologics available on the market (Figure 25.2). The main driver of this advancement has been the development of technologies that allow MAbs to contain greater percentages of human sequences, ultimately resulting in fully human MAb drugs. As we have discussed, MAbs are the most successful class of antitumor biologics; annual sales of these agents have well exceeded $7.3 billion, over 70% of total anticancer biologic sales.

The success of existing agents has prompted many drug developers to develop new antitumor protein drugs (mostly MAbs) that will improve upon current therapies. We anticipate the anti-EGFR MAb drug panitumumab will be the next agent to reach the market, and we expect numerous new biologics will launch over the next five to ten years. Further, we anticipate that drug developers will begin using MAb technology to target new pathways as understanding of the pathways increases.

In addition to developing new agents, corporate and academic researchers, especially clinical oncologists, are attempting to identify new indications for current antitumor biologics, including the use of these agents in new patient groups and in new combination therapies. These studies will not only expand the sales potential of these agents, but they will also potentially

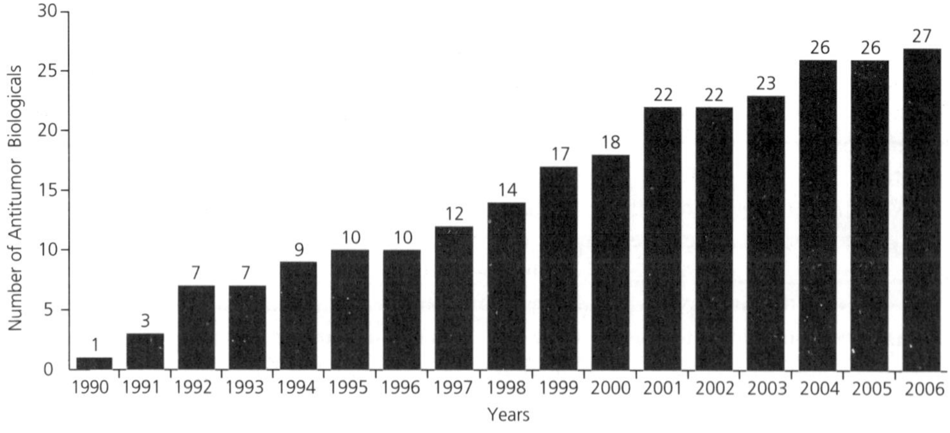

Figure 25.2 Number of Anticancer Biologics on the Market, 1995–2006

increase their efficacy. We anticipate that treatment for cancer will move toward cocktails of targeted drugs including biologics and small-molecule agents, used in addition to surgery, radiation, and cytotoxic drugs, potentially reducing the mortality associated with these diseases.

Nevertheless, the cloud on the horizon of this scenario is the expense of antitumor biologics, especially MAb drugs. The introduction of greater numbers of expensive biologics, including many that provide patients with only marginal benefits, presents a dilemma for physicians, patients, and payers, and eventually for biotechnology and pharmaceutical companies. The desire to avoid the expense of high-priced drugs is in conflict with demands of physicians, patient advocacy groups, and the general society for breakthrough treatments and cures for cancer. To help lessen this dilemma and reduce their risk in this environment, companies should aim to develop new indications for current agents as well as alternative agents that produce significant patient benefit; further, alternative agents, if possible, should have the potential for being priced lower than competitive agents while maintaining profit margins.

REFERENCES

Boudreau, N.J. and Varner, J.A. The homeobox transcription factor Hox D3 promotes integrin alpha5beta1 expression and function during angiogenesis. *Journal of Biologic Chemistry*. 2004; 279: 4862–8.

Burgess, A.W. et al. An open-and-shut case? Recent insights into the activation of EGF/ErbB receptors. *Molecular Cell*. 2003; 12: 541–52.

Cox, M.C. et al. No rational theory for drug pricing. *Journal of Clinical Oncology*. 2004; 22: 962–3.

Extra, J.M. et al. Long-term survival demonstrated with trastuzumab plus docetaxel: 24-month data from a randomized trial (M77001) in HER2-positive metastatic breast cancer. ASCO Annual Meeting, 2005. Abstract 555.

Franklin, M.C. et al. Insights into ErB signaling from the structure of the ErbB2-pertuzumab complex. *Cancer Cell*. 2004; 5: 317–28.

Hutson, T.E. and Quinn, D.L. Cytokine therapy: a standard of care for metastatic renal cell carcinoma? *Clinical Genitourinary Cancer*. 2005; 4: 155.

Nagata, Y. et al. PTEN activation contributes to tumor inhibition by trastuzumab, and loss of PTEN predicts trastuzumab resistance in patients. *Cancer Cell*. 2004; 6: 117–27.

New York Times, February 15, 2006.

Neyt, M., et al. An economic evaluation of Herceptin in adjuvant setting: the Breast Cancer International Research Group 006 trial. *Annals of Oncology*. 2006; 17: 381–90.

Romond, E.H., et al. Trastuzumab plus adjuvant chemotherapy for operable HER2-positive breast cancer. *New England Journal of Medicine*. 2005; 353: 1673–84.

Slamon, D.J., et al. Use of chemotherapy plus a monoclonal antibody against HER2 for metastatic breast cancer that overexpresses HER2. *New England Journal of Medicine*. 2001; 344: 783–92.

Tarhini, A.A., Agarwala, S.S. Interleukin-2 for the treatment of melanoma. *Current Opinion in Investigational Drugs*. 2005; 6: 1234–9.

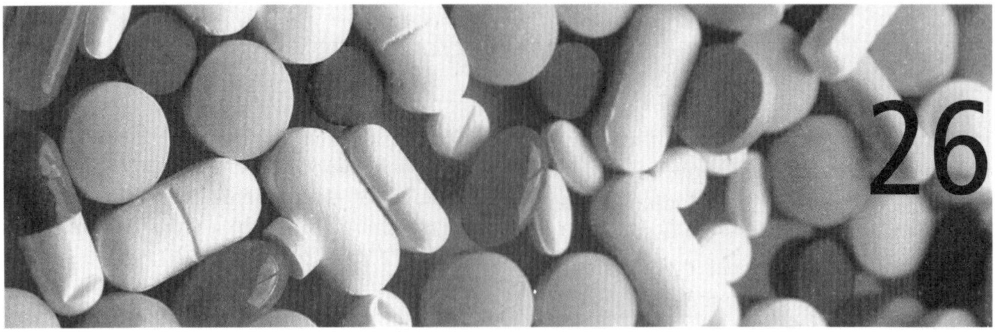

Outlook for Cancer Vaccine Development

AN ERA OF CHANGE FOR CANCER THERAPY

With the rapid incorporation of monoclonal antibodies (MAbs) into oncology therapy, an environment of acceptance of new biologic therapies – including cancer vaccines – as a viable therapeutic approach is forming. Genentech and ImClone's highly visible and successful 2004 MAb launches (bevacizumab [Avastin] and cetuximab [Erbitux], respectively) have increased anticipation for the next new therapy. Although Dendreon's long-awaited cancer vaccine, Provenge, has not yet delivered on earlier expectations, several vaccines, specifically Merck's Gardasil and GlaxoSmithKline's Cervarix, are rapidly approaching their filing dates and have the potential to initiate the therapeutic acceptance of cancer vaccines.

The gold standard for cancer treatment remains chemotherapy, but combination therapy, particularly combining chemotherapy agents with biologics, is on the rise. For many biopharmaceutical companies developing cancer therapies, including those companies developing MAbs, studies of emerging treatments as monotherapies and in combination with accepted chemotherapy regimens are an important part of their clinical trial strategies. Combination therapies consisting of multiple biologic agents are undergoing clinical study; such efforts include Cell Genesys and Medarex's investigation of a combination therapy involving MAbs and cancer vaccines. Because biologic therapies for cancer are often targeted at upregulating the immune system, these combination therapies have the potential to significantly improve outcomes with fairly low side-effect profiles compared with the often profound, long-term side effects and toxicities of chemotherapy agents.

In this chapter, we discuss the unmet needs in the cancer therapeutic market and identify how cancer vaccines may fulfill those needs. We outline the types of cancer vaccines and profile several vaccines in late-stage development. We identify challenges and opportunities facing cancer vaccines in view of their short history and discuss the outlook for the vaccine market.

CANCER VACCINES MAY FULFILL AN UNMET NEED

An Underserved Market

Today, more than 9.8 million people in the United States are living with cancer or have survived the disease, and about one in three (about 95 million people) will develop cancer. Cancer of all types results in more than 500,000 deaths in the United States each year, making the disease the second-leading cause of death in this country. In addition to surgery and radiotherapy, more than 100 FDA-approved drug therapies are available for the treatment of a variety of cancers. However, important unmet needs remain: many of these therapies cause severe side effects and many types of cancer still lack effective therapies. There is enormous potential for cancer vaccine products that offer both palliative and curative solutions.

Most cancer patients are treated with some combination of surgery, radiation, and chemotherapy. Each year in the United States, more than 800,000 patients with cancer undergo chemotherapy. Radiation and chemotherapy have the disadvantage of destroying healthy as well as malignant cells and thus can cause debilitating side effects, including nausea, vomiting, and risk of infection from the suppression of the immune system.

Of the approximately 1.4 million new cases of cancer diagnosed in the United States each year, more than 90% are solid tumors. Solid tumors, in general, are the least susceptible to conventional treatments; in 2005, an estimated 39% of diagnosed cases are expected to end in death.

Nearly one-third of cancer patients diagnosed with localized disease will experience recurrence following surgical removal of the tumor. Although the goal of resection is to remove the entire tumor and some of the surrounding tissue, this end is not always achieved. Research has demonstrated that if even a small amount of tumor remains, tumor regrowth will occur. Systemic chemotherapy and radiation are the current standards of care to reduce postoperative tumor regrowth, but more precisely targeted therapies are needed. Cancer vaccines fight tumor cells and the environment supportive of tumor-cell growth by harnessing the specificity of immune mechanisms.

Cancer vaccines are designed to stimulate the immune system to identify and remove aberrant cancer cells from the body. Vaccines targeting cancer are meant to treat existing disease and/or prevent the resurgence of disease in the future. They may contain cells, parts of cells, or antigens along with formulation ingredients and an adjuvant.

The short history of cancer vaccines to date involves false starts, little real treatment benefit, and disappointing outcomes, but, fortunately, it has displayed none of the side effects or dramatic failures that have plagued the development of gene therapy. The initial excitement about cancer vaccines developed in the early 1990s with the discovery of cytotoxic T-cell (CTL) response, providing insight into how the immune system is activated to upregulate its response against cancer cells. Cancer vaccines may emerge from a difficult start and be incorporated into standard treatment regimens by the end of the decade (Table 26.1) by addressing the many challenges of cancer treatment.

Demand for cancer vaccines is fueled by the prospect of avoiding the toxicities (and hence side effects) associated with standard chemotherapy regimens. Initially, attempts

Table 26.1 Late-stage Cancer Vaccines: Anticipated Regulatory Filings

Vaccine	*Indication*	*Company*	*Country/Region*	*Earliest Filing Date*
Gardasil	HPV infection, cervical cancer, genital warts	Merck	Europe	Late 2005
Cervarix	HPV infection, cervical cancer	GlaxoSmithKline (MedImmune)	Europe	2006
Provenge	Prostate cancer	Dendreon	United States	2006
GVAX	Prostate cancer	Cell Genesys	United States	2007
Insegia	Pancreatic cancer	Aphton (Sanofi-Pasteur)	Switzerland, Canada, Australia	2004
PanVac-VF	Pancreatic cancer	Therion Biologics	United States	2006
Canvaxin	Melanoma	CancerVax (Serono)	Europe, United States	2007
Oncophage	Melanoma	Antigenics	United States	2006

HPV = Human papillomavirus

were made to incorporate single tumor antigens or just a few tumor antigens into a vaccine. As more antigens have been identified and some autologous tumor vaccines have shown positive results, new vaccine designs tend to be multivalent. Incorporating complexity into the vaccine is a means of addressing the changing expression of cancer-cell antigens as the disease progresses. Vaccines may also address the tumor-cell environment as well as the tumor itself, further confounding the tumor's ability to remain viable.

Cancer Vaccine Varieties

Several types of cancer vaccines are under development: subunit, DNA, autologous cell, and allogeneic cell. The vaccine designs can be described as follows:

- Subunit vaccines for cancer have grown out of expanded discovery programs that identified numerous antigens that were sequenced and subsequently produced for incorporation into vaccines.
- DNA vaccines generally utilize a viral vector to deliver the genetic material needed to elicit the desired immunological response but can also use synthetic vectors, including a variety of lipid systems, as well as plasmids and naked DNA.
- Autologous cell vaccines utilize tumor cells, T cells, and other immune cells that are derived from the patient. These cells are treated ex vivo by a proprietary process that imparts therapeutic qualities to the cells and are then returned to the patient as an activated vaccine.
- Allogeneic cell-based vaccines are generally created from established tumor cell lines that are derived from a master cell bank and may be genetically altered to provide specific capabilities such as additional antigens or cytokine release.

Table 26.2 compares the advantages and disadvantages of these vaccines.

PREVENTIVE CANCER VACCINE LAUNCHES

HPV Prevention: A Multibillion-dollar Opportunity

In contrast to traditional vaccines against infectious agents that are designed to prevent infection, most cancer vaccines under development will be used as therapeutic agents with the patient receiving doses of the vaccine over a specified time period to maintain immune system vigilance. However, certain types of cancers are linked to infectious agents, and the first cancer vaccines that will have global launches will be preventive and directed against a specific virus. Therefore, these vaccines will substantially reduce the incidence of the associated cancer.

Alterations in the immune system contribute to the development and progression of cancer.

Table 26.2 Types of Vaccines

Vaccine Type	*Description*	*Advantages*	*Disadvantages*	*Examples*
Subunit	Single or multiple tumor-specific or tumor-associated antigens	Standard vaccine product Clear regulatory path Existing manufacturing technology	Immunological escape	PanVac-VF (Therion Biologics)
DNA	DNA vectors used to deliver tumor-associated antigens and/or stimulate immune system	Targeted Produces a highly specific, persistent response	Viral vector alteration to eliminate infection and gene loading	Oncolytic Virus Therapy (Cell Genesys)
Autologous cell	Cells collected from patient, modified ex vivo, returned to patient as vaccine	Multivalent Short lead time Less costly development	Difficult quality control Challenging regulatory and business environment	Provenge (Dendreon)
Allogeneic cell	Modified cells from cell lines	Multivalent Capacity for innovative cell modification Clear regulatory path	Long lead time to establish master cell bank Costly development	GVAX (Cell Genesys) Canvaxin (CancerVax)

Worldwide, about 17% of incident cancer is the result of inadequate immunity to infection. A key example is cervical carcinoma, in which nearly 100% of the cases are associated with human papillomavirus (HPV) infection. Currently, Merck and GlaxoSmithKline (GSK) are developing vaccines to prevent HPV infection. The peak-year sales for each of these emerging products is estimated at more than $1 billion.

HPV Vaccines in Development

Both Merck and GSK's HPV vaccines are progressing through Phase III clinical studies and have reported positive data from all trials to date. We discuss these vaccines in the following sections.

Merck's Gardasil

Merck is developing Gardasil, a vaccine for the prevention of HPV infection related to cervical cancer and genital warts. Gardasil is formulated with the adjuvant alum and is a quadravalent HPV vaccine, targeting four different HPV subtypes: 6, 11, 16, and 18. HPV types 16 and 18 cause approximately 70% of cervical cancers, and HPV types 6 and 11 cause approximately 90% of genital warts. Gardasil is expected to be the first cervical cancer vaccine approved worldwide and to be the only vaccine against both cervical cancer and genital warts. Merck plans to file a biologics license application (BLA) in the later part of 2005.

Merck's Phase III trial is studying the effect of the vaccine on all four HPV subtypes. Analysis of two years of data for the vaccine demonstrated that it is effective against the HPV 16 subtype and showed it to be 100% effective in preventing infection in patients who had not been previously exposed to the virus.

CSL exclusively licensed a portfolio of intellectual property to Merck in 1995 that became the basis of Gardasil. A patent was issued to CSL in Australia in 2002 covering the methods of manufacturing virus-like particle (VLP) HPV and the vaccine itself; the US patent was issued in 2003. Subsequent to a patent cross-license and settlement agreement in February 2005 between Merck and GSK regarding HPV intellectual property, Merck will pay GSK a fee and royalties on sales upon product development and launch of Gardasil. CSL will receive milestone payments and royalties from both Merck and GSK. Merck will market Gardasil in partnership with Sanofi-Aventis.

GlaxoSmithKline's Cervarix

Cervarix, GSK's recombinant HPV vaccine for the prevention of cervical cancer, is undergoing Phase III clinical trials, which began in 2004. Cervarix (formerly MEDI-517) is a VLP vaccine designed to elicit an immune response against HPV.

Results from Phase II studies showed 100% efficacy in preventing persistent HPV infection by the two HPVs associated with the highest risk of cervical cancer: HPV types 16 and 18.

GSK is developing Cervarix with MedImmune, following a December 1997 agreement that gave GSK an exclusive license for certain patents and know-how for the development of an HPV vaccine. Subsequent to the patent cross-license and settlement agreement discussed in the previous section, GSK sublicensed the rights to MedImmune's HPV patents to Merck. Cervarix is manufactured using insect recombinant technology that GSK licensed from CSL and the formulation incorporates Corixa's Monophosphoryl Lipid A (MPL) adjuvant. On April 29, 2005, GSK announced that it would acquire Corixa in a stock transaction valued at approximately $300 million.

Gardasil and Cervarix: Competitive Positioning

Although both vaccines are anticipated to prevent the majority of cervical cancers, Gardasil is expected to be positioned as a sexually transmitted disease (STD) vaccine to prevent both HPV infection and genital warts while GSK is expected to position

Cervarix as a preventive vaccine for cervical cancer. By marketing its product as a vaccination against an infectious disease, Merck may be able to gain an initial advantage for its product. This strategy places Gardasil in the same category as hepatitis B and MMR (measles, mumps, rubella) vaccines, opening up the possibility of incorporating Gardasil into a standard vaccination regimen.

Merck is also projected to have a market launch lead of six months to one year over GSK. Although this lead gives Merck market exclusivity for a period of time, it also entrusts and requires Merck to take the lead in educating the marketplace – a time-consuming and expensive proposition from which GSK will ultimately benefit. GSK will enter a primed market with Cervarix and will be able to focus its efforts on garnering market share based on the agent's potential efficacy and cost advantages.

Gardasil's adjuvant, alum, compares poorly next to Corixa's MLP adjuvant used in Cervarix. In a study comparing the effectiveness of these adjuvants at 210 days, the antibody levels for both HPV16 and HPV18 using MLP were more than double the antibody concentration of alum for HPV16 and more than quadruple that for HPV18. GSK uses insect recombinant manufacturing in Cervarix, which may offer certain cost advantages of production scale.

The acquisition of Corixa will boost GSK's profit margins on Cervarix by eliminating milestone fees and royalties, giving the company an additional competitive edge over Merck's Gardasil. In addition, based on vaccine design, formulation, and manufacturing, GSK appears to have the long-term advantage; however, Merck can make up its revenue share with the expanded market breadth of Gardasil.

NO IMMEDIATE LAUNCH FOR THERAPEUTIC VACCINES

Therapeutic cancer vaccines, which are designed to give the immune system a boost to stave off the disease, have hit road blocks in clinical trials. Patients in clinical trials continue to benefit from the administration of therapeutic cancer vaccines, but often the benefit is not enough to meet the primary end point(s).

Several therapeutic cancer vaccines are undergoing Phase III clinical trials, but the results have been mixed. CancerVax's Canvaxin stage IV melanoma trial was recently discontinued and Dendreon's Provenge has not moved beyond Phase III. The regularity of disappointments in late-stage trials is cause for concern and demands a certain caution when viewing this market segment in the near term. Yet, promise remains that these therapeutic cancer vaccines will have an important treatment role in the not-too-distant future. In the following subsections, we review the leading Phase III therapeutic cancer vaccines by indication.

Prostate Cancer

Dendreon's Provenge

Provenge, Dendreon's therapeutic vaccine targeting dendritic cells, received fast-track designation from the FDA for the treatment of men diagnosed with asymptomatic, metastatic, androgen-independent prostate cancer and a Gleeson score of seven or less. (Gleeson score is a measure of the aggressiveness of a patient's tumor ranging from 2 to 10.) Provenge is an autologous vaccine prepared from a patient's dendritic cells obtained via leukopheresis (cells are removed from an individual and later transferred back into that individual) and combined, ex vivo, with Dendreon's delivery system. The cells are then returned to the patient in an intravenous infusion. Provenge is based on Dendreon's proprietary Antigen Delivery Cassette technology, a delivery system that incorporates PAP protein fragments. The vaccine activates the immune system's T cells to identify and destroy prostate cancer cells containing PAP, which are present on approximately 95% of prostate cancer cells.

Provenge is being evaluated in a Phase III clinical trial (D-9902B) under a Special

Protocol Assessment agreement with the FDA. The study is still enrolling patients at this time. D-9902A was a Phase III study that was stopped in 2002 when analysis of D-9901, an earlier original Phase III trial, showed no significant improvement in time to disease progression. Preliminary data from D-9902A were released in mid-January 2005, and the analysis of the primary end point, time to disease progression, was not statistically significant. The secondary end point, overall survival, showed improvement that was similar to that shown in D-9901. There was, however, a benefit observed in a subgroup of patients who had Gleason scores of 7 or less; the D-9902A protocol was amended to include only this subgroup and became D-9902B.

The results of the three-year intent-to-treat analysis of D-9901 were first reported in October 2004 and showed a statistically significant survival benefit. Patients receiving Provenge had a median survival of 25.9 months compared with 21.4 months for patients receiving placebo independent of Gleason score. At 36 months, 34% of the patients receiving Provenge remained alive versus 11% of patients receiving placebo. This survival analysis included 127 patients who had asymptomatic, metastatic, androgen-independent prostate cancer. Patients receiving Provenge experienced an improvement of 4.5 months over the median survival rate and, compared with patients receiving placebo, had a threefold improvement in survival.

Cell Genesys's GVAX

Cell Genesys's GVAX prostate cancer vaccine is undergoing Phase III clinical trials in hormone-refractory patients who have failed surgical intervention and chemotherapy and are experiencing disease recurrence. GVAX is a cell-based vaccine consisting of tumor cells obtained from a tumor cell line that have been irradiated and genetically modified to secrete granulocyte-macrophage colony-stimulating factor (GM-CSF). The vaccine stimulates the immune system by exposing dendritic cells to multiple antigens at the vaccination site, resulting in the production of antibodies against the patient's tumor. GVAX is not patient-specific and is manufactured in a process similar to that of other approved biologics in a current good manufacturing process (cGMP) facility.

The first of two planned Phase III clinical trials is taking place: Vaccine ImmunoTherapy with Allogeneic Prostate Cancer Cell Lines 1 (VITAL-1) (G-0029), which is expected to enroll 600 patients with metastatic hormone-refractory prostate cancer. Patients must have radiologic evidence of metastatic disease and no prior exposure to chemotherapy. The multicenter US trial will include patients with any Gleason score as well as metastatic disease in both skeletal and nonskeletal sites although patients must be asymptomatic with respect to pain. The trial will compare the GVAX vaccine with Sanofi-Aventis's Taxotere (docetaxel) chemotherapy, currently considered the standard of care for prostate cancer treatment. The study's primary end point is a demonstration of at least 33% improvement in survival duration. The trial is being conducted under a Special Protocol Assessment from the FDA.

In Cell Genesys's second Phase III clinical trial of GVAX in prostate cancer, VITAL-2, GVAX plus chemotherapy will be compared with chemotherapy alone. The trial was expected to begin during the first half of 2005. It will include patients experiencing bone pain and will provide clinicians with information regarding the use of GVAX with docetaxel.

Data reported in June 2004 from Cell Genesys's second Phase II clinical trial of GVAX in hormone-refractory prostate cancer confirmed the clinical activity of the vaccine. Dose response was confirmed along with the demonstration of prostate cancer antibody induction. The highest dose level evaluated in the trial resulted in the best immune response and was well tolerated by patients; the same dose level is being used in the Phase III trials. The bone scans of patients with positive metastatic prostate cancer were shown to stabilize in 43% of patients (31 of 72), and 62% of patients (34 of 55) experienced improvement or stabilization in bone metastatic activity as measured by carboxy-terminal telopeptide of type I collagen (ICTP), a biochemical marker used to measure bone destruction. Two patients showed normal bone scans following treatment.

In the first Phase II clinical trial of GVAX monotherapy in hormone-refractory prostate cancer patients, 34 of 55 patients had metastatic disease with radiologic evidence. Patients were assigned to either a low-dose or high-dose group. Patients who received the high dose had a median survival of 34.9 months and patients receiving the low dose had a survival time of 24 months compared with an 18-month median survival for docetaxel-treated prostate cancer patients with bone metastases.

Pancreatic Cancer

Aphton's Insegia

Aphton's antigastrin 17 vaccine (Insegia) for gastrointestinal cancers is in Phase III clinical trials. In the European Union (EU) and North America, the vaccine is being developed in partnership with Sanofi-Pasteur. Insegia is made up of a portion of the gastrin 17 hormone conjugated to diphtheria toxoid. The diphtheria toxoid is used as a carrier and provides a means of internalization by B cells and subsequent production of antibodies. The diphtheria toxoid-bound gastrin 17 is combined with a proprietary delivery system to provide sustained antibody response. The vaccine targets and neutralizes G17 and the hormone Gly-G17. Production of Insegia involves standard vaccine-manufacturing technology and is not patient-specific.

Sanofi recently completed a randomized, double-blind Phase III clinical trial of Insegia versus placebo for the treatment of patients with advanced pancreatic cancer. In June 2004, at the Annual American Society of Clinical Oncology (ASCO), data from the completed trial were reported. Results showed that patients treated with Insegia had a median survival of 150 days versus 83 days with placebo. Insegia-treated patients also had a significantly longer time to deterioration, a median of 138 days compared with 78 days for patients receiving placebo. Additionally, patients who generated antigastrin 17 antibodies (Insegia responders) had a median survival of 176 days versus 63 days for nonresponders and 83 days for placebo.

In a second Phase III clinical study in advanced pancreatic cancer, Insegia was administered with gemcitabine versus a control group, who received gemcitabine and placebo. Preliminary data from the Insegia/gemcitabine trial were released in February 2005. Although approximately 70% of patients demonstrated an antibody response and showed prolonged survival, the primary end point of improving overall survival was not achieved.

Based on data from the Insegia monotherapy trial, Aphton has filed for marketing approval for the treatment of patients with advanced pancreatic cancer who are either intolerant to or refuse chemotherapy.

Therion Biologics' PanVac-VF

PanVac-VF is in Phase III clinical trials for patients with metastatic pancreatic cancer who have failed a gemcitabine-containing regimen. The vaccine targets two antigens, carcinoembryonic antigen (CEA) and mucin-1 (MUC-1), found on more than 90% of pancreatic tumor cells. The vaccine incorporates Therion's proprietary costimulatory molecules, TRICOM. TRICOM consists of three costimulatory molecules (B7.1, ICAM-1, and LFA-3) known to elicit strong cellular immune responses and provide a sustained effect.

Therion's PanVac-VF Phase III pancreatic cancer clinical trial is being conducted under a Special Protocol Assessment from the FDA. The study will enroll 250 patients at up to 60 centers in the United States. The site investigator chooses whether patients receive PanVac-VF in combination with GM-CSF, supportive care, or palliative chemotherapy. The primary end point is overall survival; secondary end points include quality of life, changes in levels of serum CEA and CA19–9, response rate, and safety. Two Phase I clinical trials of PanVac-VF demonstrated a median overall survival of 5.3 months and 7.9 months, respectively, compared with 3 months for historical controls. If results from this Phase III clinical trial are positive, Therion anticipates filing a BLA in 2006.

Melanoma

CancerVax's Canvaxin

CancerVax and its development partner, Serono, are investigating Canvaxin in a Phase III clinical trial involving patients with stage III melanoma. Canvaxin is a whole-cell tumor vaccine that contains at least 38 tumor-associated antigens. The polyvalent vaccine uses irradiated cells from an allogeneic tumor-cell line to create an off-the-shelf product manufactured under cGMP. Canvaxin is administered with bacillus Calmette-Guerin (BCG), a vaccine adjuvant. In December 2004, CancerVax entered into a development and commercialization agreement with Serono that included US copromotion rights for CancerVax.

In 2004, the enrollment of 1,160 patients for the stage III melanoma trial was completed. An interim analysis is planned for the third quarter of 2005. The vaccine has proven safe in trials to date. CancerVax anticipates filing with regulatory authorities in the European Union and United States in 2007.

On April 5, 2005, CancerVax announced that its Phase III clinical trial of Canvaxin for stage IV melanoma would be discontinued. The decision follows the recommendation by the independent Data and Safety Monitoring Board (DSMB), which completed its second interim analysis of the Phase III trial for stage IV melanoma. The DSMB concluded that it was unlikely that additional data would show a survival benefit compared with patients receiving placebo. Enrollment of 496 patients of the planned 670 patients for this trial had been completed, but further enrollment was discontinued.

Antigenics' Oncophage

Antigenics' lead cancer vaccine candidate, Oncophage (HSPPC-96), is an autologous vaccine in Phase III clinical trials for renal carcinoma and metastatic melanoma. The vaccine is produced by harvesting tumor cells from the patient that are then shipped to Antigenics' facility. Using its proprietary process, the company isolates the heat shock protein gp96 and its associated peptides. Following extraction, purification, and sterilization via filtration, the autologous product is placed in vials, frozen, and shipped back to administration for injecting into the patient.

Enrollment for a Phase III melanoma trial (Study C-100–21) was completed in 2004. The final analysis for the study is expected in mid-2005 and will commence once a prespecified number of events (recurrence or death) occur. The Phase III trial involves sites in the United States, Canada, Europe, Israel, and Russia. In September 2003, citing concerns over Antigenics' manufacturing processes, the FDA halted all Phase III clinical trials involving Oncophage. Antigenics was able to resume trials in November 2003. Further details regarding the FDA's clinical hold are discussed in a later section (Regulatory Obstacles).

In a Phase II clinical trial of Oncophage combination therapy with GM-CSF and interferon-alpha in patients with stage IV melanoma, treatment was given postsurgery to 18 evaluable patients. One patient remained disease-free for 419 days. Ten of sixteen patients with residual melanoma following surgery showed disease stabilization that lasted 97–372 days. Six of the sixteen patients demonstrated an increase in antimelanoma immune response and all of these patients experienced disease stabilization.

Other Vaccines

Oncophage for Renal Carcinoma

Antigenics is also sponsoring clinical studies of Oncophage for use in renal-cell carcinoma. Results of a Phase II clinical trial showed that 21 of the 61 patients with renal carcinoma who received at least one dose of Oncophage were clinically responsive. Of the 21 patients, one patient remains disease-free after 2.5 years. Patients who progressed during

Oncophage treatment received interleukin 2 (IL-2). Seven of the sixteen patients with disease progression stabilized following administration of IL-2. For patients who received Oncophage, the median progression-free survival was 18 weeks; for patients who also received IL-2, progression-free survival was 25 weeks. After two years, 30% of all patients have survived.

Enrollment for the renal carcinoma Phase III clinical trial (Study C-100–12, Part I) was completed in 2004.

In February, following a meeting with the FDA regarding the proposed registration plan for Oncophage in renal-cell carcinoma, Antigenics initiated Part II of its Phase III clinical studies and began patient enrollment. The company plans to consult the FDA regarding acceptance of Part I data for filing a BLA, while Part II of the Phase III trial continues.

Aphton's IGN-101 for Non-small-cell Lung Cancer

Aphton's recent acquisition of Igeneon, which closed on March 24, 2005, gave the company its second vaccine candidate, IGN-101, which is in Phase II/III clinical trials for the treatment of advanced non-small-cell lung cancer (NSCLC). IGN-101 triggers an immune response to epithelial cell adhesion molecule (EpCAM), a membrane protein that can be expressed on epithelial cancer cells. It selectively destroys disseminated tumor cells and so may prevent or delay the formation of metastases. EpCAM is overexpressed in most epithelial cancers, which account for approximately 70% of all cancers. IGN-101 is an off-the-shelf product comprising the murine anti-EpCAM MAb 17 1-A adsorbed on aluminum hydroxide.

Phase I studies found a significant reduction in the number of circulating tumor cells in the blood. A Phase II trial showed that the vaccine induces a strong immune response (95% seroconversion rate) despite concomitant chemotherapy. In 2001, the company launched a placebo-controlled Phase II/III study involving 750 subjects with NSCLC; the study is ongoing.

Future of Near-term Therapeutic Vaccines

Two key factors among these late-stage clinical development programs warrant caution regarding near-term therapeutic cancer vaccine development: regulatory obstacles associated with autologous vaccines and the potential for marginal efficacy. Both factors affect the likelihood of approval as well as the longer-term commercialization potential.

Regulatory Obstacles

The production of autologous cancer vaccines presents issues of product characterization and reproducibility that reduce the likelihood that this type of vaccine will become widely used. During the 1990s, many companies began developing autologous cell vaccines, particularly in Europe, where hospital-based therapies provided by physicians are not subject to the same tight regulatory scrutiny as in the United States. However, evolving regulations of biologics manufacturing, particularly in the United States, challenge manufacturers to meet the standards for quality and reproducibility. The FDA's actions in scrutinizing the practices of autologous vaccine production have made it clear that decentralized manufacturing must meet the same standards for quality control as other biologics manufacturing.

One of the first companies to come under FDA scrutiny in the 1990s for its autologous vaccine production was Avax, whose vaccine manufacturing process was completed locally in a hospital laboratory. More recently, similar circumstances have surrounded Antigenics' autologous vaccines regardless of the fact that the company's manufacturing is centralized. In Antigenics' Phase III clinical trials for melanoma, as much as 30% of its vaccine production failed and the FDA cited the company for its lack of quality and reproducibility. In September 2003, the FDA imposed a clinical hold on both Antigenics' melanoma (Study C-100–21, Part I) and renal carcinoma (Study C-100–12, Part I) Phase III clinical trials on the grounds that inadequate data supported specifications for product purity, identity, potency, and pH. Antigenics submitted its response on October 22, 2003, and on November 24, 2003, the FDA lifted the clinical hold, advising the company to reduce variability among assay readings and suggesting additional quality control improvements.

In February, following a meeting with the FDA regarding the proposed registration plan for Oncophage in renal-cell carcinoma, Antigenics initiated Part II of its Phase III clinical studies and began patient enrollment. Antigenics plans to consult the FDA regarding acceptance of Part I data from the renal carcinoma trial for filing a BLA while Part II of the Phase III clinical continues. The company does not plan to use the Part I Phase III clinical study in melanoma in a registration document because of the high failure rate of its vaccine-manufacturing process.

In contrast to autologous vaccines, allogeneic vaccines are created from cells derived from master cell banks and follow the traditional biopharmaceutical model for both regulatory path and manufacturing. Production of allogeneic vaccines, as with other biologics, is centralized in a GMP facility. By meeting the standards established for biotherapeutics manufacturing, allogeneic vaccines can follow a regulatory path that is consistent with industry practices, and drug developers can focus on efficacy rather than on creating new regulatory procedures and standards – a time-consuming activity that incorporates more obstacles into the regulatory process.

Potential for Marginal Efficacy

Cancer vaccines studied to date have not provided remarkable efficacy in clinical trials and have often resulted in failed clinical end points. Although several factors may contribute to this problem, vaccine design is certainly a key element in improving efficacy. For example, cancer vaccines may include a specific antigen type, like Antigenics' Oncophage, or multiple antigens, as seen in Dendreon's Provenge vaccine. Multivalent vaccines may increase the likelihood of providing the desired immune response in the complex and changing tumor-cell environment. In addition, vaccine designs are increasingly including a mechanism for further boosting the immune system, such as delivering an upregulating stimulus of GM-CSF that is incorporated into the vaccine, as in Cell Genesys's GVAX cancer vaccine.

As the gatekeepers of the immune system via their antigen-presenting role, dendritic cells remain a focus in cancer vaccine development. A key challenge with dendritic cell vaccines is antigen loading and maturation, which give rise to limited immunogenicity. Dendreon uses a strategy to enhance dendritic vaccines via stimulation of the maturation processes of ex vivo cytokines including GM-CSF, IL-4, tumor necrosis factor-alpha (TNF-alpha), IL-6, and IL-beta. Another approach is to use altered viruses to introduce the appropriate genes in vivo into dendritic cells. BioVex has developed technology to enhance antigen loading into dendritic cells using viruses. BioVex uses the inactivated herpes simplex virus (HSV) to infect dendritic cells and deliver antigen-encoded genes.

The incorporation of SOCS1, an inhibitory protein that limits the immunogenicity of dendritic cells, can also improve the effectiveness of dendritic-cell vaccines. Using siRNA to silence SOCS1, Baylor researchers were able to increase the immunogenicity and effectiveness of dendritic vaccines. Viral loading may make it possible to transfect dendritic cells with both siRNA targeting SOCS1 and tumor antigens, resulting in a vaccine that could have improved therapeutic value.

EMERGING APPROACHES TO CANCER VACCINE DEVELOPMENT

Harnessing the immune system to remove cancer cells via vaccines presents an array of opportunities for innovation. Although many types of vaccines can be utilized, there is a preference for allogeneic, or "druggable," vaccines, both from a regulatory and business model standpoint. Technologies that enhance the effectiveness of these off-the-shelf vaccines, moving further away from an approach requiring autologous therapy, will remain central to the ultimate success of vaccine development.

Three emerging strategies could help therapeutic cancer vaccines progress beyond the challenges they currently face in clinical trials:

- Using therapeutic vaccines in combination therapies, particularly with other biologics such as MAbs.
- Administering the therapeutic vaccine earlier in the course of the disease.
- Focusing on combination designs that both boost the immune system and suppress its specific dysfunctions.

Emergence of Combination Therapy

Using multiple therapeutic approaches to treat cancer makes sense given the complexity of the disease. Currently, combination treatments are being incorporated into single vaccines with success. In the clinic, using more than one therapy is the emerging standard of care as new biologics are studied in combination trials with chemotherapy and other biologics. In addition, combination approaches that produce cytokines (e.g., GM-CSF) and upregulate the immune system have potential, as seen with Cell Genesys's GVAX vaccine.

Cell Genesys is also studying its GVAX vaccine in combination with Medarex's MDX-010, a fully human anti-CTLA-4 antibody. CTLA-4 is a molecule found on T cells that is thought to suppress the immune system. This combination therapy demonstrated an antitumor effect when used in Phase I clinical trials in patients with ovarian cancer and melanoma. Cell Genesys is studying the combination therapy in a Phase I trial in patients with prostate cancer. The combination of removing immune system suppression via MDX-010 with upregulation via GVAX may be an approach that will be used in the future.

In February 2005, Dendreon reported results from its National Cancer Institute-sponsored proof-of-concept Phase II clinical trial (P-16) that combines Provenge with Genentech's Avastin (bevacizumab). The study involved 22 androgen-dependent patients who had relapsed following surgery and radiation treatment and found that prostate-specific antigen doubling time (PSADT) had increased. (PSADT is used as a measure of prostate cancer disease biology.) The study investigator suggests that the combination of Provenge and Avastin, or other combinations of immune therapies, may be useful in the treatment of prostate cancer.

Importance of Therapeutic Timing

The timing of cancer vaccine administration (i.e., when vaccines are used in the course of disease and treatment) could make a difference in their effectiveness. In a study in mice, researchers at Johns Hopkins showed that the mice became accustomed to having cancer and their immune systems adjusted to the presence of cancer. As a result, their immune systems recognized the disease but failed to mount an attack because they had become tolerant to slow-growing cancer. The researchers found that vaccines used early in the disease course activated the immune system and the tumor shrunk in response. For prostate cancer, the study suggested administering hormone therapy followed by a vaccine, thus allowing the immune system time to adjust and upregulate, rather than giving the vaccine at the height of the disease process when the cancer has already progressed. The Hopkins researchers stated that less than 20% of men with prostate cancer respond to vaccines alone (Drake, 2005).

Multitarget Design Enhancements

Target structures for cytotoxic T lymphocytes were recently well characterized via expression cloning. These targets include tumor-antigen proteins that are overexpressed such as HER-2, P53, and CEA; differentiation antigens such as tyrosinase and MAGE; mutant tumor proteins such as CDK4R24C; and viral oncoproteins like HPV-E6 and HPV-E7. All of these targets are available for cancer-vaccination trials, and newer allogeneic vaccines may incorporate multiple specific antigens along with a means of boosting cytokine production or silencing immune suppression caused by the cancer. Such a multivalent, multipathway design could increase the potential for cancer vaccine efficacy.

The effect of identifying these targets has been shown to date in MAb trials where increased efficacy has been seen in patients expressing specific antigens associated with specific types of cancer. Assays have been developed to identify responders versus nonresponders, and clinical trials have verified the correlation of response versus nonresponse to treatment compared with antigen expression.

MARKET OUTLOOK FOR CANCER VACCINES

In 2003, the market for solid tumor cancer therapeutics totaled $28 billion worldwide; by 2009, the market could exceed $60 billion (Figure 26.1). We project that growth in the cancer therapeutics market will be fueled by the following market drivers:

- Increased incidence and prevalence of cancer in developed countries.
- The introduction of treatments for previously untreated cancers.
- The availability of new, higher-value, premium-priced biologic therapies (Figure 26.2), including cancer vaccines.

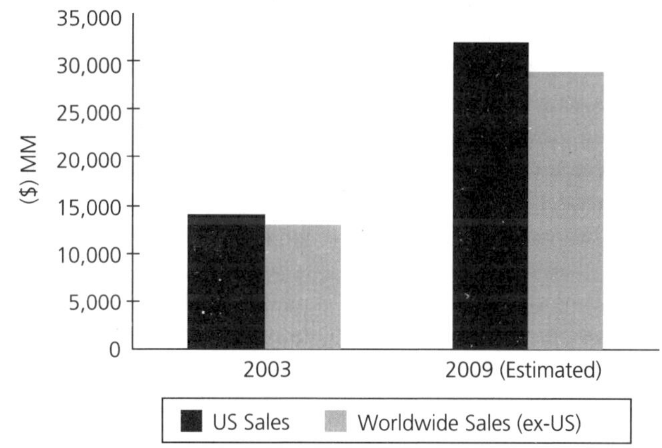

Figure 26.1 Sales of Solid Tumor Therapeutics

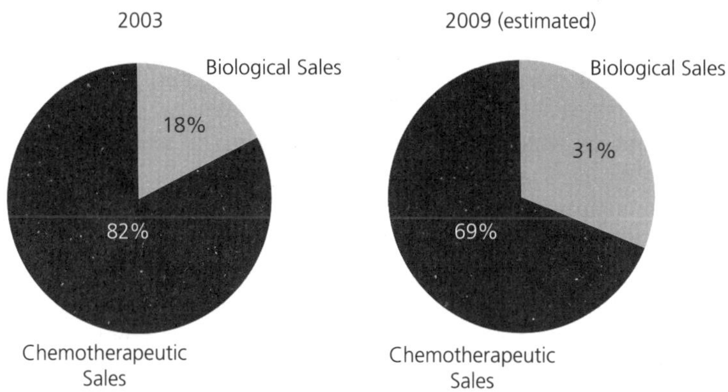

Figure 26.2 Growth in Sales of Biologics as Cancer Therapeutics

Although companies such as Dendreon are succeeding in their development of an autologous vaccine like Provenge, we believe that the use of autologous vaccines will be short-lived. The pharmaceutical industry's lack of interest in the business model of providing individualized therapies has, in part, contributed to the shift in focus toward allogeneic vaccine designs. Companies like Dendreon that have autologous products in late-stage development have had difficulty securing commercialization partners. As a result, more of the cancer vaccines currently under development follow the standard biologic product model using allogeneic components derived from cell lines to ensure quality, reproducibility, and cost-effective production, preferably using existing production facilities.

However, even companies developing allogeneic cancer vaccines that follow standard off-the-shelf product manufacturing have gone to the partnering table late in the course of clinical development. For example, CancerVax closed its development and commercialization agreement with Serono in December 2004, late in its Phase III clinical trials of Canvaxin. This trend is in stark contrast to pharma's historical partnering entry point of Phase IIb or earlier due to the increasingly competitive partnering environment. This late-stage partnering points to a wait-and-see perspective among many pharma companies toward cancer vaccines as a viable platform technology. Two notable exceptions are Sanofi-Pasteur and GSK, both of which are less at risk entering the cancer vaccine area given their established, leading biological development programs, and both have cancer vaccines in development.

The one positive trend with respect to commercialization of the autologous vaccines is that medical device companies may develop an interest. Increasingly, medical device companies have been focusing on adding biopharmaceuticals to their franchises. For example, major medical device companies, including Medtronic, Boston Scientific, and Guidant, all have cardiovascular cell therapy programs under way with biotech partners. These companies and others may look to successful autologous cancer programs as another means of adding both products and technology to their portfolios. In particular, companies such as Dendreon that have created devices aiding in the production process, serving as delivery systems, or acting in other roles in cancer-vaccine therapies may attract the interest of medical device companies.

Despite a development path marred by disappointing results, the focus on cancer vaccines has been expanding over the past five years. In part, this growing focus is due to the exponential expansion of the immunology knowledge base, although transforming this science into commercially useful technology is a process that is still evolving. Some types of cancer vaccines are more likely to become commercially successful owing to their likelihood of clinical effectiveness, preferred regulatory path, and use of standard industry manufacturing and distribution channels. Many are being evaluated for cancers that currently have no satisfactory treatments, such as pancreatic and head and neck cancers; should such vaccines achieve regulatory clearance, the cancer therapeutic market will expand. These cancer vaccines may enter the market later than several MAb products already close to submission, and, consequently, cancer vaccine companies may need to conduct head-to-head trials or, more likely, combination therapy trials with any MAbs that are successfully launched, even for cancers associated with significant unmet need.

Some vaccines, such as those in development for cervical cancer, are preventive and are targeted at the persistent viral infection that is directly linked to the progression of cancer. In this case, preventing this cancer is even more compelling than treating the disease, and no preventive vaccines against the infection or the cancer yet exist. We anticipate that a rapid ramp-up in sales of HPV vaccines will fuel substantial market expansion.

We believe that combination therapies given as early as possible in disease progression will be the new paradigm for using therapeutic vaccines. Ultimately, cancer vaccines could find their place among other chemotherapy and biologic treatments incorporated in first- through third-line treatment regimens as well as in the adjuvant setting. We predict that cancer vaccines will be market additive, rather than serving as replacements for current therapies, and will therefore expand the overall market for cancer therapies.

REFERENCE

Drake, C. et al. Androgen ablation mitigates tolerance to a prostate/prostate cancer-restricted antigen. *Cancer Cell.* March 14, 2005; 7: 239–49.

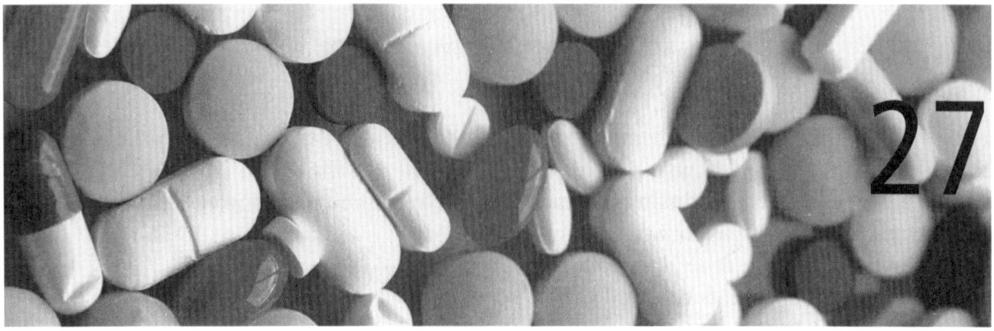

Advances Imminent in Antiangiogenesis Therapeutics

INTRODUCTION

Angiogenesis inhibitors have interested cancer researchers since 1971, when scientist and angiogenesis pioneer Judah Folkman first presented his finding in the *New England Journal of Medicine* that tumor growth depends on angiogenesis. Despite many efforts to develop angiogenesis inhibitors, this class of drugs has experienced a long and difficult road to market. After more than 30 years of research, angiogenesis inhibitors finally experienced a series of breakthroughs in 2004 and 2005, which began with the approval of Genentech's bevacizumab (Avastin).

The Food and Drug Administration's (FDA's) approval of bevacizumab for colon and rectum cancer in 2004 marked the entry of a new class of powerful drugs into the cancer market. Shortly thereafter, the FDA approved Eyetech Pharmaceuticals' pegaptanib (Macugen), demonstrating that angiogenesis inhibitors also impact ocular disease. Since the approval of these drugs, which essentially proved the concept of angiogenesis, interest in developing angiogenesis inhibitors has increased; in January 2005, for example, Pfizer announced plans to acquire Angiosyn, a company focused on developing angiogenesis inhibitors. Other Big Pharma have entered into agreements with smaller companies in order to enter this field. We expect to see more of these deals in the future.

As knowledge about angiogenesis has increased, researchers have discovered that several drugs already in the market (that work by other mechanisms of action) also have anti-angiogenic activity. Select examples of these drugs include Pfizer's celecoxib (Celebrex), ImClone Systems/Bristol-Myers Squibb/Merck KGaA's cetuximab (Erbitux), Genentech/Roche's trastuzumab (Herceptin), and AstraZeneca's gefitinib (Iressa). This chapter covers only the current and emerging therapies that are being developed and positioned as antiangiogenesis agents; it does not cover the many additional therapies that have been found to have antiangiogenic activities in addition to their primary mechanisms of actions.

OVERVIEW OF ANGIOGENESIS

Angiogenesis, or the formation of new blood vessels, is an essential element of human reproductive processes such as egg maturation, ovulation, rebuilding of the uterine lining after menstruation, and circulation between mother and fetus during pregnancy. In adult life, angiogenesis is involved in wound repair – it restores blood flow following injury (including ischemic injury) – and occurs in exercised muscle to increase blood supply. Angiogenesis also plays a key role in certain disease processes (cancer and other diseases) that are characterized by abnormal growth of blood vessels.

The family of vascular endothelial growth factors (VEGFs) and their receptors (VEGFRs) are key molecules in the angiogenesis process. The VEGF family includes VEGF-A, VEGF-B, VEGF-C, VEGF-D, and VEGF-E. VEGF-A is the most angiogenic, and the term *VEGF* is commonly used to refer to VEGF-A. In addition, multiple isoforms of VEGF have been identified. VEGF receptors include VEGFR-1 (also called flt-1) and VEGFR-2 (also called flt-1/KDR). These receptors are found on the surface of endothelial cells.

The angiogenic process begins with the production of VEGF. When VEGF (originally known as tumor-vascular permeability factor [VPF]) binds its receptors, gene expression is altered and the endothelial cells are activated. The existing blood vessels become vasodilated, and their permeability increases. In addition, the endothelial cells secrete enzymes that dissolve the basement membrane surrounding the blood vessels. New vessels begin to sprout as endothelial cells proliferate and migrate through newly formed holes in the existing vessels toward the source of the angiogenic stimulus. Their passage is aided by specialized molecules called cell adhesion molecules (CAMs). In addition, CAMs serve as anchoring molecules for endothelial cells as they migrate through the extracellular matrix (ECM; the tissue surrounding the blood vessel).

As the sprouting vessel migrates through the ECM, the ECM is remodeled to accommodate it. Matrix metalloproteinases (MMPs), secreted by the leading edge of migrating endothelial cells, degrade the ECM and thus aid cell movement. The migrating endothelial cells change shape to form vessel tubes. Ultimately, these tubes link up to form loops that can fully circulate blood (i.e., they can support both the supply of oxygenated blood and venous drainage). This process of angiogenesis is shown in Figure 27.1.

Potential targets for antiangiogenesis therapies include VEGF, VEGFR, the receptor tyrosine kinases of VEGFR (which are involved in the signaling process following

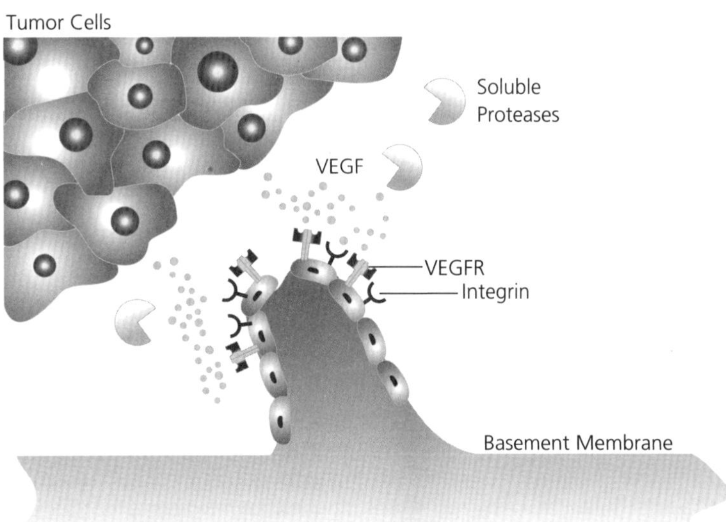

VEGF = Vascular endothelial growth factor
VEGFR = Vascular endothelial growth factor receptor

Figure 27.1 The Angiogenic Process

Table 27.1 Key Endogenous Activators of Angiogenesis

Angiogenic Factor	*Function*
Vascular endothelial growth factor (VEGF)	Mitogenic and motogenic for endothelial cells in vivo. Permeabilizes capillaries VEGF expression induced by *ras* oncogene and HIF-1α
Basic fibroblast growth factor-2 (bFGF-2)	Stimulates endothelial cell mitosis and migration in vitro. Mitogenic for fibroblasts, smooth-muscle cells, and neurons. Function may depend in part on VEGF
Acidic fibroblast growth factor-1 (aFGF-1)	Stimulates endothelial cell mitosis and migration in vitro
Platelet-derived endothelial cell growth factor (PD-ECGF)	Stimulates VEGF expression
Platelet-derived growth factor-BB (PDGF-BB)	Stimulates endothelial cell proliferation and migration
Hepatocyte growth factor (HGF)	Stimulates endothelial cell proliferation and migration
Epidermal growth factor (EGF)	Stimulates VEGF expression
Placental growth factor	Stimulates endothelial cell proliferation
Granulocyte-macrophage-colony stimulating factor (GM-CSF)	Mobilizes bone marrow endothelial precursor cells into the circulation. Increases endothelial cell-tube formation
Tumor necrosis factor-alpha (TNF-α)	Stimulates VEGF expression (derived from monocytes in synovial fluid, but not from fibroblasts)
Transforming growth factor-alpha (TGF-α)	Stimulates VEGF expression
Transforming growth factor-beta (TGF-β)	Stimulates VEGF expression
Interleukin-1-beta	Stimulates VEGF expression
Interleukin-6	Stimulates VEGF expression
Proliferin	Stimulates endothelial cell migration
Angiogenin	Mode of action unclear
Angiopoietin-1	Induces endothelial cell pericyte and smooth-muscle-cell recruitment into the vessel wall
Leptin	Mitogenic for endothelial cells
Thrombospondin 1	Destabilizes cell-ECM interaction, thereby promoting capillary sprout movement
Secreted protein acidic and rich in cysteine (SPARC)	Destabilizes cell-ECM interaction, thereby promoting capillary sprout movement
Tenascin C	Destabilizes cell-ECM interaction, thereby promoting capillary sprout movement
Developmental endothelial locus-1 (Del-1)	Promotes endothelial cell:integrin attachment and migration
Follistatin	Involved in endothelial cell migration
Pleiotrophin (PTN)	Stimulates endothelial cell proliferation and migration
Ras oncogene	Stimulates VEGF expression, decreases thrombospondin-1 expression

ECM = Extracellular matrix; HIF-1α = Hypoxia-inducible factor-1alpha

binding of VEGF to VEGFR), integrins, and the MMPs. In addition, researchers have identified numerous endogenous molecules that regulate the angiogenesis process. Table 27.1 lists examples of endogenous activators of angiogenesis; Table 27.2 shows endogenous inhibitors of angiogenesis. Blocking the endogenous activators of angiogenesis or upregulating the endogenous inhibitors of angiogenesis represent potential strategies that could be used in the development of antiangiogenesis therapies.

POTENTIAL THERAPEUTIC INDICATIONS

Angiogenesis is involved in the pathogenic disease process of several disorders, including cancer, age-related macular degeneration (AMD), diabetic retinopathy, rheumatoid arthritis, and psoriasis. Today, the two disorders that companies developing antiangiogenesis therapies target most frequently are cancer and AMD because these indications offer the largest market potential.

Table 27.2 Key Endogenous Inhibitors of Angiogenesis

Antiangiogenic Factor	*Function*
p53	Antiangiogenic tumor suppressor gene; upregulates thrombospondin-1 and downregulates VEGF and possibly IL-8
Interferon-beta (IFN-β)	Circulating angiogenesis inhibitor
Interferon-alpha (IFN-α)	Inhibits endothelial cell proliferation and migration
Interferon-gamma (IFN-γ)	Inhibits endothelial cell proliferation, migration, and tube formation
Platelet factor-4 (PF-4)	Circulating angiogenesis inhibitor; inhibits VEGF and EGF receptor binding
Angiostatin	Circulating angiogenesis inhibitor; cleaved from plasminogen by factors released from tumor cell. Inhibits endothelial cell proliferation and migration
Endostatin	Angiogenesis inhibitor; released from the ECM. Inhibits endothelial cell proliferation and migration
Thrombospondin-1	Angiogenesis inhibitor; released from the ECM. Inhibits endothelial cell proliferation and migration
Tissue inhibitors of metalloproteinases (TIMPs)	Angiogenesis inhibitors; released from ECM
Farnesyl transferase inhibitors	Inhibit expression of *ras* oncogene, which upregulates VEGF expression
Von Hippel-Lindau (VHL) protein	Tumor suppressor gene; inhibits VEGF expression
Prolactin fragment	Inhibits endothelial cell proliferation and migration
Antithrombin III	Inhibits endothelial cell proliferation
Interleukin-12 (IL-12)	Inhibits endothelial cell proliferation
Inducible protein-10 (IP-10)	Inhibits IL-8 and bFGF-induced angiogenesis
Vasostatin	Inhibits endothelial cell proliferation and migration
Canstatin	Inhibits endothelial cell migration and tube formation
Troponin I	Inhibits angiogenesis and tumor metastasis
2-Methoxyestradiol	Inhibits endothelial cell proliferation
Proliferin-related protein (PRP)	Inhibits endothelial cell migration
TNF-α	Downregulates expression of VEGFR-1 and VEGFR-2 on endothelial cells
Fibronectin fragment	Blocks endothelial cell attachment to the ECM, preventing cell migration
Plasminogen activator inhibitor (PAI)	Blocks endothelial cell migration through the ECM

bFGF = Basic fibroblast growth factor; ECM = Extracellular matrix; EGF = Epidermal growth factor; FGF = Fibroblast growth factor; IL = Interleukin; VEGF = Vascular endothelial growth factor; VEGFR-1 = Vascular endothelial growth factor-receptor-I; VEGFR-2 = Vascular endothelial growth factor-receptor-2

In this report, we focus on these two disease areas.

Cancer

Owing to the aforementioned work of Dr Judah Folkman, it is now known that tumor growth requires blood vessels to provide oxygen and nutrients to the tumor and to remove waste. Also, cancers must have access to blood vessels in order to metastasize. Formation of new blood vessels is necessary not only for solid tumors but also for hematological cancers, in which increased blood flow in the bone marrow can be seen. Figure 27.2 shows the key steps in tumor angiogenesis.

Angiogenesis inhibitors represent a promising new class of drugs for the treatment of cancer. These drugs offer several potential benefits for cancer treatment, compared with traditional chemotherapy. Angiogenesis inhibitors are typically less toxic than chemotherapeutic agents, and therefore it may be possible to treat patients with angiogenesis inhibitors on a longer-term basis to prevent tumor growth. In addition, because the antiangiogenesis agents work by a completely different mechanism than chemotherapy, it is possible to use angiogenesis inhibitors in combination with chemotherapy to enhance the activity of the cancer treatment. Finally, researchers have hypothesized that there is less risk of cancers developing resistance to antiangiogenesis inhibitors. Table 27.3 presents estimated cases of select cancers being targeted for treatment by the angiogenesis inhibitors that are currently on the market or in clinical development.

For several reasons, cancer represents a potentially significant market opportunity

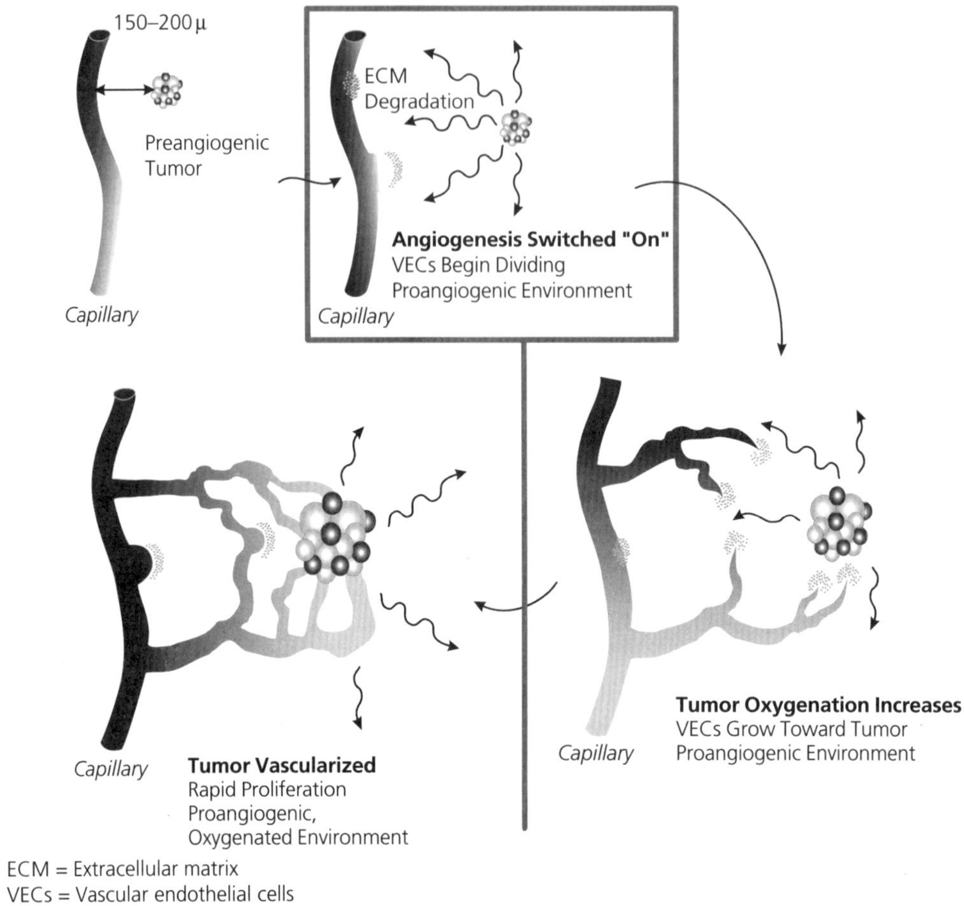

Figure 27.2 Steps in Tumor Angiogenesis

Table 27.3 Estimated Numbers of New Cases of Select Cancers Currently Targeted for Treatment with Angiogenesis Inhibitors in Development, 2005

Cancer	*Estimated New Cases*
Breast	212,930
Colorectal	145,290
Brain and other nervous system	18,500
Leukemia	34,810
Liver	17,550
Lung	172,570
Lymphoma	63,740
Melanoma	59,580
Multiple myeloma	15,980
Ovarian	22,220
Pancreatic	32,180
Prostate	232,090
Thyroid	25,690

for companies developing angiogenesis inhibitors. First, because a single antiangiogenic agent may target many different types of tumor, there is potential for a company to develop and market one drug for many cancer indications. Second, the cancer market is large and growing. The American Cancer Society reports that an estimated 1,372,910 new cases of cancer will be diagnosed in the United States in 2005 and that, as of January 2001, approximately 9.8 million people in the United States were living with a history of cancer. Finally, oncology drugs typically command premium pricing.

Age-related Macular Degeneration

AMD is an incurable disease of the eye that affects the macula (the central part of the retina in the back of the eye). As the cells in the macula deteriorate, the patient experiences a blurring of the central vision that can progress to blindness. AMD has two forms (dry and wet) and three stages (early, intermediate, and advanccd). In some patients, dry AMD converts to wet AMD over time, and all patients with wet AMD originally had dry AMD. Dry AMD is much more common than wet AMD, accounting for more than 85% of all cases of intermediate and advanced AMD. However, approximately two-thirds of all patients with advanced AMD have wet AMD, and wet AMD causes more cases of blindness than dry AMD.

An early sign of dry AMD is the presence of yellow deposits (known as *drusen*) under the macula. In patients with wet (or exudative) AMD, a condition called choroidal neovascularization (CNV) occurs in which abnormal blood vessels grow under the macula. The blood vessels behind the macula can leak, resulting in an accumulation of blood and fluid that causes the macula to rise up, or bulge. This leakage can quickly destroy a patient's vision. Researches have identified two types of CNV: classic and occult CNV. Vision loss is greater in patients with classic CNV than in patients with occult CNV.

Options for treating wet AMD are limited. Laser surgery or photodynamic therapy (using Novartis's Visudyne) are currently available, but these therapies only slow the progression of wet AMD – they do not cure the disease. Because the pathogenesis of wet AMD involves the abnormal growth of blood vessels, angiogenesis inhibitors represent a potential new strategy for treating this disease. The first angiogenesis inhibitor approved for the treatment of AMD was pegaptanib (Eyetech Pharmaceutical's Macugen), which was launched in January 2005.

Significant market opportunity exists for AMD treatments because of the significant unmet need and the size of the market. The risk of developing AMD increases with age, and AMD is the leading cause of blindness in people aged 55 or older. The National Eye Institute reports that an estimated 1.8 million adults aged 40 or older have AMD with associated vision loss and that a projected 2.9 million will have AMD in 2020. In addition, an estimated 7.3 million people have drusen that are at least 125 mm in size and are therefore at risk of developing AMD. These statistics are from a recent study on the prevalence of AMD (Friedman et al., 2004).

CURRENT THERAPIES

Bevacizumab (Avastin)

Genentech's bevacizumab (Avastin) was the first antiangiogenic therapy to be approved by the FDA. In February 2004, it was approved for use in combination with 5-fluorouracil-based chemotherapy as a first-line treatment in patients with metastatic colon cancer or rectum cancer. Bevacizumab is an intravenously administered, humanized monoclonal antibody (MAb) that binds to and blocks the activity of VEGF. Researchers at Genentech cloned VEGF in 1989 and published an article in 1993 demonstrating that an antibody targeted to VEGF could inhibit angiogenesis in preclinical models of cancer.

In 2000, Phase III trials with bevacizumab were initiated: one trial evaluated bevacizumab in combination with 5-fluorouracil/leucovorin/CPT-11 (IFL) for the treatment of metastatic colorectal cancer; another series of trials evaluated bevacizumab in combination with capecitabine (Roche's Xeloda) for the treatment of relapsed metastatic breast cancer. The Phase III trial evaluating bevacizumab in combination with capecitabine for the treatment of breast cancer did not meet the primary end point of improving survival, but the trial evaluating bevacizumab in combination with IFL did exceed the primary end point of improving survival. The median survival of patients who received the bevacizumab/IFL therapy was 20.3 months, compared with 15.6 months for patients treated with IFL alone.

Additional clinical trials have been conducted with mixed results. In 2001, for example, a National Cancer Institute (NCI) trial evaluating bevacizumab for treatment of kidney cancer was stopped early because the efficacy end point was achieved earlier than expected. However, a trial that tested the efficacy of bevacizumab as a monotherapy for treatment of colorectal cancer by comparing bevacizumab with the chemotherapy regimen 5-fluorouracil/leucovorin/oxaliplatin (FOLFOX4) was stopped early because of evidence that patient survival was inferior in the bevacizumab arm of the study.

Genentech continues to evaluate bevacizumab in clinical trials to further expand the approved labeling for this agent. Eighty ongoing or completed clinical trials are listed on ClinicalTrials.gov (a database maintained by the National Institute of Health [NIH]), including trials sponsored by Genentech and other organizations such as the NCI and academic groups. Genentech reports that bevacizumab is currently in Phase III clinical trials for adjuvant colorectal cancer, metastatic breast cancer, non-small-cell lung cancer (NSCLC), ovarian cancer, pancreatic cancer, and renal cell carcinoma. In March 2005, Genentech announced that an interim analysis of the Phase III study of bevacizumab plus paclitaxel (Bristol-Myers Squibb's Taxol, generics) and carboplatin (Bristol-Myers Squibb's Paraplatin, generics) in first-line treatment of NSCLC showed that the study had met its primary efficacy end point of improving overall survival.

In January 2005, Genentech announced preliminary results of a Phase III trial evaluating bevacizumab in combination with FOLFOX4 versus FOLFOX4 alone for the second-line treatment of metastatic colorectal cancer. Again, the results were positive: patients who received the bevacizumab/FOLFOX4 combination had a 26% reduction in the risk of death, compared with patients treated with FOLFOX4 alone.

The combination of bevacizumab and erlotinib (Genentech/OSI Pharmaceuticals' Tarceva) is being evaluated in Phase II clinical trials for treatment of renal cell carcinoma and NSCLC.

Sales of bevacizumab have been strong; Genentech reports that sales were $554.5 million in 2004, with sales of $200.4 million during the fourth quarter alone. The response to bevacizumab demonstrates the strong market potential for antiangiogenic drugs for treatment of cancer.

Pegaptanib (Macugen)

Eyetech Pharmaceutical's pegaptanib sodium injection (Macugen) was approved by the FDA for neovascular (wet) AMD in December 2004. Pegaptanib is a pegylated aptamer (a chemically synthesized oligonucleotide that is specific to a desired target) that binds specifically to VEGF. Pegylation of the oligonucleotide increases the half-life of the molecule in the body, thereby allowing less-frequent dosing.

Pegaptanib is a selective VEGF antagonist that binds specifically to an isoform of VEGF that is present in the eye and believed to be required for development of angiogenesis in the retina. The clinical data supporting approval of pegaptanib were gathered in two clinical trials in patients with wet AMD. In these trials, patients were randomized to receive the control (sham treatment) or one of three different doses of pegaptanib. The drug is delivered to the eye via intravitreous injection. Patients who received the lowest dose of pegaptanib (0.3 mg) experienced a slower rate of vision loss than patients who received the control treatment. Higher doses of pegaptanib did not improve the benefit, and pegaptanib was not as effective during the second year of treatment as it was during the first year of therapy.

As the result of a December 2002 agreement, Eyetech Pharmaceuticals and Pfizer are copromoting pegaptanib in the United States. Pfizer also has exclusive rights to develop and commercialize pegaptanib outside of the United States. Under the terms of the agreement between Pfizer and Eyetech, Pfizer paid an initial licensing fee of $75 million and has made equity investments in Eyetech that total $35 million. Future payments to Eyetech, contingent on milestones being met, include an additional equity purchase of $15 million, a milestone payment of up to $195.5 million based on achievement of worldwide submissions and approvals, and up to $450 million based on attainment of agreed-on sales levels for pegaptanib.

Pfizer and Eyetech agreed to share profits and losses from commercialization of pegaptanib in the United States, with Eyetech booking all US sales. For sales outside the United States, Pfizer will pay Eyetech a royalty on net sales. Pfizer also agreed to fund the costs of developing pegaptanib further for AMD as well as for treatment of diabetic macular edema (DME), retinal vein occlusion, and certain other ophthalmic indications.

Eyetech Pharmaceuticals is evaluating pegaptanib in additional clinical trials to further expand the indications for this drug. Currently, clinical trials are evaluating pegaptanib for treatment of DME and retinal vein occlusion; preclinical studies have evaluated the drug for other ophthalmic indications. In addition, Eyetech indicates that pegaptanib is being evaluated in preclinical studies for treatment of non-ophthalmic diseases such as cancer and psoriasis. These nonophthalmic indications are not within the scope of Eyetech's collaboration with Pfizer. Eyetech has indicated that if pegaptanib proves to be a promising therapy in these nonophthalmic diseases, it expects to pursue collaboration or outlicensing opportunities for the additional indications.

Thalidomide

Thalidomide was introduced in Europe in the 1950s as a sedative and antiemetic agent for pregnant women. Following reports that associated maternal use of thalidomide with severe limb-growth defects in babies, thalidomide was withdrawn from the European market in the early 1960s (it had not been approved in the United States). When thalidomide was withdrawn from the market, the mechanism behind the drug's teratogenic effects was unknown. Research later established that thalidomide inhibits angiogenesis and thereby inhibits formation of the new blood vessels that are essential to the formation of fetal limbs.

Thalidomide is now known to have multiple mechanisms of action. In addition to having angiogenic properties, it is also an immunomodulatory agent that can lower or raise levels of tumor necrosis factor-alpha (TNF-α). The specific effect varies under different conditions. For example, thalidomide reportedly lowers levels of TNF-α in the blood of patients with erythema nodosum leprosum (ENL), which can occur in patients with leprosy, but raises levels of TNF-α in HIV-positive patients. Researchers now know that thalidomide's mechanism of action is complex and affects multiple targets, not all of them known.

In 1998, thalidomide (Celgene's Thalomid) was approved by the FDA for treatment of ENL. (Owing to the severe birth defects associated with use of thalidomide by pregnant women, use of this drug is controlled under a "Restricted Distribution for Safety" regulation.) The antiangiogenesis effect of thalidomide has generated considerable interest in potential use of this drug for treatment of cancer. Celgene has reported that thalidomide is being or has been evaluated in more than 200 clinical trials for treatment of solid tumors and hematological cancers.

Thalidomide has proved to be a promising emerging therapy for treatment of multiple myeloma, and Celgene submitted a supplemental new drug application (NDA) to the FDA for this indication in December 2003. It received an approvable letter in 2004 requesting additional data. Thalidomide is also being evaluated in Phase II clinical trials for treatment of renal cell carcinoma, prostate cancer, and melanoma, and it has been shown to have activity in the treatment of AIDS-related Kaposi's sarcoma. Celgene reported sales of $308.6 million in 2004 for thalidomide; 2003 sales were $223.7 million.

Celgene is also developing two classes of thalidomide analogues called IMiDs (immunomodulatory drugs) and SelCIDs (selective cytokine inhibitory drugs). Celgene reports that IMiDs inhibit TNF-α production with a potency that is 10,000 times greater than that of thalidomide. The IMiDs are small molecule, orally available immunomodulatory drugs based on the activity and structure of thalidomide; the SelCIDs inhibit phosphodiesterase-4 (PDE-4), which blocks production of TNF-α. Product candidates in both classes are being positioned as immunomodulatory agents and are not discussed in detail here. However, it has been reported that IMiDs and SelCIDs also have antiangiogenesis activity.

EMERGING THERAPIES

Angiogenesis is now widely recognized as an important process in several diseases, and many pharmaceutical and biopharmaceutical companies are developing novel therapies to inhibit angiogenesis. The approaches followed are based on a wide range of technologies and potential targets. For example, many of the new therapies in development are orally available, small-molecule compounds, but others are based on technologies such as antibodies and peptides. Some emerging therapies attack angiogenesis directly by targeting VEGF, VEGFR, or the receptor tyrosine kinases associated with VEGFR; others attack angiogenesis less directly by targeting angiogenic factors involved in activating the process of angiogenesis or by focusing on targets that are involved in angiogenesis after the initial interaction between VEGF and its receptor. Several emerging antiangiogenesis therapies affect multiple targets involved in angiogenesis.

This section reviews antiangiogenesis therapies in later-stage development: agents in Phase III development plus certain emerging therapies in Phase II trials. Table 27.4 presents select angiogenesis inhibitors in development.

ABT-510

Abbott's ABT-510 is a thrombospondin-mimetic nonapeptide that was developed to mimic the antiangiogenesis activity of the endogenous angiogenesis inhibitor thrombospondin-1. ABT-510 reportedly works by inhibiting the activity of angiogenic growth factors such as VEGF.

Few clinical data are available for ABT-510. In June 2003, at the American Society of Clinical Oncology (ASCO) meeting, data were presented on a Phase I study of ABT-510 in 37 patients with different types of cancer (breast, colorectal, lung, melanoma, sarcoma, and other cancers). In this dose-ranging study, no dose-limiting toxicities were found. In addition, tumor shrinkage was seen in one patient with soft-tissue sarcoma, and disease stabilization for at least six months was seen in three other patients. Additional dose-finding data and pharmacokinetic data on ABT-510 were presented at the June 2004 ASCO meeting. Again, some evidence of antitumor activity was seen. ABT-510 is currently in Phase II clinical trials for multiple types of cancer; Abbott has reported that ABT-510 is being evaluated in lung cancer, kidney cancer, sarcoma, and lymphoma. The results of these trials are not yet available.

AE-941 (Neovastat)

AE-941 (Neovastat) is an orally bioavailable angiogenesis inhibitor derived from shark cartilage; it acts by inhibiting MMP-2 and MMP-9. In addition, AE-941 has anti-VEGF activity. AEterna Zentaris (formerly AEterna Laboratories) has been developing AE-941, but the development process has not proceeded smoothly. In September 2003, AEterna reported results of a Phase III clinical trial evaluating AE-941 in patients with renal-cell carcinoma who were refractory to immunotherapy. Although the drug did demonstrate a good safety profile, it did not meet the primary end point of improving overall median survival time. In December 2003, AEterna announced that it was discontinuing the development of AE-941 for this indication.

AEterna is currently conducting a second Phase III clinical trial that is evaluating

Table 27.4 Select Angiogenesis Inhibitors in Clinical Development, 2005

Company	*Product/Technology*	*Latest Development Phase (indication)*	*Mechanism*
Abbott Laboratories	ABT-510	Phase II (multiple cancers)	Thrombospondin-mimetic nonapeptide developed to mimic the antiangiogenesis activity of the endogenous angiogenesis inhibitor thrombospondin-1
AEterna Zentaris and Atrium Biotechnologies	AE-941 (Neovastat)	Phase III (NSCLC)	Inhibits MMP-2 and MMP-9 and has anti-VEGF activity
Alchemgen Therapeutics and Children's Medical Center Corporation	Angiostatin	Phase II (NSCLC)	Protein-based angiogenesis inhibitor that is a fragment of the clotting factor plasminogen
Alchemgen Therapeutics and Children's Medical Center Corporation	Endostatin	Phase II (melanoma, neuroendocrine tumors)	Protein-based angiogenesis inhibitor that is a fragment of collagen XVIII
Amgen	AMG-706	Phase II (GIST)	Small-molecule drug that inhibits multiple kinases involved in angiogenesis
Angstrom Pharmaceuticals	A6	Phase II (ovarian cancer)	Eight-amino acid, uPA-derived peptide that inhibits the activity of uPAR, thereby inhibiting angiogenesis
Antisoma	AS-1405	Phase I (glioblastoma multiforme)	Radiolabeled version of the murine monoclonal antibody BC1, which targets a form of fibronectin found specifically on new blood vessels
Ariad Pharmaceuticals	AP-23573	Phase II (hematological cancers and solid tumors)	An mTOR inhibitor
AstraZeneca	ZD-6474	Phase II (NSCLC, SCLC, myeloma)	Orally available VEGFR-2 tyrosine kinase inhibitor that also has activity against EGFR tyrosine kinase
AstraZeneca	AZD-2171	Phase I (solid tumors)	Orally available VEGFR tyrosine kinase inhibitor
Attenuon	ATN-161	Phase I (solid tumors)	Five-amino acid peptide derived from fibronectin that binds to several integrins
Bayer and Onyx Pharmaceuticals	BAY-43-9006 (sorafenib)	Phase III (renal cell carcinoma and advanced hepatocellular carcinoma)	Multiple-action Raf kinase and VEGFR inhibitor
Bayer	BAY-57-9352	Phase I (solid tumors)	VEGFR-2 tyrosine kinase inhibitor
Callisto Pharmaceuticals	Atiprimod	Phase I/II (multiple myeloma)	Orally available, small-molecule drug candidate with both antiangiogenic and antiproliferative properties
Celgene	Thalidomide (Thalomid)	Preregistration (multiple myeloma)	Has both immunomodulatory and antiangiogenesis properties Marketed for ENL
Centocor	CNTO-95	Phase I (solid tumors)	Fully human monoclonal antibody against alpha-v integrin receptors
Cephalon and Sanofi-Aventis	CEP-7055	Phase I (solid tumors)	Orally active small molecule VEGFR tyrosine kinase inhibitor
ChemGenex Therapeutics	Homoharringtonine (Ceflatonin)	Phase II (chronic myeloid leukemia, myelodysplastic syndrome)	Small-molecule drug candidate, affects several pathways in the cell, including regulation of genes associated with apoptosis and angiogenesis
CollaGenex	CMT-3 (Metastat)	Phase II (Kaposi's sarcoma)	MMP inhibitor
EntreMed	Panzem Capsule and Panzem NCD (2-methoxyestradiol [2ME2])	Phase II (multiple myeloma and prostate cancer)	Naturally occurring estrogen metabolite with little estrogenic activity Inhibits angiogenesis and induces apoptosis
Exelixis	XL-647	Phase I (multiple cancers)	SSKI that inhibits multiple RTKs
Exelixis	XL-999	Phase I (multiple cancers)	SSKI that inhibits multiple RTKs

(*continued*)

Table 27.4 Continued

Company	*Product/Technology*	*Latest Development Phase (indication)*	*Mechanism*
Genaera	Squalamine (Evizon)	Phase II (AMD, recurrent advanced ovarian cancer, prostate cancer, NSCLC)	Blocks multiple angiogenic factors, including VEGF, cytoskeleton formation, and integrin expression
Genentech and Novartis	Ranibizumab (Lucentis)	Phase III (AMD)	Humanized monoclonal antibody fragment targeted to VEGF
GenVec	AdPEDF	Phase I (AMD)	Uses an adenovector to produce pigment epithelium-derived factor (PEDF), a natural inhibitor of angiogenesis
ImClone Systems	IMC-1C11b	Phase I (solid tumors)	Human monoclonal antibody that targets VEGFR-2
Eli Lilly	Enzastaurin (LY-317615)	Phase II (non-Hodgkin's, mantle cell, and B-cell lymphomas)	Acyclic bisindolylmaleimide that is a potent inhibitor of protein kinase C-beta2
MedImmune	Vitaxin (LM-609)	Phase II (melanoma and prostate cancer)	Monoclonal antibody that targets the alpha-v beta-3 integrin
Merck KGaA (Germany)	Cilengitide (EMD-121974)	Phase II (glioblastoma, NSCLC, pancreatic cancer)	Cyclic peptide that is an alpha-v integrin antagonist
Novartis and Schering AG	Vatalanib (PTK-787/ ZK-222584)	Phase III (metastatic colorectal cancer)	Oral, small-molecule drug that inhibits all known VEGFR tyrosine kinases
Novartis	Midostaurin (PKC-412)	Phase II (multiple cancers)	Inhibits multiple signaling proteins, including specific receptor tyrosine kinases, and targets that are part of signal transduction pathways
Novartis	AEE-788	Phase I (multiple cancers)	Inhibits multiple receptor tyrosine kinases including the EGFR, HER2, and VEGFR RTKs
Pfizer	SU-11248 (Sutent)	Phase III (GIST, renal cell carcinoma)	Orally available molecule Inhibits PDGFR, VEGFR, Kit, and Flt2 tyrosine kinases
Pfizer	AG-013736	Phase II (multiple cancers)	Inhibits VEGF and PDGF RTKs
Pfizer	CP-547,632	Phase II (ovarian cancer)	Selective inhibitor of VEGFR-2 tyrosine kinase
Pfizer	CP-868,596	Phase I (multiple cancers)	Selective inhibitor of PDGFR
Progen Industries (Australia)	PI-88	Phase II (melanoma, liver cancer, NSCLC)	Three mechanisms of action: inhibits heparinase (blocking release of angiogenic factors from extracellular matrix); binds to VEGF, FGF-1, and FGF-2; and stimulates release of TFPI
Protein Design Labs	M200 (volociximab)	Phase II (renal cell carcinoma)	Chimeric monoclonal antibody targeted against alpha-5 beta-1 integrin
Regeneron Pharmaceuticals	VEGF Trap	Phase I (solid tumors, non-Hodgkin's lymphoma, AMD)	Regions of VEGFR1 (Flt-1) and VEGFR2 (KDR) fused to human immunoglobulin Fc domain Binds VEGF-Z 100- to 1,000-fold more tightly than antibodies
Sirna Laboratories (formerly Ribozyme Pharmaceuticals)	Sirna-027	Phase I (AMD)	Chemically modified SiRNA targeting VEGFR-1
VasGene Therapeutics	VEGF-AS (Veglin)	Phase I (relapsed and refractory malignancies)	VEGF-antisense compound that targets VEGF-A, VEGF-C, and VEGF-D Blocks production of VEGF

AMD = Age-related macular degeneration; EGFR = Epidermal growth factor receptor; ENL = Erythema nodosum leprosum; FGF = Fibroblast growth factor; GIST = Gastrointestinal stromal tumors; HER2 = Human epidermal growth factor receptor 2; mTOR = Mammalian target of rapamycin; MMP = Matrix metalloproteinases; NSCLC = Non-small-cell lung cancer; PDGF = Platelet-derived growth factor; PDGFR = Platelet-derived growth factor receptor; RNA = Ribonucleic acid; RTK = Receptor tyrosine kinase; SCLC = Small-cell lung cancer; SiRNA = Short interfering RNA; SSKI = Spectrum-selective kinase inhibitor; TFPI = Tissue factor pathway inhibitor; UPA = Urokinase plasminogen activator; UPAR = Urokinase plasminogen activator receptor; VEGF = Vascular endothelial growth factor; VEGFR = Vascular endothelial growth factor receptor

AE-941 in patients with NSCLC. This trial differs from the first, failed Phase III trial in two respects: (1) AE-941 is being administered in combination with chemotherapy and radiotherapy, and (2) this trial includes the newly diagnosed patients who are being given AE-941 as part of their first-line therapy. The NCI is sponsoring this trial. Enrollment appears to be proceeding slowly. As of December 2003, 300 patients (of a planned total of 760 patients) had been enrolled.

AEterna has entered into several agreements for the commercialization of AE-941, including agreements with Gruppo Ferrer (to market AE-941 in southern Europe, France, Benelux, and Latin America); Mayne Pharma (to market AE-941 in Australia, New Zealand, Canada, and Mexico); and LG Life Sciences (to market AE-941 in Korea). In December 2004, AEterna announced that it was granting marketing rights (excluding North America) for AE-941 to Atrium Biotechnologies, a partially owned subsidiary of AEterna. With this agreement, AEterna will increase its equity in Atrium Biotechnologies from 60.2% to 61.1%. Atrium Biotechnologies will manage AEterna's agreements with Gruppo Ferrer, Mayne Pharma, and LG Life Sciences.

Endostatin and Angiostatin

Endostatin and angiostatin are protein-based angiogenesis inhibitors. Endostatin is a fragment of collagen XVIII; angiostatin is a fragment of the clotting factor plasminogen. Angiostatin reportedly inhibits vascular endothelial cell proliferation.

These agents were formerly under development at EntreMed; however, in February 2004, EntreMed announced a three-way agreement under which it transferred all rights to endostatin and angiostatin to Alchemgen Therapeutics and Children's Medical Center Corporation (Boston, Massachusetts). This agreement is part of EntreMed's change in strategy to focus on development of small-molecule drugs for treatment of cancer. Under the agreement, Alchemgen was granted rights to market endostatin and angiostatin in Asia, while Children's Medical Center received the rights for these two proteins in the rest of the world. If Children's Medical Center licenses endostatin and/or angiostatin to any company, EntreMed is to receive 20% of all proceeds.

When EntreMed transferred rights to endostatin and angiostatin, both agents were in Phase II clinical trials. Endostatin was in Phase II for melanoma and neuroendocrine tumors, and the FDA has granted orphan drug status for these two indications. Angiostatin is being evaluated in a Phase II trial for treatment of NSCLC in combination with paclitaxel and carboplatin. In June 2004, researchers from EntreMed and Indiana University presented preliminary results of the Phase II trial of angiostatin. In this study, 24 patients were treated with angiostatin, paclitaxel, and carboplatin (23 patients were evaluable). The partial response rate was 39.1%, with one patient experiencing a partial response for 14.5-plus months. Survival data are not yet available.

Both endostatin and angiostatin were early product candidates in the field of angiogenesis inhibitors and are considered highly promising candidates for treatment of cancer. However, their future now seems uncertain.

AMG-706

Amgen's AMG-706 is a small-molecule enzyme inhibitor that inhibits multiple kinases that are involved in angiogenesis. Currently, it is being evaluated in a Phase II clinical trial in patients with gastrointestinal stromal tumors (GIST) that are resistant to imatinib mesylate (Novartis's Gleevec); this Phase II trial is an open-label study that is currently enrolling patients. AMG-706 has received fast-track status from the FDA.

A6

Angstrom Pharmaceuticals is focusing on the urokinase plasminogen activator (uPA) and its receptor (uPAR). The company's lead drug candidate, A6, is an eight-amino acid uPA-derived peptide that inhibits the activity of uPAR, thereby inhibiting neovascularization and angiogenesis.

Currently, A6 is being evaluated in a randomized, double-blind, placebo-controlled Phase II clinical trial in asymptomatic patients with CA125 progression of ovarian cancer (progression seen only with the tumor marker CA125). This trial, which started in June 2004, is expected to enroll 48–60 patients who were successfully treated with first-line therapy but still have elevated levels of the CA125 tumor marker in their blood.

AP-23573

Ariad Pharmaceuticals' AP-23573 is an intravenously administered rapamycin analogue that inhibits mammalian target of rapamycin (mTOR), a cell-signaling protein that regulates the response of cancer cells to nutrients and growth factors. Inhibiting mTOR essentially starves the cancer cells. In addition, mTOR affects VEGF and represents a potential target for antiangiogenesis therapy. Ariad plans to evaluate AP-23573 in both hematological and solid cancers. AP-23573 is currently in Phase II clinical trials as a single agent in hematological cancers (leukemias and lymphomas) and solid tumors and in Phase Ib clinical trials for glioblastoma multiforme.

Potentially, an antiangiogenesis therapy such as AP-23573 could also be used to prevent restenosis following angioplasty. In January 2005, Ariad announced a nonexclusive agreement with the medical device company Medinol to develop and commercialize stents and other medical devices to deliver AP-23573 for the prevention of restenosis following stent-assisted angioplasty. This indication is currently in preclinical development.

ZD-6474

AstraZeneca's ZD-6474 is an orally delivered drug candidate that inhibits the VEGF receptor-2 (VEGFR-2) tyrosine kinase. In addition, ZD-6474 is active against epidermal growth factor receptor (EGFR) tyrosine kinase. Owing to its dual mechanism of action, ZD-6474 has both antiangiogenic and cytostatic/cytotoxic activity.

AstraZeneca is evaluating ZD-6474 in Phase II clinical trials in NSCLC and small-cell lung cancers and myeloma. In October 2004, the company reported that ZD-6474 was approaching completion of clinical trials as a monotherapy (compared with gefitinib [AstraZeneca's Iressa]) and in combination with cytotoxic chemotherapy. In June 2004, researchers presented data from an ongoing Phase II clinical trial evaluating ZD-6474 in combination with docetaxel (Sanofi-Aventis's Taxotere) for treatment of NSCLC patients.

In addition to ZD-6474, AstraZeneca has other VEGFR tyrosine kinase inhibitors in development, including AZD-2171, a candidate in Phase I clinical development that inhibits only VEGFR tyrosine kinase.

BAY-43-9006 (Sorafenib)

Bayer/Onyx Pharmaceuticals' BAY-43-9006 (sorafenib) is a novel drug candidate that the two companies are codeveloping. BAY-43-9006 has multiple mechanisms of action: it inhibits Raf kinase (thereby inhibiting tumor cell proliferation); it inhibits angiogenesis by blocking VEGFR-2; and it binds to and blocks the platelet-derived growth factor receptor (PDGFR), which also has a role in angiogenesis.

BAY-43-9006 is being evaluated for treatment of renal-cell carcinoma in a large Phase III clinical trial called Treatment Approaches in Renal Cancer Global Evaluation Trial (TARGETs). This trial is being conducted at 123 sites in 20 countries and will include more than 800 patients with unresectable and/or metastatic renal-cell carcinoma. TARGETs is a randomized, double-blind, placebo-controlled trial. Patient recruitment for this study is ongoing. In March 2005, Bayer and Onyx announced the initiation of a Phase III study of BAY-43-9006 in patients with advanced hepatocellular carcinoma. The FDA has granted BAY-43-9006 fast-track status for treatment of metastatic renal-cell carcinoma. In addition, the FDA and the European Medicines Agency (EMEA) have granted BAY-43-9006 orphan drug status for treatment of renal-cell carcinoma.

In October 2004, Bayer and Onyx announced positive results from a recently completed randomized, discontinuation Phase II trial of BAY-43-9006 as a single agent for treatment of patients with progressive kidney cancer. In this study, 65 patients (who had been treated with BAY-43-9006 for 12 weeks) were randomized into two groups and then received either BAY-43-9006 or placebo. After an additional 12 weeks, there was a statistically significant, higher percentage of patients in the experimental group whose cancer did not progress than in the placebo group. In addition, after the initial 12 weeks, 70% of patients had experienced either tumor shrinkage or disease stabilization. In October 2004, Bayer and Onyx reported that they anticipate a 2006 launch of BAY-43-9006 in the United States.

BAY-43-9006 is also being evaluated in Phase II clinical trials for treatment of several other cancers, including breast cancer and NSCLC. In September 2004, the companies announced results of a Phase II clinical trial in which BAY-43-9006 was evaluated as a single agent in patients with advanced primary liver cancer (hepatocellular carcinoma). These data were presented at the American Association for Cancer Research-National Cancer Institute-European Organization for Research and Treatment of Cancer (AACR-NCI-EORTC) meeting. In this study, 9% of patients experienced tumor shrinkage, and an additional 43% experienced stable disease for at least four months. Median survival for all patients was 9.2 months; median time to tumor progression was 4.2 months. BAY-43-9006 was reportedly well tolerated, with manageable side effects.

Panzem Capsule/NCD (2-Methoxyestradiol)

The agent 2-methoxyestradiol (2ME2; EntreMed's Panzem Capsule and Panzem NCD) is a naturally occurring estrogen metabolite being developed for treatment of certain cancers. EntreMed reports that 2ME2 has multiple mechanisms of action, including inhibition of angiogenesis and induction of apoptosis. Other mechanisms of action (which may be important for potential non-cancer indications) include disruption of the formation of microtubules, downregulation of hypoxia-inducible factor-1alpha (HIF-1α), and inhibition of osteoclasts (involved in bone resorption). Even though 2ME2 is an estrogen metabolite, this molecule binds poorly to estrogen receptors and therefore has limited estrogenic activity.

2ME2 is currently in Phase II clinical trials for multiple myeloma and in a Phase I trial for advanced solid tumors. 2ME2 also has been evaluated in a Phase II trial for prostate cancer, two Phase I trials for metastatic breast cancer (both as a single agent and with docetaxel), and a Phase I trial for advanced solid tumors. In December 2004, EntreMed released preliminary data from the Phase II trial of 2ME2 in patients with multiple myeloma. EntreMed reported that 2ME2 was well tolerated and had stabilized disease in patients with plateaued or relapsed multiple myeloma. EntreMed has also announced positive findings in earlier studies.

EntreMed has developed a reformulated, liquid version of 2ME2 (Panzem NCD) in order to increase plasma levels of 2ME2; the liquid suspension has been optimized using Elan Drug Delivery's proprietary NanoCrystal Colloidal Dispersion (NCD) technology. The start of a Phase Ib trial evaluating Panzem NCD in patients with advanced cancer was announced in January 2005. Meanwhile, EntreMed is also developing analogues of 2ME2 to increase the antitumor and antiangiogenic properties of the agent and to decrease the drug's rate of metabolism. These 2ME2 analogues are in preclinical development.

Additional small-molecule product candidates that EntreMed has developed that also inhibit angiogenesis are in earlier stages of development. Although EntreMed was an early developer of anti-angiogenesis therapies in its work on the proteins endostatin and angiostatin (see Section "Endostatin and Angiostatin"), the company has changed its strategy and now focuses on the development and commercialization of small-molecule drugs.

Squalamine

Genaera's squalamine (Evizon), discovered in the tissues of the dogfish shark, is a member of a class of naturally occurring small molecules called aminosterols. Squalamine lactate is a synthetic compound that Genaera is developing for treatment of CNV in AMD. In addition, squalamine is being evaluated for treatment of cancer. Squalamine blocks multiple angiogenic factors, including VEGF, cytoskeleton formation, and integrin expression.

Genaera is currently conducting three Phase II clinical trials to evaluate squalamine in patients with AMD. In January 2005, Genaera announced positive preliminary results from one of the Phase II trials; these early data included results from six patients, each of whom had wet AMD in both eyes. Genaera reported that 100% of the eyes had either preserved or improved vision at week three and week five (when therapy was ended) and at two months after initiation of the therapy. Genaera also reported that these results were comparable to previously reported Phase I/II data.

Genaera plans to start a Phase III trial evaluating squalamine in AMD in 2005; this trial will run concurrently with the longest Phase II trial. Squalamine has been selected for participation in the FDA's Continuous Marketing Application Pilot 2 program, and the FDA has granted it a fast-track designation for AMD. For cancer, squalamine has been evaluated in a Phase II trial for treatment of recurrent advanced ovarian cancer and is currently being evaluated in Phase II trials for treatment of prostate cancer and NSCLC. A Phase IIa trial in NSCLC has been completed.

Ranibizumab (Lucentis)

Genentech has been developing ranibizumab, formerly called rhuFab V2 (Lucentis), for treatment of the wet form of AMD. In June 2003, Genentech announced an agreement with Novartis that granted Novartis Ophthalmics an exclusive license to develop and market ranibizumab outside North America for indications relating to diseases of the eye. Genentech retained rights to market ranibizumab in the United States, Canada, and Mexico. Under this agreement, Genentech is to receive an up-front fee, milestone payments, and royalties on sales of ranibizumab outside North America. Novartis currently anticipates filing for regulatory approval of ranibizumab in 2006.

Ranibizumab is being evaluated in two Phase III clinical trials in the United States in patients with the wet form of AMD. The MARINA trial is a randomized, multicenter, double-masked, sham-injection-controlled trial that is designed to evaluate two different doses of ranibizumab in approximately 720 patients with minimally classic or occult wet AMD. The ANCHOR trial is a randomized, multicenter, double-masked, active treatment-controlled trial that has been designed to compare two different doses of ranibizumab with verteporfin photodynamic therapy in approximately 426 patients who predominantly have classic wet AMD.

In August 2003, Genentech announced positive preliminary data from the extension phase of a Phase Ib/II, open-label study of ranibizumab. In this study, most patients reported improvement in vision with six months or more of ranibizumab treatment. This randomized, single-agent study compared ranibizumab with standard care (no ranibizumab). Of the 53 patients who received ranibizumab therapy, 50 (94%) experienced either stable or improved vision at day 98, compared with the baseline.

Enzastaurin

Eli Lilly's enzastaurin (LY-317615) has a novel mechanism of action as an angiogenesis inhibitor. The agent is an acyclic bisindolylmaleimide that is a potent inhibitor of protein kinase C-beta2. This enzyme is part of the signaling cascade for VEGF; therefore, inhibiting this enzyme blocks angiogenesis. Enzastaurin is in Phase II trials for treatment of non-Hodgkin's lymphoma (NHL), mantle-cell lymphoma, and diffuse large B-cell lymphoma. In June 2004, data from an ongoing Phase II trial in patients with recurrent high-grade gliomas were presented at the ASCO meeting. At that time, 32 patients had been enrolled in the trial, and data from 28 of these patients could be evaluated. The treatment was reportedly well tolerated, and objective radiographic responses had been seen in five patients.

Vitaxin (LM-609)

MedImmune's Vitaxin (LM-609) is a MAb that targets the alpha-v beta-3 integrin. This integrin is expressed on the surface of newly formed blood vessels and is involved in angiogenesis. It is also found on the surface of certain cancer cells (including melanoma, prostate cancer, and tumors with bone metastasis) and on mature osteoclasts. During 2003, MedImmune initiated two Phase II clinical trials to evaluate Vitaxin in patients with melanoma and prostate cancer.

Vitaxin was previously evaluated in a Phase I/II clinical study in advanced colorectal cancer, but MedImmune no longer appears to be pursuing that cancer indication. MedImmune has also evaluated Vitaxin for treatment of immunological disorders, specifically in Phase II trials for rheumatoid arthritis and psoriasis. However, in August 2004, the company announced that it was terminating those two trials based on preliminary data that did not indicate a clinical benefit of Vitaxin. The company's focus for Vitaxin now appears to be treatment of cancer.

Cilengitide

Merck KGaA's cilengitide (EMD-121974), a cyclic peptide, is an alpha-v integrin antagonist, inhibiting both the alpha-v beta-3 and alpha-v beta-5 integrins. These integrins are required for endothelial cell proliferation and migration during the angiogenesis process.

Cilengitide had been one of the more advanced angiogenesis inhibitors in development, but development has progressed slowly over the last few years. In 1999, Merck announced the start of Phase I clinical trials evaluating cilengitide for treatment of solid tumors, Kaposi's sarcoma, and brain cancer; the company also announced Phase II clinical trials in Europe for treatment of NSCLC and pancreatic cancer. In addition, Merck initiated Phase II trials for glioblastoma in October 2004. Phase I trials for glioblastoma conducted by the NCI demonstrated positive results: of the 51 patients in the study, 2 patients showed complete response, 3 exhibited partial response, and 4 had stable disease for more than six months.

Vatalanib

Novartis/Schering AG's vatalanib (PTK-787/ZK-222584) is an oral, small-molecule angiogenesis inhibitor that the two companies are codeveloping. This molecule works by inhibiting all known VEGFR tyrosine kinases, thereby blocking angiogenesis.

Vatalanib is currently being evaluated in two Phase III clinical trials for treatment of patients with metastatic colorectal cancer. These trials are called Colorectal Oral Novel Therapy for the Inhibition of Angiogenesis and Retarding of Metastases in First-line (CONFIRM 1) and Colorectal Oral Novel Therapy for the Inhibition of Angiogenesis and Retarding of Metastases in Second-line (CONFIRM 2). In the CONFIRM 1 trial, treatment with vatalanib in combination with the FOLFOX4 therapy regimen (5-fluorouracil/leucovorin/oxaliplatin) is being compared with treatment with FOLFOX4 plus placebo as a first-line therapy for colorectal cancer.

In CONFIRM 2, the two regimens (FOLFOX4 plus vatalanib and FOLFOX4 plus placebo) are being compared for treatment of patients with metastatic colorectal cancer that has progressed after first-line treatment with irinotecan (Pfizer's Camptosar, Yakult/Pfizer's Campto, Daiichi's Topotecin). These are very large trials: combined, they will enroll approximately 2,000 patients worldwide, which indicates that Novartis and Schering have high hopes for this product candidate. In June 2004, encouraging early safety and efficacy data from the CONFIRM 1 trial were presented at the ASCO meeting.

SU-11248

Pfizer's SU-11248 (Sutent) is one of the most promising angiogenesis inhibitors in development. This orally active tyrosine kinase inhibitor, which inhibits PDGFR, VEGFR, Kit, and Flt2 tyrosine kinases, was originally developed by Sugen, which Pfizer acquired (through its acquisition of Pharmacia). In February 2005, Pfizer announced that following a review of interim data from a Phase III trial of SU-11248 in patients with imatinib-resistant GIST, an independent panel of experts determined that the trial had demonstrated safety and efficacy seven months ahead of schedule. The panel has recommended that the trial be stopped; patients who received placebo in the trial have been given the option to receive SU-11248.

SU-11248 is also in Phase III trials for renal-cell carcinoma. At the June 2004 ASCO meeting, results were presented from a Phase II clinical trial evaluating SU-11248 as a second-line therapy for treatment of patients with metastatic renal-cell carcinoma. Of the 63 patients treated with SU-11248 in the trial, 24% achieved a partial response, 46% had stable disease, and 30% experienced disease progression.

SU-11248 is Pfizer's most advanced antiangiogenesis product candidate, but Pfizer has other antiangiogenesis agents in development, discussed in the following sections and listed in Table 27.4. In addition, Pfizer announced in January 2005 that it will acquire Angiosyn, a start-up company focusing on angiogenesis and currently developing a product for macular degeneration. Clearly, angiogenesis inhibition is an important part of Pfizer's oncology pipeline.

AG-013736

Pfizer is testing AG-013736, a selective oral inhibitor of the VEGF and PDGF receptor tyrosine kinases, in Phase II clinical trials for breast and renal cell cancers. In June 2004, data were presented at the ASCO annual meeting from the first Phase I study of AG-013736 in patients with advanced solid tumors. In this study, the primary objectives were to determine the maximum tolerated dose and safety, but efficacy data were also evaluated. A total of 36 patients were treated in six cohorts. Two patients achieved durable partial responses, and seven patients had stable disease for more than four months. Pharmacokinetic and tumor vascular response data were also presented. The researchers concluded that AG-013736 showed sufficient safety and activity to warrant Phase II trials. In addition, Pfizer will likely conduct Phase II clinical trials in NSCLC, thyroid cancer, and melanoma.

CP-547,632

Pfizer's CP-547,632 is a selective inhibitor of VEGFR-2 tyrosine kinase that was discovered during Pfizer's collaboration with OSI Pharmaceuticals. OSI reports that this collaboration has expired and that Pfizer is continuing to develop certain drug candidates produced by the collaboration.

At the June 2004 ASCO, data were presented on a Phase I trial of CP-547,632. In this study, CP-547,632 was administered in combination with paclitaxel and carboplatin to patients with advanced NSCLC. The authors concluded that CP-547, 632 could be combined with these two chemotherapy drugs.

PI-88

Progen Industries' PI-88 is a low-molecular-weight compound that mimics the activity of heparin sulfate. This antiangiogenic compound reportedly works via three mechanisms to block the growth of new blood vessels: (1) PI-88 inhibits the enzyme heparanase, thereby blocking release of angiogenic growth factors from the ECM (heparanase is also thought to be involved in tumor metastasis); (2) PI-88 binds with VEGF, fibroblast growth factor (FGF)-1, and FGF-2; and (3) PI-88 stimulates release of tissue factor pathway inhibitor (TFPI), which has both antiangiogenesis and anticoagulation activities.

PI-88 is currently being evaluated in the United States and in Australia as a monotherapy for treatment of advanced melanoma, as an adjuvant to surgery for primary liver cancer, and in combination with docetaxel for treatment of advanced NSCLC. In addition, a protocol is under review for a Phase II trial to evaluate PI-88 in combination with dacarbazine (Bayer's DTIC-Dome) for a first-line treatment of patients with advanced melanoma. Progen expects this trial to start by the end of the second quarter of 2005. A Phase II trial evaluating PI-88 in 19 patients with multiple myeloma has been completed. Progen reports that 41% of the evaluable patients in this trial achieved disease stabilization for eight weeks or longer. In the United States, PI-88 has been granted orphan drug status for treatment of patients with malignant melanoma.

M200

Protein Design Labs' M200 (volociximab) is a chimeric MAb targeted against the alpha-5 beta-1 integrin. This antibody blocks binding of fibronectin to the alpha-5 beta-1 integrin, thereby inhibiting angiogenesis. Protein Design Labs acquired M200 in 2003 through its acquisition of Eos Biotechnology.

At the June 2004 ASCO meeting, preclinical data were presented that demonstrated the anti-angiogenic activity of M200. In September 2004, data from a Phase I trial of M200 in patients with solid tumors were presented at the AACR-NCI-EORTC Symposium on Molecular Targets and Cancer Therapeutics. This dose-escalation trial was ongoing at the time, but preliminary data demonstrated no dose-limiting adverse effects. Of the 15 evaluable patients, 10 had stable disease as the best response. In addition, five of the six patients who received the highest dose achieved stable disease.

Protein Design Lab's focus for M200 appears to be treatment of cancer, but the company also conducts research on AMD and currently has an antibody fragment (F200) that targets the alpha-5 beta-1 integrin in preclinical development.

MARKET OUTLOOK

The FDA approval of Genentech's bevacizumab served as a "proof of principle" that therapeutic agents designed to inhibit angiogenesis are effective in treating disease. Bevacizumab has not only reached the market but has done extremely well, bringing in sales of $554.5 million within a span of slightly more than 10 months on the market. Genentech is conducting many additional trials with this product, and it is likely to be approved for other indications in the near future.

Now that the road to market has been paved, we expect several additional angiogenesis inhibitors to reach the market in the next five years. The market potential for angiogenesis inhibitors in oncology is significant. According to IMS Health, the worldwide market for anticancer agents was $24 billion in 2004. Yet, there is still significant unmet need because many current therapies are highly toxic and because drug resistance is widespread. Angiogenesis inhibitors can address toxicity and resistance issues and can be used in combination with currently marketed therapies to increase efficacy.

Oncology compounds with blockbuster potential include Pfizer's SU-11248 and

Bayer/Onyx Pharmaceuticals' BAY-43-9006. SU-11248 has demonstrated efficacy in imatinib-resistant GIST, and imatinib had worldwide sales of $1.6 billion in 2004, its fourth year on the market. BAY-43-9006 has demonstrated significant potential for renal-cell carcinoma and is currently in Phase III for this indication.

Unmet need is also high in AMD; prior to the January launch of Eyetech's pegaptanib, laser surgery and photodynamic therapy were the only treatment options. In addition, the AMD market will grow rapidly as the population continues to age.

REFERENCE

Friedman, D.S. et al. Prevalence of age-related macular degeneration in the United States. *Archives of Ophthalmology*. April 2004; 122(4): 564–72.

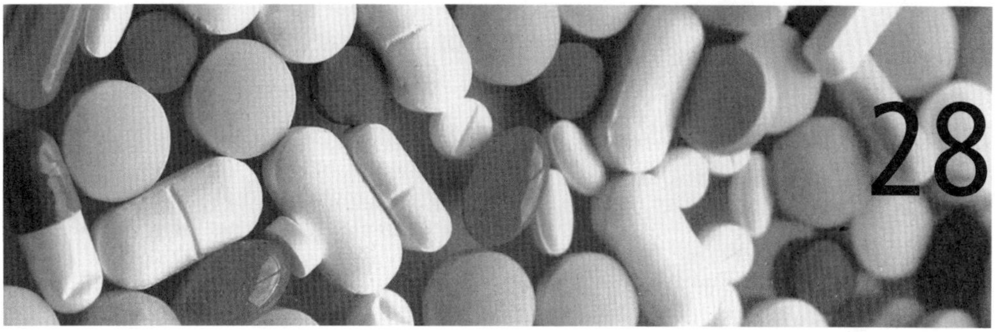

28

Discoveries and Challenges in Early-stage Apoptosis Drug Development

INTRODUCTION

Apoptosis is the major and best-studied pathway of programmed cell death, and its pathway is conserved across most multicellular organisms. Programmed cell death is the process whereby regulated cell destruction occurs to control cell numbers and eliminate cells that may be harmful to the organism. Apoptosis plays an important role in embryonic development and in the function of the immune system as well as in protection against the results of DNA damage, such as deleterious mutations and cancer. As such, it is an intriguing area for drugmakers as they decide how to allocate their drug development resources.

Several diseases are characterized by abnormal apoptosis, including neurodegenerative diseases and liver damage resulting from alcoholic cirrhosis or chronic hepatitis C. For this reason, drug companies have been interested in apoptotic pathways when searching for potential drug targets to treat these and other diseases, such as cancer and ischemic injury. Their research has paid off with the identification of several potential drug targets; some agents have even reached the clinic. Nevertheless, the development of apoptosis modulators faces significant challenges, including difficulties developing agents that target intracellular protein-protein interactions and managing the induction of other programmed cell-death mechanisms. For this reason, researchers are striving to gain a better understanding of these mechanisms, which have only been recently discovered.

Drug companies recognize that, because of apoptosis's role in many diseases, there is significant benefit to developing apoptosis modulators and inhibitors. In this chapter, we provide an overview of apoptosis, including the pathways involved and its role in several diseases. We identify several proteins within the apoptotic pathways that may represent potential targets for drug development; we discuss apoptosis modulators and inhibitors in development, particularly as cancer therapies; and we analyze some of the challenges associated with developing the agents that target this pathway, especially those associated with caspase inhibitors. Finally, we provide an overview of the future potential of these agents.

AN OVERVIEW OF APOPTOSIS

Characteristics of Apoptosis

Apoptosis is an adenosine triphosphate (ATP)-dependent, programmed, and orderly process of cellular suicide. Cells undergoing apoptosis exhibit characteristic morphological changes, including focal cell-surface protrusions (blebs), cell shrinkage and loss of intercellular contacts, chromatin condensation, and cellular fragmentation into small apoptotic bodies. Also, early in apoptosis, phosphatidylserine (PS) is transferred from the cytoplasmic surface of the cell membrane to the outer leaflet. PS and other signals are recognized by neighboring cells and macrophages, which rapidly phagocytize apoptotic bodies. This process prevents cytoplasmic contents from being released into the intercellular medium, where they can provoke inflammation and additional cell damage. Apoptosis differs from necrosis, a type of cell death that is not programmed by cellular mechanisms but that occurs as the result of toxin action, severe deprivation of oxygen, ATP depletion, or massive insult and results in the release of cell contents. A definitive biochemical feature of apoptosis is fragmentation of DNA (or DNA laddering) into internucleosomal-length fragments of 185 base pairs.

Detecting Apoptosis

Cell surface PS and DNA laddering are the basis of two assays that can detect apoptosis in cells. The first, the terminal deoxynucleotide transferase-mediated deoxyuridine triphosphate-biotin nick end labeling (TUNEL) assay, utilizes gel electrophoresis to detect DNA laddering. The second assay uses fluorescently conjugated annexin V, which has a high affinity for PS, to identify that compound on cell membranes. Both assays can be used to detect cells in the early stages of apoptosis.

Role of Apoptosis in Human Development

Apoptosis is a common feature of the development of multicellular animals. During early development, certain cells are needed that are not required during later stages, so they are programmed to die via apoptosis – for example, the excess of neurons in the developing human central nervous system (CNS). Apoptosis is also of key importance in the development and maintenance of the human immune system. The vast majority of the precursors of T and B cells that are generated throughout a person's life die via apoptosis. Apoptosis is part of the process that selects lymphocytes that react to non-self-antigens and eliminates lymphocytes that react to self-antigens. Moreover, cytotoxic T lymphocytes that recognize virus-infected cells or transplanted cells from an incompatible donor (e.g., after bone marrow or organ transplants) kill the cells that they recognize by inducing apoptosis in these cells.

Apoptosis is also involved in protection against damage to cellular DNA resulting from errors that occur during normal processes of DNA replication, recombination, or mitosis, or exposure to DNA-damaging agents such as ionizing radiation or certain toxic chemicals. DNA damage in a cell can result in the accumulation of undesirable mutations and chromosomal changes if the cell is allowed to replicate, a process that can lead to tumorigenesis. Human cells have a complex set of mechanisms to interrupt cell division in cases of DNA damage that allow cells to repair the damage before proceeding with the cell cycle or to self-destruct via apoptosis. These responses to DNA damage are initiated and coordinated by the tumor suppressor protein p53.

Role of Apoptosis in Disease

As already mentioned, abnormal apoptosis plays a role in various diseases such as alcohol-related cirrhosis and hepatitis C. Abnormal apoptosis also plays an important role in neurodegenerative diseases such as Alzheimer's disease; various studies indicate that amyloid protein can trigger apoptosis in certain neurons. In addition, apoptosis plays a role in tissue damage resulting from ischemic events, such as myocardial infarction

(MI) and stroke, as well as in ischemic injury during liver transplantation. In the heart muscle or the brain after an ischemic event (MI and stroke, respectively), cell death occurs in regions where blood flow has been interrupted. Although some of this cell death (especially in the area of the initial lesion) is due to necrosis, apoptotic processes increase the area of cell damage in the heart and brain tissues beyond the initial injury. Evidence also exists for the role of apoptosis in cellular damage in reperfusion injury and in heart failure. In addition, certain viruses have evolved mechanisms to inhibit apoptosis to counteract the initiation of apoptosis in infected cells, resulting in the interruption of viral replication.

The uncontrolled growth characteristic of cancer can result from defects in the control of cell proliferation, cell differentiation (terminally differentiated cells typically do not proliferate), and/or via blockage of cell-death pathways. In most human cancers, p53 is either mutated or otherwise rendered nonfunctional, hindering the initiation of apoptosis (Moll et al., 1992). And, as discussed later in this chapter, in many cases of cancer, apoptotic pathways themselves are deregulated, resulting in blockage of apoptosis that is a significant factor in the lack of control of cell growth. Because cytotoxic drugs used in chemotherapy typically kill cancer cells by triggering apoptosis, blockage of apoptotic pathways often renders tumor cells resistant to chemotherapy. Even when chemotherapy is initially successful, tumor cells in which apoptotic pathways are blocked may become resistant to the treatment, resulting in recurrence of disease.

The Apoptotic Pathways

The two central pathways of apoptosis are intrinsic and extrinsic. Figure 28.1 is a basic

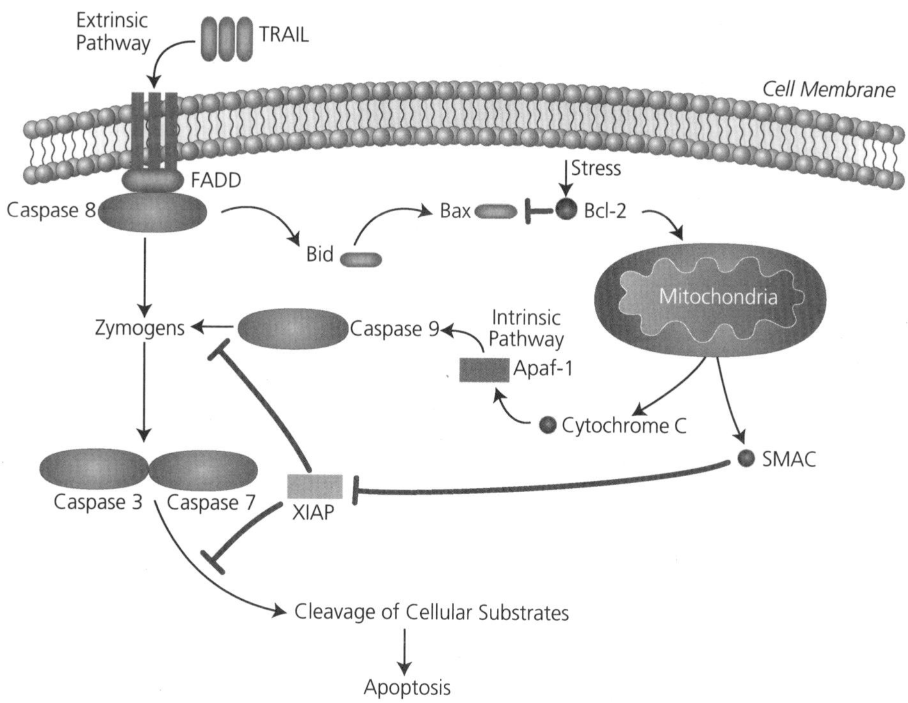

Apaf-1 = Apoptotic protease-activating factor-1
FADD = Fas-associated death domain protein
SMAC = Second mitochondria-derived activator of caspase
TRAIL = TNF-related apoptosis-inducing ligand
XIAP = X-linked inhibitor of apoptosis protein

Figure 28.1 Diagram of Central Apoptosis Pathways

diagram of these pathways; it highlights the roles of apoptotic modulators that are targets for development. In reality, the apoptotic pathway is much more complex than shown in Figure 28.1, and research continues in this area.

The following sections outline both the intrinsic and extrinsic apoptotic pathways and detail potential drug development targets. Apoptosis is also modulated by other pathways; for example, the intrinsic pathway of apoptosis is modulated by other signal transduction pathways, such as the Akt/PTEN pathway (which, when dysregulated, is a factor in several types of cancer) and the proteasome pathway for the degradation of unwanted or defective proteins within the cell. In this report, we focus on those agents that directly modulate either the intrinsic or extrinsic pathways rather than on those agents that modulate apoptosis by affecting other pathways. The most advanced apoptosis drugs in development are oncology drugs that target the intrinsic pathway.

Intrinsic Pathway

The intrinsic pathway centers on the mitochondria and is triggered by such factors as cellular stress (i.e., deprivation of growth factors needed for survival or treatment with various drugs or ionizing radiation) and DNA damage that results in p53-mediated apoptotic signals. Triggers of the intrinsic pathways work principally by modulating members of the B-cell lymphoma-2 (Bcl-2) family of apoptosis regulatory proteins. The 25 members of this family in the human genome are divided into three subfamilies:

- Antiapoptotic proteins, such as Bcl-2, Bcl-X_L, and Mcl-1, possess four conserved domains, called BH1, BH2, BH3, and BH4, which function in protein-protein interactions.
- Multidomain proapoptotic proteins, such as Bak and Bax, contain three of the domains of the antiapoptotic proteins – BH1, BH2, and BH3 – and thus are known as BH-123 proteins.
- BH3-only proapoptotic proteins, such as Bid and Bad, possess only the BH3 protein.

BH-123 proteins complex with each other and are thought to form pores in the outer membranes of the mitochondria. This process triggers mitochondrial outer-membrane permeabilization (MOMP), which results in the release of cytochrome c from the mitochondria (Green and Kroemer, 2004). Cytochrome c is best known for its function in oxidative phosphorylation, the principal means by which the cell derives its energy. Once released into the cytoplasm, cytochrome c complexes with apoptotic protease-activating factor-1 (Apaf-1) and caspase 9 to form a complex called the apoptosome (Danial and Korsmeyer, 2004).

Caspases (or cysteine aspartyl proteases) are a class of serine proteases that function in apoptosis (as we will discuss later in this chapter, some of them have nonapoptotic functions as well). Caspases are synthesized as inactive zymogens (inactive enzyme precursors), which must be activated by specific proteolysis events to display enzyme activity. In the apoptosome, caspase 9 undergoes autocatalytic activation in the presence of ATP or deoxy ATP (dATP). Caspase 9, known as an initiator caspase, activates other caspases, especially “effector caspases” or “executioner caspases” such as caspases 3 and 7. These caspases catalyze a series of proteolytic events that result in all the hallmarks of apoptosis, such as DNA fragmentation, blebbing, and the eventual formation of apoptotic bodies.

The other Bcl-2 subfamilies, antiapoptotic proteins and BH3-only proteins, modulate apoptosis by their effect on BH-123 proteins. The antiapoptotic proteins localize to the mitochondria and inhibit apoptosis by specifically binding and sequestering proapoptotic multidomain family members. The BH3-only proteins are thought to work principally by binding to antiapoptotic family members and releasing BH-123 proteins from their complexes with the antiapoptotic proteins.

The intrinsic pathway of apoptosis can be inhibited by a class of proteins known as the inhibitor of apoptosis proteins (IAPs). IAPs were originally identified in baculovirus as encoded proteins that the virus uses as a defense against apoptosis in infected cells; however, cellular members of this family are found in several groups of organisms, including mammals. IAPs contain characteristic domains known as baculovirus IAP repeats (BIRs), which are essential to the antiapoptotic activity of these proteins. Mammalian IAPs, such as X-linked IAP (XIAP), inhibit the ability of the initiator caspase 9 to activate downstream caspases. They also inhibit the effector caspases 3 and 7 by binding their active sites. Conversely, IAPs are inhibited by a class of proapoptotic proteins that are released from the mitochondria after MOMP, including second mitochondria-derived activator of caspase (Smac). Smac possesses a tetrapeptide sequence called the IAP-binding motif (IBM), which binds to the BIR2 domain of XIAP and thus enables caspase activity.

An IAP that is a particular focus as a drug target by academic and corporate laboratories is survivin. Survivin, identified by Dario C. Altieri (University of Massachusetts Medical School, Worcester, Massachusetts) and his colleagues, is a bifunctional protein that is involved in both regulation of mitosis and inhibition of apoptosis (Dohi et al., 2004). It is expressed in the developing fetus and in the vast majority of human cancers; however, in mature differentiated tissues, it is expressed at nearly undetectable levels. This characteristic suggests that agents that target survivin may promote apoptosis in tumor cells without affecting normal cell function.

Researchers have found that survivin localizes to both the cytoplasm and to mitochondria in tumor cells. The mitochondrial level of survivin increases in response to cellular stress, such as hypoxia, heat shock, and exposure to chemotherapeutic drugs. In response to triggers of apoptosis, survivin is released from the mitochondria and specifically inhibits activation of initiator caspase 9. In contrast to mitochondrial survivin, cytoplasmic survivin does not appear to inhibit apoptosis and may even impair cancer-like cellular behavior. Researchers hypothesize that this ability may be due to survivin's mitotic function.

Significant research has been done regarding the relationship between heat shock protein 90 (Hsp90) and survivin. The molecular chaperone Hsp90 binds to the Bir domains of survivin; this interaction may occur as well between Hsp90 and other IAPs. The inhibition of the Hsp90-surviving interaction results in proteasomal degradation of survivin, increased activity of effector caspases, and mitochondrial-dependent apoptosis (Fortungo et al., 2003). The development of a cell-permeable peptidomimetic drug, shepherdin, designed using sequences found in survivin Bir repeats, induced apoptosis in tumor cells in vitro and had no effect on normal cells or on in vitro hematopoietic differentiation. In xenograft-mouse models injected with a prostate tumor-cell line, shepherdin inhibited tumor growth with no apparent toxicity. However, the drug inhibited Hsp90 interactions with multiple-client proteins, including the signal transduction protein Akt and the cyclin-dependent kinases CDK-4 and CDK-6, which are involved in the cell cycle, and it induced the proteasomal degradation of these client proteins (Plescia et al., 2005). Despite this lack of selectivity, several companies are developing Hsp90 inhibitors as anticancer agents, but because the focus of this report is on agents that directly affect the apoptotic pathways, we do not discuss these agents in detail.

Extrinsic Pathway

The extrinsic apoptotic pathway involves signal transduction pathways that are activated by the tumor necrosis factor-receptor (TNFR) family of cell surface receptors and their corresponding tumor necrosis factors (TNFs), including TNFR/TNF-alpha, Fas/FasL (Fas ligand), and TNF-related apoptosis-inducing ligand (TRAIL) receptor/TRAIL. Of this group, TRAIL is of particular interest to cancer biologists and oncology drug developers because it has been found to selectively induce apoptosis in cancer cells independent of p53, which is usually inactivated in human cancers. Evidence suggests that TRAIL may be involved in tumor surveillance by natural killer cells and in defense against viral infection, although the physiological role of TRAIL is not well understood.

The binding of a specific ligand to a TNFR on the cell surface results in the clustering of the receptors. The intracellular domains of these receptor complexes then bind to multiple copies of death-adaptor proteins, such as Fas-associated death domain (FADD) protein. The death-adaptor proteins bind to caspase 8 (an initiator caspase), which is autocatalytically activated. Caspase 8 then activates effector caspases such as caspases 3 and 7, triggering apoptosis. Caspase 8 can also initiate the intrinsic program of apoptosis via cleavage of Bid, leading to MOMP via proapoptotic Bcl-2 family proteins like Bak and Bax.

In many cases, engagement of TNFRs can lead to survival and cell proliferation rather than apoptosis. This result is in part regulated by the complexing of the intracellular domains of the clustered receptors with adaptor proteins other than death-adaptor proteins (e.g., adaptor proteins which couple TNFR1 to the proinflammatory nuclear factor kappa B [NFκB] pathway). The result is cellular survival, as well as cell proliferation and/or production of proinflammatory cytokines. Moreover, the NFκB pathway modulates induction of apoptosis via the extrinsic pathway; for example, inhibitors of this pathway are under study as possible apoptosis enhancers in cancer treatment.

APOPTOSIS ACTIVATORS IN DEVELOPMENT FOR CANCER

Most corporate activity in apoptosis-based therapeutics is focused on the development of apoptosis activators for the treatment of cancer. Most of these drug candidates target the intrinsic pathway of apoptosis, although we do discuss TRAIL receptor agonists and the extrinsic pathway. Table 28.1 lists leading drug candidates now in clinical trials.

Bcl-2 Inhibitors

Bcl-2 is overexpressed in most common types of solid tumors and hematologic cancers, making it an attractive target for cancer treatment. In vitro studies and animal models indicate that overexpression of Bcl-2 blocks apoptosis in cancer cells, enhances their metastatic potential, and promotes resistance to chemotherapeutic agents (which typically work by triggering apoptosis). They also indicate that inhibiting Bcl-2 promotes apoptosis in cancer cells and results in tumor

Table 28.1 Leading Apoptosis Activators in Clinical Trials for the Treatment of Cancer

Target	*Company*	*Drug*	*Stage*
Bcl-2 inhibitors	Genta	Genasense (oblimersen, G-3139), Bcl-2 antisense compound	Preregistration for chronic lymphocytic leukemia in the United States and for melanoma in Europe
	Ascenta Therapeutics	(-) Gossypol, small-molecule inhibitor of antiapoptotic Bcl-2 proteins	Phase I
	Gemin X	GX-15-070, small-molecule inhibitor of antiapoptotic Bcl-2 proteins	Phase I/II for chronic lymphocytic leukemia Phase I for solid tumors
IAP inhibitors	Aegera Therapeutics	AEG-35156, XIAP antisense compound	Phase Ib for locally advanced metastatic solid tumors
	Avi BioPharma	XIAP NeuGene antisense compound	Phase I
	Isis/Eli Lilly	LY-2181308/ISIS-23722, survivin antisense compound	Phase I
TRAIL receptor agonists	HGS/GSK	HGS-ETR1 (mapatumumab), MAb to TRAIL receptor	Phase I, Phase II, various cancers
	Genentech/Amgen	Recombinant Apo2L/TRAIL	Phase I

IAP = Inhibitor of apoptosis protein; MAb = Monoclonal antibody; TRAIL = Tumor necrosis factor (TNF)-related apoptosis-inducing ligand; XIAP = X-linked inhibitor of apoptosis protein regression or ablation, especially in concert with treatment with standard chemotherapeutic drugs. Three companies have Bcl-2 inhibitors in active development. The lead agent, Genta's Genasense, is an antisense compound. The other two companies, Ascenta Therapeutics (San Diego) and Gemin X (Montreal), are investigating small-molecule Bcl-2 inhibitors derived from natural products.

Genta's Genasense

The Bcl-2 inhibitor that is most advanced in clinical development is Genta's Genasense (oblimersen, G-3139). It is an antisense compound – a single-stranded nucleic acid designed to specifically bind to a messenger RNA (mRNA) molecule that codes for the drug's target protein. Oblimersen is a synthetic 18-base oligonucleotide with a phosphorothioate backbone, a type of modified deoxyribose backbone that results in greater stability and longer half-life in the bloodstream than DNA oligonucleotides with an unmodified backbone (Dove, 2002). It is designed to bind to the first 18 bases in the portion of Bcl-2 mRNA that codes for the protein; the resulting stretch of double-stranded DNA is targeted within the cell by ribonuclease H, which degrades the complementary mRNA while releasing the modified antisense strand. The antisense compound is then free to target additional Bcl-2 mRNAs. Antisense compounds have had difficulties in clinical trials, independent of the types of molecules and cells that they target; researchers attribute these difficulties mainly to drug delivery issues.

Genta has been developing oblimersen as a therapy for several solid and hematologic cancers, in combination with various standard chemotherapies. In May 2004, an advisory committee of the FDA recommended the rejection of Genta's new drug application (NDA) for the treatment of metastatic melanoma by a combination therapy of oblimersen and dacarbazine because the combination therapy did not show a significant increase in survival over dacarbazine alone, which was the study's primary end point. Genta then withdrew its NDA, and its development partner for the drug, Aventis (now Sanofi Aventis), terminated its agreement. Genta is continuing development of oblimersen on its own.

The basis of the NDA in CLL is a Phase III study that achieved its primary end point, a significant increase in the proportion of patients in the oblimersen plus chemotherapy group (as compared with chemotherapy alone) who achieved either a complete response or a nodular partial response. (A complete response is the disappearance of all detectable signs of cancer; a nodular partial response is a partial response with residual lymphoid nodules in bone marrow.) The complete responses and nodular partial responses were durable, lasting six months or more, and the rate of relapse among patients who achieved these responses was significantly lower than in patients treated with chemotherapy alone. In September 2005, Genta reported that extended follow-up studies indicated that oblimersen plus chemotherapy resulted in significantly longer durations of remission and significantly lower rates of relapse as compared with chemotherapy alone. The company has initiated an NDA for accelerated approval of Genasense in CLL and requested a meeting with the FDA to discuss plans for a confirmatory postapproval study.

The basis for the European application was a Phase III clinical trial, the results of which were presented at the American Society of Clinical Oncology (ASCO) meeting in May 2005. The trial showed a significant increase in overall response, complete response, and progression-free survival in patients treated with oblimersen plus chemotherapy, as compared with patients treated with chemotherapy alone. A 24-month follow-up showed a significant increase in durable responses (i.e., responses lasting six months or more). The study also showed a near-significant trend toward increased overall survival, the primary end point. Prior to randomization, the patients were stratified in terms of their blood concentration of lactate dehydrogenase (LDH). High serum levels of

LDH in advanced melanoma patients have been linked to poor outcome. In the two-thirds of patients without elevated LDH at baseline, treatment with oblimersen plus chemotherapy showed a significant increase in overall survival as compared with chemotherapy alone.

Ascenta Therapeutics' (−) Gossypol

(−) Gossypol is derived from cottonseed and is the negative optical isomer of gossypol. (Optical isomers, or enantiomers, are non-superimposable mirror images of one another. Organic small-molecule compounds that have right-handed [positive] and left-handed [negative] optical isomers are called "chiral compounds"). S. Wang and colleagues at the University of Michigan in Ann Arbor have been studying (−) gossypol as a compound for the treatment of cancer. Dr Wang is a cofounder of Ascenta.

(−) Gossypol is a BH3 mimetic and binds to the BH3-binding groove of the antiapoptotic proteins Bcl-XL and Bcl-2. As a result, it induces apoptosis by working directly at the mitochondria in cells in which either of these proteins is overexpressed, resulting in the release of cytochrome c and triggering the activation of caspase 9 (Oliver et al., 2005). The Michigan researchers showed that (-) gossypol induced apoptosis and improved sensitivity to chemotherapy in cultured head and neck squamous-cell carcinoma (HNSCC) cells, which typically overexpress Bcl-XL and are often resistant to chemotherapy with such agents as cisplatin (Bauer et al., 2005).

Gemin X's GX15-070

Gemin X is another university spin-off, cofounded by Philip Branton and Gordon Shore of McGill University in Montreal. The company has developed a series of derivatives of the natural product prodigiosin, a bright red pigment produced by the bacterium *Serratia marcescens.* Gemin X's lead compound, GX15–070, binds to the BH3-binding groove of Bcl-2 proteins. It activates apoptosis in vitro in several cancer cell models that overexpress antiapoptotic Bcl-2 family proteins, and it shows antitumor activity in animal models. Gemin X researchers and their academic collaborators presented initial results of the ongoing Phase I trials at the 2005 ASCO meeting. At that time, the drug showed very preliminary evidence of clinical activity.

IAP Inhibitors

Three IAP inhibitors, all of which are antisense compounds, are in development. Aegera Therapeutics and Avi BioPharma are developing XIAP antisense compounds, and Isis, in collaboration with Lilly, is developing a survivin antisense compound.

Aegera Therapeutics' AEG-35156

Aegera's lead therapeutic, the XIAP antisense compound AEG-35156, is the result of research of one of its scientific founders, Robert Korneluk of the University of Ottawa (Ontario). It is a second-generation antisense compound that uses proprietary antisense chemistry licensed from Hybridon. Hybridon's second-generation antisense chemistries are designed to have significant advantages over first-generation phosphorothioate antisense chemistries because they offer the potential for oral delivery and are designed to have fewer side effects, greater potency, and a longer half-life. These antisense compounds contain a central core of DNA residues, flanked on either side by modified RNA residues. The antisense chemistries are thus known as hybrid or mixed backbone chemistries. Aegera reports that AEG-35156 has shown efficacy in preclinical models of several different cancers.

Avi Biopharma's XIAP NeuGene Antisense Compound

Avi Biopharma has developed another proprietary type of third-generation antisense compound known as NeuGenes. The backbones of these nucleic acids are based on morpholino antisense chemistry, in which the ribose or deoxyribose rings found in natural nucleic acids are replaced by morpholine rings, and the phosphate groups are replaced with phosphorodiamidate groups. In contrast to natural nucleic acids and most other antisense compounds, which are negatively charged, morpholino antisense compounds (or "morpholinos") are uncharged. They are resistant to degradation in the body due to nucleases, which do not recognize the morpholinos. Unlike several other types of antisense compounds, morpholinos work by blocking translation of mRNA targets into protein, rather than triggering degradation by RNAse H. Avi states that its NeuGenes are superior to phosphorothioate antisense compounds in efficacy, stability, drug delivery, and safety characteristics.

At the June 2005 meeting of the Endocrine Society, Avi reported that its anti-XIAP NeuGenes produced a significant reduction in XIAP expression in an ovarian cancer model, resulting in increased susceptibility to radiation. In an earlier presentation, at the American Association for Cancer Research (AACR) meeting in April of the same year, the company reported that its anti-XIAP NeuGenes gave similar results in a prostate cancer model.

Isis/Eli Lilly's LY-2181308

As discussed previously, the IAP survivin appears to be a particularly attractive target in oncology. Isis, a company that focuses on the development of antisense drugs, has been developing the antisurvivin drug ISIS-23722. Isis licensed the drug to Lilly in April 2003, and it is now known as LY-2181308. This drug is part of a broad strategic alliance between the two companies and is the first drug from the alliance to move into the clinic.

LY-2181308 is based on Isis's proprietary second-generation 2'-methoxyethyl (2'MOE) antisense chemistry, which adds the 2'MOE modification of sugar moieties to the original phosphorothioate backbone. Moreover, the second-generation compounds are composed of both RNA-like and DNA-like nucleotides, in contrast to the all-DNA structure of Isis's first-generation compounds. Isis reports that its second-generation antisense compounds have increased affinities for their mRNA targets, as well as greater resistance to degradation. The company also reports that these properties enable the compounds to be active at lower doses and to have longer half-lives. They also have the potential for oral delivery.

Lilly selected LY-2181308 for entry into clinical trials based on its antitumor activity in mouse xenograft models representing a variety of human cancers. The drug also showed selective inhibition of survivin protein based on an antisense mechanism of action, and it demonstrated an additive antitumor effect with several chemotherapy drugs.

TRAIL Receptor Agonists

As discussed previously, the TRAIL/TRAIL receptor system, which is involved in the extrinsic apoptosis pathway, is of special interest as a cancer target because of its apparent high degree of tumor specificity. Two corporate collaborations have TRAIL receptor agonists in clinical trials – a collaboration between Human Genome Sciences (HGS) and GlaxoSmithKline (GSK) and a collaboration between Genentech and Amgen. Both of these agents are protein drugs that target the TRAIL receptor.

Human Genome Sciences/GlaxoSmithKline's HGS-ETR1

HGS developed its monoclonal antibody (MAb) TRAIL receptor agonist HGS-ETR1 (mapatumumab) in collaboration with Cambridge Antibody Technology (Cambridge, United Kingdom) using the latter company's fully human antibody technology. HGS obtained an exclusive license to the drug. In August 2005, GSK exercised an option to codevelop and copromote HGS-ETR1 on a 50/50 basis. This collaboration came about as a result of a June 1996 agreement with HGS allowing GSK to exercise options to certain HGS products that complete Phase IIa clinical trials.

HGS-ETR1 specifically binds to TRAIL receptor 1 (TRAIL-R1), which is expressed on the surface of many types of human solid and hematologic cancers. In preclinical studies, the agent triggered apoptosis and inhibited tumor growth in a variety of cancers. HGS entered the drug into three Phase II clinical studies: in non-Hodgkin's lymphoma (NHL), non-small-cell lung cancer (NSCLC), and colorectal cancer. In 2005, the company reported the results of the NSCLC trial and interim results of the NHL trial. In the NCSLC trial, the drug was well tolerated, and stable disease was observed in 9 of 32 (29%) patients treated. The drug was also well tolerated in the NHL trial and showed evidence of clinical activity.

Genentech/Amgen's Recombinant Apo2L/TRAIL

Genentech is developing its recombinant Apo2L/TRAIL product in collaboration with Amgen and its subsidiary, Immunex. Preclinical studies involving a variety of mouse xenograft models demonstrated that the compound is active as a single agent and has additive activity with several chemotherapies or radiotherapy (Kelley and Ashkenazi, 2004). Apo2L/TRAIL entered Phase I trials in the last quarter of 2004.

Other Intrinsic Pathway Drug Discovery Methods

Despite the identification of several well-validated targets in the intrinsic pathway of apoptosis, drug discovery and development in this area have been difficult because all of these targets are located intracellularly and work via protein-protein interactions. Thus, they are considered, for purposes of small-molecule drug discovery, "undruggable." (The TRAIL system, which involves a cell-surface receptor, makes the extrinsic pathway of apoptosis accessible to well-proven protein-drug strategies.)

The development of an effective antisense drug would eliminate these difficulties, which accounts for the focus on antisense drugs by several companies working on several different targets. However, only one antisense drug (fomivirsen [Isis/Novartis's Vitravene]), which is administered locally for cytomegalovirus (CMV) retinitis (a disease of the eye) in AIDS patients, has reached the market. Despite the development of several different types of second-generation antisense drugs that appear to be improvements over antisense compounds that have failed in the clinic, the antisense strategy remains unproven.

Meanwhile, several companies have been devising strategies to discover small-molecule drugs for "hard targets" in the intrinsic pathway. One such strategy, represented by the drugs from Ascenta and Gemin X, discussed previously, involves developing a suitable screening assay and screening libraries of natural products or synthetic chemical libraries. Aegera is attempting to develop small-molecule IAP inhibitors. Nevertheless, it is difficult to design chemical libraries that will contain compounds that modulate protein-protein interactions, which are the prototypic "hard targets," so it is not surprising that the most advanced small-molecule drug candidates in this area are derivatives of natural products. Infinity Pharmaceuticals, however, has a chemical library platform that involves the development of "natural product-like" synthetic small organic molecules. By screening these libraries, it has discovered IPI-983L, an early-stage inhibitor of the antiapoptotic Bcl-2 family proteins.

Several research groups and companies are developing peptidomimetic drugs that act as Smac mimics and overcome IAP inhibition of caspases. Novartis reports that it has a peptidomimetic in the preclinical stage, and an academic group at the University of Texas Southwestern Medical Center in Dallas published a study on the design and properties of such a molecule (Li et al., 2004).

Stephen Fesik's group at Abbott has been collaborating with Idun (acquired by Pfizer in 2005) to develop small-molecule Bcl-2 family inhibitors using nuclear magnetic resonance-based screening and structure-based drug design. ABT-737, which was discovered in these studies, is in the preclinical stage (Oltersdorf et al., 2005). The Fesik group has also been developing small-molecule nonpeptidic Smac mimetics using similar methods (Park et al., 2005).

CASPASE INHIBITORS AS ANTIAPOPTOTIC AGENTS

Because of their role in both the intrinsic and extrinsic pathways of apoptosis, caspases have been viewed as a potential target in apoptosis drug development. However, the uses of caspase inhibitors may be more limited than originally thought, although they still have potential in the treatment of liver diseases such as alcoholic cirrhosis, viral hepatitis, biliary atresia (the closure of the biliary ducts in infants via inflammatory processes), and primary nonfunction in transplanted livers where apoptosis is a major factor. In the following sections, we discuss some of the significant challenges associated with the use of caspase inhibitors as therapeutic agents. As we explain, these challenges have led researchers into new avenues of discovery. We also examine IDN-6556, the lead caspase inhibitor in development that aims to bypass some of these difficulties.

Challenges to Caspase Inhibitor Development

Nonapoptotic Programmed Cell Death

Until recently, researchers believed that programmed cell death was synonymous with apoptosis. However, recent evidence reveals the existence of alternative, nonapoptotic pathways that do not involve caspase activation (Kroemer and Martin, 2005). The existence of these alternative pathways of cell death complicates attempts to develop caspase inhibitor drugs as apoptotic inhibitors. Figure 28.2 represents a basic schematic

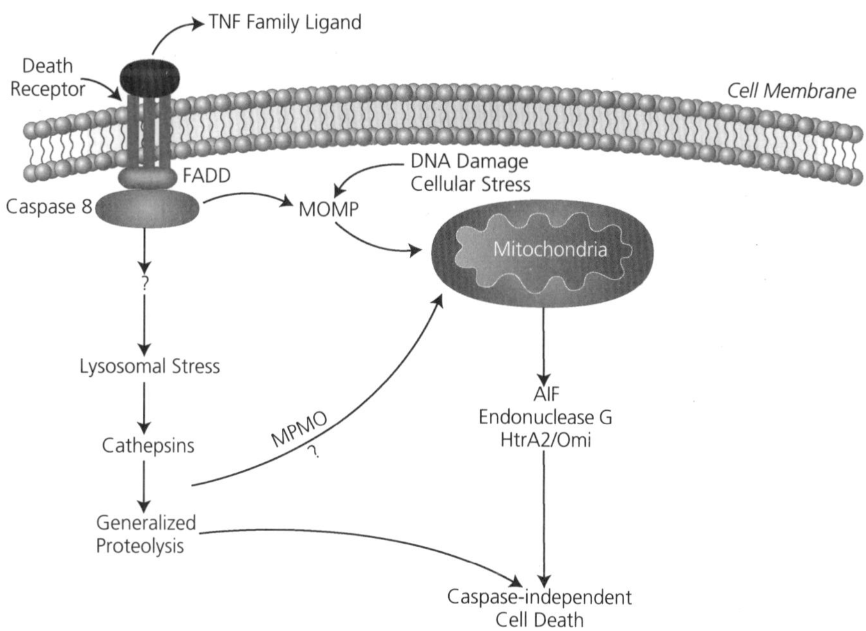

AIF = Apoptosis-inducing factor
FADD = Fas-associated death domain protein
MOMP = Mitochondrial outer membrane permeabilization
TNF = Tumor necrosis factor

Figure 28.2 Schematic of Pathways for Caspase-independent Cell Death

diagram of pathways for the induction of caspase-independent cell death and their relationship to apoptotic pathways. Especially in neuronal loss in neurodegenerative diseases and ischemic stroke, there is evidence that multiple pathways of cell death beyond apoptosis and nonprogrammed necrosis may occur (Yakolev and Faden, 2004). These alternative pathways are only partially understood and complicate strategies for the discovery and development of cell-death inhibitors for the treatment of traumatic brain and spinal-cord injury and neurodegenerative diseases.

When MOMP occurs, in addition to the release of cytochrome C and SMAC, several proteins that promote caspase-independent cell death are released from the mitochondria. Among these proteins are apoptosis-inducing factor (AIF), endonuclease G, and HtrA2/Omi. MOMP also results in the release of reactive oxygen species (ROS), which are highly toxic and can induce cell death. Under normal circumstances, the caspase activation via the intrinsic apoptotic pathway predominates over the action of these caspase-independent mitochondrial effectors, and apoptosis occurs. However, if caspase activation is blocked (e.g., by a caspase inhibitor) caspase-independent cell death occurs.

Another mechanism of caspase-independent cell death is mediated by proteases called cathepsins and calpains. Cathepsin B is released into the cytoplasm as a result of lysosomal damage (e.g., from oxidative stress). It can both trigger MOMP and act on its own, via generalized proteolysis, to trigger cell death. Calpains are proteases found in neurons and are activated by endoplasmic reticulum damage. Both cathepsin B and calpains have been implicated, for example, in neural cell death in stroke and traumatic injury.

Nonapoptotic cell death results in morphology that is different from that which is characteristic of apoptosis. "Apoptosis-like cell death" resembles apoptosis but lacks such features as nuclear fragmentation, the characteristic DNA laddering seen with apoptosis, and/or the formation of apoptotic cell bodies. Autophagic cell death involves the formation of membrane-bound vacuoles that target proteins and organelles to lysosomes for degradation. Necrosis, with swelling of cytoplasmic organelles, is a third type of nonapoptotic cell death.

In many cases, treatment with caspase inhibitors merely shifts cell death to an alternative pathway, resulting in no therapeutic benefit. This situation is especially true when MOMP is induced; attempting to stop cell death via caspase inhibitors is generally ineffective. Using or developing caspase inhibitors to block the extrinsic pathway of apoptosis by inhibiting initiator caspases such as caspase 8 has a greater probability of success. However, in some types of cells, death mediated via the TNFR family may still occur as a result of caspase-independent pathways. This situation suggests that caspase inhibitors may offer protection against cell death only in a limited number of cases.

Drugs that inhibit various pathways of caspase-independent cell death, if successful, would provide alternatives to caspase inhibitors, or they might be used in combination with caspase inhibitors. Researchers are working on several strategies for inhibiting caspase-independent cell death, all of which are in early stages of development. This work includes the discovery of drugs that may, for example, inhibit MOMP or inhibit calpains or cathepsins for use in preventing cell death in neurological disease and trauma and in ischemic heart damage (Kroemer and Martin, 2005).

Indeed, inhibiting MOMP seems like a good strategy for inhibiting major pathways of both apoptotic and nonapoptotic cell death. Some studies indicate that several drugs approved for other conditions may be MOMP inhibitors that can be used to treat diseases in which excess apoptosis is a factor. For example, the HIV protease inhibitor nelfinavir (Pfizer's Viracept) has been shown to reduce apoptosis and have therapeutic effects in several mouse models of nonviral disease associated with an apoptotic mechanism, including a model of ischemic stroke. It appears to work by inhibiting mitochondrial pore function and thus preventing MOMP (Weaver et al., 2005). Other potential MOMP inhibitors that are under investigation and that may be useful in treating neurodegenerative disease include the generic antibiotic monocycline and the Parkinson's disease monoamine oxidase inhibitor rasagiline (Teva's Agilect), which is in preregistration in the United States and marketed as Azalect in the United Kingdom (Green and Kroemer, 2004).

Nonapoptotic Functions of Caspases

Another factor that limits the prospect of caspase inhibitors acting as therapeutics is the nonapoptotic function of several caspases in essential physiological functions. In humans, caspases 1, 4, and 5 are "inflammatory caspases" that are involved in the maturation of the cytokines interleukin-1 and interleukin-18; these caspases are not involved in apoptosis. Caspases are also involved in the development of the lens of the eye and the differentiation of platelets and erythrocytes. In addition to its role in apoptosis, caspase 8 is involved in T-cell activation and in macrophage differentiation, and caspase 3 is involved in skeletal-muscle differentiation and in the differentiation of bone marrow stromal stem cells in mice.

Caspase inhibitors, especially if used to treat chronic or long-term conditions such as neurodegenerative disease, may, therefore, have a high potential for side effects because they block normal physiological functions. In some cases, caspases even increase cell survival under conditions of stress; in these cases, treatment with caspase inhibitors may cause cell death. For example, TNF toxicity in vivo was found to be mediated by a caspase-independent pathway mediated via ROS. Treatment with a pan-caspase inhibitor exacerbated TNF toxicity, resulting in kidney failure and death. In this case, caspases appear to protect against this toxicity (Cauwels et al., 2003).

IDN-6556

Idun led the industry in the discovery and development of caspase inhibitors and acquired an extensive portfolio of patents in that area. In February 2005, Pfizer acquired Idun and is now developing Idun's first-in-class pan-caspase inhibitor, IDN-6556, which targets the liver. In several liver diseases, such as alcoholic cirrhosis, viral hepatitis, biliary atresia, and primary nonfunction in transplanted livers, apoptosis is mediated by upregulation of Fas and TNF-α. Apoptosis in these diseases is therefore initiated by the extrinsic apoptotic pathway, eliminating the concerns associated with MOMP induction and making these diseases attractive candidates for a pan-caspase inhibitor. This strategy is aimed at bypassing the difficulties in developing caspase inhibitors as apoptosis inhibitors, which were discussed previously.

IDN-6556 is an oral small-molecule drug that traffics to the liver. It is in Phase II clinical trials for the treatment of hepatitis C and patients who have undergone liver transplantation. In preclinical studies, oral administration of IDN-6556 was found to be efficacious in reducing liver injury and preventing death in two rodent models of liver apoptosis induced via the extrinsic pathway (Hoglen et al., 2004). In a Phase IIa trial reported in early 2005, orally administered IDN-6556 was well tolerated and significantly improved levels of serum liver enzymes (which are markers of liver damage) in patients infected with the hepatitis C virus.

OUTLOOK

In 2002, S. Brenner, J. Sulston, and H.R. Horvitz received the Nobel Prize for Medicine for their groundbreaking work in the identification of apoptotic pathways. Their research began in the mid-1980s, and corporate activity to develop drugs that modulate apoptosis began in the early 1990s. Despite more than a decade of drug discovery, not a single drug that modulates the central pathways of apoptosis has yet reached the market.

As we have discussed, the key obstacles that companies face in developing apoptosis drugs are "undruggable" targets and caspase-independent cell death pathways (see Table 28.2). In oncology, attempts to

Table 28.2 Problems and Potential Solutions in Developing Apoptosis-based Drugs

Problem	*Potential solutions*
"Undruggable" protein–protein interaction targets in the intrinsic pathway, for development of oncology drugs that induce apoptosis	• Develop antisense drugs • If first-generation antisense drugs do not work, develop new antisense chemistries with improved potency and delivery characteristics • Develop small-molecule drugs by screening natural product or natural product-like libraries • Develop peptidomimetic Smac mimics, which inhibit IAPs and thus can potentiate apoptosis • Develop small-molecule drugs via structure-based drug design • Develop protein drugs that target the extrinsic pathway via the TRAIL receptor, which is accessible to this strategy because it is a cell surface receptor • Develop drugs that act on signaling pathways that modulate apoptotic pathways (e.g., Akt/PTEN, nuclear factor kappa B [NFκB], the proteasome pathway, Hsp90, various growth factors)
Caspase-independent cell death pathways complicate efforts to develop caspase inhibitors as apoptosis inhibitors, especially of the intrinsic pathway	• Target conditions that involve the extrinsic pathway using a drug that trafficks to a specific organ to reduce side effects (e.g., Idun/Pfizer's IDN-6556) • Develop drugs that inhibit MOMP, or that inhibit cathepsins and calpains, as alternatives or adjuncts to caspase inhibitors • Develop drugs that act on signaling pathways that induce apoptosis via the intrinsic or extrinsic pathway (e.g., the amyloid pathway in Alzheimer's disease, excitotoxic amino acids in stroke)

Hsp90 = Heat shock protein 90; IAP = Inhibitor of apoptosis protein; MOMP = Mitochondrial outer-membrane permeabilization; Smac = Second mitochondria-derived activator of caspase; TRAIL = Tumor necrosis factor (TNF)-related apoptosis-inducing ligand

overcome undruggable targets have led to the development of antisense drugs, but these agents are often hindered by drug delivery issues. To circumvent problems with drug delivery, companies are developing small-molecule drugs and protein drugs that target the TRAIL receptor. Several of these drugs have reached the clinic. Another strategy that some companies are exploring is the development of drugs that target other pathways that interact with apoptotic pathways, an approach that is particularly viable in oncology.

The existence of caspase-independent pathways of cell death, especially those that are triggered by MOMP, remains the primary difficulty in the development of caspase inhibitors to treat conditions that involve excessive apoptosis. Idun has attempted to bypass this problem in its development of IDN-6556 by carefully targeting a condition that involves the extrinsic pathway with a drug that traffics to a specific organ. Researchers are also attempting to develop agents that inhibit MOMP and other caspase-independent death pathways. Alternatively, drugs that target the signaling pathways that induce either the intrinsic or extrinsic pathway of apoptosis can circumvent issues with caspase-independent cell death.

The second-generation IAP antisense drugs still need to show that they are more efficacious than antisense compounds based on first-generation chemistries, and HGS/GSK's HGS-ET1 TRAIL receptor agonist and Idun/Pfizer's IDN-6556, as all these compounds remain in early-phase clinical trials and have not yet proved their efficacy in humans. Despite the obstacles associated with this field of study, we believe that because of the key role apoptosis plays in cell development, the immune system, and DNA repair, it is likely to remain a promising opportunity for drug development research.

REFERENCES

Bauer, J.A. et al. Reversal of cisplatin resistance with a BH3 mimetic, (–)-gossypol, in head and neck cancer cells: role of wild-type p53 and Bcl-XL. *Molecular Cancer Therapeutics.* 2005; 4: 1096–104.

Cauwels, A. et al. Caspase inhibition causes hyperacute tumor necrosis factor-induced shock via oxidative stress and phospholipase A2. *Nature Immunology.* 2003; 4: 308–10.

Danial, N.K. and Korsmeyer, S.J. Cell death: critical control points. *Cell.* 2004; 116: 205–19.

Dohi, T. et al. Mitochondrial survivin inhibits apoptosis and promotes tumorigenesis. *Journal of Clinical Investigation.* 2004; 114: 1117–27.

Dove, A. Antisense and sensibility. *Nature Biotechnology.* 2002; 20: 121–4.

Fortungo, P. et al. Regulation of survivin functions by Hsp90. *Proceedings of the National Academy of Sciences USA.* 2003; 100: 13791–6.

Green, D.R. and Kroemer, G. The pathophysiology of mitochondrial cell death. *Science.* 2004; 305: 626–9.

Hoglen, N.C. et al. Characterization of IDN-6556 (3-[2-(2-*tert*-butyl-phenylaminooxalyl)-amino]-propionylamino]-4-oxo-5-(2,3,5,6-tetrafluoro-phenoxy)-pentanoic acid): a liver-targeted caspase inhibitor. *Journal of Pharmacology and Experimental Therapeutics.* 2004; 309: 634–40.

Kelley, S.K. and Ashkenazi, A. Targeting death receptors in cancer with Apo2L/TRAIL. *Current Opinion in Pharmacology.* 2004; 4: 333–9.

Kroemer, G. and Martin, S.J. Caspase-independent cell death. *Nature Medicine.* 2005; 11: 725–30.

Li, L. et al. A small-molecule Smac mimetic potentiates TRAIL- and TNF-alpha-mediated cell death. *Science.* 2004; 305: 1471–4.

Moll, U.M. et al. Two distinct mechanisms alter p53 in breast cancer: mutation and nuclear exclusion. *Proceedings of the National Academy of Sciences USA.* 1992; 89: 7262–6.

Oliver, C.I. et al. (–) Gossypol acts directly on the mitochondria to overcome Bcl-2 and Bcl-X(L) mediated apoptosis resistance. *Molecular Cancer Therapeutics.* 2005; 4: 23–31.

Oltersdorf, T. et al. An inhibitor of Bcl-2 family proteins induces regression of solid tumors. *Nature.* 2005; 435: 677–81.

Park, C.M. et al. Nonpeptidic small-molecule inhibitors of XIAP. *Bioorganic and Medicinal Chemistry Letters.* 2005; 15: 771–5.

Plescia, J. et al. Rational design of shepherdin, a novel anticancer agent. *Cancer Cell.* 2005; 7: 457–68.

Weaver, J.G. et al. Inhibition of adenine nucleotide translocator pore function and protection against apoptosis in vivo by an HIV protease inhibitor. *Journal of Clinical Investigation.* 2005; 115: 1828–38.

Yakolev, A.G. and Faden, A.I. Mechanisms of neural cell death: implications for development of neuroprotective treatment strategies. *NeuroRx.* 2004; 1: 5–16.

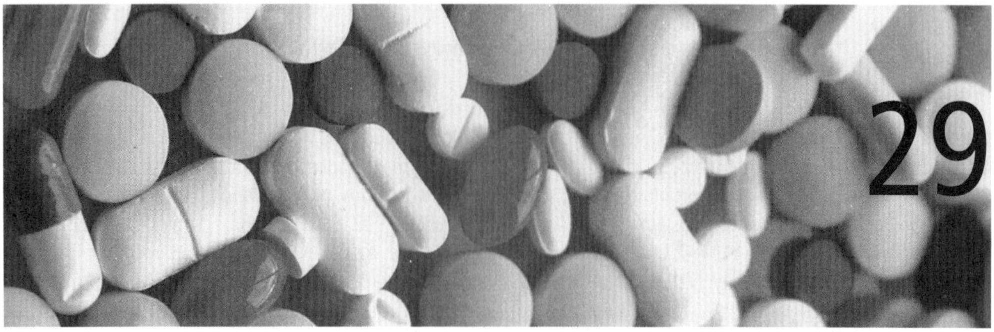

Chronic Lymphocytic Leukemia: Monoclonal Antibodies Will Drive Steady Growth

INTRODUCTION

Chronic lymphocytic leukemia (CLL), which is considered incurable, is the most common leukemia in the Western world. Current research is focusing on the urgent unmet need for agents that improve survival, particularly for patients with advanced disease. Improved responses from treatment regimens that combine targeted biological agents with established chemotherapy, as well as increased drug therapy for early-stage patients who are likely to progress based on potential prognostic markers, have already begun and will continue to create market opportunities and propel steady growth of the CLL market.

In this chapter, we provide an overview of CLL, including its staging, epidemiology, and biological markers. We focus on the US market for this chapter because the United States accounts for approximately 80% of CLL market sales, largely because of the higher cost of CLL agents in this market compared to other markets. We discuss the current treatments and promising late-stage agents in development for CLL.

OVERVIEW OF CHRONIC LYMPHOCYTIC LEUKEMIA

Disease Characteristics

Etiology and Pathophysiology

Leukemia is a cancer that arises from blood-forming cells, in which blood cells mature incompletely or abnormally, resulting in uncontrolled cell proliferation and disruption of the normal functioning and balance of blood cells in the bone marrow, blood, and lymphoid organs. Leukemias are classified as acute or chronic, depending on the maturity of the malignant cells involved (as determined by blood cell counts, microscopic examination of blood cells, and bone marrow aspiration and biopsy), and as lymphocytic or myelogenous based on the lineage of the malignant cell.

CLL, the most prevalent form of leukemia, is a slowly progressing disease in which the malignancy occurs in either a T or B lymphocyte, causing too many lymphocytes to be produced within the body. In 95% of CLLs, the affected cells are B lymphocytes; in the remaining 5%, T lymphocytes are affected.

No etiologic factors have been clearly defined for CLL. Most CLL cases occur arbitrarily, but approximately 1 in 20 patients has a familial form of the disease. The presence of familial cases clearly suggests that inherited genetic factors contribute to the development of the disease, although the specific abnormal genes connected to CLL have not yet been identified. The incidence of CLL in first-degree relatives is three times greater than in the general population (3 in 10,000, compared with 1 in 10,000).

CLL has no single pattern of progression – approximately one-third of patients never require treatment and die from causes unrelated to CLL; one-third have an initial indolent phase followed by progression; and the remaining one-third have aggressive disease at the outset, requiring immediate therapy. In 3–10% of CLL patients, the disease transforms into a more aggressive condition distinct from CLL. The transformation is usually into large-cell lymphoma (also known as Richter's syndrome), and the prognosis for these patients is poor – median survival is six months.

Symptoms

The onset of CLL is usually insidious, and most patients are asymptomatic during the early stages of the disease. Diagnosis is often made following routine blood tests or investigations for an unrelated disease. The median age of onset of CLL is 65–68 years, but approximately 20% of cases occur in people younger than age 55.

In symptomatic patients, the most frequent clinical findings are fatigue, loss of appetite, weight loss, and enlarged lymph nodes. CLL's progressive symptoms are related to leukocyte infiltration of the bone marrow, spleen, and lymphoid tissue. This infiltration, together with disruptions in normal hematopoietic function, results in anemia, neutropenia, thrombocytopenia, and immunological dysfunction. The most severe immunological dysfunction is the lack of immunoglobulins (hypogammaglobulinemia), a condition that occurs in up to 60% of patients with advanced disease. This condition leaves the patient more susceptible to infection, which is a primary cause of death and morbidity.

Autoimmune disease, an immune response against the body's own cells and tissues, occurs in 10–35% of untreated CLL patients. The autoimmunity usually manifests as autoimmune hemolytic anemia. Immune thrombocytopenia, pure red-cell aplasia, and immune neutropenia occur less frequently. Autoimmunity is usually successfully treated with corticosteroids; steroid-refractory patients may need to undergo a splenectomy.

Staging and Survival

CLL is classified using three major staging systems. These systems are described in Table 29.1. The original Rai system, consisting

Table 29.1 Common Staging Systems Used in the Treatment of CLL

System	*Stage*	*Definition*
Rai staging system	0	Lymphocytosis only
	I	Lymphocytosis and lymphadenopathy
	II	Lymphocytosis, spleen or liver enlargement
	III	Lymphocytosis and anemia (hemoglobin <11 g/dL)
	IV	Lymphocytosis and thrombocytopenia (platelet count <100,000 mL)
Modified Rai staging system	Low risk of progression	Rai stage 0
	Intermediate risk of progression	Rai stage I or II
	High risk of progression	Rai stage III or IV
Binet staging system	A	Lymphocytosis, with enlargement of <3 lymphoid areas[a]; no anemia or thrombocytopenia
	B	Lymphocytosis, with enlargement of ≥ 3 lymphoid areas
	C	Lymphocytosis and either anemia (hemoglobin <10 g/dL) or thrombocytopenia (platelet count <100,000/mL), or both

[a]The following lymphoid areas are included: cervical, axillary, inguinal (whether unilateral or bilateral), spleen, and liver

of stages 0-IV, is based on the presence of lymphadenopathy (disease or swelling of the lymph nodes), organomegaly (organ enlargement), and cytopenia (reduction in the number of blood cells) and demonstrates a correlation between Rai stage and survival (Rai et al., 1975). In the modified Rai system, which has three (as opposed to five) tiers, patients are still categorized based on the presence of the aforementioned characteristics in Rai stages 0-IV but are classified as having a low (corresponding to stage 0), intermediate (stages I and II), or high (stages III and IV) risk of disease progression. The Binet classification system (stages A, B, and C) was devised based on a retrospective analysis of disease burden that draws a correlation between the number of nodal groups involved with disease and bone marrow failure (Binet et al., 1981). The original and modified Rai systems are used throughout the United States; all three systems are used in Europe.

The median survival of patients with Rai stage 0 exceeds 12 years and may reach 20 years, with a 10-year overall survival rate of 70–75%. Patients with Rai stages I and II have a median survival of 8–10 years and 5–8 years respectively. Recent data show a median survival of 2–5 years in Rai stages III and IV patients.

Role of Biological Markers in Prognosis

Because the majority of CLL patients have an indolent disease course, identification of patients whose disease is likely to progress plays an important part in treatment recommendations. Particularly in patients who are classified as having a low risk of disease progression, many of whom do not initially receive treatment, biological markers allow physicians to identify those patients more likely to progress based on prognostic markers and other factors.

Researchers have found several biological markers that are associated with more-aggressive disease:

- A rapid (less than 12 months) lymphocyte doubling time (LDT; calculated as the number of months it takes the absolute lymphocyte count to double in number) is associated with decreased median survival (61 months) compared with a slow LDT, which is associated with a longer median survival (118 months) (Montserrat et al., 1986). In several studies, this factor has been confirmed as a prognostic indicator that is independent of disease stage (Shanafelt et al., 2004).
- Elevated serum beta 2-microglobulin is an adverse prognostic feature in CLL, although data supporting this marker as a strong predictor of survival have been inconsistent across studies.
- CD38 (a cell-surface molecule expressed by mature B cells) expression on CLL cells has been shown to have prognostic significance and is easily measured, but it is limited by differences in expression over time in individual patients (Shanafelt et al., 2004).
- The absence of immunoglobulin heavy (IgVH) chain mutations is associated with a high risk of early progression, but the test is not widely available (Damle et al., 1999; Hamblin et al., 1999).
- ZAP-70 (a signaling molecule involved in transducing intracellular signals from the T-cell receptor to the nucleus in T lymphocytes) is aberrantly expressed in malignant CLL B cells that have unmutated *Ig* genes. Studies suggest that ZAP-70's expression is predictive of patients with more-rapid disease progression and death. ZAP-70 is detectable through a test that is easier to perform than the IgVH test (Crespo et al., 2003; Wiestner et al., 2003).

CURRENT TREATMENT OPTIONS FOR CHRONIC LYMPHOCYTIC LEUKEMIA

Despite relatively good long-term survival rates, CLL is considered incurable; patients ultimately relapse and die of their disease. The overall CLL population is elderly and has a low tolerance for toxic chemotherapy regimens. Therefore, the aim of current drug regimens is to obtain the highest possible rate and duration of remission in CLL patients while balancing the associated toxicity and infection rate. Table 29.2 describes the current agents used to treat CLL, including their mechanisms of action and sales.

Drug regimens for CLL are complex and can involve either monotherapy or a combination of drugs. Some of the commonly used

Table 29.2 Select Current Therapies Used for Treatment of Chronic Lymphocytic Leukemia, 2006

Generic Name	*Company/Brand*	*Mechanism of Action*	*2005 Sales (millions of dollars)*[a]
Alkylating agents			
Chlorambucil (single agent)	GlaxoSmithKline's Leukeran	Alkylation of DNA results in breaks in the DNA molecule as well as cross-linking of the twin strands, thus interfering with DNA replication and transcription of RNA and ultimately causing cell death	0.6
Cyclophosphamide	Bristol-Myers Squibb's Cytoxan; Bristol-Myers Squibb/Baxter's Endoxan, Endoxana; Pfizer's Cyclostin; generics	Alkylate DNA bases, thereby producing cross-links that covalently link the two DNA strands and prevent cell replication	0.3
Purine analogues			
Fludarabine (single agent)	Berlex/Schering AG's Fludara, generics	Metabolized rapidly to F-Ara-ATP, which inhibits DNA synthesis by inhibition of DNA polymerases and prevents elongation of DNA strands through direct incorporation into the DNA molecule	22.2
Pentostatin	SuperGen/Wyeth/Pfizer's Nipent	Potent, irreversible inhibitor of adenosine deaminase (ADA), a vital enzyme in the purine salvage pathway. Inhibition results in depletion of the nucleotide pool and inhibition of DNA synthesis and subsequent toxicity to the cell	1.5
Cladribine	Ortho-Biotech's Leustatin	Cladribine closely resembles fludarabine; it inhibits DNA synthesis by interfering with DNA polymerases, thereby preventing elongation of DNA strands	N.M.
Cytotoxic antibiotics			
Doxorubicin	Pfizer's Adriamycin, Adriblastine; generics	Anthracycline interacts with several cellular targets, most important the DNA regulation enzyme topoisomerase II, thereby exerting a cytotoxic effect	0.1
Vinca alkaloids			
Vincristine	Eli Lilly's Oncovin, generics	Vinca alkaloids interact with tubulin and disrupt microtubular function in the mitotic spindle. This action leads to metaphase arrest, resulting in mitotic arrest and cell death	0.1
Corticosteroids			
Prednisone	Prednisone (generics)	Reduce inflammatory responses and suppress the immune system	N.M.
Prednisolone	Prednisolone (generics)	Reduce inflammatory responses and suppress the immune system	N.M.
Monoclonal antibodies			
Alemtuzumab	Berlex/Genzyme's Campath; Schering's MabCampath	A chimeric, humanized MAb directed against the cluster of differentiation (CD) molecule 52, a molecule expressed on all mature lymphocytes and monocytes. Binding of alemtuzumab to CD52 results in results in cell death	56.1

[a]Due to the level of off-label prescribing, sales are estimates
N.M.: Not Measurable

agents and treatment regimens are described in the following sections. In addition to these pharmacotherapeutic options, stem cell transplantation (SCT) is being used experimentally in some patient populations. Further details on SCT can be found in the sidebar, "Stem Cell Transplantation: A Potential Cure for CLL?"

Stem Cell Transplantation: A Potential Cure for CLL?

Occasionally, autologous or allogeneic stem cell transplantation (SCT) is used as a first-line therapy in a minority of CLL patients. SCT is the only treatment currently available for CLL that offers the possibility of a cure; however, the morbidity and mortality associated with the treatment are considerable. This course of action is considered experimental and is generally reserved for young patients (< 55) who have poor prognostic factors or as a last-chance option for patients with advanced disease.

There are two main types of SCT: (1) autologous, in which the patient's own stem cells are harvested and then returned to the patient, and (2) allogeneic, in which a related or unrelated donor is the source of stem cells. Allogeneic SCT carries the risk of the patient developing graft-versus-host disease (GVHD), a potentially fatal condition in which the donated stem cells trigger an immune response against the patient. Indeed, allogeneic SCT carries a high mortality risk – but it offers a higher chance of cure than autologous SCT. This advantage is due, in part, to the graft-versus-leukemia (GvL) effect, whereby the donor's stem cells trigger an immune response against the patient's leukemia cells. Autologous SCT, which eliminates the risk of GVHD, does not trigger GvL, which reduces its effectiveness. In addition, stem cells harvested from the patient may be contaminated by tumor cells, and the relapse rate for autologous SCT is high.

Current research is investigating allogeneic SCT in a nonmyeloablative rather than fully ablative setting. Nonmyeloablative SCT uses less-intensive conditioning regimens that rely on immunosuppression rather than cytotoxicity. The chemotherapy or irradiation given immediately prior to a transplant is called the conditioning regimen. The purpose is to help eradicate the patient's disease prior to the infusion of the transplant cells and to suppress immune reactions. In myeloablative allogeneic transplants, cyclophosphamide and total body irradiation is commonly employed as a conditioning regimen that results in eradication of the patient's bone marrow cells. This treatment also has an immunosuppressive effect that prevents rejection of the transplant by the recipient's immune system.

Compared with a fully ablative approach, nonmyeloablative allogeneic transplantation uses lower doses of chemotherapy and radiation (such as immunosuppressive doses of purine nucleotide analogues and relatively low doses of either an alkylating agent or irradiation). These doses are too low to eradicate all of the recipient's bone marrow cells. Therefore, this approach does require high doses of immunosuppressive agents in the early stages of treatment, which results in a state of mixed chimerism early after transplant in which recipient cells and donor cells coexist in the bone marrow space. The dose of the immunosuppressive therapy is then decreased, allowing donor T cells to eradicate the remaining recipient stem cells and to induce GVHD and the GvL effect.

Because it offers patients the best chance of a full recovery, use of SCT as a treatment for CLL is likely to become increasingly more common, particularly as the mortality rates decline with improved conditioning regimens.

Treatment Decisions

In making treatment decisions, physicians consider the disease burden as determined by the Rai clinical staging system and many other factors, including prognostic factors, molecular and clinical factors, age, performance status (a measure that attempts to quantify a cancer patient's general well-being), and hospital-specific policies. The majority of patients with Rai low-risk CLL do not initially receive drug therapy but are monitored regularly. Approximately 50% of patients with low-risk disease eventually progress and require treatment. Studies show that treating early-stage patients before the disease progresses does not confer any survival benefit and may, in fact, be associated with an increased risk of secondary malignancies (Chronic Lymphocytic Leukemia Trialists' Collaborative Group, 1999). However, 5–10% of low-risk CLL patients show signs of disease progression and/or poor risk factors. These patients do require and receive treatment.

In many cases, the decision to treat patients in the Rai intermediate- and high-risk categories is based on clinical and biological symptoms (such as enlarged lymph nodes, rapid lymphocyte doubling time (LDT), increasing anemia) as well as performance status and age. The majority of patients in these stages do receive treatment.

The identification of new biomarkers that help determine prognosis has led to improvements in risk stratification of patients, which, in turn, has led to better approaches to initial management of patients. Physicians follow the National Cancer Institute (NCI) guidelines in determining when to treat. To determine whether a patient has responded to therapy, clinicians apply the NCI criteria for response guidelines, listed in Table 29.3.

First-line Therapies

First-line therapy for CLL consists of treatment with either the oral alkylating agent chlorambucil (GlaxoSmithKline's Leukeran) or with the purine analogue fludarabine (Schering AG/Berlex's Fludara, generics). Chlorambucil has been the most widely used first-line approach to managing CLL for the past 40 years. Fludarabine was approved in 2000 and is indicated only for patients previously treated with alkylating agents, but a significant proportion of hematologists are using it off-label as the first-line agent, particularly to treat younger patients (aged < 55) with stage III or IV disease. Chlorambucil does have a less-toxic side-effect profile and is therefore the preferred therapy for older patients (65 or older) and for patients with a poor performance status who cannot tolerate the severe myelosuppression caused by fludarabine.

Recent trials have shown that first-line fludarabine therapy provides superior response rates compared with chlorambucil (a 20% complete response [CR] and 43% partial response [PR] with fludarabine versus 4% and 33%, respectively, with chlorambucil) as well as a longer duration of remission than chlorambucil (Rai et al., 2000). However, the two compounds' long-term survival rates are not significantly different. Two factors inhibit the use of fludarabine as first-line therapy: first, fludarabine has greater toxicity than chlorambucil (severe infections are more common with fludarabine because of its greater immunosuppressive activity); second, although fludarabine is an efficacious second-line therapy in patients with chlorambucil-resistant disease, the reverse is not true.

Second-line Therapies

For patients who have failed first-line treatment, various options are available. Fludarabine may also be used in the second-line setting in the case of nonresponse to

Table 29.3 NCI Definition of Response to Treatment in CLL Patients

Complete response	Normal physical examination
	No symptoms
	Lymphocytes $\leq 4x10^9/L$
	Neutrophils $\geq 1.5x10^9/L$
	Platelets $>100x10^9/L$
	Hemoglobin >11g/dL (untransfused)
	Bone marrow lymphocytes <30% with no nodules
Partial response	50% decrease in size of lymph nodes and/or liver/spleen upon physical examination
	Plus one or more of the following:
	Neutrophils $\geq 1.5x10^9/L$
	Platelets $>100x10^9/L$
	Hemoglobin >11g/dL or 50% improvement
Stable disease	Patients who have not achieved a complete or partial response and do not have progressive disease
Progressive disease	≥50% increase in lymph node, spleen, or liver size
	≥50% increase in circulating lymphocytes
	Transformation to Richter's syndrome

NCI = National Cancer Institute

chlorambucil or early relapse. Physicians also prescribe fludarabine combinations as second-line therapy, including fludarabine/cyclophosphamide (Bristol-Myers Squibb's Cytoxan, BMS/Baxter's Endoxan/Endoxana, Pfizer's Neosar/Cyclostin, generics) and fludarabine/cyclophosphamide/mitoxantrone (Serono/Wyeth/Takeda's Novantrone, Baxter's Onkotrone, generics).

Additional second-line therapies include the combination regimens CHOP (cyclophosphamide, doxorubicin [Pfizer's Adriamycin/Adriblastine, generics], vincristine [Eli Lilly's Oncovin, generics], and prednisone [generics]) or CVP (cyclophosphamide, vincristine, and prednisone). These combination regimens are alternative second-line therapies because of their poorer response rates in the first-line setting and higher toxicities compared with fludarabine-based regimens.

Third-line Therapies

The prognosis of patients who relapse after two courses of therapy is very poor, but many patients receive a third line of therapy to relieve symptoms and delay disease progression by a few months. Alemtuzumab (Schering AG's MabCampath, Genzyme/Berlex's Campath) was launched for the third-line therapy of CLL in the United States and Europe in 2001. Alemtuzumab is approved for single-agent use in fludarabine-refractory CLL patients. Alemtuzumab is a chimeric, humanized MAb directed against the cluster of differentiation (CD) molecule 52, a glycosylphosphatidylinositol-anchored glycoprotein expressed on all mature lymphocytes, monocytes, and spermatozoa but not on hematopoietic stem-cell progenitors. Binding of alemtuzumab to cell-surface CD52 results in complement-mediated lysis, antibody-dependent cellular cytotoxicity (ADCC), and opsonization, resulting in cell death. Alemtuzumab is associated with severe hematologic toxicities and subsequent high-infection rates. In addition, alemtuzumab is very expensive, a disadvantage that limits its widespread use in countries with predominantly public healthcare systems. Despite these disadvantages, and because of a lack of alternative options, alemtuzumab is a popular therapy choice in the third-line setting.

The FDA granted approval for alemtuzumab largely on the basis of an international study that investigated the efficacy of alemtuzumab as a single-agent treatment in CLL patients who had failed at least one alkylating-based regimen and fludarabine treatment. In the pivotal trial, alemtuzumab administered to fludarabine-refractory patients achieved a response in 33% of patients (2% CR and 31% PR). Median time to progression (TTP) in responders was 9.5 months, with a median survival of 16 months in all patients, which is longer than historical controls. Infusion-related reactions were commonly reported adverse events that included rigors, fever, vomiting, and rash; these events declined over time of treatment. Most patients experienced transient cytopenias. Notable infections occurred in a little more than one-quarter of the patients (Keating et al., 2002). Overall, treatment with alemtuzumab provided a benefit for patients with a very poor prognosis.

Although alemtuzumab is approved only for use in the third-line setting, it has been under investigation for use in earlier treatment settings. High response rates were observed in previously untreated patients who received alemtuzumab as first-line therapy (19% CR and 68% PR, giving an overall response rate of 87%). Acute administration-related reactions such as rigor, nausea, hypotension, and bronchospasm were rare or absent. These reactions are commonly seen when alemtuzumab is administered intravenously; the reason for the discrepancy is unclear. Hematologic toxicity included transient grade IV neutropenia in 21% of patients (Lundin et al., 2002).

Alemtuzumab has also been under investigation for use in combination with chemotherapy. The FluCam regimen consists of fludarabine in combination with alemtuzumab. In previously treated patients, this combination resulted in CR and PR rates of 29% and 56% respectively (overall response of 85%). This response rate is one of the best seen in previously treated patients to date. Elimination of residual disease from blood was achieved in 44% of patients (Elter et al., 2003). These data suggest that FluCam is a promising regimen for previously treated CLL patients.

EMERGING THERAPIES FOR CHRONIC LYMPHOCYTIC LEUKEMIA

Several pharmaceutical and biotechnology companies are developing new treatments for CLL. Some of these treatments are aimed at previously defined targets or have mechanisms of action similar to current treatments; others have novel targets and/or mechanisms of action. Agents in development include immune system modulators (such as MAbs and immunotoxins), cell-cycle inhibitors, proteasome inhibitors, apoptosis inducers, and angiogenesis inhibitors. Some treatments are being developed as single agents; others are being developed as combinations with existing therapies and in various settings. Agents that have reached at least Phase II clinical trials for CLL in the United States are listed in Table 29.4. Emerging therapies that have reached late-stage clinical trials for CLL (at least Phase III) and several passive immunomodulation treatments (MAbs and immunotoxins) are discussed in greater detail in the following sections.

Monoclonal Antibodies

MAbs target cell-surface proteins and can interfere with receptor/ligand interactions, thereby affecting downstream signaling and subsequent growth and proliferation. They can also alert the immune system to target the cell for death via cell ADCC. The launch of alemtuzumab for the treatment of CLL has clearly paved the way for the success of MAbs in this disease.

Rituximab

Biogen Idec/Genentech's mouse/human chimeric MAb rituximab (Rituxan, MabThera) is intended for the treatment of CLL as both a single agent and in combination with chemotherapy. The agent has already been approved for treatment of non-Hodgkin's lymphoma and sees significant, extensive off-label use for treatment of CLL in the United States, mainly in the first- and second-line settings in combination with chemotherapy. The clinical trial results reviewed in the following paragraphs suggest that this agent has great potential when used in combination with chemotherapy for treatment of CLL but not as a single agent.

Rituximab targets CD20, a calcium channel expressed on both normal and malignant B cells that interacts with the B-cell immunoglobulin receptor complex. Because CLL is primarily a B-cell disorder, rituximab's mechanism of action is more specific than that of the current therapy, alemtuzumab, whose target molecule (CD52) is also expressed on other immune cells, such as monocytes and lymphocytes.

Limited Phase II data suggest that rituximab as a monotherapy may be more effective when used as a first-line therapy than as a second- or third-line therapy. In one Phase II trial, 51% of previously untreated CLL patients who received rituximab achieved an objective response after six weeks, and 49% had stable disease. The response rate rose to 58% at the 24-month follow-up, with 9% experiencing a CR (Hainsworth et al., 2003). Median progression-free survival was 18.6 months. Trials with rituximab as a second- or third-line therapy were less successful, with response rates ranging from 11% to 35% (Huhn et al., 2001; Winkler et al., 1999). Although the response rate as a first-line therapy is encouraging, the low CR indicates that single-agent rituximab will not result in long-term survival in CLL (Lin et al., 2003).

The most active and promising area of research involves rituximab in combination with chemotherapy. In a randomized Phase II study of previously untreated CLL patients, patients received six courses of sequential or concurrent fludarabine plus rituximab, followed two months later by an additional four weeks of single-agent rituximab for

Table 29.4 Select Emerging Therapies for Treatment of Chronic Lymphocytic Leukemia in the United States, 2006

Drug	*Company*	*Status (U.S.)*	*Notes*
Monoclonal antibodies			
Rituximab (Rituxan, MabThera)	Biogen Idec/ Genentech	Phase III	Mouse/human chimeric MAb directed against the calcium channel CD20 Thought to deplete B cells in a number of ways, including antibody-dependent cellular cytotoxicity (ADCC), complement-dependent cytotoxicity (CDC), and alteration of calcium flux and factors involved in apoptosis
Lumiliximab (IDEC-152)	Biogen Idec	Phase II	A macaque-human chimeric antihuman CD23 MAb. CD23, the low-affinity IgE receptor, is expressed constitutively on CLL cells
Apolizumab	National Cancer Institute	Phase II	Binds to an epitope on the MHC class II molecule, HLA-DR. Believed to target CLL B cells by inducing apoptosis in these cells
Anti-CD40 (CHIR-12.12)	Chiron/Xoma	Phase I	Fully humanized anti-CD40 MAb Induces apoptosis in primary CLL B cells as well as facilitates ADCC against CD40 positive cells
Ofatumumab (Humax-CD20)	Genmab	Phase I/II	Fully human high-affinity antibody targeted against CD20 antigen on B cells Mechanism of action is similar to rituximab
Immunotoxins			
Denileukin diftitox (Ontak)	Ligand	Phase II	Interleukin-2 (IL-2) diphtheria toxin fusion protein designed to direct the cytocidal action of diphtheria toxin to cells that express the IL-2 receptor Upon internalization, the toxin is cleaved into an active form and causes cell death
Cell-cycle inhibitors			
Alvocidib (Flavopiridol)	National Cancer Institute/Sanofi-Aventis	Phase III	Inhibition of the enzymes involved in key cell-cycle checkpoints can result in cell-cycle arrest and, ultimately, cell death, usually by apoptosis
Antisense oligonucleotides			
Oblimersen (Genasense)	Genta	Pre-registered	Designed to block production of the bcl-2 protein from bcl-2 (a proto-oncogene) Inhibition of bcl-2 allows cells to progress through the cell death pathway By reducing the amount of bcl-2 protein in cancer cells, oblimersen may enhance the effectiveness of conventional anticancer treatments
Immunotherapeutics			
IL-2/CD40-expressing leukemia vaccine	Baylor College of Medicine/ MaxCyte	Phase I/II	Autologous skin fibroblasts from patients are transduced with adenoviral vectors encoding IL-2 and CD40 ligand and injected back into the patient to stimulate T cell immune responses
Apoptosis inducers			
Motexafin gadolinium (Xcytrin)	Pharmacyclics	Phase II	A texaphyrin known to target cells that have increased rates of metabolism, such as cancer cells Promotes oxidative stress by generating reactive oxygen species, and tumor cells treated with this agent undergo apoptosis through the mitochondrial-mediated intrinsic pathway
SDX-101	Cephalon	Phase II	Small-molecule, orally administered, proapoptotic agent that is the R-isomer of etodolac, a marketed anti-inflammatory drug Induces apoptosis in primary CLL and multiple myeloma cells as well as in various lymphoma cell lines

Table 29.4 Continued

Drug	*Company*	*Status (U.S.)*	*Notes*
Proteasome inhibitors			
Bortezomib (Velcade)	Millennium Pharmaceuticals	Phase II	Works through multiple pathways, including those that influence apoptosis and angiogenesis Has high selectivity for the 26S proteasome over other proteases (e.g., thrombin) Has demonstrated in vitro cytotoxicity against a wide range of tumor cell lines
Antimetabolites			
Clofarabine (Clorar)	Bioenvision/ Genzyme Oncology	Phase II	A second-generation purine nucleoside analogue Nucleoside analogues are antimetabolites that inhibit DNA production necessary for cancer cell growth
Angiogenesis inhibitors			
Lenalidomide (Revlimid)	Celgene	Phase II	A thalidomide-derived immunomodulatory drug Thalidomide exhibits both immunomodulatory and antiangiogenic effects. Thalidomide stimulates the proliferation of cytotoxic T cells able to destroy tumor cells. Lenalidomide exerts potent antiangiogenic activity by blocking two growth factors that control angiogenesis – VEGF and bFGF The compound increases secretions of cytokines such as IFN-gamma and IL-2; both exhibit an antitumor effect
Alkylating agents			
Bendamustine (Treanda)	Cephalon	Phase II	Alkylation of DNA results in breaks in the DNA molecule as well as cross-linking of the twin strands, thus interfering with DNA replication and transcription of RNA and ultimately causing cell death
Fibroblast activation protein antagonists			
Talabostat	Point Therapeutics	Phase II	Orally active compound that interacts with a target enzyme believed to be fibroblast activation protein Interaction increases immune effector cell expansion and facilitates cytotoxicity against tumor cells
Purine nuclesoside phosphorylase inhibitors			
Forodesine	BioCryst Pharmaceuticals	Phase II	Functions by blocking T cells' ability to synthesize DNA

responders and patients with stable disease. Concurrent administration of these two agents demonstrated superior response rates when compared with the sequential arm: 47% CR in the concurrent arm versus 28% CR in the sequential arm and 43% PR versus 49% PR. Neutropenia was more common in the concurrent arm, but infectious complications occurred at similar frequencies in both arms. This encouraging study establishes that concurrent administration of rituximab and fludarabine produces CR rates superior to those achieved with fludarabine alone.

To date, the impact of rituximab on improving progression-free survival and overall survival compared with fludarabine monotherapy has not been analyzed in a randomized trial. A retrospective comparison with data from 179 patients enrolled in the North American Intergroup Study CALGB 9011 who received fludarabine monotherapy showed that CR, PR, and two-year performance-free and overall survival rates were significantly superior in the fludarabine/rituximab group (Byrd et al., 2003).

The triple-drug regimen fludarabine/cyclophosphamide/rituximab (FCR) is also under intense investigation. In one study, previously untreated CLL patients received the FCR regimen; fludarabine and cyclophosphamide were administered in combination with rituximab. The CR rate with this regimen was 70% and the overall response rate was 95%, with most patients having no detectable disease by flow cytometry evaluation of the bone marrow at the end of therapy (Keating et al., 2005). The projected failure-free survival at four years was 69%, which was the highest response rate reported for any regimen in previously untreated CLL patients. The FCR regimen has also had success in patients with relapsed or refractory CLL. In previously treated patients with a median of two prior therapies, 25% achieved CR and the overall response rate was 73%. Approximately one-third of the CRs tested had no detectable disease in the bone marrow by polymerase chain reaction evaluation. The estimated median survival for all 177 study participants was 42 months (O'Brien et al., 2005).

In an attempt to improve the success seen in FCR, the M.D. Anderson Cancer Center has pioneered a trial examining a regimen that consists of cyclophosphamide, fludarabine, alemtuzumab, and rituximab (known as the CFAR regimen) for previously treated CLL patients. An early evaluation of 31 heavily pretreated patients who had a median of four prior treatments reported CR in 14% of patients and an overall response rate of 52%. Despite the increase in the incidence of myelosuppression and thrombocytopenia in patients treated with CFAR, these patients did not experience a significant increase in major infections compared with patients treated with FCR. The addition of alemtuzumab caused an increase in cytomegalovirus reactivation with CFAR (O'Brien et al., 2004).

The purine analogue pentostatin has shown significant activity and minimal toxicity when combined with cyclophosphamide in CLL patients. Rituximab added to this combination (known as the PCR regimen) is being tested in both untreated and previously treated patients. In one study, 32 previously treated CLL patients received this regimen as well as granulocyte colony stimulating factor (G-CSF) support and were assessable for response. In this subgroup, 75% of patients responded; 25% were CR. This regimen was well tolerated, with the principal toxicity being myelosuppression (Lamanna, 2006). A similar regimen with a lower dose of pentostatin, also with G-CSF support, was used to treat chemotherapy-naive patients with CLL (Lamanna et al., 2004). In a study of 33 previously untreated patients who received this regimen, 33% achieved CR, 21% achieved nodular partial response (nPR), and 39% achieved PR, for an overall response rate of 97% (Geyer et al., 2004).

Lumiliximab

Lumiliximab is a macaque-human chimeric antihuman CD23 MAb that is being developed by Biogen Idec for the treatment of CLL. CD23, the low-affinity IgE receptor, is expressed constitutively on CLL cells and is therefore a target of interest for MAb therapy in this disease. Unlike rituximab, lumiliximab, as a macaque-human chimera, does not contain a mouse component, which should minimize immunogenicity.

This treatment was evaluated in a Phase I clinical trial for previously treated patients with CLL. The trial investigated increasing doses of lumiliximab up to 500 mg/m^2 three times weekly for four weeks (O'Brien et al., 2005). The study identified no dose-limiting toxicities, and 90% of patients experienced decreases in absolute lymphocyte counts; more than one-quarter of patients experienced a 50% reduction or more. A reduction in lymph node size occurred in 59% of patients. However, there were no complete or partial responders according to NCI criteria in this Phase I trial. Lumiliximab is currently being evaluated in combination chemoimmunotherapy regimens.

Other Monoclonal Antibodies

Other MAbs in various development stages include the following:

- An anti-MHC II antibody (apolizumab) by the NCI.
- A fully humanized anti-CD40 MAb (CHIR-12.12) by Chiron/Xoma.
- HuMax-CD20 (ofatumumab), a fully human, high-affinity antibody targeted against CD20 antigen on B cells, whose mechanism of action is similar to that of rituximab, by Genmab. The agent was granted fast-track status in the United States in December 2004 for patients with refractory CLL.

Immunotoxins

Ligand is developing denileukin diftitox (Ontak) for the treatment of CLL. Phase II trials are under way in the United States. This agent is likely to launch for CLL in 2008 if approved. It has already been launched in the United States for the treatment of cutaneous T-cell lymphoma.

Denileukin diftitox is an interleukin-2 (IL-2) diphtheria toxin fusion protein designed to direct the cytocidal action of diphtheria toxin to cells that express the IL-2 receptor (including activated T and B lymphocytes and activated macrophages). The growth factor IL-2 directs the toxin to the IL-2 receptor on cells, similar to the mechanism of action of MAbs, which are also specifically directed to their target on a cell. However, the diphtheria toxin brings about the death of the cells that express the IL-2 receptor directly, unlike the mechanism of action of unconjugated MAbs (such as alemtuzumab and rituximab), in which cell death is mediated by mechanisms such as ADCC and complement-dependent cytotoxicity (CDC).

In April 2006, interesting data on a Phase II study investigating the use of denileukin diftitox in patients with recurrent or refractory CLL were released (Frankel, 2006). Of the 22 patients who received denileukin diftitox and could be evaluated, 4% achieved a CR and 23% achieved a PR. These results suggest that this agent has some biological activity in this difficult-to-treat group of patients. However, toxicities seen in earlier studies, while moderate, are significant. Therefore, further analysis is needed to weigh response against this therapy's toxicity profile.

Cell-cycle Inhibitors

The NCI and Sanofi-Aventis are developing alvocidib (Flavopiridol) for treatment of CLL. This synthetic flavenoid inhibits cyclin-dependent kinases (CDKs), enzymes involved in key cell-cycle checkpoints. Inhibition of these enzymes can result in cell-cycle arrest and, ultimately, cell death, usually by apoptosis.

Results in early clinical trials of alvocidib using a continuous infusion regimen (50 mg/m^2/day for 72 hours every two weeks) were disappointing because patients showed no response to this treatment. However, more recent results using a bolus treatment regimen in previously treated CLL patients showed a response. In the bolus regimen, patients received 50 mg/m^2/day as a one-hour bolus daily for three days, repeated every three weeks. Patients received up to eight cycles of this treatment. Eleven percent of patients showed PR, 53% showed stable disease, and 36% showed progressive disease. The median progression-free survival was three months; median overall survival was 24 months. Toxicity included myelosuppression, infections, fatigue, and diarrhea and was considered manageable (Byrd et al., 2005). This demonstration of activity has renewed interest in this agent based on optimum dosing and administration.

Antisense Oligonucleotides

Genta's oblimersen (Genasense) is an antisense oligonucleotide specific for messenger RNA (mRNA) transcribed from the *bcl-2* gene. This binding, or hybridization, triggers enzymatic degradation of the mRNA, thereby blocking the translation of the mRNA and the generation of the corresponding protein. In 2001, the FDA awarded oblimersen orphan drug status for CLL.

In a February 2006 press release, Genta reported the results of a Phase III study with oblimersen. The randomized Phase III study compared fludarabine and cyclophosphamide, with or without oblimersen, in patients with relapsed or refractory CLL. The addition of oblimersen increased the proportion of patients who achieved a CR or nPR from 7% in the fludarabine/cyclophosphamide arm to 17% in the fludarabine/cyclophosphamide/oblimersen arm. Furthermore, the duration of CR/nPR was significantly longer in patients treated with oblimersen (22 months) compared with patients who received fludarabine/cyclophosphamide only (median not reached).

Grade 3 or 4 adverse events that occurred during treatment or within 30 days of last treatment included, but were not limited to, thrombocytopenia, nausea, and intravenous-catheter complications. Adverse events resulted in discontinuation of therapy in an equal percentage of patients in both groups. While the trial met its primary end point, the results are inferior to those observed with rituximab in the same combination and setting. Therefore, oblimersen is unlikely to significantly challenge chemoimmunotherapy with rituximab in this setting.

MARKET OVERVIEW

In 2005, sales of drugs used to treat CLL exceeded $153 million in the United States, including estimated off-label sales of rituximab for this indication. The United States accounts for 80% of total sales in the seven major markets (United States, France, Germany, Italy, Spain, United Kingdom, and Japan), a reflection of both the large number of prevalent cases of CLL in the United States and the higher price point for these agents in the United States. Because a significant number of prescriptions to treat CLL are off-label, US sales include both approved and off-label sales.

The US CLL market is small ($153 million in 2005), but CLL drug development in the United States is driven by various other factors that temper the relatively low sales potential of this indication:

First, agents for this indication have had certain regulatory advantages. The FDA has granted fast-track status to CLL drugs in development. This designation has been most commonly assigned to third-line treatments for refractory patients with low survival. Also, the FDA has granted orphan drug status to many CLL agents in development; this status is reserved for use when a disease has a prevalence of less than 200,000 in the United States.

Second, although some emerging agents such as MAbs are expensive, their cost is not a significant barrier to entry in the United States. The CLL population is largely elderly and therefore mainly covered by Medicare. Medicare is required to cover the cost of these higher-priced drugs, even if used off-label.

Third, the significant off-label use of an oncology treatment builds up sales as well as clinical experience before an agent is officially FDA-approved and serves as an entry into other oncology markets, even when the agent is still in clinical development.

As discussed at the beginning of this chapter, the most urgent unmet need in CLL is for an agent that will improve survival, particularly in patients with advanced disease. At present, patients with intermediate- and high-risk CLL who are treated with chemotherapy achieve a survival of approximately three to eight years. Because of the relatively long survival in CLL, improvement in CR is used as a guide for efficacy. Results to date show that the addition of rituximab to fludarabine and to fludarabine/cyclophosphamide increases response rates, which may ultimately translate into increased survival. Recent long-term studies analyzing the newer chemotherapy agents, such as fludarabine, report an increased complete remission rate; however, for reasons that remain unclear, this response has not translated into an improved median survival. Analysis of long-term survival data is difficult because of the way in which the studies have been designed. Patients who do not respond to the initial first-line therapy are moved to an alternate arm of the study (a procedure known as "crossover"), thus obscuring survival based on regimen. Further investigation into how these agents affect survival is necessary to ensure the greatest benefit for patients.

REFERENCES

Binet, J.L. et al. A new prognostic classification of chronic lymphocytic leukemia derived from a multivariate survival analysis. *Cancer.* 1981; 48(1): 198–206.

Byrd, J.C. et al. The addition of rituximab to fludarabine significantly improves progression-free and overall survival in previously untreated chronic lymphocytic leukemia (CLL) patients. *Proceedings of the American Society of Hematology.* 2003. Abstract 245.

Byrd, J.C. et al. Treatment of relapsed chronic lymphocytic leukemia by 72-hour continuous infusion or 1-hour bolus infusion of flavopiridol: results from Cancer and Leukemia Group B study 19805. *Clinical Cancer Research.* 2005; 11(11): 4176–81.

Chronic Lymphocytic Leukemia Trialists' Collaborative Group. Chemotherapeutic options in CLL: a meta-analysis of the randomized trials. *Journal of the National Cancer Institute.* 1999; 91(10): 861–8.

Crespo, M. et al. ZAP-70 expression as a surrogate for immunoglobulin-variable-region mutations in chronic lymphocytic leukemia. *New England Journal of Medicine.* 2003; 348: 1764–75.

Damle, R.N. et al. IgV gene mutation status and CD38 expression as novel prognostic indicators in chronic lymphocytic leukemia. *Blood.* 1999; 94(6): 1840–7.

Elter, T., et al. Development of new four-weekly schedule (FluCam) with concomitant application of Campath-1H and fludarabine in patients with relapsed/refractory CLL. *Proceedings of the American Society of Clinical Oncology.* 2003. Abstract 2331.

Frankel, A.E. Phase II clinical studies of denileukin diftitox diphtheria toxin fusion protein in patients with previously treated chronic lymphocytic leukemia. *Cancer.* May 15, 2006; 106(10): 2158–64.

Geyer, S.M. et al. Combination chemotherapy with pentostatin, cyclophosphamide and rituximab induces high rate of remissions including complete responses and achievement of minimal residual disease in previously untreated B-chronic lymphocytic leukemia. *Blood.* 2004: 100a. Abstract 339.

Hainsworth, J.D. et al. Single-agent rituximab as first-line and maintenance treatment for patients with chronic lymphocytic leukemia or small lymphocytic lymphoma: a phase II trial of the Minnie Pearl Cancer Research Network. *Journal of Clinical Oncology.* 2003; 21(9): 1746–51.

Hamblin, T.J. et al. Unmutated Ig V(H) genes are associated with a more aggressive form of chronic lymphocytic leukemia. *Blood.* 1999; 94(6): 1848–54.

Huhn, D., et al. Rituximab therapy of patients with B-cell chronic lymphocytic leukemia. *Blood.* 2001; 98(5): 1326–31.

Keating, M.J., et al. Early results of a chemoimmunotherapy regimen of fludarabine, cyclophosphamide, and rituximab as initial therapy for chronic lymphocytic leukemia. *Journal of Clinical Oncology.* June 20, 2005; 23(18): 4009–12.

Keating, M.J., et al. Therapeutic role of alemtuzumab (Campath-1H) in patients who have failed fludarabine: results of a large international study. *Blood.* 2002; 99: 3554–61.

Lamanna, N. Pentostatin, cyclophosphamide and rituximab is an active, well-tolerated regimen for patients with previously treated chronic lymphocytic leukemia. *Journal of Clinical Oncology.* 2006; 24: 1575–81.

Lamanna, N. et al. Pentostatin and cyclophosphamide with or without rituximab has significant activity in patients with previously treated chronic lymphocytic leukemia and other low grade lymphoid neoplasms. *Blood.* 2004; 104: 950a. Abstract 3484.

Lin, T.S. et al. Rituximab in B-cell chronic lymphocytic leukemia. *Seminar in Oncology.* 2003; 30(4): 483–92.

Lundin, J. et al. Phase II trial of subcutaneous anti-CD52 monoclonal antibody alemtuzumab (Campath-1H) as first-line treatment for patients with B-cell chronic lymphocytic leukemia (B-CLL). *Blood.* 2002; 100: 768–73.

Montserrat, E. et al. Lymphocyte doubling time in chronic lymphocytic leukemia: analysis of its prognostic significance. *British Journal of Hematology.* 1986; 62(3): 567–75.

O'Brien, S. et al. Chemoimmunotherapy with fludarabine, cyclophosphamide, and rituximab for relapsed and refractory chronic lymphocytic leukemia. *Journal of Clinical Oncology.* 2005; 23: 4070–8.

O'Brien, S. et al. Combined cyclophosphamide, fludarabine, alemtuzumab, and rituximab (CFAR) is active for relapsed and refractory patients with CLL. *Blood.* 2004; 104: 101a. Abstract 340.

Rai, K.R. et al. Clinical staging of chronic lymphocytic leukemia. *Blood.* 1975; 46(2): 219–34.

Rai, K.R. et al. Fludarabine compared with chlorambucil as primary therapy for chronic lymphocytic leukemia. *New England Journal of Medicine.* 2000; 343(24): 1750–7.

Shanafelt, T.D. et al. Prognosis at diagnosis: integrating molecular biologic insights into clinical practice for patients with CLL. *Blood.* 2004; 103(4): 1202–10.

Wiestner, A. et al. ZAP-70 expression identifies a chronic lymphocytic leukemia subtype with unmutated immunoglobulin genes, inferior clinical outcome, and distinct gene expression profile. *Blood.* 2003; 101: 4944–51.

Winkler, U. et al. Cytokine-release syndrome in patients with B-cell chronic lymphocytic leukemia and high lymphocyte counts after treatment with an anti-CD20 monoclonal antibody (rituximab, IDEC-C2B8). *Blood.* 1999; 904(7): 2217–24.

SECTION B

CNS

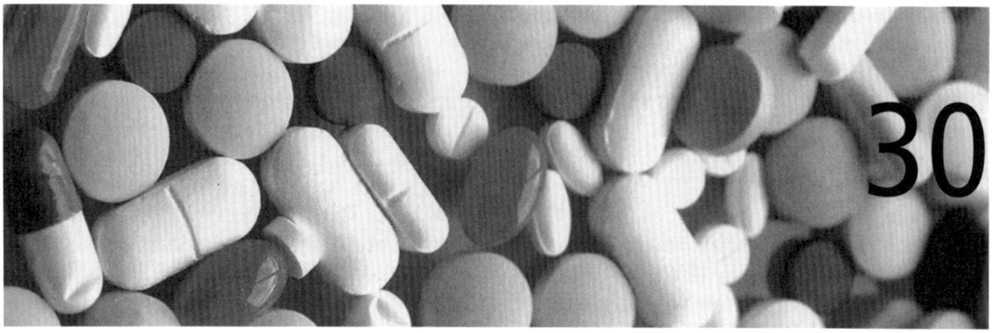

Opportunities in the Pharmacotherapy of Addiction

SOCIETAL AND PHARMACOTHERAPY TRENDS IN ADDICTION

Substance abuse – including the inappropriate use of alcohol, illegal and prescription drugs, and nicotine – is a significant societal and healthcare issue in the United States. In 2003, almost 18 million people in the United States abused or were dependent on alcohol, and almost 20 million were illicit drug users. (Note that there is considerable overlap in these numbers because many people abuse both alcohol and drugs.) The National Institute on Drug Abuse (NIDA) and the National Institute on Alcohol Abuse and Alcoholism (NIAAA) report that the economic cost of alcohol and drug abuse was \$328.4 billion in 1998, encompassing treatment and prevention costs, other healthcare costs, reduced productivity and lost wages, and other costs to society. Drug abuse accounted for \$143.4 billion of this amount, and \$185 billion resulted from alcohol abuse.

Despite the significant need for improved therapies, treatment of alcohol and drug addiction historically has attracted limited attention from the pharmaceutical industry. However, this trend has been changing in recent years, and several novel therapies for drug and alcohol addiction are in development.

According to the Centers for Disease Control and Prevention (CDC), smoking is the single most common avoidable cause of morbidity and mortality in the United States, resulting in more than 440,000 deaths and more than \$75 billion in direct medical costs each year. The CDC estimates that 46.2 million adults (i.e., people aged 18 or older) in the United States smoke cigarettes and that 70% of those smokers have a desire to quit, representing a large potential market for smoking cessation products. Although many products are already available to help people quit smoking, several new therapies are being developed in response to a demand for more efficacious treatment.

This chapter provides an overview of substance abuse and dependency and reviews current and emerging therapies for the treatment of addiction to alcohol, illicit drugs, and nicotine. In addition, we discuss market prospects for pharmacotherapeutic treatments for addiction.

OVERVIEW OF SUBSTANCE ABUSE

As we detail in the following subsections, the abuse of alcohol, drugs, and nicotine affects a significant percentage of people in the United States. This section provides an overview of the use and abuse of these substances as well as a description of the deleterious effects these substances have on health.

Alcohol

Alcohol is a commonly consumed beverage in today's society. According to findings from the 2003 National Survey on Drug Use and Health (NSDUH), 119 million people (or 50.1% of the population) in the United States aged 12 or older had at least one drink within the previous 30 days in 2003. This statistic includes all levels of consumption and encompasses approximately 10.9 million people aged 12–20 (Substance Abuse and Mental Health Services Administration, 2004). Although many people drink light or moderate amounts of alcohol, some people abuse alcohol and/or suffer from alcoholism, defined by the NIDA as dependence on alcohol. According to information from the NSDUH, approximately 17.9 million people abused or were dependent on alcohol in the United States in 2003.

Alcoholism is now recognized as a disease that can result in tissue/organ damage, such as cirrhosis of the liver, damage to the brain, peripheral neuropathy, and cardiomyopathy. Consumption of high levels of alcohol also can cause impairment of functioning in social or work environments, referred to as alcohol abuse. In addition, regular consumption of high levels of alcohol may lead to tolerance and, if consumption of alcohol is stopped, a potentially dangerous alcohol withdrawal syndrome that causes symptoms such as tremor, sweating, gastrointestinal symptoms, seizures, alcoholic hallucinosis, and delirium tremens. People who develop tolerance and withdrawal symptoms are considered to be alcohol dependent.

Alcohol is absorbed into the body primarily through the small intestine and accumulates when it is absorbed more rapidly than it is excreted or oxidized. The neurological basis of alcohol's activity is its ability to bind to hydrophobic pockets of certain proteins, thus changing their structure and function. These proteins include ion channels and neurotransmitter receptors in the cell membranes of the brain. Neurotransmitters whose receptors are affected by alcohol include gamma-aminobutyric acid (GABA), glutamate (and the *N*-methyl-D-aspartate [NMDA] receptor), serotonin, dopamine, neuropeptide-Y (NPY), and cannabinoid receptor-1 (CB1).These and other receptors represent potential pharmacological targets for treatment of alcohol dependence.

Abused Drugs

A wide range of drugs, including illegal drugs and several legal prescription drugs, can be abused, leading to drug addiction. Examples of addictive drugs include marijuana, heroin, cocaine, and hallucinogens such as lysergic acid diethylamide (LSD) as well as prescription drugs such as pain relievers, stimulants, and depressants. The 2003 NSDUH, which includes both illegal drugs and nonmedical use of prescription drugs, estimates that 19.5 million people in the United States aged 12 or older, or 8.2% of the population, used an illicit drug within the previous 30 days in 2003. Approximately 35% of these people (6.8 million) were dependent on illicit drugs (Substance Abuse and Mental Health Services Administration, 2004).

Use of illicit drugs can affect several neurotransmitters and their receptors, including GABA, glutamate, serotonin, dopamine, acetylcholine, the CB1 receptors, and the opioid receptors. Although it is not within the scope of this report to discuss in detail the effect of each type of drug that is commonly abused, these types of neurotransmitters and their receptors represent potential targets for treatment of drug addiction.

Smoking

According to the CDC, an estimated 46.2 million adults in the United States smoke cigarettes, and more than 8.6 million people in the United States have one or more serious illnesses caused by smoking, resulting in more than 440,000 deaths each year. Diseases that result in deaths attributable to smoking include lung cancer, chronic lung disease (including emphysema), and cardiovascular diseases.

The addictive compound in cigarettes is nicotine, a colorless alkaloid molecule that turns brown when burned and has several effects on the brain and body, including increasing levels of dopamine in the brain. According to the CDC, more than 70% of current smokers have expressed a desire to quit smoking, but long-term success rates are low, partly because of nicotine- withdrawal symptoms including irritability, loss of ability to focus, sleeplessness, and increased appetite that often results in weight gain. Potential targets for the treatment of nicotine dependence include nicotine receptors and the CB1 receptor.

CURRENT PHARMACOLOGICAL TREATMENTS FOR ADDICTION

Although many current treatment programs for alcohol or drug addiction involve psychotherapy or counseling and support groups such as Alcoholics Anonymous, the use of medications can increase a patient's likelihood of success and abstinence. The following sections review the medications currently available for the treatment of alcohol, opioid, and nicotine dependence.

Alcohol

According to findings from the 2003 NSDUH, an estimated 2.4 million people were treated for alcohol abuse in the United States in 2003; 1.3 million people received treatment for both alcohol and illicit drug abuse, and another 1.1 million received treatment for alcohol abuse alone. These treatment estimates include people treated with psychotherapy, pharmacotherapy, or a combination of the two. Because the focus of this report is the pharmacotherapy of addiction, we discuss only briefly the pharmacological treatment of alcohol withdrawal and psychotherapeutic treatment of alcoholism.

Drug therapy for alcohol withdrawal is generally focused on alleviating the condition's physical symptoms. Drugs used to treat alcohol withdrawal include the benzodiazepines (chlordiazepoxide and others) and sometimes anticonvulsants or agents such as beta blockers or alpha agonists. Following alcohol withdrawal, treatment of alcohol addiction typically involves some form of psychotherapy, often group therapy.

In the United States, only three drugs are approved for treatment of alcohol dependence (Table 30.1). Disulfiram (Antabuse) was introduced more than 50 years ago. Odyssey Pharmaceuticals, a subsidiary of Pliva D.D. of Croatia, markets this agent, which was developed by Wyeth. Disulfiram works by affecting the body's ability to metabolize alcohol. Alcohol is metabolized in the body in a two-step process: (1) it is metabolized by the enzyme alcohol dehydrogenase (ADH) to form acetaldehyde, and (2) it is then metabolized to acetic acid (acetate) by the enzyme aldehyde dehydrogenase (ALDH). Disulfiram inhibits ALDH, causing a build-up of acetaldehyde, which results in unpleasant physical symptoms that provide an incentive for patients to avoid alcohol. Symptoms of excess acetaldehyde include flushing of the face, throbbing in the head and neck, headache, nausea and vomiting, thirst, sweating, chest pain, and tachycardia. One of the major drawbacks of

Table 30.1 FDA-approved Drugs for Treatment of Alcohol Dependence, 2005

Generic Name	*Company/Brand Name*	*2003 US Sales, Branded and Generic Drugs ($MM)*
Disulfiram	Odyssey Pharmaceuticals' Antabuse	9
Naltrexone	Barr Pharmaceuticals' ReVia, generics	15
Acamprosate calcium	Forest Laboratories' Campral	N.A.[a]

[a]Campral was launched in the United States in 2005
N.A. = Not available

this treatment is that many patients are not compliant in taking disulfiram. In addition, the overall usefulness of this drug for treatment of alcohol dependence has not been clearly established.

The second drug approved in the United States for treatment of alcohol dependence is naltrexone (Barr Pharmaceuticals' ReVia, generics). The Food and Drug Administration (FDA) first approved this opioid receptor antagonist in 1984 and approved it for treatment of alcoholism in 1994. The structure of naltrexone is related to the structure of the opioid analgesic oxymorphone, but a methyl group on oxymorphone is replaced by a cyclopropylmethyl group. Naltrexone is available in a once-daily oral tablet formulation. Clinical studies evaluating naltrexone have demonstrated that it is more effective than placebo in reducing alcohol cravings and relapse rates in heavy drinkers. However, it is not effective for all patients, and patient compliance can be a problem because heavy drinkers do not always remember to take a pill each day. Use of naltrexone to treat opioid drug addiction and dependence is discussed later in this chapter.

The FDA approved Forest Laboratories' acamprosate calcium (Campral) delayed-release tablet in July 2004 for maintaining abstinence in alcohol-dependent patients who stopped drinking before treatment initiation. Acamprosate was developed by Merck Sante (a subsidiary of Merck KGaA) and licensed to Forest Laboratories in 2001 for the United States; Forest launched the agent in January 2005. Acamprosate is a synthetic compound with a structure similar to that of homotaurine, an endogenous amino acid that is a structural analogue of the neurotransmitter GABA and the amino acid neuromodulator taurinc. Although researchers do not know acamprosate's mechanism of action for treating alcoholism, they believe it acts by interacting with the glutamate and GABA neurotransmitter systems.

Data supporting US approval of acamprosate came from three double-blind, placebo-controlled clinical trials that involved a total of 998 alcohol-dependent patients who had undergone detoxification and were abstinent from alcohol at the start of the study. Study durations ranged from 90 to 360 days. A greater percentage of patients who received acamprosate were reportedly continuously abstinent during the treatment period compared with patients who received placebo, although the precise percentages have not been revealed. In a fourth study, involving patients who had not undergone detoxification and were not required to be abstinent from alcohol at the start of the clinical trial, acamprosate did not demonstrate any benefits compared with placebo.

Although current therapies offer benefits in the treatment of alcoholism, a clear need exists for more efficacious treatments. One possible approach, given that naltrexone and acamprosate work by different mechanisms of action, is to combine the two drugs. In 2001, the NIAAA announced the start of the Combining Medications and Behavioral Interventions (COMBINE) study, a multicenter, randomized, placebo-controlled study with the objective of evaluating treatment with naltrexone and acamprosate together. This study is expected to include 1,375 alcohol-dependent patients who will be treated with either one of the drugs, a combination of both drugs, or a placebo. The patients will be treated in outpatient sessions for 4 months and then followed for 12 months. Patient accrual in this trial is now complete, and the study is ongoing. In addition to the COMBINE study, the NIAAA is conducting other clinical trials to further evaluate naltrexone and acamprosate individually for treatment of alcoholism.

Abused Drugs

According to findings from the 2003 NSDUH, an estimated 1.8 million people were treated for illicit drug abuse in the United States in 2003, with 1.3 million people receiving treatment for both alcohol and illicit drug abuse and another 500,000 receiving treatment for drug abuse alone. The NSDUH also estimates that 557,000 people were treated for cocaine abuse in 2003, which is a significant decrease from the estimated 796,000 who were treated for cocaine dependence or abuse in 2002. Only a limited number of pharmacotherapies are currently available in the United States for treatment of drug dependence (Table 30.2).

The first pharmacological-based therapy to reach the market was methadone (Roxane Laboratories' Dolophine, generics), which has been available for decades. Methadone is a synthetic, long-acting mu-opioid receptor agonist with pharmacological activities that are similar to those of morphine and heroin. Methadone is used as an opiate substitute in maintenance programs, preventing the symptoms of withdrawal and decreasing cravings for opiates, allowing people who are addicted to function in society.

A second opiate agonist, levomethadyl hydrochloride acetate (Roxane Laboratories' Orlaam), often called Laam, was approved by the FDA and introduced to the market in 1995; the drug is now discontinued. Levomethadyl was indicated for management of opiate dependence and reserved to treat patients who did not show an acceptable response to other treatments. After launching this drug, Roxane Laboratories received increasing reports of severe cardiac-related adverse effects, including QT interval prolongation. As a result, changes were made to the US package insert in 2001, and levomethadyl was removed from the European market in March 2001. Use of levomethadyl in the United States reportedly decreased dramatically after these events, and, in August 2003, Roxane Laboratories announced that the sale of levomethadyl in the United States would be discontinued.

Naltrexone (Barr Pharmaceuticals' ReVia, generics), a synthetic opioid antagonist that has no opioid agonist properties, was first approved in 1984 for treatment of opioid dependence. As discussed earlier, naltrexone is also used to treat alcohol dependence. Naltrexone blocks the effects of opiates, including the euphoric effect of illicit opiates. The expectation is that the suppression of these euphoric effects will, over time, break the habit of opiate addiction. However, the suppression of these effects is a large part of the reason naltrexone therapy has such a low rate of compliance, and use of naltrexone is generally most beneficial to patients who have made a commitment to stop using opiates.

In 2002, buprenorphine (Reckitt Benckiser's Subutex) was approved for treatment of opioid dependence. Buprenorphine is a partial agonist at the mu-opioid receptor and an antagonist at the kappa opioid receptor. This agent is available as a sublingual tablet alone or in combination with naloxone (Reckitt Benckiser's Suboxone), an antagonist

Table 30.2 FDA-approved Drugs for the Treatment of Opioid Dependence/Addiction, 2005

Generic Name	*Company/Brand Name*	*2003 US Sales, Branded and Generic Drugs ($MM)*
Methadone	Roxane Laboratories' Dolophine, generics	43
Levomethadyl hydrochloride acetate	Roxane Laboratories' Orlaam (discontinued)	71
Naltrexone	Barr Pharmaceuticals' ReVia, generics	15
Buprenorphine	Reckitt Benckiser's Subutex	22
Buprenorphine/naloxone	Reckitt Benckiser's Suboxone	10

at the mu-opioid receptor. Before the approval of Subutex and Suboxone, both buprenorphine and naloxone were already on the market for other indications. Reckitt Benckiser markets an injectable formulation of buprenorphine (Buprenex) for treatment of moderate to severe pain, and Endo Pharmaceuticals' naloxone (Narcan) is FDA approved for complete or partial reversal of opioid depression. Use of buprenorphine provides benefits associated with both methadone (suppression of withdrawal symptoms and craving) and naltrexone (blocking the effects of other opiates).

The approval and introduction of buprenorphine marked a major shift in how pharmacological-based treatment of drug dependence can be administered. Subutex and Suboxone were the first two drugs to benefit from the Drug Abuse Treatment Act of 2000 (DATA, 2000), which allows qualified physicians to treat opioid-dependent patients in office-based settings. DATA 2000 lifted the restrictions of the Harrison Act of 1914, which prohibited physicians in the United States from prescribing narcotic medications to patients who were dependent on narcotics. The Harrison Act also helped shape the impression that drug dependence was primarily a criminal rather than a medical problem. For these reasons, most physicians were reluctant to treat narcotics addicts, and the pharmacological treatment of drug addiction occurred primarily at specialized clinics. At this time, Subutex and Suboxone are the only two medications that the FDA has classified for office-based treatment of opioid dependence.

Smoking

Treatment of smoking cessation can involve counseling and/or the use of medications (Table 30.3). Most medications for smoking cessation are nicotine replacements; several such products are available, including over-the-counter (OTC) products based on gum, transdermal patch, and lozenge delivery technology as well as a nasal spray and inhaler-based system available by prescription. Currently, bupropion (GlaxoSmithKline's Zyban) is the only non-nicotine therapy available by prescription.

The objective of nicotine replacement therapy is to relieve withdrawal symptoms. These products generally provide a lower dose of nicotine than obtained from tobacco, do not generate the pleasurable effects associated with tobacco products, and do not contain the carcinogens associated with cigarettes and other tobacco products. Each delivery system has different advantages and drawbacks. For example, use of the gum allows patients to self-titrate the desired amount of nicotine absorbed from the therapy; however, some patients do not enjoy the taste of the gum or the need for chewing it. Also, adverse effects such as hiccups, soreness of the mouth, or throat irritation can occur. The transdermal patch can be more convenient to use; however, titration on a daily basis is not possible, and skin irritation at the site of the

Table 30.3 Select FDA-approved Products for Smoking Cessation, 2005

Generic Name	*Company/Brand Name*	*Formulation*	*2003 US Sales ($MM)*
Nicotine polacrilex			
	GlaxoSmithKline's Nicorette	Gum (OTC)	59
	GlaxoSmithKline's Commit	Lozenge (OTC)	7
Nicotine			
	GlaxoSmithKline's NicoDerm CQ	Transdermal patch (OTC)	38
	Pfizer's Nicotrol	Transdermal patch (OTC)	3
	Pfizer's Nicotrol NS	Nasal spray (prescription)	4
	Pfizer's Nicotrol	Inhaler (prescription)	19
Bupropion			
	GlaxoSmithKline's Zyban	Tablet (prescription)	60

OTC = Over the counter

patch can occur. The choice between these or the other formulations for nicotine replacement therapy should be based on patient preference.

Zyban is the only non-nicotine product that is currently FDA approved for smoking cessation. This agent is a sustained-release tablet formulation of bupropion and is indicated as an aid to smoking cessation treatment. (GlaxoSmithKline markets its tablet formulation of bupropion for treatment of depression under the trade name Wellbutrin.) Researchers do not completely understand bupropion's mechanism of action for treatment of nicotine addiction; the agent is a dopamine and norepinephrine reuptake inhibitor. Bupropion can ameliorate the symptoms of withdrawal, and its effectiveness is not limited to patients with symptoms of depression. In a comparative trial, bupropion was more effective than a nicotine patch, and these two therapies were most effective when used together – cessation rates of approximately 50% were achieved. Bupropion can cause seizures and is contraindicated in patients with seizure disorders and in patients who are taking monoamine oxidase inhibitors (MAOIs).

As stated, bupropion is currently the only antidepressant that is FDA approved for smoking cessation; however, its success has stimulated interest in evaluating other types of antidepressants for this indication. The tricyclic antidepressants (TCAs) may help in smoking cessation, and nortriptyline (Ranbaxy's Aventyl, Mallickrodt's Pamelor) had demonstrated some efficacy in multiple clinical trials. However, this class of antidepressants can cause significant side effects. The selective serotonin reuptake inhibitors (SSRIs) do not appear to be useful as aids for smoking cessation.

EMERGING THERAPIES FOR TREATMENT OF ADDICTION

Although currently available medications and other programs for treating alcohol, opioid, or nicotine dependence can increase a patient's likelihood of success, these medications are not successful for many patients. A clear need exists for safe, nonaddictive, more effective medications for these indications. Several companies have entered this field and are developing new medications for treating addiction. Select examples of later-stage product candidates are discussed in the following sections.

Alcohol

At least three companies have late-stage emerging therapies for treating alcohol dependence. Table 30.4 summarizes these and other products. Bristol-Myers Squibb (BMS)

Table 30.4 Emerging Pharmacological Therapies for Treatment of Alcohol Dependence, 2005

Compound	*Company*	*Development Status*	*Comments*
Aripiprazole (Abilify)	BMS	Phase IV	• A partial agonist for dopamine D2 and serotonin (5-HT1A) receptors, and an antagonist for 5-HT2A receptors • On the market for treatment of schizophrenia, acute manic, and mixed episodes associated with bipolar disorder
Naltrexone (Vivitrex)	Alkermes	Phase III	• Long-acting injection version of naltrexone
Naltrexone depot	DrugAbuse Sciences	Phase III	• An extended-release, injectable formulation of naltrexone • Based on the company's LACTIZ drug delivery technology, which is based on a poly (D,L-lactide) polymer matrix
Rimonabant (Acomplia)	Sanofi-Aventis	Phase II	• A cannabinoid receptor-1 (CB1) receptor antagonist • The National Institute on Alcohol Abuse and Alcoholism (NIAAA) is evaluating rimonabant in a Phase II trial to assess its use in reducing alcohol consumption

is evaluating aripiprazole (Abilify) in a Phase IV trial for alcohol-dependent patients who want to stop using alcohol. Also, two of the late-stage products are long-acting formulations of naltrexone, which is already used for treatment of alcohol dependence. The introduction of monthly dosing formulations may increase use of this drug and patient compliance.

Bristol-Myers Squibb's Aripiprazole

Aripiprazole (Abilify) is a psychotropic drug that interacts with both the dopamine and the serotonin receptors. BMS is sponsoring a multicenter Phase IV clinical trial to evaluate aripiprazole for treating alcohol-dependent patients who want to stop using alcohol. Aripiprazole was first approved in the United States for treating schizophrenia, and in October 2004, it was approved for treating acute manic and mixed episodes associated with bipolar disorder. At the time of this second approval, BMS reported that more than 2.4 million prescriptions had been written for Abilify in the United States. BMS and Otsuka Pharmaceuticals, which originally developed Abilify, are collaborating on the commercialization of aripiprazole in the United States and major European countries. Both BMS and Otsuka are conducting additional clinical trials evaluating Abilify for treatment of other neurological conditions.

Alkermes' Naltrexone (Vivitrex)

Vivitrex is a long-acting, injected formulation of naltrexone, which is currently used for treating alcohol dependence and is available as a generic drug, as discussed earlier. Alkermes has designed Vivitrex for dosing once monthly. The agent uses the Alkermes Medisorb sustained-release technology, a microsphere-based system in which the active drug molecule is incorporated into a bioabsorbable polymer consisting of poly-DL-lactide-co-glycolide (PLG). Alkermes has completed a Phase III clinical trial of Vivitrex and, in a December 2003 press release, reported that patients treated with the higher of two doses of Vivitrex achieved an approximately 25% reduction in the rate of heavy drinking compared with patients taking placebo. Alkermes is also evaluating Vivitrex in a 12 month, open-label safety study in more than 400 patients. Enrollment in this Phase III extension study was completed in April 2004.

DrugAbuse Sciences' Naltrexone Depot

DrugAbuse Sciences is a biopharmaceutical company that is focusing on development of agents for treating alcohol and substance abuse and dependence. Its lead product in development, naltrexone depot, is an extended-release, injectable formulation of naltrexone. Naltrexone depot uses the company's LACTIZ drug delivery technology, which is based on a poly (D,L-lactide) polymer matrix. This agent is designed for once-monthly administration, as opposed to the once-daily administration of the currently available naltrexone. DrugAbuse Sciences reports that naltrexone depot is in Phase III clinical trials for alcohol dependence, and in May 2003, the company reported data from a Phase III trial in which patients who had received naltrexone depot for 12 months experienced 73% more drink-free days compared with patients taking placebo.

Other Drugs under Evaluation for Treating Alcohol Dependence

In addition to activity at pharmaceutical companies to develop new pharmacotherapies for alcohol addiction, government agencies and academic researchers are conducting clinical trials to evaluate whether drugs developed for other indications are useful in the treatment of alcohol dependence. These studies may lead to additional marketing or licensing possibilities for pharmaceutical companies and represent an interest on the part of the healthcare community in identifying better pharmacological options for the treatment of alcoholism. The following are examples of additional drugs being evaluated for treating alcoholism in ongoing or completed trials sponsored by the NIAAA:

- Rimonabant (Sanofi-Aventis's Acomplia), a CB1 receptor antagonist for treating obesity and smoking cessation.
- Fluoxetine (Eli Lilly's Prozac, generics), an SSRI that is currently FDA approved for treating depression, obsessive compulsive disorder, bulimia nervosa, and panic disorder.
- Sertraline (Pfizer's Zoloft, generics), an SSRI that is currently FDA approved for treating depression, obsessive compulsive disorder, panic disorder, posttraumatic stress disorder, and premenstrual dysphoric disorder.
- Ondansetron (GlaxoSmithKline's Zofran, generics), a selective serotonin (5-HT2) receptor antagonist that is currently FDA approved for preventing nausea and vomiting associated with chemotherapy as well as postoperative nausea and vomiting.

In addition, academic researchers are evaluating topiramate (Ortho-McNeil Pharmaceuticals' Topamax) for treating alcohol dependence. Topiramate is a sulfamate-substituted monosaccharide that modulates certain GABA receptors and also the AMPA and kainite glutamate receptors. Topiramate is currently FDA approved for treating epilepsy and migraine headaches.

Abused Drugs

Several new pharmacological-based therapies are in development for treating drug addiction (Tables 30.5 and 30.6). Most of the company activity in this field is focused on opiate dependency (sometimes focusing even more specifically on cocaine and/or heroin addiction). Many of these agents are still in early-stage development, and companies have revealed limited information about their new therapies. Three agents in at least Phase II development for treating drug addiction are discussed in detail in the following sections.

DrugAbuse Science's Adrogolide

Adrogolide (also called ABT-431 and DAS-431) is a pro-drug of a compound called A-86929, which is a dopamine D1 receptor agonist. Abbott Laboratories originally developed adrogolide and licensed the agent to DrugAbuse Sciences in September 2000.

Early clinical trial data have shown that adrogolide reduces both cocaine cravings and the intent to use. DrugAbuse Sciences reports that a Phase II trial in cocaine-dependent patients has been completed and that additional studies are under way for chronic addiction, schizophrenia, and cognitive impairment in the elderly. The formulation that has reached Phase II trials for cocaine dependence is an intravenous (IV) formulation. Because adrogolide has poor solubility, an aerosolized formulation is being evaluated in preclinical studies.

DrugAbuse Sciences' Naltrexone (Naltrel)

DrugAbuse Sciences is developing Naltrel, an injectable suspension formulation of naltrexone depot for treating opiate dependence. Phase IIb clinical trials have been completed, and Naltrel reportedly was successful in blocking the effects of the opiate hydromorphone over a six-week treatment period. Like naltrexone depot, Naltrel has been designed for once-monthly administration.

Xenova's TA-CD

TA-CD is a therapeutic vaccine under development for treating cocaine addiction. It consists of a nicotine derivative coupled to recombinant cholera toxin B. This protein conjugate is then adsorbed onto an aluminum hydroxide gel adjuvant. The agent is administered by injection. The objective is to stimulate the body to generate antibodies against cocaine. These antibodies bind to the cocaine, preventing the drug molecules from crossing into the brain, which in turn prevents or reduces the euphoric effect that results from taking cocaine.

In April 2003, Xenova announced the start of a Phase IIa clinical trial that included 10 patients. Later, in October 2003, Xenova

Table 30.5 Early-stage Emerging Pharmacological Therapies for the Treatment of Drug Addiction, 2005

Compound	*Company*	*Development Status*	*Comments*
GBR-12909 (vanoxerine)	National Institute of Drug Abuse	Phase I	• Presynaptic dopamine transporter inhibitor • For treatment of cocaine abuse
Lobeline	Yaupon Therapeutics	Phase I	• Dopamine-modulating agent • In Phase I for methamphetamine addiction • Is neuroprotective to dopamine-producing nerves and is therefore a potential treatment for Parkinson's disease • May also be a potential treatment for attention deficit hyperactivity disorder (ADHD)
CPP-109 (vigabatrin to treat addiction) \	Catalyst Pharmaceutical Partners	FDA has accepted an investigational new drug application; start of U.S. Phase I trial planned for first quarter of 2005	• Being developed to treat cocaine addiction • Inhibits the enzyme that breaks down the dopamine-modulating neurotransmitter gamma-aminobutyric acid (GABA) • Licensed from Brookhaven National Laboratory • Has been evaluated in two early-stage clinical trials in Mexico
Buprenorphine (Buprenorphine Depot)	DrugAbuse Sciences	Preclinical	• Extended-release injectable form of buprenorphine that uses the LACTIZ drug delivery technology • For treatment of heroin dependence
COC-AB (equine F[ab])2 cocaine antibody)	DrugAbuse Sciences	Preclinical	• For emergency treatment of cocaine overdose
InterveXin-PCP	InterveXion Therapeutics	Preclinical	• Monoclonal antibody for treatment of phencyclidine (PCP) abuse. Can bind to and absorb the toxin (PCP) from the blood • 1/05: InfleXion Therapeutics announced that it had received a $3 million business development grant from the National Institute on Drug Abuse (NIDA) to conduct clinical trials on InterveXin-PCP
InterveXin-METH	InterveXion Therapeutics	Preclinical	• Monoclonal antibody for treatment of methamphetamine abuse. Can bind to and absorb the toxin (methamphetamine) from the blood
NRP-104	New River Pharmaceuticals (in partnership with Shire Pharmaceuticals)	Preclinical	• Prodrug of amphetamine Initial indication is for treatment of ADHD • 8/04: announcement that the FDA had designated NRP-104 as a fast-track product for treatment of cocaine dependence • In discussion with the NIDA to design preclinical and clinical programs for cocaine dependence At this time, New River and Shire have not determined whether they will pursue this agent for treatment of cocaine dependence
G-protein-coupled receptor (GPCR) products	14TM	Research	• Company focus is on GPCR structure and function, including a discovery program in biogenic (mono)amine receptors (including receptors for dopamine and serotonin), which are related to substance addiction. 14TM has additional GPCR programs • 11/04: announcement of a collaborative venture between 14TM and the NIDA for the design, synthesis, and assay of agents for treatment of drug abuse and dependency

Table 30.6 Late-stage Emerging Pharmacological Therapies for the Treatment of Drug Addiction, 2005

Compound	*Company*	*Development Status*	*Comments*
Adrogolide (ABT-431, DAS-431)	DrugAbuse Sciences	Phase II	• Dopamine D1 receptor agonist • Originally developed by Abbott Laboratories; exclusive license granted to DrugAbuse Sciences in 2000 • Potential therapy for a range of conditions, including chronic addiction • Phase II trial of DAS-431 intravenous (IV) in cocaine-dependent patients completed; additional clinical trials ongoing for chronic addiction • DAS-431 aerosol in preclinical trials for cocaine relapse
BP-897	Bioprojet	Phase II	• A dopamine D3 receptor ligand • Being developed to treat cocaine abuse and craving
Modafinil (Provigil)	Cephalon	Phase II	• Being evaluated in a National Institute on Drug Abuse (NIDA)-sponsored Phase II clinical trial for reducing cocaine use in patients who are cocaine dependent Plan for this trial is to enroll 210 patients; started in October 2004 • FDA approved to improve wakefulness in patients with excessive sleepiness associated with narcolepsy, obstructive sleep apnea/hypopnea syndrome, and shift work sleep disorder
Naltrexone (Naltrel)	DrugAbuse Sciences	Phase IIb complete Preparing for Phase III	• An injectable suspension formulation of naltrexone depot • For treatment of opiate dependence
TA-CD	Xenova	Phase II	• Therapeutic vaccine for treating cocaine addiction • Consists of a cocaine derivative coupled to recombinant cholera toxin B • Stimulates the immune system to produce anticocaine antibodies
Tetrodin	WEX Pharmaceuticals	Phase IIa	• A non-narcotic agent • Being developed to reduce pain and other symptoms associated with withdrawal in opioid-dependent patients (for heroin and other opiate addiction) • Tetrodin reportedly has shown no addictive properties • The Phase IIa trial includes 20 opiate-dependent patients who are receiving methadone in a treatment program • Results from the trial are expected in spring 2005

announced the start of a Phase IIb clinical trial that will include up to 132 methadone-dependent cocaine addicts being treated for drug dependency. The early data on TA-CD are promising. In June 2004, results of two dose-escalation trials were presented at the College of Problems of Drug Dependence annual scientific meeting. Patients who were administered TA-CD developed cocaine-specific antibodies that persisted for at least six months. The maximum mean response was seen between 70 and 90 days following vaccination. Use of TA-CD reduced the likelihood that patients would use cocaine, and it reduced the euphoric effects of cocaine in many patients who relapsed (88% in one study and 63% in another study).

Smoking

Several additional non-nicotine therapies for smoking cessation are under development (Table 30.7). These include two therapeutic vaccines, plus agents that work via other

Table 30.7 Emerging Pharmacological Therapies for Smoking Cessation, 2005

Compound	*Company*	*Development Status*	*Comments*
Rimonabant (Acomplia)	Sanofi-Aventis	Phase III	• In Phase III trials for smoking cessation and obesity • A cannabinoid-1(CB1) endocannabinoid receptor antagonist
Varenicline	Pfizer	Phase III	• Targets the alpha4-beta2 nicotinic receptors in the brain
468816	GlaxoSmithKline	Phase II	• Glycine antagonist
NicVAX (nicotine conjugate vaccine)	Nabi Biopharmaceuticals	Phase II	• For treatment of nicotine addiction and as an aid to smoking cessation
CP-945598	Pfizer	Phase I trials completed	• Targets the CB1 receptor • One of four CB1 candidates being developed by Pfizer • Inhibits appetite and is a potential treatment for obesity
TA-NIC	Xenova	Phase I	• Therapeutic vaccine to treat nicotine addiction • Consists of a nicotine derivative coupled to recombinant cholera toxin B • Stimulates the immune system to produce anti-nicotine antibodies
Nornicotine	Yaupon Therapeutics	Preclinical	• Second-generation smoking cessation agent that comes from the plant *Nicotiana tobaccum.* Reportedly has a longer half-life and improved side-effect profile compared with nicotine replacement therapy

novel mechanisms. Examples of agents that have reached at least Phase II clinical development are discussed in the following subsections.

Sanofi-Aventis's Rimonabant

Sanofi-Aventis is developing the CB1 receptor antagonist rimonabant (Acomplia) for treating obesity and for smoking cessation both as an aid to quit smoking and for long-term maintenance of abstinence from smoking. Rimonabant is in Phase III clinical trials for both obesity and smoking cessation. The Phase III clinical program for smoking cessation was started in 2002 and includes more than 6,500 patients worldwide in three clinical trials. The Phase III trials in obesity were started in 2001 and include more than 6,600 patients worldwide in four clinical trials.

In March 2004, researchers presented results from two pivotal studies of rimonabant at the American College of Cardiology meeting. These studies were Rimonabant In Obesity (RIO-Lipids) and the Studies with Rimonabant And Tobacco Use (STRATUS-US). The STRATUS-US trial, reported in March 2004, included 787 smokers at 11 clinical trial sites in the United States. In this double-blind, placebo-controlled trial, patients were treated with rimonabant or placebo for ten weeks. Each person was allowed to smoke for the first two weeks but was given a target quit date at day 15 of their treatment. Abstinence from smoking for the last four weeks of the study was reported by the patients and confirmed by measurements of carbon monoxide concentrations in expired air. Results were that 36.2% of patients treated with rimonabant quit smoking, compared with 20.6% of patients who received placebo. Rimonabant was reportedly well tolerated. The results reported in March 2004 from the RIO-Lipids (obesity) trial also were positive.

Pfizer's Varenicline

Varenicline is a novel compound in late-stage development that, unlike many other current or emerging therapies for smoking cessation, is neither a nicotine derivative nor an antidepressant medication. Varenicline selectively targets the alpha4-beta2 nicotine receptors, which stimulate the release of dopamine in the brain. Treatment with varenicline has two effects: (1) reducing a person's craving for nicotine and (2) blocking the positive rewards experienced from smoking. Pfizer reports that in a Phase II clinical trial, nearly half of the smokers who were treated with varenicline quit smoking. Varenicline is currently being evaluated in Phase III trials.

GlaxoSmithKline's 468816

GlaxoSmithKline is already a major player in the smoking cessation market, with both prescription and nonprescription products available. In addition, the company has a glycine antagonist called 468816 in Phase II development for smoking cessation. At this time, limited information is available about 468816.

Nabi Biopharmaceuticals' NicVAX

Nabi Biopharmaceuticals is applying its expertise and knowledge of the immune system to the development of products for nicotine addiction and smoking cessation. Nabi is developing NicVAX, which consists of a nicotine derivative conjugated to the carrier protein recombinant exotoxin protein A (rEPA) from *Pseudomonas aeruginosa.* This vaccine stimulates the patient's body to produce antibodies that bind to nicotine, thus preventing the nicotine from reaching the brain and providing the positive stimulus that usually results from nicotine.

A Phase I clinical trial was started in August 2002. In February 2003, a Phase I/II trial was started in the Netherlands to evaluate the safety of the vaccine and to determine nicotine-specific antibody levels. This placebo-controlled trial included smokers, exsmokers, and nonsmokers. Nabi reports that the vaccine was well tolerated and that use of the vaccine resulted in production of nicotine-specific antibodies.

In August 2003, Nabi started a double-blind, placebo-controlled, randomized Phase II trial in the United States. Positive results from this trial were reported in September 2004. The study included 68 smokers who were randomized to receive up to four injections of NicVAX (at one of three doses) or placebo. Nabi reports that the vaccine was well tolerated, and smokers who received the highest dose level had a 33% quit rate compared with the placebo group. Nabi plans to conduct an additional dosing study to evaluate NicVAX at even higher doses.

PROSPECTS FOR ADDICTION PHARMACOTHERAPY

For many decades, progress in the pharmacotherapy of addiction has been slow. Alcohol and drug abuse traditionally have not been principal research areas for most major pharmaceutical companies, although some of these companies have been and continue to be active in the somewhat larger smoking-cessation market. We expect that growth in the alcohol and drug dependence market will be slow; however, there is an unmet need in the smoking-cessation market that represents an opportunity for new products. As we will discuss, several factors have contributed to this situation.

Alcohol/Drug Dependence Pharmacotherapy Markets

We anticipate some growth in the market for pharmacotherapeutic treatment of drug and alcohol abuse but expect that this market will expand slowly. The market size will remain small; although the number of people who abuse drugs and alcohol each year is high, only a small number of these people seek treatment. One of the main reasons is that many of these people do not realize that they require treatment. According to the 2003 NSDUH, 19.3 million people in the United States older than age 12 with a drug or alcohol abuse problem did not think they needed to seek treatment.

Moreover, people who do seek treatment face a variety of barriers to receiving it. Approximately 1 million people in the United States believed they needed treatment in 2003 but did not receive it, citing issues such as cost, insurance, social stigma, and emotional issues. Another factor limiting the market size is the type of treatment sought; of the 3.3 million people who received treatment, 1.9 million obtained treatment from a specialized treatment facility that did not focus on the use of medications (Substance Abuse and Mental Health Services Administration, 2004). Additional factors constraining the market include limited efficacy of available medications for many patients and problems with patient compliance when the medications are prescribed.

Despite the issues that restrict the market, we forecast changes in the market that will increase opportunities for drug developers:

- Awareness is growing that alcoholism is a disease and that medications can be important aids for treating patients who are addicted to alcohol or drugs.
- The Drug Abuse Treatment Act of 2003 that makes it possible to treat drug addiction in the physician's office should further expand the availability of medications to patients.
- As we have discussed, several novel therapies for treating addiction are being developed, and the introduction of more effective medications should expand this market even further, particularly if these agents achieve a classification that allows drug administration in a doctor's office rather than a treatment facility. The presence of major pharmaceutical companies with their considerable marketing strength should increase awareness of drug treatment options among both physicians and patients.

These market drivers should counteract some of the issues restricting market growth and may increase the percentage of people who seek pharmacotherapeutic treatment.

Smoking-cessation Pharmacotherapy Market

The smoking-cessation market is larger than the market for treating alcohol and drug dependence; more than 32 million people in the United States have expressed a desire to quit smoking. Growth of this market is fueled by the large number of smokers who have indicated their desire to quit as well as various programs and efforts to motivate smokers to quit smoking. This market is highly competitive, and companies marketing the branded OTC smoking-cessation products face significant competition from one another and from store-brand products.

Sales of GlaxoSmithKline's prescription drug Zyban have been limited, with only $60 million in US sales in 2003; however, we expect the market for prescription products for smoking cessation to change rapidly in the near future. Significant market potential exists for a highly efficacious smoking-cessation product. Both Sanofi-Aventis (rimonabant) and Pfizer (varenicline) have promising candidates in Phase III clinical trials, and additional agents are in earlier stages of development. If any of these products proves to be more effective than current therapies or is available in a formulation that is more likely to encourage compliance, it is likely to claim a large portion of the smoking-cessation market.

REFERENCE

Substance Abuse and Mental Health Services Administration. *Overview of Findings from the 2003 National Survey on Drug Use and Health* (Office of Applied Studies, NSDUH Series H-24, DHHS Publication No. SMA 04–3963). Rockville, MD; 2004.

SECTION C

Immunology

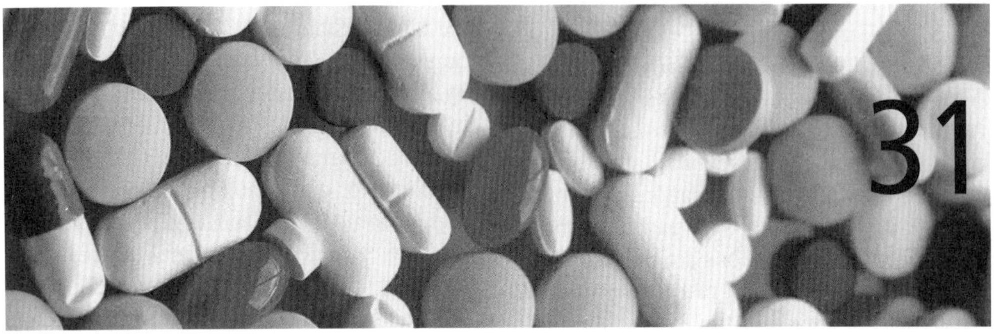

Prevention of Organ Transplant Rejection: Current Therapies and Novel Strategies

THE NEED FOR NEW ANTIREJECTION DRUGS

The practice of organ transplantation has expanded substantially since the first successful kidney transplant, more than 40 years ago. According to the Scientific Registry of Transplant Statistics (SRTR), about 25,000 transplants were performed in the United States in 2002, a 38% increase since 1993 (Organ Procurement and Transplant Network [OPTN]/SRTR 2004 Annual Report). Despite improvements in the rate of acute organ rejection following transplantation, organ loss remains a problem. Figure 31.1 shows graft survival rates for commonly transplanted organs over 10 years posttransplantation. Approximately 50% of the $5 billion spent annually in the United States on organ transplants is used for posttransplantation immunosuppressive therapy and/or complications following transplantation, including rejection. In addition, the strides made in managing acute organ rejection (which occurs immediately following transplantation) have not been paralleled in chronic organ rejection (which occurs over time despite immunosuppressive therapy), and stemming the long-term organ loss remains a substantial unmet need. In this environment, where the demand for organs continues to exceed the supply, reducing the need for retransplantation due to organ rejection is critical. Fortunately, evolving knowledge of the immune system is spawning new approaches to the management of both acute and chronic rejection.

Significant reductions in acute rejection and associated morbidity and mortality following organ transplantation have been achieved

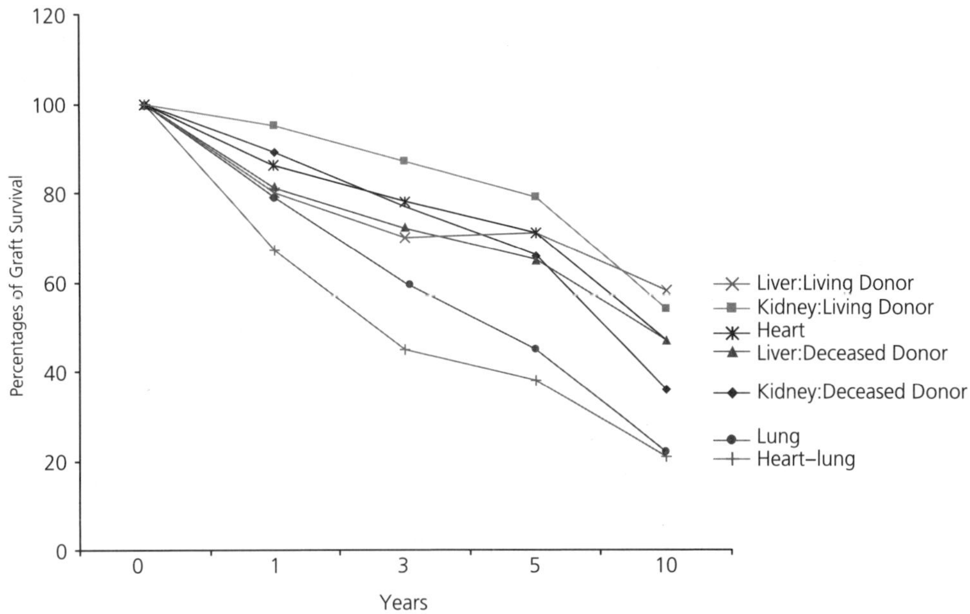

Figure 31.1 Graft Survival Rates Over 10 Years for Select Transplant Organs

since the introduction of cyclosporine (Novartis's Sandimmune) in 1982. Since that time, newer antirejection drugs have been launched, including Roche's mycophenolate mofetil (CellCept), Wyeth's sirolimus (Rapamune), and tacrolimus (Astellas Pharma's Prograf). Today, the most common antirejection treatments are drug regimens that combine these newer therapies with traditional immunosuppressants, which have reduced the incidence of acute organ rejection.

Although numerous challenges remain in the effort to reduce acute organ failure, preventing chronic organ rejection has proved even more difficult. Posttransplant vasculopathy (disease of the blood vessels) is one of the most common causes of late organ failure. In patients whose transplanted organs survive more than five years, approximately 40–60% of graft loss has been attributed to vasculopathy (Subbotin et al., 1999). Lifelong immunosuppressant therapy has enabled patients to live with donor organs, but these regimens are far from ideal. Immunosuppressive regimens have numerous side effects that contribute to morbidity and mortality because they depress the immune system, an effect that leaves transplant patients vulnerable to infections and potential malignancies. The hope remains that newer drugs with improved safety and side-effect profiles will replace these regimens.

In this chapter, we examine the causes of both acute and chronic organ rejection and discuss the benefits and drawbacks of current treatment options. We review emerging targets for rejection therapies and discuss the transition from immunosuppression to immunomodulation in emerging therapies. Finally, we profile several drugs in clinical development that we expect will change the standard of care for transplant patients by 2010.

CAUSES OF TRANSPLANT REJECTION

Before a patient undergoes an organ transplantation, technicians must determine a match between the patient and an organ donor based on blood type (A, B, or O), human leukocyte antigen (HLA; tissue antigen) type, or major histocompatibility antigens (MHAs).

The match, however, is never 100%, except in cases of identical twins. Once the patient receives the transplant, the patient's immune system identifies the organ as foreign based on its MHAs. To avoid transplant rejection, the patient must begin immunosuppressant therapy, which will continue for the remainder of his or her life.

HLA molecules are cell surface molecules with four immunoglobulin domains that play a role in the activation of T cells, the primary immune system cells that cause rejection of organ transplants. HLA molecules found on the surface of antigen-presenting cells (APCs) bind with antigens for presentation to the T-cell receptor. These HLA molecules, categorized as Class I and Class II alloantigens, can induce transplant immunity (which ultimately results in rejection) via two pathways:

- The direct pathway, in which the T cells of the recipient respond to the APCs of the donor that are expressing HLA donor antigens. In this case, organ rejection is caused by cell-mediated cytotoxicity.
- The indirect pathway, in which HLA antigens from the donor are processed by the transplant recipient's APCs and are presented to their T cells along with the recipient's own HLA molecules. Organ rejection is ultimately caused by delayed hypersensitivity (DHT).

Because the transplanted organ is a constant source of HLA antigens, the potential for organ rejection is continuous from the time of transplantation.

Even with immunosuppressant therapy, complications from organ transplantation can result, including loss of organ or tissue function, infections, and side effects from medication. Certain organs are more successfully transplanted than others, but even organs that have high success rates, such as kidneys, can be rejected; kidney transplants from living donors have a rejection rate of almost 50% within 10 years (Figure 31.1).

The processes of acute and chronic rejection involve different mechanisms that have recently become better understood. The primary mechanism of *acute rejection* is the graft-versus-host reaction, which is characterized by the infiltration of mononuclear cells into the allograft and subsequent hemorrhage and edema. Following resolution of acute rejection, the allograft can achieve prolonged survival even with low-level immunosuppressive therapy. In contrast, *chronic rejection*, which can proceed slowly and despite high therapy levels, is thought to involve cell-mediated responses. In this process, the endothelium of the artery to the allograft becomes occluded as a result of tissue proliferation, an event that finally causes ischemia and fibrosis of the allograft.

CURRENT THERAPIES

Physicians use several types of immunosuppressant drugs in various combinations to manage patients post-transplantation. The 2004 immunosuppressant market for organ transplantation was more than $1 billion in the United States (Table 31.1). In the following paragraphs, we review the key drugs used in current antirejection therapy regimens.

Immunosuppressant drugs act on a large number of targets, and therefore all have some side effects. These drugs block cells from dividing, thereby preventing lymphocytes from becoming activated and expanding; however, they have some of the same toxic side effects as many chemotherapy drugs (e.g., nausea, muscle pain, weakness). In addition, because these drugs suppress the patient's whole immune system, the patient has a reduced defense against bacterial and viral infections and may develop lymphoma cancers. Other complications that can result from immunosuppressant therapy are as follows:

- Nephrotoxicity.
- Neurotoxicity.
- Posttransplantation diabetes with therapy initiation.
- Hypertension.
- Hyperlipidemia.

Researchers are examining new drug-combination strategies in clinical trials in the

Table 31.1 US Sales of Select Antirejection Therapies, 2004

Generic Name	*Brand/Manufacturer*	*Mechanism of Action*	*US Sales ($MM)*
Tacrolimus	Prograf/Astellas	Inhibits T-cell activation	480
Mycophenolate mofetil	CellCept/Roche	Cytostatic effect on T and B lymphocytes	300
Cyclosporine	Neoral/Novartis	Inhibits activation of T and B cells	126
Sirolimus	Rapamune/Wyeth	Suppresses T-cell proliferation	125
Anti-thymocyte globulin (rabbit)	Thymoglobulin/Genzyme	Depletes T cells	74
Cyclosporine	SandImmune/Novartis	Inhibits activation of T and B cells	45
Daclizumab	Zenapax/Roche	IL-2 inhibitor	19
Mycophenolic acid	Myfortic/Novartis	Cytostatic effect on T and B lymphocytes and inhibits activation of T and B cells	18
Basiliximab	Simulect/Novartis	IL-2 inhibitor	17
Azathioprine	Imuran/Prometheus Products, generics	Inhibits activation of T and B cells	7
Prednisone	Deltasone/Pfizer, generics	Inactivates NF-κB	3

hope that effective regimens can be created that will eliminate the need for long-term immunosuppressant therapy and its associated side effects. Given the serious need for transplants, however, these drugs are currently the only hope for many patients to avoid rejection of their new organs.

First-generation Immunosuppressants

Cornerstone immunosuppressants that have been used after organ transplant include corticosteroids (e.g., prednisone), azathioprine (GlaxoSmithKline's [GSK's] Imuran), and cyclosporine. Naturally occurring glucocorticoids include hydrocortisone and cortisone; prednisone is a synthetic glucocorticoid analogue that has potent anti-inflammatory effects. Corticosteroid use can cause infection, whose signs can be masked by the therapy's use. Azathioprine is an immunosuppressive agent used as adjunct therapy to prevent renal transplant rejection. The use of azathioprine reduces the need for chronic steroid treatment and therefore limits the related adverse events associated with steroid treatment. However, chronic use of azathioprine, a purine antimetabolite, increases cancer risk. Cyclosporine was the first drug approved (in 1982) for transplant patients. It inhibits B and T lymphocytes from becoming activated, an action that results in general immune-system suppression. Cyclosporine essentially shields the transplanted organ from recognition by the patient's immune response. Novartis's Sandimmune is the original cyclosporine formulation that is used to prevent organ rejection in kidney, heart, and liver transplant patients. Novartis reformulated cyclosporine in 1995 to create a microemulsion-modified version (Neoral) with improved drug-absorption properties. Immunosuppressive therapy often involves using cyclosporine in combination with other drugs.

Next-generation Immunosuppressants

In the 1990s, several new immunosuppressant drugs became available to manage organ transplantation, including drugs from Novartis, Astellas Pharma, Roche, and Genzyme. Although these drugs have shown improvements in outcomes – such as longer patient- and organ-survival times – when used in various combination therapy regimens, the generalized immunosuppressive effects of these drugs, like their predecessors' effects, result in an increased risk of infection and malignancy.

Astellas's tacrolimus, a macrolide immunosuppressant, was launched for the treatment of liver transplantation in Japan first, in 1993, and subsequently in the United States in 1994. Currently, tacrolimus is available in approximately 40 countries and is indicated for patients receiving kidney and liver transplants. Tacrolimus suppresses cell-mediated reactions and, to some extent, humoral immunity. The mechanism by which tacrolimus inhibits T-cell activation in not known; however, experimental data suggest that the action may occur via binding of tacrolimus to FKBP-12, an intracellular protein. The FKBP-12/tacrolimus complex triggers a series of steps that result in calcineurin inhibition, which ultimately may prevent the nuclear factor involved in the initiation of lymphokine formation (e.g., IL-2, which stimulates T-cell activation). By blocking this action, tacrolimus prevents T-cell activation that results in immunosuppression. Tacrolimus is administered with low-dose corticosteroids to diminish its risk of anaphylaxis. Like patients taking other immunosuppressive drugs, patients taking tacrolimus are more susceptible to infection and to development of lymphoma.

Three years of data from a multicenter European clinical trial in liver transplant patients have shown tacrolimus to be more effective in preventing acute rejection than cyclosporine: 55.1% versus 45.4%. Similar results were found in the four-year data of the European multicenter clinical trial in kidney transplantation, in which tacrolimus also reduced the incidence of rejection compared with cyclosporine: 25.9% versus 45.7%. The improvement appears to be related to action on the renal vasculature in addition to action on the organ itself.

More than 80% of kidney transplant patients take Roche's mycophenolate mofetil (MMF) (CellCept), launched in 1995 for the prevention of acute rejection. Mycophenolate has a cytostatic effect on T and B lymphocytes that are dependent on purine synthesis, and the drug may also inhibit the recruitment of leukocytes to the graft site. Like other immunosuppressive agents, MMF used long term as part of an immunosuppressive regimen increases the risk of malignancy.

In May 2004, the SRTR presented data on more than 25,000 patients receiving MMF that demonstrated better patient and organ survival for liver- and kidney-transplant patients than other therapy regimens. One study compared the use of MMF with tacrolimus and corticosteroids versus tacrolimus and corticosteroids alone in 11,670 adult primary liver-transplant recipients. At four years, the group receiving MMF showed statistically significant improvements in patient survival (81.4% versus 77.2%), graft survival (77.7% versus 74.2%), and death-censored graft survival (87.0% versus 83.9%). In addition, the MMF group experienced a decrease in the risk of death due to bacterial infection (Lake et al., 2004).

A second study evaluated 21,017 patients and compared patients receiving sirolimus and cyclosporine in combination with patients receiving mycophenolate with cyclosporine. Four-year graft survival and death-centered graft survival rates were lower for the sirolimus/cyclosporine combination group compared with the MMF/cyclosporine microemulsion group: 74.6% versus 79.3%, four-year graft survival; 83.7% versus 87.2%, death-centered graft survival (Meier-Kriesche, 2004).

Novartis's Myfortic, a delayed-release formulation of mycophenolic acid with cyclosporine microemulsion (Neoral), is a new treatment option for kidney-transplant patients. The delayed-release formulation can be useful in diminishing side effects that can occur with mycophenolate and cause physicians to lower the dose, which increases the risk of rejection. Myfortic was approved in the United States in March 2004. It has been approved in 40 countries, including Switzerland (first approval in 2003), Germany, France, the United Kingdom, Austria, India, Brazil, and some Latin American countries.

In 1995, Roche's daclizumab (Zenapax) was approved for the prevention of acute rejection following kidney transplantation. Additional indication approvals followed in 1998 for heart transplants, in 2000 for liver transplants, and in 2001 for pancreas transplants. Daclizumab is a recombinant humanized IgG1 monoclonal antibody (90% human, 10% murine) that binds to the interleukin-2 (IL-2) receptor that is expressed on activated lymphocytes, thereby inhibiting

IL-2 binding. The transplanted organ is protected from the cellular immune response that is caused by IL-2-mediated activation of lymphocytes. However, daclizumab also impairs the ability of the immune system to respond to the challenge made by other antigens and therefore increases the risk of infection.

In 1998, Novartis introduced basiliximab (Simulect), a two-dose, high-affinity, chimeric monoclonal antibody to the IL-2 receptor. Basiliximab suppresses interleukin-driven proliferation of T cells and is used for induction therapy. By blocking the cellular immune response, basiliximab prevents acute rejection of kidney transplants when used in combination with cyclosporine and corticosteroids. In US/Canadian and European studies, basiliximab reduced acute rejection during the four- to six-week period following transplantation by 28% and by 32%, respectively.

Genzyme's Thymoglobulin (antithymocyte globulin [rabbit]) is a polyclonal antibody that suppresses T cells and is used to manage acute rejection as part of a solid organ-transplant immunosuppression regimen. Thymoglobulin is approved in the United States for treatment of acute kidney transplant rejection, in Canada for prevention and treatment of acute kidney-transplant rejection, and in many European countries for prevention and treatment of acute graft rejection, prevention and treatment of acute graft-versus-host disease, and treatment of aplastic anemia. Thymoglobulin is registered in 56 countries, and the product has already been filed with regulatory authorities in Japan for severe aplastic anemia and graft-versus-host disease. Genzyme is currently studying the safety and efficacy of Thymoglobulin as a kidney induction agent and in a regimen that involves reduced immunosuppressive maintenance dosing. Additional pilot clinical trials, begun in 2005, are under way to explore the use of Thymoglobulin induction in liver transplantation and in bone marrow transplantation.

With the acquisition of Ilex Oncology in December 2004, Genzyme added the human monoclonal antibody therapy alemtuzumab (Campath) to its growing oncology franchise. As a T-cell depleter that targets CD52 positive lymphocytes, alemtuzumab is indicated for B-cell chronic lymphocytic leukemia (B-CLL). Data presented at the 2005 American Transplant Congress supported the safety and efficacy of alemtuzumab for induction of immunosuppression in renal-transplant patients. The data analyzed three outcomes and showed no documented cases of chronic rejection and minimal infection and malignancy complications. Schering AG has exclusive worldwide marketing and distribution rights to the product; Schering affiliate Berlex Laboratories is responsible for US sales. The Federal Trade Commission (FTC) required Genzyme to transfer all development and commercialization responsibility for alemtuzumab in solid organ transplantation to Schering as a requirement of the acquisition for competitive reasons. Therefore, Genzyme will not receive the portion of alemtuzumab sales attributed to solid organ transplant induction therapy.

The Newest Immunosuppressants: mTOR Therapies

The newest immunosuppressive agents target the kinase mammalian target of rapamycin (mTOR), inhibiting its activity and suppressing T-cell proliferation. By preventing T cells from proliferating, the possibility of near-term rejection is reduced, thereby improving the organ's chance of long-term survival as well. These agents, indicated for both acute and chronic rejection, include sirolimus and everolimus (Novartis's Certican).

Sirolimus is an orally active, novel immunosuppressant designed to prevent acute rejection in kidney-transplant patients. The product was launched in May 2001 and is approved and marketed worldwide. Sirolimus is used in combination with cyclosporine and corticosteroids, after which cyclosporine should be eliminated – two to four months following kidney transplantation. The pivotal Rapamune Maintenance Regimen study demonstrated superior renal function, less-chronic allograft nephropathy, better blood pressure control, and fewer malignancies in patients undergoing cyclosporine withdrawal versus those who continued on cyclosporine.

The FDA issued a Safety Alert for sirolimus in 2003, reporting warnings for use in de novo liver and lung transplantation. When sirolimus was used in combination with cyclosporine or tacrolimus in de novo liver transplant patients, hepatic artery thrombosis, organ loss, and mortality increased. In de novo lung-transplant recipients, fatal bronchial anastomotic dehiscence has been reported when sirolimus was used in the immunosuppressive regimen.

Clinical studies in additional patient populations (renal, liver) are under way. Ongoing Phase III clinical studies include conversion to sirolimus in maintenance renal and liver populations, as well as the newly initiated calcineurin inhibitor free study comparing sirolimus plus MMF and corticosteroids with cyclosporine plus MMF and corticosteroids in de novo kidney transplant patients.

Everolimus is a novel proliferation-signal inhibitor that targets the primary causes of chronic organ rejection (also called allograft dysfunction), including acute rejection and vascular remodeling. Everolimus is approved in more than 40 countries. In August 2004, Novartis received an approvable letter from the FDA for everolimus to be used in combination with Neoral, Novartis's reformulation of cyclosporine, for the prevention of rejection episodes following heart or kidney transplantation. The FDA requested additional information in support of safe and effective dosing regimens for the combination. The agency had previously issued an approvable letter for everolimus, in October 2003, with a request for additional clinical data on dosing regimens. Novartis submitted data in response to the first approvable letter in February 2004.

NEW APPROACHES TO ANTIREJECTION DRUG DISCOVERY

The ultimate solution to preventing the rejection of transplanted organs may be the induction of tolerance. With this solution in mind, several companies and research institutes are investigating novel strategies for addressing transplant rejection. As a result, the next generation of transplant drugs will use immunomodulation rather than immunosuppression to achieve improved transplantation outcomes with fewer side effects. This approach involves training the patient's immune system to accept the presence of the organ, thereby creating a new environment in which conventional immunosuppression would no longer be needed. Key strategies for inducing tolerance are discussed in the following sections. Some of these strategies have already produced agents now in commercial development. These agents and other emerging treatments are detailed under Section "Emerging Drug Therapies" of this chapter.

Costimulatory Blockers

The National Institute of Allergy and Infectious Diseases (NIAID) has supported research on immune tolerance for decades, including the study of the costimulatory receptors involved in T-cell activation. In addition to the presentation of antigen via APCs to the T cell for recognition, a signal from a costimulatory pathway is required for T-cell activation to occur normally (Figure 31.2). If this signal is absent, the T cell enters a state of anergy (immune unresponsiveness), inhibiting T-cell proliferation. In the early 1990s, researchers identified two key costimulatory molecules involved in organ-transplant rejection: CD28 and CD40.

The interactions between CD28 and B7 and between CD40 and CD154 has stimulated research on a strategy to induce immune tolerance by blocking these costimulatory molecules. These pathways can be manipulated by using monoclonal antibodies or fusion proteins such as cytotoxic T leukocyte antigen 4 immunoglobulin (CTLA4Ig), a recombinant fusion protein of CTLA-4. However, a simple blockade of these pathways will not necessarily produce tolerance. For example, there are reports of

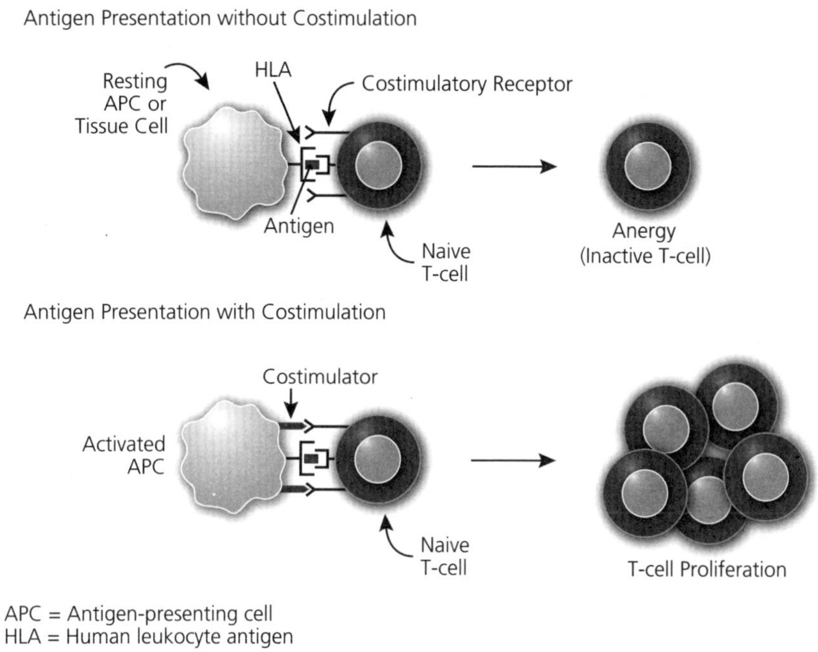

Figure 31.2 Role of Costimulatory Receptors in T-cell Activation

a refractory population of CD8+ lymphocytes that proliferate when the CD28 and CD40 pathways are blocked. Nevertheless, the blocking of these costimulatory pathways remains a promising approach to the induction of tolerance (Adams, 2002).

Mixed Chimerism

Mixed chimerism, whereby the transplant recipient receives cells from the donor's immune system in addition to the solid organ, is being investigated as a potential strategy to reduce organ transplant rejection. Mixed chimerism involves depletion of the patient's lymphocytes (before transplantation) followed by a transfer of the donor's bone marrow cells. The objective is to remove antibodies capable of immunoreaction to the donor organ and thereby induce tolerance to the donor organ. This approach develops tolerance centrally. Newer methods of T-lymphocyte depletion, such as non-myelosuppressive strategies, are milder and less challenging to the patient than older methods, which have significant toxicities. These newer methods have significantly improved the potential of mixed chimerism as a treatment. Mixed chimerism plays a central role in Novartis's tolerance induction agent FTY-720, discussed in the section "Emerging Drug Therapies," and several research centers are studying the benefits of this approach in stimulating tolerance.

A NIAID Immune Tolerance Network Phase I clinical trial is enrolling patients to determine whether a combined bone marrow and kidney transplant will be effective in treating stage II or greater multiple myeloma and associated kidney failure. The organ-transplant recipient will receive both the kidney and bone marrow from the same donor to determine whether the underlying malignancy can be cured. This method may allow the recipient to accept the kidney transplant without the need for chronic immunosuppression. The study began in June 2003. The 10 patients anticipated for enrollment will be followed for at least two years posttransplantation.

Clinical research is also under way at the Thomas E. Starzl Transplantation Institute, affiliated with the University of Pittsburgh. The protocol, instituted in July 2001, involves giving the transplant patient an infusion of donor bone marrow or stem cells. A large dose of Thymoglobulin and a relatively low dose of tacrolimus are given prior to transplant surgery. Steroids are given before the dose of Thymoglobulin and during surgery only, unless the organ is rejected; otherwise, no immunosuppressive drugs are used. By month three or four post-transplantation, if the patient appears to be doing well, the tacrolimus dose is decreased to once daily, and tapering of the dose continues. A biopsy is completed to verify that the organ is not undergoing rejection. To date, this approach has been used successfully in patients undergoing kidney, pancreas, liver, or intestinal transplantation. Clearly, long-term results will be required to determine whether this protocol can replace lifelong immunosuppression.

Toll-like Receptors

Until now, the adaptive immune system has been the primary target for preventing organ rejection. However, in the case of lung transplants, which have a high rate of acute rejections even with immunosuppressant therapy, new treatments that target the innate immune system instead could be particularly useful. Because the lung is constantly exposed to pathogens and toxins from the environment, innate immunity provides the first critical component of protection, and toll-like receptors (TLRs) provide the rapid response continually required to protect lung function. Researchers at Duke University Medical Center found that TLR4 plays a role in the rejection of transplanted lungs. At the 100th International Conference of the American Thoracic Society on May 24, 2004, the Duke team presented research indicating that the lung-transplant recipients with variants of the *TLR4* gene were substantially protected from acute organ rejection.

The Duke researchers had previously found two variants of *TLR4* that linked patients to a reduced response to bacterial toxins by the lung. Furthermore, patients with the *TLR4* variants also showed a reduction in acute organ rejection: 28% versus patients with other forms of the *TLR4* gene who suffered acute rejection of 58%. They found no impact on the rejection rate related to the gene type of the donor.

Agents That Induce Peripheral Tolerance

Peripheral tolerance is the mechanism that prevents autoreactivity of lymphocytes to proteins within the body that are not expressed in the thymus or serum. Four mechanisms generate peripheral tolerance:

- Lymphocytes do not respond to the presence of autoantigens because their concentration is too low, or they are located in an immunologically privileged site, such as the central nervous system (CNS), testis, or eye.
- Suppression, or dominant regulation, occurs when T cells that are capable of reacting to antigen are prevented from doing so by the presence of other T cells.
- Split tolerance occurs when some lymphocytes are not activated in the presence of antigen when others are, thereby inhibiting the overall immune response. For example, a T cell may have established tolerance although B cells may remain autoreactive. In this case, the B cells will be unable to mount an immune response without T-cell activation.
- Anergy develops when normal cells that lack costimulatory molecules (B7.1/B7.2, CD40, or both) present antigen to T cells. The T cells then enter a state of anergy, in which they no longer react to the same antigen at a later time even in the presence of costimulatory molecules.

Novartis is working with the United States' National Institutes of Health (NIH) to develop agents that induce peripheral tolerance through T-cell depletion by anti-CD3 immunotoxin. A conjugated antibody that combines a CD3 monoclonal antibody linked to genetically engineered diphtheria toxin is used to deplete T lymphocytes at the local transplant site. This immunotoxin has produced positive results in primate renal allografts. Following depletion of the T lymphocytes by the immunotoxin, any remaining T lymphocytes are retrained to tolerate the transplant, resulting in peripheral tolerance induction.

Gene Therapy

Novartis is also investigating the use of ex vivo gene therapy to prevent transplant rejection. By modifying genes in the donor organ prior to transplantation, Novartis has found that the immune system response from the recipient can be altered to prevent recognition of the transplanted organ. The genes that are modified are involved very early in the acute rejection response. By activating and/or suppressing these specific genes, the organ can be shielded from the recipient's immune system, avoiding the subsequent damage that results from acute rejection. Additionally, an increased margin of safety can be achieved by treating the organ ex vivo rather than the patient systemically, thereby limiting any exposure and potential immunogenicity to the viral vector used in the gene therapy. This research is in the preclinical stages of development.

EMERGING DRUG THERAPIES

Several therapies are currently in clinical development for managing acute and chronic organ rejection (Table 31.2). These therapies include improvements on existing agents, achieved through combination therapy and/or improved drug delivery, as well as novel agents, including some that incorporate one or more of the strategies discussed in the previous section.

Combination Therapies

Researchers are investigating combination therapies to try to further reduce the rate of transplant rejection and potentially eliminate the need for immunosuppressants. In addition to the studies already discussed, the NIAID Immune Tolerance Network has initiated Phase I and II clinical trials to study alemtuzumab in combination with tacrolimus and sirolimus for kidney transplantation.

The primary goal of the study is to reduce the overall rate of rejection following kidney transplantation. A secondary goal is to determine whether the combination therapy will allow patients to be weaned off lifelong immunosuppressive therapy. The study began in November 2003, and patients will be followed for four years following kidney transplantation. Alemtuzumab and tacrolimus are given as induction therapy, followed by sirolimus monotherapy for maintenance. Patients who meet the necessary study criteria will be weaned off sirolimus over a three-month period; periodic kidney biopsies will monitor their progress.

Data from another study involving sirolimus were presented on May 23, 2005, at the American Transplant Congress. These four-year data from the Rapamune

Table 31.2 New Antirejection Drugs in Development for Organ Transplantation, 2005

Drug Candidate	*Company*	*Mechanism of Action*	*Indication*	*Development Status*
Pulminiq (cyclosporine, USP inhalation solution)	Chiron	Immunosuppression	Lung transplant	U.S. filing, October 2004
FTY-720	Novartis	Sphingosine-1-phosphate receptor (S1P-R) agonist	Acute kidney rejection	Phase III
LEA-29Y	Bristol-Myers Squibb	Costimulatory T-cell blocker	Acute kidney rejection	Phase II
CP-690,550	Pfizer	JAK3 inhibitor	Acute and chronic kidney rejection	Phase II
Alemtuzumab (Campath)	Schering-Plough	T-cell depletion via CD52	Acute kidney rejection	Phase II
AGI-1096	Atherogenics & Astellas Pharma Inc.	Bind VCAM-1 proteins	Solid organ transplant	Phase I

Maintenance Regimen study showed that kidney-transplant patients on an immunosuppressive regimen of sirolimus plus cyclosporine had significantly better graft survival than patients who remained on a cyclosporine regimen; this benefit appeared to be related to the significantly improved kidney function these patients experienced. Poor kidney function is the most accurate predictor that a transplant patient will lose his or her transplanted kidney. Calcineurin inhibitors, such as cyclosporine, while protecting the transplanted kidney from rejection, are also toxic to the kidney.

In this study, calcineurin inhibitor toxicity was associated with deteriorating kidney function in transplant patients receiving the agent and was almost universal more than ten years post-transplantation. In this, the largest cyclosporine withdrawal trial, 430 eligible patients were randomized to remain on cyclosporine, sirolimus, and steroids ($n = 215$) or to have the cyclosporine withdrawn and remain on a maintenance regimen of sirolimus and steroids ($n = 215$). The study examined the long-term impact on baseline renal function, calculated by glomerular filtration rate (GFR) when withdrawing cyclosporine. Overall, at four years, graft survival was significantly better in patients who had cyclosporine withdrawn and remained on a maintenance regimen of sirolimus and steroids than in patients who were maintained on cyclosporine: 91.5% versus 84.2% ($p = 0.024$).

Chiron's Pulminiq

In April 2003, Chiron acquired the exclusive worldwide rights to Novartis's aerosolized cyclosporine, Pulminiq (cyclosporine, USP inhalation solution), which the company is developing for use in lung transplantation. Although other types of organ transplantation, such as the pancreas and liver, have experienced improved survival rates, lung transplantation survival remains at the same levels achieved in the late 1980s. According to 2004 registry data compiled by the International Society for Heart and Lung Transplantation (which examined the current status of patients who had received lung transplants from January 1998 through June 2002), survival one year after lung transplantation was 75%; after five years, it dropped to 50%. Current drugs available to prevent transplant rejection have not been effective for lung transplantation; developers hope that if cyclosporine can be formulated for delivery directly to the transplant site, its efficacy can be improved.

Chiron filed the new drug application (NDA) for Pulminiq in mid-October 2004 for the treatment of chronic lung-transplant rejection; the FDA granted orphan drug status to Pulminiq in November 2003. Phase III clinical trial data were presented at the 18th Annual North American Cystic Fibrosis Conference in October 2004. The randomized, double-blind, placebo-controlled study included patients who had received both single- and double-lung transplants. One study arm received standard immunosuppressive therapy; the other arm received Pulminiq. The study measured the estimated survival duration hazard ratio of 0.213, which translated to a 79% reduction in morbidity risk. Fewer Pulminiq-treated patients died or developed broncholitis obliterans syndrome grade 1 or higher (allograft dysfunction not related to immediate acute rejection, a leading cause of death one or more years following lung transplant): 39% versus 70% for patients taking placebo. The combined incidence of broncholitis obliterans or morbidity was 60% in the placebo group and 19% in patients receiving Pulminiq. Although its effect on chronic transplantation is evident, Pulminiq did not affect the development or prevention of acute transplant rejection.

Novartis's FTY-720

Novartis has a substantial program devoted to the development of new drugs to manage organ transplantation, including research on costimulatory molecules, mixed chimerism, peripheral tolerance, and gene therapy. The company's lead transplant-drug candidate,

FTY-720, is a novel immunomodulator in Phase III clinical development. FTY-720 was discovered by Yoshitomi Pharmaceutical Industries (now Mitsubishi Pharma) during the company's efforts to identify new cancer drugs. Instead of showing antitumor activity, the compound showed immune activity.

FTY-720 is derived from myriocin, a potent immunosuppressant isolated from the fungus *Isaria sinclairii*. FTY-720 is a sphingosine-1-phosphate receptor (S1P-R) agonist; if approved, it would be the first agent of this class indicated for organ transplantation. FTY-720 induces lymphopenia (a reduction in the number of lymphocytes in the blood) by sequestering circulating lymphocytes into secondary lymphoid tissues. Therefore, instead of inactivating the lymphocytes, which impairs the whole immune response, FTY-720 appears to keep lymphocytes restricted to the lymphatic system (i.e., lymph nodes, thymus, and Peyer's patches in the intestine).

FTY-720 is being studied for the prevention of acute organ rejection and graft loss in renal-transplant patients. In clinical trials, patients have been treated with single or multiple doses of FTY-720 in de novo renal transplantation; the results suggest that the compound is generally well tolerated. There has been no sign of increased infection rates versus other immunosuppressive regimens, and FTY-720 has demonstrated that it can prevent rejection of kidney transplants without causing the gastrointestinal toxicity common with other immunosuppressive drugs. Phase II clinical trials have also evaluated FTY-720 in combination with cyclosporine and everolimus at different dose levels. Combination therapy may allow dose reduction of cyclosporine and everolimus, a step that could improve the tolerability of the immunosuppressive regimen.

In a Phase II, one-year, multicenter clinical trial that was randomized and partially blinded, the safety and efficacy of FTY-720 was studied in combination with corticosteroids and cyclosporine microemulsion in either a full dose or a reduced dose in adult patients undergoing de novo renal transplantation. The study involved 43 centers in 15 countries. The study objective was to compare FTY-720, in combination with corticosteroids, with a full dose and a reduced dose of cyclosporine microemulsion in biopsy-confirmed rejection, graft loss, death, or premature study discontinuation for 6- and 12-month periods.

The four study arms included two groups that received a loading dose of FTY-720 followed by two different maintenance regimens: one group received a higher dose of daily FTY-720, the second group received a lower dose of FTY-720, and both groups were given a reduced dose of cyclosporine microemulsion and corticosteroids. In the third study arm, patients received a loading dose of FTY-720 followed by a reduced dose of FTY-720 with a full dose of cyclosporine microemulsion and corticosteroids. The fourth arm of the study received a loading dose of mycophenolic acid followed by a maintenance regimen that included mycophenolic acid with a full dose of cyclosporine microemulsion and corticosteroids.

At 12 months, the study group receiving the higher dose of FTY-720 with full doses or reduced doses of cyclosporine microemulsion and corticosteroids showed noninferiority to the control arm receiving mycophenolic acid, measured by the incidence of biopsy-confirmed acute rejection. However, the lower dose of FTY-720 with reduced doses of cyclosporine microemulsion and corticosteroids did not adequately protect patients from rejection after six months and was discontinued.

Bristol-Myers Squibb's LEA-29Y

Bristol-Myers Squibb is developing LEA-29Y (also called BMS-224818) for the prevention of acute solid organ transplant rejection. LEA-29Y is a costimulatory blocker that prevents one of the two signals required for T-cell activation once the organ is recognized by the immune system as foreign but does not inhibit the T cells' ability to respond to pathogens. The agent arose out of NIH-funded research on immune tolerance at the University of California at San Francisco's Diabetes Center Immune Tolerance Network. The researchers showed that CTLA4Ig, a precursor to LEA-29Y, could induce tolerance.

In a Phase II clinical trial conducted in 20 centers involving kidney transplantation, LEA-29Y was shown to be as effective as cyclosporine, and patients exhibited better kidney function, blood pressure, and total cholesterol levels after six months. The 221 patients in the study all received standard immunosuppressive therapy, including MMF, corticosteroids, and basiliximab; 148 patients also received LEA-29Y, and 73 received cyclosporine. Both groups had comparable acute kidney rejection at six months: 19% for the study group taking LEA-29Y and 18% for the control group receiving cyclosporine. However, the patients receiving LEA-29Y had better kidney function and fewer side effects than cyclosporine-treated patients.

Pfizer's CP-690,550

Pfizer is developing CP-690,550, a Janus tyrosine kinase (JAK3) inhibitor to prevent kidney-transplant rejection. JAKs were discovered in a National Institute of Arthritis and Musculoskeletal and Skin Diseases (NIAMS) Intramural Research Program laboratory in 1995. JAK3 plays a critical role in the development and function of T cells and is therefore considered an attractive target for antirejection drugs. It is expressed primarily in T cells and B cells and is activated by cytokines – including IL-2, IL-4, IL-7, IL-9, IL-15, and IL-21 – via their common gamma chain, IL-2R. CP-690,550 was originally identified and developed following screening of the company's chemical library for JAK3 inhibitors. CP-690,550 is in Phase II clinical trials for kidney transplantation. In October 2003, researchers reported the results of studies in murine and primate models (Changelian et al., 2003). Although anemia was seen at high-dose levels in primate models, other dose-limiting side effects were not observed. CP-690,550 was found to significantly increase graft survival, compared with cyclosporine, in a primate kidney transplant study.

A key characteristic of CP-690,550 that differentiates the drug from other immunosuppressive drugs, according to the NIAMS, is that it acts specifically on JAK3, and unlike other immunosuppressive drugs, it does not have an effect on enzymes located outside the immune system that contribute to toxicities. CP-690,550, a protein kinase, may be the first drug candidate of this type that offers the potential for a more targeted means of immune regulation rather than overall immunosuppression.

Atherogenics' AGI-1096

In collaboration with Astellas Pharma (formerly Fujisawa), Atherogenics is developing AGI-1096 for the prevention of solid organ-transplant rejection. AGI-1096 uses Atherogenics' proprietary V-Protectant technology platform to target the accelerated inflammation that occurs in chronic rejection. Drugs using V-Protectant block the oxidant class of signals that are generated within the endothelial cells. When genes are activated by oxidant signals, inflammatory proteins are produced, including vascular cell adhesion molecule-1 (VCAM-1), which is responsible for attracting lymphocytes to the chronic inflammation site. By acting as antioxidants, V-Protectant compounds reduce the number of VCAM-1 proteins available on cell surfaces. The first Phase I clinical trial in healthy volunteers commenced in February 2002. AGI-1096, administered orally, was found to be safe and tolerable, with no drug-related adverse events.

THE FUTURE OF ANTIREJECTION THERAPY

Currently, the organ transplantation antirejection drug segment is in transition away from immunosuppressive drugs, on which physicians have historically relied. This transition is being accomplished through the use of new drug combinations that support the elimination of immunosuppressants and the development of new immunomodulatory drugs.

Numerous strategies involving clinical trials whether to eliminate the use of cyclosporine and/or reduce the use of immunosuppressive drugs is under investigation. As clinical outcome data from drug-data registries are analyzed, positive reports continue to support the reduction of long-term immunosuppressive drug use by means of novel combination therapies. Based on these analyses, change in immunosuppressive drug use in the near term is likely to move slowly toward a decrease in use. A sudden shift to limiting or eliminating immunosuppressive therapies is unlikely, given the risk of organ loss.

The primary catalyst for a more dramatic move away from immunosuppressive drugs will be the availability of an entirely new means of achieving protection for transplanted organs that poses less risk of the toxicities associated with immunosuppressive drugs, but we do not expect that shift in treatment paradigm to occur until the introduction of immunomodulators, which have an entirely new mechanism of action. When immunomodulators offer a safer alternative, one that does not include side effects such as the infections and malignancies that contribute to morbidity in transplant patients, then we expect to see immunosuppressive drug usage begin to decrease.

Bristol-Myers Squibb's LEA-29Y and Pfizer's CP-690,550 could launch closer to the end of the decade. These key drugs, along with ongoing clinical trials focused on the elimination of immunosuppressive drugs, are expected to permanently alter the landscape of antirejection regimens by 2010.

The treatment of chronic rejection or posttransplant vasculopathy remains a substantial unmet need. Currently available immunosuppressive drugs have little effect, with the possible exception of tacrolimus: certain emerging data from studies of this agent suggest some impact on kidney vasculature. Should Astellas provide more positive data on the use of tacrolimus to treat posttransplant vasculopathy, the company would become positioned to own the chronic vasculopathy segment of the market, provided that newer immunomodulators do not show an improvement in posttransplant vasculopathy.

Novartis is particularly well positioned to expand its market share, both in the near term and in the long term. The company's introduction of Myfortic in 2004 provides Novartis with a near-term product life-cycle management and sales-growth vehicle by selling against Roche's MMF, which claims 80% of sales in the US kidney-transplant market. By increasing Novartis's visibility and sales as it moves into the late-stage development of FTY-720, the company can prime the market for a rapid launch and market penetration of FTY-720. It is important for Novartis to gain market share rapidly to establish a firm foothold prior to the anticipated launches of Pfizer's CP-690,550 and Bristol-Myers Squibb's LEA-29Y later in the decade.

REFERENCES

Adams, A.B. et al. Costimulation blockade and tolerance. *Current Opinion in Organ Transplantation.* March 2002; 7(1): 7–12.

Changelian, P. et al. Prevention of organ allograft rejection by a specific Janus kinase 3 inhibitor. *Science.* 2003; 302(5646): 875–8.

Lake, J.R. et al. Efficacy of triple therapy with mycophenolate mofetil (MMF), tacrolimus (TACRO) and corticosteroids (CS) compared to TACRO and CS immunosuppression in liver transplantation: An analysis of the US liver transplant experience. *American Journal of Transplantation.* 2004; 4(Suppl 8): 266.

Meier-Kriesche, H.-U. Sirolimus in combination with cyclosporine microemulsion versus mycophenolate mofetil with cyclosporine microemulsion is associated with decreased graft survival in renal transplant recipient. *Transplantation.* July 27, 2004; 78(2) Supplement 1: 3.Subbotin, V. et al. Marked mitigation of transplant vascular sclerosis in FasLglg (CD95L) mutant recipients. The role of alloantibodies in the development of chronic rejection. *Transplantation.* May 27, 1999; 67(10): 1295–300.

SECTION D

Cardiovascular

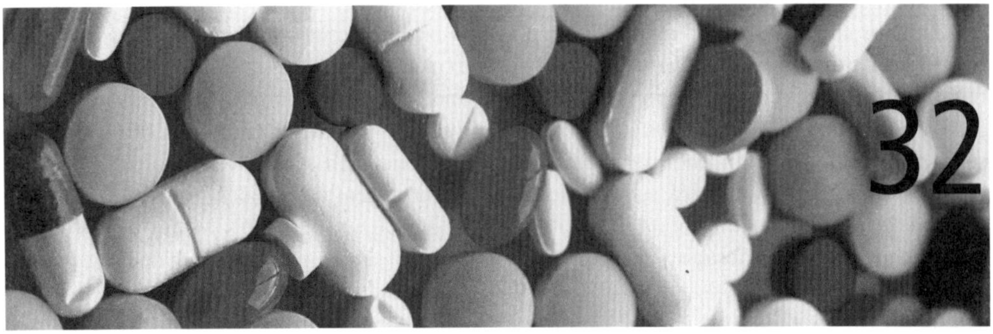

Cardiovascular Drugs and Devices Market: Some Successes and Setbacks in Recent Years

INTRODUCTION

Recent years have been a period of conspicuous change for the cardiovascular market. Several significant events affected drugs and devices on the market and in the pipeline. By examining some of the most noteworthy of these events (ones of 2005, just as an example), this chapter offers a snapshot of important forces driving the cardiovascular market and an analysis of their implications. The "flurry" of activities and important developments, all of which were observed to occur during merely one sample year of 2005 (even during one quarter of that year, the third quarter), is indeed indicative of the almost unbelievable pace of extensive changes of the market situation in this field. Even if from a somewhat historical perspective now, it is of interest to analyze the fascinating dynamics in the market of that indicative period.

We begin by looking at events in the cardiac stent market, whereby several third-quarter events of that year played a key role in shaping this field. Then, based on this analysis, we will discuss successes and setbacks for specific agents as they gained regulatory approvals or faced challenges owing to the emergence of study findings or potential generics competition.

COMPETITION INTENSIFIES IN CARDIAC STENT MARKET

Recent years (and the year 2005 in particular) saw a flurry of activity in the field of drug-eluting stents. Issues surrounding Boston Scientific's market-leading Taxus Express[2] continued to limit the company's financial success. Medtronic introduced its anticipated addition to the drug-eluting stent market, and Guidant initiated late-stage trials of its Xience V drug-eluting stent. In addition, the acquisition of Guidant by competitor Johnson & Johnson moved forward another step when the two companies received approval for the merger from the European Commission and began to divest holdings to meet the requirements for that approval.

This activity has stepped up the competition for the companies that currently market or are developing these devices. Since the approval in April 2002 of Cordis/Johnson & Johnson's (J&J's) Cypher stent in Europe, many companies have tried to gain a strong share of this lucrative market. (Figure 32.1 shows select milestones in the drug-eluting stent market.) Physicians hope that a major effect of the increasing competition in this field will be lower prices for drug-eluting stents. The events that affected this market and their possible impact are discussed in greater detail in the following sections.

Difficulties Build for Boston Scientific's Taxus

Since its first full quarter on the US market (the second quarter of 2004), Boston Scientific's Taxus stents have led the market. However, already in the third quarter of 2005, Taxus's sales dropped below the sales of its primary competitor, Cordis/J&J's Cypher (Figure 32.2), a reflection perhaps of continuing questions regarding Taxus's efficacy compared with Cypher. Although studies have shown that both the Taxus Express[2] stent and the Cypher stent show marked benefit over bare metal stents, head-to-head trials published in the third quarter of 2005 generally favored Cypher over Taxus. Such studies, together with issues concerning Taxus's quality control and a $598 million expense for a legal settlement, led to persistent woes for Boston Scientific in the quarter. We discuss each of these events in the following sections.

Despite the various study results for these stents, many experts see these products as essentially equally effective in most patients. In the case of both stents, the drug coatings discourage tissue from reclogging the vessel

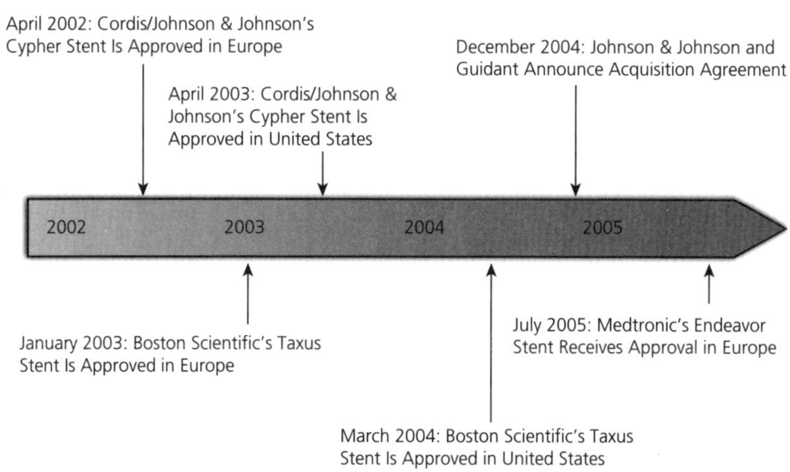

Figure 32.1 Select Milestones in the Drug-Eluting Stent Market

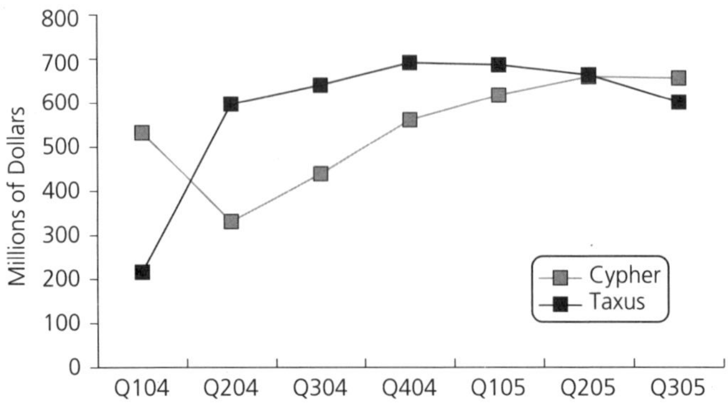

Note: The second quarter of 2004 was the first full quarter on the US market for Taxus

Figure 32.2 Sales Comparison: Boston Scientific's Taxus Stent versus Cordis/Johnson & Johnson's Cypher Stent (millions of US dollars)

by growing through the wire-mesh stent tubes, although Taxus elutes paclitaxel (Bristol-Myers Squibb's Taxol), while Cypher elutes sirolimus (Wyeth's Rapamune). Nonetheless, the overall effect of the 2005 third-quarter events was a $279 million third-quarter loss for Boston Scientific and declining sales of Taxus; the company earned $347 million in the third quarter of 2005 versus $404 million in the same quarter in 2004. Taxus had its highest sales in the fourth quarter of 2004 at $691 million versus Cypher sales of $561 million. In the third quarter of 2005, Taxus sales had declined to $601 million versus $656 million for Cypher.

Taxus versus Cypher: Study Results

Results of three randomized, head-to-head comparisons between Cypher and Taxus could be found in subsequent publications (e.g., August 2005). In all of these studies, Cypher was associated with less tissue ingrowth, and, consequently, the incidence of reblockage was lower with Cypher, as was, consequently, the need for repeat procedures.

An article in the *New England Journal of Medicine* gave results for the Sirolimus-Eluting Stent Compared with Paclitaxel-Eluting Stent for Coronary Revascularization (SIRTAX) study, which enrolled 1,012 patients undergoing percutaneous coronary intervention (Windecker et al., 2005). The study found that use of Cypher versus Taxus resulted in significantly fewer major adverse cardiac events (at a rate of 6.2% versus 10.8%), primarily because Cypher was associated with less need for repeat procedures.

A second study, Intracoronary Stenting and Angiographic Results – Do Diabetic Patients Derive Similar Benefits from Paclitaxel-Eluting and Sirolimus-Eluting Stents (ISAR-DIABETES), was published in the same issue of the *New England Journal of Medicine* (Dibra et al., 2005). It involved 250 patients with diabetes and coronary artery disease. In these patients, the Cypher stent was associated with reblockage in 6.9% of patients versus 16.5% for Taxus.

The third study with results favoring Cypher was a meta-analysis of six trials including 3,669 patients with coronary artery disease (Kastrati et al., 2005). The researchers found that patients receiving the Cypher stent had a significantly lower risk of restenosis (9.3% versus 13.1%) and target vessel revascularization (5.1% versus 7.8%) than those who received Taxus. The study found similar rates of myocardial infarction (MI) and stent thrombosis (blood clots) between the two stents.

On August 16, 2005, however, Boston Scientific published a press release citing results of a study in the August 1 edition of the *American Journal of Cardiology* that the company stated favored Taxus (Andrew et al., 2005). According to the company, the study found that Taxus had better results than Cypher in two of three major adverse cardiac event (MACE) areas in 293 patients with diabetes and de novo coronary artery disease and essentially was the same in a third MACE component. The results favored Taxus over Cypher in the cumulative rates of target vessel revascularization (or re-treatment rate) (5.9% for Taxus versus 10.3% for Cypher) and MI (10.0% for Taxus versus 14.1% for Cypher). For the third component, cumulative mortality, the results were basically equivalent at 7.2% for Taxus versus 7.7% for Cypher.

Manufacturing Issues

On August 10, 2005, Boston Scientific received its third warning letter from the FDA since May of the same year concerning quality problems with the company's products, including stents. The letter addressed the shipping of defective Taxus stents from Boston Scientific's Quincy, Massachusetts, facility. It highlighted a January 2005 incident in which eight Taxus stents were sent to hospitals after they had been placed in a quality assurance quarantine area because they had failed kinetic drug-release testing. Boston Scientific discovered the error soon after shipping and found that although an employee had marked the products as blocked from shipping, another employee had overridden the block in the company's computer system.

The FDA states that Boston Scientific's investigation into the incident did not adequately identify ways to avoid shipping defective products in the future. Although some financial analysts were cautious about how the incident would affect sales of Taxus, others said that the impact may be minimal if Boston Scientific is able to address the FDA's concerns about its quality procedures.

Also in the area of manufacturing, Boston Scientific announced on September 21, 2005, that it had settled a dispute with the Israel-based firm Medinol over an unfulfilled contract to jointly make stents. Medinol filed a lawsuit in 2001 charging that Boston Scientific had violated intellectual property laws by copying Medinol's stent-manufacturing equipment without permission. Boston Scientific agreed to pay a $750 million legal settlement and stated that the after-tax cost of the agreement in the third quarter of 2005 was $598 million.

Medtronic Launches Endeavor Stent

On July 31, 2005, Medtronic announced that it had received Conformité Européenne (CE) mark approval to market its Endeavor stent in the European Union. The stent is not yet approved in the United States. Endeavor elutes the sirolimus analogue ABT-578 (which Abbott licensed to Medtronic) and is coated with phosphorylcholine (PC), a polymer designed, according to Medtronic, to "simulate the outside surface of a red blood cell and mimic the structure of the natural cell membrane." Based on strong clinical results, we believe Endeavor will enjoy significant uptake among physicians. Endeavor's presence in the market may add to the erosion of Taxus's market share, although it will probably affect Cypher's market share and eventually help drive down prices in the competitive drug-eluting stent market. The ongoing (at the time) Endeavor III and IV trials were comparing Endeavor with the Cypher and Taxus stents, respectively, and the results of these trials were expected to have a significant effect on Endeavor's penetration in this market.

However, on October 17, 2005, Medtronic announced that Endeavor III had found no statistically significant differences between Endeavor and Cypher in terms of clinical outcomes. The study did find a significant procedure success rate in favor of Endeavor for deliverability and a lower rate of inhospital MIs. Additionally, on October 10, Medtronic filed the first in a series of premarket approval [PMA] modules with the FDA, the beginning steps in gaining US approval for the Endeavor stent.

Johnson & Johnson's Acquisition of Guidant

On August 24, 2005, the European Commission (EC) approved J&J's planned $25.4 billion acquisition of Guidant subject to J&J divesting specific products or businesses to preserve fair competition in the stent market. First announced in December 2004, the acquisition will merge Guidant with J&J's Cordis subsidiary. The acquisition strengthens J&J's position as a supplier of cardiac devices and removes a potential competitor from the drug-eluting stent market.

Although Guidant's business is primarily based on products and services that aim to provide less-invasive care for various conditions, the company first entered the drug-eluting stent market through a February 2004 agreement with Cordis that granted Guidant copromotion rights in the United States for the Cypher stent. In addition, the company has been developing Xience, a drug-eluting stent that uses the company's cobalt chromium Multi-Link Vision coronary stent system platform. Xience elutes everolimus (Novartis's Certican), which Novartis licensed to Guidant for this application. Guidant made several announcements during the third quarter of 2005 regarding the then continuing enrollment of patients in its Spirit II and III trials evaluating Xience, which were to compare Xience with Taxus in coronary artery disease patients.

On November 7, 2005, Guidant announced that it had filed a lawsuit in a US federal court in an attempt to force J&J to complete its acquisition of the company. In days prior to the announcement, J&J had warned that it was no longer obligated to go through with the acquisition because of recent recalls of or warnings about Guidant's heart defibrillator and pacemaker products as well as regulatory investigations. On November 16, J&J agreed to acquire Guidant for $21.5 billion, 15% less than its initial offer.

However, Boston Scientific has joined the fray. On December 5, it offered to buy Guidant for $25 billion in cash and stock, nearly matching J&J's original offer. J&J responded to Boston Scientific's offer by stating that it is committed to the transaction; however, J&J did not raise its offering price.

APPROVALS OF NEW DRUGS/ INDICATIONS EXPAND TREATMENT OPTIONS

Table 32.1 lists important approvals or submissions of new drugs as well as new indications for marketed drugs during the third quarter of 2005.

NitroMed's BiDil (Isosorbide Dinitrate/Hydralazine) Launched for African-Americans

On June 23, 2005, NitroMed announced in a press release that the FDA had approved its drug BiDil (isosorbide dinitrate/hydralazine) for heart failure in African-American patients. It launched the drug on July 1. BiDil, approved as an adjunct to standard heart failure therapy, is the first agent ever to receive FDA approval based on its performance in a particular race. On August 16, the American College of Cardiology (ACC) and the American Heart Association (AHA) released updated guidelines supporting the use of the combined drugs in BiDil as an adjunct to current standard heart failure therapy for African-American patients.

The approval was based primarily on results from the African-American Heart Failure Trial (A-HeFT), a randomized, double-blind, placebo-controlled study involving 1,050 self-identified African-American patients with New York Heart Association (NYHA) classes III or IV heart failure (Taylor et al., 2004). Patients taking BiDil in addition to standard current therapy experienced a 43% reduced risk of mortality and a 39% reduction in risk of first hospitalization for heart failure versus placebo patients. The trial was

Table 32.1 Important Approvals/Submissions for New Drugs and for New Indications for Marketed Drugs, Third-quarter 2005

Drug (Brand/Generic Name)	*Company*	*Date of Approval, Submission, or Launch/Market*	*Comments*
BiDil (isosorbide dinitrate/hydralazine)	NitroMed	July 1/United States	• New drug approved for heart failure in African-American patients • Approved on June 23
Revatio (sildenafil)	Pfizer	July 27/Europe	• EMEA granted initial marketing authorization for new drug to treat patients with pulmonary arterial hypertension (PAH) • Sildenafil is the active ingredient in the marketed erectile dysfunction drug Viagra
Procoralan (ivabradine)	Servier	July 27/Europe	• EMEA granted initial marketing authorization for new drug to treat chronic stable angina in patients with normal sinus rhythm with a contraindication to, or an intolerance of, beta blockers • Servier is seeking a US partner to commercialize ivabradine in the United States
Thelin (sitaxsentan)	Encysive Pharmaceuticals	July 28/Europe	• Marketing authorization application (MAA) completed for new drug to treat PAH • Company filed a new drug application (NDA) with the FDA on May 25
Diovan (valsartan)	Novartis	August 4/United States	• Approved for new indication to reduce cardiovascular death in patients at high risk (with left-ventricular failure or left-ventricular dysfunction) following myocardial infarction • Available in the US market for hypertension since 1997 and for heart failure since 2002 • Approved in Europe for various indications
Aceon (perindopril erbumine)	Solvay Pharmaceuticals/ CV Therapeutics	August 23/ United States	• Approved for new indication to reduce the risk of cardiovascular mortality or nonfatal myocardial infarction in patients with stable coronary artery disease • Received FDA approval to treat essential hypertension in 1999

stopped early so that patients taking placebo could be switched to BiDil. BiDil's availability is particularly significant because African-Americans aged 45–64 are 2.5 times more likely to die from heart failure than whites in the same age-group, according to the Centers for Disease Control and Prevention (CDC). In addition, African-Americans present with heart failure die from it at an earlier age than whites.

The approval has set a precedent for licensing drugs on a race-specific basis. However, despite the benefits shown in the A-HeFT trial, the targeting of this drug to a specific ethnic group has been controversial. Critics comment that it enforces biological notions of race and that, because the trial did not include whites, it did not provide any scientific evidence that the drug is more beneficial to African-Americans than whites. It could be noted that guidelines for hypertension already carry race-specific guidance because African-American patients may be refractory to some commonly used antihypertensives (e.g., angiotensin-converting enzyme [ACE] inhibitors). From that perspective, BiDil can be seen as addressing an unmet need in a specific patient population.

Pfizer's Revatio (Sildenafil) Receives Initial Marketing Authorization

On July 27, 2005, the Committee for Medicinal Products for Human Use (CHMP) of the European Medicines Agency (EMEA) recommended granting an initial marketing authorization for Pfizer's Revatio (sildenafil), a phosphodiesterase (PDE) inhibitor, for the treatment of patients with pulmonary arterial hypertension (PAH). This opinion will be sent to the EC, which is responsible for transforming it into a market authorization valid for the entire European Union. Pfizer had already announced FDA approval of the agent for this indication on June 6. Sildenafil is the active ingredient in the erectile dysfunction drug Viagra. The marketing authorization was based on the results of a large, randomized, double-blind, placebo-controlled study. At the October 2005 meeting of the American College of Chest Physicians (ACCP), Pfizer unveiled data from the Phase III Sildenafil Use in Pulmonary Arterial Hypertension (SUPER-1) study. The study randomized 278 patients to placebo or to 20, 40, or 80 mg of sildenafil three times a day for 12 weeks. After 12 weeks, patients on the 80 mg dose demonstrated an increase in the six-minute walk distance of up to 50 meters, while those on 40 mg and 20 mg showed improvements of 46 meters and 45 meters, respectively, versus placebo. Treated patients also experienced improvements in mean pulmonary artery pressure among other cardiac function measures. The drug was well tolerated.

Data from the SUPER-1 study indicated that Revatio will be ideally positioned to treat New York Heart Association (NYHA) class II patients.

On November 4, 2005, Revatio received marketing approval from the EMEA to treat PAH.

Servier's Procoralan (Ivabradine) Receives Initial Marketing Authorization

On July 27, 2005, the CHMP of the EMEA recommended granting a marketing authorization for Servier's Procoralan (ivabradine) for the treatment of chronic stable angina in patients with normal sinus rhythm who have a contraindication to, or an intolerance of, beta blockers.

Ivabradine is the first of a new class of drugs called I_f inhibitors; the agent inhibits I_f channels on the sino-atrial node of the heart. It lowers heart rate without other cardiovascular effects. The lack of blood-pressure-lowering effects makes ivabradine an attractive therapeutic option in patients who may already have been treated with several agents that all reduce blood pressure, such as an ACE inhibitor, a beta blocker, and a calcium-channel blocker (CCB), leading to a risk of hypotension.

The CHMP states that it based its marketing authorization on data from more than 5,000 patients gathered in double-blind, randomized trials using exercise testing and comparing ivabradine with placebo as well as antianginal treatments such as atenolol (AstraZeneca's Tenormin, generics) and amlodipine (Pfizer's Norvasc).

Per the authorized indication, initial use of ivabradine will be restricted to stable angina patients who are contraindicated for, or intolerant of, beta blockers. However, physicians are enthusiastic about the arrival of a new weapon in their armamentarium after decades without any innovative therapies for stable angina, especially one that seems to have a marked lack of such side effects as the sexual dysfunction seen with beta blocker use. We believe ivabradine will enjoy significant uptake as the baby boomer population ages and people expect to remain active into old age. For these patients, the side effects of agents such as the beta blockers will be less acceptable, prompting requests for alternatives.

On November 3, 2005, Servier received marketing approval from the EMEA for ivabradine for the previously described indication.

Encysive Pharmaceuticals' Thelin (Sitaxsentan) Completes Marketing Authorization Application

On July 28, 2005, Encysive Pharmaceuticals reported that it had completed a marketing authorization application (MAA) with the EMEA for the endothelin-A (ETA) antagonist Thelin (sitaxsentan) for use as a once-daily, oral treatment in PAH patients. The company filed an NDA with the FDA for the PAH indication on May 25, 2005. On July 14, 2005, Encysive announced that the FDA target action date for completing its review of the NDA is March 24, 2006, in accordance with the Prescription Drug User Fee Act (PDUFA), under which industry provides funding in exchange for the FDA's agreement to meet drug-review performance goals. The FDA also requested a plan for the study of sitaxsentan in pediatric PAH patients. These filings in Europe and the United States contain the largest database ever assembled for regulatory filings for the PAH indication, including data on approximately 900 patients.

Encysive has evaluated sitaxsentan in two randomized, placebo-controlled pivotal studies: Sitaxsentan to Relieve Impaired Exercise (STRIDE)-1 and STRIDE-2. Following positive results in STRIDE-1, the 18-week STRIDE-2 trial enrolled 246 patients randomized to receive one of four treatments: 50 mg sitaxsentan once daily, 100 mg sitaxsentan once daily, placebo once daily, or bosentan (Actelion's Tracleer) twice daily. Bosentan was the first ETA antagonist to be launched for PAH in the United States and Europe.

In a February 14, 2005, press release reporting on results from STRIDE-2, Encysive announced that sitaxsentan met the primary end point of improved six-minute walk distance, demonstrating an improvement superior to that achieved with bosentan. Sitaxsentan 100 mg showed a statistically significant increase of 31.4 meters over placebo, while bosentan increased the six-minute walk distance over placebo by 29.5 meters. Sitaxsentan also demonstrated a potential safety advantage over bosentan; it was associated with a 3% rate of liver function abnormality, compared with 6% for placebo and 11% for bosentan.

Label Expanded for Novartis's Diovan (Valsartan)

Novartis announced on August 4, 2005, that the FDA had approved its angiotensin II receptor antagonist (AIIRA) Diovan (valsartan) for an additional indication. Valsartan, which has been on the market since 1997 for hypertension and was approved to treat heart failure in 2002, is now approved in the United States to reduce cardiovascular death in patients at high risk (with left-ventricular failure or left-ventricular dysfunction) following MI. In addition, the FDA expanded valsartan's heart failure labeling; it can now be prescribed to a broader range of heart failure patients and is no longer restricted to patients who cannot tolerate ACE inhibitors.

Valsartan is also available in Europe for hypertension; on June 13, 2005, the EC approved the agent for a new indication to treat symptomatic heart failure when an ACE inhibitor cannot be used or as add-on therapy to ACE inhibitors when beta blockers cannot be used.

The new US approval was based on results from the Valsartan in Acute Myocardial Infarction (VALIANT) trial, which compared valsartan and the ACE inhibitor captopril (Bristol-Myers Squibb's Capoten, generics) as well as a combination of the two drugs (Pfeffer et al., 2003). With 14,703 patients and a median follow-up of 24.7 months, VALIANT was one of the largest long-term studies of people experiencing an MI. The researchers found that valsartan improves survival and reduces cardiovascular events, including recurrent MI and hospitalizations for heart failure. The study reported no differences in overall mortality among the treatment groups.

The FDA's new approvals will boost valsartan's market share with respect to other marketed AIIRAs. However, it is unlikely to expand the use of AIIRAs in high-risk patients outside of those who are ACE-intolerant (about 10% of total heart failure patients) because clinical trials failed to show that AIIRAs are superior to the well-established and less expensive ACE inhibitors.

Label Expanded for Solvay Pharmaceuticals/CV Therapeutics' Aceon (Perindopril Erbumine)

On August 23, 2005, Solvay Pharmaceuticals and CV Therapeutics announced that the

FDA had approved the ACE inhibitor Aceon (perindopril erbumine) to reduce the risk of cardiovascular mortality or nonfatal MI in patients with stable coronary artery disease. The two companies have copromoted the drug since 2004. Perindopril received FDA approval to treat essential hypertension in 1999.

The label extension is based on the European Trial on Reduction of Cardiac Events with Perindopril in Patients with Stable Coronary Artery Disease (EUROPA) study. This multicenter, double-blind, placebo-controlled, randomized trial of 12,218 patients with stable coronary disease and no heart failure found a 20% reduction in the combined end point of cardiovascular mortality, nonfatal MI, and cardiac arrest compared with placebo (Fox et al., 2003).

This additional approval is likely to increase market share of this aggressively marketed ACE inhibitor and will strengthen the case in general for use of this drug class in the approved patient population.

CURRENT DRUGS FACE CHALLENGES TO INITIAL MARKET SUCCESS

In the third quarter of 2005, several currently marketed drugs confronted new challenges. These challenges derived from two main sources: controversial study findings and emerging generics competition.

Momenta Pharmaceuticals Files ANDA for Enoxaparin (Sanofi-Aventis's Lovenox)

Momenta Pharmaceuticals filed an abbreviated new drug application (ANDA) for its M-enoxaparin generic drug on August 30, 2005. On June 16, 2005, the US District Court for the Central District of California granted Teva Pharmaceuticals and Amphastar Pharmaceuticals a judgment essentially invalidating Sanofi-Aventis's patent for the low-molecular-weight heparin (LMWH) Lovenox (enoxaparin). The patent had been set to expire in 2012. Both Teva and Amphastar have filed ANDAs for enoxaparin; however, as shown below, Momenta is the company that seems to have the most potential to take advantage of Lovenox's potential patent vulnerability.

Lovenox is widely used to prevent and treat deep vein thrombosis (DVT) as well as to treat acute coronary syndromes (ACS). It was Sanofi-Aventis's best-selling drug in 2004, generating estimated worldwide sales of more than $2 billion. The drug is a biological, a fact that poses a significant challenge for generics companies. The FDA demands that generic agents show equivalence – a drug must be chemically equivalent to the proprietary drug to be approved as a generic. Lovenox, like all LMWHs, is a heterogeneous mixture of complex sugar chains, making its exact chemical composition difficult to determine.

An examination of the court's ruling in favor of Teva and Amphastar reveals why Momenta may be the winner in this scenario – at least in the near term. The ruling does not invalidate the patent protecting Lovenox; rather, the court found that the patent does not provide protection against the particular generic drugs that Teva and Amphastar are developing. The ruling, therefore, brought the Teva and Amphastar drugs' equivalence to Lovenox into question.

Momenta, however, has expertise in the area of complex sugar sequencing that will help it develop a drug equivalent to the complicated mixture involved in producing Lovenox. The company, which is working in partnership with generic drugmaker Sandoz (the generics division of Novartis), reports that it has proprietary technology that is enabling it to analyze Lovenox and produce an agent with the same active ingredients.

Troubles Abound for Scios's Natrecor (Nesiritide)

A July 2005 article in the *New England Journal of Medicine* cited studies showing a higher association of mortality and renal failure with Scios's Natrecor (nesiritide), a recombinant form of human B-type natriuretic peptide (BNP), than with standard therapies used to treat patients with acute heart failure (AHF) who have dyspnea at rest with minimal activity. Given these findings and the fact that the drug costs 50 times as much as standard therapies, the author found how nesiritide, which received FDA approval in August 2001 for this indication in hospitalized patients, had widespread, off-label use in the United States in outpatient populations who used it once or more per week for several months to avoid a recurrence of AHF. His reasoning was that Scios (a subsidiary of J&J) had used an aggressive marketing campaign suggesting to physicians that they could use intravenously administered nesiritide in this capacity and bill Medicare in the same way they bill for chemotherapy infusions.

As a result of the controversy generated by the article, other leading US cardiologists questioned how nesiritide was being used, and, in July 2005, the US attorney's office in Boston issued a subpoena to J&J relating to the sales and marketing of nesiritide. Scios updated the product label to include information that nesiritide may be associated with adverse effects on survival and renal function and issued a "dear doctor" letter to alert healthcare providers to this information. These changes highlighted the fact that the agent should not be used in the outpatient setting. In 2004, Natrecor had sales of approximately $400 million, including off-label use, but these sales have fallen since the publication of the studies as mentioned above.

This controversy suggested that nesiritide was unlikely to become standard therapy for patients with AHF. J&J initially expected nesiritide to be launched in Europe in late 2004. However, the EMEA issued guidance in 2004 stating that 30-day and 6-month mortality data and data on worsening renal function are required for all NDAs for AHF. This requirement delayed the launch of nesiritide in Europe.

German Study and Generics Competition Challenge Pfizer's Lipitor (Atorvastatin)

A study released in early September 2005 by Germany's Institute for Quality and Efficiency in Healthcare (IQWiG) (www.iqwig.de) found that Pfizer's Lipitor (atorvastatin) is no more effective than other statins and may be associated with worse side effects. The study was not based on any new data but rather on a survey of previous studies of statins conducted worldwide. Pfizer had already encountered difficulty in Germany in mid-2004 when the government proposed a new reference- pricing system to reduce costs. In response, Pfizer excluded its drug (marketed as Sortis in Germany) from the reference-pricing system, a move that backfired because patients decided they were unwilling to contribute the copay for the drug.

Atorvastatin is Pfizer's best-selling product and the top-selling statin; in 2004, sales exceeded $10 billion worldwide. (Table 32.2 shows the 2004 sales for the top-selling statins.) Events in Germany highlight the difficulties that Pfizer is facing as it tries to defend Lipitor against increased competition from generic versions of other statins. Germany's position reflects worldwide government efforts to reduce healthcare costs. In particular, government initiatives in Europe will continue to place an emphasis on reducing pharmacy costs by prescribing generic agents. Pfizer will need to support Lipitor with an expanded marketing campaign if the company hopes to maintain the drug's strong sales.

A ruling from the United Kingdom's High Court of Justice on October 12, 2005, upheld the main patent covering atorvastatin until November 2011.

ASCOT Study Results Could Help Boost Sales of Some Drugs

Results from the Anglo-Scandinavian Cardiac Outcomes Trial (ASCOT) were presented at the European Society of Cardiology 2005 Congress on September 4, 2005. Final results

Table 32.2 Worldwide Sales of Leading Statins, 2004

Generic Name	*Company/Brand Name*	*2004 Worldwide Sales ($MM US)*
Atorvastatin	Pfizer/Lipitor	10,862
Simvastatin	Merck & Co./Zocor	5,197
Pravastatin	Bristol-Myers Squibb/Pravachol	2,635
Rosuvastatin	AstraZeneca/Crestor	908
Fluvastatin	Novartis/Lescol	758

of the Blood Pressure-Lowering Arm (BPLA) of ASCOT were published in the *Lancet* (Dahlöf et al., 2005). The study included more than 19,000 patients with high blood pressure who were at moderate risk of stroke and MI. Patients received either a standard antihypertensive regimen of a beta blocker (atenolol) plus or minus a thiazide-type diuretic (bendroflumethiazide) or a combination of newer drugs – a calcium-channel blocker (CCB) (amlodipine) plus or minus an ACE inhibitor (perindopril).

Overall, major cardiovascular events were reduced by 16%, new-onset diabetes by 30%, stroke by 23%, and mortality by 11% in the amlodipine (plus or minus perindopril) group compared with the atenolol (plus or minus bendroflumethiazide [generics]) group. Statin therapy using atorvastatin in conjunction with antihypertensive therapy further reduced cardiovascular events. A nearly 50% reduction in coronary and stroke events was found in the amlodipine (plus or minus perindopril) plus atorvastatin arm compared with standard diuretic therapy without a statin.

These findings contradicted those from the Antihypertensive and Lipid-Lowering Treatment to Prevent Heart Attack Trial (ALLHAT) study, which began in February 1994 and ended in March 2002, with patient follow-up averaging 4.9 years. Results of ALLHAT, published in several journal articles, found that traditional diuretics were more effective than newer medicines at lowering high blood pressure and preventing some forms of heart disease. It seems that the ASCOT study results may slow or counteract some of the erosion seen in CCB sales as a result of the ALLHAT study because physicians will feel less pressure to prescribe less-expensive diuretics. As noted previously, the ASCOT findings may help boost sales of the ACE inhibitor perindopril, as part of a successful combination therapy.

REFERENCES

Andrew, T.L. et al. Comparison of short- (one month) and long- (twelve months) term outcomes of sirolimus-versus paclitaxel-eluting stents in 293 consecutive patients with diabetes mellitus (from the RESEARCH and T-SEARCH Registries). *American Journal of Cardiology.* August 1, 2005; 96(3): 358–62.

Dahlöf, B. et al. Prevention of cardiovascular events with an antihypertensive regimen of amlodipine adding perindopril as required versus atenolol adding bendroflumethiazide as required, in the Anglo-Scandinavian Cardiac Outcomes Trial-Blood Pressure-Lowering Arm (ASCOT-BPLA): a multicentre randomised controlled trial. *Lancet.* September 10, 2005; 366: 895–906.

Dibra, A., et al. Paclitaxel-eluting and sirolimus-eluting stents to prevent restenosis in diabetic patients. *New England Journal of Medicine.* August 18, 2005; 353(7); 663–70.

Fox, K.M. et al. Efficacy of perindopril in reduction of cardiovascular events among patients with stable coronary artery disease: randomised, double-blind, placebo-controlled, multicentre trial (the EUROPA study). *Lancet.* September 6, 2003; 362(9386): 782–8.

Kastrati, A. et al. Siroliumus-eluting stents vs. paclitaxel-eluting stents in patients with coronary artery disease. *Journal of the American Medical Association.* August 17, 2005; 294(7): 819–25.

Pfeffer, M.A. et al. Valsartan, captopril, or both in myocardial infarction complicated by heart failure, left-ventricular dysfunction, or both. *New England Journal of Medicine.* November 13, 2003; 349(20): 1893–906.

Taylor, A.L. et al. Combination of isosorbide dinitrate/hydralazine in blacks with heart failure. *New England Journal of Medicine.* November 11, 2004; 351(20): 2049–57.

Windecker, S. et al. Sirolimus-eluting and paclitaxel-eluting stents for coronary revascularization. *New England Journal of Medicine.* August 18, 2005; 353(7): 653–62.

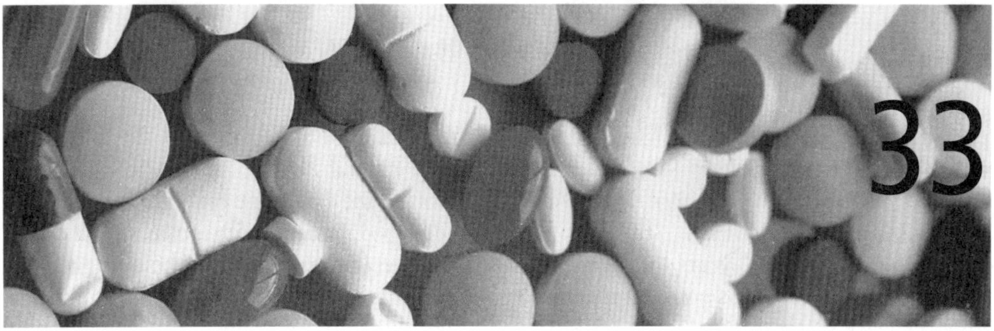

Renin Inhibitors: A Novel Approach to Hypertension

INTRODUCTION

Hypertension, or high blood pressure (BP), is a significant health concern worldwide. It is a major risk factor for cardiovascular disease (CVD), and poorly controlled hypertension, especially if prolonged, can damage target organs, such as the heart, kidneys, the retina of the eye, and the brain. Over time, this target organ damage can result in heart failure, end-stage kidney disease, retinopathy, stroke, and vascular dementia.

Essential hypertension (hypertension with no known cause) accounts for approximately 90% of hypertension and is usually treated with oral antihypertensive drugs. In 2005, the market for these agents exceeded $25 billion in the seven major pharmaceutical markets under study (United States, France, Germany, Italy, Spain, United Kingdom, and Japan). Overall, the treatment of hypertension represents one of the largest markets for prescription drugs.

Renin inhibitors are a novel class of drugs in development for the treatment of hypertension. The first of these agents, aliskiren (Novartis/Speedel's Rasilez), is preregistered in the United States. If approved, it will be the first of a new class of antihypertensive drugs to enter the market in more than a decade.

In this chapter, we present an overview of hypertension, focusing on the role of the renin-angiotensin-aldosterone system (RAAS) pathway in the control of BP. We briefly review agents currently used to treat hypertension and discuss the unmet need that remains in this mature market. We then review the potential of renin inhibitors as treatments for this disease, including an in-depth discussion of aliskiren. We conclude with our outlook for the future of these agents in this market.

OVERVIEW OF HYPERTENSION

Definition of Hypertension

According to the Joint National Committee-7 (JNC-7) guidelines, normal BP is characterized by systolic blood pressure (SBP, the pressure in the arteries when the heart contracts and pumps blood into the tissues of the body) less than 120 millimeters of mercury (mm Hg) and diastolic blood pressure (DBP, the pressure in the arteries when the heart relaxes and fills with blood) less than 80 mm Hg. Blood pressures are written as SBP/DBP, for example, 120/80.

Under the JNC-7 guidelines, people with BPs between 120/80 and 139/89 are considered prehypertensive. People with higher BPs are classified as having stage 1 hypertension (between 140/90 and 159/99) or stage 2 hypertension (higher than 160/100). In people more than 50 years of age, SBP higher than 140 mm Hg is considered a more important risk factor for CVD than DBP. The risk of essential hypertension increases with a family history of the condition and increasing age. In addition, obesity or being overweight, lack of exercise, smoking, and excessive salt or alcohol intake increase the risk of developing hypertension.

Physiological mechanisms for controlling BP principally involve the sympathetic nervous system (SNS) and the kidneys. In response to stress (as in the "fight or flight" response), the SNS stimulates the adrenal glands to release the hormones epinephrine and norepinephrine. These hormones cause BP to rise via several mechanisms:

- Stimulating the heart to beat more rapidly and forcefully, thereby increasing blood volume.
- Causing most arterioles to constrict, thereby increasing resistance to blood flow.
- Dilating arterioles in skeletal muscle, thereby increasing blood flow to this tissue.

The SNS also stimulates the kidneys to reduce excretion of salt and water, which increases blood volume. Under normal circumstances, when BP rises because of exercise (which results in increased blood flow and therefore elevated BP), these mechanisms trigger dilation of blood vessels and increased renal excretion of salt and water in order to maintain BP in the normal range. The kidneys and the adrenal glands also control BP via RAAS, discussed in the next section. In essential hypertension, these normal physiological functions are disrupted by largely unknown mechanisms.

Importantly, hypertension is a component of the metabolic syndrome, a constellation of CVD risk factors that includes, in addition to elevated BP, abdominal obesity, dyslipidemia, and elevated fasting-blood glucose. Patients with three or more of these risk factors are deemed to have metabolic syndrome. Researchers identify insulin resistance (the inability of tissues to use insulin efficiently in the uptake of glucose from the blood) as being central to the metabolic syndrome; however, the syndrome remains only partially understood. Patients with metabolic syndrome are generally considered to be at higher risk of developing both CVD and type 2 diabetes. Approximately one-third of patients with primary hypertension and without type 2 diabetes have metabolic syndrome.

The Renin-Angiotensin-Aldosterone System

Figure 33.1 depicts the RAAS, an important physiological pathway for the control of BP. Renin is an aspartic protease enzyme that is released into the bloodstream by the kidneys in response to underperfusion or stimulation by the SNS. Renin cleaves the plasma protein angiotensinogen, producing the peptide angiotensin I. Another enzyme, angiotensin-converting enzyme (ACE), then cleaves angiotensin I to release angiotensin II, a hormone and vasoconstrictor. Angiotensin II causes arterioles to constrict, thereby increasing BP, and stimulates the adrenal glands to release aldosterone into the bloodstream. Aldosterone causes the kidneys to retain salt and water and to excrete potassium, resulting in elevated BP. All the various steps in this pathway are potential targets for control of BP.

In addition to the systemic RAAS, there are local tissue renin-angiotensin systems, which involve the expression and activity of tissue ACE, angiotensin II, and at least in some cases, renin within specific cells and tissues (Re, 2004). In particular, excessive production of angiotensin II in endothelial cells is involved in endothelial-cell dysfunction that leads to atherogenesis. Other tissues, such as adipose tissue, skeletal muscle, and the pancreas, appear to have local renin-angiotensin systems with potential importance in metabolic diseases such as type 2 diabetes and obesity.

Prevalence

In 2005, the prevalence of hypertension in the markets under study exceeded 201 million. Prevalence appears to be higher

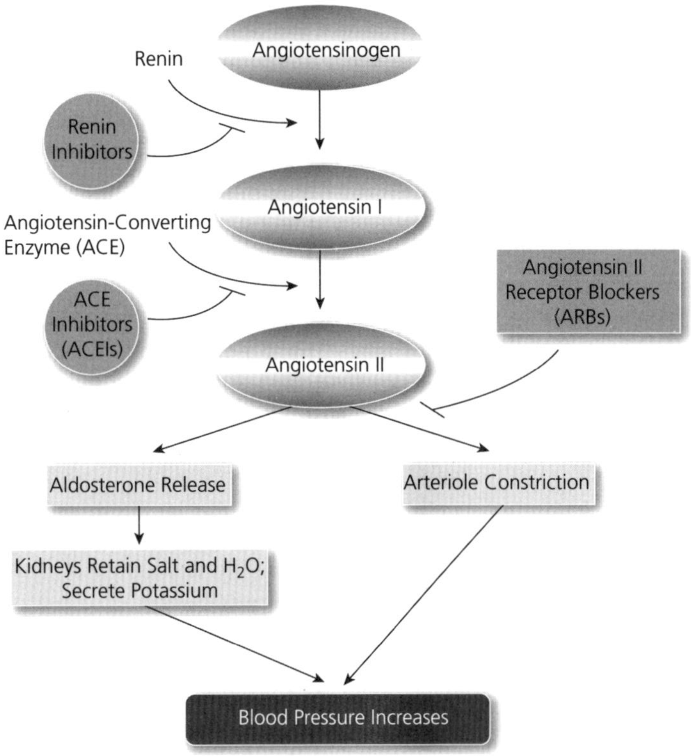

Figure 33.1 The Renin-Angiotensin-Aldosterone System (RAAS)

in African-Americans than in whites and slightly higher in men. The number of people whose hypertension has been diagnosed is significantly smaller; the JNC-7 estimates that during the most recent period surveyed (1999–2000) 30% of people with hypertension were undiagnosed.

Worldwide, the prevalence of hypertension is growing as a result of changing diets and an increasingly sedentary lifestyle. In 2000, more than 26% of the worldwide adult population had hypertension. The hypertensive population is expected to increase by 60%, to 1.56 billion, by 2025 (Kearney et al., 2005).

CURRENT TREATMENT FOR HYPERTENSION

Under the JNC-7 guidelines, prehypertensive patients are generally treated with lifestyle modification, including diet, exercise, and weight loss. Patients with stage 1 or 2 hypertension must be treated with antihypertensive drugs in addition to lifestyle modification. The large, mature hypertension drug market comprises several classes of drugs that include many branded and generic agents. In the following sections, we discuss currently available treatment options and the remaining unmet patient need in the hypertension market.

Current Therapies

Table 33.1 lists the major classes of drugs commonly prescribed for hypertension (and recommended in the JNC-7 guidelines for uncomplicated cases of hypertension), together with examples of the leading agents. These drugs are also the most commonly prescribed antihypertensives for patients with complicating indications such as diabetes, high coronary disease risk, postmyocardial infarction (PMI), and heart failure. In addition to lowering BP, the listed drugs (used alone

Table 33.1 JNC-7 Recommended Drug Classes for Treatment of Uncomplicated Hypertension

Class	*Physiological Effect*	*Select Drugs*
Thiazide diuretics	Stimulate the kidneys to secrete salt and water, decreasing blood volume	Chlorothiazide (Merck's Diuril, generics) Hydrochlorothiazide (Merck's HydroDiuril, generics) Chlorthalidone (generics)
Beta blockers	Block the response of the sympathetic nervous system to stress	Atenolol (AstraZeneca's Tenormin, generics) Metoprolol tartrate (Novartis's Lopressor, generics) Propranolol (Wyeth's Inderal, generics)
ACE inhibitors (ACEIs)	Inhibit RAAS	Captopril (Bristol-Myers Squibb's Capoten, generics) Enalapril (Merck's Vasotec, generics) Lisinopril (Merck's Prinivil, AstraZeneca's Zestril, generics) Ramipril (King Pharmaceuticals/Sanofi-Aventis's Altace)
Angiotensin II receptor blockers (ARBs)	Inhibit RAAS	Irbesartan (Bristol-Myers Squibb/Sanofi-Aventis's Avapro) Losartan (Merck's Cozaar) Valsartan (Novartis's Diovan) Candesartan (AstraZeneca's Atacand)
Calcium-channel blockers	Cause arterioles to dilate by inhibiting the entry of calcium ions into vascular smooth muscle cells	Diltiazem (Biovail's Cardizem, Watson Pharmaceuticals' Dilacor, Forest's Tiazac, generics) Verapamil (Pfizer's Calan, Abbott's Isoptin, generics) Amlodipine (Pfizer's Norvasc, generics)

Note: All drugs listed in this table are single compounds. Fixed-dose combinations of these drugs are also used to treat hypertension
ACE = Angiotensin-converting enzyme

or in combination) have been shown in clinical trials to reduce the incidence of complications of hypertension, such as CVD and target organ damage.

The goal of drug treatment is to reduce BP to less than 140/90 for most patients and to less than 130/80 in patients with diabetes or chronic kidney disease. However, because the risk of CVD increases when BP is higher than 120/80, achieving BPs well below the goal of 140/90 – ideally, near normal BP (120/80) – is desirable. Most hypertensive patients, especially those with stage 2 hypertension, require combination therapy to control their BP. Combination therapy consists of two or more drugs of different classes and usually includes a thiazide diuretic. The use of alternative drugs or classes of drugs may be necessary because of side effects experienced by particular patients with a given drug and/or by the ability of particular drugs or combinations to control a patient's BP.

The JNC-7 guidelines recommend that thiazide diuretics be the first agents prescribed for most patients with stage 1 hypertension. However, physicians and patients may consider the use of other agents, such as ACE inhibitors (ACEIs), angiotensin II receptor blockers (ARBs; also known as angiotensin II antagonists), beta blockers, and calcium-channel blockers (CCBs). In some cases, patients may have "compelling indications," in which case the JNC-7 recommends treatment with one or more antihypertensive drugs of particular classes that specifically address the complications – for example, chronic kidney disease treatment includes ACEIs or ARBs. Treatment of hypertension in diabetics may involve combinations of drugs, including thiazide diuretics, ACEIs, ARBs, and/or CCBs, based on evidence that ACEIs and ARBs can slow the progression of diabetic nephropathy and prevent development of this complication.

Diuretics control BP by increasing the excretion of sodium and water, thereby reducing plasma volume, cardiac output, and peripheral resistance. The emphasis on diuretics, particularly thiazide diuretics, as a first-line therapy is based especially on the results of the Antihypertensive and Lipid-Lowering to Prevent Heart Attack Trial (ALLHAT), which concluded that thiazide diuretics were superior to other antihypertensives in preventing CVD, including coronary heart disease, stroke, heart failure, and peripheral artery disease (ALLHAT Officers and Coordinators for the ALLHAT

Collaborative Research Group, 2002). However, some researchers cite evidence that thiazide diuretics may have adverse effects on glucose and lipid metabolism and may exacerbate the metabolic syndrome.

Beta blockers inhibit sympathetic innervation of the heart via the beta adrenoreceptor. Beta blockers are preferentially prescribed as a first-line therapy for hypertensive patients who have heart failure, angina, and/or ischemic heart disease, and they are often used as add-on therapies with ACEIs and diuretics. However, there is some evidence that beta blockers, like thiazide diuretics, may have adverse effects on glucose and lipid metabolism and may exacerbate the metabolic syndrome.

Available for more than 20 years, CCBs have proved to be effective both as monotherapy and in combination with other agents. These agents induce vasodilation by inhibiting the entry of calcium ions, which mediate cellular contraction, via L-type calcium channels into vascular smooth-muscle cells. CCBs are particularly well suited for patient subpopulations such as elderly patients and black patients, who often do not respond well to other antihypertensive medications, particularly those that modify RAAS. The most common side effects associated with CCBs are caused by excessive vasodilation: dizziness, hypotension, headache, flushing, and edema.

ACEIs and ARBs inhibit RAAS. ACEIs inhibit the enzymatic activity of ACE, thereby preventing the formation of angiotensin II from angiotensin I; ARBs inhibit the binding of angiotensin II to its receptors on arterioles, thereby preventing vasoconstriction. ACEIs are a popular first-line therapy, particularly in patients with dyslipidemia or diabetes. They have a relatively benign side-effect profile, but use of ACEIs can lead to the accumulation of bradykinin, a vasodilator, that results in a cough. ARBs are the newest class of hypertension drugs. Their principal advantage over ACEIs is that they do not cause a buildup in bradykinin.

ACEIs and ARBs also have clinical benefits beyond their antihypertensive effects, which may in part be explained by their effects on tissue renin-angiotensin systems. Drugs that inhibit the RAAS may be beneficial in preventing CVD and the development of type 2 diabetes in hypertensive patients with metabolic syndrome (Leiter and Lewanczuk, 2005; Kurtz, 2006). In addition, they may provide cardioprotection and renal protection in patients at risk for cardiac or kidney disease because of hypertension, diabetes, or certain other conditions (Dzau et al., 2001). More recently, researchers obtained evidence that these drugs reduce the incidence of new-onset type 2 diabetes in patients at risk for that disease (e.g., patients with metabolic syndrome) (Jandeleit-Dahm et al., 2005). Based on animal models and human studies, researchers attribute these benefits to effects on endothelial and/or tissue renin-angiotensin systems, but the biology of these systems is not completely understood. Large, long-term clinical trials designed to prove this hypothesis are in progress. For a list of conditions other than hypertension for which ACEIs and/or ARBs are used, see Table 33.2.

Unmet Needs in the Treatment of Hypertension

According to the JNC-7, the most significant unmet need in the treatment of hypertension is the ability to achieve and maintain control of BP. In the most recent period surveyed (1999–2000), 59% of patients with hypertension were treated, but only 34% (58% of treated patients) achieved control. Controlling systolic BP in patients older than 50 is especially difficult. Clinical trials have demonstrated that the majority of hypertensive patients can achieve control, usually with two or more agents; therefore, the JNC-7 attributes the suboptimal control to clinicians' failure to prescribe adequate drug doses and/or appropriate drug combinations and patients' failure to modify their lifestyles sufficiently.

Patient compliance with drug regimens and crucial lifestyle changes is an important factor when evaluating a patient's ability to

Table 33.2 Other Conditions Treated with ACE Inhibitors (ACEIs) and Angiotensin II Receptor Blockers (ARBs)

Condition	*Effects of ACEI or ARB Treatment*
Diabetic nephropathy	Slows disease progression
Asymptomatic left ventricular dysfunction	Slows progression to heart failure Reduces mortality
Congestive heart failure	Slows disease progression Reduces mortality
Cardiovascular disease (coronary heart disease, diabetes, other vascular disease)	Reduces mortality and cardiovascular events, including myocardial infarction and heart failure
Metabolic syndrome[a]	Reduces the incidence of new-onset diabetes

[a]The efficacy of ACEIs and ARBs for this indication is not yet definitively established by the appropriate clinical trials. All other uses of drugs in this table are approved by the FDA and other regulatory agencies
ACE = Angiotensin-converting enzyme

achieve BP control. The inability of some patients to tolerate some hypertension medications hinders compliance and makes prescription of adequate drug regimens more challenging for physicians. The need for polypharmacy also plays a role: as the number of drugs required to achieve the desired result increases, patient compliance often declines. In addition, although weight control and exercise are important factors in BP control, most overweight patients find it difficult to maintain long-term weight loss, and many patients find it difficult to get enough exercise, owing to time constraints, ill health, and/or disability.

Even in controlled clinical trial settings, where appropriate drugs and patient compliance can be assured, significant numbers of patients still fail to achieve or maintain BP control. In one clinical trial, titration of medication was forced by computerized recommendations to increase the dose or number of agents when a patient had not achieved goal BP, and 84.8% of patients achieved goal BP (<140/90). Over two years of treatment, 67–69% of patients maintained goal BP. Thus, even under these controlled conditions, approximately one-third of patients failed to maintain control over the two-year period (Black et al., 2001). Such results indicate a need to identify novel treatments that can be used in patients whose disease proves refractory to currently available drug regimens.

RENIN INHIBITORS

The unmet needs described in the previous section have prompted pharmaceutical companies to continue to develop new drugs for this mature market. Their goal is to develop an agent that will improve BP control through either a better side-effect profile or a reduction in the need for polypharmacy, either of which could improve patient compliance. In addition, an agent with improved pharmacokinetics may enable 24-hour dosing (existing treatments may lose effectiveness during the 24-hour period and therefore require multiple daily doses), thereby enabling a significant number of patients to achieve better BP control throughout the day.

One novel class of agents, the renin inhibitors, has compelling theoretical mechanistic advantages over current agents, including agents that inhibit the RAAS. Clinical trials suggest that renin inhibitors offer better side-effect profiles, potency, and pharmacokinetics. We discuss the development of this promising class of agents, including the first-in-class drug aliskiren (Speedel/Novartis's Rasilez), in the following sections.

The Development of Renin Inhibitors

The action of renin on angiotensinogen is the first and rate-limiting step in the systemic RAAS pathway. For this reason, plus the fact that renin is specific for angiotensinogen as a substrate, renin is a logical target when developing compounds that inhibit the RAAS. Consequently, researchers have been pursuing the discovery and development of renin inhibitors for about 20 years; however, in part because the interaction between renin and angiotensinogen has the characteristics of a protein-protein interaction, the discovery of renin inhibitors by means of conventional medicinal chemistry has been difficult.

To avoid the challenges associated with the development of agents that target protein-protein interactions, early work on renin inhibitors involved studies of peptide and peptidomimetic compounds, especially analogues of the relevant amino acid sequences of the substrate, angiotensinogen. These compounds were potent competitive inhibitors of renin, but they were poorly bioavailable and therefore not clinically useful. Meanwhile, the development of ACEIs and eventually ARBs made the commercial success of peptidomimetic renin inhibitors seem unlikely (Fisher and Hollenberg, 2005).

However, since this early work, the development of marketed agents that inhibit another aspartic protease, the HIV-1 protease (for the treatment of HIV/AIDS), has lent further support to the idea that renin should be a druggable target. HIV-1 protease inhibitors were discovered by means of X-ray crystallography and structure-based drug design; these technologies also enabled the development of small-molecule inhibitors that bind to the active site of renin, which is a deep cleft. This generation of renin inhibitors – all of them oral, small-molecule agents – is listed in Table 33.3.

With the exception of aliskiren, discussed in detail in the next section, all the agents listed in Table 33.3 are in the early stages of development, and most were discovered by small biotechnology companies. However, because the antihypertensive market is a highly competitive primary care market that requires large salesforces, many of these small biotechs have sought out partnerships with large pharmaceutical companies. In addition to Novartis's partnership with Speedel on the development of aliskiren, GlaxoSmithKline (GSK) has partnered with Vitae Pharmaceuticals, and Merck has partnered with Actelion to develop early-stage renin inhibitors that the smaller companies discovered in-house. The interest of large pharmaceutical companies in partnering for compounds that are only in the preclinical stage demonstrates the high potential that they see in renin inhibitors. The exception to this model is Pfizer, which sponsors its own in-house renin inhibitor program, thereby lending further credence to the potential of these agents.

Speedel/Novartis's Aliskiren

In April 2006, the FDA accepted Novartis's new drug application (NDA) for aliskiren as a monotherapy and in combination with other hypertension medications. Speedel (Basel, Switzerland) inlicensed aliskiren in the late discovery stage from Novartis in 1999 and developed the compound through Phase II. At that point, in the fall of 2002, Novartis exercised its call-back option for aliskiren.

Table 33.3 Renin Inhibitors in Development

Compound	*Company*	*Stage*
Aliskiren (Rasilez; formerly SPP-100)	Speedel/Novartis	Preregistration
Aliskiren + valsartan	Novartis	Phase II
SPP-635	Speedel	Phase I
Unnamed compound	Actelion/Merck	Preclinical (Phase I planned before mid 2006)
SPP-1100	Speedel	Preclinical (Phase I planned for late 2006/early 2007)
Unnamed compound	Pfizer	Preclinical
Unnamed compound	Vitae Pharmaceuticals/ GlaxoSmithKline	Preclinical

Early clinical studies of aliskiren showed that the agent has a half-life in the bloodstream of 24 hours and a sustained antihypertensive effect over 24 hours (Stanton et al., 2003). This finding suggests that once-a-day dosing with aliskiren will be sufficient to maintain effective BP lowering over the course of 24 hours. Such is not the case with many current BP medications, some of which must be given more than once a day, thereby hindering patient compliance.

In November 2005, the results of a Phase II open-label study sponsored by Speedel were presented at the American Heart Association Scientific Sessions in Dallas (O'Brien et al., 2005). The trial examined aliskiren in combination with irbesartan (Bristol-Myers Squibb/Sanofi-Aventis's Avapro). The 23 patients in the trial received once-daily treatment with irbesartan 150 mg for three weeks, followed by irbesartan 150 mg plus aliskiren 75 mg for three weeks, followed by irbesartan 150 mg plus aliskiren 150 mg for three weeks. Ambulatory BP was measured continuously in all patients. Irbesartan monotherapy was found to lower BP throughout a 24-hour period. The addition of aliskiren was associated with significantly greater reductions in night-time BP than that achieved by irbesartan monotherapy. There was also a trend toward increased daytime BP lowering with the irbesartan-aliskiren combination therapy, compared with irbesartan monotherapy, but the results were not statistically significant, a determination that researchers attributed to the small number of patients in the trial. The results of this small, open-label study must be confirmed by large, placebo-controlled, double-blind Phase III clinical trials.

The Speedel-sponsored trial also examined plasma renin activity. High essential plasma renin activity has been associated with the development of CVD and renal disease in hypertensive patients (Alderman et al., 1997; Baldoncini et al., 1999). As researchers have observed in earlier studies with both ARBs and ACEIs, irbesartan significantly increased plasma renin activity by an average of 2.4-fold compared with baseline readings. The addition of aliskiren at both doses significantly reduced this rise in plasma renin activity. The researchers therefore hypothesized that aliskiren may protect against damage to such end organs as the heart and the kidneys. This hypothesis is supported by an animal model study of end-organ damage caused by an overactive RAAS; in this study, rats that are transgenic for both renin and angiotensinogen genes develop heart and kidney damage if untreated. Both high-dose valsartan and lower-dose aliskiren ameliorated end-organ damage and prevented death due to this organ damage (Pilz et al., 2005). The hypothesis that aliskiren may protect against end-organ damage must be proven in appropriate clinical trials.

Aliskiren has also shown promising results in Phase III trials both as monotherapy and in combination with other antihypertensives. In March 2005, Novartis and its academic collaborators published the results of a randomized Phase III study that compared treatment of hypertensive patients with aliskiren in one of three doses (150, 300, or 600 mg), irbesartan 150 mg, or placebo over an eight-week period (Gradman et al., 2005). Patients in this study had mild-to-moderate hypertension; mean BPs were 152/99.

Trial results showed that all three doses of aliskiren significantly lowered BP. The lowest dose of aliskiren was comparable to the irbesartan treatment in terms of mean BP lowering and the percentage of patients reaching target BP levels. Aliskiren at the two higher doses was superior to irbesartan, but the 600 mg dose was no more effective than the 300 mg dose. The researchers concluded that a 300 mg dose of aliskiren could be used in patients who are not brought to target BP by a 150 mg dose and that this higher dose would likely help more patients achieve target BP.

At all doses tested, aliskiren showed a low incidence of adverse effects, similar to the adverse-effect profiles of placebo and irbesartan 150 mg. Irbesartan, like all marketed ARBs, has a placebo-like adverse-effect profile. The finding in this and other studies that aliskiren has an adverse-effect profile comparable to the profiles of placebo and ARBs suggests that aliskiren will not have the tolerability issues that limit patient use of and compliance with other classes of antihypertensives. These results are supported in further, longer-term (one-year) Phase III trials. In a September 2005 press release, Novartis reported the results of two placebo-controlled clinical trials in which aliskiren as a monotherapy continued to demonstrate the BP-lowering and safety profile seen in the published Phase III study, including sustained 24-hour BP lowering.

A study investigating the benefits of aliskiren given in combination with the thiazide diuretic hydrochlorothiazide (Merck's HydroDiuril, generics) showed that the combination treatment resulted in significantly greater BP lowering than either agent given alone. In addition, the combination had excellent responder rates – measured by the percentage of patients who experienced a reduction in BP of more than 10 mm Hg or a diastolic BP of less than 90 mm Hg – and a good safety profile.

In a January 2006 press release, Novartis reported the results of Phase III clinical trials of aliskiren in combination with the ACEI ramipril (King Pharmaceuticals/Sanofi-Aventis's Altace, generics) and the CCB amlodipine (Pfizer's Norvasc, generics). In the trial of aliskiren plus ramipril in hypertensive diabetic patients, aliskiren monotherapy showed double-digit reductions in SBP and DBP, and the combination therapy resulted in additional statistically and clinically significant declines in SBP and DBP. The addition of aliskiren to ramipril was also reported to lower the incidence of dry cough, a common adverse effect of ACEIs. Both the aliskiren monotherapy and the combination therapy with ramipril resulted in excellent responder rates; safety and tolerability were also excellent. The trial of aliskiren in combination with amlodipine in hypertensive patients showed increased benefits in BP control, compared with monotherapies, and excellent safety and tolerability. Combination treatment with aliskiren and amlodipine was also reported to reduce the rates of edema, a common side effect of CCBs.

The clinical trial results for aliskiren indicate that this agent may have several advantages over existing antihypertensives (see Table 33.4). In addition to possible advantages as a monotherapy, aliskiren may improve BP control when used in combination with other agents and may offer a new option to patients who have been unable to achieve their goal BP using current therapies. To this end, Novartis is developing a fixed-dose combination of aliskiren and valsartan, which is in Phase II trials. Please note that the Phase III clinical trials of aliskiren have used BP reduction as their only end point; therefore, many of the possible advantages listed in Table 33.4 are theoretical and will need to be proven in the clinic. Moreover, aliskiren is the only renin inhibitor with Phase III study data; it is not known whether its effects will be replicated by other renin inhibitors in development. However, results with earlier agents in animal models and in small human studies suggest that many of these results may be effects of renin inhibitors as a class.

The Potential for Renin Inhibitors in Other Diseases

As discussed earlier, ACEIs and ARBs have therapeutic benefits that extend beyond their ability to lower BP. In large, controlled clinical trials, ACEIs and ARBs conclusively demonstrated their ability to slow the progression of several serious cardiovascular conditions and to reduce the rates of mortality and morbidity in patients with these conditions. Specifically, the landmark Heart Outcomes Prevention Evaluation (HOPE) trial showed that the ACEI ramipril reduced the incidence of cardiovascular events, the development of heart failure, and death in high-risk patients more than 55 years old who had vascular disease and/or diabetes (Yusuf et al., 2000).

An important issue for renin inhibitors and their market potential is whether they offer the same or greater safety and efficacy than

Table 33.4 Potential Advantages of Renin Inhibitors over Other Antihypertensives

- Aliskiren[a] has an apparently lower incidence of adverse effects than most other classes of antihypertensives; its side-effect profile resembles that of the ARBs
- Aliskiren provides true 24-hour BP lowering and high response rates (i.e., clinically meaningful BP lowering), depending on the dose used
- Unlike other antihypertensives (ACEIs, ARBs, diuretics, and calcium-channel blockers), aliskiren does not elevate plasma renin activity. Lower plasma renin levels and more complete blocking of the RAAS may, at least in theory, translate into better end-organ protection
- Aliskiren blocks the generation of angiotensin I, thereby enabling more complete blocking of angiotensin II and its physiological effects
- Aliskiren shows increased and more prolonged inhibition of aldosterone production than ACEIs or ARBs
- Combination therapies of aliskiren with ACEIs or ARBs are expected to effect more complete blockade of the RAAS and may result in increased BP control in patients who do not reach goal BP with one agent alone
- Renin inhibitors appear to achieve larger increases in renal plasma flow than ACEIs[b]

[a]Aliskiren is the only renin inhibitor so far that has been extensively tested in human clinical trials. Most of the data on which this table was based were obtained in human studies with aliskiren. It is not yet determined whether the effects of aliskiren can be considered class effects

[b]Studies were done with early renin inhibitors in healthy human volunteers

ACEI = Angiotensin-converting enzyme inhibitor; ARB = Angiotensin receptor blocker; BP = Blood pressure; RAAS = Renin-angiotensin-aldosterone system

that of ACEIs and ARBs in these additional cardiovascular conditions and whether renin inhibitors might be used in combination with other agents to achieve even greater efficacy. Thus far, no clinical evidence suggests that aliskiren or any other renin inhibitor has the beneficial effects of ACEIs and ARBs on any of these conditions, although, in theory, renin inhibitors would be expected to have the same beneficial effects. However, the incomplete knowledge of the biology of tissue-renin-angiotensin systems suggests caution in predicting such benefits from renin inhibitors without definitive clinical evidence.

Novartis indicated that it is conducting long-term studies to establish the benefits of aliskiren in cardiovascular indications; it may be some time before definitive clinical evidence of aliskiren's efficacy in the treatment of these indications is available. Similar trials for ACEIs and ARBs have lasted several years. For example, the HOPE trial examined the effects of ramipril on high-risk cardiovascular patients over a mean five-year period; the Valsartan Heart Failure Trial (VAL-HEFT), which investigated the benefit of valsartan treatment in heart failure patients who were not receiving ACE inhibitors, had a mean follow-up period of 23 months; and the Candesartan in Heart Failure Assessment of Reduction in Mortality and Morbidity (CHARM) trial, which investigated candesartan (AstraZeneca's Atacand) in heart failure patients who were receiving ACE inhibitors or could not tolerate them, had a follow-up period of two to four years. We expect that equivalent trials of aliskiren will take as long as these trials, and other renin inhibitors will need to reach late-stage trials in hypertension, their primary indication, before trials in additional indications can begin.

OUTLOOK FOR RENIN INHIBITORS

The hypertension market is a mature, highly competitive, primary care market with many treatment options and many agents available generically. It includes two well-established classes of drugs that inhibit the RAAS – ACEIs and ARBs. The nature of this market raises the question whether a new class of drugs, such as renin inhibitors, is really needed. Are they likely to be merely expensive alternatives to ACEIs and ARBs with limited utility? Several leading ACEIs are available generically, and if patients cannot tolerate ACEIs, ARBs are available and efficacious, though more expensive than generic ACEIs.

The information available on renin inhibitors is limited. The only extensive clinical data available are from trials of aliskiren, and the data on that compound are limited to its efficacy in reducing BP as a monotherapy or in combination with other agents. Even certain proven advantages of renin inhibitors over ACEIs (e.g., the low incidence of adverse effects) do not translate into advantages over ARBs. Moreover, many of the potential advantages of this drug class, listed in Table 33.4, are still theoretical; clinical data are required to support them. The efficacy of renin inhibitors in treating other indications (for which ACEIs and ARBs are already prescribed) has not been established, and it will be some time before these data are available.

Although the role that renin inhibitors will play in the hypertension market remains unclear, hypertension experts compare the prospects of this drug class with those of ARBs when they were first developed. Initially, they appeared to be expensive alternatives to ACEIs, but, ultimately, their different side-effect profile made them an alternative treatment for patients who cannot tolerate ACEIs. Moreover, they can be used in combination with ACEIs to effect more complete blockage of the RAAS and enable patients to reach their goal BPs. Consequently, ARBs have found their place in the antihypertensive market and become a successful drug class. In 2005, their total sales were estimated at $13 billion.

Aliskiren has a low incidence of side effects and potent, 24-hour efficacy in reducing BP. We therefore expect it to become another option for physicians in search of a drug or combination of drugs that is well tolerated and will enable patients to reach goal BPs. Combination therapies of the renin inhibitor aliskiren and ARBs look particularly promising, both with respect to available data and from a theoretical mechanistic standpoint, that is, obtaining more complete blockage of the RAAS without stimulating it. As data come in over the next several years on the effects of aliskiren on the end-organ damage prevention and other effects beyond BP reduction, we expect increasing acceptance of the agent by the medical and patient communities and by third-party payers and a corresponding increase in sales.

The early-stage deals signed by Merck and GSK for renin inhibitors discovered by Actelion and Vitae, respectively, demonstrate that these Big Pharma companies see significant potential for follow-on renin inhibitors despite Novartis's long lead.

REFERENCES

Alderman, M.H. et al. Plasma renin activity: a risk factor for myocardial infarction in hypertensive patients. *American Journal of Hypertension.* 1997; 10: 1–8.

ALLHAT Officers and Coordinators for the ALLHAT Collaborative Research Group. Major outcomes in high-risk hypertensive patients randomized to angiotensin-converting enzyme inhibitor or calcium-channel blocker vs. diuretic: the Antihypertensive and Lipid-Lowering to Prevent Heart Attack Trial, (ALLHAT). *Journal of the American Medical Association.* 2002; 288: 2981–97.

Baldoncini, R. et al. High plasma renin activity is combined with elevated urinary albumin excretion in essential hypertension patients. *Kidney International.* 1999; 56: 1499–504.

Black, H.R. et al. Baseline characteristics and early blood pressure control in the CONVINCE trial. *Hypertension.* 2001; 37: 12–18.

Dzau, V.J. et al. The relevance of tissue angiotensin-converting enzyme: manifestation in mechanistic and end point data. *American Journal of Cardiology.* 2001;88: 1L–20.

Fisher, N.D. and Hollenberg, N.K. Renin inhibition: what are the therapeutic opportunities? *Journal of the American Society of Nephrology.* 2005; 16: 592–9.

Gradman, A.H. et al. Aliskiren, a novel orally effective renin inhibitor, provides dose-dependent antihypertensive efficacy and placebo-like tolerability in hypertensive patients. *Circulation.* 2005; 111: 1012–18.

Jandeleit-Dahm, K.A. et al. Why blockade of the renin-angiotensin system reduces the incidence of new-onset diabetes. *Journal of Hypertension.* 2005; 23: 463–73.

Kearney, P.M. et al. Global burden of hypertension: analysis of worldwide data. *Lancet.* 2005; 365: 217–23.

Kurtz, T.W. New treatment strategies for patients with hypertension and insulin resistance. *American Journal of Medicine.* 2006; 119: S24–30.

Leiter, L.A., and Lewanczuk, R.Z. Of the renin-angiotensin system and reactive oxygen species: type 2 diabetes and angiotensin II inhibition. *American Journal of Hypertension.* 2005; 18: 121–8.

O'Brien, E. et al. Aliskiren, an orally effective renin inhibitor, suppresses plasma renin activity and improves blood pressure lowering in combination with irbesartan in patients with hypertension. 2005 American Heart Association Scientific Sessions. November 13–16, 2005. Dallas, TX.

Pilz, B. et al. Aliskiren, a human renin inhibitor, ameliorates cardiac and renal damage in double-transgenic rats. *Hypertension.* 2005; 46: 569–76.

Re, R.N. Tissue renin angiotensin systems. *Medical Clinics of North America.* 2004; 88: 19–38.

Stanton, A. et al. Blood pressure lowering in essential hypertension with an oral renin inhibitor, aliskiren. *Hypertension.* 2003; 42: 1137–43.

Yusuf, S. et al. Effects of an angiotensin-converting-enzyme inhibitor, ramipril, on cardiovascular events in high-risk patients. The Heart Outcomes Prevention Evaluation Study Investigators. *New England Journal of Medicine.* 2000; 342: 145–53.

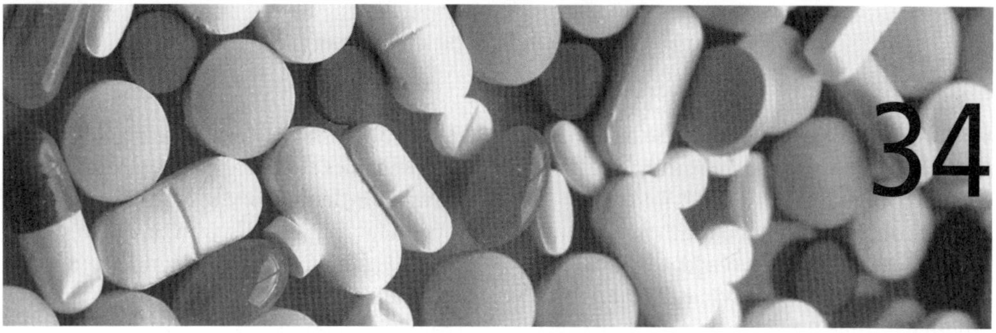

Future of VLA-4 Antagonist Drugs and Implications for the Regulatory Process

INTRODUCTION

Several companies have been investigating the potential of very late activation antigen-4 (VLA-4, also known as α4β1 integrin), located on the surface of T cells, as a drug target in a variety of inflammatory diseases. However, in March 2005, in response to difficulties with Biogen Idec and Elan's natalizumab (Tysabri, formerly Antegren) – a marketed monoclonal antibody (MAb) directed against this integrin – the FDA decided to place a clinical hold on another VLA-4 acting drug in clinical trials, and a second company voluntarily withdrew its VLA-4 drug from development while an investigation into the safety of this drug class is conducted. These safety concerns have affected drugs in development for the treatment of multiple sclerosis (MS), Crohn's disease (CD), asthma, and others.

Natalizumab's regulatory journey shows how this promising new drug class has come to encounter difficulty. Prior to the FDA's March 2005 decision, the agency granted expedited approval of natalizumab in November 2004 for treatment of MS. Natalizumab was the first MS treatment to begin the approval process after one year of clinical trial data, and Biogen Idec and Elan submitted second-year data in the same month that the drug was approved. Analysts predicted that the drug would become the new breakthrough treatment for MS. (Biogen Idec and Elan were also investigating natalizumab for treatment of CD and rheumatoid arthritis [RA].)

On February 28, 2005, however, Biogen Idec and Elan announced that they were voluntarily removing natalizumab from the market after two MS patients who had been taking the drug developed progressive multifocal leukoencephalopathy (PML), a rare and often fatal viral infection. The patients had been enrolled in a clinical trial studying the effects of the drug in combination with Biogen Idec's interferon-beta-1a (IFN-β-1a; Avonex), and initially, there was speculation that it was the combination of these drugs that allowed the infection to take hold. This theory was called into question when it was determined that a third patient, who had been taking natalizumab for treatment of CD, had died from PML in December 2003. This patient had also been taking azathioprine (GlaxoSmithKline's Imuran, generics); however, that treatment had been halted in late 2002. After the diagnosis of the initial two cases of PML, physicians, in cooperation with Biogen Idec and Elan, examined the CD viral load and determined that the level of the JC virus (the virus responsible for PML) in the patient had risen 12-fold after his second round of treatment with natalizumab (Van Assche, 2005). Two additional cases of PML in patients receiving Tysabri were reported in June 2005; these cases have yet to be confirmed.

This chapter covers the mechanism of VLA-4 and discusses its potential as a drug target. In addition, we identify the therapeutic markets most likely to be affected by the hold on VLA-4 development and comment on the likelihood of success for VLA-4 drug candidates currently being investigated in clinical trials. We will also cover potential long-term implications for the overall drug approval process in the wake of the problems with natalizumab.

VLA-4 AS A THERAPEUTIC TARGET

Because alpha (α)4 integrin plays an important role in the body's inflammatory response (Figure 34.1), it has been an intriguing target for companies focusing on therapeutic areas where an inflammatory response is a crucial component of the disease, including MS, CD, and asthma. The α4 integrin subunit can combine with either the β1 or β7 subunit to create a functional cell surface adhesion molecule, which is found on the surface of most white blood cells with the exception of neutrophils. The role of α4 integrins is to mediate cell-to-cell and cell-to-extracellular matrix interactions. VLA-4 binds to vascular cell adhesion molecule-1 (VCAM-1), a receptor found on the surface of the endothelium lining blood vessels; α4β7 binds to the mucosal addressin cell adhesion molecule-1 (MadCAM-1), found in the endothelium of the intestine.

As stated, α4 integrins play an important role in the body's inflammatory response. For leukocytes to migrate to the site of inflammation, they must traverse the endothelial layer. Under normal circumstances, leukocytes flow within the blood stream, rolling along endothelial cells and

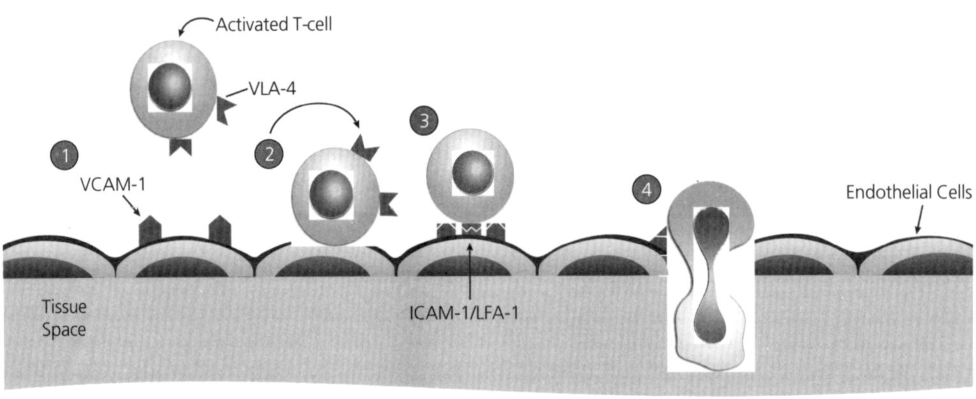

(1) The expression of various CAMs (i.e., selectins and VCAM-1) is upregulated in the presence of proinflammatory cytokines such as TNF-α and IL-1. (2) Early weak adhesion, or "rolling," is caused by the low affinity binding of selectins to their ligands. (3) The binding of VLA-4 to VCAM-1 and ICAM-1 to its ligands causes firm adhesion of the T-cell to the epithelial cells and initiates the secretion of various chemokines and (4) the migration of the T-cell across the endothelial layer (diapedesis)

CAM = Cell adhesion molecule
ICAM-1 = Intercellular adhesion molecule-1
IL-1 = Interleukin-1
LFA-1 = Lymphocyte function-associated antigen-1
TNF-α = Tumor necrosis factor-alpha
VCAM-1 = Vascular cell adhesion molecule-1
VLA-4 = Very late activation antigen-4

Figure 34.1 Schematic of VLA-4's Role in Transendothelial Migration

binding weakly to the cells' surface. During the initial stages of inflammation, VCAM-1 is upregulated on the surface of the endothelium at the site of inflammation. The α4 integrin molecule binds to VCAM-1, encouraging firm adhesion of the leukocyte to the endothelium, which in turn allows the cell to migrate through the layer. The binding of VLA-4 to VCAM-1 also stimulates the production of cytokines, which leads to the proliferation of leukocytes, thus increasing the overall inflammatory response. Blocking the interaction between VCAM-1 and VLA-4 effectively limits inflammation by preventing activated T cells from migrating across the endothelium to their target and by limiting the proliferation of leukocytes. Currently, the FDA has put a hold only on drugs that target VLA-4; therefore, we focus most of our discussion on compounds that directly affect this molecule.

MULTIPLE SCLEROSIS

In multiple sclerosis, myelin (a sheath of cells known as oligodendrocytes that insulates nerves) is the target of an autoimmune attack in which several immune components, especially activated T cells, are believed to be key players. The disease destroys myelin, leaving behind well-demarcated hypocellular areas – that is, areas with lower than normal oligodendrocyte cell counts. These hypocellular areas are called plaques. The MS market is currently dominated by IFN-β treatments from various companies and Teva Pharmaceuticals' altered peptide ligand glatiramer acetate (Copaxone) (Table 34.1).

Endothelial cells lining cerebral blood vessel walls express the VCAM protein in response to proinflammatory cytokines. Simultaneously, activated T cells begin expressing the VLA-4 protein on their surface. The VLA-4 binds to V-CAM on endothelial cells lining blood vessels; this interaction allows activated T cells to migrate through the vessel lining into the central nervous system (CNS). Currently, three drugs that are launched or in clinical development for MS target the interaction between VLA-4 and V-CAM, thereby preventing activated T-cell migration into the CNS and the subsequent destruction of myelin: Elan/Biogen Idec's natalizumab, GlaxoSmithKline/Tanabe Pharmaceuticals' 683699, and Antisense Therapeutics' ATL-1102.

Natalizumab

Natalizumab, a humanized MAb produced in murine myeloma cells, was originally developed by Elan's subsidiary, Athena Neurosciences, for treatment of MS. Natalizumab targets the α4 integrin subunit specifically, meaning it prevents the binding of both VLA-4 and α4β7 to their ligands.

In 2000, Elan and Biogen Idec (then Biogen) agreed to collaborate exclusively on development, manufacturing, and marketing of natalizumab. Elan and Biogen Idec created a stir in the MS market by announcing in February 2004 that they would file for FDA approval of natalizumab in 2004, a year earlier than expected, after evaluating preliminary, one-year results from two Phase III trials. The FDA accepted the early filing, marking the first time an MS drug was filed based on one year of results. The FDA reviewed these data rapidly – in six weeks, instead of the anticipated four to five months – and allowed Elan and Biogen Idec to submit a biologics license application (BLA). The

Table 34.1 Top-Selling Multiple Sclerosis Drugs, 2004 Worldwide Sales

Drug	*Brand/Company*	*Drug Type*	*Sales ($ MM)*
Interferon-beta-1a	Avonex/Biogen Idec	Recombinant interferon	1,415
Interferon-beta-1a	Rebif/Serono and Pfizer	Recombinant interferon	1,090
Interferon-beta-1b	Betaseron/Schering and Berlex	Recombinant interferon	970
Glatiramer acetate	Copaxone/Teva Pharmaceuticals	Altered peptide ligand	920
Mitoxantrone	Novantrone/Serono and Amgen	Chemotherapeutic agent	80

companies filed the BLA in May 2004; in June 2004, they filed a marketing authorization application (MAA) with the European Medicines Agency for the Evaluation of Medicinal Products (EMEA). The FDA granted the BLA priority review and accelerated review status; in November 2004, the company submitted second-year trial data, and the drug was approved that same month.

As part of their filing for FDA approval, Elan and Biogen Idec submitted data from two multicenter, randomized, placebo-controlled, double-blind Phase III trials of natalizumab for relapsing-remitting MS (RRMS). The first was a two-year study known as Antegren Safety and Efficacy in RRMS (AFFIRM), which aimed to determine whether natalizumab monotherapy is effective in reducing the number of relapses and slowing the rate of disability in RRMS patients; the second was the two-year safety and efficacy of natalizumab in combination with Avonex (SENTINEL) trial, which sought to determine whether treatment with natalizumab in combination with Avonex is more effective in reducing the number of relapses and slowing the rate of disability in RRMS patients than treatment with Avonex alone.

In February 2005, two patients in the SENTINEL trial who had been receiving natalizumab and Avonex for two years developed PML. Consequently, Elan and Biogen Idec chose to withdraw natalizumab from the market until a determination of the potential health risk associated with treatment could be made.

After the withdrawal, in April 2005, the two-year results from the AFFIRM trial and the one-year results from the SENTINEL trial were published. Both trials met all primary and secondary end points. The AFFIRM trial showed a reduction of 67% in the rate of relapses relative to placebo and a reduction of 42% in disability progression at two years compared with placebo; the SENTINEL trial showed that natalizumab plus Avonex produced a 54% reduction in clinical relapses at one year over Avonex alone. No information was released on the reduction of disability in the SENTINEL trial. In comparison, other MS drugs reduce the relapse rate by approximately one-third (18–32%) in clinical trials. Natalizumab as a monotherapy also showed a slightly better reduction of disability than other MS drugs. Neither study showed any severe safety issues, although the AFFIRM trial showed a slight increase in the risk of infection over placebo; the patients who developed PML had not developed the disease within the first year of treatment. Biogen Idec and Elan's reinvestigation of the natalizumab studies is ongoing; the companies hope to have the results in late summer 2005.

Ultimately, the mechanism that makes natalizumab so effective is likely to be the reason patients may be at risk for developing opportunistic infections. By blocking VLA-4, activated T cells are prevented from reaching the site of infection, making the patient more vulnerable to opportunistic infection.

683699/T-0047

GlaxoSmithKline (GSK) and Tanabe Pharmaceuticals have been developing 683699 (also known as T-0047) for the treatment of MS and inflammatory bowel disease (IBD). 683699 is being developed as an oral formulation; if approved, it would become one of the first oral treatment options for MS. 683699 targets the α4 integrin subunit, thereby blocking leukocyte trafficking into disease tissues. GSK and Tanabe have stated that while 683699 has the same molecular target as natalizumab, 683699 is in a different class of agents and is chemically unrelated. However, the safety issues associated with natalizumab are likely due to the blocking of the α4 integrin subunit; therefore, the safety concerns would seem to apply to 683699 as well. Early clinical trials showed that 683699 has pharmacodynamic activity comparable to that of natalizumab. In late 2004, GSK initiated Phase II trials for MS and CD, and the company expected to file for approval in 2008. In March 2005, a GSK spokesman stated that the FDA was taking the precautionary measure of halting all clinical trials of VLA-4 antagonist drugs. The Phase II trial was halted as a result of the FDA clinical hold, as the FDA assessed the cases of PML in natalizumab-treated patients. At this time, there has been no evidence of opportunistic infections (including PML) in patients taking 683699.

ATL-1102

Antisense Therapeutics is developing ATL-1102 for treatment of MS and other inflammatory diseases. ATL-1102 is an antisense nucleotide therapy that targets the α4 integrin mRNA. Antisense Therapeutics exclusively licensed the agent from Isis Pharmaceuticals in December 2001, and Phase IIa trials were initiated in December 2004. Preliminary data from the Phase I trials showed that the agent has a favorable safety profile and is generally well tolerated by patients. In response to safety concerns, Antisense has suspended clinical trials of ATL-1102 and has assembled an advisory committee to determine the agent's future in the treatment of MS.

The Future of VLA-4 Antagonists in MS

The future development and commercialization of VLA-4 antagonists for MS rests first in the hands of the FDA, which will need to determine whether to allow natalizumab to reenter the market and whether to lift its hold on clinical trials of drugs in development. Given the need for more efficacious treatments to slow the progression of MS and natalizumab's considerable level of efficacy, and assuming the FDA does determine that it will approve drugs in this class, we believe it is likely that natalizumab will return as a treatment for MS, albeit as a second-line therapy with a restricted patient population and a black-box warning. The recent suggestion that the JC virus could be monitored for appearance in patients' bloodstreams and natalizumab treatment halted in time to prevent the PML virus from infecting the CNS has slightly increased the drug's chances of returning to the market for treatment of MS (Berger and Kolnalwick, 2005).

While it is unlikely that natalizumab will return to the market as a first-line therapy for patients with RRMS, the drug will likely become an alternative for patients who are not responding to interferon therapy and/or those who are rapidly progressing toward the secondary progressive stage of the disease. In addition, screening for the JC virus may be a requirement for patients prior to beginning treatment with natalizumab and throughout the therapy, and the agent may be contraindicated for use with other immunosuppressants. Natalizumab's efficacy in reducing the debilitating effects of MS is superior to that of available therapies; physicians and patients will need to determine on a case-by-case basis what constitutes an acceptable risk.

Given that current MS treatment options are all injectables, an oral formulation is likely to have a strong competitive advantage owing to its convenience. For this reason, we believe that GSK and Tanabe will continue with the development of 683699, provided the FDA releases its hold on the clinical trials. If the drug can demonstrate efficacy comparable to that of natalizumab, its improved formulation makes it likely that 683699 will claim a portion of natalizumab's sales, and the companies have enough capital and strong-enough pipelines to wait out the clinical hold. In contrast, the mechanism of action pursued by Antisense Therapeutics' ATL-1102 may create greater health risks, given that preventing the transcription of the α4 subunit mRNA will eliminate the formation of several α4β dimers (e.g., α4β7), not just β1, and affect multiple biological functions in the body. For this reason, the compound may have trouble gaining any significant market share over both natalizumab and 683699. Therefore, as a smaller company with a less-robust pipeline (four compounds in development, including ATL-1102), it seems unlikely that Antisense Therapeutics will choose to expend its resources to develop and market an agent with significant competition and increased safety concerns.

Should the FDA decide that it will not approve VLA-4 antagonists, or if patients and physicians are unwilling to accept the risks associated with natalizumab, we believe that treatment for MS will continue in the short term as it has in the past, with the IFN-β class of drugs (Biogen Idec's Avonex, Schering/Berlex's Betaseron, Serono/Pfizer's Rebif) and glatiramer acetate (Teva Pharmaceuticals' Copaxane) taking the largest percentage of the MS market. Biogen Idec will continue to be a significant player in this market, but Avonex will progressively lose patient share to Rebif, perceived as more efficacious among the IFN-β agents, and the company will no longer have the sales of natalizumab to maintain its overall MS market share. Chemotherapeutics such as mitoxantrone (Serono/Amgen's Novantrone), which are an option for patients in advanced stages of MS, would likely have been negatively impacted by the VLA-4 antagonists because these agents would theoretically reduce the number of patients whose disease progresses within a given time period. Without the VLA-4 antagonists, the market share of these agents is likely to stay stable. Currently, no other MS drug in late-stage development is likely to have the same impact on disease therapy as the VLA-4 antagonists.

CROHN'S DISEASE

Crohn's disease is a chronic, relapsing/remitting inflammatory disease of the gastrointestinal (GI) tract. Common symptoms of the disease include diarrhea, abdominal pain, rectal bleeding, and weight loss; complications include intestinal abscesses, fistulas, and intestinal obstructions. The cause of CD is unclear, but one hypothesis holds that it is caused by an overreaction of the immune system to the presence of antigens in the GI tract. The human GI tract is routinely exposed to antigens through food and through the body's natural flora; in normal persons, this exposure generally results in an undetectable immune response. The inflammatory response associated with CD is believed to be driven by the activation of T cells, which are assisted through the GI tract's epithelial layer by α4β7 molecules. Drugs that inhibit integrin α4β7 are viewed as potential therapeutic candidates for CD. Treatment for CD is aimed at either inducing remission (induction) or preventing future attacks (maintenance). CD is most often treated with aminosalicylates, immunosuppressants, or corticosteroids; occasionally, a tumor necrosis factor-alpha (TNF-α) inhibitor is used to treat patients with severe, treatment-refractory disease (Table 34.2).

Because natalizumab targets the integrin α4 subunit, Biogen Idec and Elan were investigating the drug as a potential treatment for CD; prior to its withdrawal, it was in Phase III clinical trials. Results from earlier studies in CD patients had shown a positive effect in eliminating symptoms, but its efficacy did not surpass that of the TNF-α inhibitor infliximab (Centocor/Schering-Plough/Tanabe Seiyaku's Remicade), currently the only biological agent approved for treatment of CD. Physicians have expressed concerns about the long-term safety of infliximab and the possibility of opportunistic infections such as tuberculosis. Because initial studies of natalizumab had shown an improved safety profile compared with infliximab, natalizumab had the potential to position itself as a safer, if slightly less effective, biological treatment option. At this time, natalizumab will likely be marketed for treatment of CD in the United States but is less likely to launch in

Table 34.2 Top-Selling Crohn's Disease Therapies, 2004 Worldwide Sales

Drug	*Brand/Company*	*Drug Type*	*Sales ($ MM)*
Infliximab	Remicade/Centocor, Schering-Plough, and Tanabe Seiyaku	TNF-α inhibitor	2,960
Enteric-coated mesalamine	Asacol/Procter & Gamble	Oral mesalamine	430
Ethylcellulose-coated mesalamine	Pentasa/Shire Pharmaceuticals and Ferring Pharmaceuticals	Oral mesalamine	295
6-Mercaptopurine	Purinethol/GlaxoSmithKline and Teva	Immunosuppressant	35
Budesonide	Entocort /AstraZeneca	Corticosteroid	30

other markets for treatment of this indication. Treatment with this agent will most likely be reserved for patients who have failed all other treatment options; its use with other immunosuppressants may be contraindicated and JC virus screening may be required prior to beginning treatment. Natalizumab's chances of success will be most enhanced if the drug is positioned as a treatment for induction of remission rather than for long-term maintenance. Marketing natalizumab as an induction therapy will address some of the primary concerns associated with this agent – specifically, its cost and the risk of opportunistic infections associated with long-term use.

Initially, physicians were optimistic about the potential of anti-integrin for treatment of CD, and other agents in this class were in development for this indication. GSK and Tanabe were testing 683699 in Phase II clinical trials for the treatment of CD, and Millennium Pharmaceuticals was developing MLN-02, an integrin α4β7 antagonist, for the treatment of ulcerative colitis (UC) and CD. However, at this time, the future of α4 antagonist drugs as a therapeutic option for CD is uncertain. Although natalizumab showed positive efficacy in treating CD, MLN-02 failed to meet its primary end point (inducing remission) in Phase II clinical trials for treatment of CD, which may indicate that this agent has insufficient therapeutic effect to replace existing therapies. In addition, one of the principal reasons infliximab remains a third-line therapy for CD is the high cost of the treatment. It is unlikely that any new biological agent will be marketed at a price point low enough to lure physicians and patients away from the existing first- and second-line therapies.

ASTHMA

Asthma is a chronic lung disorder in which inflammation causes bouts of breathlessness, wheezing, and coughing. Asthma is thought to be caused by both genetic and environmental factors, with the majority of cases exhibiting a hypersensitivity to an environmental allergen that results in a heightened immune response and increased inflammation of the airways. T-cell migration into the airways via the interaction of VLA-4 with its ligand is a necessary step in the inflammatory response and therefore has been under investigation by several companies as a potentially new mechanism for treating asthma. VLA-4 and α4β7 receptors have been shown to be more highly expressed in asthmatic patients. The most common current asthma therapies include corticosteroid/beta-2 agonist combinations, inhaled corticosteroids, and leukotriene antagonists (Table 34.3).

Roche's R-411 is a dual antagonist, targeting both VLA-4 and α4β7. The drug is slated to be a once-daily oral treatment, a formulation physicians prefer to inhalants because it improves patient compliance. The agent began Phase II clinical trials in 2002, including a dosing study, a study comparing R-411 with inhaled corticosteroids, and a pediatric safety and pharmacokinetics in chronic asthma study. Phase II studies of the drug had been completed prior to the FDA hold, and Roche announced its intention to continue with a Phase IIb trial of the drug, based on the Phase II efficacy results and

Table 34.3 Top-Selling Asthma Therapies, 2004 Worldwide Sales

Drug	*Brand/Company*	*Drug Type*	*Sales ($ MM)*
Fluticasone	Advair/GlaxoSmithKline	Corticosteroid/beta-2 agonist combinations	4,470
Montelukast	Singulair/Merck	Leukotriene antagonists	2,620
Budesonide	Pulmicort/AstraZeneca	Inhaled corticosteroid	1,050
Fluticasone propionate	Flovent/GlaxoSmithKline	Inhaled corticosteroid	1,130
Omalizumab	Xolair/Genentech, Novartis, Sankyo, and Tanox Biosystems	Anti-IgE agent	185

R-411's safety and tolerability profile. No major adverse effects were found during the trial. Because the drug is an α4 integrin antagonist, any continuing concerns about its safety will likely delay the progression of this agent into Phase IIb trials. Although Roche has not made any statements regarding the safety concerns raised by the FDA, the company had earlier stated that it would be filing for approval in 2007; however, in May 2005, the company projected a post-2008 filing.

Currently, more α4 integrin antagonists are under development for the treatment of asthma than for any other indication. However, progress on these agents has been slow. Prior to its merger with Sanofi-Synthélabo, Aventis had two VLA-4 antagonists in Phase II clinical trials: IVL-745 and 1031, both inhaler formulations. Both agents entered Phase IIa clinical trials in 2002, but no new information on these studies or the status of these compounds has been released since then. Ranbaxy has RBx-7796 (clafrinast) in Phase I proof-of-concept studies; in January 2005, the company announced that no safety or tolerability issues had been reported. In addition, Encysive Pharmaceuticals has several VLA-4 antagonists in development for the treatment of asthma, including an oral compound licensed by Schering-Plough in 2002.

The size of the asthma market (approximately 20 million people in the United States, according to the American Lung Association) and the fact that the disease is chronic, requiring long-term therapy, makes it an attractive candidate for drug development. The challenge for developers is that most physicians view the level of unmet need in this area as relatively low because existing therapies are highly effective and have well-documented safety profiles. Therefore, physicians tend to be conservative about prescribing new products. To draw a significant number of physicians away from proven therapies, any product new to the asthma market will need to prove either improved dosing convenience that enhances compliance or success in treating the subset of patients who respond poorly to inhaled corticosteroids. VLA-4 antagonists offer a novel strategy for treatment of asthma, but the strategy is as yet untested; some physicians – prior to the report of problems associated with natalizumab – expressed concerns about the possibility of opportunistic infection based on the agents' mechanism of action. The concern about infection, especially associated with long-term use of VLA-4 antagonists, will need to be thoroughly addressed by any company attempting to market such a drug for asthma. Despite this concern, we believe that the development of VLA-4 antagonists for the treatment of asthma is likely to continue, provided that the FDA chooses to approve these agents. However, at the least, the safety concerns may slow the progress of these agents to market or make companies more likely to abandon candidates that show only modest efficacy for this indication.

THE REGULATORY PROCESS: INCREASED SCRUTINY WILL LEAD TO CHANGE

The decision to place a hold on another drug in the VLA-4 antagonist class due to complications associated with natalizumab is an unusual move for the FDA. At this time, there has been no definitive evidence that the problems associated with natalizumab are a class effect, and the agent placed on hold has shown no evidence of PML. While the severity of adverse events associated with natalizumab suggests caution when evaluating agents in this class, the FDA's decision to halt the trials entirely was likely influenced by the criticism it has received as a result of other recent, high-profile drug withdrawals, such as the withdrawals of the cyclooxygenase (COX)-2 inhibitors rofecoxib (Merck's Vioxx) and valdecoxib (Pfizer's Bextra). These problems have increased the scrutiny of the FDA approval process, causing legislators and public interest groups to question whether significant reform is necessary. The subsequent public discussion has generated a variety of recommendations for changing the regulatory process:

- Slow down the approval process by reducing the number of accelerated approvals and fast-tracked drugs.
- Make information associated with clinical trials more transparent to the public.
- Increase the FDA's control over drug labeling and require approval for direct-to-consumer (DTC) advertising.
- Control the number of industry-sponsored physicians on FDA advisory boards.

Since 2001, in part due to previous criticism that the FDA was not approving drugs quickly enough for life-threatening illnesses such as HIV infection and cancer, the number of new drug applications (NDAs) approved by the FDA has increased by 36%, while the average time for approval has declined by 29% (Figure 34.2). Although many factors influence the speed and the volume of approvals, proponents of FDA reform claim that this trend indicates reduced analysis of the compounds requesting approval. If a drug receives accelerated approval, it is likely that the review process began prior to completion of all Phase III clinical trials, as it did for natalizumab, which submitted one year of Phase III data in May 2004 and did not submit second-year data until November 2004, the same month the drug was approved.

It is possible that the FDA will begin demanding more clinical trial data prior to review, greatly reducing the number of drugs that receive accelerated approval. In addition, the FDA may begin demanding an increased number of postmarketing studies and begin putting improved systems in place to track and review the data gathered from approved drugs. Given the evidence that fewer than half of postmarketing studies are completed, Congress will likely review the FDA's handling of postmarketing studies and has proposed the Patient Protection Act of 2005, which will impose a fine of up to $10,000 a day on companies that do not comply with FDA-mandated postmarketing studies.

The implication in demanding increased amounts of clinical trial data is that more data, obtained either by increasing the number or length of clinical trials, will increase the likelihood that rare adverse events will be caught. However, the benefit of increasing the number of clinical trials is debatable. While it is possible that an increased number of adverse events may be detected by gathering more clinical trial data, it is unlikely that truly rare events will be identified with increased regularity. Increasing the length of clinical trials will

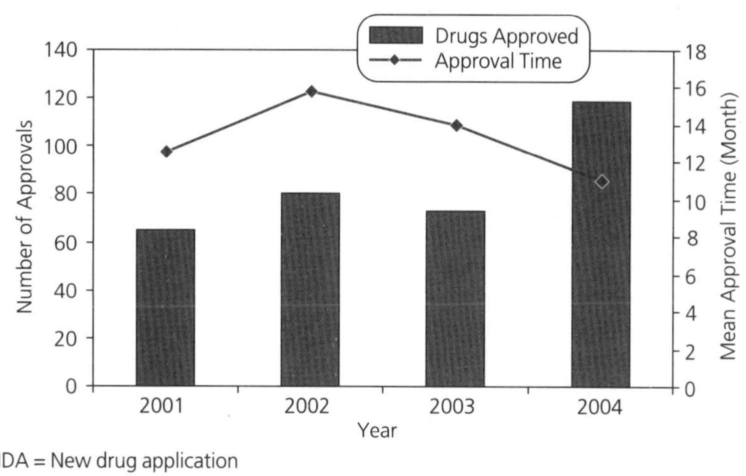

Figure 34.2 Yearly NDA Approvals and Approval Time

greatly raise the cost of bringing a drug to market, particularly for indications for which clinical trial time is historically shorter (such as asthma) and reduce the amount of time a drug is on the market under patent protection. Demanding long-term clinical data may be enough of a financial burden to dissuade drug companies from pursuing novel therapeutic options. Perhaps most importantly, the length of time necessary for new therapies to reach the patient will be increased. The consequences of demanding increased clinical trial data will be seen most frequently in therapeutic areas where there is a high unmet need for treatments. Currently, emerging drugs in these areas are more likely to receive fast-track approval than drugs indicated for diseases where many efficacious treatments are already available, such as asthma. Nonetheless, we believe that in the short term, the FDA will begin demanding more Phase III data prior to review.

The issues surrounding natalizumab come on the heels of other setbacks for the pharmaceutical industry (specifically, the questions about antidepressant use and the problems associated with the COX-2 inhibitors), which have created the perception that the public is not being fully educated in the risks associated with emerging therapies. One solution proposed for this issue is to increase the transparency of clinical trial data. Historically, pharmaceutical companies have been reluctant to fully disclose all clinical trial data, primarily to prevent competitors from using the data. This attitude has been changing over the past year, with large pharma companies, including Eli Lilly, Roche, and GSK, creating Web sites where clinical trial information can be seen by the public. Lawmakers in the United States and the United Kingdom have proposed bills mandating that all clinical trial data be publicly available. In June of 2005, the state of Maine passed one of the first bills of this type: the governor of Maine signed a bill that requires all drug companies that do business in the state to fully disclose all clinical trial data back to 2002. Given patients' demands to fully understand the risks associated with therapies and the pharmaceutical companies' need to maintain their reputations and minimize their vulnerability to litigation, we expect that the amount of clinical trial data that is made available to the public will continue to increase.

The role of DTC advertising in educating the public about the risks involved in a therapy is also a matter of concern for consumer groups, physicians, and legislators. DTC advertising has proved to be a successful marketing approach for drug companies – but critics believe that DTC ads do not provide enough information about dangers that may be associated with a therapy and call for increased scrutiny by the FDA. Currently, the FDA reviews all DTC advertisements prior to their release, and according to a 2002 congressional report by the Government Accountability Office (GAO), the FDA is generally effective in enforcing the removal of misleading information from advertisements it reviews. However, the agency does not have the resources to expunge all misleading information, and given the success of this marketing strategy, it seems likely that DTC advertising will continue to increase. A Kaiser Family Foundation study released in June 2003 estimated that for every dollar spent in DTC advertising for prescription drugs, sales increased by $4.20. DTC advertising was responsible for 12% of the overall growth in pharmaceutical sales in 2000.

It seems unlikely that the FDA will be in position to increase its review of DTC advertising. However, we believe that drug companies will be increasingly cautious in their design of DTC ads. Recent problems with drugs such as rofecoxib and valdecoxib have generated an increasingly negative view of the drug development industry. This trend is likely to motivate drug companies to fully educate patients about the possible risks associated with a therapy in order to mitigate the possibility of negative publicity and expensive lawsuits resulting from adverse events.

THE FUTURE OF VLA-4 ANTAGONISTS

Although VLA-4 antagonists present a novel therapeutic approach for many indications, the future of their clinical development and commercialization remains uncertain. The development of opportunistic infections as a result of treatment with natalizumab did not come as a surprise to researchers; many have acknowledged that the possibility always existed with this type of immune suppression. The future of natalizumab and other VLA-4 antagonists will depend on several factors:

- Determination of the level of risk associated with natalizumab and the rest of this class of drugs.
- Changes in the FDA regulatory process intended to decrease the risks associated with approved drugs while continuing to make new treatments available for diseases with high unmet need.
- Examination of the risk/benefit ratio associated with the use of VLA-4 therapy vis-à-vis the unmet needs of a particular indication.

For natalizumab, provided it is allowed to reenter the market, its efficacy in the treatment of MS means it is likely to remain a therapeutic option for some patients, particularly when combined with increased education of patients and physicians about the potential risks. The interest of MS patients in seeing this agent return to the market is highlighted by the positions of special interest groups such as the small but well-organized National Multiple Sclerosis Society, a research organization that supports the drug's return. For other indications, the efficacy of the drug may not be sufficient to overcome the potential risks. Ultimately, the drug will be unlikely to achieve the potential anticipated by both its developers and analysts when it was launched.

For compounds in development, the future hinges on whether the adverse reactions seen with natalizumab use are associated with natalizumab specifically or with use of any drug in this class. In addition, it remains to be seen whether significant risk exists only when these agents are used in combination with other immunosuppressants. Should the problems be associated only with natalizumab or with its use as combination therapy, VLA-4 antagonists will likely remain attractive candidates for drug development, with potential applications to a wide range of diseases in which inflammation plays a critical role. If, however, the adverse effects are determined to be class-related, we believe that development will continue – but in areas of high unmet need where the risks of not receiving treatment outweigh the risks of therapy.

REFERENCES

Berger, J. and Kolnalwick I. Progressive multifocal leukoencephalopathy and natalizumab – unforeseen consequences. *New England Journal of Medicine.* 2005;352 www.nejm.com (electronic).

Van Assche, G. Progressive multifocal leukoencephalopathy after natalizumab therapy for Crohn's disease [electronic]. *New England Journal of Medicine.* 2005; 352 www.nejm.com.

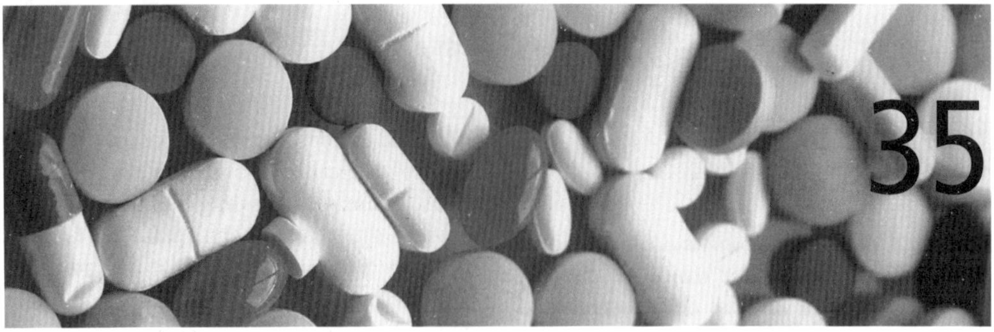

Impact of Inhaled Insulin on the Insulin Market

INTRODUCTION

There is considerable need for an insulin delivery system that will eliminate the requirement for multiple daily injections in type 1 and type 2 diabetes patients. Recognition of this need has prompted several companies to begin developing less-invasive methods of insulin administration. The first of these alternative methods is an inhaled formulation of rapid-acting insulin, Pfizer's Exubera, launched in the US market in September 2006. The advent of this technology has the potential to impact the insulin market significantly by adding new players and may change medical practice as barriers to the initiation of insulin therapy are lowered.

This chapter provides an overview of current insulin therapy, including various delivery devices, and a review of insulin use in the treatment of diabetes. We provide detailed information on Exubera, the first inhaled-insulin product to come to market. Several other inhaled-insulins are in late-stage development; we discuss each of these agents, including details of crucial business transactions associated with each agent. Finally, we describe inhaled insulin's likely effect on the overall insulin market.

OVERVIEW OF INSULIN THERAPY

Mechanism of Action

Insulin is an endocrine hormone secreted by the beta cells of the pancreatic islets of Langerhans in response to elevated blood levels of glucose, fatty acids, ketone bodies, and amino acids. Insulin has two key functions in maintaining health: it signals the body that it has been fed, and it promotes efficient storage and consumption of energy sources and nutrients. It carries out the latter function by controlling the transport of glucose, amino acids, and fatty acids across cellular membranes. Insulin also promotes the synthesis of several important substances, including glycogen (the form in which glucose is stored in the liver), proteins, and lipids. In diabetics, an insulin deficit (most common in type 1 diabetes) or insulin resistance (most common in type 2 diabetes) results in a hyperglycemic state that can engender microvascular and macrovascular complications (retinopathy, nephropathy, metabolic syndrome). In diabetic patients, exogenous insulin replaces or augments the action of endogenous insulin, but manufactured insulin cannot mimic the pancreas's response to changes in blood glucose levels.

Types of Insulin Manufactured

To achieve and maintain glycemic control, insulin therapy generally has two components: treatment with a long-acting agent to maintain basal levels of insulin during fasting periods and a bolus treatment of faster-acting insulin taken before meals. Manufactured insulins can be categorized by their onset of action: long-acting, intermediate-acting, and short-acting; we describe each type in detail in the following sections.

The first insulins to reach the market were derived from animals, specifically cows and pigs. Since the advent of recombinant technology, however, these early insulin products have been replaced by recombinant human products manufactured in genetically engineered bacteria. The human insulin produced by these bacteria is altered to achieve the desired onset of action. Most recently, companies have developed insulin analogues, recombinant products in which key amino acids are substituted for other amino acids in order to achieve a specific release profile. Currently, insulin analogues are available only in long-acting and short-acting formulations.

Long-acting Insulins

Long-acting insulin and insulin analogues are used to maintain basal levels of insulin throughout the day. In recent years, the use of long-acting human insulin (such as Eli Lilly's Humulin U) has been overtaken by use of a long-acting insulin analogue, Sanofi-Aventis's Lantus (insulin glargine). Lantus has shown considerable benefit compared with long-acting human insulins: its onset of action is considerably shorter (one hour versus more than six hours), and its flat absorption rate and consistent duration of action make Lantus the most predictable of the long-acting insulin products. The success of Lantus compared with other products in this category is highlighted by Lilly's 2005 decision to discontinue production of Humulin U, citing declining sales and a dwindling patient share.

Intermediate-acting Insulins

Intermediate-acting insulins are also intended to maintain basal levels of insulin. These insulins generally contain zinc or NPH (Neutral Protamine Hagedorn) in order to delay the product's release. In general, these products have a duration of action of 14–18 hours and an onset of activity of 1–3 hours. Intermediate-acting insulins gained popularity because of their predictability of release compared with long-acting insulins, but insulin glargine (Lantus) has proved to be more predictable than the intermediate-acting products.

Most marketed intermediate-acting products use NPH to regulate their release. Although products that use zinc have a better release profile and fewer adverse allergic reactions, they are incompatible with regular human insulin (short-acting), which is generally required for bolus treatments before meals. Lilly discontinued its zinc product (Humulin L) and Humulin U at the same time. Both Lilly and Novo Nordisk market NPH insulins: Humulin N and Novolin N, respectively. Although there are combination products (fixed-dose combinations of short- and intermediate-acting insulins) that contain intermediate-acting insulin analogues, no intermediate-acting insulin analogues are currently available as monotherapies.

Short-acting Insulins

Short-acting insulins are the best mimic of the form of insulin found in the body. These agents have a duration of action of 4–8 hours and are most often used as a bolus dose of insulin before meals. Recombinant human insulin (or regular insulin) is identical to the insulin naturally produced by a healthy pancreas, but because it is stored in a container rather than secreted directly into the bloodstream, the insulin molecules may cluster into dimers or hexamers. Because the body absorbs these aggregates more slowly than single insulin molecules, onset of action is delayed. Therefore, patients must administer regular human insulin 30–60 minutes before a meal to ensure that sufficient levels of insulin will be available when glucose from the meal reaches the bloodstream.

The two short-acting insulin analogues on the market, Lilly's Humalog (insulin lispro) and Novo Nordisk's NovoLog (insulin aspart), prevent the creation of dimers and hexamers, thereby shortening the time to onset of action. Clinical trials have shown these agents to be comparable if not slightly superior to regular human insulin. In addition, the short onset of action allows patients to take the insulin immediately before eating, which increases the convenience of these agents.

Drug Delivery

Insulin is measured in international insulin units; 22 units have the activity equivalent of 1 mg of zinc-insulin crystals. Insulin bottles are labeled according to the number of units in one milliliter of liquid: a 100U bottle contains a concentration of 100 units/mL. Before Exubera became available, all insulin products were administered by subcutaneous injection. (The one exception is Generex Biotechnology's Oral-lyn, an orally administered insulin approved only in Ecuador.) Injections can be administered using one of three devices:

- *Syringes*: Syringes are the most common and economical method of administration. Syringes can be disposable, and the most recent versions come with a specially coated needle that minimizes the pain of the injection. Bottled insulin is used with syringes.
- *Pens*: A variation on the syringe, pens use prefilled cartridges of insulin. Patients set dosage by using a dial on the side of the pen. Pen injections are considered less painful than traditional syringe injections. Pens come in both disposable and reusable forms and are more expensive than syringes.
- *Pumps*: Pumps deliver insulin injections throughout the day through a catheter into the abdomen. They can be programmed to deliver bolus injections before meals or small injections throughout the day to maintain a basal insulin level. Only short-acting insulins and insulin analogues can be used in pumps.

Insulin pens are steadily gaining popularity because of their small size and less-painful injections. There are also short- and intermediate-acting combination cartridges that may reduce the number of injections required each day. Pumps are considered a significant step forward in delivery technology; they do not require multiple needle sticks throughout the day, and they provide the tightest control over insulin levels. However, the expense of these devices is a drawback, and they are well suited only for patients who are willing to monitor their insulin levels and pump activity regularly throughout the day.

Use of Insulin in the Treatment of Diabetes

Type 1 Diabetes

Insulin is the primary therapy for patients with type 1 diabetes. Although some adjunct medications (such as Amylin's Symlin) are available, and physicians advise patients to make appropriate diet and lifestyle changes, the lack of endogenous insulin requires the use of exogenous insulin. The most common form of insulin therapy is the bolus-basal approach: bolus injections of rapid-acting insulin prior to meals and one or two daily injections of an intermediate- or long-acting insulin. Dosage varies from patient to patient; the goal is to achieve a level of insulin that best mimics the activity of a healthy pancreas. Patients with type 1 diabetes are required to monitor their blood glucose levels daily to ensure maintenance of healthy levels.

Type 2 Diabetes

For type 2 diabetics, insulin therapy is not a first-line treatment. Initial treatments for type 2 diabetics include weight control, lifestyle modifications, and treatment with an oral antidiabetic agent such as a sulfonylurea, biguanide, or peroxisome proliferator-activated receptor-gamma (PPAR-gamma) agonist. Insulin therapy is generally initiated only after failure to achieve glycemic control with two or three oral antidiabetics. Historically, physicians have hesitated to begin type 2 patients on insulin therapy because they worry that insulin resistance might increase or because they want to postpone the need for daily injections. However, evidence continues to support the use of insulin in type 2 patients to mitigate some of the long-term complications of the disease.

The 2005 launch of Amylin and Eli Lilly's glucagon-like peptide-1 (GLP-1) analogue Byetta (exenatide) could significantly alter the course of insulin therapy in type 2 diabetics. Byetta stimulates insulin secretion and has been shown to preserve pancreatic beta-cell mass in animal models. The agent has the additional benefit of promoting patient weight loss, thereby greatly increasing its benefit. Byetta is indicated for patients who cannot maintain glycemic control with metformin or sulfonylureas. Treatment with this agent may delay or eliminate the need to begin insulin therapy in some patients. Although the agent is injectable, like insulin, Byetta's additional benefits overcome the inconvenient formulation, and Byetta has experienced wide uptake since its launch. Additionally, Amylin and Lilly are developing an extended-release version of Byetta that would require injection only once a week, thereby lowering remaining physician barriers to prescribing the agent.

THE INSULIN MARKET

According to the 2005 data, worldwide sales of insulin products exceeded $7.5 billion in 2005, accounting for approximately 45% of the overall antidiabetic market. Growth of the insulin market over the last five years has been considerable: 18% per year since 2000, outpacing the overall antidiabetic market by approximately 6% (Figure 35.1). This strong market growth does not appear to reflect a significant increase in the number of patients taking insulin; more likely, it indicates that a larger percentage of patients are switching to the comparatively more expensive insulin analogues, particularly insulin glargine,

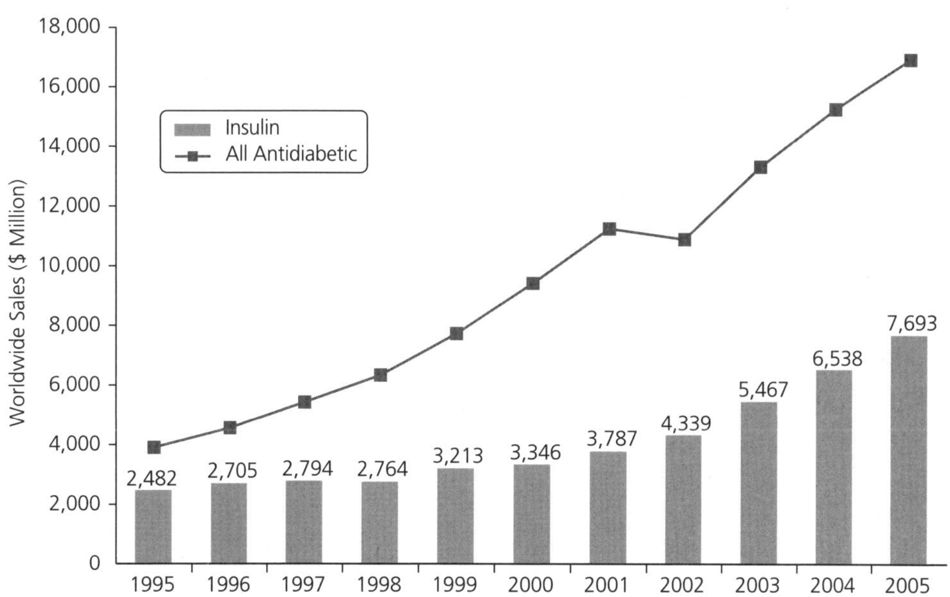

Figure 35.1 Growth of the Insulin and Antidiabetic Markets, 1995–2005

Table 35.1 Top-Selling Insulin Products, 2005

Product	*Company*	*2005 Worldwide Sales ($MM)*
Lantus (insulin glargine)	Sanofi-Aventis	1,510
Humalog (insulin lispro)	Eli Lilly	1,198
Insulin analogues (Novolin, NovoRapid/NovoLog, NovoMix)	Novo Nordisk	1,130
Humulin R (human insulin)	Eli Lilly	1,005
Insuman (human insulin)	Sanofi-Aventis	218
Levemir (insulin detemir)	Novo Nordisk	88
Iletin (bovine and porcine insulin)	Eli Lilly	18
Apidra (insulin glulisine)	Sanofi-Aventis	16

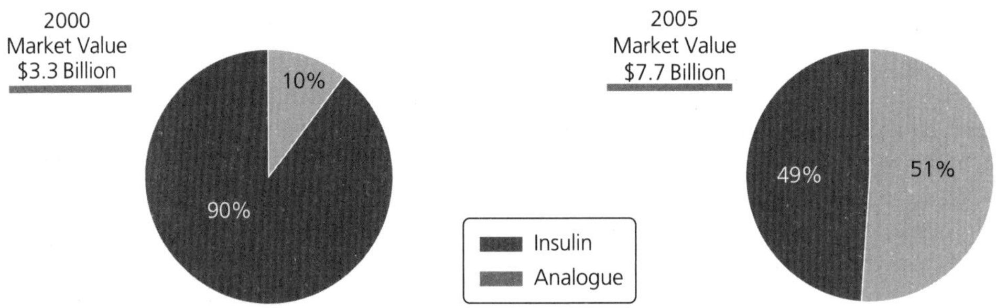

Figure 35.2 Expansion of Sales of Insulin Analogues, 2000–5

which has had strong adoption since its launch in 2000.

Sales of the top-selling insulin products in the same year 2005 can be seen in Table 35.1. Sales of insulin analogues have grown steadily over the past five years, increasing from 12% of insulin sales in 2000 to 51% of sales in 2005 (Figure 35.2). Of the insulin analogues, Sanofi-Aventis's Lantus (insulin glargine) was the best-selling product, with $1.5 billion in 2005 sales worldwide.

Novo Nordisk dominates the insulin product market; the company has maintained a 48% market share for the past 10 years. Eli Lilly is also a strong presence in the market; after the launch of Humalog in 1996, the company's market share rose steadily, reaching its peak in 2002 with 45% of market share. Since then, however, Lilly's share has fallen to pre-Humalog levels (about 38%). The most likely cause of this decline is the launch of Lantus in 2000, which has established Sanofi-Aventis as a significant competitor in the market.

EXUBERA

How Exubera Works

Pfizer's Exubera is a fast-acting recombinant human insulin intended for use as bolus insulin prior to meals. The agent is formulated as a dry powder that is inhaled through a specifically designed inhaler. Pfizer describes the inhaler as being "the size of an eyeglasses case" when closed; however, it is considerably larger when opened and in use (about 12 inches long). The insulin is packaged in 1 mg and 3 mg "blisters." The user inserts the insulin into the inhaler; presses a button, thereby converting the powder to a vapor; and then inhales slowly. In clinical studies, Exubera was absorbed as quickly as rapid-acting insulin analogues; therefore, it should be taken within 10 minutes before eating.

Development History

The Exubera delivery system was initially developed by Nektar Therapeutics (formerly

Inhale Therapeutic Systems). In January 1995, Nektar announced that it would collaborate with Pfizer on the development and marketing of Exubera. According to the agreement, Pfizer would manage the clinical development of the product and provide financial support for R&D, with Nektar supplying both the inhaler and the insulin powder. Pfizer acquired all commercialization rights to Exubera, with Nektar receiving milestone payments and royalties on product sales.

Exubera began Phase II clinical trials in the first quarter of 1996 (details of clinical trials are given in the following section). In 1998, Pfizer and Hoechst Marion Roussel (now Sanofi-Aventis) announced an agreement to codevelop and copromote Exubera worldwide. Under the terms of the agreement, Hoechst provided Nektar with insulin to be converted to powder form, and Hoechst and Pfizer jointly built an insulin-manufacturing facility in Germany. In January 2006, Pfizer announced that it had reacquired all development and promotion rights to Exubera from Sanofi-Aventis and the manufacturing facility as well, paying Sanofi-Aventis $1.3 billion.

Pfizer conducted numerous Phase III trials to support Exubera's safety and efficacy, including a long-term study that investigated its pulmonary effects. Pfizer filed a market authorization application (MAA) with the European Medicines Agency (EMEA) in early 2004; a new drug application (NDA) to the FDA followed in early 2005. The Exubera review date was initially planned for fall of that year, but the FDA delayed its decision in order to review additional data. In late January 2006, Exubera received approval from both the FDA and the EMEA. The FDA required that Pfizer conduct several postmarketing studies to determine Exubera's long-term effect on lung function.

Exubera's introduction to the market has not gone smoothly. Its launch was initially intended for July of 2006, but in late July, Pfizer announced that it was delaying the launch to allow sufficient time to train physicians and patients. The launch was rescheduled for September. In addition, the US Institute for Safe Medication Practices (a nonprofit watchdog group) issued a warning about Exubera concerning the possibility of confusion about dosing: unlike injectable insulin, Exubera measures its doses in milligrams instead of units. Potentially, the biggest roadblock to Exubera's launch was Novo Nordisk's patent-infringement lawsuit, filed in August. In addition to requesting compensatory damages, the lawsuit requested that Pfizer be blocked from launching Exubera until the lawsuit is settled. Exubera is now available to US patients.

Clinical Trials

The first program of Phase III trials of Exubera was completed in mid-2001. At the 62nd Scientific Sessions of the American Diabetes Association (ADA) in June 2002, Nektar presented the results of a Phase III trial. The three-month multicenter study investigated the efficacy of inhaled insulin in patients who had not achieved sufficient glycemic control with oral antidiabetic agents. The study compared Exubera – as monotherapy or in combination with oral antidiabetic agents – with oral antidiabetic agents alone. Patients taking Exubera exhibited HbA_{1c} reductions of 1.4% (monotherapy) and 1.9% (combination therapy) from baseline, compared with a 0.2% reduction in patients treated with oral agents alone. The Exubera patient groups experienced postprandial glucose reductions of 43 mg/dL (monotherapy) and 24 mg/dL (combination therapy), compared with a 2 mg/dL reduction in the oral antidiabetics group. Hypoglycemia occurred more frequently with Exubera than with oral antidiabetic agents, and there was some evidence of weight gain with Exubera use (average 2.8 kg) (Rosenstock et al., 2002).

At the 63rd Scientific Sessions of the ADA in June 2003, results of a trial comparing Exubera with rosiglitazone in type 2 diabetics showed that Exubera was more efficacious in maintaining glycemic control than rosiglitazone: 83% of Exubera patients achieved $HbA_{1c} < 8\%$, compared with 58% of rosiglitazone-treated patients. This study also showed that Exubera caused weight gain and increased incidence of hypoglycemic events (DeFronzo, 2003).

A six-month trial that compared Exubera (in combination with basal insulin) with subcutaneous mixed insulin in type 2 diabetics showed Exubera to be slightly superior in achieving healthy glucose levels. Patients who received Exubera experienced 0.7% reductions in HbA_{1c} levels, compared with a 0.6% reduction in patients who received subcutaneous insulin. Furthermore, 47% of the Exubera-treated patients reached $HbA_{1c} < 7\%$, compared with 32% of the subcutaneous insulin patients. Adverse events, including hypoglycemia, were similar in the two groups, with the exception of coughing, which was higher in the Exubera group. No difference in pulmonary function was detected (Hollander, 2004).

The potential for a long-term pulmonary damage (pulmonary fibrosis) with Exubera use concerns many physicians. The study discussed in the previous paragraph and another study presented at the 2001 meeting of the American Thoracic Society in San Francisco showed no evidence of increased lung function impairment with Exubera use. However, in May 2001, Pfizer and Aventis (now Sanofi-Aventis) announced that 1 patient out of the 1,000 patients who had participated in the six-month Phase III trials had developed pulmonary fibrosis. To better determine whether Exubera use correlates with pulmonary fibrosis, Pfizer and Aventis decided to conduct several additional long-term trials to collect more long-term pulmonary safety data.

In June 2006, Pfizer announced that interim data from these long-term trials would be presented at the 66th Annual Scientific Sessions of the ADA. In a press release dated June 10, 2006, Pfizer stated that in a trial that compared Exubera with injectable insulin in type 2 diabetics, both types of insulin showed similar positive results in achieving and maintaining glycemic control, but Exubera patients exhibited slightly better fasting blood-sugar levels. In a similar trial in type 1 diabetes patients, Exubera and injectable insulin showed similar results in achieving and maintaining good glucose levels. In both trials, decreases in lung function were slightly worse in Exubera patients, but these decreases occurred early in the treatment, and lung function was restored when therapy was discontinued. Adverse events associated with the two types of insulin were similar except for cough, which occurred more often in the Exubera group.

OTHER INHALED INSULINS IN DEVELOPMENT

Exubera is the first inhaled insulin to reach the market, but several other inhaled insulins are in late-stage development. Table 35.2 lists inhaled insulins that have reached clinical development; late-stage agents are described in detail below.

Eli Lilly and Alkermes' AIR Inhaled Insulin System

Eli Lilly and Alkermes are collaborating on the development of inhaled-insulin products that use AIR, the Alkermes pulmonary delivery system. The AIR system uses a small handheld inhaler, described as "about the size of a marker." Unlike the Exubera system, the AIR system is breath activated, meaning it does not require any motors or fans to operate. The unit uses a dry powder insulin packaged in capsules of various unit strengths.

Table 35.2 Inhaled Insulins in Development

Product	*Company*	*Status*
AIR Inhaled Insulin System	Alkermes/Eli Lilly	Phase III
AERx-iDMS	Aradigm/Novo Nordisk	Phase III
Technosphere Insulin	MannKind	Phase III
Inhaled insulin	Kos Pharmaceuticals	Phase I/II
Alveair	Coremed	Phase I
Inhaled insulin	QDose	Phase I

The two companies signed the first collaboration agreement in 2001. Under the terms of that agreement, Eli Lilly assumed all responsibility for clinical development, regulatory filings, manufacturing, and marketing of the agent. Alkermes received funding for development of the inhaler system, milestone payments, and royalties on sales. In February 2002, the two companies announced they were building a facility dedicated to the manufacture of inhaled products. In late 2002, the original agreement was expanded; Eli Lilly made a $30 million equity investment in Alkermes in return for Alkermes funding the development of the product through 2004. The royalty rate for Alkermes was increased, but Eli Lilly retained an option to exchange equity for a lower royalty rate.

Although the initial agreement between Eli Lilly and Alkermes covered the development of long-acting and rapid-acting insulins, most development up to this point has focused on the latter formulation. The agent entered Phase III clinical trials in July 2005, when a study was initiated in type 1 diabetics to evaluate the efficacy and safety of preprandial insulin delivered by the AIR system compared with the efficacy and safety of injected insulin. A second study began in August 2005 to compare the safety and efficacy of preprandial inhaled insulin in type 1 and type 2 diabetics who have mild to moderate asthma or chronic pulmonary obstructive disease (COPD). In April 2006, a safety and efficacy trial was initiated to compare preprandial inhaled insulin with rapid-acting injectable insulin in type 2 diabetes patients.

In a press release dated September 12, 2005, Alkermes released Phase II data on the efficacy of the rapid-acting inhaled insulin compared with injected insulin (these data were originally presented at the 41st Annual Meeting of the European Association for the Study of Diabetes). The results showed that the HbA_{1c} levels achieved with inhaled insulin (7.9) were similar to those achieved with injected insulin (8.0). The agents also showed similar safety profiles. Perhaps more importantly, 80% of the patients in the study expressed a preference for the AIR system instead of premeal injections. Other early trial results showed that the inhaler was easy to use, needing only written instructions, and that large-dose capsules (6U) could be replaced by multiple smaller-dose capsules (2U). Data from a Phase I trial in COPD patients showed that absorption and action of the inhaled insulin was reduced in patients with COPD compared with patients without COPD, but the reduction was consistent and the agent was well tolerated in this patient population (Alkermes, press release, June 2006).

Novo Nordisk and Aradigm's AERx-iDMS System

Novo Nordisk and Aradigm are developing an inhaled-insulin treatment using Aradigm's AERx Insulin Delivery Management System (iDMS). The AERx-iDMS is a handheld electronic delivery system (the only electronic system in late-stage development) that directs patients to breathe at a rate and depth that will ensure delivery of the right dose of insulin. Additionally, the system offers single-unit increment dosing (allowing patients to tailor doses more closely to their insulin needs) and can track dosing data. The AERx-iDMS also uses liquid insulin – not the powdered form used in other inhaled devices in late-stage development – which is less expensive to manufacture.

Novo Nordisk and Aradigm began their collaboration on an inhaled-insulin system in 1998. The initial agreement gave Novo Nordisk exclusive worldwide marketing rights to the product, with Aradigm receiving a share of revenue from sales. Novo Nordisk assumed responsibility for funding development of the insulin, but the companies shared the cost of developing the delivery system. Aradigm agreed to handle all manufacturing and receive milestone payments throughout the development life cycle; Novo Nordisk agreed to provide funding through equity investments. Later amendments to this agreement resulted in Novo Nordisk gaining full development and manufacturing rights (2004) and gaining relevant patents associated with the product (2006) in exchange for cash and equity investments in Aradigm.

Phase III clinical trials of the AERx-iDMS system began in 2002 in type 1 diabetes patients. The study was designed to compare the effectiveness of the inhaled insulin with Novo Nordisk's rapid-acting insulin analogue NovoLog/NovoRapid. Interim results from this trial were released in April 2004. In a press release dated April 30, 2004, the companies announced that AERx-iDMS had achieved its primary end points: comparable HbA_{1c} lowering by the two insulins, no change in pulmonary function, and no adverse effects. However, the interim analysis revealed an unexpected result – postprandial glucose levels were higher and nighttime glucose levels were lower in the inhaled-insulin group than in the subcutaneous insulin group. The trial was halted to analyze the data. Phase III clinical trials were reinitiated in May 2006 in type 1 diabetes patients.

Phase II data showed that the AERx-iDMS system is comparable to subcutaneous insulin in lowering Hb1Ac levels as a bolus treatment in type 2 diabetics. AERx-iDMS was shown to be safe and well tolerated. Novo Nordisk also ran Phase II trials in smokers and asthma patients. Although the amount of insulin absorption was different in these subpopulations than in nonsmokers and nonasthmatics (absorption is higher in smokers, lower in asthmatics), the AERx-iDMS system was safe and well tolerated and did not pose a specific risk to these patient populations.

MannKind's Technosphere

Mannkind is developing an inhaled-insulin system that administers powdered insulin (Technosphere insulin) via a palm-sized mechanical inhalation device (MedTone inhaler). Mannkind has stated that Technosphere insulin's more-rapid onset of action closely mimics the first release of endogenous insulin that nondiabetic persons experience during a meal. This insulin spike, which signals the liver to stop releasing glucose, is not achieved by any of the existing subcutaneous rapid-acting insulins.

Technosphere insulin entered Phase III clinical trials in late 2004 in Europe; pivotal US Phase III trials began in June 2005. In September 2006, Mannkind released data on a Phase III trial in type 2 diabetics that compared Technosphere insulin with a rapid-acting insulin analogue. The trial showed that patients receiving Technosphere insulin showed improvements in glycemic control similar to the improvement effected by the injectable insulin. Patients receiving Technosphere insulin also experienced weight loss, whereas patients receiving the injectable insulin experienced some weight gain. No loss of pulmonary function was associated with Technosphere insulin use.

Phase II data in type 2 diabetes patients showed that preprandial treatment with Technosphere insulin was more efficacious than placebo in reducing Hb1Ac levels. In a Phase II trial in patients with type I diabetes, Technosphere insulin was comparable to subcutaneous rapid-acting insulin analogues in improving Hb1Ac levels and slightly superior in controlling the postprandial glucose rise. In all clinical trials reported, no deterioration in lung function was detected. Also, compared with other insulin therapies, Technosphere insulin did not appear to cause weight gain.

THE OUTLOOK FOR INHALED INSULINS

Although the need for insulin formulations that will eliminate the need for multiple daily injections has long been established, inhaled insulin products will have to overcome several challenges before they can gain a significant share of the insulin market. Perhaps the most significant challenge will be reimbursement from third-party payers. Most analysts agree that Exubera is likely to cost about $4 per day – approximately twice the current cost of insulin therapy for type 1 diabetics – and it is likely that other emerging inhaled insulins will also be priced at a premium. Recently, the United Kingdom's National Institute for Health and Clinical Excellence (NICE) stated that there was no clear difference in efficacy between Exubera and available insulins and recommended that Exubera be prescribed only for patients with diagnosed "needle phobia" (belonephobia) and patients who have persistent problems with injection sites; this recommendation is perhaps the first indication that payers may resist reimbursement of this premium-priced product's cost. Many special interest groups have expressed displeasure about this potential resistance, but it remains to be seen what effect pressure from these groups will have on reimbursement policy.

Another issue is the safety concern about long-term use of inhaled insulin. Clinical data for Exubera show a decline in lung function, which would limit the treatment population to patients with normal lung function. Early trials on other inhaled insulins did not identify any pulmonary effects, but longer-term data are necessary to clearly establish the effects of these agents on lung function. The possibility of long-term effects may dissuade physicians from prescribing inhaled insulins, particularly to younger patients.

An additional challenge to the long-term success of inhaled insulins will be the launch of other alternative methods of insulin administration. Generex is developing its oral insulin, Oral-lyn, for approval in the United States and Europe, and both Emisphere and Biocon have an oral insulin in the pipeline. (Biocon had been developing this agent with Nobex, but Biocon acquired all intellectual property rights to this agent when Nobex declared bankruptcy in December 2005.) Oral insulin delivery is considered preferable because it is more convenient and more closely mimics the natural pathway of insulin secretion. Nasal and transdermal formulations of insulin that offer more convenient administration are also in early stages of clinical development.

Inhaled insulin products will likely claim only a small share of the rapid-acting insulin market, appealing primarily to needle-phobic patients who would normally delay insulin treatment. The availability of inhaled insulin may prompt physicians to begin type 2 patients on insulin treatment earlier in the disease because the elimination of injections will reduce patient resistance. Few patients who are already using injectable insulin are likely to switch to the inhaled version, particularly because reimbursement could be an issue – these patients have already established their ability to use injected insulin. Although none of the inhaled insulins discussed in this chapter has been studied in pediatric populations, this population may be an opportunity for developers of inhaled insulin because children are more likely to resist needles. However, other alternate delivery devices in development – oral, transdermal – are less complicated than inhaled versions and will probably be more successful in pediatric populations. Ultimately, the overall success of these agents will depend on their long-term safety, a positive reimbursement policy, and patients' perception of convenience.

REFERENCES

Alkermes, press release, June 2006.

DeFronzo, R.A. et al. Efficacy and safety of inhaled insulin (Exubera) compared with rosiglitazone in type 2 diabetes patients not optimally controlled on diet and exercise: results of a 3-month, randomized, comparative trial. *63rd Scientific Sessions of the American Diabetes Association. Abstracts.* 2003; 52(suppl. 1). Abstract 162-OR.

Hollander, P.A. Efficacy and safety of inhaled insulin (Exubera) compared with subcutaneous insulin therapy in patients with type 2 diabetes. *Diabetes Care.* 2004: 2356–62.

Rosenstock, J. et al. Mealtime rapid-acting inhaled insulin (Exubera) improves glycemic control in patients with type 2 diabetes failing combination oral agents: a three-month, randomized, comparative trial. *Diabetes.* 2002; 51(suppl. 2). Abstract 535-P.

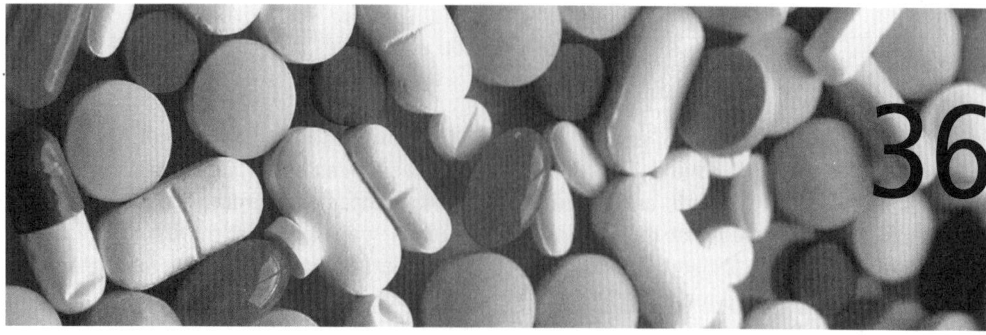

36

Impact of the PROactive Study on the Treatment of Type 2 Diabetes

INTRODUCTION: PROMISING RESULTS IN THE RECENT PROACTIVE STUDY

Type 2 diabetes is a chronic and progressive disease that is frequently linked with long-term microvascular events that cause morbidity (neuropathy, nephropathy, retinopathy, microangiopathy) as well as macrovascular events that cause morbidity and mortality (coronary artery disease, stroke, peripheral vascular disease). Moreover, type 2 diabetes is the primary cause of end-stage renal disease worldwide. The life-threatening complications of this disease constitute a significant unmet medical need worldwide, particularly because the prevalence of type 2 diabetes has soared in recent years as a result of changing eating habits and lifestyles.

The therapeutic goals with every type 2 diabetes patient are maintenance of euglycemia (a normal level of glucose in the blood) and evasion of long-term diabetic complications, including the prevention of cardiovascular events. Several classes of oral antidiabetic drugs, including insulin, are available to manage glycemic control and the aforementioned microvascular complications. However, these agents neither provide a cure for type 2 diabetes nor have a significant effect on the disease's macrovascular complications.

Although several clinical trials in type 2 diabetes patients have demonstrated that some of these antidiabetic drugs decrease the risk of cardiovascular events, until recently there were no data correlating the use of an antidiabetic agent with the actual incidence of cardiovascular disease (CVD) in patients at high risk of a fatal cardiovascular result. The Prospective Pioglitazone Clinical Trial in Macrovascular Events (PROactive) study, the results of which were released in late 2005, was the first large-scale clinical trial to report on the efficacy of a specific antidiabetic drug, pioglitazone (Takeda/Eli Lilly's Actos), in suppressing risk factors for macrovascular morbidity and mortality and the actual incidence of fatal and nonfatal cardiovascular events in type 2 diabetes patients who had previously experienced a cardiovascular episode (Dormandy et al., 2005).

Results of the PROactive study suggest that pioglitazone, a peroxisome proliferator-activated receptor-gamma (PPAR-γ) agonist that was approved for diabetes in 1999, may, in contrast with most other antidiabetic treatments, not only control blood glucose levels but, importantly, mitigate the occurrence of cardiovascular events in type 2 diabetes patients with a history of CVD. This additional benefit to pioglitazone treatment may represent new commercial opportunities for the drug and enable it to establish an advantage in the competitive therapeutic market for diabetes drugs.

This chapter discusses the PROactive study, focusing on the study's results. To provide a context for how large an impact this study may have on diabetes treatment and sales, we begin with an overview of type 2 diabetes, including information on its increasing prevalence and associated comorbidities, particularly cardiovascular complications, and available therapies. Next, we discuss pioglitazone's pharmacological profile as well as the design, results, and possible shortcomings of this breakthrough trial. Finally, we forecast the potential effect of the PROactive study on sales of pioglitazone and the commercial opportunities for other antidiabetic agents.

TYPE 2 DIABETES: DISEASE BACKGROUND AND PREVALENCE

Pathophysiology and Risk Factors

Type 2 diabetes (also called insulin-independent diabetes mellitus or adult onset diabetes) is a chronic and complex metabolic disorder characterized by insulin resistance (attenuated responsiveness of peripheral tissue to insulin) and diminished insulin secretion by the beta (β) cells in the pancreatic islets of Langerhans. Figure 36.1 displays this process and the complications of the disease. Insulin is a principal anabolic

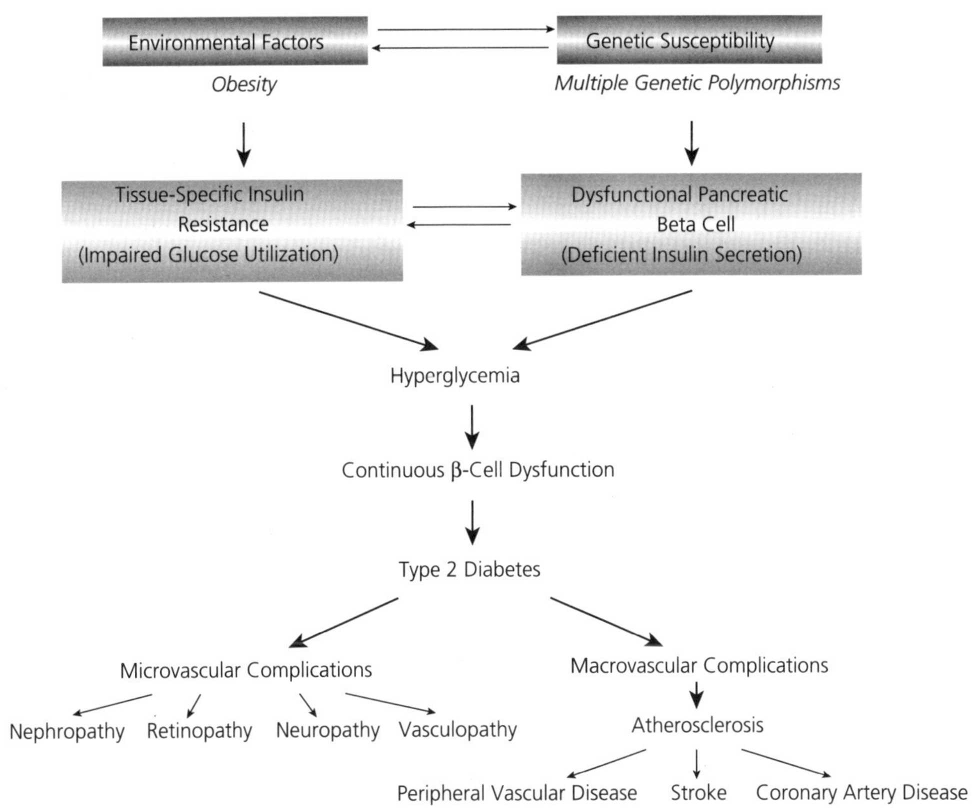

Figure 36.1 Onset and Complications of Type 2 Diabetes

hormone that is necessary for the homeostatic regulation of carbohydrate, fat, and protein metabolism.

Multiple genetic defects that respond to environmental factors (e.g., obesity, lack of physical activity) initiate the diabetic process in susceptible persons. Insulin resistance in liver, skeletal muscle, and adipose tissue is the first indication of disease in prediabetic individuals. Researchers believe that the insulin resistance in these tissues occurs at the level of the insulin receptor and/or post-receptor signaling pathways for insulin. In addition to insulin resistance, dysfunctional pancreatic β cells are central to the pathophysiology of type 2 diabetes. The progressive loss in insulin secretion from β cells, as a consequence of impaired glucose-stimulated insulin secretion, places added stress on these cells to produce additional insulin so as to overcome the insulin-resistant state in type 2 diabetes patients. Over time, the pancreas becomes unable to secrete sufficient insulin to overcome the resistance, leading to impaired glucose tolerance and hyperinsulinemia (abnormally high levels of insulin in the blood). Ultimately, chronically impaired insulin secretion by dysfunctional β cells results in sustained hyperglycemia and full-blown type 2 diabetes.

Obesity has emerged as a principal risk factor for type 2 diabetes; the American Diabetes Association (ADA) has estimated that approximately 90% of people with newly diagnosed type 2 diabetes in the United States are obese. In addition, the Association for Weight Management and Obesity Prevention estimates that 64% of people in the United States are either overweight or obese. The steadily rising numbers of people who are obese is of significant concern to public health organizations. An additional concern is the rising prevalence of obesity in the pediatric population. According to the Centers for Disease Control and Prevention (CDC), 16% of children and adolescents were overweight in 2002; triple the percentage seen in 1980. Although type 2 diabetes is seen predominantly in adults older than age 40, this increase in pediatric obesity could lead to an increase in the development of type 2 diabetes in younger populations.

Type 2 Diabetes and Cardiovascular Disease

Patients with type 2 diabetes have a greater risk of CVD than nondiabetic individuals, since they are prone to lipid abnormalities and hypertension, conditions that greatly increase the risk of mortality from cardiovascular complications such as heart attack and stroke. In fact, a prospective study of nearly 350,000 men in the Multiple Risk Factor Intervention Trial (MRFIT) indicates that type 2 diabetes is a stronger predictor of CVD risk than classic CVD risk factors such as hypertension, high total serum cholesterol, and history of smoking tobacco (Stamler et al., 1993). Atherosclerosis, the buildup of plaque (a mix of lipids, inflammatory cells, and extracellular matrix components) on the artery linings, is the principal cause of cardiovascular and peripheral vascular disease in type 2 diabetes. Myocardial infarction (MI) caused by rupture of atherosclerotic plaques in the coronary arteries is the most common cause of death in diabetes patients.

Obesity enhances the risk for cardiovascular comorbidity and other long-term complications of type 2 diabetes. Aside from fat content or degree of obesity, the distribution of fat within the body is predictive of insulin sensitivity. Visceral fat and upper body fat is more resistant to insulin than subcutaneous fat and lower-body fat, and visceral fat cells produce and release inducers of insulin resistance and proinflammatory adipocytokines, the latter contributing to atherosclerosis.

Although the medical community continues to debate the relative contributions of hyperglycemia and hyperinsulinemia in the development of CVD, it has become widely accepted that even prediabetic patients who have borderline laboratory values for some of the metabolic complications that accompany diabetes (dyslipidemia and hypertension) are at increased risk for CVD. This cluster of comorbidities is known as metabolic syndrome, a disorder comprising abdominal obesity, insulin resistance, hypertension, elevated triglycerides, and low high-density lipoprotein (HDL) cholesterol. Researchers estimate that 84% of type 2 diabetic patients meet the World Health Organization's (WHO's) criteria for metabolic syndrome (Isomaa et al., 2001). In addition, the elevated cardiovascular risk in type 2 diabetics stems in part from insulin resistance, which is associated with elevated plasma levels of C-reactive protein (CRP), fibrinogen, plasminogen activator inhibitor-1 (PAI-1), resistin, interleukin-6 (IL-6), and tumor necrosis factor-alpha (TNF-α). The elevated levels of these proteins and hormones increase the risk of CVD by promoting inflammation, atherosclerosis, and thrombosis.

Prevalence of Type 2 Diabetes

The high prevalence of type 2 diabetes worldwide is of great concern to medical professionals. According to the WHO, more than 150 million people worldwide have type 2 diabetes. The WHO projects that worldwide prevalence is growing annually at almost 3% and will reach 300 million by 2030. Diabetes is the sixth-deadliest disease in the United States, with death rates due to heart disease two to four times higher in adults with the disease than those without it, according to the CDC. The CDC estimates that more than 17 million people are type 2 diabetics and that another 41 million between ages 40 and 74 have prediabetes.

OVERVIEW OF CURRENT DRUG THERAPIES

Diet, exercise, and an overall healthy lifestyle can, on a patient-specific basis, lessen or eliminate the chances of developing type 2 diabetes. These measures also lessen the severity and chances of long-term complications in patients diagnosed with the disease; often, however, patients must utilize antidiabetic medications, either as monotherapies or in combinations, to manage their disease. Drug treatment is used in patients with type 2 diabetes in order to achieve consistent glycemic control and decrease the possibility of a cardiovascular event. A broad spectrum of oral antidiabetic drugs, including pioglitazone (the focus of the PROactive study), target the known components of type 2 diabetes; sales of these agents are shown in Table 36.1.

In addition to the oral antidiabetic agents discussed in the following sections, some patients require insulin therapy to approach or maintain a euglycemic state. Short-acting (insulin lispro) and long-acting (insulin glargine) insulin formulations are typically used in combination with other medications or alone following an unacceptable response of type 2 diabetes patients to previous treatments.

Sulfonylureas

Sulfonylureas are insulin secretagogues that stimulate insulin secretion from the pancreatic islet β cells and lower plasma glucose levels. This class of agent, used as a monotherapy or in combination with other oral antidiabetic agents or insulin, has been a popular choice as a first-line therapy since its introduction in the 1950s. Since that time, three generations of sulfonylureas have been developed. The first-generation agents, which include tolbutamide (generics), tolazamide (generics), acetohexamide (generics), and chlorpropamide (Pfizer's Diabinese, generics), are rarely used today.

The second-generation agents, which include glyburide (Pfizer's Micronase, Sanofi-Aventis's Diabeta, generics), glipizide (Pfizer's Glucotrol, Glucotrol XL, generics), and gliclazide (Servier's Diamicron, Molteni & C.F. LLI Alitti's Diabrezide, Dainippon's Glimicron, generics), are far more potent than the first-generation agents and are considered efficacious and safe. In the United States, a micronized version of glyburide (Pfizer's Micronase) is also available; this agent has enhanced absorption characteristics that enable a faster onset of action compared with

Table 36.1 US and Worldwide Sales of Select Antidiabetic Agents, 2005

Drug Class	*Generic Name*	*Company/Brand*	*US Sales (millions $US)*	*Worldwide Sales (millions $US)*
Sulfonylureas	Gliclazide	Servier/Diamicron; Dainippon Sumitomo/ Glimicron; generics	Not marketed	506
	Glimepride	Sanofi-Aventis/Amaryl	225	842
	Glipizide	Pfizer/Glucatrol XL; generics	381	411
	Glyburide	Sanofi-Aventis/Diabeta; Pfizer/ Micronase; generics	45	45
Class total			651	1,804
Meglitinides	Mitiglinide	Kissei-Takeda/Glufast	N.A.	27
	Nateglinide	Novartis/Starlix; Daiichi Sankyo/ Fastic; Astellas/Starsis	86	265
	Repaglinide	Novo Nordisk/Prandin; NovoNorm	129	285
Class total			215	577
Alpha-glucosidase inhibitors	Acarbose	Bayer and Schering-Plough/ Precose; Glucobay	25	392
	Miglitol	Bayer, Pfizer, Sanofi-Aventis/Glyset	Not marketed	24
	Voglibose	Takeda/Basen	Not marketed	569
Class total			25	985
Biguanide	Metformin	Merck/Glucophage; Bristol-Myers Squibb/Glucophage IR, XR; First Horizon, Andrx/Fortamet; Dainippon Sumitomo/Melbin; generics	297	704
Class total			297	704
PPAR-γ agonists	Pioglitazone	Takeda, Eli Lilly, Abbott/Actos	1,713	2,111
	Rosiglitazone	GlaxoSmithKline/Avandia	1,500	2,003
Class total			3,213	4,114
Insulin	Insulin lispro	Eli Lilly/Humalog	740	1,198
	Insulin glargine	Sanofi-Aventis/Lantus	892	1,510
Class total			1,632	2,708
GLP-1 analogue	Exenatide	Amlyin, Eli Lilly/Byetta	75	75
Class total			75	75
Amylin analogue	Pramlintide acetate	Amylin/Symlin	12	12
Class total			12	12
Combination therapy	Metformin/glipizide	Bristol-Myers Squibb/Metaglip	24	24
	Metformin/glyburide	Bristol-Myers Squibb/Glucovance; generics	131	134
	Metformin/rosiglitazone	GlaxoSmithKline/Avandamet	196	303
Class total			351	461
Market total			6,446	11,440

N.A. = Information not available

nonmicronized glyburide. A drawback of these second-generation agents is their short half-life; most of these agents only have periods of activity between two and ten hours. In addition, these agents can cause potentially serious hypoglycemia.

There is currently only one third-generation sulfonylurea available, glimepiride (Sanofi-Aventis's Amaryl). This agent has a longer half-life than the second-generation agents, allowing once-daily administration and making it more advantageous than other drugs for patients who have difficulty complying with multiple daily doses. Double-blind, randomized, one-year, placebo-controlled trials of glimepiride have demonstrated 1.4–2.5% reductions in glycosylated hemoglobin (HbA_{1c}), which indicates the level of glucose attachment to hemoglobin in red blood cells compared with placebo; this result is similar to that achieved with other, older sulfonylureas. Glimepiride also carries the potential for severe hypoglycemia, although it appears that the incidence of this side effect is less than with other agents in this class.

Meglitinides

Meglitinides stimulate pancreatic β cells to release insulin, in a manner similar to that of the sulfonylureas. This drug class includes repaglinide (Novo Nordisk's Prandin/NovoNorm), the first in its class; nateglinide (Novartis's Starlix/Starsis); and mitiglinide (Kissei/Takeda's Glufast), the newest member. These agents, characterized by rapid onset and short duration of action, target postprandial hyperglycemia and are commonly used as adjunct therapies with other antidiabetic agents. In particular, nateglinide has shown enhanced efficacy in combination with metformin (Bristol-Myers Squibb's [BMS's] Glucophage and Glucophage XR, Biovail/DepoMed's Glumetza, generics) (discussed in detail in a later section). Meglitinides and sulfonylureas reduce HbA_{1c} to a comparable extent; however, because meglitinides exert their effects only in the presence of elevated glucose levels, they minimize the risk of hypoglycemia, providing an advantage over sulfonylurea therapy.

Alpha-Glucosidase Inhibitors

Alpha-glucosidase inhibitors (AGI) interfere with the rate of carbohydrate digestion by delaying the completion of carbohydrate digestion in the gastrointestinal tract. The AGIs on the market today are acarbose (Bayer's Precose/Glucobay, generics), miglitol (Bayer/Pfizer/Sanofi-Aventis's Glyset), and voglibose (Takeda's Basen). Compared with other oral antidiabetic agents, the efficacy of this drug class is modest, causing a 0.5–1.0% decrease in HbA_{1c} (Holman et al., 1999). These agents are also considered particularly safe, and when taken with meals they offer an alternative means to reduce postprandial hyperglycemia and lower levels of insulin in patients who are prone to hypoglycemia or lactic acidosis. However, their modest efficacy combined with gastrointestinal side effects (including flatulence, abdominal pain, and/or diarrhea) and a higher price point have limited the use of AGIs.

Biguanides

The only biguanide available for the treatment of type 2 diabetes is metformin. The agent targets insulin resistance in type 2 diabetes and is defined as an insulin sensitizer. Although metformin's exact mechanism of action is unknown, it appears to inhibit hepatic glucose production and stimulate glucose uptake in skeletal muscle and adipose tissue, leading to a long-term glucose-lowering effect. Metformin's nonhypoglycemic properties, combined with its ability to normalize lipid levels and its safety profile, have resulted in the agent becoming the therapy of choice for overweight and obese type 2 diabetes patients.

The drug may be used as a monotherapy or in combination with any other class of antidiabetic drug or insulin. Specifically, combination therapy with a sulfonylurea (an insulin secretagogue) and metformin (an insulin sensitizer) in certain type 2 diabetes patients may reduce insulin resistance and permit the sulfonylurea-stimulated insulin secretion to exert glycemic control. Currently, four single-pill combination therapies include metformin. BMS's Glucovance (metformin/glyburide) and Metaglip (metformin/glipizide) combine sulfonylureas with metformin, while GlaxoSmithKline's (GSK's) Avandamet (metformin/rosiglitazone) and Takeda's Actoplus Met (metformin/pioglitazone) combine metformin with a PPAR-γ agonist.

The clinical efficacy of metformin requires the presence of insulin in quantities sufficient to maintain blood glucose levels close to normal limits. Therefore, patients whose β-cell function supplies insufficient insulin levels must use insulin in combination with metformin. Unlike sulfonylureas and meglitinides, metformin does not cause hypoglycemia and therefore can be used in populations that are more likely to develop this side effect (such as the elderly).

The most serious adverse effect associated with metformin therapy is lactic acidosis, which is rare but fatal in 50% of the patients who develop it. Therefore, metformin is contraindicated in patients who are prone to lactic acidosis and unable to metabolize lactate, and the occurrence of lactic acidosis mandates stoppage of treatment.

Peroxisome Proliferator-activated Receptor-Gamma Agonists

PPAR-γ agonists are a newer class of insulin sensitizers that mitigate insulin resistance. PPARs are ligand-activated transcription factors belonging to the nuclear receptor superfamily. To date, three PPAR genes (α, β/δ, and γ) have been cloned. PPAR-γ, which is expressed in hepatic, adipose, and skeletal muscle tissue, activates insulin-sensitive genes.

PPAR-γ agonists are also sometimes referred to as thiazolidinediones (TZD, glitazones), although several PPAR agonists that are nonthiazolidinedione agents are in development. PPAR-γ agonists improve insulin sensitivity and glycemic control in type 2 diabetes patients and reduce hyperglycemia by increasing glucose uptake by skeletal muscle and decreasing hepatic glucose production. In addition, PPAR-γ agonists have also been reported to preserve pancreatic β-cell function as indicated by a decrease in the proinsulin/insulin ratio and restoration of the first-phase insulin response (Li et al., 2003; Pfutzner et al., 2005). These actions of pioglitazone suggest that it may mitigate the need for insulin therapy in certain type 2 diabetes patients. Figure 36.2 illustrates the mechanisms by which PPAR-γ agonists improve glycemic control and mitigate cardiovascular complications in type 2 diabetes patients.

Pioglitazone and rosiglitazone (GSK's Avandia) are the currently approved PPAR-γ agonists for the treatment of type 2 diabetes. These agents can be used in combination with metformin, sulfonylureas, or insulin. As with metformin, adequate insulin concentrations are needed for PPAR-γ agonists to achieve an acceptable level of efficacy. As discussed in the previous section, PPAR-γ agonists are used in the single-pill combination treatments Avandamet (metformin/rosiglitazone) and Actoplus Met (metformin/pioglitizone). In clinical trials, the two agents showed similar efficacy in reducing HbA_{1c} levels (approximately 1–1.5% reduction). The efficacy of each of these agents was improved by combining it with another oral antidiabetic agent.

PPAR-γ agonists are generally well tolerated, with moderate weight gain, edema, and fluid retention the most common side effects. There is some question about the potential for liver toxicity with agents in this drug class, mainly owing to the withdrawal of troglitazone (Warner-Lambert's [now part of Pfizer] Rezulin, GSK's Romozin, Sankyo's Noscal) from the market because of the fatal development of liver toxicity in patients. However, given that neither of the available agents has shown a similar side effect, researchers and physicians generally believe that liver toxicity is not a class effect.

Glucagon-like Peptide-1 Analogues

Exenatide (Eli Lilly/Byetta) is a synthetic analogue of the intestinal hormone glucagon-like peptide-1 (GLP-1). GLP-1 is a member of the incretin family of intestinal peptides that displays a spectrum of glucoregulatory activities, including stimulation of the pancreas to produce insulin in a glucose-sensitive manner, inhibition of pancreatic glucagon release, slowing of the nutrient absorption rate, and reduction of food intake. Exenatide improves plasma glucose control by decreasing both postprandial and fasting glucose levels, resulting in improved long-term glycemic control.

Exenatide received approval in April 2005 for type 2 diabetes patients who have not achieved adequate glycemic control on metformin and/or a sulfonylurea. Although the drug shows significant efficacy in patients who have exhibited resistance to other first-line therapies, the agent does have

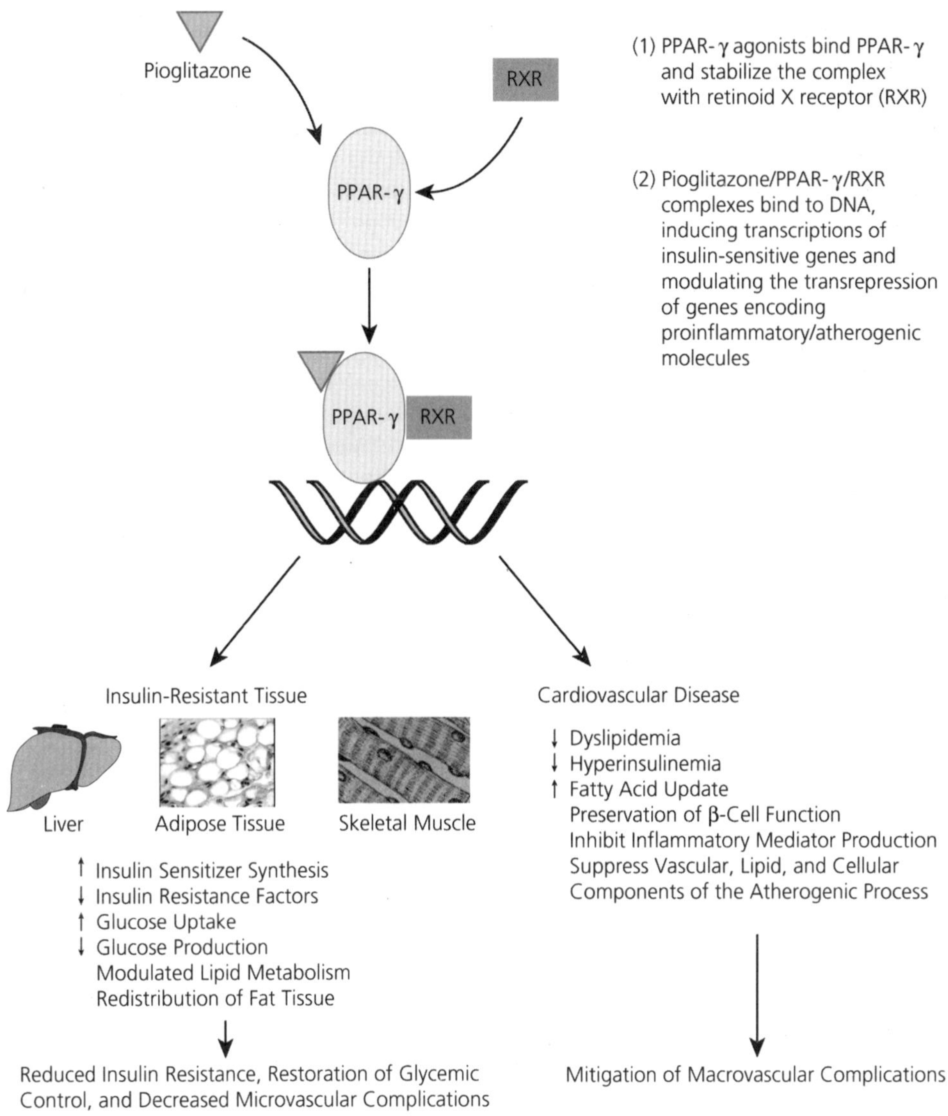

PPAR-γ: Peroxisome proliferator-activated receptor gamma

Figure 36.2 Mechanism of Action for PPAR-γ Agonists in Type 2 Diabetes

some drawbacks. Unlike many other agents used to treat type 2 diabetes, exenatide must be administered via a subcutaneous injection. In addition, the agent has a short duration of activity, requiring multiple daily doses. Amylin is developing a controlled-release version of exenatide (Byetta LAR) in collaboration with Alkermes and Eli Lilly to address this issue.

Amylin Analogues

In March 2005, Amylin Pharmaceuticals received market approval for a synthetic analogue of human amylin, pramlintide acetate (Symlin), to be used as adjunct therapy with insulin in type 2 diabetes patients who are unable to achieve or maintain glucose control with insulin therapy alone. The hormone amylin, contained and released by pancreatic β cells, functions with insulin to maintain glycemic control. Replacement of insulin does not replace the action of amylin or normalize postprandial glucagon concentrations in the blood, which can exacerbate the hyperglycemic state in type 2 diabetes.

Data from short-term clinical trials involving both type 1 and type 2 diabetes patients using insulin show that pramlintide acetate prevented the postprandial rise in glucagon, slowed the rate of gastric emptying, and reduced the range of postprandial fluctuations in blood glucose levels. In a 26-week, 166-patient clinical trial, adjunctive therapy with pramlintide acetate resulted in significant reductions in HbA_{1c} levels and body weight. However, the agent's injectable formulation may limit its success.

THE PROACTIVE STUDY: REVEALING A POTENTIAL BREAKTHROUGH TREATMENT FOR CARDIOVASCULAR DISEASE IN TYPE 2 DIABETES

Although established oral antidiabetic agents and insulin are able to improve glycemic control and mitigate microvascular complications, they are less successful in reducing macrovascular complications. The landmark UK Prospective Diabetes Study provided data showing the benefit of some antidiabetic medications on glycemic control and microvascular complications, with a much smaller impact on cardiovascular risk factors and macrovascular complications (UK Prospective Diabetes Study [UKPDS] Group, 1998). These results are supported by the absence of a reduction in cardiovascular mortality with most other traditional medications in more than 30 years (Gu et al., 1999).

The UKPDS showed that a metformin/sulfonylurea or metformin/insulin combination treatment significantly reduces the risk of fatal and nonfatal cardiovascular events compared with diet changes. However, these combination therapies showed only marginal benefit over sulfonylurea or insulin monotherapies. In addition, a modest increase in cardiovascular events occurred in obese patients receiving metformin as an adjunct to sulfonylurea.

The results of several clinical studies have cited the relationship between insulin resistance, metabolic syndrome, and the risk of CVD in type 2 diabetes. Numerous data from these studies support the hypothesis that pioglitazone's effects extend beyond glycemic control and impact cardiovascular risk factors of metabolic syndrome, including modifying dyslipidemia. However, until recently, no clinical outcomes study had been published in which the principal clinical objective was the impact of a medication on clinically meaningful end points such as the incidence of actual cardiovascular events and mortality in type 2 diabetes patients. Moreover, no study was published with type 2 diabetes patients who had a history of CVD.

In October 2005, the PROactive study published data on the efficacy of pioglitazone in type 2 diabetes patients at high risk for CVD. Earlier observations had shown that PPAR-γ agonists cause a reduction in risk factors for macrovascular disease (i.e., elevated lipid levels in the blood); however, no clinical data were available that correlated these effects with the actual incidence of CVD in type 2 diabetes patients. The PROactive study sought to demonstrate that pioglitazone treatment in type 2 diabetes patients reduces total macrovascular mortality and morbidity. In the following sections, we discuss the PROactive study in detail, including the study design and results.

(Note that, unless otherwise specified, all study results in the following sections come from the following source: Dormandy J, et al. Secondary prevention of macrovascular events in patients with type 2 diabetes in the PROactive study [PROspective pioglitAzone Clinical Trial In macroVascular Events]: a randomized controlled trial. *Lancet*. 2005; 366: 1279–89.)

The Role of PPAR in Cardiovascular Disease

As discussed previously, although oral antidiabetic drugs and insulin achieve glycemic control and manage long-term microvascular complications of the disease, most do not have an appreciable impact on the atherosclerotic macrovascular complications and mortality in type 2 diabetes patients. Like other agents, such as the biguanide metformin, PPAR-γ agonists target insulin resistance; however, several studies have shown that pioglitazone – in addition to exerting glycemic control and mitigating hyperglycemia – normalizes the dysfunctional metabolic components of diabetes. This pharmacological profile suggests that pioglitazone has nonglycemic properties in addition to its antihyperglycemic actions, which may negatively impact the development of CVD in type 2 diabetes patients.

In type 2 diabetes patients, skeletal muscle, liver, and adipose tissue – all of which express PPAR-γ – are resistant to insulin. Insulin resistance can cause the dysregulated carbohydrate and lipid metabolism that lead to dyslipidemia, a significant risk factor in the development of CVD. PPAR-γ transcriptionally activates and transrepresses insulin-inducible genes that encode various components of carbohydrate and lipid metabolic pathways. Previous clinical studies have shown pioglitazone to correct the aberrant lipid metabolism in type 2 diabetes patients, perhaps acting via PPAR-γ-mediated events.

In addition, there is some clinical evidence to suggest that pioglitazone has antiatherosclerotic effects. As discussed previously, visceral fat produces and releases proinflammatory adipocytokines that contribute to atherosclerosis. Adipose tissue expresses the highest levels of PPAR-γ, and pioglitazone, a PPAR-γ agonist, upregulates insulin-sensitizing molecules (adiponectin) and transrepresses genes encoding inflammatory molecules (e.g., TNF-α) in adipose tissue (Figure 36.2). Also, in vitro studies have shown that pioglitazone suppresses the formation of advanced glycosylation end products (AGEs), which are formed under hyperglycemic conditions. AGEs are formed by the interaction of glucose with interstitial tissue and vascular wall proteins, and researchers believe that the excessive formation of these products contributes to the microvascular complications of diabetes. In addition, AGE receptors are expressed on cellular components of the atherosclerotic process, contributing to the development of atherosclerosis, making it likely that they play a role in the development of macrovascular complications of diabetes.

PROactive Study Design

The PROactive study was a 34.5-month prospective, randomized, double-blind, placebo-controlled trial in 5,238 type 2 diabetes patients. The trial took place in 321 clinical centers in 19 European countries. Participants in the trial were between 35 and 75 years of age and had evidence of previous macrovascular disease.

Patients were assigned to either a treatment or placebo arm. Patients in the treatment arm received pioglitazone at 15 mg per day for the first month, 30 mg per day for the second month, and 45 mg per day thereafter to achieve the maximum tolerated dose. If patients were being treated with other antidiabetic agents (metformin, sulfonylureas, insulin), they continued to use those medications concomitantly until no longer necessary to adequately control their disease. Throughout the study, concomitant antidiabetic therapies could be prescribed if deemed necessary. Table 36.2 shows the percentage of patients in the study who were taking antidiabetics in addition to pioglitazone when enrolled and when the study completed. Patients also continued with their prescribed antihypertensive drugs, lipid-altering agents, and antithrombotic drugs.

At the onset and throughout the trial, HbA_{1c}, lipids, liver enzymes, creatinine, and albumin concentration were measured. The

Table 36.2 Number of Patients Using Concomitant Medication During the PROactive Study

Drug	*Beginning of Trial*	*End of Trial*
Metformin	2,971	1,990
Sulfonylureas	2,955	2,947
Insulin	1,584	2,551

Note: Numbers include patients taking combination therapies primary end point of the study was the time elapsed between randomization and any of the following events:

- Death from any cause.
- Nonfatal myocardial infarction (MI) (including silent MI).
- Stroke.
- Acute coronary syndrome.
- Endovascular or surgical intervention on the coronary or leg arteries.
- Amputation above the ankle.

Secondary end points included time elapsed between randomization and death (by any cause), nonfatal MI (excluding silent MI), and stroke; time elapsed between randomization and cardiovascular death; and time elapsed between randomization and the individual components of the primary end point.

PROactive Study Results

A summary of the results from the PROactive study can be seen in Table 36.3. Although there was no significant difference between pioglitazone and placebo in the composite primary end point, fewer individuals in the pioglitazone group than the placebo group experienced a minimum of one cardiovascular event. However, for the principal secondary end point, there were significantly fewer mortalities (127 in the pioglitazone group compared with 136 with placebo), MIs, and strokes in the pioglitazone group than the placebo group. Pioglitazone-treated patients experienced a reduced first occurrence of MI, stroke, acute coronary syndrome, and cardiac intervention, as well as a reduced total number of events reported compared with the placebo-treated patients.

Table 36.3 PROactive Trial: Summary of the Effects of Pioglitazone on the Study Parameters

Clinical Target	*Therapeutic Outcome*
Primary composite end point	There was no significant difference ($p = 0.095$) between the pioglitazone group and the placebo group in terms of the proportion of patients experiencing a cardiovascular event within the primary composite end point (Hazard Ratio = 0.90)
Principal secondary end point	Significantly fewer ($p = 0.027$) pioglitazone- than placebo-treated patients experienced at least one cardiovascular event (Hazard Ratio = 0.84)
Frequency of first events within the primary composite end point	Death, MI, and stroke occurred with greater frequency in the placebo group compared with the pioglitazone group
Frequency of first events within the main secondary end points	Death, MI, and stroke occurred with greater frequency in the placebo- versus pioglitazone-treated patients
Components of the primary composite end point	Pioglitazone-treated patients demonstrated a markedly reduced incidence of first event (nonfatal MI [including silent MI], stroke, acute coronary syndrome, and cardiac intervention) compared with the placebo group; 514 and 572 total first events were recorded in the pioglitazone and placebo groups, respectively
Use of concomitant medications	At the conclusion of the trial, significantly fewer pioglitazone-treated patients had maintained metformin ($p = 0.0001$) or insulin ($p < 0.0001$) medications compared with placebo-treated patients. Oscillations in use of all other medications remained the same for both groups
Insulin use	With no prior use of insulin, 11% (pioglitazone) and 21% (placebo) of these patients initiated insulin treatment during the 34.5-month trial ($p < 0.0001$)
Hyperglycemia	Pioglitazone (–0.8) significantly reduced ($p < 0.0001$) the HbA_{1c} concentration compared with placebo (–0.3)
Dyslipidemia	Pioglitazone caused a significant decrease in triglyceride concentrations ($p < 0.0001$), a rise in HDL cholesterol concentrations ($p < 0.0001$), and a decrease in the LDL/HDL ratio ($p < 0.0001$) compared with placebo values. Pioglitazone stimulated an increase ($p = 0.003$) in LDL-C concentrations versus placebo
Serious adverse events	Slightly fewer serious adverse events occurred in pioglitazone-treated patients compared with placebo-treated patients
Heart failure	Pioglitazone increased the rate of edema without heart failure, but mortality related to heart failure was comparable in the pioglitazone and placebo groups

HDL = High-density lipoprotein; LDL = Low-density lipoprotein; MI = Myocardial infarction

Only 4% of patients were not taking concomitant antidiabetic medication before the start of the study, so it is difficult to determine the effect on macrovascular events of pioglitazone as a monotherapy versus as a combination therapy. However, fewer patients in the pioglitazone group (11% versus 21% in the placebo group) began permanent insulin use during the course of the study. In addition, the study showed that pioglitazone use caused a significant reduction in plasma HbA_{1c} concentrations.

As discussed earlier, dyslipidemia is an independent risk factor for the development of CVD, and patients with type 2 diabetes have an increased chance of developing dyslipidemia. Patients treated with pioglitazone demonstrated a significant reduction in triglyceride levels, increased HDL cholesterol (HDL-C) levels, and a decreased low-density lipoprotein cholesterol (LDL-C)/HDL-C ratio compared with placebo-treated patients. There was a slight increase in LDL-C levels; however, the decreased LDL/HDL ratio suggests this increase may not result in an overall adverse effect.

Shortcomings of the PROactive Study

While the PROactive study demonstrated pioglitazone's increased overall therapeutic benefit to type 2 diabetes patients at high risk for a cardiovascular event and death, certain aspects of this study have been a cause for concern among members of the medical community. Chief among these is the question of whether the main secondary end point (which contained only a few of the outcomes measures used in the primary composite end point) would still have shown pioglitizone to have a statistically significant effect if more factors had been added. Given this question, some experts have suggested that the study may not accurately predict pioglitazone's effects.

In addition to this issue, there have been several criticisms regarding the trial design:

- Despite the large number of trial participants, questions have been raised regarding the diversity of the study participants, suggesting that the mostly Caucasian patients may have been less insulin-resistant than other populations.
- Because the mechanism of action of pioglitazone is unknown, assessment of the effects of pioglitazone on markers of inflammation, atherosclerosis, and other parameters of CVD should have been performed to support the conclusion that pioglitazone, and not the concomitant medications, was responsible for the reduction in macrovascular events.
- The 45 mg daily dose of pioglitazone is not approved for use in combination with other therapies. Some critics have questioned whether the study results would have been different had the recommended combination dose of 30 mg been used.

It is important to note that in order to address many of these issues, study investigators would have needed to greatly expand the scope of the already expansive trial. The objective of the PROactive study was to "ascertain whether pioglitazone reduces macrovascular morbidity in high-risk patients with type 2 diabetes." Although this trial does provide significant evidence that pioglitazone reduces the incidence of macrovascular events, it is apparent that further study on the effects of this compound and other PPAR-γ agonists will be beneficial to understanding the potential benefit of this class of drugs.

OUTLOOK

While diet and exercise will remain the first-line treatment for prediabetic and type 2 diabetic patients, the use of oral antidiabetic agents continues to rise. The market for these agents grew 15% worldwide from 2000 to 2004. We expect this growth to continue, particularly given the increase in obesity worldwide. However, while drugs in the current armamentarium of oral antidiabetic therapy have shown strong efficacy in maintaining glycemic control and mitigating the microvascular complications of type 2 diabetes, the effective long-term management of macrovascular complications is a significant unmet need.

The PROactive study was the first study to specifically correlate the incidence of cardiovascular events with the use of an antidiabetic drug. Although the primary end point of the study (reduction in the time to a cardiovascular event) was not achieved with statistical significance, the study still provided significant evidence that use of pioglitazone reduces the incidence of adverse cardiovascular events and fatalities in diabetes patients.

PPAR-γ agonists are one of the fastest growing drug classes in the treatment of diabetes, with sales growing at a significantly higher rate than those of many other agents. Figure 36.3 shows the sales growth of antidiabetic drug classes from 2000 to 2004. In part, the high sales of PPAR-γ agonists are reflective of their higher price compared with agents in other drug classes; however, PPAR-γ agonists captured 17% of the prescribing volume in the United States in 2004, according to PDDA Verispan. The drug was most often used in combination with other antidiabetic agents, and the growth of this agent may be reflective of physicians' recognition of the benefits of PPAR-γ agonists as adjunct therapies. Now, with the data from the PROactive study, use in patients at clear risk for an atherosclerotic cardiovascular event represents an emerging market opportunity for pioglitazone.

Currently, in the United States, pioglitazone is prescribed concomitantly with other antidiabetics more than 60% of the time. During the PROactive study, 96% of the trial population was taking concomitant medications. These facts indicate a demand for single-pill combinations of PPAR-γ and other antidiabetics, providing the improved efficacy of multiple medications while eliminating the need for polypharmacy. GSK's combination therapy Avandamet has seen significant uptake since its introduction in 2002. In addition, in November 2005, Takeda launched a single-pill combination of pioglitazone and metformin (Actoplus Met) and filed an NDA for a single-pill combination of pioglitazone and glimepiride. It seems likely that this type of agent may see a boost in sales as a result of the PROactive study, although the competition between

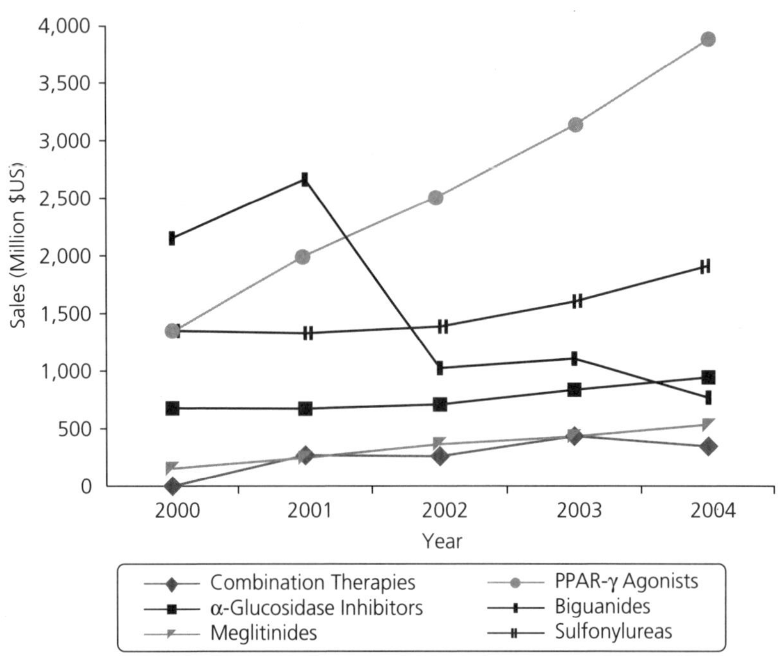

Figure 36.3 Sales Growth of Antidiabetic Drug Classes, 2000–4

combination therapies (particularly the PPAR-γ/metformin combinations) is likely to be significant.

The results of the PROactive study also raise questions about the potential of other PPAR receptors as targets in the treatment of type 2 diabetes and its macrovascular complications. For example, PPAR-α agonists (fibrates) activate genes that regulate atherogenic dyslipidemia. The development of a dual PPAR-α/γ agonist, therefore, would appear to have both enhanced therapeutic potential and commercial appeal.

Many companies have been developing PPAR-α/γ agonists; however, the drug class has been plagued with serious side effects, including edema and tumor formation, prompting most companies to discontinue development of such agents. The lead agent in this drug class, BMS's muraglitazar (Pargluva), had received an approvable letter from the FDA for treatment of diabetes, pending further clinical data. However, in clinical trials, muraglitazar showed a higher incidence of death, major adverse cardiovascular events (major MIs, stroke), and congestive heart failure, prompting study investigators to state, "Muraglitazar should not be approved to treat diabetes based on laboratory end points until safety is documented in a dedicated cardiovascular events trial" (Nissen et al., 2005). Therefore, the future of this drug class as a treatment for diabetes remains uncertain.

Although sales of pioglitazone are likely to benefit from the results of the PROactive study, the extent of that benefit is difficult to determine. It remains to be seen whether the cardiovascular benefits seen in the PROactive study are specific to pioglitazone and PPAR-γ agonists or whether the same results can be achieved with other antidiabetic treatments. For example, the UKPDS indicated that metformin use had some positive effect on cardiovascular health in type 2 diabetes patients, although the agent did not appear to have as significant an impact on cardiovascular events. Should further studies show that another agent has a similar effect to pioglitazone, the positive benefit for sales of pioglitazone resulting from the PROactive study are likely to be mitigated.

REFERENCES

Dormandy, J. et al. Secondary prevention of macrovascular events in patients with type 2 diabetes in the PROactive study (PROspective pioglitAzone Clinical Trial In macroVascular Events): a randomized controlled trial. *Lancet*. 2005; 366: 1279–89.

Gu, K. et al. Diabetes and decline in heart disease mortality in US adults. *JAMA*. 1999; 281:1291–7.

Holman, R.R. et al. A randomized double-blind trial of acarbose in type 2 diabetes shows improved glycemic control over 3 years (UK Prospective Diabetes Study 44). *Diabetes Care*. 1999; 22: 960–4.

Isomaa, B. et al. Cardiovascular morbidity and mortality associated with the metabolic syndrome. *Diabetes Care*. 2001; 24: 683–9.

Li, J. et al. Effect of pioglitazone on first phase insulin secretion in type 2 diabetes mellitus and impaired glucose intolerance. *Diabetes*. 2003; 52(suppl. 1): A130. Abstract 556-P.

Nissen, S.E., et al. Effect of muraglitazar on death and major adverse cardiovascular events in patients with type 2 diabetes mellitus. *JAMA*. 2005; 294: 2633–5.

Pfutzner, A. et al. Pioneer Study: PPAR gamma activation results in overall improvement of clinical and metabolic markers associated with insulin resistance independent of long-term glucose control. *Hormone Metabolic Research*. 2005; 37: 510–15.

Stamler, J. et al. Diabetes, other risk factors, and 12-yr cardiovascular mortality for men screened in the Multiple Risk Factor Intervention Trial. *Diabetes Care*. 1993; 16(2): 434–44.

UK Prospective Diabetes Study (UKPDS) Group. Intensive blood-glucose control with sulphonylureas or insulin compared with conventional treatment and risk of complications in patients with type 2 diabetes (UKPDS33). *Lancet*. 1998; 352: 837–53.

PART IV

Diagnostics

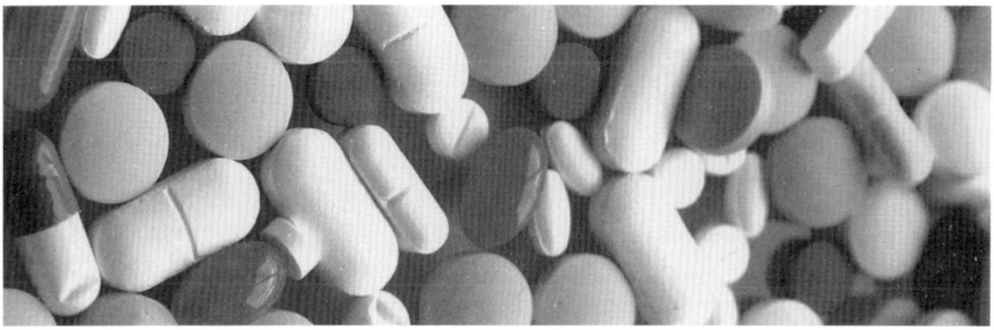

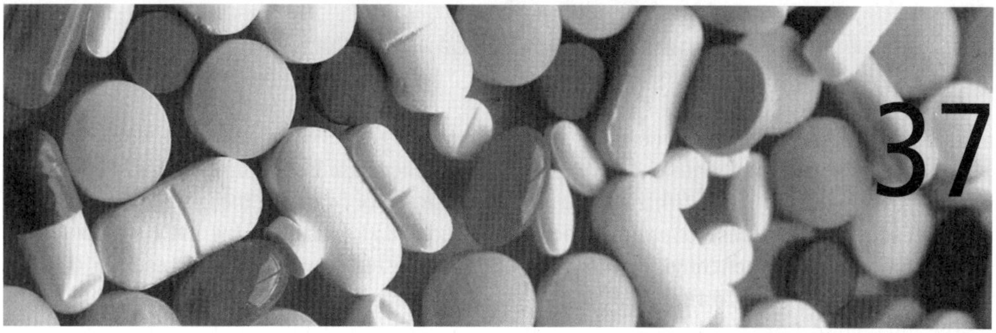

Integrating Diagnostics and Therapeutics for Targeted Therapies – Part 1: Optimizing the Comarketing Plan

OVERVIEW OF DIAGNOSTICS AND PHARMACEUTICAL COMARKETING EFFORTS

The era of paired diagnostics and pharmaceuticals is upon us. Throughout pharmaceutical R&D, diagnostics (in the guise of molecular and genetic testing) and therapeutics are being integrated with considerable productivity benefits. As T. Nagle and colleagues described: "Not only can pharmacogenetic analysis reduce the size and cost of many clinical trials, it also allows researchers to predict which patients will benefit most" (Nagle et al., 2003). The FDA also understands how the industry is evolving. Its officials have noted that: "Major advances in basic research have identified many opportunities for the development of personalized treatments for individuals identified by genomic tests. However, the integration of these tests into routine clinical practice remains a major multidisciplinary challenge" (Lesko and Woodcock, 2004).

With a broad range of targeted therapies requiring the use of a diagnostic coming to market, the comarketing (joint promotion and sales) of diagnostics and therapeutics will become routine. Even as theranostics (combined diagnostics and therapy) and personalized medicine (targeted therapy) promise to change the pharmaceutical business model, pharmaceutical companies still lack an understanding of how to commercialize or market a diagnostic. Despite the many clinical benefits that diagnostics bring (e.g., fewer adverse events, more-appropriate patient selection, home therapy monitoring), many pharma companies see this area as too complex and unfamiliar. Pharmaceutical marketers are understandably wary of embracing diagnostics as part of their brands' life-cycle management.

This chapter, the first in a two-part series, is not designed to create a comprehensive marketing plan for diagnostics teamed with therapeutics. Instead, it is intended to help pharmaceutical marketers facilitate the optimum design of their comarketing plans. Herein, we separate fact from fiction in the diagnostics-marketing arena, explain the benefits pharma can expect to gain by becoming intimately involved in this process, and provide three logical hypotheses to start planning and negotiation with a diagnostics partner. In the second part of this series, we will present a new case-based financial model on which to benchmark return on investment (ROI) and refine the overall marketing plan in a financial context. We will focus on quantifying incentives for CEOs, CFOs, and boards of directors and explore why the creation of new marketing core competencies makes financial sense.

Cultural Differences between Pharmaceutical and Diagnostics Companies

Pharmaceutical and diagnostics companies have different perspectives on this multidisciplinary challenge. When each perspective is viewed more closely, it is easy to understand why the idea of collaboration seems so alien to both sides.

Pharmaceutical marketing has arguably been refined into a science all its own. Marketing departments use a range of resources to determine what it takes to build value (and brand awareness) in the eyes of the primary target audience of clinicians and the secondary target audience of third-party payers (e.g., insurers, HMOs), professional bodies, and consumers. Examples of pharmaceutical marketing resources include the following:

- Case studies.
- Market research programs.
- Consumer acceptance studies.
- Opinion leader analysis.
- Trade-off analysis of key benefits.
- Longitudinal prescription data.
- Pharmacy benefit (PBM) management company data.
- Reimbursement studies.

Marketing managers aim to build up demand for their products in as many as 60,000–70,000 physicians and obtain requests by brand name from millions of patients without resorting to lower prices. Within the United States, the annual cost of marketing a new drug (even in a minor drug class) to this customer base is seldom less than \$100–\$200 million. For example, the impending launch of Merck and GlaxoSmithKline's two potential blockbuster cervical cancer vaccines (GSK's Cervarix; Merck's Gardasil) will most likely require more than \$1 billion in sales and marketing. This new category of drug is estimated to be worth many billions of dollars.

In contrast to the pharmaceutical industry's marketing strategy, the majority of the diagnostics industry's marketing efforts are geared toward promoting a test to a relatively small number of very technically oriented customers (e.g., 6,000–7,000 US laboratories) and maintaining market share by *discounting* prices. To date, few diagnostics garner annual sales of more than \$40 million, and the majority takes in less than \$1 million (Leon, 2004).

Budgets to launch novel diagnostics and address marketing issues seldom reach the levels of spending that accompany the launch of a drug. To command this level of spending would require a fundamental change in perspective on the part of diagnostics investors, who are used to limited marketing spends and modest returns.

Consider, for example, the exceptional efforts of Digene in exclusively promoting a novel marker (the $p53_{arg}$ gene) as a potential indicator for the increased risk of cervical cancer associated with human papillomavirus (HPV). Merck and GlaxoSmithKline anticipate that this same market will support billion-dollar pharmacotherapies. Yet it has taken 13 years for Digene's HPV diagnostic test to be recommended by the American College of Obstetricians and Gynecologists (ACOG), the key milestone in broaching this market. In 2004, Digene spent approximately \$34 million marketing its test, which yielded only \$88 million in sales.

Another barrier to overcome is that diagnostics are rarely marketed directly to physicians. Marketers of novel diagnostics simply have no reservoir of experience in marketing to physicians, let alone promoting test-and-treatment protocols. Thus, the pharmaceutical industry cannot rely on a diagnostics-industry marketing model to promote widespread adoption of a therapy to the much broader pharmaceutical customer base (e.g., physicians). To effectively market a new targeted therapy that is enabled by a particular diagnostic, it is in the interests of both pharmaceutical and diagnostics companies to distribute and heavily promote diagnostic tools as widely as possible.

Past Collaborations

Despite the polar opposite approaches taken to marketing a diagnostic versus a therapy, specific diagnostic/therapy copromotion deals are not necessarily new. However, these agreements have often been limited in scope and resulted in failed or aborted comarketing programs. Because so few comarketing agreements have succeeded, there is no benchmark to follow when building this type of agreement. Thus, the comarketing of a diagnostic and a therapy is viewed by pharmaceutical and diagnostics companies as a daunting task. Lack of experience with comarketing has led to a variety of myths about diagnostics within the pharmaceutical industry. These myths (which we discuss later) have warded off many potential drug marketers from aligning the launch and marketing of their products with an "alien" technology. They view this type of alliance with suspicion because of the partner product's unfamiliar and possibly unpredictable course after launch.

Ongoing and Future Collaborations

More than 50 targeted therapies are in Phases II and III in the drug development pipeline (Leon, 2004). In this context, many marketers will need to learn how to drive the use of related diagnostics in their target audience if their therapeutics are to reach their full potential. The first such interdependent therapy and diagnostics relationship has emerged in DakoCytomation and Genentech's comarketing of HercepTest. HercepTest is a diagnostic for the assessment of human epidermal growth factor receptor-2 (HER2) overexpression, which identifies patients who will benefit from the cancer therapy trastuzumab (Genentech's Herceptin).

We believe that the need for adaptability is a second, and equally important, reason pharmaceutical/diagnostic (Rx/Dx) comarketing skills will become a new core competency in the pharmaceutical industry. In the past, marketers of therapeutics have demonstrated their ability to address new challenges in a structured and well-planned manner; this ability was seen during the rapid growth of managed care in the 1980s and the transition to direct-to-consumer (DTC) marketing in the early 1990s. Eventually, pharmaceutical companies will learn how the novel diagnostics market works and begin to understand that sales of diagnostics (like therapeutics) respond to long-range planning, branded marketing strategies, and direct selling. Also, diagnostics can enhance a therapy's life-cycle management in a wide range of circumstances; they may even provide more predictable return on marketing investment, which is the mainstay of therapy marketing.

Such insights may be grasped soonest by companies that have both diagnostics and pharmaceutical business segments. For example, Roche and Abbott Laboratories have both invested in pairing tests and treatments in indications such as hepatitis, HIV, and diabetes. And even traditional pharmaceutical companies such as Eli Lilly and GlaxoSmithKline have appointed senior managers and diagnostics experts to the formulation of corporate strategy. These experts will help each company understand how it can comarket the diagnostic-dependent therapies in its pipeline.

BARRIERS TO COMARKETING: SEPARATING FACT FROM FICTION

Three common myths have developed around marketing diagnostics and, in turn, have served to ward off potential collaboration with the pharmaceutical industry.

Myth #1: Many Diagnostic Competitors Are Good for Therapy

Many pharmaceutical marketers avoid becoming directly involved in the distribution of a diagnostic within a specific therapeutic area, hoping that free-market forces and multiple diagnostic companies will create an efficient market (i.e., one with few barriers) for their therapy. However, the belief that multiple markers and multiple tests are all that is required should be reexamined in the light of past experience.

It is true that areas such as diabetes and antithrombosis therapy, which have enjoyed 30–40 years' worth of multiple technologies and diagnostic companies, have facilitated the growth of multibillion-dollar therapeutic categories. However, on another level, these therapeutic areas have failed to result in truly efficient diagnosis of much of the prevalent population or to optimize therapy. In 2002, for example, an estimated 18.2 million people in the United States were living with diabetes. Of this group, 5.2 million were undiagnosed (Centers for Disease Control and Prevention, 2003). Only 60% of the prevalent population was being managed with therapy, despite the hundreds of diagnostic companies and laboratories in diabetes disease management. Clearly, market forces are not enough to optimize therapy for a given population.

Another problem is that competition among multiple diagnostics companies has historically served to drive down the price of tests that enable therapy. Low market prices make it uneconomical for any single diagnostics company or laboratory to promote its test with sufficient momentum to close the clinical gaps. In addition, since the mid-1980s, various trade organizations have been unable to protect laboratories from Medicare payment cuts. For example, a test paid at $10 in 1984 receives only $8.55 today; in 2002, the same test would have been reimbursed at $16.57 if inflation increases had been applied over the past 18 years. Today, a glucose test costs only a few cents.

Although the availability of many tests drives down prices (despite growing demand), the adoption of a novel test or medical intervention would be valuable to a wide population of patients. It would also generate new demand for products and, therefore, new markets for the developers and manufacturers. However, for companies to access an untapped patient population, the market requires new and expensive forms and channels of communication to consumers who may not recognize they are at risk for the disease but for whom early diagnosis and intervention would benefit long-term prognosis. The major investments required to reach these patient pools are traditionally found in the budgets of over-the-counter (OTC)/consumer goods companies, whose R&D expenses are low, rather than biotechnology or diagnostics companies.

We believe that the auspicious arrival of proprietary molecular and genetic diagnostics will go a long way to help revive the economics of promoting an individual marker. New genetic markers now command entry-level prices ranging from $100 to $850. These prices are significantly higher than those seen by the diagnostics industry in the past decade.

Commercial and hospital laboratories constantly assess the profitability of novel tests. They make commercial decisions that are key to promoting or inhibiting the dissemination of a diagnostic. Without a compelling reason to adopt a new test in the clinic, laboratories are left to assess profitability levels on their own. This assessment may be valid for a well-known disease marker but is not encouraging for a test whose price-to-profit ratio has declined over time, or a test that is perceived as esoteric or rarely required. For example, Factor V Leiden testing in Virginia Commonwealth University's laboratories costs $71.98 to run but receives reimbursement of only $67.77; immunoglobulin gene testing costs $276.37 but is reimbursed at $164.49 (Ferreira-Gonzalez, 2004). Understandably, products that lose money for laboratories are not often at the top of these laboratories' promotional agenda.

Inadequate reimbursement is more acute in the physician's office, where on-site testing requires new resources, including lab technicians, equipment, quality control (QC) monitoring, and possibly counseling services. In the physician's practice, reimbursement codes may be in place, but if managed care's response to these codes is varied, or the correct procedural code (CPT) is new, then the test's uptake may be in jeopardy. Questions of when and how often to use it and who will pay all dampen the early dissemination of diagnostics in the market. The point-of-care (POC) diagnostics market, which focuses on promoting novel tests directly to physicians, has promised much in changing the healthcare paradigm, but it remains a minor player and represents less than 10% of overall diagnostics revenues. This situation is not the result of a failure of technology or the lack of clinical need but a failure on the part of marketing executives to recognize the huge costs involved in shifting physician behavior. The poor track record of the physician-based POC market is a window onto tomorrow's theranostics market unless there is a drastic change in approach.

Considering the aforementioned challenges, the comarketing plan should include certain aspects to ensure that positive incentives for product adoption (on behalf of laboratories or physicians) are in place and working. The plan should involve creating new reimbursement codes if required, clarifying existing codes, and negotiating with third-party payers to ensure adequate contribution to overhead for both labs and physician offices. Executives who are planning comarketing campaigns need to understand the long-term profit chain of a diagnostic within the particular therapeutic area they are targeting. Both parties should pay attention to creating financial incentives for the diagnostics partner or partners and enabling them to spend their marketing dollars on broadening clinical use.

We are not arguing for an exclusive dedication to one diagnostics partner because there may be other reasons why multiple diagnostics competitors are necessary over the life cycle of the therapy. However, partnerships and proactive distribution planning are much more likely to create efficient markets for diagnostics than are the cannibalizing economics that have been a hallmark of the diagnostics market.

Myth #2: Diagnostic Intellectual Property Cannot Be Defended

A second myth is that diagnostics intellectual property (IP) lacks the strength to support dedicated partnerships built around core platform technologies or biomarkers. Historically, this belief about the diagnostics market has been true because the patents surrounding a new marker or technology were often ignored or circumvented. However, this way of thinking may no longer be valid because of the wide range of new platform technologies (multiplexes), biomarkers, and molecular and genetic tests for which IP is rigorously created and defended. With the advent of defensible diagnostics IP, a viable licensing and cross-licensing environment has emerged. Recently, Chiron actively defended its hepatitis C virus (HCV) patents and earned new revenues by outlicensing its technology to companies like Roche. A similar change is taking place in the traditional immunoassay market with companies such as Inverness, which is investing in IP acquisitions from Abbott Laboratories and Unilever while leading a very successful campaign to defend patents from Acon Laboratories, Pfizer, and Quidel.

This trend toward building up and defending diagnostics IP is good for the diagnostics industry and, in turn, for the pharmaceutical industry. However, it is not a substitute for the evolutionary development of a diagnostics program for staying ahead of the technology curve. Such a program could harness the complementary protection offered by effective branding, as is the case with pharmaceutical products.

Many pharma marketers fear those aspects of the diagnostic market that are most alien to them. For example, multiple biomarkers and platforms for a single disease are often flexible qualities in diagnostics; however, they contrast greatly with the single chemical entity focus demonstrated by the pharma industry. We believe that the ability to meet the technical needs of different end users should be seen as a benefit. As a therapy moves through its life cycle, it may evolve from requiring diagnosis by an analyte-specific test conducted in one national reference laboratory, to a broadly available enzyme-linked immunosorbent assay (ELISA) screening test used by 4,000–5,000 laboratories, to a home-monitoring kit for patients (Table 37.1). These evolving needs can be met only by a variety of testing technologies, each of which may be subject to its own licensing and sublicensing restrictions.

We believe that a diagnostics/therapy comarketing plan should consider diagnostics IP in the context of enabling the broader use of the target therapy. At one stage, it may be appropriate to focus on one technology, thereby allowing the diagnostics partner to invest in marketing. At another stage, it may be preferable to concentrate on promoting the availability of tests in multiple channels (e.g., esoteric tests, mainstream laboratory tests, rapid POC tests, OTC home tests). This strategy, rather than a preoccupation with tomorrow's winning technology, will better serve the interests of optimizing therapy.

Myth #3: No Diagnostic Is Worth Spending $50 Million at Launch

The third myth is that there can be no return on investing $50 million per year to market a diagnostic. Although the current structure of the diagnostics industry does not allow for this type of spending, that does not mean it cannot or should not happen in the future.

Diagnostics and pharmaceutical marketers have functioned with tunnel vision in this area. Each has focused narrowly on their own marketing plans while failing to see the combined ROI possible for both partners. For example, in scenario A of Figure 37.1, a venture-backed diagnostics company might launch a new genetic test for neck cancer. The company could persuade its venture capitalists to back a major $5 million annual expenditure (a major sum for a diagnostics company) to promote the test by proving that it would enable a specific therapy. Meanwhile, the launch budget for the enabled therapy is $242 million, which will be spent to ensure appropriate uptake by those diagnosed patients. Therefore, of the total marketing budget spent on this clinical issue, 2% ($5 million) is spent on the patient-finding mechanism (diagnosis), represented by the narrow part of the hourglass in Figure 37.1, and 98% ($237 million) is spent on ensuring that those diagnosed patients receive the right therapy. At best, this

Table 37.1 Planning Stages for a Parallel Evolution of a Therapeutic and a Diagnostic

Stage	*Premarketing*	*Market Development*	*Peak-Sales Optimization*	*Patent Expiry Strategies*
Assessing marketing needs	• Promoting use in clinical trials; publicizing among opinion leaders	• Launch promotion • Generating initial use in a target population	• Pursuing new indications • Compliance programs	• OTC switch • Reduced-price brand • Select high-value-indication marketing
Enabling proprietary markers	• Predisposition tests	• Predisposition tests • Screening tests • Therapeutic differentiation	• Dose-titration-levels test • Therapeutic monitoring tests	• Indication-specific tests
Choosing diagnostic technology options	• Laboratory tests • Proprietary diagnostic services	• Laboratory tests • Proprietary diagnostic services • POC tests	• Laboratory tests • POC tests • OTC diagnostics • Home monitoring tests	• Laboratory tests • Proprietary diagnostic services • POC tests • OTC tests • Home monitoring tests

OTC = Over the counter; POC = Point-of-care

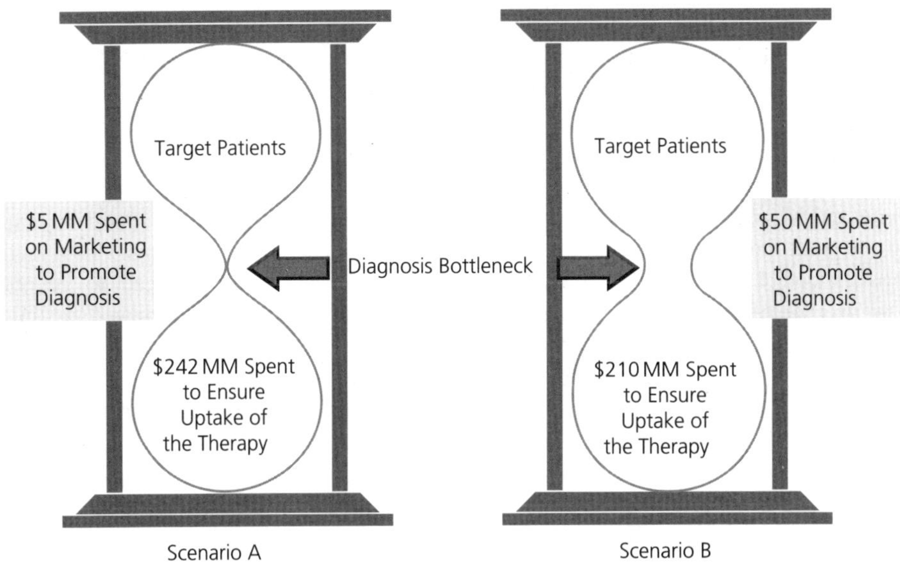

Figure 37.1 Comparison of Promotional Spending Plans for a Targeted Therapy Enabled by a Diagnostic

approach seems out of balance; at worst, and in the case of specific markers for specific therapies, it is definitely the wrong way around.

In scenario B of Figure 37.1, a reallocation of promotional spending (24%) may be more appropriate because it focuses on addressing the diagnostic bottleneck. From this example, we can see that a greater flow of patients through the bottleneck will lead more quickly to peak sales, even in a situation where therapeutic competition is lively.

The main lesson here is that comarketing strategies should feature joint budgets that will break down key barriers to disseminating a new technology and not rely on marketing silos. With a properly focused marketing strategy, the problems of how to allocate spending and drive market growth can be addressed. In an upcoming section – "Hypothesis 3: Funding the Plan" – we explore this issue in more detail.

THE NEED FOR NEW THINKING

Many other authors have written about the radically divergent marketing cultures in the pharmaceutical and diagnostics industries (Keeling and Meade, 2003). Their visions of how to market within a specific therapeutic area diverge in terms of selling, budgeting, distribution, marketing strategy, and economic return. To reach an era of maximized comarketing campaigns, these gaps must be closed. In the following sections, we explore three principal frameworks for achieving this goal: becoming involved early in the process, creating a shared marketing vision, and financing common goals.

Hypothesis 1: Early Proactive Involvement Is Essential

The long time frame associated with the adoption of a new marker or novel diagnostic standard makes early involvement in diagnostic planning essential. For example, low-density lipoprotein/high-density lipoprotein (LDL/HDL) markers for serum cholesterol were cited in the literature as early as 1950. After languishing for years and promoted by only a few diagnostics companies, these markers came into their own with the arrival of the statin therapy class in the early 1990s. The launch of TV campaigns, such as Merck's "Know your number," were also helpful in raising awareness of these markers, which have since become mainstays of primary care practice.

However, further work done in 2002 differentiated diagnostics that were not commercially driven from those that were (Keeling and Meade, 2003). Several authors suggested that adoption time frames for diagnostics could be shortened drastically, from an average of ten years (for acceptance of a new marker) to three or four years – well within the time frame for premarketing a therapy.

Typically, the pharmaceutical industry segments market development into something to be done either after the company has the lion's share of the existing market (i.e., when it can afford to) or when every dollar spent on it (e.g., for DTC advertising) has had a predictable impact on market share. Even though diagnostics can increase the overall market for a therapy, the focus on them is delayed until well after the drug has been on the market and diagnosis bottlenecks have appeared, therefore curbing the potential of the therapy during its patent life.

A key benefit of diagnostic alliances would be to help a drug that is equivalent to another succeed in the marketplace. It is important to note that equivalent therapies, launched in the same class in which two to three competitors exist, will typically result in market share of 10% or less for each one. Conversely, therapies with a perceived clinical advantage (e.g., a more convenient dosing regimen) can more easily cannibalize market share from competitors. If positioned as a clinical advantage, a combined test-and-treatment approach to a medical condition is likely to elevate the market share of such a drug.

Ironically, the dedicated molecular or genetic markers that will create tomorrow's enabling diagnostics have some of the greatest market-diffusion hurdles to surmount and will require not only early commercial involvement but also smart planning. Recent research in primary care suggests that the clinical market is poorly prepared for the issues that new diagnostics bring (Carroll et al., 2003). Complicating the uptake of new diagnostics are the lack of guidelines on patient counseling, the lack of educational tools, uncertainty over reimbursement, and a dearth of procedural terminology. One survey of more than 1,200 clinicians suggested that less than a third felt equipped to explain genetic predisposition testing. This reluctance is neither new nor confined to genetic or molecular testing; it has persisted in clinically sensitive infectious diseases from herpes to HIV for several years.

As one leading expert described the market readiness for novel molecular tests: "We are in good shape as far as I can see for widespread testing: we have no standards, no counseling, no informed consent, adverse discrimination, and no way to pay for it. Other than that, we are ready to go" (Caplan, 2002).

Two main attitudes are holding back peak drug sales potential:

1. Many diagnostic markers come to a market that is unprepared for their arrival and not ready to promote the use of a therapy.
2. Many pharmaceutical marketers hide behind the lengthy adoption time frame as an excuse to bypass addressing the diagnostic element altogether.

Because multiple stakeholders are involved in making decisions about reimbursing diagnostics, companies formulating comarketing plans will need to be sensitive to the financial incentives and disincentives at work. Instead of forming a minimal, defensive marketing plan, proactive marketing programs can be tailored to the needs of both industries.

In short, with the right partner and marketing objectives in focus, a marketing program for the product's entire life cycle can be developed that will enhance clinical use and market share. This type of comprehensive evolution will require in-depth planning with one or more diagnostic partners. However, it can play a significant role in expanding the market in a timely way and can narrow the focus to key indications as well as evolving the competitive landscape.

All these objectives can be achieved through an early effort at understanding and planning around key technical and marketing issues (discussed further on).

Hypothesis 2: Unifying Copromotion Brand Objectives

Abbott recently focused a working party on the planning aspects of joint diagnostic/therapy commercialization. One of the greatest challenges the group cited is the lack of a common language. It is a strange fact that two sister industries, which rely on the same target customers, have evolved corporate languages that so drastically differ. If these two industries are to work together, there is undoubtedly a reason for creating a common dialect. But more important, the two industries should focus on unifying their polar opposite approaches to branding.

Pharmaceutical companies undertake extensive market research and spend millions of dollars preparing for a drug to enter the market. The end point of that investment is to identify the core brand value(s) for the therapy, which in turn provide the drug with its clinical and competitive positioning. Brand values are an essential element driving the behavior of central and regional pharmaceutical marketing departments, and they influence material sent to advertising agencies and professional relations groups that interact with key opinion leaders and professional bodies. This influence makes brand values and equity the heart of a pharmaceutical product marketing campaign.

Diagnostics companies lack the branding and marketing skills of many pharmaceutical companies. Figure 37.2 shows the comparative marketing spending of two companies that focus on the same clinical area: Innogenetics, a molecular diagnostics company, and Gilead Sciences, a biopharmaceutical company. Both companies were founded within 12 months of each other in the late 1980s and have focused their product development and marketing strategies on the high-value antiviral

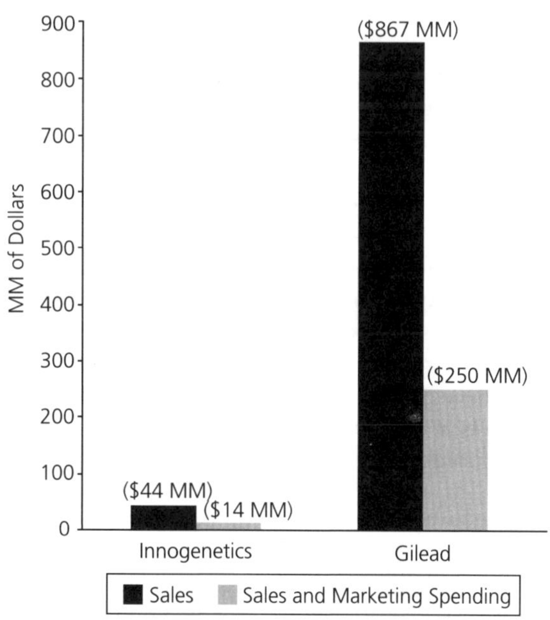

HBV = Hepatitis B virus; HIV = Human immunodeficiency virus
Note: Based on 2003 financial reports

Figure 37.2 Diagnostics versus Pharmaceuticals in the Small-Cap HIV/HBV Market—Comparison of Innogenetics with Gilead Sciences

(HIV/HBV) therapeutic areas. Both companies are public and utilize a combination of sales partners to help commercialize their own products; both spend approximately 30% of their sales revenues on sales and marketing. Despite these similarities, it is apparent that the relative scale of sales and marketing spending differs widely between the two industries.

Traditionally, building brand equity among physicians has not been a priority of diagnostics-marketing plans. Reasons for this position include the following:

- *Budget limitations.* As previously discussed, there are perceived limits for marketing within a competitive diagnostics field. Investors in the diagnostics industry also share this perception.
- *Longevity of tests.* Once a novel test has been established as a laboratory standard, the heavy focus on building brand equity is perceived to be unnecessary. This opinion comes about because the test has no ROI benefit to the diagnostics company, and the laboratory manager's focus is on a lower price per test.

Of course, a few companies have invested in brand-name awareness to differentiate their particular product or technology platform from that of competitors (Table 37.2). Even so, brand equity (i.e., investing in a major value proposition) is underserved within the diagnostics industry.

Any manager's definition of brand equity will reveal that establishing brand-name awareness for a diagnostic should not be mistaken for building the type of equity that has become the mainstay of a drug's competitive profile. Instead, brand equity for a diagnostic requires a more-comprehensive spending approach to cover all aspects of the product's uptake, dissemination, and sales.

Table 37.2 Select Companies Investing in Brand-Name Awareness

Diagnostics Company	*Primary Brand Name*
DakoCytomation	HER2 FISH pharmDx
Roche Diagnostics	TaqMan
Cytyc	Thin Prep
Focus Diagnostics	HerpeSelect

FISH = Fluorescence in situ hybridization; HER2 = Human epidermal growth factor receptor-2

To enable joint marketing and avoid the expensive need to build separate diagnostic brand equity, pharmaceutical companies should ask their diagnostic partners to orient their marketing spend toward the brand objectives of the therapy. This step will become the central plank for building long-term brand equity in the joint franchise. If therapy companies achieve this, several marketing advantages will be attained:

- A shared vocabulary is achieved early on.
- A common goal for planning is established while retaining the individuality of each partner's contribution toward common goals.
- The pharmaceutical company (the licensor) lets the diagnostic partner inside its "thought process," sharing valuable research data on key barriers to prescribing. This information sharing, in turn, can determine the technical development or regulatory pathway a test will take, which will support the drug's life-cycle objectives (Table 37.1).
- Physician goodwill is generated by creating seamless clinical tests and treatment protocols in the face of ever-increasing disease management options.

Next, we present two scenarios to show how this step will work in practice.

Scenario 1

A combined analysis identifies a therapy that requires early administration but whose brand values are "fastest acting." The result is physicians regarding diagnosis as a drain on their existing resources that would necessitate additional investment in patient counseling. The physician's resistance to the diagnosing process will hinder the uptake of the drug – from creating a delay in prescribing to causing a bottleneck in disease management. If the diagnostics partner focuses on the need to deliver on the value of *fast acting*, then a rapid diagnostic for use in the physician's office could lead to higher reimbursement for additional time dedicated to diagnosis. The rapid diagnostic could also obtain better reimbursement to allow for educational tools and information services to ease the diagnostic's transition into use.

Scenario 2

A drug that is likely to attract widespread and rapid use and become the leader of its therapeutic class might have *enhanced performance* as its core value. However, the product might face strong competitors and see only 50% repeat use (also known as *therapeutic adherence*) by patients. This lack of adherence to the recommended drug regimen suggests that some patients do not perceive the benefit of *enhanced performance*. In this instance, the diagnostics comarketing program might include a second-line or follow-up home test (or testing service) for certain patients to facilitate longer-term use and competitively differentiate the new drug from others in its class.

We are beginning to see this type of joint marketing in complementary treatment areas (e.g., hepatitis, HIV, and diabetes). In these areas, the clinical "face" of therapy, diagnosis, and counseling is unified around common treatment goals even though multiple companies are involved.

Building a comarketing partnership around brand values not only affects issues of positioning and customer service but also influences the selling process. The pharmaceutical sales model is designed to deliver brand values directly to clinicians and consumers. To date, the industry has found no better substitute for the delivery of complex messages over time than deploying an army of direct sales and detailing representatives. Therefore, if a pharmaceutical company would not entrust a third-party distributor to deliver its core brand values, the same company should consider nothing less for the diagnostics mission.

Diagnostics companies that are marketing products for their own economic return resort to a distribution model that relies on third-party distributors. Novel diagnostics marketing messages may be just as complex as those of the therapy they enable, or they may require early insertion into the patient management regimens. Given this fact, direct promotion must be considered essential. It would be inefficient for a comarketing program to delegate diagnostics distribution to third-party general distributors; instead, joint marketing programs must be delivered as a team and in the most efficient manner.

Currently, there is no basis from which to measure comarketing success because not enough joint sales programs have been undertaken. The recent growth in targeted therapy (e.g., trastuzumab, imatinib mesylate) has seen a closer alliance between the delivery of diagnostics and therapeutics to the physician's office, but joint sales teams are still not widely employed. Until the economics of a shared salesforce is explored in the field, the responsibility for organizing direct detailing of the diagnostic must rest on the shoulders of the diagnostics partner.

In the United States, funding 60 direct representatives in the field requires an investment of approximately $10 million. Higher comarketing spending may be sufficient to enable peak sales of a drug by building core brand values and delivering a diagnostics program. However, such an investment may reach too far into the budgets of most diagnostic companies. Rather than accept this inevitability, we need to revisit ways to fund sales and marketing spending in comarketing programs – which leads us to the third hypothesis.

Hypothesis 3: Funding the Plan

Venture capitalists have invested in new and novel diagnostics companies for more than 25 years, but historically, funding marketing programs has not been a priority. Instead, the primary focus has been on getting the technology to work and ensuring that it fits well in existing sales channels. This objective is managed within a tight budget that is approximately one to two times the cost of developing the technology. In the era of molecular and genetic diagnostics, the primary goal of venture capital funding needs to be overhauled.

Building comarketing plans around the therapy's core brand values is a strong argument for the joint allocation of spending. However, it does not answer the question of which party should fund what. This question is perplexing, considering that partners arguing over such spending are very likely to reach an impasse. The diagnostics partner faces the greater challenge in creating a common marketing platform centered on the concept of brand values because it needs to fund this effort with additional spending. Diagnostics companies retort that Big Pharma needs to pick up the tab for the additional marketing spend because it has the most to gain. This way of thinking has done little to strengthen the position of diagnostics with pharma partners because it breaks an important rule in business: bring your partner a solution, not a problem.

In practice, it makes the most sense to combine the total budgeted market spending to better focus on key hurdles to dissemination in the market. A joint budget can allocate resources toward total market development (in particular, to diagnosis or monitoring bottlenecks), not only to uptake of the therapy. We argue that, in most diagnostics markets, there already exists a measurable relationship between therapeutics and diagnostics sales that can be used as a valid benchmark to strengthen funding formulas.

Table 37.3 shows the percentage of pharmaceutical sales in a range of long-standing (e.g., diabetes) to more recent (e.g., HIV) diseases. The last column shows diagnostic revenues as a percentage of therapy sales. Clearly, the relationship between diagnosis and treatment revenues reflects many different dynamics at work in these therapeutic classes, including age of the segment, size of the key players, and levels of reimbursement. Nonetheless, such a relationship (whether it be disease-specific or generic) can be used to guide who should contribute what to the comarketing budget. By agreeing to a fixed-financial-equation approach, real market data can be accounted for and the company likely to be rewarded for the efforts it puts forth can be acknowledged. In addition, the equation can forestall disagreement with regard to marketing investment, helping to decide which company should invest in what part of the comarketing program.

To further demonstrate a fixed financial equation, Table 37.4 depicts three potential scenarios. In each one, the ratio of marketing spend for the therapy and the diagnostic is similar, at 30%. (This figure, of course, can

Table 37.3 Relationship between Therapy and Diagnostics Markets, 2003

	Therapy Sales ($US millions)	*Diagnostics Sales ($US millions)*	*Diagnostics Sales as a % of Therapy Sales*
Diabetes	12,000	3,600	30
Anticoagulation	2,700	400	15
HIV viral load	5,000	306	6

Table 37.4 Potential Scenarios for Marketing Expenditures on a Diagnostic versus a Therapy

	Therapy A	*Therapy B*	*Therapy C*
Therapeutics			
Sales ($MM)	150	300	700
Marketing expenditures ($MM)	45	90	210
Sales devoted to sales and marketing[a] (%)	30	30	30
Diagnostics			
Sales ($MM)	9	36	168
Marketing expenditures ($MM)	2.7	10.8	50.4
Sales spent on sales and marketing[b] (%)	30	30	30
Relationship of diagnostics to therapeutics sales (%)	6	12	24
Total marketing expenditures ($MM)	47.7	100.8	260.4
Share of marketing budget spent on diagnostics (%)	5.7	10.7	19.4

[a]Typically, the pharmaceutical industry spends 30% of its sales revenue on sales and marketing
[b]Typical marketing ratios in the diagnostic industry range from 20% to 40%

vary depending on the profitability of the individual products.)

For Therapy A, 6% of its revenues typically arise from its diagnostic component. Therefore, 6% of the total marketing budget should be supported by the diagnostic company and 94% by the therapy company. For Therapy C, 24% of therapy revenues typically arise from its diagnostic component. Thus, 19% of the total marketing budget should be supported by the diagnostic company and 81% by the therapy company.

By using the simple formula (marketing spend of diagnostic companies/total marketing spend of both pharma and diagnostic companies), these ratios can be applied to specific therapy/disease situations built around a simple premise. That is, growing therapeutic revenues is a direct result of increasing the efficiency of the diagnostics market. In other words, a larger number of patients will undergo therapy if the diagnostics market is more efficient. This dynamic creates a symbiosis that can be financially modeled. But more significantly, it can help remove contentious issues of which company should fund what aspect of the comarketing program and instead focus attention on fixing the bottlenecks (see Figure 37.1).

However, this formula may solve only half the problem. Because diagnostics companies are not used to operating with major marketing budgets, they may be unable to fund what they perceive as risky marketing investments. Under their own steam, one could imagine the same diagnostics investors balking at proposed levels of spending unseen elsewhere in the industry because they are used to modest marketing budgets that are one to two times greater than development spending.

To their detriment, most pharmaceutical companies abide by the philosophy of encouraging multiple competitors and keeping diagnostics relationships at arm's length financially. This thinking denies the diagnostics company access to third-party sources of capital to fund peak sales growth. Most diagnostics companies and their investors would welcome targeted alliances with pharmaceutical companies that center on a comarketing initiative. To see the value placed in these initiatives, one only has to look at the news releases of small to midsize diagnostics companies when they secure a business relationship with a large pharma company. When a diagnostics company is public, such an alliance can add 10–15% to the market value of the company.

With the aid of clear comarketing agreements and formulaic spending requirements, investors will be more willing to fund diagnostics companies more generously. In turn, few other investors will consider expending money to support loose marketing relationships that have no clearly defined partnership arrangements. Pharmaceutical marketers should help themselves by negotiating tightly conceived comarketing deals that will allow them to make the most of their investment and their investors.

CONCLUSION: INTEGRATION OF DIAGNOSTICS AND THERAPEUTICS

The arrival of more new tests and pharmaceuticals and the prospect of ever more therapies based on a patient's particular diagnostic response will highlight the need for clear clinical diagnostic standards. Because professional bodies often lag in their response to the need for new diagnostic standards, the responsibility falls on the player with the most resources – the pharmaceutical company – to address it appropriately. We argue that, with the aid of adjustments in thinking, techniques, and use of resources, such standards would facilitate more appropriate and earlier use of therapy.

Although more mature and better-integrated medical solutions are in place in indications such as diabetes, it is important to note that it took more than 40 years for testing, treatment, and monitoring to become fully integrated into this billion-dollar treatment market. To enhance peak-market development, the pharmaceutical industry does not need to micromanage all aspects of providing the diagnostic, but it does need to take total ownership of joint efforts to disseminate the test among clinicians, labs, and patients.

Such a shift in behavior will require new thinking and training at the marketing level but will undoubtedly redefine the marketplace in favor of the companies that can solve problems of integrating care in simple, innovative ways. By taking a logical approach to the partnership, care can be integrated in ways that expand the market, help patients, and provide better economic returns for both pharmaceutical and diagnostics companies. The pharma industry, which has earned so much competitive advantage from a first-to-market strategy, should not hesitate to take a similar approach to the delivery of integrated care.

If both the pharma and diagnostics industries built new core competencies on both sides, in 10 years' time the comarketing landscape could be drastically altered. As seen from a customer/physician point of view, this landscape might manifest itself in a marked increase in protocols in which diagnosis, treatment, and monitoring are intimately linked and target a preselected, clinically appropriate patient population. Such a landscape would provide pharmaceutical companies with working examples of comarketing programs from which to benchmark and further improve. In addition, there will be a growing group of diagnostics companies with comarketing experience to call on.

There are no shortcuts for reaching this ideal paradigm. Bringing novel diagnostics to market in a way that enhances the long-term return of a therapy requires diligence and planning similar to that used in a new drug launch. In addition, it requires that marketing professionals grasp the diagnostics issues relating to development, reimbursement, regulatory approval (or rejection), and the clinic. Paradoxically, these issues will be more important to effective comarketing plans than if the diagnostic were being developed as a stand-alone product.

For their part, diagnostics companies will have to profoundly change their current business model. They will have to move away from financing and servicing a lone product marketing plan, and become an industry skilled at helping solve clinical issues and getting therapy to patients who need it.

REFERENCES

Caplan, A. Are we ready for mass genetic testing? Presented at the Women in Biotechnology Meeting; October 16, 2002; Baltimore, MD.

Carroll, J.C. et al. Genetic susceptibility to cancer. Family physicians' experience. *Canadian Family Physician.* 2003; 49: 45–52.

Centers for Disease Control and Prevention. National diabetes fact sheet: general information and national estimates on diabetes in the United States, 2003. Rev ed. Atlanta, GA: U.S. Department of Health and Human Services, Centers for Disease Control and Prevention, 2004.

Ferreira-Gonzalez, A. A laboratorian's insights on reimbursement of molecular diagnostics. The Center for Business Intelligence Conference on Molecular Diagnostics; November 19, 2004; Arlington, VA.

Keeling, P. and Meade, P. How to make Rx-Dx alliances work [electronic]. *Pharmaceutical Executive.* July 2003. www.pharmexec.com.

Leon, J.A. Select the right molecular diagnostic product portfolio and secure market success – it is not just about money or about science. Presented at the CBI Molecular Diagnostics Meeting; November 18, 2004; Arlington, VA.

Lesko, L.J. and Woodcock, J. Translation of pharmacogenomics and pharmacogenetics: a regulatory perspective. *Nature Reviews Drugs Discovery.* 2004; 3: 763–9.

Nagle, T. et al. The further evolution of biotech. *Nature Reviews Drug Discovery.* 2003; 2: 75–9.

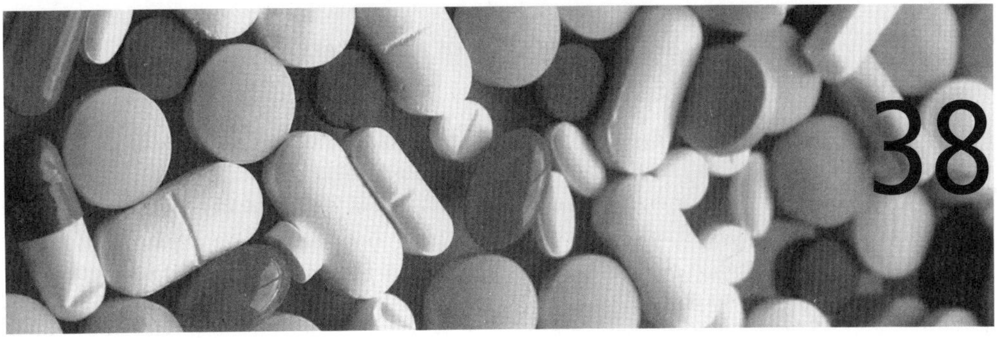

Integrating Diagnostics and Therapeutics for Targeted Therapies – Part 2: The Importance of Calculating the Return on Investment

INTRODUCTION

As the promise of diagnostic/therapeutic combinations is increasingly recognized, pharmaceutical companies must determine best practices in terms of comarketing these combinations. This two-part series is designed to showcase fundamental considerations in diagnostic/drug comarketing plans. Part 1 of this series examined the potential benefit that drug companies can gain from entering into well-planned marketing collaborations with diagnostics companies and presented a framework on which to build these collaborations. In this chapter, Part 2, we focus on the importance of the financial justification for those collaborations. To highlight the importance of this analysis, we discuss the variables that must be considered when quantifying the expected return. We review three hypotheses often encountered when determining the benefit of a diagnostic, applying to them historical cases in which the relationships between diagnosis and treatment can be measured or analyzed and used as benchmarks when estimating the financial return on new ventures.

The use of historical data is critical when developing a financial model meant to quantify the economic benefit that diagnostics have on pharmaceutical life cycles. Using these benchmarks allows pharmaceutical marketers and investors to assess the sales impact associated with the perceived improvement in clinical service associated with diagnostic use. This assessment will help marketers and investors determine where partnering with diagnostics companies makes the most sense and drive the decision to expend resources on the appropriate biomarker development program.

REASONS FOR CALCULATING THE RETURN ON INVESTMENT

The potential reduction in R&D costs associated with pairing diagnostics with pharmaceuticals has been widely discussed and recorded. The ability to identify patients more likely to respond to a therapy prior to enrollment can have a significant impact on the cost of a clinical trial. A 2004 article in *Nature Drug Discovery* suggested that a 10% improvement in predicting failure before beginning a large-scale Phase III clinical trial could save approximately $100 million in development costs. (Lesko and Woodcock, 2004). Other quantitative analyses have suggested that diagnostics could cut the time from target identification to drug launch from 10–12 years to 3–5 years, thus reducing prelaunch development costs per drug to about $200 million – a quarter of some recent estimates (Arlington et al., 2002; Di Masi et al., 2003).

In contrast to the growing number of estimates and formulas addressing the impact that diagnostics will have on pharmaceutical R&D costs, there has been no published assessment of the specific impact on future drug revenues using the extensive history of diagnostics and pharmaceuticals working in individual disease areas. As a result, investors making decisions regarding targeted therapies do not have available to them one of the critical investment tools that accompany most other aspects of the pharmaceutical business model.

This lack of quantitative assessment is the basis of one of the principal financial fears surrounding the involvement of diagnostics with a therapy: that identifying the specific populations for which a therapy is beneficial will have the effect of reducing the potential patient pool and therefore the earning power of the therapy. Steve Arlington, head of IBM's pharmaceutical consulting division, has stated that pharma companies are understandably wary of the personalization of medicine. In an industry where companies rely on blockbuster products to support their R&D efforts, the possibility of reducing a blockbuster drug's market size by 80% by prescreening patients with a diagnostic potentially means significant damage to a company's revenue stream.

When considering whether to comarket a diagnostic with a therapy, decision makers must assess the financial benefit – that is, the impact that the decision will have on the financial returns of the pharmaceutical model. The lack of precedents or role models makes it difficult to construct likely returns on investment (ROI) with the degree of certainty required to change a whole investment behavior away from the traditional model of the segregated marketing of diagnosis and therapy. The recently launched targeted therapies trastuzumab (Genentech/Roche's Herceptin), imatinib mesylate (Novartis's Gleevec), and cetuximab (ImClone's Erbitux), all of which have related diagnostics, are too new to be exclusively relied upon to fill this financial assessment gap.

However, failure to thoroughly assess the impact of diagnostics on a therapy while following the traditional pharmaceutical model can hurt a company's revenues. An example of the risk from avoiding diagnostics can be seen in the recent FDA refusal to approve AstraZeneca's new antithrombotic therapy, ximelagatran (Exanta), based, in part, on concerns regarding liver toxicity. FDA experts indicated that safe use of ximelagatran could be improved through use of individualized dosing rather than fixed doses for all patients. Phase II clinical trials for ximelagatran showed evidence of elevated liver enzymes in patients taking ximelagatran compared with the placebo group, indicating that some form of liver function testing would probably be necessary. After the FDA verdict, shares in AstraZeneca tumbled, suggesting that the strategy to proceed with development without incorporating a monitoring test had cost the company dearly.

Pharmaceutical companies are still reluctant to comarket new therapies with diagnostics, even in situations where they help develop them. An example can be seen in the ongoing court battle between Sanofi-Aventis and PharmaNetics over the marketing of Sanofi-Aventis's heart therapy enoxaparin sodium (Lovenox). In early 2003, PharmaNetics announced a collaborative marketing program with Sanofi-Aventis (then Aventis) to promote the use of PharmaNetics' Enox test. The Enox test would allow physicians to monitor the activity of enoxaparin (an anticoagulant) and adjust dosages based on patient response. Sanofi-Aventis had funded the development of the Enox test and, under the marketing agreement, the two companies would coordinate worldwide advertising, marketing, and educational efforts, including joint calls on qualified hospital leads within 600 top hospitals. Ultimately, however, Sanofi-Aventis's advertising campaign de-emphasized the importance of pre-screening with the Enox test by claiming that the drug did not require monitoring, and in November 2003, PharmaNetics filed suit against Aventis claiming false and misleading advertising. PharmaNetics has appealed a judgment against it; no date for the trial has been set.

ESTIMATES OF RETURN

As stated earlier, one of the primary concerns associated with the partnering of diagnostics and therapeutics is the possibility of limiting a potential blockbuster's market size; however, many industry experts believe that such collaborations could have the opposite effect and that developing personalized therapies that are less likely to result in treatment failures but instead significantly improve the chances of success can help maximize profits, particularly courtesy of their ability to demand a premium price.

Although opinions such as this one seem intuitively correct and are based on key industry insights, pharmaceutical companies will need to calculate a quantifiable return to motivate a shift toward paired therapeutics and diagnostics. Several formulas have been developed to illuminate the financial impact that diagnostics will have on future pharmaceutical revenues.

One such model was suggested by Dr. Stan Bernard in a report for *Pharmaceutical Executive* (Bernard, 2003). Bernard states that when evaluating the effect that a diagnostic will have on the market share of a specific therapy, pharmaceutical companies must take into account not only the variables that will reduce market share (such as the identification of patients who will have adverse effects or little to no response) but also variables that could have a potentially positive effect on the drug's market share:

- More-efficient clinical trials will allow the drug to be introduced to the market sooner.
- Patients can potentially be recruited away from less-efficacious competitors.
- Patients who chose to remain untreated given the low efficacy of existing treatments may choose to begin treatment if they can be more confident of the outcome.
- Diagnostics (and their associated genomic information) can be used to identify new diseases that can be treated with the same drug, thus increasing patient share.
- Patients who have not developed a disease but carry a biomarker may wish to begin preventive treatment.
- Patient compliance can improve based on increased perceived value.
- The improved chance of efficacy offers the potential for premium pricing.

Bernard goes on to suggest that the net benefit of incorporating a diagnostic could be an overall gain. However, without benchmark data to determine the relative values within the formula, Bernard's approach is best used, as its originator intended, as merely a useful mathematical way of looking at the relationship. Without benchmark data, individual companies must assign their own values to each of these variables based on their own best guess, and those values may not reflect what is actually occurring in the marketplace. For example, a market forecaster may determine that a drug will have a 39% revenue advantage associated with improved patient compliance, but the complexities and inefficiencies of the diagnostic market would suggest a market share advantage of only 13%.

Another model, developed by Integrated Medicines, calculates the value of a diagnostic test by examining the impact on both revenue and R&D costs. The benefit of this model is that it incorporates a net present value (NPV) of savings associated with reduced development costs (fewer patients will need to be enrolled in clinical trials) into the overall calculation of return. The model also assumes that improved clinical trials will result in an earlier launch and incorporates an associated impact on sales revenue. However, this model does not rely on a real-life determination of the relationship between diagnostic and therapy and is therefore unable to provide much insight except as a theoretical perspective on the potential of a therapy/diagnostic marriage.

Axis Shield has gone one step further to model the likely impact of diagnostics over time in a specific therapeutic area for use with its Diastat anticyclic citrullinated peptide antibody (anti-CCP) test, which detects proteins associated with the incidence and severity of rheumatoid arthritis (RA).

The assumption that anti-CCP in theranostics can accomplish the following is the basis of Axis Shield's case study (Axis Shield. Theranostics: exploring the utility of Dx/Rx partnering in drug development and marketing):

- Detect early onset of RA disease.
- Measure severity and erosiveness of RA.
- Predict arthritis outcome.
- Differentiate between autoimmune diseases.
- Stratify RA patients for treatment with disease-modifying antirheumatic drugs (DMARDs).
- Measure the effectiveness of treatment.

If diagnostics can effect any or all of the above treatment dynamics in a financially favorable manner, Axis Shield's conclusion is that diagnostics can increase the $15 billion RA market size (or individual drug revenues) by approximately $3 billion (or 20%).

This case example is an extremely useful insight into the potential impact of a diagnostic on therapy in an individual disease scenario based on Axis Shield's experience in the field and will have utility in assessing a commercial relationship in the RA treatment area. A drawback, however, is that it focuses on the theoretical upsides of the incorporation of a diagnostic, such as the savings associated with reduced development time and the increased sales associated with product differentiation, and it does not necessarily take into account the inefficiencies of the relationship around and between therapy and diagnostic that work to distort straight-line financial theory.

Published insights and formulas available to quantify the likely benefit of diagnostics estimate increases of 17–85% over the equivalent revenues expected from a therapy-only strategy. These estimates appear to overinflate the impact of a diagnostic and assume a perfect and efficient interaction of diagnostic with therapy. However, pharmaceutical companies are often skeptical of the value of diagnostics and are aware that this type of efficient interaction is not often seen in the marketplace. Pharmaceutical executives will need a model that accounts for both the efficiencies and inefficiencies of the relationships around and between therapy and diagnostic to make a well-informed estimate of the ROI.

USING CASE-BASED REASONING TO CALCULATE THE RETURN ON INVESTMENT

Case-based reasoning (CBR) first appeared in commercial tools in the early 1990s; since then, it has been used in a wide number of applications both in academic and commercial fields. Dr. Janet Kolodner, a professor at the Georgi Institute of Technology who has done significant research on CBR, cites three instances in which CBR is relevant (Kolodner, 1993):

- Adapting an old solution to a new problem.
- Identifying possible failures when adapting old solutions to new problems.
- Interpreting the present situation by comparing it with many past situations.

CBR is of particular use to decision makers when there are significant historical data (cases) that can be called on to help solve a problem. For instance, CBR is used to build knowledge-based diagnostics in medical diagnosis where previous patient histories are relevant to diagnosing new patients. In the following sections, we discuss a model that uses CBR when evaluating the expected ROI associated with a diagnostic/therapy collaboration by using known cases to determine values for key variables.

The Diaceutics Model

This CBR approach is constructed around base cases (a seven-year revenue stream for a blockbuster drug and a nine-year revenue stream for a specialty therapy), which provide the constant against which a diagnostic impact is measured. The model uses seven variables (Table 38.1) that can affect these revenue streams in order to identify past cases that can be used as benchmark data when analyzing a new scenario. These variables and their importance to calculating ROI are discussed in the following section. Historical data can be used to apply appropriate values to the variables and to create a ballpark solution that serves as a first-pass value for the effect that a diagnostic will have on a therapy's sales. Refinements to the calculation are made by making additional adjustments to the relevant variables until a solution that best fits the new scenario is achieved. The solution can be validated by testing the scenario against the historical cases.

Variables

The seven variables in Table 38.1 are values that drive the revenue stream of a drug. These values can be either direct or indirect. Direct variables are those whose overall value can be influenced by the availability of a diagnostic, such as the level of patient compliance. Indirect variables are those whose overall value is not affected by the availability of a diagnostic, such as the number of patients who will respond to a drug, but who may perceive greater value to a therapy with an attached diagnostic. The sections below discuss the relevance and importance of each of these variables when calculating a ROI.

Table 38.1 Direct and Indirect Variables Used in Case-Based Reasoning

Indirect Variables	*Direct Variables*
Responders	Presenting patients
Pricing	Competitive market share advantage
	Patient compliance with therapy
	Early adoption
	Off-patent erosion

Responders

The majority of therapies used today are effective in only about 40–70% of the available patient population; traditionally, physicians have had to determine patient response after the therapy has been administered. However, breakthroughs in molecular medicine and more-accurate diagnostic techniques offer the opportunity to identify those patients most likely to benefit from a drug prior to initiating therapy. This ability to identify responders can have both positive and negative effects on a drug's profitability.

On the positive side, identifying responders prior to enrollment in a clinical trial offers the potential for pharmaceutical companies to reduce both the size and duration of expensive late-stage trials. As stated earlier in this chapter, an improved response rate in patients enrolled in clinical trials can save $100 million in development costs and reduce time to launch by five or more years, both of which would have a beneficial effect on a drug's profitability.

On the other hand, prescreening reduces the potential patient population, particularly if third-party payers begin to mandate screening in an effort to control high drug costs. This practice has been the main reason cited for pharmaceutical companies' hesitance to incorporate diagnostics into their therapies. However, it is critical that both the positive and negative effects of this driver be taken into account when calculating an ROI.

Presenting Patients

The ability to properly diagnose patients and begin therapy is a critical variable in the market size of a drug. A diagnostic that is targeted toward a disease area that remains underdiagnosed, or where diagnosis occurs at a later stage than is optimal, can have a positive effect on the overall market size of a therapy. Diagnostics that help identify candidates earlier or with greater accuracy, such as Digene's HPV test or Orasure's rapid HIV test, are already beginning to show their value in the clinic. Although the ability to improve diagnosis would in theory have an equally positive effect on all drugs that treat a particular disease, the incorporation of the test used to diagnosis the disease with the therapy used to treat it can provide a competitive advantage for a pharmaceutical company and drive revenue growth.

Pricing

Since the mid-1980s, emerging therapies have used extensive pharmacoeconomic analysis when determining pricing. In fact, formularies today seldom include therapies on their lists without clear justification of economic benefit. As a result, only drugs that can demonstrate clear economic benefit through improved clinical response can justify premium prices. The pharmaceutical industry particularly has been able to achieve these prices in new or redefined therapeutic classes; however, the association of a diagnostic that improves the likelihood of positive clinical benefit also represents an opportunity.

Pricing is a driver when analyzing the benefit of a diagnostic because improved clinical and economic outcome is likely to translate into niche premium pricing. This approach is already evidenced by the treatment cost differences of 40–70% for Herceptin, Erbitux, and Gleevec over the older established cancer regimens. Therefore, despite the loss of market size from a targeted therapy that might work in only 25% of a patient population, there is an opportunity to demonstrate significant therapeutic advantage to this smaller group. This advantage will also have a clear economic benefit to public and private payers and can therefore support premium pricing.

Competitive Market Share Advantage

In drug classes or therapeutic areas where competitors are many and products are little differentiated (such as in antibiotics or type 2 diabetes), companies are in a constant struggle to earn or maintain market share. Often, companies use direct-to-consumer advertising or increased sales promotion to urge physicians to increase the prescribing of a therapy. Targeted therapies offer companies an opportunity to gain an advantage in the competition for market share that is not tied to promotional strategies.

Targeted therapies, particularly those that include a specific test in their label, offer physicians a clinical basis from which to determine the best treatment option for their patients. In addition to this clinical validity, providing the means to identify a subset of patients who will respond specifically to a given therapy increases the switching costs (away from that given therapy) for both patient and physician, reducing the likelihood of losing market share to similar drugs. In smaller therapeutic areas, or areas that feature less competition, a targeted therapy offers the potential to gain market share from the drugs that arrived earlier to the market and as such are likely to hold the greatest share of the market.

Patient Compliance with Therapy

Patient adherence to a therapy has a clear impact on a drug's revenue potential. Along with issues such as inconvenient formulations and side effects, a significant factor in patient compliance is the perception of benefit from a therapy. For example, patients take cholesterol-lowering drugs to reduce their long-term risk of cardiac events. However, many patients stop taking their therapy because they do not perceive the lack of a negative outcome (in this case, a cardiac event) as a significant positive benefit.

Clinical evidence in diabetes, HIV, and coagulation management suggests that when diagnostic monitoring tools make patients aware of clear progress in their therapeutic goals, particularly when combined with education and healthcare worker interaction, compliance improves. It can be beneficial for a pharmaceutical company to seek a closer alignment with just such diagnostic monitoring tools either to help achieve the correct therapeutic dose or to make visible to patients that they are "in control" or improving, thus encouraging patient compliance and driving revenue.

Early Adoption

When determining how an emerging therapy will be received in the market, the pharmaceutical industry classifies its target physicians by their behavior in response to a new therapy:

- Early adopters, who will try a new therapy shortly after its launch.
- Early followers, who await an understanding of who to treat and when to treat as well as clearer evidence of the new drug's effectiveness.
- Physicians who are the last to adopt a novel therapy.

The process of adoption of a novel therapy can take two to three years. It has a direct impact on when a drug will reach its peak-year sales. To optimize the rate of adoption, pharmaceutical companies strive to continuously provide new and more reassuring clinical information to convert nonprescribers to prescribers.

The availability of a diagnostic that clearly identifies a patient's candidacy for treatment or demonstrates the value of treatment through post-treatment monitoring removes some of the uncertainty associated with a novel therapy. This benefit can be seen in the change in prescribing behavior for Herceptin after the launch of the HER2 test; physicians were more willing to use the therapy based on clear evidence of clinical relevance. Therefore, the incorporation of a diagnostic can influence the adoption rate and affect the revenue of a new therapy.

Off-patent Erosion

The generics-manufacturing industry in the United States has grown in size and sophistication over the past 15 years. Today, in blockbuster treatment categories, branded pharmaceutical companies expect that 50–80% of their revenues will be lost the year following patent expiry. A proprietary diagnostic linking a new indication to a therapy prior to patent expiry offers the potential to minimize the sales erosion resulting from patent expiry. Companies such as Prometheus Labs are already utilizing this strategy and have built niche therapeutic revenues in treatment areas identified by proprietary diagnostics. Pharmaceutical companies that explore this approach can minimize the loss of sales to generic competition and positively affect their revenues.

ANALYZING SCENARIOS USING CASE-BASED REASONING

Although it is not possible within the context of this chapter to address the many scenarios that can be analyzed by using CBR, the following sections present scenarios in which existing cases are used to evaluate three hypotheses often encountered when determining the benefit of a diagnostic.

Hypothesis 1: A Related Diagnostic Will Accelerate the Uptake of a Novel Drug in Clinical Areas Where Diagnosis Is Difficult

Historically, pharmaceutical companies try to recruit early adopters to a therapy and have focused a large portion of their marketing budget on prelaunch marketing initiatives and on sales representation in the first six months after launch. The investment in the prelaunch and launch effort is critical because it is a determinant of the market reception to the new drug and the ultimate peak-year sales. Achieving early adoption of a new therapy is critical in order to maximize sales prior to patent expiry. The following are two ways in which an associated diagnostic can affect the adoption of an emerging therapy:

- A diagnostic may identify specific responders to a therapy or may highlight beneficial differences between therapies not seen before.
- A diagnostic available 9–12 months before the launch of a related therapy may help condition the market to the need for the new therapy, thereby accelerating the adoption of the novel therapy.

Highlighting the potential effect of a diagnostic on adoption, some of the more recent targeted therapies launched with diagnostics have been witnessing a rapid uptake in the market. Table 38.2 lists therapies and their associated diagnostics. The colon-cancer drug bevacizumab (Roche and Genentech's Avastin), in its second full quarter of sales, had sales of $183 million. Imatinib mesylate (Novartis's Gleevec) experienced immediate market uptake and acceptance, achieving sales of $153 million for Novartis in its first eight months on the market. Sales of trastuzumab (Genentech/Roche's Herceptin) grew by 26% in the United States and by 140% outside of the United States in 2001, exceeding $500 million (United States). This rapid uptake can be attributed to the strong clinical data associated with these therapies, clinical data that are predicated on the use of the associated diagnostic tests to select patients most likely to derive benefit from the therapy. In addition, these drugs have seen significant adoption despite exhibiting many of the characteristics that are cited as concerns for the pharmaceutical industry: restricted patient responders, reimbursement issues, and the additional counseling burdens associated with new and novel molecular or genetic tests.

From these examples, it can be seen that the incorporation of a diagnostic can have a positive impact on the adoption rate of a new therapy and boost sales during the critical six months immediately following launch. This experience does not indicate that every new therapy would benefit in this way from a closely tied diagnostic, but it does show that marketers should ask themselves if the availability of a related diagnostic would increase success when introducing the product.

Hypothesis 2. A Related Monitoring Test Will Improve Patient Compliance with a Drug That Requires Long-term Use

Patient compliance with long-term prescribed therapies for indications such as diabetes, high cholesterol, HIV, and epilepsy is a major concern for both clinicians and the pharmaceutical industry. The problems of poor patient compliance can be seen in several studies of statin regimens. A study presented in 2003 at the European Society of

Table 38.2 Select Therapies and Associated Diagnostic Tests

Therapy	*Indication*	*Diagnostic*	*Diagnostic Manufacturer*	*Notes*
Bevacizumab (Genentech/ Roche's Avastin)	Colorectal and endometrial cancer	Colaris	Myriad Genetics	Launched in September 2000 Detects disease-causing mutations in two genes, *MLH1* and *MSH2*
Imatinib mesylate (Novartis's Gleevec)	Gastrointestinal stromal tumors	VentanaDX	Ventana Medical Systems	Approved in August 2004 c-KIT rabbit monoclonal antibody diagnostic test that detects overexpression of the c-KIT protein
Trastuzumab (Genentech/ Roche's Herceptin)	Breast cancer	HercepTest	DakoCytomation	Approved in September 1998 Tests for overexpression of the HER2/neu protein in breast cancer patients
		PathVysion	Abbott/Vysis	Approved in December 2001 Tests for overexpression of the *Her-2/neu* gene in breast cancer patients

Cardiology Congress showed that of 19,898 patients in the United Kingdom initiated on lipid-lowering therapy from 1998 to 2001, researchers found that overall less than 30% of patients were titrated to a higher dose; 18% of patients discontinued therapy within less than three months of initiation; and 60% allowed prescriptions to lapse for 60 days or longer. Researchers from the University of Michigan Health System and Cleveland Clinic reported similar findings: almost half of those patients who were prescribed a statin did not adhere to the treatment, and about half of first-time users discontinued taking the drug within four years (Ellis, 2004).

As stated earlier in this chapter, one reason that patients discontinue therapy is the lack of perceived benefit from a drug. Therefore, there is an opportunity for diagnostics that monitor a drug's effect to provide quantitative evidence of the benefits of a treatment. This evidence would then positively affect patient compliance and the overall revenue potential of a therapy. Figure 38.1 shows the potential revenue gain for select available long-term therapies based on hypothetical improvements in compliance.

It is important to note, however, that the benefit derived from a diagnostic monitoring test is enhanced by regular interaction with healthcare workers. A number of studies have examined therapeutic compliance in patients with whom there is an ongoing medical interaction. In one such study, the impact of a continuous quality improvement (CQI) intervention on glycemic control was studied in patients with diabetes mellitus attending a primary care clinic. This study used a diagnostic test to measure glycosylated hemoglobin (HbA1c) levels and compared the compliance rates between a clinic that utilized CQI techniques in conjunction with the monitoring test and a similar clinic that did not implement CQI techniques. The study concluded that involvement of nurses, physicians, and managers in a CQI process can improve patients' glycemic control in some health maintenance organization primary care settings, without increasing utilization or charges (O'Connor et al., 1996).

The financial benefit of increased compliance compared with the additional cost of funding a diagnostically enabled patient interaction program varies depending on the disease area and the therapy. In blockbuster therapies such as diabetes control, the financial benefits may clearly outweigh the cost; however, in a specialty area, the cost of the

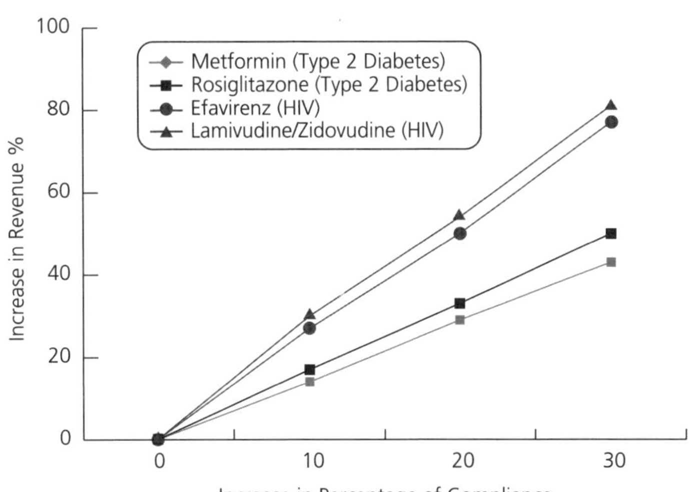

Note: Compliance increases are hypothetical: figure shows potential revenue improvements over 2004 revenues

Figure 38.1 Effect on Revenue of Select Therapies from Increased Patient Compliance

program needs to be closely compared with the potential for increased revenues to justify a return on investment.

Hypothesis 3. A Well-managed Diagnostic Program Can Justify Premium Pricing, Offsetting Restrictions in the Size of the Patient Pool

Some 56 new targeted therapies are expected to reach the market over the next 10 years, primarily (although not exclusively) in specialty drug areas. Some of these products have already been launched and are enjoying rapid uptake and increasing clinical use. These newly launched and emerging therapies are representative of a new way to manage patient care. For example, a special report in *The Economist* predicts that the targeted drugs now appearing on the market for cancer should be the first wave of new anticancer therapies. The number of targeted therapies will expand rapidly over the next five years as more targets are identified and new classes of drug are approved by regulators.

For pharmaceutical companies, the targeted nature of these therapies is cause for concern in terms of revenue potential. Despite the clinical advantages of a targeted therapy, the impact of fewer responders on potential revenue streams is significant. For example, high-dose imatinib has shown significantly longer progression-free survival in gastrointestinal stromal tumor (GIST) patients; however, this benefit is seen only in patients with the Philadelphia chromosome, a group that encompasses only about 25% of the total patient population. The inability to effectively market this therapy to the entire patient population (given its lack of efficacy in 75% of patients) certainly limits the drug's revenue potential. One method of counteracting this restriction on market size is through the use of premium pricing, a strategy that, although highly criticized, would appear to be an essential part of maintaining a return on investment for the pharmaceutical industry, particularly in specialty markets such as cancer.

However, the incorporation of a diagnostic can be beneficial when justifying the premium pricing often seen in these therapeutic specialty areas. The ability to identify responders prior to beginning treatment allows physicians to be more confident of the outcome of the therapy; in general, physicians will be more likely to prescribe an expensive therapy if there can be some assurance of success. This confidence will increase adoption and potentially encourage physicians to switch patients to the targeted therapies, resulting in a market advantage over competition. The incorporation of a diagnostic that has strong clinical relevance can therefore be used to maximize a drug's market potential, by helping establish the therapy as highly efficacious within its subpopulation.

EVALUATING A DIAGNOSTIC PARTNERSHIP

The key disadvantage of the CBR approach is the potential for bias in the use of old cases, blindly relying on previous experience without criticizing or validating it in the context of the new situation. When determining the benefit of an associated diagnostic, it is important to take into account the limitations of a given diagnostic as well as the efficacy of the therapy compared with its competitors. Notwithstanding these limitations, however, we believe that when developing a model that calculates the potential ROI of a companion biomarker strategy or diagnostic partner, the incorporation of historical data is critical. By developing a model of this kind to provide an essential financial assessment of the incentives to comarket a drug with a diagnostic, it is likely that some of the concerns often associated with diagnostic-drug combinations can be reversed.

When considering whether to comarket a diagnostic with an emerging therapy, it will be important for pharmaceutical companies to consider the following key points:

- A return on investment for comarketing with a diagnostic is not necessarily clear-cut in some cases – such as specialty therapies – and its usefulness has been underestimated in blockbuster therapies.

- The ultimate usefulness of a diagnostic is to enable clinical decisions. In some instances, those decisions will reduce the use of a drug and, in others, promote it. A proactive comarketing strategy can embrace both dimensions in a way that improves the clinical validity to use the therapy and engineers financial return into the life cycle.
- Joint therapeutic/diagnostic pricing strategies will be a critical part of building long-term value into the franchise and should be considered early. The first chapter in this series focused further on the essential need to consider diagnostic as well as therapeutic pricing strategies.
- Successful biomarker strategies have a critical financial as well as clinical bearing on the long-term potential for a drug; development of the diagnostic should begin early in order to avoid diagnostic bottlenecks hindering peak sales.

Calculating the impact on revenue is only one aspect of an informed decision regarding collaboration between pharmaceutical and diagnostic companies. Key to the success of these collaborations is the identification of models and processes that provide a quantitative assessment of the value of integrating a diagnostic with a therapeutic. By developing these tools, pharmaceutical companies will be able to look past some of the traditional concerns associated with integrated programs and begin developing joint therapeutic/diagnostic products that can benefit both industries as well as patients and third-party payers.

REFERENCES

Arlington, S. et al. Pharma 2010: the threshold of innovation. *IBM Consulting Services Future Series*. 2002.

Bernard, S. 5 myths of pharmacogenomics. *Pharmaceutical Executive*, October 2003.

Di Masi, J.A. et al. The price of innovation: new estimates of drug development costs. *Journal of Health Economics*. 2003; 22: 151–85.

Ellis, J. Suboptimal statin adherence and discontinuation in primary and secondary prevention populations. Should we target patients with the most to gain? *Journal of General Internal Medicine*. June 2004; 19(6): 638.

Kolodner, J. *Case-Based Reasoning*. Morgan Kaufmann Publishers, 1993. San Mateo, California.

Lesko, L. and Woodcock, J. Translation of pharmacogenomics and pharmacogenetics: a regulatory perspective. *Nature Drug Discovery*. September 2004; 3(9): 763.

O'Connor, P.J. et al. Continuous quality improvement can improve glycemic control for HMO patients with diabetes. *Archives of Family Medicine*. 1996; 5(9): 502–6.

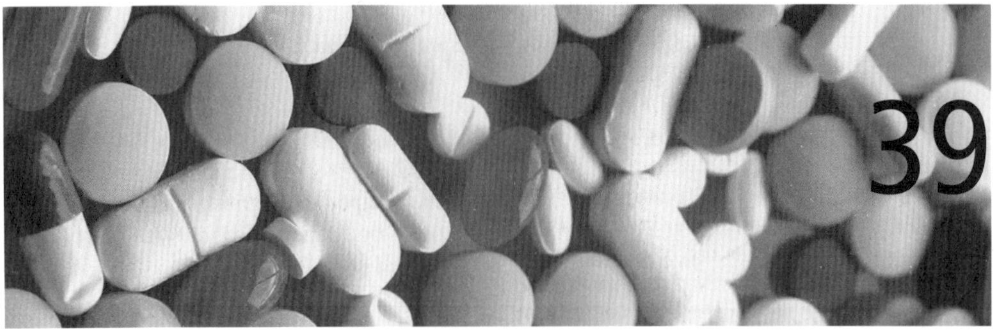

Emerging Diagnostic Markers in Alzheimer's Disease

INTRODUCTION

Alzheimer's disease (AD) is a neurodegenerative disease. During its course, neurons die progressively because of the accumulation of neurotoxic proteins that form Aβ-amyloid plaques and neurofibrillary tangles (NFTs). Unlike other cells, neurons do not self-renew; consequently, the number of functioning brain cells in an AD patient's brain decreases as the disease progresses. The decrease in the number of brain cells accounts for the severity of AD symptoms at moderate and late stages of the disease. The accumulation of Aβ-amyloid plaques and NFTs begins years before the disease symptoms become apparent. Several drugs that prevent or slow the accumulation of Aβ-amyloid plaques are in development for treatment of AD, and we expect two of these drugs to launch in the United States during the next 10 years. However, to be most effective, these treatments must be initiated in patients as soon as possible. Early intervention will preserve a higher number of functioning neurons and help maintain patients' cognitive function – but early intervention requires early diagnosis of AD, and no AD diagnostic marker is currently available. As the US population ages, AD will become a significant public health burden because currently, no therapy is available to alter the course of the disease. By the year 2050, if AD is left untreated, its prevalence in the United States is expected to reach 13.2 million (Hebert et al., 2003).

Currently, AD is diagnosed based on the patient's clinical history and the exclusion of other neurological disorders. On average, specialists achieve 80–90% diagnostic accuracy (Knopman et al., 2001), but this percentage drops for primary care physicians – who typically see the majority of AD patients – because early signs of AD are subtle and not easily distinguished from the normal signs of aging. By the time most cognitive deficits have progressed to the point where a physician diagnoses AD, neuronal damage is extensive. A diagnostic marker would provide physicians with an objective way to diagnose AD and begin drug treatment.

As stated previously, no AD diagnostic markers are currently available, but several are in development. Researchers are investigating the following areas for the diagnosis of AD: the imaging of Aβ-amyloid plaque, the measurement of the shrinkage rate of certain brain regions by magnetic resonance imaging (MRI), the measurement of new biochemical marker levels in serum or cerebrospinal fluid (CSF), and the identification of genes that predispose to or cause the disease. Thus far, experts say, none of these markers adequately fulfills the criteria (e.g., specificity, sensitivity) for diagnostic agents. However, several markers now in development hold great promise for the diagnosis of AD. In this chapter, we review AD diagnostic markers currently in use and in development, the main players in the AD diagnostics arena, and the impact these markers will have on the US AD market over the next 10 years.

PATHOPHYSIOLOGY OF ALZHEIMER'S DISEASE

AD is characterized by the inexorable death of neurons, striking first the cholinergic neurons (neurons that produce the neurotransmitter acetylcholine [ACh]). Because the cholinergic system is involved in learning and memory pathways, the first symptom of the disease is cognitive impairment, especially in memory. As the disease progresses, cognitive decline becomes more marked, and higher functions – such as judgment, planning, organization, and reasoning – are affected. As neurons from other classes begin to die (e.g., neurons from the serotonergic or norepinephrine systems), patients start exhibiting behavioral symptoms such as aggression or wandering. Eventually, the patient enters a vegetative state, which is the end stage of the disease, characterized by the inability to use or understand language, obliviousness, and complete loss of independent functioning. The patient usually dies from complications due to this vegetative state. Typically, most patients die 8–10 years after diagnosis of the disease.

Controversy surrounds the cause of neuronal death. Some researchers believe that extracellular accumulations of a protein fragment, the Aβ-42 peptide, that form amyloid plaques (Aβ-amyloid plaques) are the cause of neuronal death. Other researchers believe that neuronal death is due to intracellular accumulations of the tau protein, which is normally involved in maintaining the cell structural framework. Currently, the diagnosis of AD is most often reached at autopsy, when the presence of both Aβ plaques and NFTs formed by tau aggregations is confirmed (Figure 39.1). Alternatively, a diagnosis could be made from a biopsy of brain tissue, a risky and invasive procedure for elderly patients that is rarely used.

The progression of the disease – more specifically, whether Aβ plaques or NFTs appear first – is controversial. All genetic mutations associated with inherited forms of AD have been shown to stimulate increased production of the toxic Aβ-42 peptide. Transgenic mouse models indicate that increased Aβ plaque load correlates with learning and memory deficits, but a correlation

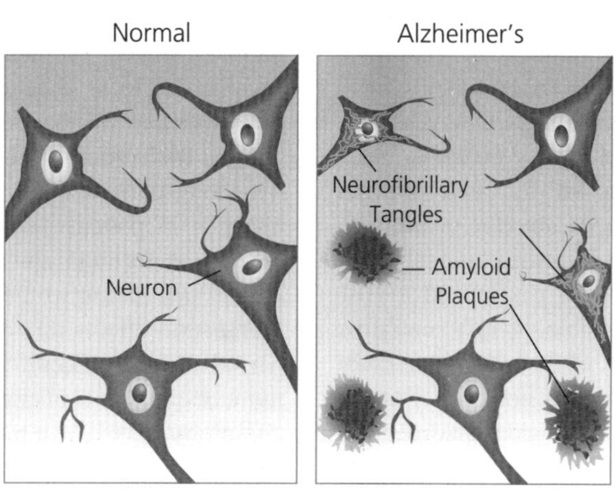

Figure 39.1 Amyloid Plaques and Neurofibrillary Tangles in Alzheimer's Disease

between Aβ plaque load and cognitive decline has not been established in humans. Also, autopsies have shown that the sequence of NFT accumulation correlates better than Aβ-amyloid load with symptom progression in AD patients. Increasingly, researchers believe that short stretches of Aβ peptides, known as amyloid-derived diffusible ligands (ADDLs), account for the neurotoxicity of Aβ. ADDLs have recently been shown to affect cognition negatively (Cleary et al., 2005); therefore, the relationship between the hallmarks of AD (Aβ plaques and NFTs) and dementia remains unclear. The development of a marker capable of tracing the accumulation of Aβ or NFTs would not only shed light on the natural progression of the disease and the cause of cognitive decline, but would also mean an increase in diagnosis and drug treatment rates.

VALUE OF A BIOMARKER FOR ALZHEIMER'S DISEASE

In addition to elucidating the progression of AD, a biomarker for AD would increase patients' drug-treatment rates and therefore increase revenues for drug companies with marketed AD therapies. The increase in drug-treatment rates would result from earlier diagnosis of more patients and longer durations of disease treatment. The diagnosis of AD is most often based on the guidelines published by the National Institute of Neurologic and Communicative Disorders and Stroke – Alzheimer's Disease and Related Disorders Association (NINCDS-ADRDA). A patient diagnosed with "probable AD" (showing symptoms of the disease, but without confirmation by autopsy or biopsy), has a 65% sensitivity value (capable of detecting AD in 65% of cases) and a 70% specificity value (capable of differentiating AD from other forms of dementia in 70% of cases). Currently, most physicians rely on the exclusion of other neurological disorders. In addition, neuropsychological tests such as the Mini-Mental State Examination (MMSE) are used to test cognitive function, but because these tests require expertise in their interpretation, GPs are reluctant to use them and therefore hesitant to broach an early diagnosis of AD.

A diagnostic marker would give the physician a more objective means of diagnosing AD (increased sensitivity) and differentiating AD from other diseases (increased specificity). Such a diagnostic marker would cause diagnosis rates to rise rapidly, especially if disease-modifying therapies had reached the market, because physicians would begin treatment with disease-modifying therapies as early in the disease as possible, when such therapies would have the greatest impact on disease progression. Primary care physicians typically do not diagnose early AD because its symptoms are often mistaken for those of "normal aging." As stated previously, AD is mostly diagnosed by specialists. However, a survey commissioned by Pfizer and Eisai (the "Facing Dementia Survey") noted that, according to physicians interviewed, approximately 35% of specialists do not accurately diagnose the disease.

In addition, a biomarker could lessen the cost of developing AD therapies by reducing the number of patients necessary to detect a drug's therapeutic effect and by decreasing the length of clinical trials. Currently, patients are selected for clinical trials based on the suspicion of having plaques and therefore represent a heterogeneous patient population. Because a biomarker would allow the selection of a more homogeneous patient population, a smaller number of patients would be necessary to detect a treatment effect. In addition, owing to the heterogeneity of the patient population in clinical trials, these trials must be conducted over long periods of time before significant changes in patients' cognitive performance become detectable. A more homogeneous patient population would enable detection of therapeutic effects on cognition in a shorter period of time. Therefore, by reducing the number of patients in clinical trials and shortening clinical trials, a biomarker will enable smaller, more cost-effective pivotal trials for AD therapies. Currently, the FDA clinical gold standard for drugs in development for AD is an effect on cognition, determined by use of psychometric tests. Experts caution that this end point is not sensitive or accurate enough to measure changes in cognition, but they believe that an amyloid marker would provide direct evidence of a reduction in amyloid plaque deposition by a disease-modifying therapy.

A genetic biomarker would also enable researchers to carry out AD preventive studies. Such studies are currently impractical because the small effect of therapies necessitates a huge number of patients and requires a long follow-up period. Because a genetic biomarker would allow more rigorous patient selection that would result in a more homogeneous patient population, preventive effects could be assessed more readily.

Finally, a biomarker would enable much faster assessment of a therapy's efficacy, thereby allowing drug developers to streamline the decision-making process during drug development. The FDA will likely refuse to accept a surrogate marker to demonstrate the efficacy of an AD therapy (e.g., the correlation between clearing Aβ plaques and restoring cognitive function is not established) and will likely insist on the demonstration of cognitive stabilization. The possibility of assessing a compound's efficacy at the earliest opportunity in the pipeline will encourage drug developers to decide quickly and confidently whether to abandon or pursue the compound's development.

NECESSARY ATTRIBUTES OF ALZHEIMER'S DISEASE BIOCHEMICAL MARKERS

Several biochemical and genetic markers for the diagnosis of AD have been tested, but many fail to meet the requirements for an adequate agent. Most have examined the levels of the Aβ peptide as a measure of the Aβ plaque load in the brain or the tau protein as a marker for NFTs. Because none have proved ideal, physicians do not rely exclusively on these biochemical markers, using them instead as supplemental tests to support their decision making. The limitations of the currently available markers and the large unmet need for an AD diagnostic marker underscore the large commercial value of such a diagnostic. Table 39.1 lists current biochemical markers used in the diagnosis of AD; Table 39.2 lists select companies that are pursuing AD diagnostics.

Sensitivity and Specificity

Like any biomarker, a biochemical marker must have adequate sensitivity (ability to detect AD) and specificity (ability to distinguish AD from other forms of dementia). The requirements for an adequate AD biomarker have been outlined by the National Institute on Aging Working Group on Biological Markers of Alzheimer's Disease in conjunction with the Ronald and Nancy Reagan Institute of the Alzheimer's Association. These requirements state that a biomarker for AD should have a diagnostic sensitivity greater than 80% and specificity greater than 80%. In other words, the biomarker would detect AD in 80 cases out of 100 and would distinguish AD from other forms of dementia – for example, fronto-temporal dementia (FTD), vascular dementia (VaD), or Lewy body dementia (LBD) – and from diseases such as stroke or depression in 80 cases out of 100. Many biomarkers currently used for research purposes are sensitive enough to distinguish between a normal elderly person and an AD patient. For example, the ratio of CSF Aβ-42 to tau and levels of phosphorylated tau have proved useful in some prospective studies to identify MCI patients who convert to AD. Such sensitivity permits earlier detection and earlier treatment. However, most of the current biomarkers lack the specificity to distinguish AD from other forms of dementia or other brain insults – for example, levels of the Aβ-42 peptide are increased in all forms of dementia, brain trauma, and stroke, and levels of the tau protein are increased in AD, FTD, and VaD.

According to the consensus group, the biomarker should detect a "fundamental feature of neuropathology" that should not be present in normal aging brains. Some pitfalls of the biochemical markers include a significant overlap of biomarker levels in AD

Table 39.1 Current Markers Used in the Diagnosis of Alzheimer's Disease

Biomarker	*Parameters Assessed*	*Origin*	*Limitations*
Genetic markers			
ApoE ε4	Presence of the apolipoprotein E ε4 genetic allele, a risk factor for sporadic AD	DNA extracted from blood	The gene is a risk factor and does not necessarily indicate that the patient will progress to AD
Presenilin 1 and 2	Presence of mutations in the presenilin 1 or 2 genes; some mutations in these genes have been associated with FAD	DNA extracted from blood	FAD represents only approximately 5% of AD cases
Amyloid markers			
sAPPα	Levels of the soluble portion of the APP after cleavage with α-secretase	CSF	Methods to measure this marker are not quantitative. There is too much overlap between control and AD sAPPα levels for the marker to be useful in clinical practice
sAPPβ	Levels of the soluble portion of the APP after cleavage with β-secretase	CSF	Methods to measure this marker are not quantitative. There is no difference in sAPPβ levels between control and AD patients
Aβ-42	Levels of the amyloidogenic Aβ-42 peptide	CSF or serum	The test is sensitive for dementia but not specific for AD (levels also increase in other dementias and in brain trauma or stroke patients). Large interpatient variability implies that the marker is useful for longitudinal follow-ups of one patient but not for screening of a population. Large variability reported in the literature; some researchers measuring CSF Aβ-42 levels have not seen an increase in AD patients. Significant overlap in Aβ-42 levels of AD patients and normal control patients. No correlation between Aβ-42 levels and disease severity
Aβ-42/Aβ-40	Ratio of the levels of amyloidogenic Aβ-42 peptide to levels of the nonamyloidogenic Aβ-40 peptide	CSF or serum	The test is sensitive for dementia but not specific for AD (levels of Aβ-42 also increase in other dementias and in brain trauma or stroke patients)
Amyloid-derived ligands (ADDLs)	Levels of Aβ-42 peptides aggregated in groups of two to three	CSF	Need for highly specialized equipment Levels are too low to be detected in the serum
Tau markers			
Total tau	Levels of the tau protein	CSF or serum	Sensitive but not specific for AD (e.g., tau levels also increase in stroke, FTD, and VaD patients) Total tau levels increase with age in normal patients; before tau can be used as a marker in a clinical setting, age-specific standardization of tau levels is necessary.
Phosphorylated tau (P-tau)	Levels of tau protein abnormally phosphorylated at various residues (e.g., threonine 181)	CSF	Sensitive and relatively specific (levels are not elevated in FTD, VaD, LBD, or patients with depression). Not detectable in blood or urine
P-tau/Aβ-42	Ratio between levels of abnormally phosphorylated tau protein and levels of Aβ-42	CSF	Although this measurement is sensitive and appears to discriminate better between AD and other dementias, these proteins are not detectable in blood or urine

Table 39.1 Continued

Biomarker	*Parameters Assessed*	*Origin*	*Limitations*
Other markers			
Choline acetyl transferase (CAT)	Levels of the CAT enzyme		Too much overlap between AD patients and normal controls. Levels of the enzyme are not affected in patients with mild cognitive impairment (MCI), and these patients have high loads of beta-amyloid
Acetylcholinesterase (AChE) levels	Levels of the AChE enzyme		The test is not sensitive enough; too much overlap between AD patients and normal controls. Levels of the enzyme are not affected in patients with MCI, and these patients have high loads of beta-amyloid
Neuronal thread protein (NTP)	Levels of the neuronal thread protein, often associated with NFTs	CSF	The relevance of NTP in AD is still unclear. The marker is not specific enough because Parkinson's disease and multiple sclerosis patients also have elevated levels of NTP. There is significant interpatient variability in the levels of NTPs

AD = Alzheimer's disease; APP = Amyloid precursor protein; CSF = Cerebrospinal fluid; FAD = Familial Alzheimer's disease; FTD = Fronto-temporal dementia; LBD = Lewy body dementia; NFT = Neurofibrillary tangles; VaD = Vascular dementia

patients and in normal elderly persons – for instance, some studies have found that CSF Aβ-42 could distinguish between controls and AD patients in only 42% of cases, and no difference has been shown in the serum Aβ-42 levels of AD patients and normal elderly persons. A biomarker should also indicate the progression of the disease – that is, its levels should change as the disease worsens. Levels of Aβ-42 peptide, for instance, fail to correlate with the severity of AD.

Consistency

The marker should also be consistent (i.e., reliable and reproducible). Many of the current biochemical markers show significant inter-patient variability; while such a marker could be used to monitor disease progression in a single patient, it would not be useful as a screening tool for a large population. In addition, levels of a biomarker should not change when taken with other drugs that are not treating AD; this is an especially important issue for elderly people because they are typically taking several drugs for several indications.

Other Requirements

Ideally, the marker should be present in body fluid samples that are easily obtained from a patient. A biomarker found in blood or urine would have a significant commercial advantage over a biomarker found in samples that are harder to obtain. For example, CSF samples require more invasive techniques, a drawback in treatment of a frail, elderly patient population.

Finally, the lack of assay standardization between laboratories has hindered the use of current biochemical markers. Biomarker studies have used select patient populations that have little in common with populations encountered in the clinical setting. These studies have mostly excluded patients with non-AD forms of dementia and, for the most part, have not been prospective; consequently, few asymptomatic AD patients have been included.

Limitations of Genetic Markers

Most genetic markers are sensitive enough to detect variations (mutations) in the order (sequence) of genes, but many current

Table 39.2 Select Companies Pursuing Alzheimer's Disease Diagnostics

Company/Partner	*Company Description*	*Technology*
Genomics screening		
deCode Diagnostics/ Roche Diagnostics	deCode is an Icelandic genomics discovery company based in Reykjavik; Roche Diagnostics, a Switzerland-based diagnostic company, commands one of the largest worldwide market shares in the medical diagnostics arena	deCode, founded on a genomics discovery-based platform, has become a company capable of taking gene candidates into preclinical development. Roche Diagnostics was to acquire commercial rights to any DNA-based diagnostic agent issuing from its collaboration with deCode. However, in February 2002, the companies no longer appeared to be collaborating in AD
Athena Diagnostics	Athena Diagnostics, based in Worcester, Massachusetts, was a subsidiary of Elan that specialized in AD diagnosis. In 2002, Behrman Capital, a private equity investment firm, acquired the company from Elan	Athena markets two AD tests: one measures the tau protein to Aβ-42 ratio (see under "Biochemical Markers") and the presence of the ApoE ε2, ε3, or ε4 alleles; the second test detects genetic mutations in the presenilin 1 gene that indicate predisposition to FAD
Perlegen Sciences/ National Institute on Aging (NIA)	Perlegen Sciences is based in Mountain View, California; the NIA is a branch of the U.S. government's National Institutes of Health (NIH)	Perlegen will identify genome-wide SNPs from LOAD patients in exchange for a grant from the NIA
Translational Genomics Research Institute (TGen)/ Kronos Science Laboratories	TGen is a nonprofit biomedical research institute; Kronos Science Laboratories provides clinical reference laboratory services. Both TGen and Kronos are located in Phoenix, Arizona	TGen will identify genome-wide SNPs from more than 1,000 LOAD patients; Kronos will have an exclusive worldwide license to all resulting intellectual property. Kronos plans to develop a diagnostic test to diagnose AD and a test to determine genetic predisposition to AD
Imaging markers		
Avid Radiopharmaceuticals	Avid Radiopharmaceuticals, a molecular imaging company based in Philadelphia, is developing radiopharmaceuticals for imaging AD pathology	Avid is developing radiolabeled Aβ-amyloid markers for use in PET or single photon emission computed tomography (SPECT) imaging
Biochemical markers		
Applied Neurosolutions/ BioMérieux	Applied Neurosolutions of Vernon Hills, Illinois, focuses on diagnosis and treatment of AD; BioMérieux, headquartered in Marcy L'Etoile, France, specializes in in vitro diagnostics	Applied Neurosolutions is developing an assay to detect tau protein phosphorylated at residue 231and levels of isoprostane as diagnostic biochemical markers of AD in CSF; the company will also develop a similar, serum-based assay. BioMérieux will obtain regulatory approval of the test and exclusive commercial rights to any diagnostic agent issuing from the agreement in exchange for milestone payments and royalties
Athena Diagnostics	Athena Diagnostics, based in Worcester, Massachusetts, was a subsidiary of Elan that specialized in AD diagnosis. In 2002, Behrman Capital, a private equity investment firm, acquired the company from Elan	Athena markets an AD test that measures the tau protein to Aβ-42 ratio and the presence of the ApoE ε2, ε3, or ε4 alleles
Dyax/AstraZeneca	Dyax, based in Cambridge, Massachusetts, is focused on inflammation and oncology; AstraZeneca, based in London, is a global pharmaceutical company	Dyax uses its phage display technology (where thousands of antibody targets can be translated to protein and used to select antibodies) to identify, characterize, and optimize antibodies binding to an undisclosed target for the treatment of AD

Table 39.2 Continued

Company/Partner	*Company Description*	*Technology*
Innogenetics/Takeda Chemical Industries	Innogenetics, based in Ghent, Belgium, is a specialty diagnostics company focused on infectious diseases, genetic testing, and neurodegeneration; Takeda Chemical Industries, based in Osaka, Japan, is a global pharmaceutical company	Innogenetics has entered into a license agreement for use of Takeda's anti-Aβ-amyloid antibodies as an AD diagnostic
Power3 Medical Products/Baylor Medical College	Power3 Medical Products, located in The Woodlands, Texas, is a proteomics company focused on chemotherapeutic drug resistance and early detection of breast cancer and neurological diseases; Baylor Medical College is located in Houston	Power3 is testing NuroPro, a panel of nine serum proteins released into the bloodstream after the death of neurons for the diagnosis of AD and differentiation of AD from Lou Gehrig's disease and Parkinson's disease; the nine proteins were identified from patient samples by protein purification and mass spectroscopy techniques
Proteome Sciences	Proteome Sciences, located in Cobham, United Kingdom, focuses on applied proteomics and uses high-sensitivity technologies to detect biomarkers	Proteome Sciences is expanding a panel of biomarkers that focuses on Aβ-amyloid and NFT markers, originally inlicensed from Bayer for diagnosis of AD
Brain activity monitoring devices		
Aspect Medical Systems	Aspect Medical Systems, based in Newton, Massachusetts, focuses on brain monitoring and develops technology that can measure the direct effects of drugs and diseases on the brain	Aspect intends to use its Bispectral Index platform and electroencephalography (EEG) technology for early diagnosis of AD; the technology monitors electrical brain waves induced by external stimuli
Izalex	Izalex, based in Santa Barbara, California, develops medical devices that help physicians to diagnose and treat psychiatric disorders	Izalex intends to use its proprietary Neurograph platform to diagnose AD and mild cognitive impairment; the technology monitors electrical brain waves induced by external stimuli, such as patterns of sound or light

AD = Alzheimer's disease; FAD = Familial Alzheimer's disease; LOAD = Late-onset Alzheimer's disease; MCI = Mild cognitive impairment; NFT = Neurofibrillary tangles; PET = Positron emission tomography; SNP = Single nucleotide polymorphism

markers of sporadic AD lack specificity. For instance, the *ApoEε4* allele of the *ApoE* gene is a risk factor for AD. Patients with this allele have a three- to eight-times greater risk of developing AD, but not all of them will develop AD. Genetic markers for certain genes, such as the *presenilin* or the *APP* genes, are quite specific for inherited forms of AD (familial AD [FAD]). Because FAD represents only 5% of all AD cases, however, the usefulness of such markers is limited, as is their market share.

EMERGING IMAGING AGENTS FOR DIAGNOSIS OF ALZHEIMER'S DISEASE

Currently, no imaging agents are available in the clinical setting for the diagnosis of AD. An imaging agent used as a biomarker for AD must specifically bind a pathological hallmark of AD. For example, an imaging agent against amyloid plaques must bind only Aβ in plaques, not soluble Aβ or non-Aβ amyloid structures. The agent must also be sensitive – for example, an anti-Aβ agent will bind Aβ-amyloid at very small doses.

Imaging agents face additional requirements, compared with biomarkers, before they can be used in AD. They must be capable of crossing the blood-brain barrier (BBB) to penetrate the brain from the blood stream. To cross the BBB, an agent must have a small molecular weight (less than 400–600 kDa) and be fairly soluble in cell membranes (lipophilic). In addition, the agent must be nontoxic and capable of being labeled – e.g., with a radioactive tag. A radioactively labeled compound should have a radioisotope with a short half-life. This combination of attributes will enable detection of enough radiation to increase the sharpness of the image and reduce imaging time while clearing rapidly from the patient's brain and bloodstream.

Researchers have tested three imaging agents in AD patients. We discuss the two most promising agents in the sections that follow as well as a compound developed for multiple sclerosis (MS) that may have potential for AD diagnosis.

Pittsburgh Compound B

The most promising imaging agent for AD is Pittsburgh Compound B, which is being developed by researchers at the University of Pittsburgh in collaboration with Sweden's Uppsala University, Karolinska Institute, and Huddinge University. Pittsburgh Compound B is derived from the Aβ-amyloid-binding agent thioflavin-T, labeled with radioactive carbon. In April 2004, the University of Pittsburgh licensed the agent to Amersham, a British company that was subsequently acquired by GE Healthcare, a subsidiary of General Electric.

In a small clinical trial, Pittsburgh Compound B labeled the cortex (a region of the brain that typically has high Aβ-amyloid load at autopsy) of AD patients (Klunk et al., 2004); the agent did not label the cortex of normal elderly patients or young healthy persons. However, the trial raised two caveats associated with the agent. First, the highest levels of the agent were found in the frontal cortex region of the brain in AD patients, a region that typically does not have the highest levels of Aβ-amyloid. Researchers speculated that the lesser labeling of regions that typically have the highest Aβ-amyloid loads (e.g., the entorhinal, parietal, and temporal cortices) is due to the reduced cerebral blood flow to these regions. Second, the agent nonspecifically labeled regions of the brain that typically do not have high Aβ-amyloid loads (e.g., subcortical white matter, the pons, the cerebellum); the labeling was nonspecific because the same region of the brain in normal elderly patients was labeled with similar intensity. These two caveats aside, the agent penetrates the brain rapidly and most nonspecific binding is cleared rapidly, thereby enabling a signal-to-noise level high enough to detect labeling easily.

The researchers did not see a correlation between high levels of Pittsburgh Compound B labeling and low scores on the Mini-Mental State Exam (MMSE), a neuropsychological exam typically used to measure cognitive decline in AD patients. However, this lack of correlation could be due to the fact that many patients in the trial had very early AD and scored well on the MMSE, which lacks the sensitivity to cognitive change in the higher ranges of the test. In addition, the small number of patients in the trial could explain the lack of correlation between labeling and MMSE scores. However, such a correlation assumes the validity of the hypothesis – as yet unproven – that Aβ-amyloid plaques cause cognitive decline.

^{18}F-FDDNP

^{18}F-FDDNP is a radioactive, fluorine-labeled, amyloid-binding agent derived from the Aβ-amyloid-binding agent DDNP (2-(1-[6-(dimethylamino)-2-naphthyl]ethylidene) malononitrile). Researchers at the University of California, Los Angeles, developed ^{18}F-FDDNP, and the university is seeking to outlicense the agent so that it may be used to evaluate the efficacy of anti-amyloid therapeutics. The agent is in Phase I clinical trials and has been tested in nine AD patients and seven controls (Shoghi-Jadid et al., 2002).

^{18}F-FDDNP shows great promise because, unlike Pittsburgh Compound B, the agent's levels of labeling appear to correlate with cognitive decline as measured by MMSE scores. In postmortem brain slices of AD patients, ^{18}F-FDDNP also appears to specifically label Aβ-amyloid and, to a lesser degree, NFTs. One advantage of ^{18}F-FDDNP is that, unlike Pittsburgh Compound B, the agent appears to show good specificity and can be retained in vivo for a longer period of time in regions of the AD brain (i.e., the hippocampus/amygdala/entorhinal cortex region) that have the greatest Aβ-amyloid plaque and NFT load. The agent did show some interpatient variability: one AD patient and one control patient did not show predominant labeling in the hippocampus/amygdala/entorhinal region. However, as with Pittsburgh Compound B, some nonspecific ^{18}F-FDDNP labeling occurs both in AD and in control brains. Finally, the difference between the highest-staining regions and the regions that should not stain is very small (30%), and a specific signal is hard to differentiate from the nonspecific background. If ^{18}F-FDDNP can be modified to clearly differentiate specific signaling from the nonspecific background, the agent will have great commercial promise.

BX-471

Berlex and its parent company, Schering, are developing BX-471, a chemokine receptor-1 (CCR-1) antagonist, as an anti-inflammatory agent for treatment of MS and psoriasis. BX-471 is in Phase II trials for both of these indications and in Phase I/II studies as a diagnostic agent in AD. The CCR-1 protein has been shown to accumulate around Aβ-amyloid plaques owing to the inflammatory response generated by microglial cells in the AD brain in response to cellular damage caused by Aβ-amyloid plaques. CCR-1 is detectable in MCI patients, and levels of CCR-1 increase with the progression of AD. Therefore, the agent may have promise as a diagnostic marker of Aβ-amyloid plaques. However, the presence of Aβ-amyloid plaques is not specific to AD (the plaques are also seen in patients with VaD); therefore, the agent would lack some specificity (VaD can be differentiated from AD by MRI) but would nevertheless be useful in evaluating AD patients and MCI patients who have plaques.

KEY PLAYERS IN ALZHEIMER'S DISEASE DIAGNOSTICS

The search for markers in an indication with such high unmet need is intensive. Current strategies include the development of Aβ-amyloid imaging agents for use in positron emission tomography (PET) scans, genomic screens for identification of genes or combinations of genes associated with AD, and the discovery of biochemical markers in the CSF or serum of AD patients. In this section, we discuss the most promising approaches; other, select collaborations in AD diagnostics are described briefly in Table 39.3.

Imaging Agent Alliances

Imaging agents for Aβ-amyloid or NFTs would allow physicians to visualize the extent and location of these pathological features by PET scanning and to assess their progression. The commercial uptake of these agents will be limited by the availability of the expensive equipment: there are approximately 1,000 PET scanners in the United States, and a PET scan currently costs $2,000 (compared with $800 for an MRI), which third-party payers may balk at reimbursing. However, in September 2004, the Centers for Medicare and Medicaid Services (CMS) approved the reimbursement of PET scans, under certain circumstances, for patients suspected of having AD, a provision that may facilitate the uptake of imaging agents.

GE Healthcare

GE Healthcare is developing Pittsburgh Compound B, the most promising imaging diagnostic for AD. GE Healthcare, headquartered in the United Kingdom, is a $14 billion unit of General Electric. The company comprises two business units: GE Healthcare Technologies and GE Healthcare Bio-Sciences. GE Healthcare Technologies, an $11 billion business, specializes in medical-imaging technologies, information technology, and patient-monitoring systems. GE Healthcare Bio-Sciences develops diagnostics, drug discovery systems, and protein separation platforms. In April 2004, GE Healthcare acquired Amersham, a British company that specializes in diagnostics, discovery systems, and protein separation.

Table 39.3 Select Collaborations in Alzheimer's Disease Diagnostics

Company	*Partner*	*Comments*
Genomic screening		
deCode Diagnostics	Roche Diagnostics	• In 1998, the two companies agreed to collaborate to discover genes involved in 12 indications, including AD • In August 2000, the companies announced the discovery of a gene implicated in LOAD; the gene was not identified • In February 2002, the companies signed a three-year extension of their collaboration for 4 of the 12 indications agreed on in 1998 The companies are no longer collaborating in AD
Perlegen Sciences	National Institute on Aging (NIA)	• In September 2004, Perlegen began a collaboration with the NIA to identify SNPs associated with LOAD • Presumably, the SNPs uncovered in this screen will enter the public domain
Translational Genomics Research Institute (TGen)	Kronos Science Laboratories	• TGen is a nonprofit research institute • In February 2005, Kronos and TGen initiated a collaboration. Kronos will have exclusive worldwide license to all intellectual property resulting from the screening to identify genes involved in the development of AD. Kronos plans to develop a diagnostic test for AD and a test to determine genetic predisposition to AD
Biochemical markers		
General Electric (GE)	Eli Lilly	• In April 2005, General Electric entered a collaboration with Eli Lilly whereby GE Healthcare would have access to Lilly's molecular libraries to develop diagnostic imaging agents against Aβ plaques • Eli Lilly will be able to use any resulting diagnostic agent to accelerate the discovery and development of anti-Aβ therapeutics
Applied Neurosolutions	BioMérieux S.A.	• In December 2004, the two companies agreed to research AD diagnostics • The test the companies are developing will need to demonstrate interpatient stability and ability to reproduce the results obtained from CSF in serum, a significant technical hurdle
Dyax	AstraZeneca	• In May 2002, AstraZeneca and Dyax entered a collaboration wherein Dyax would use its page display technology to identify, characterize, and optimize antibodies to an undisclosed AD target • AstraZeneca will retain the rights to develop and commercialize the antibodies developed by Dyax for therapeutic and diagnostic purposes, in exchange for milestone payments and royalty payments to Dyax in the event of successful commercial launch of any product issuing from the collaboration • AstraZeneca will fund the screening undertaken by Dyax
Innogenetics	Takeda Chemical Industries	• In June 2004, Innogenetics entered a licensing agreement with Takeda Chemical Industries by which Innogenetics gains access to Takeda's patent rights for the diagnostic and research use of Aβ antibodies. Specifically, Innogenetics may develop a diagnostic test based on Aβ levels in combination with their antibodies to tau and phosphorylated tau
Power3 Medical Products	Baylor Medical College	• In August 2004, Power3 Medical secured worldwide licensing rights from Baylor Medical College for Baylor's panel of biomarkers used in AD. Power3 paid Baylor a licensing fee and will make milestone payments. Baylor is also entitled to royalties associated with the commercialization of any diagnostic • The test so far has a sensitivity level between 86% and 99%, but its specificity level is still low, between 60% and 70% • The test has the advantage of monitoring proteins in serum instead of CSF • The proteins monitored in this test are released in the bloodstream after irreversible neuron death, when therapeutic intervention is of little value

AD = Alzheimer's disease; CSF = Cerebrospinal fluid; LOAD = Late-onset Alzheimer's disease; SNP = Single nucleotide polymorphism

Amersham Health, one of two business units of Amersham, specialized in the development of imaging reagents, particularly in the fields of cardiovascular, neurology, and oncology research. Amersham Health had also established a network of PET centers, the Imanet subsidiary of Amersham, which included two PET imaging centers, one at Uppsala, Sweden, and the other at Hammersmith Hospital in London. PET technology provides diagnostic imaging information at the sub-cellular level, data that is critical to drug development, but PET is costly and requires expertise that is often unavailable in companies that do not specialize in diagnostics. The Imanet network gave academic centers and companies access to PET imaging and expertise. A collaboration between the University of Pittsburgh and Imanet for the testing of Pittsburgh Compound B at the Uppsala facility allowed Amersham Health to enter an agreement with the University of Pittsburgh and inlicense the imaging agent.

The acquisition of Amersham added several imaging agents to GE Healthcare's diagnostics portfolio. The Amersham Health division had a strong background in innovation and had developed several novel tracers, including MRI imaging and radiolabeled agents used in neurology and oncology. GE Healthcare also acquired an ultrasound agent used in cardiology and imaging agents for X-ray and computed tomography (CT).

Through the acquisition of Amersham and its portfolio of neurology imaging agents, GE Healthcare gained a solid foothold in the field of neurology. The addition of Pittsburgh Compound B to GE Healthcare's pipeline will give the company a strong advantage in the race to develop AD diagnostics because of the expertise, capital, and facilities that both companies bring to the table. In addition, the reputation of both companies in large academic centers that specialize in AD research will facilitate further research and development of Pittsburgh Compound B and will likely promote uptake of the imaging agent by AD specialists.

Berlex/Schering

Berlex and Schering are developing the CCR-1 antagonist BX-471 as a diagnostic agent for AD and as an anti-inflammatory agent for relapsing-remitting MS and psoriasis. Berlex, based in Montville, New Jersey, is the US subsidiary of the German pharmaceutical company Schering AG. In addition to diagnostic imaging and radiopharmaceuticals, Berlex Biosciences (the research division of Berlex) focuses on dermatology, female healthcare, and oncology.

The diagnostics in the Berlex/Schering portfolio include several MRI contrasting agents and a radiolabeled vascular contrasting agent. In addition, Berlex and Schering have some presence in the neurology field. In 1994, the companies launched their interferon-β-1b therapy (Betaseron), which is indicated for treatment of MS. The companies' continued presence in neurology is underscored by the development of BX-471 for MS.

We expect Berlex and Schering to leverage their reputations and neurology infrastructures to continue the in-house development of BX-471 as a diagnostic agent for AD. We believe that the companies will consider the launch of BX-471 as a diagnostic agent worthwhile because of the lower up-front costs associated with its development, due to the completion of Phase I clinical trials of BX-471 in MS and psoriasis, and to the companies' established sales force in neurology.

Genetic Marker Alliances

A person's genes or combination of genes may predict an increased susceptibility to AD. In people with familial AD, variations in certain genes (mutations), compared with genes in the rest of the population, have been identified; however, FAD cases make up only approximately 5% of prevalent AD cases. Current genetic screens for mutations in AD focus on late-onset AD (LOAD), which constitutes 95% of prevalent AD cases. Problems associated with this approach include the uncertainty about whether certain gene combinations are necessarily associated with development of the disease or are simply risk factors for AD. In the latter case, a person with those genes will not necessarily develop AD. Certain gene combinations may also predict the course of disease progression, its severity, or the patient's response to particular therapies – but the small number of therapies available to AD patients makes this last factor less important in AD. One commercial risk associated with this approach is the possibility that a drug manufacturer will see its patient population, and therefore market share, limited by the genetic makeup of the population.

Merck/Celera Diagnostics

Formed in 2001, Celera Diagnostics is a joint venture of the Celera Genomics group and Applied Biosystems; both Celera Genomics and Applied Biosystems are part of the Applera Corporation. Celera Diagnostics discovers and commercializes diagnostics, based on genome-wide scans in disease-association studies performed in-house and at Celera Genomics. Celera Diagnostics also provides genetic discovery services to client companies, such as Merck. The Merck pipeline encompasses multiple disease areas and includes agents for the treatment of AD: C-7617 and C-9138 are in Phase I trials, and C-9136 is in Phase II trials; it is unclear what mechanism of action is targeted by these drugs.

In July 2004, Celera Diagnostics and Merck entered into a collaboration to identify single nucleotide polymorphisms (SNPs) as targets for drug discovery and diagnostic markers for LOAD. In October 2003, Merck and Celera entered a similar agreement for development of prognostic tests and drugs for certain cancers. SNPs are single nucleotide changes in a gene that can alter its normal function and cause disease or susceptibility to a disease. According to the terms of the agreement, Celera will test the cellular function of candidate genes, and Merck will fund the scan and receive rights to any AD therapy identified during the collaboration. Celera will retain the rights to any diagnostic marker identified. In January 2005, Celera received a milestone payment from Merck.

In a scan of a portion of chromosome 12 that compared samples from 1,089 LOAD patients with samples from 1,196 normal persons, Celera has identified several SNPs associated with LOAD, including the gene for glyceraldehyde-3-phosphate dehydrogenase, an enzyme involved in glucose metabolism and neuronal programmed cell death (apoptosis), and a gene of similar function on chromosome 19. In addition, SNPs were identified on the amyloid-beta binding protein 2 (ABBP-2) and in regions of chromosome 10; so far, the function of these genes is unknown.

The collaboration between Celera Diagnostics and Merck is fraught with risk for Merck, but the payoffs could be significant if the company develops a therapy based on a genetic candidate identified by Celera. In addition, if AD biomarkers are identified during the collaboration, Merck could also stand to benefit from the acceleration of its decision-making process in the clinical development of AD compounds now in its pipeline and the development of any candidates discovered through the collaboration with Celera. The two companies have considerable expertise and the assets necessary to collaborate successfully. If diagnostic markers can be identified through the collaboration, Celera stands to profit from a marketed diagnostic for LOAD.

Celera Diagnostics collaborates with Abbott Laboratories to market its diagnostics, and the companies have already commercialized several diagnostic products, including an HIV genotyping assay and several Analyte Specific Reagents (ASRs; sets of reagents used to identify mutations associated with a particular disease), in particular, ASRs for cystic fibrosis and for the measurement of viral load in hepatitis C. In addition, Celera has established collaborations with Quest Diagnostics and LabCorp, the two major clinical laboratories in the United States. Despite having the infrastructure necessary to market a diagnostic for AD, Celera must overcome additional hurdles to bring its diagnostic successfully to market. The company must convince physicians of the utility of the test – which will be difficult with no disease-modifying drug available to treat AD – and convince third-party payers to reimburse the cost of the test.

Biochemical Marker Alliances

Several companies have formed alliances to identify combinations of protein markers found in the CSF or serum that can be used in the diagnosis of AD (Table 39.3). Many rely on the detection of Aβ-peptide levels and phosphorylated tau protein, but the use of these biomarkers has so far been fraught with limitations. Researchers at Northwestern University (Evanston, Illinois) have developed one approach that holds great promise, which we discuss in the following section, but it is in very early, proof-of-concept stages.

The Bio-Barcode Assay

Researchers at Northwestern University developed the "Bio-Barcode assay" for the detection of ADDLs (small aggregates of Aβ-amyloid) in the CSF of AD patients (Georganopoulou et al., 2005). Although the technology appears to have been licensed, it is unclear at this juncture which company may have acquired the technology. Because ADDLs, which aggregate into Aβ-amyloid plaques, may be more neurotoxic than the Aβ-42 peptide, and because ADDLs appear before Aβ-amyloid plaques form, the assay may be measuring a more relevant biochemical marker for AD and detecting an earlier step in the formation of Aβ-amyloid plaques.

The Bio-Barcode assay makes use of antibodies against ADDLs attached to magnetic microparticles and ADDL antibodies attached to 30-nanometer gold particles (Figure 39.2, step 1). The gold particles have hundreds of short strands of "barcode" DNA attached to their surfaces, which can be "melted off" at higher temperatures. The ADDLs will bind to the antibodies on the magnetic microspheres and gold nanospheres so that a complex of magnetic microparticle/ADDL/gold nanoparticle and DNA will form (Figure 39.2, step 2). The complexes can be purified out of the CSF by placing the sample in a magnetic field (Figure 39.2, step 3). The DNA associated with the gold nanoparticles in the complex can then be melted away from the complex at high temperatures into single strands of DNA (step 4). The free, single-stranded DNA can be purified and detected by several methods, including the widely available polymerase chain reaction (PCR). The technique is very sensitive because one ADDL is associated to hundreds of Bio-Barcode DNA molecules; therefore, the signal from one ADDL complex is amplified 100-fold. The developers of the Bio-Barcode assay are confident that the test has not reached its lower detection limits, which means that ADDLs may also be purified from the serum of AD patients, where they are present in much lower concentrations than in the CSF.

The developers of the Bio-Barcode assay demonstrated that ADDLs could be purified from the CSF of AD patients and that their levels were consistently higher than in control patients. Although the study was small – only 15 AD patients and 15 control patients – the results are encouraging (Georganopoulou et al., 2005). Should Bio-Barcode assay results continue to be consistent, if there is little interpatient variability, and if ADDL concentrations are shown to change with disease progression, the technique could be commercially successful. The Bio-Barcode assay has the advantage of being faster and less expensive than imaging methods. Therefore, it may surmount the hurdle of third-party payer reimbursement, which could prove to be the downfall of several other diagnostic approaches.

MARKET IMPLICATIONS

The development of an AD biomarker is of growing interest to pharmaceutical companies,

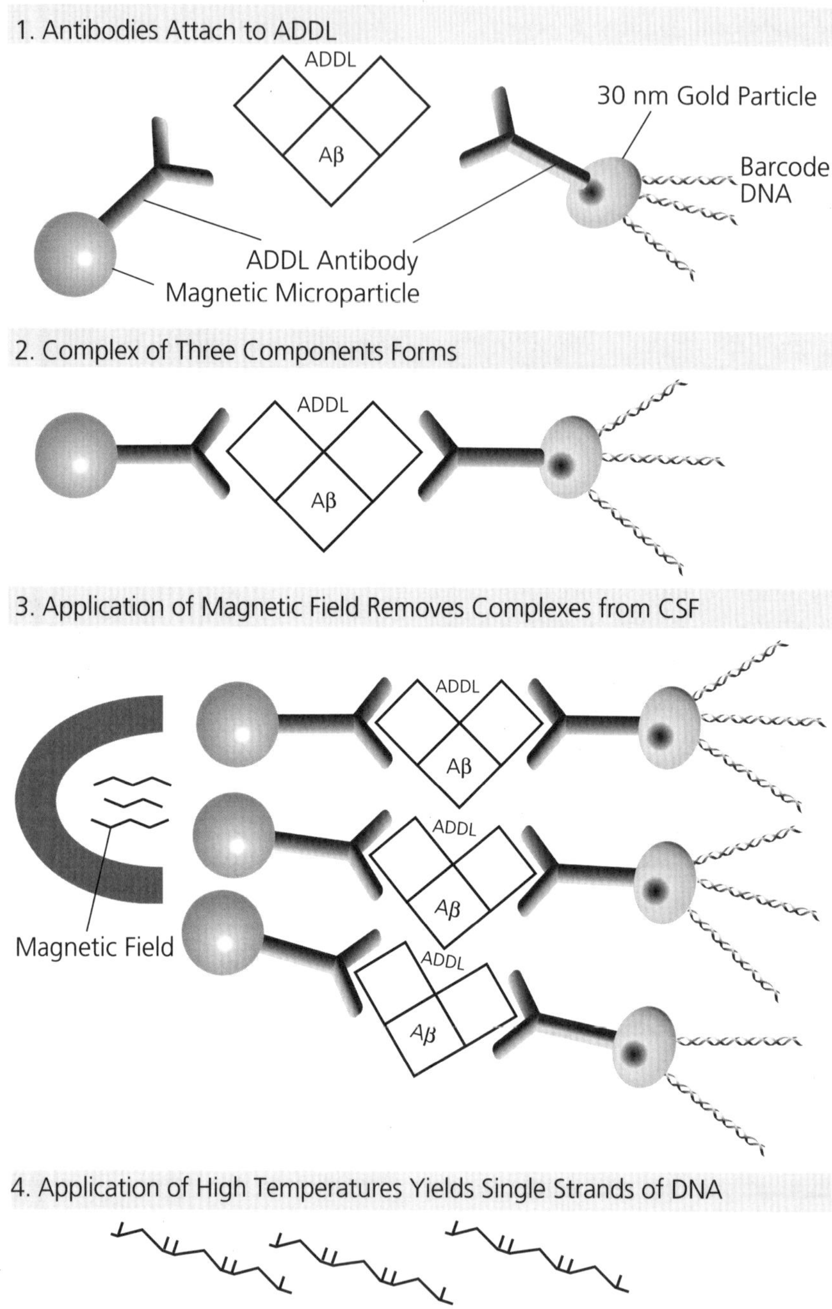

Figure 39.2 The Bio-barcode Assay

which are forming alliances with diagnostic companies in an effort to develop such markers. The development of the biomarker per se has been less interesting to pharmaceutical companies than the potential impact of an AD biomarker on the AD therapeutic market should a therapy become available.

Pharmaceutical companies view the development of diagnostic agents for AD as risky because such ventures would yield little return on their investment. Indeed, while diagnostics must undergo years of the same rigorous validation and testing as therapies and are associated with the same risks, they have not traditionally commanded comparable prices. In addition, the FDA has not yet delineated the necessary attributes of an AD biomarker; the agency could change its position during development of the diagnostic. Also, a diagnostic for AD would be used at the time of initial diagnosis and at follow-up intervals, but not chronically, like an AD therapy. Given the risks and drawbacks of diagnostics development, large pharmaceutical companies, for the most part, have not devoted many in-house resources to development of an AD diagnostic agent.

Instead, pharmaceutical companies have formed discovery alliances with diagnostic companies because of their expertise and in-house resources. Pharmaceutical companies are also hopeful that new drug targets will emerge from screens for diagnostic agents, particularly in the case of genetic screens. Many alliances between pharmaceutical companies and diagnostic companies stipulate that the pharmaceutical company will fund the search for drug targets that could serve as diagnostic agents and retain the rights to any therapeutic agent emerging from the search, while the diagnostic company will retain the rights to any diagnostic agent that emerges from screens. The potential for sales of an AD diagnostic agent could be significant, due to the increasing prevalence of the disease and the possibility that a novel diagnostic agent could command better pricing than a traditional diagnostic, given the large unmet need for a diagnostic agent in this indication. Indeed, diagnostic markers have become more widely accepted as part of treatment practices: according to the August 2003 issue of *The Wall Street Transcript*, the molecular diagnostic market has been estimated to "generate over $1.2 billion in revenue and is growing very rapidly, somewhere between 15% and 25% per year."

The success of a diagnostic agent hinges on the availability of a therapeutic agent because physicians will be unwilling to order the diagnostic test if no therapy is available to treat the patient, and patients will have little incentive to obtain a diagnosis they fear. A survey commissioned by Eisai and Pfizer (the Facing Dementia Survey) found that diagnosis rates in Europe (France, Germany, Italy, Poland, Spain, and the United Kingdom) were influenced by patient and caregiver fears of the AD diagnosis. The survey canvassed 2,500 caregivers, physicians, policy makers, and members of the general population; 48% acknowledged that fear of the disease prevented their talking to their physicians about the condition. The survey found that patients delayed consulting a doctor about their symptoms for nearly two years, owing in part to fear of the diagnosis.

Similarly, the commercial success of an AD therapy hinges on the availability of a biomarker. Because of the large unmet need in AD, sales of a therapy that slows cognitive decline will be significant, but they will be limited unless a biomarker is available. Indeed, diagnosis rates will not increase significantly without a biomarker, and drug treatment will not begin earlier. If a biomarker is available when a therapy launches, diagnosis rates will increase and treatment will begin earlier; thereby prolonging the time a patient is on a chronic therapy and significantly increasing drug sales. In addition, if the therapy is disease-modifying, progression of the disease will likely slow, which will further prolong the time during which a patient receives drug therapy and potentially increase drug sale revenues significantly (Figure 39.3).

If a biomarker is accepted as an efficacy end point by the FDA, several significant advantages would be available to pharmaceutical companies that are developing AD drugs. First, if a drug is in early development stages, it might be screened for its ability to alter the levels of a biomarker, thus providing evidence of efficacy. Consequently, drug development would be accelerated because decisions could be made earlier about a compound's therapeutic potential. If a drug is further in development, a biomarker would enable faster, more efficient Phase III clinical

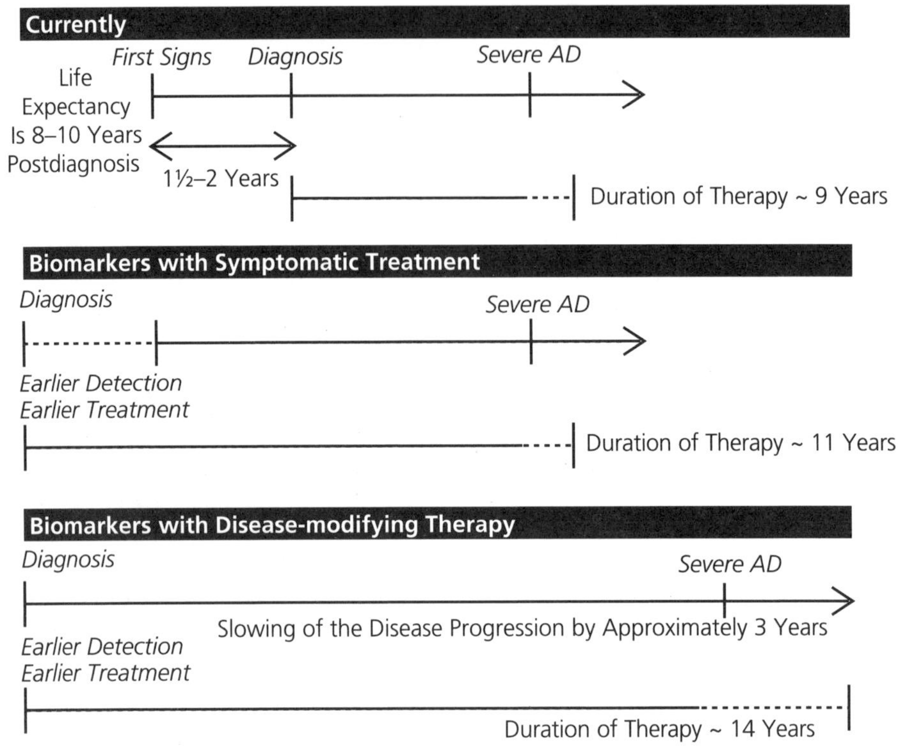

Currently, the diagnosis of Alzheimer's disease (AD) patients is delayed by approximately 1½ year and 2 years. Life expectancy after diagnosis is 8–10 years. The use of current therapies is suspended once the patient enters severe stages of the disease, resulting in a therapy duration of approximately 9 years.

If a symptomatic treatment for AD launched in a market in which a biomarker were available, diagnosis and treatment would occur earlier, thus increasing the duration of therapy by approximately 2 years.

If a disease-modifying treatment for AD launched in a market in which a biomarker were available, diagnosis and treatment would occur earlier and the progression of the disease would be slowed, thereby prolonging the time before a patient enters severe stages of the disease and therapy is suspended. The duration of therapy would therefore lengthen by 3 years in our example.

Figure 39.3 Duration of Therapy for Alzheimer's Disease Drugs

trials because patient selection could be more homogeneous and the efficacy of a disease-modifying drug would be easier to assess. Furthermore, if a drug could demonstrate disease modification based on a biomarker diagnostic test, the drug would command a premium in the market. If a disease-modifying drug were launched before a biomarker is accepted as an end point, sales would likely decrease because the developers would have to show efficacy according to the biomarker in Phase IV, postmarketing trials, with no possibility of raising its price.

OUTLOOK

We forecast that the biomarker Pittsburgh Compound B and two disease-modifying therapies, the Aβ-amyloid aggregation inhibitor NC-758 (Neurochem's Alzhemed) and R-flurbiprofen (Myriad Genetics' Flurizan) will reach the US market before 2013 (Figure 39.4). These launches will grow the market at a compound annual rate of approximately 8% from 2003 to 2013; sales of new therapies will account for approximately 70% of the market. The earlier diagnosis of

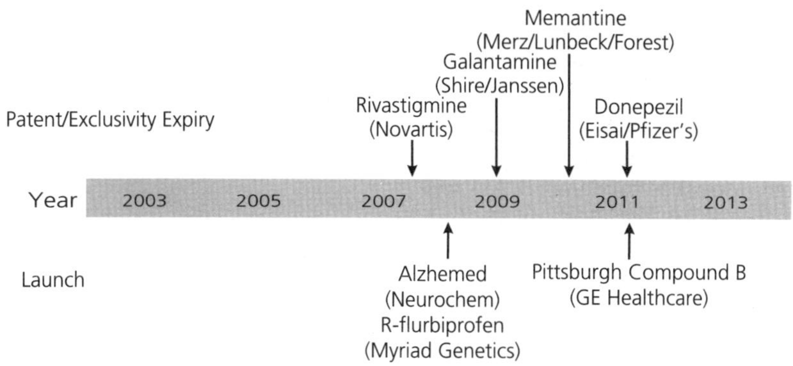

Figure 39.4 Major Events Shaping the Alzheimer's Disease Market, United States

AD due to Pittsburgh Compound B, which we forecast will launch in 2011, will contribute to the rapid market expansion. We expect that AD disease-modifying drugs launched after 2011 will have to demonstrate an effect on Aβ-amyloid plaque load as gauged by Pittsburgh Compound B labeling – and if such drugs demonstrate a reduction in amyloid plaque levels as measured by Pittsburgh Compound B, we forecast that they will command significant premiums.

However, diagnostic biomarkers for AD must surmount several hurdles if they are to achieve market uptake. First, diagnostics manufacturers must forge alliances with the medical community to ensure that physicians understand the value of biomarker tests and use them in diagnosing their AD patients. Second, diagnostics manufacturers must convince third-party payers (e.g., private insurers) and the CMS of the utility of their diagnostic tests so that patients will be reimbursed for the costs. (See the sidebar CMS Reimburses Cost of PET for Early Detection of AD.)

CMS REIMBURSES COST OF PET FOR EARLY DETECTION OF AD

The Centers for Medicare and Medicaid Services (CMS), recognizing the potential cost savings associated with early detection of AD, recently agreed to reimburse Medicare patients for the cost of PET scans, beginning in September 2004. Consequently, PET scans may become more widely available, especially if anti-amyloid therapies now in development demonstrate a delay in AD progression. According to a 2004 report by the Lewin Group commissioned by the Alzheimer's Association, costs currently incurred by Medicare beneficiaries with AD are disproportionately high: although AD patients are only 12.8% of the population older than 65 years, they account for 34% of Medicare spending. However, for a patient to be reimbursed for a PET scan, the AD diagnosis must otherwise be uncertain or the patient must agree to enroll in a CMS-approved clinical trial. Medicare beneficiaries who have already developed the symptoms of dementia are not covered under this Medicare reform law.

Third, diagnostics manufacturers must convince AD patient advocacy groups of the utility of biomarker tests so that patients will pressure physicians to use them and third-party payers to reimburse their costs. Finally, it is unclear whether the FDA will accept biomarkers as efficacy-end points for submission of an NDA; acceptance would significantly cut the drug development risks, time, and costs currently ventured by drug manufacturers attempting to bring an AD therapy to market.

A further caveat for drug manufacturers surfaces with the use of genetic markers. Genetic markers will ensure that patients with particular genetic makeups are monitored by physicians for signs of AD and potentially treated with preventive drugs, but the market share of drug manufacturers could become more limited than it currently is if the genetic composition has a low prevalence – for example, a marker for familial AD will have a maximum market share of approximately 5%, similar to the prevalence of familial AD in the AD population.

Diagnostic tests for AD will increase the potential of the AD market, but both a diagnostic marker accepted by the FDA and a disease-modifying drug will have to be available for the market to reach its full potential. The AD market will greatly expand at the end of our forecast period due to the increase in prevalence of AD, higher diagnosis and drug treatment rates, and longer treatment of AD patients. We forecast that the launch of Pittsburgh Compound B in 2011 will greatly increase the market potential for AD drugs and that the market will grow at 8% compound annual growth rate from 2003 to 2013. The market holds tremendous potential because of the large unmet need for an AD therapy, but realizing that potential requires the introduction of a reliable AD diagnostic agent.

REFERENCES

Cleary, J.P. et al. Natural oligomers of the amyloid-beta protein specifically disrupt cognitive function. *Nature Neuroscience*. 2005; 8(1): 79–84.

Georganopoulou, D. et al. Nanoparticle-based detection in cerebral spinal fluid of a soluble pathogenic biomarker for Alzheimer's disease. *Proceedings of the National Academy of Sciences of the United States of America*. 2005; 102: 2273–6.

Hebert, L.E. et al. Alzheimer disease in the US population: prevalence estimates using the 2000 census. *Archives of Neurology*. 2003; 60: 1119–22.

Klunk, W.E. et al. Imaging brain amyloid in Alzheimer's disease with Pittsburgh Compound-B. *Annals of Neurology*. 2004; 55: 306–19.

Knopman, D.S. et al. Practice parameter: diagnosis of dementia (an evidence-based review). Report of the Quality Standards Subcommittee of the American Academy of Neurology. *Neurology*. 2001; 56: 1143–53.

Shoghi-Jadid, K. et al. Localization of neurofibrillary tangles and beta-amyloid plaques in the brains of living patients with Alzheimer disease. *American Journal of Geriatric Psychiatry*. 2002; 10: 24–35.

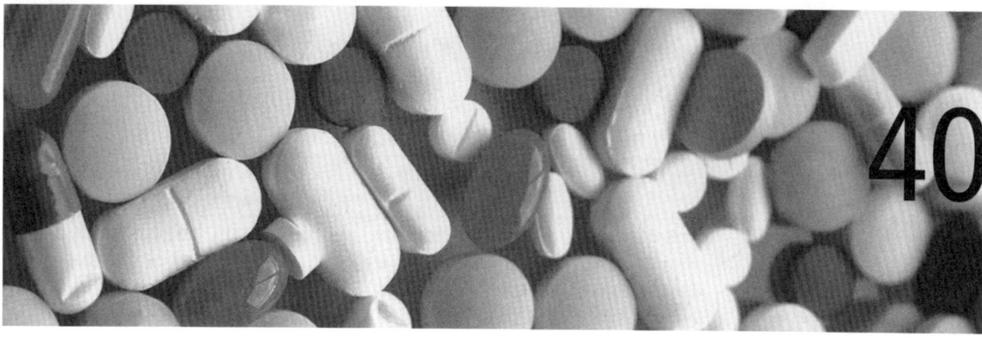

How Are Translational Medicine Biomarkers Impacting Industry?

THE DAWN OF TRANSLATIONAL MEDICINE

Many experts believe that the future of the pharmaceutical industry hinges upon the development of new and better translational approaches. Failure rates for the development of new drugs will continue to rise if basic research findings cannot be quickly turned into valuable medicines. The result of increasing drug failures will be a pharmaceutical industry that is unsustainable; an industry that will not be able to refresh lean drug development pipelines merely by pushing more preclinical projects into development. As a result, translational medicine is one of the fastest growing areas of drug discovery and development today. Biomarkers are at the heart of this effort. Today, companies want to understand more about how drugs actually work before putting them into pivotal clinical trials, let alone onto the market. Because biomarkers can be used to actually confirm hypotheses and even to bridge preclinical and clinical results, they are considered the central tool in translational medicine. A biomarker can be anything from an X-ray (showing bone erosion) to a gene expression signature. The most important thing, however, is that somehow it can be used across various experiments to help researchers gain certainty about how drugs work.

Within the pharmaceutical industry, the emphasis on translational medicine is fueled by two major factors: the decline in overall productivity of the drug industry and the increase in the number of drug failures (Table 40.1). In response to these trends, companies are increasingly engaging in translational studies, not only to better ensure that animal findings are predictive of what will be seen in humans but also to better anticipate unexpected biological effects. At the same time, a common goal is to speed projects.

On the public side, translational medicine (or translational research) grew out of the genomics revolution. Many of the original genome projects focused on basic research to better understand genes, expressed proteins, and biological pathways. There has been a growing desire to see these findings "translated" into clinical applications. From the academic perspective, this desire has meant engaging in more clinical research projects in addition to ongoing projects in basic research. Indeed, a growing number of academic centers are even becoming

Table 40.1 Select Safety-based Drug Withdrawals, 1997–2006

Drug	*Brand Name*	*Company*	*Approved Use*	*Approved/ Withdrawn*	*Safety Concern(s)*
Alosetron[a]	Lotronex	Glaxo Wellcome	Irritable bowel syndrome	2000/2000	Ischemic colitis, severe constipation
Astemizole	Hismanal	Janssen-Cilag	Antihistamine	1988/1999	Fatal arrhythmia
Bromfenac	Duract	Wyeth-Ayerst	Pain relief	1997/1998	Liver toxicity
Cerivastatin	Baycol	Bayer	Cholesterol reduction	1997/2001	Muscle damage leading to kidney failure
Cisapride	Propulsid	Janssen/Johnson & Johnson	Heartburn	1993/2000	Fatal arrhythmia
Co-proxamol[b]	Paracetamol/ dextropro-poxyphene combination	Various generic companies	Pain relief	1960s/2005	Overdose, suicide
Dexfenflura-mine	Redux	Wyeth-Ayerst/ Interneuron	Appetite suppression	1996/1997	Heart value disease
Droperidol[c]	Droleptan	Janssen-Cilag	Anti-psychotic	1995/2001	Fatal arrhythmia
Etretinate	Tegison	Hoffmann-La Roche	Psoriasis	1986/1999	Birth defects
Fenfluramine	Pondimin	Wyeth-Ayerst	Appetite suppression	1973/1997	Heart valve disease
Grepafloxacin	Raxar	Glaxo Wellcome	Antibiotic	1997/1999	Fatal arrhythmia
Levomethadyl	Orlaam	Roxane Laboratories	Opiate dependence	1993/2003	Fatal arrhythmia
Mibefradil	Posicor	Roche	Blood pressure reduction	1997/1998	Fatal arrhythmia
Natalizumab[d]	Tysabri	Biogen Idec/Elan	Multiple sclerosis	2004/2005	Rare demyelinating disease
Rapacuronium	Raplon	Organon Akzo Nobel	Anesthetic	1999/2001	Severe breathing difficulty
Rofecoxib	Vioxx	Merck & Co.	Pain relief	1999/2004	Heart attack, stroke
Terfenadine	Seldane	Hoechst Marion Roussel	Antihistamine	1985/1998	Fatal arrhythmia
Tolcapone[e]	Tasmar	Hoffmann-La Roche	Parkinson's disease	1997/1998	Liver toxicity
Troglitazone	Rezulin	Warner-Lambert/ Pfizer	Diabetes	1997/2000	Liver toxicity
Trovafloxacin[f]	Trovan	Pfizer	Antibiotic	1998/1999	Liver toxicity
Valdecoxib	Bextra	Pfizer	Pain relief	2001/2005	Skin reactions, poor cardiovascular safety
Ximelagatran[g]	Exanta	AstraZeneca	Anticoagulant	2003/2006	Liver toxicity

[a]Remarketed in 2002 with restrictions
[b]Phased withdrawal in the United Kingdom
[c]Marketed with black-box warnings in the United States by Akorn Pharmaceuticals under the name Inapsine
[d]Voluntarily withdrawn in 2005. In February 2006, the FDA withdrew its hold on clinical testing; in March 2006, the FDA's Peripheral and Central Nervous System Drugs Advisory Committee unanimously recommended reintroduction of Tysabri
[e]Marketed in the United States with restrictions; European Union marketing approval withdrawn
[f]Marketed in the United States with restrictions; European Union marketing approval withdrawn
[g]Marketed in Europe and South America; failed to be approved in the United States in 2004

involved in drug-discovery-like activities. For example, the Harvard Center for Neurodegeneration and Repair's Laboratory for Drug Discovery in Neurodegeneration was established specifically to discover new drugs for diseases such as Alzheimer's.

From the perspective of the pharmaceutical industry, the challenge is quite different. Pharmaceutical companies have seen firsthand the problems associated with pursuing drug targets that are not well understood. For instance, genomics brought the pharmaceutical industry a flood of new targets, but some experts believe that these poorly validated targets decreased productivity rather than increased it. Genomics-derived targets are proving much less predictable than expected. Rather than pushing even more of these targets into clinical trials, pharmaceutical companies now want better validated targets and more evidence that drugs against any of their targets will have a predictable biologic effect.

Hence, drugmakers want to translate biological targets, and the drugs that address them, into wellunderstood biological phenomena. As a result, more and "smarter" studies are needed. In particular, better tools for correlating a drug's effect in animal models and in humans – one of the most challenging aspects of drug development – must be developed, as well as much better tests for predicting a drug's potential toxicity.

Speaking at the Post-Approval Summit at Harvard University in May 2006, Mathias Hukkelhoven (senior vice president and global head of drug regulatory affairs at Novartis) summed it up when he said, "Pharma must modernize the drug development process."

This chapter looks at the modernization of the drug development process through widespread adoption of translational studies using biomarkers. We discuss different types of biomarkers, including the potential use of new imaging technologies, and assess whether these changes are sufficient to reverse the industry's productivity decline. We review two case studies on drugs that could have benefited from having a clinic-ready biomarkers and examine what lessons can be learned. Lastly, some companies are engaged in developing biomarkers in combination with drugs. We discuss some of these companies, their products, and the role of the FDA in promoting such codevelopment activities.

RECENT FDA INITIATIVES

Over the last few years, biomarkers have become one of the most popular tools in translational research. Biomarkers are defined by the FDA as "measurable characteristics in animals or humans that can help predict the performance of a product during development, reducing uncertainties about safety or effectiveness." Largely because of all the criticism the FDA has received lately for not "protecting" the public from unsafe drugs, the agency has emerged as one of the foremost proponents of biomarker use. While the agency's main effort apparently focuses on toxicity markers, it also seems to be keenly aware of pharma's productivity problem and the role that biomarkers could play in addressing that issue.

The FDA not only is helping to define the problems that biomarkers can help solve but also is directly involved in major projects. For example, in November 2005, the agency announced a collaboration with BG Medicine – the Liver Toxicology Biomarker Study – to discover biomarkers of human hepatotoxicity. More recently, the FDA helped form the Predictive Safety Testing Consortium, a collaboration of industry, academia, and government to identify and validate drug safety biomarkers and the tests needed to measure them. The agency is an adviser to the consortium, which is headed by the new Critical Path Institute and includes Bristol-Myers Squibb, GlaxoSmithKline, Johnson & Johnson Pharmaceutical Research & Development, Merck & Co., Novartis, Pfizer, Roche Palo Alto, and Schering-Plough Research Institute.

It is not a coincidence that the FDA has paired biomarkers with animal models among its major areas of focus. One of the primary goals of translational medicine with respect to pharmaceutical development is to generate biomarkers that can be used across species or biomarkers that are at least comparable across species. The transition from animal to human studies is one of the biggest problem spots in all of drug development. Instead of simply looking at crude end points, researchers are trying to develop biomarkers that will measure specific drug or related biological activity. As described later, some of these markers are proximal to the drug/target interaction, while others may occur downstream from that point. Understanding the relationships of these biomarkers to one another and to the effects of drugs is one of the priorities of biomarkers discovery.

USES OF BIOMARKERS

Biomarkers are used for a variety of purposes and during multiple phases of drug discovery and/or development (Table 40.2). Biomarkers are characterized, in particular, by their intended use and by attributes such as their degree of acceptance (e.g., validation) within the scientific community. Different terms used to describe biomarkers include the following:

- Diagnostic biomarkers become the basis of a test that can be used clinically to diagnose a disease or decide on a treatment strategy. Tests that are paired to a particular drug are sometimes also called pharmacodiagnostics, theranostics, therapeutic diagnostics, or companion diagnostics.
- Pharmacogenetic/pharmacogenomic biomarkers correlate a single or limited number of inherited genetic variations with a response to a drug (pharmacogenetic) or many genetic variations across the genome with a response to a drug (pharmacogenomic). That response can relate to efficacy or to side effects.
- Pharmacokinetic/pharmacodynamic biomarkers measure an aspect of the uptake, distribution, or mode of action of a drug.
- Probable valid biomarkers, as defined by the FDA, are those that seem to have predictive clinical value but that have not yet been either widely accepted or replicated by others in the scientific community.
- Validated biomarkers, as defined by the FDA, are those that are accepted by the scientific community to predict a clinical outcome.
- Observational or exploratory biomarkers, according to the FDA, are markers that are under study to further establish clinical utility.
- Surrogate biomarkers can substitute for a clinical end point and can predict clinical benefit.
- Toxicity biomarkers can be used to predict drug metabolism or toxicity effects.
- Novel biomarkers are biomarkers that have never been previously used. Most of these are generated by innovative technologies. They include gene expression and proteomic signatures.

In the next subsections, we give examples of research, toxicity, and pharmacogenetic biomarkers.

Research Biomarkers

As noted earlier, by far the most common types of biomarkers are those used in early research studies (preclinical through Phase II) to verify scientific hypotheses. These include surrogate markers of drug effect and pharmacodynamics, and pharmacokinetic markers. Today, companies investigate many potential biomarkers during drug discovery and development. For example, Rules Based Medicine's Multi-Analyte Profile is a panel of immunoassays that measures protein expression patterns of more than 180 plasma analytes (everything from alpha fetoprotein through varicella zoster) that may be indicative of responses to a disease or to a drug. Researchers use such tools to literally fish for

Table 40.2 When and How Biomarkers Are Used in Drug Development

Type of Biomarker	*When Used*	*Purpose of Use*
Surrogate	Preclinical through post-marketing	• Proof of concept • Target validation • Monitoring for specific desired or undesired effects
Pharmacokinetic/ pharmacodynamic	• Preclinical • Phase I	• Lead selection • Dose determination • Toxicity indication
Pharmacogenetic/ pharmacogenomic	• Phase II • Phase III	• Selection of patients predicted to respond to a drug treatment • Identification of those at risk of side effects
Diagnostic	• Phase II • Phase III • Increasingly recommended for preclinical or Phase I use	• Disease predisposition • Disease prognosis

biomarkers associated with the biological effect they are studying.

Finding markers that are associated with a response is relatively easy; it is very difficult, however, to find markers that are truly linked to a particular biological effect. For example, the levels of many analytes fluctuate in different disease states, resulting in different observations depending on when the analytes are measured. As a result, validating both biomarkers and the results obtained from using them has become very important.

In the following subsections, we discuss examples of research biomarkers found in cancer and Alzheimer's research.

Cancer Research

Sunitinib (Pfizer's Sutent) is a multikinase inhibitor that inhibits several receptor tyrosine kinases. This field is highly competitive, and Pfizer was keen to get this drug to market in a timely fashion. Sunitinib has both antiangiogenic and antitumor activity and has been approved for gastrointestinal stromal tumors (GIST), a form of stomach cancer, and for renal-cell carcinoma, a form of kidney cancer. While developing sunitinib, Pfizer explored a range of biomarkers in preclinical animal studies and then compared those results with clinical specimens. The drug inhibits Fms-like tyrosine kinase 3 (FLT3), stem cell factor receptor (KIT), vascular endothelial growth factor receptors (VEGFR1, VEGFR2 and VEGFR3), and platelet-derived growth factor receptors (PDGFRα and PDGFRβ), among others. Through a range of studies, Pfizer determined that all of these proteins are useful markers of activity but that FTL3 levels were the most useful. These markers were studied with the intention of speeding drug development and were not developed as companion diagnostics (discussed further in the section "Theranostics/Companion Diagnostics").

The company used fluorodeoxyglucose-positron emission tomography (FDG-PET, discussed further in Section "High Hopes for New Imaging Techniques") to confirm, quickly and early on, that sunitinib was indeed inhibiting tumor metabolism in human subjects. FDG-PET is a procedure where a radioactive sugar molecule is injected into a patient followed by PET imaging. Because tumor cells grow more rapidly than normal cells, they metabolize sugar more rapidly. The extent of sugar metabolism thus becomes a surrogate marker for the effectiveness of cancer drug treatment.

Alzheimer's Disease Research

A biomarker can also be used to determine the stage of a disease. Such a biomarker is useful not just for diagnosis and treatment but also for selecting patients to take part in clinical trials. In this case, the biomarker helps to make certain that the drug is being tested in a relatively homogeneous population, so a clear correlation between drug and effect can be established. One of the biggest problems that drug developers face is selecting sufficiently homogeneous study populations.

Alzheimer's disease is one area where such markers are sorely needed. There are many types of cognitive impairment that might, or might not, be early signs of Alzheimer's. According to a 2006 study in *Lancet* (Hansson et al., 2006), biomarkers in cerebrospinal fluid might help to predict the progression of disease from mild cognitive impairment to Alzheimer's disease. Dementia currently affects approximately 40% of individuals aged 90–95 years. Previous research has shown that damage to axons and neurons in Alzheimer's disease, the most common cause of dementia, begins decades before clinical signs appear. Alzheimer's disease is also usually preceded by mild cognitive impairment, but many patients with mild cognitive impairment can have a stable form that does not progress further.

The *Lancet* study found that 42% of patients with mild cognitive impairment developed Alzheimer's disease and 15% developed other types of dementia. The rate of progression to Alzheimer's disease in patients with mild cognitive impairment was substantially increased in those who had abnormal concentrations of biomarkers for beta-amyloid (Abeta42), total tau, and phosphorylated-tau in their cerebrospinal fluid. The researchers found they could identify patients with incipient Alzheimer's with 95% sensitivity and 83% specificity using a combination of total tau and Abeta42. These findings could form the basis of a test that could be used both as part of diagnostic assessment of dementia and in the design of clinical trials for Alzheimer's disease.

Toxicity Biomarkers

Given the tremendous publicity around drug safety over the last few years, there is broad-based interest in identifying and validating biomarkers to be used as early surrogate markers of toxicity or of other unwanted drug effects. The FDA is especially interested in this application of biomarkers and is trying to encourage and expand work in this arena. One of the biggest challenges in toxicity research has been finding animal models that can accurately predict common human toxicities. As a result, researchers are trying different approaches.

Companies such as Pfizer are pioneering a type of marker identified by gene-expression signature/structure relationship analysis. In this technology, researchers identify "signatures of toxicity" by analyzing gene expression in biological samples using technologies such as microarrays on chips. A drug's signature is determined from the pattern of changes it causes in the expression of multiple genes. Once the signature for a certain type of drug-induced toxicity has been identified, it can be correlated with other expression-signatures, and the structures of different drugs can be compared to identify common toxicity-causing chemical structures. If researchers can understand which structures cause toxicities, they can try to design compounds that avoid these structures. But gene expression studies must be done carefully and systematically, or they are not reproducible (discussed further in the section "The Unique Challenges of Genomic Data"). Companies, including Iconix and Gene Logic, are building gene-expression databanks for toxicity markers in partnership with pharmaceutical clients and the FDA.

Pharmacogenetic Biomarkers

Pharmacogenetics is another growing area for biomarker development. It has long been known that genetics can influence how people metabolize drugs. Genetic variations in drug-metabolizing enzymes (e.g., cytochrome P450 [CYP] enzymes) are becoming well-characterized biomarkers for toxicity and drug dosing. One example where dire consequences can occur is in people who have inherited specific mutations in the thiopurine methyl transferase (TPMT) gene. These people metabolize the drug 6-mercaptopurine differently than most patients and can experience life-threatening side effects when treated with this medication for acute lymphocytic leukemia. These mutations have been well characterized, and there is now a genetic test available to screen for them (e.g., Prometheus Laboratories' PRO-Predict TPMT Genetics assessment test). It is worth noting, however, that physicians are not required to use this test. It is up to the physician's discretion whether or not to use it. Although the FDA considered making testing a requirement in the drug's label, physicians argued that this would be an infringement of their autonomy and that it was not warranted – very few life-threatening reactions occur, and they can usually be medically managed. Physician resistance to TPMT based on the perception that it is an unwanted complication is one sign of the difficulty that theranostics in general face.

Antidepressants, meanwhile, work poorly or not at all in people carrying certain types of mutations in drug-metabolizing enzymes. Currently, clinicians may have to prescribe multiple drugs, and the patients can spend months sequentially trying these drugs and waiting for them to take effect. Particularly in the case of severe depression, some clinicians would like to have tests for genetic variants that influence antidepressant metabolism. Clinical Data, which recently acquired Icoria and pharmacogenomics pioneer Genaissance Pharmaceuticals, has just started a clinical trial that pairs an antidepressant and a biomarker of drug response (see the upcoming Section "Clinical Data's Depression Drug Test").

THE VALUE OF CLINIC-READY BIOMARKERS

Currently, the vast majority of biomarkers are used in research rather than in clinical trials, but there is increasing discussion about the value of having biomarkers available that could quickly come into clinical use. As noted earlier, late-stage drug failure has become an increasingly common problem for drug companies. Several high-profile drugs have had to be withdrawn recently for safety reasons. In addition, other drugs have fared poorly on the market because they do not work as well as expected. Often, side effects or drug response is limited to a subset of patients – Why not test to identify these patients? Proponents of theranostics, or companion diagnostics, argue that by having biomarker-based tests ready for clinical use, companies can save drugs that would otherwise fail, improve drug performance, and possibly stave off market withdrawal. Notable examples of drugs that faced problems after reaching market are Merck's rofecoxib (Vioxx) and AstraZeneca's gefitinib (Iressa). Experience with both of these major drugs illustrates how serious repercussions can be when the full range of biological effects for a drug is not known.

Both rofecoxib and gefitinib were under study for many years, but their development occurred during a transition period when many novel targets were being quickly addressed, and companies were still mostly opposed to the idea of using theranostics: at the time, the most common view was that proving a drug works only in a subset of people would limit the drug's sales. But the lessons learned from cyclooxygenase-2 (COX-2) inhibitors and gefitinib suggest that it may be time to look beyond that concern and to recognize clinic-ready biomarkers (i.e., diagnostic grade tests) as an important strategic tool for today's drug developers. The primary lesson from both these experiences is that it is probably best to have biomarkers ready for when you need them. Of course, this represents a huge investment for uncertain gain. What if the drug gets approved and never needs a supporting test of any kind? Nonetheless, most major companies are now at least collecting samples and doing some early clinical biomarker studies in case they end up in a situation where they need to show a subpopulation effect, or they need to prove that a safety problem is restricted to a set of patients that can be easily identified.

Lessons to Be Learned from the COX-2 Inhibitor Rofecoxib (Merck's Vioxx)

The recent controversy over the safety of COX-2 inhibitors has impacted the entire drug industry. Once hailed as a breakthrough in safe, chronic pain relief, rofecoxib is associated with severe adverse effects in some patients including heart attacks, strokes, and even death. Rofecoxib-associated risks were noticed during the Adenomatous Polyp Prevention on Vioxx (APPROVe) trial for what could have been a new indication: the prevention of colon cancer (Bresalier et al., 2005). Drug withdrawals such as the rofecoxib withdrawal have rattled the drug industry: not only does Merck face the prospect of having a massive liability in this case, but in spring 2005, Pfizer also had to withdraw one COX-2 inhibitor, valdecoxib (Bextra), and put a black-box warning on the label of another, celecoxib (Celebrex). The entire field of COX-2 inhibition, which once seemed so promising, has been disrupted. In addition, many experts believe that the FDA has now become much more sensitive to drug safety issues, making it even harder to get drugs approved, even when side effects are extremely rare.

So, would it be better to have a test that determines who is at risk of such side effects, even before the drug goes to market?

Millions of people took COX-2 inhibitors, but only approximately 2% of these patients ever experienced the serious side effects. A recent study found that up to 30% of variation in response to this class of drugs can be attributed to individual genetic makeup (Fries et al., 2006). Researchers examined the variability, both within and between subjects, in response to celecoxib and rofecoxib, in a randomized, double-blind, placebo-controlled study conducted on 50 healthy volunteers between ages 21 and 43. Trial participants received a single dose of placebo, celecoxib, and rofecoxib in random order so that responses to the drugs could be compared within the same subjects. Five of the patients went through the entire protocol five times to see how much variation could be seen within the responses of a single patient.

The study illustrated that even healthy individuals without a recognized risk of disease respond quite differently to these drugs. A variety of responses were seen even in one patient dosed with the same drug at different times. This effect was seen even when researchers standardized or controlled for as many variables as possible. Approximately 30% of the variability found in patients was attributable to genetic differences, which led the authors to suggest that biomarkers might be useful to guide prescribing. Although the researchers looked at 25 different genetic variations in genes such as *COX-1* and *CYP2C9* (a major metabolizing enzyme for celecoxib), definitive biomarkers for predicting adverse responses have not yet been identified. Given the attention that has surrounded the withdrawal of rofecoxib and subsequent legal proceedings, it is unlikely this particular drug will ever reach the market again. But companies that are developing similar drugs will be trying to find ways both to avoid toxicities and to identify patients at greatest risk for them.

It is important to note, however, that even in this study, genetic differences were associated with only about one-third of all the variability seen in patients. Age, other medical conditions, and a variety of other environmental factors have a major effect on how individuals react to drugs. It may be that such environmental causes are more important than genetic variation in many cases. As a result, any test that predicts toxicity is never going to predict all cases. Determining when such a test is useful will be complicated.

Lessons to Be Learned from Gefitinib (AstraZeneca's Iressa)

A different lesson came from the travails of gefitinib, once thought to be a very promising therapy targeting the human epidermal growth factor receptor (EGFR or HER-1). Phase III trial results were discouraging, with barely 10% of patients responding to the therapy. In its favor were some remarkable responses among the few patients it did help, mainly nonsmokers and people of Asian descent. Intense investigation and debate surrounded how to select those patients. At first, it seemed as if specific mutations in *EGFR* were responsible for the variation in response. Later, it seemed like *EGFR* copy number was important. But none of that work moved quickly enough to keep gefitinib in wide use, and in summer 2005, the FDA issued a new label limiting the drug's use only to patients already shown to be benefiting from it, a move that significantly limited gefitinib's prospects.

Ironically, recent data presented at the American Association for Cancer Research's Annual International Conference on Molecular Targets and Cancer Therapeutics by researchers from the University of Colorado Cancer Center now seem to confirm the earlier findings that the best indicator of positive response to gefitinib is a fairly basic test – *EGFR* gene copy number – that can be measured by a fluorescent in situ hybridization (FISH) test. Studies using samples collected during the Phase III Iressa Survival Evaluation in Lung Cancer (ISEL) trial found that FISH-positive patients taking the drug lived about twice as long (8.3 months versus 4.5 months) as those taking placebo. Meanwhile, overall, FISH-negative patients gained little benefit from gefitinib. *EGFR* copy number does not explain all the responses to the drug: some FISH-negative patients still do well. As a result, scientists believe that other factors must be involved, and they have been looking at additional markers. In this particular ISEL-based study, EGFR expression and Akt activation status were examined, but neither of these two other biomarkers were useful.

Most interesting about the gefitinib saga is that the relationship between the targeted receptor and drug response appears to be similar to that seen with trastuzumab (Herceptin) and its target, human epidermal growth factor receptor-2 (HER-2). Trastuzumab is the poster child of targeted therapy and is a very successful product (discussed further in "Theranostics/Companion Diagnostics"). Although other factors may be involved, there appears to be a predictable relationship between *EGFR* copy number and response. This relationship could well impact other EGFR-targeting drugs, such as cetuximab (Bristol-Myers Squibb/ImClone's Erbitux) and erlotinib (Genentech/OSI's Tarceva). New entrants in this field will be evaluated from the standpoint that *EGFR* copy number is probably going to be valuable in predicting drug response.

UNIQUE CHALLENGES OF GENOMIC DATA

One reason there is so much interest in biomarkers is the emergence of new technologies to identify them. With these new tools in hand, researchers hope that perhaps novel, and more specific, biomarkers will be forthcoming. Genomics is one of the particularly promising areas of novel biomarker development. Initially, there was tremendous anticipation that genomics could quickly lead to the development of many new biomarkers. Gene expression, proteomics, metabonomics/ metabolomics, and genetic variation were the basis of many start-up companies, beginning in the late 1990s. A number of these companies focused primarily on building databanks (e.g., Variagenics and Gene Logic) or tools (e.g., Affymetrix and Sequenom) to perform such studies. Many of these companies were eventually acquired or simply shuttered, although some have survived and their products are becoming established tools in biomarker discovery and development.

Rather than "popping out" of gene chip or mass spectrometry experiments, biomarkers at first seemed to explode out. Researchers quickly identified two major problems with the wealth of new biomarker data: it is extremely difficult to reproduce, and much of it can be irrelevant. The genome is gigantic, comprising more than 3 billion base pairs, and the proteome and metabolome are even bigger. Hence, any time researchers scan any "ome" for a signal, they are likely to find many signals, and a good number of them will not be meaningful. Searching for biomarkers in gene chip or mass spectrometry data must be scrupulously done, must be reproducible, and must be clinically validated.

The FDA's Position on Pharmacogenomic Data

As noted earlier, the FDA has a strong interest in seeing industry use biomarkers both to help get more good drugs to market and to catch safety problems early. The agency has high hopes that genomics in particular will offer novel and very specific biomarkers. However, the agency is keenly aware of the problems inherent in these data. Many pharmaceutical companies have been reluctant to use genomic biomarkers during clinical trials for fear that early data could be incorrectly interpreted. What if a genomic biomarker suggests a drug will cause liver toxicity, but there is no other sign of liver toxicity? Companies worry that naïve reviewers will jump to conclusions about preliminary and unvalidated data. If companies do not do the studies, however, it will be impossible to determine the real value of such tools.

To calm companies' fears, the agency has issued its Guidance for Industry on Pharmacogenomic Data Submissions. The guidance establishes a clear pathway by which companies can share novel data with the agency early on and not be concerned that the agency will later misuse the data. This guidance, which is available on the FDA Web site, details how the agency will determine whether a biomarker is truly a "known valid" biomarker that is ready for clinical evaluation or whether the marker is still "exploratory" (Table 40.3). The agency hopes that this new approach will encourage more companies to conduct these types of studies. As companies do the studies and submit them along the "Voluntary Genomic Data Submission" process, agency reviewers will also be learning about the technical aspects of these data. It is important to note that the guidance does not cover proteomics and metabolomics and does not replace the well-established review process for any required data. It targets investigational use of genomic tools.

The process is still early, but the agency has so far received at least 25 voluntary submissions of genomic data. These submissions have related to a range of indication areas, including cancer, Alzheimer's disease, hypertension, hypoglycemia, depression, obesity, and rheumatoid arthritis. Submissions have been made related to a variety of products, including genotyping devices and analysis software.

Genomic Biomarkers in the Clinic

Even as many researchers still struggle to use omic tests in basic studies, gene expression

Table 40.3 Classification of Genomic Biomarkers and Requirements for Regulatory Submissions

Description	*Requirement for Submission of Biomarker and Pharmacogenomics Data*	*Examples of Biomarkers (drugs)*
Known valid biomarker	Submission is required by the FDA for: • INDs • New (unapproved) NDAs, BLAs, or supplements • Previously approved NDAs or BLAs	*Intended use as a safety biomarker:* • TPMT (6-MP, azathioprine) • UGT1A1 (irinotecan) • CYP2C9/VKORC1 (warfarin) • CYP2D6 (Strattera) *Intended use as an efficacy biomarker:* • EGFR status (Erbitux, Tarceva) • HER2/neu status (Herceptin) • Philadelphia chromosome – Bcr-abl (Gleevec) • c-kit (Gleevec)
Probable valid biomarkers	• Submission is not required for an IND, but the FDA welcomes a VGDS • Submission is recommended by the FDA for new (unapproved) NDAs, BLAs, or supplements • Submission is required by the FDA for previously approved NDAs or BLAs	*Intended use as a safety biomarker:* • Kim1 – preclinical (nephrotoxicity) • Gene panels for preclinical evaluation *Intended use as an efficacy biomarker:* • EGFR mutations (Iressa) • CYP2D6 (tamoxifen) • OncotypeDx gene panel (radiation therapy)
Exploratory or research biomarkers	• The FDA welcomes a VGDS for INDs • The FDA recommends submission for new (unapproved) NDAs, BLAs, or supplements but also welcomes a VGDS • The FDA welcomes a VGDS for previously approved NDAs or BLAs	*Intended use as a safety biomarker:* • Gene panels for preclinical evaluation *Intended use as an efficacy biomarker:* • APOE4 (donepezil, Alzheimer's disease) • VEGF (several anticancer agents) • Adiponectin mutations (rosiglitazone, type 2 diabetes)

6-MP = 6-mercaptopurine; APOE4 = Apolipoprotein E4; BLA = Biologics license application; EGFR = Epidermal growth factor receptor; IND = Investigational new drug; NDA = New drug application; RGDS = Required pharmacogenomics data submission; TPMT = Thiopurine methyltransferase; UGT1A1 = UDP-glucuronosyltransferase 1; VEGF = Vascular endothelial growth factor; VGDS = Voluntary pharmacogenomics data submission

Note: 25 VGDS submissions had been received by the FDA as of March 2006

signatures of drug response and toxicity are finally, but very slowly, starting to come into clinical use. One of the first such tests is Genomic Health's Oncotype DX test for breast cancer that compares the expression of 21 genes and predicts the likelihood of cancer recurrence. There is still some debate about the widespread use of genomic tests such as this one in clinical settings. These tests typically measure many more data points than do traditional tests, and it is difficult to obtain reproducible results even when highly trained personnel perform them. The Oncotype DX test addresses these concerns by using a traditional technology (polymerase chain reaction) rather than a gene chip. Also, the test is performed in a licensed Genomic Health laboratory where the assay was developed.

This test is already available but is still being studied because this is such a new field. The National Cancer Institute (NCI) has just launched the Trial Assigning Individualized Options for Treatment (Rx), also called TAILORx. All the NCI-sponsored clinical trials groups that perform breast cancer research studies have collaborated in the trial's development and are participating in this study, which will follow participants for at least 10 years. The study aims to see whether using the test can safely allow more women to skip chemotherapy.

HIGH HOPES FOR NEW IMAGING TECHNIQUES

Imaging technologies are another area where a great deal of promising new biomarker research is being carried out. Some of the most striking evidence that researchers presented to support the effectiveness of Pfizer's anticancer drug sunitinib was FDG-PET imaging data. This imaging technique showed that even when the drug did not appear to be shrinking tumors, it was shutting down their blood flow. As a result, researchers are beginning to question well-established clinical criteria for drug "success" such as time to progression. Instead, they want to use imaging techniques to evaluate the following:

- Whether a targeted drug is hitting the target.
- Whether a targeted drug is having the intended effect of downregulating a particular receptor (e.g., HER-2, EGFR).
- Whether a targeted drug is inhibiting certain key molecules in a particular pathway.
- Whether a targeted drug is having observable effects such as increasing apoptosis (cell death) or inhibiting angiogenesis.

Dynamic contrast enhanced magnetic resonance imaging (DCE-MRI), diffusion MRI, magnetic resonance spectroscopy (MRS), and FDG-PET are key imaging techniques being explored for use in drug discovery and development. Most importantly, some of these new modalities are allowing researchers to actually visualize metabolic activity so that they can associate clinical observations with molecular activity. This field is in the early stages, and imaging studies are still expensive enough that they are done on a relatively limited basis. However, there is much anticipation that imaging will emerge as a critical tool in the development of targeted therapies and in drug development in general.

THERANOSTICS/COMPANION DIAGNOSTICS

One of the biggest questions lingering about biomarkers is not who is using them – because almost everyone is – but who plans to take them into the market as companion diagnostics, or theranostics. Although most major pharmaceutical companies and a horde of smaller drug developers are engaged in biomarker-related research, very few companies have actually committed to bringing drug/diagnostic pairs to market. Instead, a lot of work is being done either to identify subset effects, without necessarily having this information included in a drug's label, or to determine if any subgroups of patients are metabolizing drugs differently and are thus at risk for potential side effects.

Trastuzumab is often held up as evidence of how successful drugs with companion diagnostics could be. Trastuzumab would not have been approved if Genentech had not been able to identify a marker (overexpression of HER-2) that identifies patients who will respond better to the drug. This drug is now extremely profitable, even though it is prescribed only to a subset of breast cancer patients.

In the past, pharmaceutical developers were wary of unearthing "subpopulation effects" where a drug behaves differently in various subgroups of people. The common perception was that such effects would harm a drug's commercial prospects by segmenting a potentially large market into smaller sectors. This attitude is starting to change for several reasons, including some costly failures (discussed earlier in the section "The Value of Clinic-Ready Biomarkers"). The tremendous success of trastuzumab demonstrates that even drugs targeted to only those patients who have specific markers (such as higher-expression levels of certain genes) can be very profitable. Novartis's imatinib (Gleevec), which targets a specific genetic mutation, also supports this idea. Now that targeted drugs are being used in a growing number of indications and in earlier-stage disease, biomarkers for drug response in subpopulations of patients are looking much less threatening to some people on the commercial side of drug development.

Nonetheless, there are still very few examples of drugs that even have a companion test available, and even fewer examples where the test is required (in the label) for use with the drug. Some recent announcements do suggest, however, that the field of drug/diagnostic co-development could be gaining ground. In the next sections, we discuss select companies that are developing biomarkers in combination with drugs.

Roche Diagnostics and Lilly Cancer Drugs

Roche Diagnostics recently partnered with Eli Lilly to investigate biomarkers that identify patients most likely to respond to certain cancer therapies. The first phase of the agreement targets biomarkers linked to Lilly's pemetrexed (Alimta) and gemcitabine (Gemzar). If successful, Roche Molecular Diagnostics (a business area of Roche Diagnostics) and Response Genetics will work with Lilly to develop appropriate companion diagnostic tests. Roche, the leading diagnostics company, recently received the FDA clearance for its AmpliChip CYP450 Test, the first microarray-based diagnostic test for the detection of genetic variations that influence drug efficacy and adverse drug reactions. Although the company is developing other commercial biomarkers, one of its major goals is to partner with pharmaceutical firms and become the "biomarker developer" of choice. The major strategic hurdle for Roche is getting other pharmaceutical companies to feel comfortable turning over these projects to an enterprise that seems very closely allied with a competitor – Roche's pharmaceutical arm.

Clinical Data's Depression Drug Test

Clinical Data recently began enrollment in a pivotal Phase III trial for vilazodone in depression and is actively looking for biomarkers that can predict which patients will respond to treatment. Vilazodone is a novel dual serotonergic antidepressant that acts both as a selective serotonin reuptake inhibitor (SSRI) and as a 5HT1A partial agonist. Clinical Data acquired rights to this compound from Merck KGaA in September 2004. Based on recent discussions with the FDA, the company decided to accelerate the development plan for vilazodone and for a companion biomarker test.

Developing a drug/diagnostic combination is a big play for a little company. But, as noted, depression has long been regarded as one of the most attractive targets for biomarker development. Because it is such a large market, it can take a long time for patients to demonstrate response to a drug. There are so many drugs to choose from in the first place, and there is concern that seriously depressed patients could commit suicide if not quickly given a drug that works for them. Since vilazodone is already in Phase III trials, it is quite possible that this drug/diagnostic could become one of the first drug/test combinations to be launched. In May, Clinical Data announced that it plans to spin out its vilazodone business as a separate company to be named Precigen Therapeutics. Precigen will be responsible for further development and commercialization of vilazodone and its companion biomarker.

In April, the company also announced that it had validated a genetic marker to identify patients at risk for clozapine-induced agranulocytosis (CIA). Plans are to develop a genetic test for this biomarker to be sold under the brand Therapeutic Diagnostics.

Bristol-Myers Squibb's Commitment

Bristol-Myers Squibb (BMS) recently completed the rolling submission of its new drug application for dasatinib to the FDA. Dasatinib, one of several multitargeted kinase inhibitors making their way to market, is being developed for the treatment of chronic myelogenous leukemia (CML) and for Philadelphia chromosome-positive (Ph+) acute lymphoblastic leukemia (ALL). Most people with CML and approximately 25% of adults with ALL carry a mutation called the Philadelphia chromosome. Many patients with CML who are treated with imatinib become resistant to this treatment over time. Dasatinib may prove useful in imatinib-refractory disease.

Dasatinib is one of BMS's key new oncology products. At the Cambridge Healthtech Institute (CHI) Clinical Biomarker Congress in May 2006, BMS presented data identifying response biomarkers for this drug, as well as more than 100 genes that, looked at together, may form a "signature" of response. It will not be necessary to use this gene signature for studies in Philadelphia chromosome-based malignancies because the chromosome mutation itself is essentially a marker. But as the drug moves into other indications, this signature could become an important feature for distinguishing dasatinib from similar products in what will be an increasingly competitive market.

Backing up BMS's commitment to biomarkers is the company's recent technology access and product development agreement with Epitome Biosystems. BMS has discovered biomarkers that it wants to integrate into its clinical development program. Epitome will develop custom antibody arrays for this purpose to measure specific proteins designated by BMS.

POTENTIAL IMPACT OF BIOMARKER USE

The pharmaceutical industry has high hopes that biomarkers will rescue it from the pipeline doldrums, and a small but vocal segment of the biotechnology industry is pressing for rapid adoption of biomarkers as theranostics, to speed personalized medicine. But biomarkers are difficult to find and to validate even for research purposes. It is even harder to apply them as diagnostics and very complicated to integrate companion diagnostics into the current medical paradigm.

One of the greatest challenges ahead is, "How easy will it be to develop clinically useful biomarkers?" Already, it is clear that human variation in response to drugs, in susceptibility to disease, and in progression of disease is influenced by a great many factors, including age, sex, nutrition, medical history, genetics, medications, and environment. It is exacting work to find any useful biomarker. Many putative biomarkers have been used or developed over the last few years, but large numbers of them have turned out to be false leads or useful in only a very small number of cases. As a result, there is no wave of biomarkers coming out of anyone's lab, either from industry or from academia, despite a significant effort to replicate and to validate them. The need to produce reliable biomarkers remains a major challenge in the pharmaceutical industry.

Companies that have access to large numbers of appropriately preserved, well-cataloged biological samples have a huge advantage when hunting for biomarkers. Unfortunately, it can be extremely difficult to collect such samples. For one thing, it is very expensive, particularly to catalogue and preserve patient samples correctly but also to annotate the samples with sufficient clinical data to make them useful. Patient data collection and storage constitute a very sensitive issue in terms of confidentiality and who will be able to access and use such data. In particular, genomic data can not only indicate an individual's risk or susceptibility of developing a debilitating or costly disease but also potentially reveal information about an individual's behavioral tendencies. Pharmaceutical companies and those academic or public research facilities that have had the foresight to begin storing clinically annotated samples should have a head start in developing really useful biomarkers. It is only by looking at many samples, in some cases tens of thousands, that certain correlations are even going to be seen: that is why serious side effects are often identified only when drugs are released to the mass market, and many more people are exposed to them.

Another challenge to developing and using biomarkers in drug development is, "How many biomarkers are enough?" There is some debate about whether the most useful biomarkers will be single markers, whether a few biomarkers will be needed per disease, or whether whole constellations of markers (such as genomic, proteomic, or metabolomic signatures) will be necessary. Some experts favor constellations of markers because it may be easier to represent a complex disease state with a more comprehensive set of markers. Others say that the most important thing is to have biomarkers that are meaningful – that is, biomarkers that represent biological mechanisms that make sense in the context of the disease being studied or evaluated. It is likely that many disease states will not be as straightforward as those seen in targeted cancer therapy, for example, where only one biomarker may be necessary to accurately select patients for treatment.

Despite all these challenges, there are signs that the industry's new emphasis on biomarkers and other translational tools is helping. A study recently released from the Tufts Center for the Study of Drug Development (CSDD) found that the number of drugs that entered clinical testing (at the 10 top-selling US drug companies) surged 52% from 2003 through the end of 2005. This is a huge reversal. In contrast, the number of drugs entering trials during 1993–7 compared with 1998–2002 showed a 21% decline at these 10 companies.

This upsurge in clinical trials does not guarantee that more polished products will reach the market – attrition in later phases has been a huge problem. However, this activity does suggest that companies are willing to make the huge investment that clinical trials require, and that suggests they may feel more confident about a growing number of drug candidates. New strategies, such as biomarkers, may be helping to advance more drugs from preclinical to clinical phases.

Biomarkers could also lead to a surge in the co-development of companion diagnostics and therapeutic drugs, which will fundamentally change the way the pharmaceutical industry develops new drugs. This application of diagnostic biomarkers will arise under two influences: the demands of regulatory agencies and those of market competition. Public concern about drug safety is growing. The public, the drug industry, and regulatory agencies all alike want more safety data and far better information about how drugs act. The FDA in particular is strongly promoting the use of biomarkers and of pharmacogenomic data in the drug development process so that safer and more effective drugs can be produced. In fact, biomarkers and drug toxicity are among the agency's first projects in its Critical Path Initiative.

From a pharmaceutical-industry perspective, it is increasingly important to identify patients at risk of toxicity and to identify patients who will respond to drugs in order to tailor drug dose and treatment to the individual. This is just starting to occur and is much easier in some fields – such as

HIV treatment or cancer – than others. Still, market competition in stratified patient markets will fuel continued biomarker development, particularly within the field of targeted therapeutics and in other hotly contested markets. As an example, multikinase inhibitors are already on the market going head-to-head for market share. Sunitinib (Pfizer's Sutent) and sorafenib (Onyx/Bayer's Nexavar) are both approved for kidney cancer. Dasatinib (Bristol-Myers Squibb's BMS-354825) and lapatinib (GlaxoSmithKline's GSK-572016) are two other multi-kinase targeting drugs that are close to market. In such circumstances, companies will want to demonstrate their drug has advantages, even if those advantages are restricted to a subpopulation (as long as the subpopulation is still a healthy market, of course). Going forward, any drug developed in association with a biomarker could provide a marketing advantage as the drug enters a crowded and competitive marketplace.

REFERENCES

Hansson, O. et al. Association between CSF biomarkers and incipient Alzheimer's disease in patients with mild cognitive impairment: a follow-up study. *Lancet Neurology.* 2006;5(3):228–34.

Bresalier, R.S. et al. Cardiovascular events associated with rofecoxib in a colorectal adenoma chemoprevention trial. *New England Journal of Medicine.* 2005; 352(11): 1092–102.

Fries, S. et al. Marked interindividual variability in the response to selective inhibitors of cyclooxygenase-2. *Gastroenterology.* 2006; 130: 55–64.

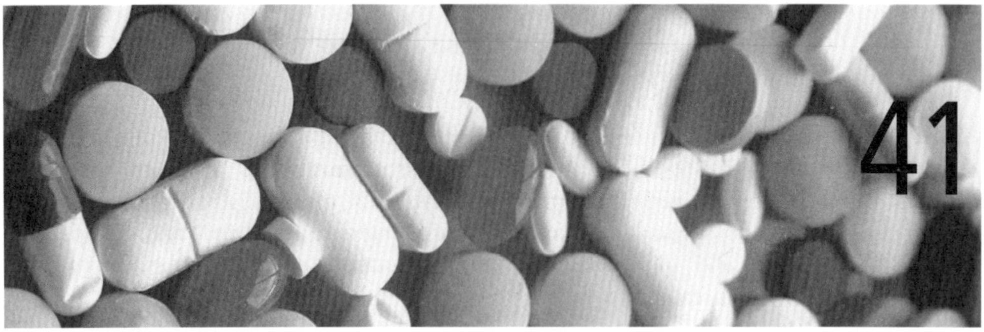

Unlocking the Potential of Biomarkers in Targeted Oncology

IMPROVED DIAGNOSTICS AS IMPORTANT AS IMPROVED THERAPIES TO OPTIMIZING CANCER TREATMENT

In Europe and the United States, close to 20 million people live with cancer today, and approximately 2.6 million new cases are diagnosed each year, a number that is increasing mainly as a result of demographic change, because most types of solid cancer are typically diseases of the elderly. More than 6 million people around the world die of cancer every year, and one of two men and one of three women will develop cancer in their lifetimes. Moreover, cancer is the leading cause of death, after cardiovascular diseases, in the major pharmaceutical markets (United States, France, Germany, Italy, Spain, United Kingdom, and Japan). The overall annual costs associated with malignancies currently amount to $107 billion.

According to the American Cancer Society's Cancer Facts & Figures 2003 publication, more than 1.3 million new cases were expected to be diagnosed in the United States in 2003. More than 550,000 Americans die of cancer each year, and 8.9 million have a history of cancer, with a significant risk of recurrence. This large market therefore offers significant opportunity not only for pharmaceutical therapies but also for diagnostics.

As a result of constantly improved surgical and pharmacological therapies, most cancers have a fairly good prognosis if they are detected at stages I or II, when they are generally still resectable and no metastases have yet formed. Typically, however, most cases – particularly in pancreatic, ovarian, and small-cell lung cancer – are detected in later stages when therapies are mostly palliative.

Tools that can provide earlier diagnosis of carcinomas and better monitoring and targeting of cytotoxic therapy could therefore be at least as beneficial in optimizing cancer treatment as better antiproliferative drugs could be. This fact has led scientists to look for biomarkers for cancer that can be detected and quantified in biopsy tissue or body fluids.

In this chapter, we describe biomarker detection technologies and the cancers to which they are most applicable. We then discuss the leading cancer indications – prostate, cervical, breast, ovarian, lung, and colorectal – and specific biomarker applications that are marketed or are in development for them.

THE CONCEPT AND PURPOSE OF CANCER BIOMARKERS

Biomarker analysis is central to personalized medicine because it enables treatment based on a patient's profile – genetic or somatic – that indicates a likely response to treatment. Biomarker analysis introduces molecular concepts of disease derived from drug discovery to cancer treatment. Identified differences between nonmalignant and malignant cells, such as regulatory mechanisms, can potentially be exploited for the detection and treatment of malignancy. A useful biomarker for cancer detection and characterization should appear early in carcinogenesis so that it can provide evidence of possible occult disease (high sensitivity), but it should also offer clear evidence of progression from normal to cancerous tissue (high specificity).

Three basic types of biomarkers are useful for somatic diagnosis, typing, and predisposition testing:

1. Genetic markers (e.g., gene amplification and mutation, oncogenes, and tumor suppressor genes).
2. Cellular markers (e.g., differentiation markers, micronuclei, and measures of proliferation, such as thymidine labeling index).
3. Biochemical and pharmacological markers (e.g., key enzymatic activities such as transcription factors, telomerase, and certain invasion-associated proteins and proteases).

All three types of cancer biomarkers can be used to monitor and optimize the state-of-the-art therapy regimens prescribed as first-line therapy. Depending on treatment success or failure, biomarkers could be used to determine whether another cytotoxic drug might be added to the cocktail or whether another, potentially more suitable regimen might be chosen.

Tumor markers are already successfully used in patients with known or suspected cancer. Research is focused on the future applications of cancer biomarkers that include staging of the disease, treatment response, disease reemergence or relapse, and broad-based screening of the general population not known to be at particular risk. Identification of a reemergence or relapse requires biomarkers that give a signal in proportion to tumor load for validity as surrogate markers. In most cases, the biomarkers that are used for diagnosis meet this requirement. In some cases, tumor markers themselves are novel drug targets.

These two strongly interlinked aspects of diagnosis and therapy monitoring and modification reflect the classical requirement profile for a biomarker that is useful for targeted oncology therapies.

Biomarkers are increasingly used in cancer drug development to understand the molecular mechanism of action of novel drugs and to decipher their pharmacological properties in vivo. In clinical trials, predefined tumor marker levels are now frequently used for patient stratification and as additional end points to clinical outcomes.

Two other functions of cancer biomarkers are genetic predisposition testing, which assesses the risk for developing cancers, and environmental testing, which reflects an individual's or population's exposure to a carcinogen. Both of these functions are outside the scope of this chapter.

BIOMARKER DISCOVERY GAINS SUPPORT

In October 1999, the National Cancer Institute (NCI) awarded $8 million in grants for the creation of the Early Detection Research Network to discover and develop new cancer biomarkers. These awards enabled the creation of 18 biomarker developmental laboratories that focus on advancing anticipated discoveries to the clinical level with the assistance of separate biomarker validation laboratories. Table 41.1 lists several of the program's pharmaceutical collaborators.

In November 2002, the Fred Hutchinson Cancer Research Center in Seattle, Washington, received a four-year, $7 million grant from the Breast Cancer Center of Excellence (funded by the US Department of Defense) and a $1 million grant from a multiyear, public-private partnership of the Avon Foundation and the NCI. The grant from

Table 41.1 Early Detection Research Network Projects with Pharmaceutical Cooperation

Institution	*Subject*	*Pharmaceutical Collaborator(s)*
University of Colorado Health Science	Use of spectral imaging technology, differential gene expression techniques, and standard genetic and biochemical techniques to identify lung cancer biomarkers	Spectral Imaging, Cobe BCT
University of South Florida	Evaluate existing and potential biomarkers in archived sputum specimens from a screening trial of smokers and former smokers	Bayer Pharmaceuticals
Robert H. Lurie Comprehensive Cancer Center of Northwestern University	Detection of early-stage ovarian cancer in asymptomatic women at increased risk using genetic changes and aberrant mRNA expression	Atairgin Technologies, Chiron
Johns Hopkins University	Identification of biomarkers in bronchoalveolar lavage and serum samples from lung cancer patients. Focus is on non-small-cell lung cancer	Research Genetics, Calbiochem-Novabiochem
University of Maryland School of Medicine	Evaluating telomerase activity in plasma of patients with a variety of cancers as aids in diagnosis and as a monitoring tool during therapy to predict relapse	Advanced Bioscience Laboratories
Duke Medical Center	Expression-based markers for breast cancer to detect circulating breast cancer cells	Abbott Laboratories
Thomas Jefferson University	Serum polypeptides as potential broad biomarkers in liver cancer and hepatitis	Oxford GlycoSciences
Eastern Virginia Medical School	Customized protein chips in proteomic analysis based on SELDI to identify biomarkers for prostate and breast cancers at different stages of progression	Ciphergen Biosciences, Arcturus Engineering
University of Washington	Develop assays to detect cancer-related proteins in body fluids and tissues and determine which secreted proteins correlate with cancerous or precancerous lesions	Orca Biosciences

SELDI = Surface-enhanced laser desorption/ionization

the Breast Cancer Center of Excellence (which involves investigators from 10 institutions in Seattle; Houston, Texas; and Los Angeles, California) established the Center for the Evaluation of Biomarkers for Early Detection of Breast Cancer, and will be used to develop a blood test to be used in conjunction with mammography to improve early detection of breast cancer. The funds will be divided equally among the Fred Hutchinson Center, the University of Alabama, the Fox Chase Cancer Center, and the M.D. Anderson Cancer Center.

Another effort is a program run by the federal National Institute for Standards and Technology (NIST) to develop faster and more efficient methods for sequencing of mitochondrial DNA. Such mutations are found in lung cancer cells but not in the normal cells of the same patients.

DETECTION TECHNOLOGIES FOR BIOMARKERS

Today's applied cancer research has enabled a high rate of discovery of potential tumor markers. Cytology, genetic analysis, and proteomics are the principal tools that today's scientists employ to accomplish this discovery. In the following sections, we describe the technologies that are used in biomarker analysis in patients.

Classical Modes of Detection in Biofluids

Many protein biomarkers in serum and urine can be detected by conventional immunodiagnostic methods, such as antigen capture assays that employ immobilized monoclonal antibodies that are directed specifically against the respective protein. The bound target is then detected by nonimmobilized antibodies that carry tags consisting of enzymes, fluorescent or luminescent markers, or in the case of the older radioimmunoassay, a radioactive label. Such immunoassays can be made very sensitive and specific. At the same time, they are generally inexpensive, rapid, and can easily be made compatible with existing automated equipment in serological or immunological laboratories.

Biomarkers on Chips

Transcriptional profiling and the protein synthesis patterns of tumors can be characterized using high-density genomic or proteomic microarrays. Nucleic acid and protein chips are ideally suited to provide fixed combinations of capture agents (nucleic acids, antibodies, or other binding proteins). Compared with a single biomarker, sets of independent, judiciously chosen biomarkers used as part of a validated test panel can offer significantly increased statistical power and superior predictive value. The output from this "wet" part of the profiling job most frequently consists of fluorescence signals or mass spectrograms (see the next section). These data can then be processed by sophisticated software, which might include neural networks, to interpret and integrate the results.

Mass Spectrometry

Increasingly sophisticated mass spectrometry (MS) methods have been broadly applied to the detection and characterization of small molecules. Analytical laboratories, both in clinical and research settings, have employed MS to elucidate the chemical nature of elution peaks from gas chromatography (GC) and high-performance liquid chromatography (HPLC) systems.

The 1990s saw a surge of MS applications in the study of biomolecules, driven by the introduction of new methodologies such as electrospray ionization (ESI), matrix-assisted (or surface-enhanced) laser desorption ionization (MALDI, SELDI), and MALDI/SELDI's combination with time-of-flight spectroscopy (TOF). These MS methods allow proteins and nucleic acids to be analyzed with high resolution and have co-evolved with genomics and proteomics, where they are integral analytical tools today.

In SELDI-TOF, which has become especially powerful in combination with chip-based proteomics, proteins with the desired properties that are present in the analytes (which could be biological fluids or tissue extract) are adsorbed to the chip surface, where specific capture agents (binding proteins, antibodies, or metals) are firmly bound. Because their interaction with the surface coating is highly specific but relatively weak, the proteins can be evaporated by a brief laser pulse.

RT-PCR Detection of Tumor Markers in Circulating Cells

The establishment of distant tumor metastases requires transport of malignant cells that the primary tumor sheds into the bloodstream. Reverse transcriptase-polymerase chain reaction (RT-PCR) may enable greater sensitivity and specificity than cytological identification. The detection of disseminated tumor cells in the peripheral blood of cancer patients by RT-PCR could therefore be an attractive method for predicting occult metastasis, detecting micrometastases, and monitoring treatment efficacy. This technology is currently under investigation for several solid tumors, including prostate, breast, and gastrointestinal (GI) cancers.

SELECT BIOMARKERS WITH POTENTIAL MULTIPLE CANCER APPLICATIONS

Although several of the following biomarkers have been linked to specific cancers, some may have potential in multiple cancer types but are at too early a stage in discovery to specify their possible applications. In the following sections, we highlight select biomarkers and identify their leading cancer applications.

p53 (the Prototypical Cancer Marker)

Loss-of-function mutations of *p53*, a ubiquitous tumor suppressor gene on chromosome 17p, are the most common gene mutations found in cancer. Normally, the p53 protein expressed from the intact gene stops cells with DNA damage from multiplying until the DNA is repaired naturally or the defective cell is eliminated through apoptosis. Mutations of the *p53* gene, which occur spontaneously or in response to carcinogen exposure, result in formation of inactive p53 protein that has a longer half-life than its wild-type counterpart. Inactive p53 can be found in biofluids (e.g., blood, urine) collected from patients with clinically overt cancer and from some people exposed to genotoxic and mutagenic agents. A wealth of studies has confirmed that such a finding is an indication of aggressive disease. Mutations of *p53* correlate most strongly with colorectal and urothelial cancers.

Carcinoembryonic Antigen

Carcinoembryonic antigen (CEA), the first tumor-associated antigen identified, is expressed in nearly 50% of all human tumors. CEA was originally developed as a marker for colorectal cancer. However, it has become widely used for adenocarcinomas in general (Ballesta et al., 1995).

Proliferating Cell Nuclear Antigen

The proliferation marker proliferating cell nuclear antigen (PCNA) has a striking ability to interact with multiple partners that are involved in DNA repair, translesion synthesis, methylation, chromatin remodeling, and cell-cycle regulation (Maga and Hubscher, 2003). Ultimately, it is a marker for DNA replication fidelity. In normal cells, PCNA undergoes poly(ADP)-ribosylation; however, in cancer cells and tissues, this post-translational modification does not occur. PCNA is being investigated for a variety of cancers.

Angiogenesis-related Markers

Angiogenesis markers are associated with tumor invasiveness and/or metastasis because their appearance indicates an actively growing tumor that requires the creation of new blood vessels. The most significant representative of this group is vascular endothelial growth factor (VEGF). Other biomarkers in this class include platelet-derived endothelial cell growth factor (PD-ECGF), thrombospondin (TSP), and angiogenin. Recent evidence has linked the ability of tumor cells to turn on angiogenesis with *p53*. Lacking a normal *p53* gene, tumor cells begin to produce VEGF and other factors that draw new blood vessels toward them. Angiogenesis-related markers would have applications in a variety of cancers.

Telomerase

Telomeres are structures found at the ends of chromosomes; they serve to stabilize and protect the chromosomes. In healthy cells, the ends of telomeres shorten during each cell cycle until a critical length is reached, leading to breakdown of the cell. Telomerase is an enzyme that maintains the telomere length and chromosomal stability. When telomerase remains activated, the telomere length is conserved through the cell cycle, potentially leading to cell immortality and tumor development. Human serum telomerase is an early cancer marker because acquisition of the capability to express this enzyme marks the "immortalization" of cell lines within precancerous tissue and thus marks a transition to malignancy. Telomerase can be detected using fluorescent label methods based on capillary electrophoresis. We discuss the application of telomerase as a biomarker in the "Cervical Dysplasia and Cancer" section.

Multiple Drug Resistance Markers

Multiple drug resistance (MDR) is a predominant cause of chemotherapy failure. Therefore, identification of MDR markers can play a critical role in the selection of treatment regimens. MDR-1 expression in cancer cells is associated with resistance to chemotherapeutic agents such as paclitaxel (Bristol-Myers Squibb's Taxol), doxorubicin (Adriamycin), and etoposide (Eposin). Applications of these markers span a number of cancers.

Epidermal Growth Factor Receptor Tests

Epidermal growth factor receptor (EGFR), a signaling tyrosine kinase that is an important component of cell-cycle control, is mutated and/or overexpressed in many cancers. Testing for EGFR is bound to become very important because several of the most-recently approved cancer drugs are EGFR blockers whose therapeutic feasibility in individual patients depends entirely on their EGFR status – that is, whether it is normal or mutated/overexpressed. These drugs include gefitinib (AstraZeneca's Iressa), cetuximab (Bristol-Myers Squibb/Merck AG's Erbitux), and erlotinib (Roche/Genentech's Tarceva).

The Dako EGFR pharmDx kit received the FDA approval in conjunction with Erbitux on February 12, 2004, as a tool required for the identification of colorectal cancer patients eligible for Erbitux therapy. This immunohistochemical assay was already being used to determine the eligibility of all patients enrolled in all Erbitux clinical trials.

Zymed Laboratories' EGFR Kit (PicTure Plus Polymer Detection) is another immunohistochemical test of this type.

In addition to testing bound EGFR, the soluble portion of the protein (known as p110) – the extracellular domains of the EGFR that are shed into the bloodstream – can be detected and quantified in serum and plasma. Increasing levels of p110 indicate cancer. Although it shows promise, this method is still experimental.

We expect that EGFR assays working on all levels (genetic, histological, and serological) will become widely used as increasing numbers of EGFR-targeted cytotoxic drugs are approved. We also expect that the commercial significance of this field will surpass that of HER2/neu expression testing in breast cancer (see the "Breast Cancer" section).

APPLICATION OF BIOMARKERS TO SELECT CANCER TYPES

Several of the biomarker technologies we described above are being applied to various cancer types. In the following sections, we describe the cancers that have generated the most activity in terms of biomarkers.

Prostate Cancer

PSA

PSA, first described in 1979 (Wang et al., 1979) is the only cancer biomarker that the FDA (and equivalent regulatory bodies in other major pharmaceutical markets) has approved for use in a screening setting; it is approved for use in conjunction with a digital rectal exam as an aid to detection of prostate cancer in men aged 50 or older. (European countries frequently set lower age limits – that is, 40 or 45 years.)

The American Cancer Society reports that the five-year survival rate for prostate cancer is 100% if the cancer is not yet metastatic. A debate is ongoing as to whether the widespread introduction of PSA testing in the early 1990s has triggered excessive follow-up testing, but patterns of incidence, survival, and mortality support the contention that increased PSA testing has resulted in earlier detection of prostate cancer, thus reducing the death rate. Current prostate cancer mortality rates in both white men and African-American men in the United States are at their lowest levels in several decades for many age groups.

PSA is a ubiquitous membrane serine protease from the kallikrein family that is massively overexpressed in prostate cancer. Its extracellular portion is sheared off and carried away by the bloodstream, where it can be detected. Most of the circulating PSA in men with prostate cancer is complexed with alpha-1-antichymotrypsin. The cutoff for normal levels is usually set at 2–4 ng/mL total (i.e., free plus complexed) PSA, depending on national standards. In men who have an elevated total PSA (4–10 ng/mL; "grey zone results") but a normal rectal exam, free PSA is also determined. The ratio of free to total PSA can be used to partially discriminate cancer patients from noncancer patients in about 40% of cases. Therefore, a prostate biopsy, which is painful and costs at least $1,200, is required for definitive diagnosis of prostate cancer.

Owing to PSA's good regulatory position in the most important markets, and because PSA is intensely used for therapy monitoring and relapse surveillance in men treated for prostate cancer, PSA tests account for as much as 40% of the entire cancer diagnostics market, and annual sales total more than $350 million, according to IBEX Technologies. The Hybritech Tandem IRMA from Beckman Coulter was the first automated test system for PSA; today, several major vendors offer such tests based on their clinical chemistry platforms (see Table 41.2). Notably, the majority of these assays have FDA approval only for prostate cancer detection.

Other Potential Biomarkers for Prostate Cancer

PSA is a prototypical tumor marker, but certainly not an ideal one. Benign prostate hyperplasia (BPH), which frequently coexists with prostate carcinoma, and prostatitis may elevate concentrations of PSA in serum. Only 20–30% of men with total PSA values between 2 and 4 ng/mL actually have prostate cancer. Up to 30% of men with histologically proven BPH have PSA levels >4 ng/mL, pushing them into the grey zone. Additional markers would therefore be valuable to keep as low as possible the number of biopsies for diagnosis of prostate cancer.

The typical early-stage prostate carcinoma produces mostly PSA. However, as the tumor undergoes mutation and starts to express more primitive-cell populations, other general tumor markers such as PAP, CGA, NSE, and CEA are produced. However, these markers are not specific for prostate carcinoma; they have gained limited importance in therapy monitoring, but not in differential diagnosis.

PSA is only one of 15 currently known members of the kallikrein family and has

Table 41.2 Selection of PSA Tests Approved by the FDA

Trade Name	*Vendor*	*FDA Approval Date*
Tandem-R free PSA	Hybritech	March 1998
Tandem-MP complexed PSA	Hybritech	October 5, 2000
Architect Total PSA	Abbott Laboratories	February 9, 2004
AxSYM Total PSA		
IMx Total PSA		
Architect Free PSA		
AxSYM Free PSA		
IMx Free PSA		
BMC Elecsys tPSA + fPSA	Roche Diagnostics	February 22, 2001
Immuno 1 PSA Assay	Bayer Diagnostics	June 25, 1999
Immuno 1 Complexed PSA	Bayer Diagnostics	September 8, 2000
ACS:180 PSA	Bayer Diagnostics	December 22, 2000
ADVIA Centaur PSA		
Immulite PSA	Diagnostic Products	June 25, 2001
Immulite 2000 PSA		
Immulite Third Generation PSA		
Immulite 2000 Third Generation PSA		

therefore been named human kallikrein 3 (hK3). Two other members of that family are gaining importance as biomarkers: human glandular kallikrein (hK2) (Rittenhouse et al., 1998; Martin et al., 2004), for which the precursor of PSA is the natural substrate, and hK11 (Nakamura et al., 2003), for which researchers at the Mount Sinai Hospital in Toronto have developed an immunofluorimetric assay. HK11 measurements can be combined with measurements of the ratio of total PSA to free PSA to distinguish benign prostatic hyperplasia from prostate cancer, further reducing the number of unnecessary prostatic biopsies. Hybritech (a subsidiary of Beckman Coulter) has developed a commercial version of an hK2 test based on a patent (US-5516639) from the Mayo Clinic. Recent reviews of the studies evaluating these tests and their combinations with established PSA tests have been published (Haese et al., 2003).

Hybritech/Beckman Coulter is also investigating Pro-PSA, the enzymatically inactive precursor of PSA that – along with some of its truncated forms – has been shown to be more closely associated with prostate carcinoma than PSA itself (Mikolajczyk and Rittenhouse, 2003).

The Ki-67 proliferation antigen is useful to determine if a prostate carcinoma is growing aggressively. Ki-67 should be very useful in stratifying patients in future clinical trials. (About 90% of prostate carcinomas are low-grade and contain few growing cells at any given time. Aggressive PC has a poorer prognosis.) The largest biomarker study conducted so far for prostate cancer patients treated with radiation therapy has found that Ki-67 staining is a strong predictor of patient outcome for patients treated with androgen deprivation plus radiotherapy: when more than 7.1% of the tumor cells stained for Ki-67, there was a significantly increased risk of distant metastasis and death due to aggressive prostate cancer (Pollack et al., 2003).

Avalon Pharmaceuticals is investigating D-PCa-2 (Dresden Prostate Carcinoma 2), a transcript that was discovered in a screen of the Avalon's GeneExpress transcriptome database (Weigle et al., 2004). D-PCa-2 is highly expressed in the human prostate; however, no clear difference in the level of expression of this gene in normal versus malignant prostate cells has been found. D-PCa-2 could nevertheless be a suitable biomarker for metastatic prostate cancer because prostate cells do not circulate in the blood and lymph nodes of healthy individuals.

EZH2 (Enhancer of Zeste Homolog 2) is a transcriptional repressor that is more actively expressed in metastatic prostate cancer than in localized prostate cancer. Significance analysis of microarrays has shown that EZH2 tops a list of 55 genes that are significantly upregulated in metastatic prostate cancer relative to localized prostate cancer (Varambally et al., 2002). EZH2 has been found to be a significantly better predictor of clinical outcome than Gleason score, tumor stage, or PSA levels. In combination with E-cadherin (ECAD; a cell adhesion molecule), EZH2 status was statistically significantly associated with prostate-cancer recurrence after radical prostatectomy and may be useful in defining a cohort of high-risk patients (Chatta, 2003).

The uPM3 test from Bostwick Laboratories, a leading private pathology reference laboratory, detects PCA3, a protein that is expressed in prostate-cancer tissue at levels about 35 times higher than in normal prostate tissue and is virtually absent from other organs (Hessels et al., 2003). The test makes use of the fact that manipulation of the prostate during the obligatory digital rectal exam causes cells to be shed into the urine, which is sent to Bostwick Laboratories for PCA3 expression testing. According to the company, the uPM3 test predicts prostate cancer with 81% accuracy in biopsy material.

Cervical Dysplasia and Cancer

The current standard of medical care in cervical disease calls for assessment of two consecutive, minimally abnormal Pap smears by colposcopy, which is both expensive ($200–500 per patient) and invasive, requiring examination and painful biopsy of suspect lesions. Although human papilloma virus (HPV) is found in 99.7% of all cervical carcinomas, HPV testing for the viral strains associated with cervical cancer has proved to be of limited clinical value. However, Digene offers the DNAwithPAP Test, which combines Pap cytology testing with HPV testing, for adjunctive cervical cancer screening in women aged 30 or older.

Telomerase expression is a potentially important marker of high-grade cervical dysplasia and squamous cell carcinoma. Because the cervical smear samples the uppermost cell layers of the cervical mucosa, which express telomerase only in cases of high-grade dysplasia, the detection of telomerase in exfoliated cells of the cervical smear may have specificity for clinically significant lesions (Jarboe et al., 2002).

Breast Cancer

Breast cancer is the carcinoma in which biomarker testing for direct therapy management has probably made the greatest inroads so far. The American Society of Clinical Oncology (ASCO) recommends that all women diagnosed with breast cancer should have tumor marker tests.

HER2/Neu Testing

Herceptin (Roche/Genentech's monoclonal antibody trastuzumab, directed at the HER2/neu [human epidermal growth factor-2/neuroblastoma] oncogene) was approved only because a test was available that detected overexpression of this biomarker in women with breast cancer. (This very time-consuming and laborious noncommercial assay, known only as the "Clinical Trial Assay" [CTA], was replaced by HercepTest, developed by Dako A/S in collaboration with Genentech, when Herceptin won the FDA approval.) HER2/neu overexpression is present in only 25–30% of breast cancer cases. Such overexpression indicates a poor basic prognosis (Slamon et al., 1987), but it also indicates that the cancer might respond to Herceptin treatment. Currently, two immunohistochemical test kits and one fluorescent in situ hybridization (FISH) assay have FDA approval for selection of patients eligible for Herceptin therapy: the HercepTest from DAKO A/S (FDA approval September 1998); Pathway HER2 from Ventana Medical Systems (FDA approval November 2000); and the PathVysion HER 2 DNA Probe Kit from Vysis, a subsidiary of Abbott Laboratories (FDA approval December 2001).

All three assays are performed on tissue obtained during biopsy or surgery. In clinical practice, HER-2 status is determined with Dako's or Ventana's immunohistochemistry to detect protein overexpression; positive findings in these tests are followed up with Abbott's FISH assay to check for the underlying gene amplification.

In May 2003, the National Comprehensive Cancer Network updated its Practice Guidelines in Oncology to indicate that FISH may be more accurate than immunohistochemistry. In January 2002, the FDA granted Abbott approval to include Herceptin in PathVysion's label, making it the only HER-2 diagnostic product to have three capability claims: prognosis (adjunct to existing clinical and pathological information in stage II, node-positive breast cancer patients), selection for doxorubicin-based therapy, and selection for Herceptin therapy.

Serum testing of this biomarker based on a 110 kDa-soluble fragment has been investigated to allow HER2/neu testing before any biopsy has been made (Kandl et al., 1994; Hoopman et al., 2003) and developed into a test kit – the Bayer Immuno 1 HER2/neu serum test – that was approved by the FDA in December 2000 for monitoring women with metastatic breast cancer. In addition, another study has shown that saliva may be a suitable biofluid for diagnostic purposes (Bigler et al., 2002).

CA 15-3

CA 15-3 (a mucin, expressed from the MUC1 gene) has become a widely recognized serum marker for breast cancer (including node-negative forms) that is equally suitable for monitoring therapy and detecting recurrence of the carcinoma after an initially successful treatment (Gion et al., 2002). In 1997, the FDA approved the use of CA 15-3 (and the related marker BR27.29) for the detection of recurrent cancer.

The original diagnostic was an immunoradiometric assay from Centocor, but diagnosis today is dominated by immunoassays with nonradioactive detection methods. Beckman Coulter has developed a test (Access BR Monitor) and implemented it on its Access and Access 2 immunoassay systems as well as the new UniCelTM DxI 800 Access immunoassay system, which can perform up to 400 tests per hour. A CA 15-3 diagnostic test is also available on the Synchron LXi 725 clinical system, which combines chemistry and immunoassay analysis technology with data management and automated sample handling on a single instrument.

Roche Diagnostics markets a sandwich immunoassay based on its Elecsys immunoassay system that uses biotinylated and ruthenylated monoclonal antibodies as capture and detection antibodies, respectively, and electrochemiluminescence as the detection technology (Steber et al., 2003). Other competing products include the Enzymun-Test CA 15-3 on ES 700 and Abbott Laboratories' AxSYM CA 15-3.

Potential Breast Cancer Markers under Investigation

TA-90, A 90 kDa glycoprotein, is an immunogenic tumor-associated antigen that is present in circulating immune complexes in the early stage of disease. TA-90 can be detected with an antigen-specific, enzyme-linked immunosorbent assay that scientists at the John Wayne Cancer Institute developed using a murine monoclonal antibody as a capture agent. Values on the TA-90 assay differed significantly in 42 patients with invasive carcinoma detected on mammography from values detected in 82 patients with benign breast lesions. Furthermore, the combination of the TA-90 assay and mammography identified 54 of 56 breast neoplasms, indicating that the TA-90 assay might be a suitable adjunct to this routine screening procedure. Because free TA-90 antigen predominates in late-stage disease, the ratio of free to complexed antigen might become a useful staging tool, similar to PSA in prostate cancer. The same research group has successfully applied this immune complex capture assay to melanoma patients (Kelley et al., 1998).

The great majority of breast cancers express estrogen receptors. However, a subset is estrogen receptor-negative, more aggressive, and particularly difficult to treat because it is unresponsive to the estrogen receptor antagonists and aromatase inhibitors that suppress estrogen production. (In this context, the estrogen receptor is the most important biomarker for breast cancer treatment; its status is determined from initial biopsy material.) Psoriasin (also known as S100A7 and HID-5), a member of the S100 gene family, might enable further subdivision of the estrogen receptor-negative subset of breast cancers because its presence seems to indicate a particularly bad prognosis (Emberley et al., 2003), which could warrant immediate aggressive treatment with non-antiestrogenic cytotoxic drugs normally reserved for later stages of therapy.

Europroteome AG (Hennigsdorf/Berlin, Germany) is performing discovery studies in breast cancer patients in collaboration with Abbott Laboratories. Europroteome will analyze serum samples from women with breast cancer using proteomic and bioinformatic technologies. The data produced will be compared to cancer markers provided by Abbott from which promising marker combinations will be further developed as diagnostics tools.

Ovarian Cancer

Ovarian cancer is the leading cause of death from gynecological malignancies. Seventy-five percent of women who are diagnosed with this cancer present with disease that has already spread outside the ovaries, and frequently outside the pelvis.

To date, levels of CA125 in the blood of ovarian cancer patients have been considered the benchmark for monitoring response to therapy and for detecting subclinical disease in women treated for ovarian cancer. Because this tumor marker is mostly restricted to the pelvic region and is derived from coelomic epithelium, it offers a limited degree of organ specificity; elevated levels are sometimes seen in benign conditions or in other malignancies. To date, CA125 assays are the only commercially available biomarker tests for ovarian cancer.

Current guidelines recommend that once remission is achieved by surgery and chemotherapy, patients should have a CA125 test every three months for two years, then every six months for five years, and then once yearly for a minimum of 10 years. This long surveillance period is required because approximately 50% of the patients with ovarian cancer who have normal CA125 levels after completing therapy have persistent disease. In addition, approximately 15% of women with advanced ovarian cancer have only insignificantly elevated CA125 levels. Together with the substantial market size, this fact has prompted a search for additional biomarkers that is being pursued with even higher intensity than for other types of cancer.

To date, the marker HE4 (a protein of unknown function) appears to be most promising. In a study conducted at the Pacific Northwest Research Institute (PNRI) in Seattle, Washington, HE4's sensitivity for ovarian carcinoma was 40% higher than that of CA125 (Hellstrom et al., 2003). To increase sensitivity, the researchers created double-determinant ELISA that employs two antibodies directed against different epitopes of the HE4 molecule. The detection technology flags only molecules where both antibodies have bound. Fujirebio Diagnostics, in a license agreement with the PNRI, is confirming the laboratory assay results and working to develop a new clinical diagnostic test.

A group working at the Roswell Park Cancer Institute found beta 1,4-galactosyltransferase (b1,4GalT), a potential biomarker for detecting early recurrence of ovarian cancer after primary therapy that might be useful in patients whose CA125 levels have normalized (Odunsi et al., 2002).

Other potential new serum biomarkers that can be detected and quantified by immunoassay methods include prostasin, a trypsin-like serine protease that is a normal secretion product of the prostate in males but is overexpressed in epithelial ovarian cancer (Mok et al., 2001); urokinase plasminogen activator receptor, a soluble urokinase plasminogen activator receptor in preoperatively obtained plasma from patients with gynecological cancer or benign gynecological diseases (Rüsbro et al., 2001); plasminogen activator inhibitor 2 (PAI-2) (Nordengrren et al., 2002); CD105/endoglin, a marker for endometrial cancer angiogenesis (Salvesen et al., 2003); and various proteins from the human kallikrein family (see Section "Prostate Cancer Biomarkers"), among which hK6 has attracted the particular attention of Ibex Technologies (Diamandis et al., 2003). HK6 identifies an additional 40% of patients with early-stage disease, compared with CA-125 alone. Another marker, osteopontin, can be demonstrated in plasma and tissue using cDNA microarrays (Kim et al., 2002).

Using Ciphergen's ProteinChips and SELDI-TOF, researchers from the UCLA School of Medicine have identified three ovarian-cancer-biomarker panels that, when used together, effectively distinguished serum samples from healthy controls and from patients with either benign or malignant ovarian neoplasia (Kozak et al., 2003).

In early 2004, the impending launch of the OvaCheck system (developed by Correlogic Systems, Bethesda, Maryland), which targets the estimated 10 million American women who have been treated for ovarian cancer or are at increased genetic risk, sparked considerable public discussion because the test might be able to circumvent the requirement for device approval by the FDA. The distributed component of the assay is merely a sophisticated blood collection device, which is mailed to the laboratories of Correlogic's competing licensees, Quest Diagnostics and Laboratory Corp. of America Holdings. In the laboratory, plasma proteins are desorbed from the carrier and analyzed for specific biomarkers using mass spectroscopy. The laboratories say they expect to begin offering the test for $100 to $200.

Lung Cancer

The American Cancer Society estimates that 171,900 new cases of lung cancer were diagnosed in 2003 and that an estimated 157,200 deaths resulted from the disease in that year, making it the leading cause of cancer death in the United States

Biomarkers have played a relatively limited role in diagnosing and monitoring lung cancer, in part because presurgery tissue samples are difficult to obtain in lung cancer patients. Nevertheless, blood tests for CEA, squamous-cell carcinoma antigen (SCC), neuron-specific enolase (NSE), and pro-gastrin-releasing peptide (proGRP) have been helpful in differential diagnosis for several years. CEA is sensitive for adenocarcinoma, SCC for squamous-cell carcinoma, and NSE and proGRP for small-cell carcinoma. Serum levels of pro-GRP reflect the disease course of patients with small-cell lung cancer more accurately than NSE or CEA (Niho and Shinkai, 2001). In the mid-1990s, a newer cytokeratin marker, CK 19 fragments (CYFRA 21-1), became popular and widely accepted for detection of the non-small-cell form of lung cancer. Commercial kits are available for this biomarker from CIS Bio-International (Gif sur Yvette, France) and other manufacturers.

Colorectal Cancer

Lack of sensitivity and specificity preclude the use of any available serum markers – such as CEA, CA 19-9, CA 242, CA 72-4, tissue polypeptide antigen (TPA), or tissue polypeptide-specific antigen (TPS) – for the early detection of colorectal cancer.

However, the European Group on Tumor Markers (EGTM) recommends in its guidelines that preoperative measurement of CEA is desirable because it may give independent prognostic information and help with surgical management (Duffy et al., 2003).

In monitoring patients with stage 2 or 3 (Dukes' B or Dukes' C) disease who may be candidates for liver resection, CEA levels should be measured every two to three months for at least three years after diagnosis. In monitoring the treatment of advanced disease also, CEA should be tested every two to three months. Currently, not enough evidence is available to recommend the routine use of other serum markers for monitoring purposes.

POTENTIAL OF BIOMARKERS HAS YET TO BE REALIZED

Biomarkers for cancer have been in clinical use for years to aid in the detection of primary or recurrent cancer and to monitor therapy response, but their true potential is unfolding only now. Genentech's monoclonal antibody for breast cancer, Herceptin, was the first-targeted cancer therapy linked to mandatory testing of a specific biomarker, the HER2/neu antigen. With the increased number of approvals of EGFR/HER1 blockers for major types of solid tumors, we expect this group of targeted therapies to grow and secure a constant stream of line extensions during the next three to five years, thereby spurring growth of the respective diagnostics market.

In addition, new tumor biomarkers are being discovered that are increasingly important in conventional therapy monitoring, where they can aid in adjusting the dose of cytotoxic drugs, adding a new cytotoxic to an existing regimen, or making protocol switching decisions. This flood of potential new biomarkers is being discovered mainly through proteomics technology. Proteomic chips might soon become useful as carriers of panels that combine the diagnostic strengths of several or many different tumor markers while eliminating the less-than-optimal specificity of most individual markers.

REFERENCES

Ballesta, A.M. et al. Carcinoembryonic antigen in staging and follow-up of patients with solid tumors. *Tumor Biology*. 1995; 16: 32–41.

Bigler, L.R. et al. The potential use of saliva to detect recurrence of disease in women with breast carcinoma. *Journal of Oral Pathology & Medicine*. 2002; 31(7): 421–31.

Chatta, G. Multiplex biomarker approach for determining risk of prostate-specific antigen-defined recurrence of prostate cancer. *Urologic Oncology*. 2003; 21(6): 488.

Diamandis, E.P. et al. Human kallikrein 6 (hK6): a new potential serum biomarker for diagnosis and prognosis of ovarian carcinoma. *Journal of Clinical Oncology*. 2003; 21(6): 1035–43.

Duffy, M.J. et al. Clinical utility of biochemical markers in colorectal cancer: European Group on Tumour Markers (EGTM) guidelines. *European Journal of Cancer*. 2003; 39(6): 718–27.

Emberley, E.D. et al. Psoriasin (S100A7) expression is associated with poor outcome in estrogen receptor-negative invasive breast cancer. *Clinical Cancer Research*. 2003; 9(7): 2627–31.

Gion, M. et al. Prognostic role of serum CA15.3 in 362 node-negative breast cancers. An old player for a new game. *European Journal of Cancer*. 2002; 38(9): 1181–8.

Haese, A. et al. Total, free and complexed PSA and hK2 for early detection of prostate cancer. *Medical Laboratory Observer*. June 2003.

Hellstrom, I. et al. The HE4 (WFDC2) protein is a biomarker for ovarian carcinoma. *Cancer Research*. 2003; 63: 3695–700.

Hessels, D. et al. DD3(PCA3)-based molecular urine analysis for the diagnosis of prostate cancer. *European Urology*. 2003; 44(1): 8–15.

Hoopman, M. et al. HER-2/neu determination in blood plasma of patients with HER-2/neu overexpressing metastasized breast cancer: a longitudinal study. *Anticancer Research*. 2003; 23(2A): 1031–4.

Jarboe, E.A., et al. Analysis of telomerase as a diagnostic biomarker of cervical dysplasia and carcinoma. *Oncogene*. 2002; 21(4): 664–73.

Kandl, H. et al. Soluble c-erbB-2 fragment in serum correlates with disease stage and predicts for shortened survival in patients with early-stage and advanced breast cancer. *British Journal of Cancer*. 1994; 70(4): 739–42.

Kim, J.H. et al. Osteopontin as a potential diagnostic biomarker for ovarian cancer. *Journal of the American Medical Association*. 2002; 287(13): 1671–9.

Kelley, M.C. et al. Tumor-associated antigen TA-90 immune complex assay predicts subclinical metastasis and survival for patients with early stage melanoma. *Cancer*. 1998; 83(7): 1355–61.

Kozak, K.R. et al. Identification of biomarkers for ovarian cancer using strong anion-exchange ProteinChips: potential use in diagnosis and prognosis. *Proceedings of the National Academy of Sciences of the United States of America*. 2003; 100(21): 12343–8.

Maga, G., and Hubscher, U. Proliferating cell nuclear antigen (PCNA): a dancer with many partners. *Journal of Cell Science*. 2003; 116(Pt 15): 3051–60.

Martin, P.J. et al. Early detection of prostate cancer in African-American men through use of multiple biomarkers: human kallikrein 2 (hK2), prostate-specific antigen (PSA), and free PSA (fPSA). *Prostate Cancer and Prostatic Diseases*. 2004, in press.

Mikolajczyk, S.D. and Rittenhouse, H.G. Pro PSA: a more cancer speci?c form of prostate speci?c antigen for the early detection of prostate cancer. *The Keio Journal of Medicine*. 2003; 52(2): 86–91.

Mok, S.C. et al. Prostasin, a potential serum marker for ovarian cancer: identification through microarray technology. *Journal of the National Cancer Institute*. 2001; 93(19): 1458–64.

Nakamura, T. et al. The usefulness of serum human kallikrein 11 for discriminating between prostate cancer and benign prostatic hyperplasia. *Cancer Research*. 2003; 63(19): 6543–6.

Niho, S. and Shinkai, T. Tumor markers in lung cancer. *Gan To Kagaku Ryoho*. 2001; 28(13): 2089–93.

Nordengrren, J. et al. High tumor tissue concentration of plasminogen activator inhibitor 2 (PAI-2) is an independent marker for shorter progression-free survival in patients with early stage endometrial cancer. *International Journal of Cancer*. 2002; 97(3): 379–85.

Odunsi, A. et al. Evaluation of beta1,4-galactosyltransferase as a potential biomarker for the detection of subclinical disease after the completion of primary therapy for ovarian cancer. *American Journal of Obstetrics and Gynecology*. 2002; 187(3): 575–80.

Pollack, A. et al. Ki-67 staining is a strong predictor of patient outcome for prostate cancer patients treated with androgen deprivation plus radiotherapy: an analysis of RTOG 92–02. *International Journal of Radiation, Oncology, Biology, Physics*. 2003; 57(2 suppl): S200–1.

Rittenhouse, H.G. et al. Human kallikrein 2 (hK2) and prostate-specific antigen (PSA): two closely related, but distinct, kallikreins in the prostate. *Critical Reviews in Clinical Laboratory Sciences*. 1998; 35(4): 275–368.

Rüsbro, R. et al. *Gynecological Oncology*. 2001; 82(3): 523–31.

Salvesen, A.B. et al. Significance of CD 105 expression for tumour angiogenesis and prognosis in endometrial carcinomas. *Acta Pathologica, Microbiologica, et Immnunologica Scandinavica.* 2003; 111(11): 1011–18.

Slamon, D.J., et al. Human breast cancer: correlation of relapse and survival with amplification of the HER2/neu oncogene. *Science.* 1987; 235: 177–82.

Steber, P. et al. Clinical evaluation of the Elecsys CA 15–3 test in breast cancer patients. *Clinical Laboratory.* 2003; 49(1–2): 15–24.

Varambally, S. et al. The polycomb group protein EZH2 is involved in progression of prostate cancer. *Nature.* 2002; 419(6907): 624–9.

Wang, M.C. et al. Purification of a human prostate specific antigen. *Investigative Urology.* 1979; 17(2): 159–63.

Weigle, P. et al. D-PCa-2: a novel transcript highly overexpressed in human prostate and prostate cancer. *International Journal of Cancer.* 2004; 109(6): 882–92.

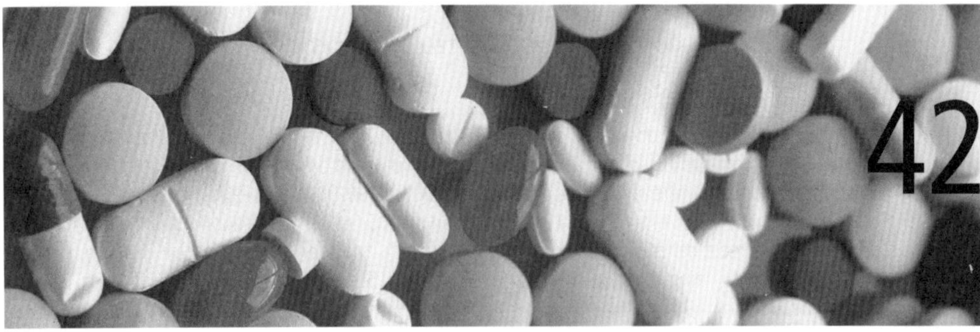

From Bioterrorism to Predictive Medicine: New Applications of Salivary Diagnostics

OVERVIEW

Salivary diagnostics are expanding into a broad range of new applications. Two major drivers fuel this growth: the advantages of this testing modality compared with traditional blood- and urine-based tools (such as their noninvasive nature, convenience, cost-efficiency, and the fact that they do not require specially trained medical personnel) and the emergence of new markets for which rapid results or inexpensive technologies are essential (such as therapeutic monitoring and predictive medicine).

This chapter will further explain the role of salivary diagnostics in emerging markets such as bioterrorism, drug monitoring (for both therapeutic drugs and drugs of abuse), and common endocrine conditions. Diagnostic tools have long been available in these markets, but the need for faster results at the point of care and a less-invasive way of obtaining repeat samples has fostered the development of saliva-based tools in these areas.

Finally, the chapter will investigate the use of salivary diagnostics in preventive medicine. These noninvasive screening techniques will offer individuals new opportunities to identify their health status at an early stage while avoiding unnecessarily complex and potentially harmful diagnostic procedures.

SALIVA AS A DIAGNOSTIC TOOL

Like blood, saliva naturally contains functional components such as enzymes, growth factors, cytokines, immunoglobulins, and hormones. Exogenous chemicals such as illegal or prescription drugs may also be present in this fluid. The detection of any of these salivary components can indicate a specific infection, disease, or condition.

Advantages

For saliva-based diagnostics to become a significant sector in the diagnostics arena, the process must have several substantial advantages over other tools that have already gained widespread acceptance among both physicians and patients. The primary hurdle is achieving accuracy comparable to that available through traditional testing methods. Convenience, safety, sample processing time, and cost-per-test are also important considerations in selecting a diagnostic test.

Accuracy is the most important attribute of a diagnostic test. In general, blood- and urine-based tests have established the standard of accuracy with which saliva-based tools are to be compared. In many instances, saliva sampling is considered as reliable

Table 42.1 Select Analytes in Saliva

Antibodies	HIV antibodies
	Anthrax antibodies
Disease markers	Biomarkers of cancer
	Risk factors for cardiovascular disease
	Glucose levels for diabetes
Drugs of abuse	Cocaine
	Marijuana
	Opiates
	Methamphetamine
Hormones	Estradiol
	Progesterone
	Testosterone
Therapeutics	Acetaminophen
	Carbamazepine
	Lithium

as blood sampling. Table 42.1 lists several analytes present in saliva that could be useful diagnostic indicators because they accurately reflect the level of these markers in the body as a whole. However, in each case, the diagnostic tool itself must be shown to be sensitive to this sample type as well. For some purposes, such as detecting the ovarian cancer biomarker CA-125, saliva is simply not an appropriate testing fluid because it does not accurately reflect the marker levels that are present in blood.

For indications for which salivary diagnostics are appropriate, they offer patients a less-invasive form of specimen collection than blood-based tests. Removing the pain, anxiety, and inconvenience from sample collection is particularly valuable for patients who are required to provide multiple samples over an extended period of time to monitor a chronic condition. Painless tests are also in high demand for testing children, as in the case of type 1 diabetes. (See the upcoming section on diabetes for more information on this application.) More-convenient tests will increase compliance rates, which, in some cases, will enhance the patient's treatment and overall health.

In addition, the process of donating test specimens is much less complicated when saliva is collected instead of blood. Collecting blood samples requires specially trained clinicians; saliva samples can be provided by patients. Saliva samples can even be collected in the privacy and convenience of the patient's home.

Another advantage of saliva diagnostics relative to blood-based tests is safety: medical personnel do not risk contracting an infectious disease from an accidental needle stick. Although saliva, like all bodily fluids, may also transmit infections, the risk of contracting a disease from a sample of saliva in a collection device is lower than the risk associated with processing whole vials of blood.

Sample processing time is always an important factor in a diagnostic test; in the case of drugs-of-abuse testing, however, it is critical to employ a tool that provides rapid results. Saliva-based tests allow the individual to provide the sample immediately. To test a potentially intoxicated individual on the road, for example, a law enforcement officer needs a reliable test that features fast and easy sampling as well as rapid results so that he or she is able to appropriately and promptly deal with the situation.

Cost is another significant concern when selecting a testing modality, especially when screening the general, symptom-free population. The storage and processing procedures associated with blood are more complex than those associated with saliva samples; thus, the cost-per-sample expense is less when saliva is used. Also, for smaller test centers or developing countries, the lower cost of saliva-testing equipment is especially attractive because cost-containment may preclude the purchase of sophisticated laboratory processing equipment that many other types of testing instruments require.

Disadvantages

Although many salivary diagnostics have been developed in recent years, few have gained FDA approval. The FDA does not require all in vitro diagnostics to obtain premarket approval, and companies do not often go through the time-consuming and expensive approval process voluntarily. Tests that do not typically go through this process include ovulation and menopause diagnostics, for example. Alternatively, the FDA does require tests to obtain premarket approval if incorrect test results could severely affect a patient's well-being. For example, viral hepatitis and HIV diagnostics cannot be marketed in the United States until the test is strictly reviewed and approved by the FDA.

In many ways, the lack of FDA approval inhibits the rate at which these tools may penetrate the mainstream diagnostics market. For example, third-party payers are less likely to cover tests that have not yet received the FDA backing. Also, many physicians are concerned about the accuracy of unapproved tests and are therefore less likely to implement them.

Another disadvantage is that physicians may have doubts about the reliability and accuracy of tests that are based on saliva samples instead of the traditional blood samples. The concentration of hormones in saliva is different from that in blood. If any blood is present in a patient's mouth during the collection of a saliva specimen (owing to a cut in the mouth or bleeding gums), the test has the potential to produce incorrect results. Additionally, patients and physicians alike may not regard salivary diagnostics as advantageous in situations where the patient must still provide a blood sample for the diagnosis of other conditions (for which no saliva-based tools are currently available).

BIOTERRORISM

Over the past three years, government agencies, diagnostics companies, and even the general population have been paying more attention to the threat of intentional use of infectious agents to harm large numbers of people – that is, bioterrorism. Bioterrorism remains a realistic threat to military personnel overseas as well – where expensive pieces of equipment and complex laboratory facilities are not always readily accessible.

Thus, the US government, through the National Institutes of Health (NIH), is responding to the harsh reality of this situation by awarding seven cooperative agreements to fund novel research in this area. In January 2003, the NIH released an announcement describing this new program, which was specifically established through the National Institute of Dental and Craniofacial Research to fund research for saliva- and other oral-fluid-based diagnostics.

In addition, the Naval Institute for Dental and Biomedical Research is collaborating with the Centers for Disease Control and Prevention (CDC) to develop a more sensitive and specific salivary diagnostic for the detection of antibodies to the anthrax bacteria in saliva samples. These tools will have a dual application as both a confirmatory tool in individuals who have been vaccinated for anthrax and as a screening tool to detect exposure to the bacteria in the general population.

The government has invested substantial funding in this field because these salivary tools are by far the most appropriate instruments for use in the battlefield or other military units such as naval ships and submarines. These enclosed vessels, where contamination with an infectious agent would rapidly infect the entire population, are particularly vulnerable to the threat of bioterrorism.

Smallpox

Although naturally occurring cases of the smallpox virus have been eliminated, this potentially lethal infectious agent remains a threat to the general population as a vehicle of bioterrorism. This virus, clinically referred to as variola, has no effective treatment. Thus, vaccination is a critical preventive measure. Unfortunately, many of the individuals who have been inoculated against the virus have experienced an assortment of adverse effects. Therefore, because the risk of exposure to the virus is relatively low, most individuals have chosen not to obtain the vaccination. Some individuals, such as smallpox response teams and military personnel, are at a higher risk of being exposed and therefore have received the vaccination.

The aversion to this vaccine underscores the importance of developing an appropriate plan of action to implement in the case of a smallpox outbreak. Rapid diagnosis of infected individuals is crucial to minimize the impact of such an event. Given the severity of the infection and the similarities between this disease and other viral infections (such as varicella and herpes simplex), highly specific diagnostic tools are required. A misdiagnosis could result in widespread unwarranted panic or rapid uncontrolled spread of the disease.

Currently available diagnostic tools are not optimal. According to the CDC, a clinical case definition of this infection occurs when a patient presents with symptoms including a fever of higher than 101 degrees Fahrenheit and a rash with firm, deep-seated vesicles. These vesicles must be at all the same stage and there must be no apparent cause for the condition. As noted, this subjective detection strategy could have deleterious ramifications.

Laboratory confirmation of the disease is also available. Polymerase chain reaction may be used to verify the presence of the virus in a clinical sample, or the virus itself may be isolated from the specimen. Although this method of diagnosis is highly specific, several drawbacks remain:

- Specialized facilities are required for these procedures, thus increasing the cost and time required for diagnosis.
- In-the-field diagnosis with these techniques is not an option.
- Accidental contamination of laboratory personnel is possible.

Although salivary diagnostics for this application have not yet been developed, such tools would shorten the process time needed to obtain results and reduce the costs for each test. During the early stages of the rash, high concentrations of the virus are present in the patient's saliva. Thus, the saliva can easily transmit the disease, but it is also a convenient way to test for its presence. These simplified tools would also be suitable for use in remote areas where complex laboratory equipment is not accessible. The National Institute of Allergy and Infectious Diseases (NIAID) is actively researching smallpox in light of recent bioterrorism activity. The institute's research focuses on the diagnosis, prevention, and treatment of the disease.

Anthrax

Caused by the *Bacillus anthracis* bacterium, anthrax infection occurs in three types: inhalation, cutaneous, and intestinal. Although treatment with an antibiotic may cure infected individuals, early diagnosis and initiation of therapy are critical for survival, particularly with inhalation anthrax, which is the most serious. An anthrax vaccine, manufactured and distributed by BioPort of Lansing, Michigan, may prevent infection; however, according to the CDC, this vaccine is not recommended for the general public. In October 2004, the US District Court for the District of Columbia issued an injunction to prevent the further distribution of the vaccine (which was recommended for people who work with the bacteria in research laboratories and for military personnel) to further verify the safety and efficacy of the agent.

Although an outbreak of anthrax infections was identified in late 2001 in the United States, the general public is not believed to be at significant risk of infection. People who may be involved in activities that are associated with an elevated risk of anthrax contamination include researchers who study the infection in the laboratory, people who work closely with animals or animal products that may come from locations where the incidence of this infection is higher than normal, and members of the armed forces.

Because postexposure therapies are highly effective in preventing the onset of full-blown disease following exposure, the major hurdle in successful treatment is the timely diagnosis of the infection. Various diagnostic methods are available, including chest X-ray (for use in people who present with symptoms consistent with the disease) and nasal swabs (for use in screening asymptomatic people who may have been exposed to the bacteria).

The shortfalls of the currently implemented testing procedures for anthrax exposure are similar to those discussed previously in the section on smallpox diagnostics. Specifically, misdiagnosis would result in widespread unnecessary alarm. Furthermore, in the case of anthrax, for which cure is possible, a delay in diagnosis would inhibit therapeutic success. Therefore, following one confirmed case of exposure, the best strategy to limit the outbreak is to quickly and accurately identify other infected individuals.

Identification of valid genetic markers will enable the development of salivary diagnostics that could easily be used to screen a large population of people who may have come in contact with this infectious agent. NIAID is researching new ways of detecting this agent in the environment and in infected individuals. The institute's current focus is on identifying which genetic markers within the bacterial genome would be best for screening.

HUMAN IMMUNODEFICIENCY VIRUS

Despite prevention efforts by the CDC and other agencies, the number of individuals infected with HIV continues to climb; in 2003, there were approximately 960,000 cases in the United States, 390,000 in Europe, and 12,000 in Japan.

Although public awareness of the disease is high, many people do not undergo HIV testing for various reasons. For example, asymptomatic individuals may be too embarrassed to visit a physician and request to be screened or may choose to avoid testing because of the discomfort associated with providing blood samples. Because early diagnosis of the disease and initiation of highly active antiretroviral therapies are critical steps to preserving the quality of life of infected individuals, more-suitable methods of screening must become available.

Diagnostics to detect HIV cover three main areas: (1) screening, (2) confirmatory diagnostics, and (3) therapeutic monitoring. Screening tools are relatively inexpensive and are employed primarily to test the symptom-free population. Confirmatory HIV diagnostics are typically more complex and are implemented as follow-up tests once a screening test yields a positive result. Therapeutic monitoring is an essential component of successful HIV treatment.

The area of therapeutic monitoring comprises quantitative determination of viral load, genotyping, and drug-resistance testing. Therapeutic monitoring has emerged as a major focal point in the treatment of HIV to assist physicians in providing the patient with effective, personalized care. The next generation of antiviral therapeutics is sure to once again solidify the necessity of therapeutic monitoring tools in HIV treatment.

Within the field of HIV diagnostics, oral-fluid diagnostics are particularly suitable for screening and therapeutic monitoring, and such tests are already on the market. Oral fluid diagnostics are slightly different from standard saliva-based diagnostic tools. For example, OraSure Technologies (profiled later in this report) tests oral mucosal transudates, which are fluids from the capillaries beneath the buccal mucosa and at the base of the crevice between the teeth and gums. This type of oral fluid contains a higher concentration of antibodies compared with whole saliva, making this fluid a better testing medium than whole saliva. Identifying the level of antibodies present in tiny samples of blood from the oral cavity is simpler than obtaining the blood through traditional blood draws. In addition, because frequent long-term testing is required for adequate therapeutic monitoring, oral-fluid diagnostics offer an approach that is less invasive than repeated blood sampling, without sacrificing accuracy of the results. The low cost of these tools and their ease of use make oral-fluid diagnostics suitable to screen large populations and individuals in developing nations, where the rate of HIV is especially high. Some of these tools have been developed for in-home use, which may be particularly beneficial to the segment of the population who may avoid visiting a physician because of embarrassment or inconvenience.

ENDOCRINE CONDITIONS

Salivary diagnostics are ideal tools for convenient in-home testing or testing that needs to be repeated daily or multiple times each day. Many endocrine conditions require such frequent monitoring for a period of time (e.g., until pregnancy is confirmed) or even for years (e.g., glucose monitoring). For the endocrine conditions described in the following sections, ideal saliva-based diagnostic tools would possess the following attributes:

- Simple sample collection (no pain).
- Short processing time.
- Easy-to-understand, accurate results.
- Multiple-use or inexpensive disposable components.

Women's Health

Salivary diagnostics also play a role in monitoring the onset of female conditions such as ovulation and menopause. Although the traditional, urine-based diagnostics in this area already allow for in-home usage, saliva-based tools provide additional advantages, which will be discussed in their respective sections.

For example, saliva measures the biologically active (free) steroids in the bloodstream, unlike blood and urine, which measure total steroid levels. Only about 1–10% of the steroids in blood are in the unbound or free form, and this fraction diffuses into target tissues of the body as well as into saliva. These "free" hormones are the hormones that move easily into target organs and fulfill their functions. Most (90–99%) steroid hormones in the blood are bound to carrier proteins and do not diffuse into target tissues; they serve more as "storage" hormones, so measurements of the total hormone level may be less useful for evaluating the impact that hormones are having on a patient's health. Figure 42.1 illustrates the relationship between the bioavailable hormone level found in the blood and that found in saliva.

Ovulation

Ovulation-cycle monitoring may increase the success rate for women trying, for an extended period of time, to conceive. For the many women who are now waiting until their mid-to late-30s or even early 40s before trying to conceive, ovulation monitoring may help to quickly identify their most fertile days.

Three options are available to women who wish to monitor their ovulation cycle and increase the likelihood of fertility. These options include saliva-based tools, urine-based tools, and more advanced and

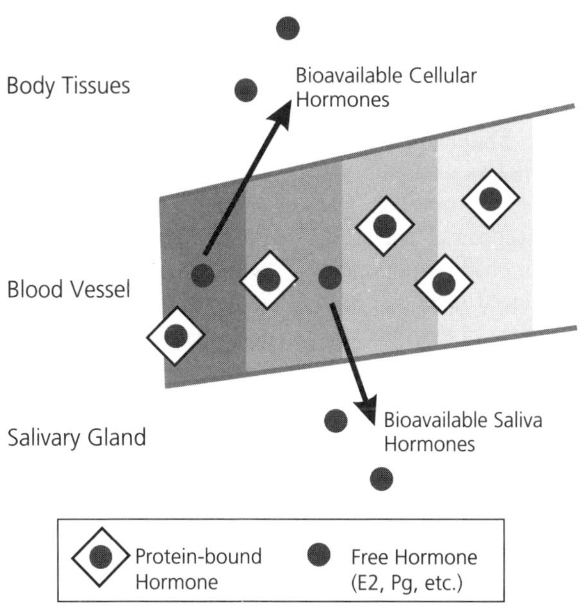

Figure 42.1 Comparison of Hormone Levels in Blood and Saliva

technical fertility-monitoring devices. Salivary diagnostics are the most appropriate tools for many women because they are simple to use and inexpensive. They are less expensive than many urine-based tools, per test, because the saliva sample may be removed from the testing device and the tool may be used again.

Available testing kits include the Ovulation-Scope (Quest Products), the Donna (Poggio Fiorito), MaybeMOM (MaybeMOM), Ovulite (Dynamic Health), Lady-Q (Kurkel Enterprises), and the TCI-31 Ovulation Tester (TCI New York).

Menopause

During menopause, women experience fluctuating hormone levels that can cause many uncomfortable side effects, such as hot flashes, sleep disturbances, and mood swings. In addition to these relatively temporary symptoms of menopause, women experience more-serious, long-term effects caused by the natural drop in hormone levels. For example, estrogen protects women against developing osteoporosis, certain kinds of cancer, tooth and gum problems, and even incontinence. One common treatment for these symptoms is hormone replacement therapy (HRT). The market for such therapies was valued at $4.4 billion in the major pharmaceutical markets (United States, France, Germany, Italy, Spain, United Kingdom, and Japan) in 2001, and we anticipate that it will grow to $5.2 billion in 2006. In 2001, we estimate, 135 million women in the major markets were aged 50 or older (the typical age-group for menopausal and post-menopausal women) or had experienced premature, surgically induced menopause; in 2006, that number will exceed 145 million.

Close monitoring of hormone levels assists a physician in determining the right treatment regimen for each patient. For example, when assessing the risk/reward potential associated with HRT, a physician may wish to monitor the decline in a woman's natural hormone levels over a period of time before prescribing such treatment. For a woman to provide multiple samples for hormone monitoring (before, during, and after therapy), in-home specimen donation is the most convenient testing method. Given their ease-of-use and low-cost attributes, salivary diagnostics are well suited for this indication. For more information on examples of marketed hormone-related salivary diagnostics, see the section "Aeron Biotechnology" later in this chapter.

Men's Health

Saliva-based diagnostic tools for hormone monitoring have not yet penetrated the men's health market to the extent seen in the women's health arena. However, as more men come to understand the relationship between balanced hormone levels and overall good health, the potential for greater acceptance will grow. For example, significantly reduced levels of testosterone may result in minor annoyances such as poor mood or more-substantial consequences such as increased risk of cardiovascular or neurological diseases. Furthermore, unhealthy levels of bioavailable dihydrotestosterone and estradiol have been linked to health problems such as benign prostatic hyperplasia (BPH) and prostate cancer.

Diabetes

Patients with type 1 diabetes must undergo multiple daily finger pricks to constantly monitor blood glucose levels. Often, these pricks are followed by yet another needle to provide the individual with an accurate amount of insulin. The process is a significant inconvenience for adults who have dealt with this condition for decades, and it is even more agonizing for the many children with the disease. Unfortunately, less-invasive saliva-based glucose- monitoring systems are not yet available.

Because glucose levels may be detected in samples of saliva – rather than samples of blood obtained via painful finger pricks – the opportunity for such diagnostics to enhance the quality of life in diabetics is significant. The number of type 1 diabetics in the major markets in 2002 was estimated at 1.67 billion and will grow to over 1.7 billion by the end of 2007; in addition, a segment of the type 2 diabetes population will advance to the point they require daily glucose monitoring and would thus benefit from less-invasive testing as well. The market for drugs to treat type 1 diabetes approached $1.1 billion in the major markets in 2002 according to our estimates, and we project it will surpass $1.2 billion in 2007.

DRUG MONITORING

Saliva diagnostics are valuable tools in drug monitoring, both for tracking therapeutic drug effectiveness and for detecting the presence of drugs of abuse. In the case of therapeutic drug effectiveness, multiple tests over a long period of time may be required. Therefore, cost, convenience, and possibly in-home use will affect the market acceptance of new diagnostics in this area. However, when testing for drugs of abuse, it is critical that the sample can be obtained and processed under a variety of conditions, including roadside testing of individuals who may be under the influence while driving. Both applications are described in the following sections.

Therapeutic Drugs

Diagnostics to monitor the therapeutic effectiveness of a prescription drug regimen are often critical for adequate patient treatment. A wide variety of tools are used; however, saliva-based diagnostics have not yet penetrated all the available markets, which include HIV, psychiatric disorders, and cancer.

In the case of HIV diagnostics, the saliva-based tools would quantitatively measure the level of HIV antibodies present in the saliva to determine if the prescription medications are adequately controlling the disease. For other indications, it may be more appropriate to use salivary diagnostics to directly monitor the concentrations of a therapeutic drug or to measure various biomarkers that are related to certain conditions.

Another example is the use of saliva diagnostics in psychiatric treatment, where one of the major barriers to achieving positive treatment results is patient compliance. It is difficult to objectively measure patient compliance when compliance testing involves frequent blood draws – procedures that are significantly uncomfortable and inconvenient for the patient to undergo. Salivary diagnostics in this area would offer patients a much more convenient alternative and therefore aid physicians in the treatment of patients with a variety of conditions such as anxiety, depression, bipolar disorder, and epilepsy.

Cancer patients would also significantly benefit from an alternative method of therapeutic monitoring that does not involve blood sample testing. Although salivary diagnostics are not currently available to monitor therapeutic levels of chemotherapeutics in cancer patients, often the side effects of these drugs are substantial and collecting additional blood samples only further weakens the patient. Thus, there is significant market potential here for salivary diagnostics. Notably, researchers have demonstrated that the anticancer agents irinotecan and cisplatin can be detected in saliva samples, indicating that saliva is a suitable means of measuring therapy concentrations.

Drugs of Abuse

Another growing area for salivary diagnostics is the drugs-of-abuse testing arena. Currently, the most common form of testing for illegal drug use and alcohol abuse is the collection of a urine sample. However, because such a sample is not collected in the presence of another individual, the risk of sample tampering is significant. By using saliva as the diagnostic fluid, testers can preserve the need for accurate test results while reducing – effectively removing – the risk of sample tampering. In addition, illegal substances can be detected in urine samples only after the substances have been metabolized by the liver. However, the same substances would appear in samples of saliva very soon after ingestion, essentially eliminating the lag time that occurs with urine samples.

Drugs-of-abuse testing is becoming increasingly popular in the workforce as well as the criminal justice system because more than 16 million people in the United States currently engage in illegal drug use, according to the 2001 National Household Survey on Drug Abuse. The costs to society are great, in terms of the economic loss due to reduced productivity and missed days of work as well as the human costs of drug abuse and addiction.

Saliva may be used to detect a variety of illicit drugs including marijuana, cocaine, opiates, and amphetamines. Unlike diagnostics to detect drugs used for therapeutic purposes, diagnostics designed for drugs-of-abuse testing typically do not provide specific information about the concentration of the drug – the mere presence of the substance provides most users with an adequate amount of information. Table 42.2 lists select salivary diagnostics currently marketed for the detection of drugs of abuse.

PREDICTIVE MEDICINE

Most of the diagnostic applications previously discussed in this report focused on the detection of current disease states or health conditions. In addition to diagnosing a disease once the individual has contracted or developed it, diagnostics companies have also begun to develop ways to predict the likelihood that an individual will develop a particular disease. This area is becoming increasingly active because more therapeutic agents are being developed for use in the early stages of disease to delay disease progression. Also, more advanced predictive tools for diseases such as cancer will enable individuals to seek out more complex diagnostic procedures earlier, thus increasing their chance of survival.

In the breast cancer diagnostics market, salivary diagnostics that provide a more sensitive testing mechanism than mammograms may enjoy rapid and widespread acceptance among physicians and patients alike. One study has shown that saliva may be a suitable biofluid for detecting the presence of the oncogene *HER2/neu*; overexpression of this biomarker is used to diagnose certain kinds of breast cancer.

Saliva diagnostic tools may also be used to help predict the onset of cardiovascular disease. Such tests would allow physicians to more closely monitor the higher-risk subset of the population sooner – possibly even preventing a major cardiac event. California-based BioHealth Diagnostics offers functional adrenaline profiles. These saliva-based tests require a series of four samples to test for two hormones produced by the adrenaline glands: cortisol and dehydroepiandrosterone (DHEA). A circadian rhythm for cortisol and an average for the sulfated form of DHEA are established to assess the

Table 42.2 Select Saliva Diagnostics for Drugs of Abuse Testing

Test	*Company*	*Time to Result*	*Drugs Detected*
ORALscreen	Avitar	15 minutes	Cocaine, marijuana, methamphetamine, opiates
On Site OraLab	Varian (formerly Ansys Technologies)	15 minutes	Amphetamines, cocaine, methamphetamines, morphine, PCP
Intercept	OraSure Technologies	24 hours	Amphetamines, barbiturates, benzodiazepines, cocaine, marijuana, methadone, methamphetamines, opiates, PCP
Q.E.D. Saliva Alcohol Test	OraSure Technologies	2–5 minutes	Alcohol
Impact Test System	LifePoint	5 minutes	Alcohol, amphetamines, cocaine, marijuana, methamphetamines, opiates, PCP

PCP = Phencyclidine
Note: These point-of-collection tests are typically priced at $10–$30

functioning of the adrenaline glands. A high level of cortisol and a low level of sulfated DHEA may indicate that the adrenaline glands are overworked as a result of stress on the body. Adrenaline exhaustion is a potential precursor to cardiac failure.

SELECT SALIVARY DIAGNOSTICS COMPANIES

In the following sections, we profile some of the companies active in the saliva-diagnostics arena and describe select products available on the market or in development. Table 42.3 presents a strategic comparison of players in the oral-fluid diagnostics market.

Aeron Biotechnology

California-based Aeron Biotechnology focuses on noninvasive methods for the detection of hormone levels. In November 2001, the company introduced the PeriPanel test through its clinical diagnostics arm, Aeron Life Cycles Clinical Laboratory. The PeriPanel is used to monitor fluctuations in hormone levels in premenopausal and peri-menopausal women. It is critical to monitor hormone levels for the adequate treatment of menopausal conditions. Such monitoring is also beneficial in the treatment of hormone-dependent breast cancer. The PeriPanel in-home test requires the woman to simply provide a saliva sample and mail it to the laboratory for processing. Results are available in three to five days.

Aeron Biotechnology also markets a salivary-based diagnostic tool to measure the bioavailable dihydrotestosterone (DHT) levels in men. The test is similar to the PeriPanel in that the patient simply collects a saliva sample in the comfort of his own home and mails the sample to the company for processing. The company has also demonstrated that measurements of salivary levels of bioavailable testosterone highly correlate with the levels found through serum testing. By helping monitor male hormone levels, Aeron Biotechnology's salivary tools can assist physicians in the treatment of hypogonadism, BPH, prostate cancer, and hair loss.

Table 42.3 Strategic Comparison of Oral Fluid Diagnostics Companies

Company	*Therapeutic Areas*	*Diagnostic Medium*	*Products*	*Annual Revenue[a] (USD)*
Aeron Biotechnology	Endocrine conditions	Saliva	PeriPanel	N.A.
Avitar	Drugs of abuse Endocrine conditions Infectious diseases	Saliva Other oral fluids	ORALscreen family of tests	4,598,025
ImmunoScience	Infectious diseases	Saliva Other oral fluids	Salivax family of tests	N.A.
LifePoint	Drugs of abuse	Saliva	Impact Test System	49,000
Medical Services International	Infectious diseases	Saliva Other oral fluids	VScan rapid test kit	420,599
OraSure Technologies	Drugs of abuse Infectious diseases	Saliva Other oral fluids	OraSure HIV-1 OraQuick Rapid HIV-1 Antibody Test UpLink System Q.E.D. Saliva Alcohol Test Intercept	40,451,000
Pacific Biometrics	Endocrine conditions	Saliva	N.A.	5,800,000
Saliva Diagnostic Systems	Infectious diseases	Saliva Other oral fluids	Saliva-Strip HIV	N.A.
VRI BioMedical	Infectious diseases Immunological diseases	Saliva	Helirad Performax and KIDSAlert	1,754,010

[a]Total annual revenue for fiscal year 2003
N.A. = Not available

Avitar

Avitar, a Massachusetts-based oral fluids diagnostics company, developed the first oral-fluid rapid-result drugs-of-abuse testing system. This system, the ORALscreen, was first marketed in April 1999. Currently, Avitar is focusing on supplying this oral-fluid-based test to both the corporate and educational sectors. Through a distribution partnership that began in April 2004 with Placement Pros, Avitar is well positioned to be a significant player in this market. Placement Pros, based in Pleasanton, California, is a full-service staffing company specializing in recruitment, placement, and background checks.

Avitar has also expanded its drug-screening platform with confirmatory tests and more-inclusive rapid tests to screen for methamphetamines, including MDMA (ecstasy), in addition to the original panel of marijuana, cocaine, and opiates. The company's complete drug-testing portfolio of oral fluid-based tools includes the following:

- ORALscreen 4, a 15-minute oral-fluid-based drug screening test.
- ORALscreen Drugometer, the second-generation product with sample collection and testing occurring within the same device.
- ORALscreen OSR, a handheld drug-testing analyzer to record and report results from the ORALscreen tests.
- ORALadvantage, a comprehensive drug-testing kit for use in small businesses.
- ORALconfirm, a follow-up test to positive results obtained with a drug-screening test. This test uses gas chromatography and mass spectrometry in the laboratory to validate and quantitate precise drug levels.

Aside from Avitar's drug-testing capabilities, the company is expanding into other areas of the clinical diagnostics arena. Building upon its proprietary polyurethane foam saliva-collection technology, additional applications will include glucose monitoring, influenza screening, and pregnancy testing. The company notes that, like its original drugs-of-abuse testing line, these new tools will be easy to use and inexpensive.

ImmunoScience

ImmunoScience is a Nevada-based biomedical products company. It markets a saliva-based immunochromatographic assay, Salivax, in developing countries and Japan and is planning to expand its distribution network to Europe and the United States. The Salivax platform is available in two versions: Salivax-HIV detects antibodies to HIV-1 and HIV-2, and Salivax-Syphilis detects antibodies to the syphilis-causing bacteria, *Treponema pallidum*. Salivax is appropriate for in-home use. Also, it is particularly well suited for markets where cost and the limited availability of highly trained medical professionals inhibit the widespread use of more-complex screening tools. ImmunoScience intends to expand the Salivax platform to include hepatitis B and C, drugs of abuse, tuberculosis, and *Helicobacter pylori.*

LifePoint

LifePoint, a California-based medical products company, launched the Impact Test System in February 2002. The system is unique because it simultaneously screens for drugs of abuse and the presence of alcohol. It is based on two proprietary technologies: (1) a flow immunosensor for more rapid results and increased sensitivity compared with that available in other diagnostic tools and (2) an aspiration component for collecting and processing the saliva. The total time needed to obtain results is approximately five minutes, including the 30 seconds to one minute necessary for sample collection.

LifePoint originally targeted the three major segments of the drugs-of-abuse testing market: law enforcement (highway safety for example), industrial workplaces, and emergency rooms. In October 2004, the company announced it was increasing its efforts to expand its market reach into the drug courts sector. According to LifePoint, the US drug courts are responsible for monitoring approximately 70,000 people for drug use. An average of two tests are administered per week, making the annual market size, in this sector alone, top 7.8 million tests each year.

The European market is another key growth area for LifePoint's technology. The company is initiating new distribution contracts and participating in a study of European driving safety to position itself in this market. In October 2004, the company announced it would be participating in the Roadside Testing Assessment (ROSITA) II Project, which will be conducted by a consortium of six European Union countries. The goal of the study is to evaluate roadside oral-fluid diagnostics over a one-year period. According to LifePoint, in 65–85% of the accidents that occur in Europe in which the driver is considered to be driving under the influence, drug use rather than alcohol abuse is the trigger. Therefore, the Impact Test System is likely to be particularly valuable in this market.

Medical Services International

The British West Indies-based holding company Medical Services International comprises two separate businesses: one operates medical facilities and the other develops diagnostic tests for infectious diseases. The company's VScan rapid test kits are used to detect HIV, hepatitis B and C, tuberculosis, West Nile virus, and Dengue fever. Highly accurate results are available in less than 15 minutes, and samples of blood, urine, or saliva are all acceptable. The VScan is available in many countries, especially in Asia, but it is not yet available in any major pharmaceutical markets other than Japan. In September 2003, Medical Services International initiated efforts with US regulatory agencies to gain marketing approval.

OraSure Technologies

Epitope and STC Technologies merged in September 2000 to form the medical diagnostics company OraSure Technologies. This Pennsylvania-based company's primary interest is the collection and testing of oral fluids for HIV antibody testing. The company also has products for substance-abuse testing and forensic toxicology. It focuses on the point-of-care (POC) testing market and offers two main oral-fluid POC platforms – OraQuick and UpLink – as well as other diagnostic platforms. OraSure Technologies is the market leader in oral-fluid diagnostics.

In November 2002, OraSure announced the launch of its POC OraQuick test for HIV-1 and HIV-2 antibodies. Using specimens of oral fluid, blood, or plasma, the assay can provide results in 20 minutes. This test is the first rapid oral-fluid POC test for HIV that has received the FDA approval and a Clinical Laboratory Improvements Amendment (CLIA) waiver. As a result of the waiver, the test can be performed in places such as hospitals, physician offices, and clinics rather than in a laboratory – expanding the product's market potential. The company has entered into a partnership with Abbott Laboratories to help sell the product to hospitals and physician offices.

The OraSure HIV-1 Oral Specimen Collection Device received the FDA approval in March 2004. It is the only FDA-approved collection device where oral fluid, instead of a blood sample, is tested for the presence of antibodies to HIV-1. Results, available in 20 minutes, are more than 99% accurate.

The HIV-1 test is not approved for use at home or direct-to-consumer sale. Rather, the tool is to be used in a physician's office where patients can be instructed on how to properly collect their oral-mucosal transudate for testing. As noted earlier, oral-mucosal transudate, which is distinct from saliva, contains a high concentration of antibodies and is therefore the more appropriate oral fluid to use in detecting HIV antibodies. The OraSure collection pad is used to collect such samples from the blood vessels in the mouth. If positive results are obtained through this method, a physician is likely to perform a confirmatory test where a blood sample would be used to verify the original finding before initiating treatment.

The OraSure Oral Specimen Collection Device may also be used for additional clinical applications such as forensic identification and paternity testing.

OraSure is also developing a new, high-sensitivity, substance- abuse detection method – the UpLink System using the company's Up-Converting Phosphor Technology (UPT) – which would allow on-site testing of oral samples, further enhancing the ability to effectively screen large populations for drugs of abuse. The UpLink System employs the company's proprietary UpLink microparticle labels to achieve detection sensitivity that rivals that of chemiluminescence immunoassays, which are currently the most sensitive immunoassay-labeling method employed in the central lab. Readout is performed at the point of care using a compact, laser-based reader. Prototype tests have been developed for the detection of drugs of abuse in saliva samples, where the high sensitivity of the system allows detection at concentrations many times lower than those in blood.

In April 2002, OraSure received the FDA approval for an oral-fluid UpLink assay to detect opiates only. This test will not be marketed as a stand-alone system, however; the company is developing several other assays (for cocaine, methamphetamine/amphetamine, phencyclidine [PCP], and marijuana) and will eventually market a multiassay UpLink panel once it receives the FDA clearance for all the assays.

In 2002, OraSure Technologies began a joint-research program with the University of Pennsylvania on the development of oral-fluid diagnostics based on the UpLink System. Funded by the National Institute of Dental and Craniofacial Research, the four-year study focuses on the development of tools for the simultaneous detection of an array of viral and bacterial infectious agents. The goal of the project is to develop a single system that can collect, process, and detect up to 200 analytes, including agents of bioterrorism such as anthrax.

OraSure Technologies also markets two products for substance abuse testing through oral-fluid sampling. The Q.E.D. Saliva Alcohol Test and the Intercept drug test provide clinicians with alternatives to the standard breath- or blood-based testing tools.

Pacific Biometrics

Pacific Biometrics supports pharmaceutical and diagnostic manufacturers through clinical trial research. This Washington-based company is also developing proprietary technology for its own diagnostics products through its wholly owned subsidiary, PBI Technology. The company is developing a line of glucose-monitoring tests that will use saliva samples instead of the traditional testing method of blood samples from painful finger pricks.

These tests will target two markets: (1) patients who have not yet been diagnosed as diabetics but wish to test their glucose levels and (2) diabetics who require daily and specific glucose monitoring. For the first patient population, the technology will be applied for the rapid detection of glucose levels through an at-home screening tool that allows patients to determine when glucose levels surpass a specific threshold, perhaps through a color-change mechanism. Once an elevated glucose level is recognized, the patient will then see a physician for further care. For the second patient population, the technology will be applied to a more sensitive tool where specific glucose levels are provided through an electronic read-out apparatus for long-term monitoring of diabetes progression. The patient can then administer medication or modify his or her diet as required.

Saliva Diagnostic Systems

New York-based Saliva Diagnostic Systems (SDS) markets the Saliva-Strip HIV test for the detection of HIV antibodies in oral- fluid specimens. The test is currently available only in the United Kingdom. In response to the market demand for simple and inexpensive testing products, this tool does not require specially trained personnel or temperature-sensitive storage. The Saliva-Strip

HIV test provides results in approximately 20 minutes. Eventually, the company hopes to expand its technology to additional markets, including oncology, cardiology, and drugs-of-abuse screening.

VRI BioMedical

VRI BioMedical, an Australia-based biotechnology company, is developing probiotics (bacterial therapeutics), diagnostics, and vaccines for infections of the immune system. The company has created three saliva-based assays in this field.

The Helirad test screens for the presence of antibodies to the stomach ulcer trigger, *H. pylori*, in a patient's sample of saliva. This test may be administered in a laboratory or at the point of care as a rapid diagnostic tool. After a patient completes a typical therapeutic regimen to overcome the bacterial infection, the Helirad test should be performed again to confirm that no signs of the bacteria remain.

VRI BioMedical is also focusing on preventive diagnoses in the immune-system arena. The Performax and KIDSAlert (the children's version of Performax) tests detect immunoglobulin A (IgA) levels in saliva samples. IgA is present in the body's mucosal barriers; its role is to protect the body against infection. Therefore, low levels of this protein may indicate a higher susceptibility to infection. Identifying low IgA levels is particularly critical in children; such measurements may indicate serious disorders that would benefit from early diagnosis.

Additionally, in March 2003, VRI BioMedical announced a collaborative research effort with Proteome Systems (an Australia-based proteomics technology and diagnostics company) and sporting authorities including the Australian Institute of Sport. The collaboration focuses on developing a diagnostic tool to evaluate the immune system of elite athletes. This tool will use Proteome Systems' DiagnostIQ platform, which rapidly and quantitatively identifies biomarkers in saliva (or other bodily fluids) to diagnose or monitor disease. VRI BioMedical is also developing probiotic products to enhance the intestinal systems of individuals with gastrointestinal disorders.

MARKET TRENDS

The potential patient population for salivary diagnostics continues to grow at a rapid pace. Key market drivers include a wide variety of factors such as new markets, as in the case of bioterrorism, and patients' increasing desire to monitor their health in a convenient way, as in the case of women's health diagnostics. In addition, emerging tools are accurate, inexpensive, and typically more convenient than many available alternatives.

The reality of bioterrorism has sparked new opportunities for diagnostics. Specific information is not yet available to assess the progress that diagnostics companies have made on this front. However, the copious funding – almost $1.6 billion – that NIAID received in 2004 to develop new vaccines, diagnostics, and therapeutics suggests the US government acknowledges that basic research efforts are essential and are likely to proceed to corporate development. We expect these efforts to result in new technologies for both civilian and military applications in the next five years.

The interdependency between diagnostics and pharmaceuticals – in the case of HIV diagnosis and therapeutic monitoring, for example – will stimulate growth in both markets. Salivary diagnostics to track the therapeutic effectiveness of HIV drugs will provide physicians with a noninvasive mechanism by which frequent convenient samplings may be used to tailor treatment regimens. Physicians will implement more complicated therapeutic regimens, and patients will quickly accept the more- convenient disease-monitoring methods. Salivary diagnostics may also be developed to diagnose and monitor other infectious diseases, such as hepatitis. For all such diseases, privacy (achieved through in-home screening) and long-term testing (necessary for chronic conditions) are particular concerns – which are well addressed with saliva-based diagnostic tools.

In the field of drug abuse, immediate results are often crucial. Law enforcement personnel are likely to prefer salivary diagnostics compared with other options because they provide an assessment of the individual's condition precisely when an incident occurs. A delay in testing, to bring the individual to a facility where a urine or blood sample may be obtained, may not accurately represent the condition of the individual at the time when the crime was committed. Therefore, we expect to see more widespread use of these tools as in-the-field trials, such as the ROSITA II Project, produce favorable results in terms of both accuracy and convenience.

In-home diagnostics to confirm pregnancy have been available for decades. Now, women are demanding more control over other aspects of their health as well. The anxiety over HRT that reached the news in 2002 brought women's health issues to the forefront. Untapped potential lies in the hormone-monitoring market for women as well as men. As the profile of salivary diagnostics increases, these tools will infiltrate this space and meet the demand.

Perhaps the most exciting avenue for salivary diagnostics is in the field of predictive medicine. Asymptomatic individuals do not wish to undergo an invasive battery of tests to determine their risk of developing diseases in the future. However, by testing a saliva sample, physicians may be able to identify higher-risk individuals long before problems arise. Salivary diagnostics are sure to contribute greatly to the trend toward earlier screening and, subsequently, the closer monitoring of individuals with specific risk factors. Although the tools in this arena are in the early stages of development, the market need for such tools and the promising technologies that are being developed in response to that need suggest that reliable saliva-based diagnostics will successfully reach the predictive-medicine market.

Index